ELSEVIER'S DICTIONARY OF ABBREVIATIONS, ACRONYMS, SYNONYMS AND SYMBOLS USED IN MEDICINE

Second, Enlarged Edition

ELSEVIER'S DICTIONARY OF ABBREVIATIONS, ACRONYMS, SYNONYMS AND SYMBOLS USED IN MEDICINE

Second, Enlarged Edition

compiled by

DR. SAMUEL A. TSUR (MANSOOR), M.D.
Bombay – London – Akko (Acre), Israel

2004

ELSEVIER

Amsterdam – Boston – Heidelberg – London – New York – Oxford
Paris – San Diego – San Francisco – Singapore – Sydney – Tokyo

ELSEVIER B.V.
Sara Burgerhartstraat 25
P.O. Box 211
1000 AE Amsterdam
The Netherlands

ELSEVIER Inc.
525 B Street, Suite 1900
San Diego,
CA 92101-4495
USA

ELSEVIER Ltd
The Boulevard, Langford Lane
Kidlington
Oxford OX5 1GB
UK

ELSEVIER Ltd
84 Theobalds Road
London WC1X 8RR
UK

First edition 1999
Second, enlarged edition 2004

Library of Congress Cataloging in Publication Data
A catalog record from the Library of Congress has been applied for.

British Library Cataloguing in Publication Data
Elsevier's dictionary of abbreviations, acronyms, synonyms
and symbols used in medicine. - 2nd enlarged ed.
1.Medicine - Acronyms - Dictionaries 2. Medicine -
Abbreviations - Dictionaries 3.Medicine - Dictionaries
4.Signs and symbols
I.Tsur, Samuel A., 1924- II.Dictionary of abbreviations,
acronyms, synonyms and symbols used in medicine
610.1'48

ISBN 0-444-51265-9

∞ The paper used in this publication meets the requirements of ANSI/NISO Z39.48-1992 (Permanence of Paper).

Printed in The Netherlands.

This book is dedicated to my wife

RACHELLE

who has been my dearest partner and constant

companion for more than 55 years

Preface to the First Edition

Abbreviations used in medical articles, papers, and scientific journals abound in every tongue, but particularly so in the English language. This dictionary covers usage in the United States, Britain and other English-speaking countries, including those of the Third World.

A vast amount of information, including abbreviations of medical terms used in the field of anatomy, bacteriology, biology, chemistry, medicine (human and veterinary), pathology, pharmacology, etc., has been meticulously catalogued since work on the project started in 1979, from medical journals, scientific dictionaries and encyclopedias, and compilations of medical abbreviations published in the U.S. and other countries.

Over 20,000 entries have been included, with especially detailed itemization of the Chemical Elements ("Elements"), Hormones ("Hormones"), Insulins ("Insulin"), Kidney Function Tests ("KFT"), Pulmonary Function Tests ("PFT"), Serological Tests for Syphilis ("STS"), Symbols used in various disciplines, such as biology, calculation, chemistry, Greek alphabet, medicine and pharmacy, numeration and signs of the zodiac (all under "Symbols"), the Vitamins ("Vitamins"), etc. Besides these, under their respective headings different names, scientific and otherwise, have been catalogued for drugs such as amphetamine ("amphet"), cocaine ("Erythoxylum"), heroin ("Diamorph HCl"), lysergic acid ("LSD"), marijuana ("Cannabis"), opium ("Papaver"), etc.

Finally it must be remembered that a dictionary, however exhaustive the information provided within its covers, has its own limitations in that the addition of new discoveries and diseases, new terminologies and treatments, and the as yet unknown trends of Medical Science into future horizons, can have only a sobering influence on the writer of this book which has been compiled and catalogued over more than two decades.

Dr. Samuel A. Tsur (Mansoor), M.D.
Akko, Israel

Preface to the Second Edition

This second, enlarged edition comprises more than 30,000 entries, including the abbreviations, synonyms and symbols from the first edition, together with new terms and material for the advancement of medical knowledge, assembled from numerous medical articles, books and encyclopedias.

These terms include (each provides numerous examples or types):

AEI - Acute ethanol intoxication; Akinesia; Amblyopia; Amnesia; Anaphylaxis; Aneurysms; Apnea; Apraxia; ASS - Apgar scoring system (for IEB or Infant evaluation at birth); Asthenia; Audiometry; etc.

Biopsy; Birth; Catheters; CCA or Congenital cardiac anomaly; Conflicts; Contraceptives; DRMs or Diabetes-related malformations; Dwarfs; etc.

GHT or Graves' hyperthyroidism (manifestations of); HMs or Humoral mediators ("spasmogens" in the allergic diatheses); HVM or Humal viral myocarditis (various types); IMC or Inflammatory Markers and Cytokines; inc (incisions); IP (inclubation period of various illnesses); etc.

Mania; OHAs or Oral hypoglycemic agents; OI/OP or Orthopedic Implants/ O. Protheses; Paranoia; Pessaries; philia: emotional (psychological) and chemical (physiological) types; phob (a greatly enlarged summation of the various phobias); PM or Pacemakers; Pneumoconiosis; etc.

Radionuclides (20-odd materials released through atomic radiation); SHT or Suspected hyperthyroidism; Soa or Signs of Anxiety; Sut (sutures).

Finally it must be said, a tome of this category has no end, no final conclusion. Medical terms and new life-affecting maladies, new drugs and more efficient methods of counteracting illness appear daily, so I humbly conclude that this second edition will not be the last!

Dr. Samuel A. Tsur (Mansoor), M.D.
Akko, Israel

Appreciation

My deep gratitude to my friend Mr. Herman Rosenfeld of West Hills, California, my younger brother Dr. Isaac A. Mansoor, FRCS (Edin., UK), Orthopedic Surgeon, my nephew Dr. Moshe J. Manor, MD, Obstetrician & Gynecologist (Kaplan Govt. Hospital), Rehovot, and my son Dr. Daniel S. Tsur, DVM (Pisa, Italy), Chief Veterinary Surgeon, Golan Heights, Israel, who all four provided me respectively, each in their own field Medical, Orthopedic, Obstetric/Gynecological and Veterinary material, from sources the world over, in the completion of the second enlarged edition of this Dictionary.

A

A Abbot Laboratories and Warner-Lambert Pharmaceutical Co code for experimental substances; Abnormal; Abortion; Absent; Absolute temperature (K preferred); Absorbance (also symb. a; the degree of absorbability of a particular substance or surface-spectrophotometry); Absorptivity (also symb. a); Acceleration (also symb. a); Acceptor; Accommodation (also symb. a; accom. - eye examination); Acetone; Acetum (e.g. A. plumbi - a "vinegar" or solution in dil. acetic acid); Acid (e.g. A. Nicotinic); Acidity-total (also symb. a): Acidophil; Acidophilic; Acidum (e.g. A. Benzoicum); Acromion; Actin; Actinomyces; Activity (radiation); Adenoma; Adenosine; Admittance; Adrenalin(e); Adult; Age; Akinetic; Alanine; Albino (guinea pig); Albumin; Alcohol (e.g. A. Dehydratum); Alive; Allergy/ist/ologist; Alpha (cell); Alveolar gas; Ambulatory; Ampere (a unit of electric current in the MKS [Meter-kilogram-second] system); Amphetamine (see Amphet); Ampicillin; Analysis; Anaphylaxis; Androsterone; Anesthetic/sia (start of); Angioplasty; Angle; Angstrom unit (a unit of wavelength of electromagnetic and corpuscular radiation [= 10^{-7} mm; 10^{-10} m]); Angulus (L.), angle (e.g. A. iridis [= A. iridocornealis] in anatomy); Annum (L.), year; Anode (also symb. a); Anopheles; Antagonism/ist; Ante (L.), before; Anterior (also symb. a); Antrectomy; Apical; Aqua (L.), water (e.g. A. Destillata [= Distilled water]) (see Aq); Aqueous; Area (of heart shadow); Argon (Z = 18); Arteria (L.), Artery (e.g. A. brachialis); Arterial blood (also symb. a); Artery (e.g. Brachial A.); Assessment (in problem-oriented medical records); Asthma; Asymmetric; Atomic weight; Atrial; Atrium (= Auricle) (e.g. A. glottidis = A. of glottis; Vestibulum laryngis); Atropine; atto- (also symb. a) 10^{-18} (e.g. ag. = attogram; 10^{-18} gram; μμμg; micromicromicrogram); Auricle (see A. Atrium); Auricula (L.), a little ear (e.g. A. dextra cordis = A. atrii dextri, right atrium of the heart); Auricular; Auscultation; Auto- (e.g. Autoanalysis; Auto-antigen); Avo- (= 10^{-24}) e.g. Ag (= Avogram; μμμμg; 10^{-24} gram); Axial (also symb. a); Axillary; Before, (L. ante); Blood type A (of the ABO system); Ear, (L. auris); Mass number (atomic weight); Subspinale; Thermodynamic activity (also symb. a); Total acidity; Vitamin A (see Vitamins); Water (L. aqua; also symb. a); Year (L. annum).

A (band) The dark-staining zone of a striated muscle.

Å Angström unit.

A+ General symbol for a positive organic ion.

A– General symbol for a negative organic ion.

A' Acetaminophen.

A1 Aortic first heart sound.

A2 Aortic second heart sound.

$\bar{A}$ Cumulated activity; antinuclear antibody.

$\bar{a}\bar{a}$ Before (L. ante).

(a) axillary temperature.

α alpha. The first letter of the Greek alphabet; reference to the carbon atom appearing next to the carbon atom bearing the active molecular group (in organic compounds); symbol, designing first.

AI, II, III Angiotensin I, II, III.

aII Equal parts of azure I and methylene blue.

A 16 Ambucetamide - an antispasmodic used in the treatment of dysmenorrhea.

A 68 Symbol for a protein found in the brains of patients with Alzheimer's disease.

A 250 5% Albumin 250 ml.

A 1000 5% Albumin 1000 ml.

A - 1981-12 Prodilidine hydrochloride (= CI 427; Merolidine HCl; Methoxidine HCl) - an analgesic used in the treatment of arthritis.

A 2371 Methramycin (= NSC 24559; PA 144) - an antimicrobial acid produced by the growth of *Streptococcus* argillaceus and *Streptomyces* tanashiensis. Has been used in clinical investigations in neoplastic diseases.

A 8103 Pipobroman (= NSC 25154) - a cytotoxic alkylating agent used in the treatment of polycythemia vera and thrombocytosis.

A 19120 Pargyline hydrochloride (= MO 911; N-Methyl-N-prop-2-ynylbenzylamine HCl) - a monoamine oxidase inhibitor, used as a hypnotic in the treatment of benign hypertension.

AA Acetic/ Adenylic/ Arachidonic acid; Achievement age (pediatrics); Acta Allergologica (journal); Acta Anatomica (journal); Activation analysis; Active alcoholic; Active assistance (range of motion); Active avoidance; Acupunctural analgesia; Acute anaphylaxis; Addicts Anonymous; Adenine arabinoside; Adjuvant arthritis; Administration on Aging (OHD); Adrenal androgen; Affirmative action; Agents and Actions (journal); Agranulocytic angina; Alcohol abuse; Alcoholics Anonymous; Allergic alveolitis; Alopecia areata; Alveolar-arterial; Alzheimer's Association; Aminoacetone; Aminoacid; Amplitude of accommodation; Amyloid A (protein); Androgenetic alopecia (see MPHL); Angular aperture (microscope); Annals of Allergy (journal); Anterior aorta; Anti-arrhythmic agent; Anticipatory avoidance; Antigen aerosol; Antinuclear antibody; Aortic aneurysm/arch; Aplastic anemia; Arabinoside cytosine (cytarabine) and Adriamycin (doxorubucin); Arm ankle (pulse ratio); Arteries; Ascending aorta; Association of Anesthetics; Atlanto-axial; Atomic absorption (laboratory method); Audiologic assessment; Audiometric assistant; Auger analysis; Australia antigen (= Hepatitis B surface antigen) (see HBsAG); Authorized absence; Autoanalyzer; Auto-antibody; Automobile accident; Axonal arborization; So much of each (Gr. ana).

aa arteries (L. arteriae); so much of each (Gr. ana)

A̅A̅; ā̄ā̄; aa Equal parts; Of each (Gr. ana) (medical orders/prescriptions).

A-A Atlanto-axial.

A-a Alveolar-arterial. Difference of gas pressure between alveolus (A) and pulmonary artery (a) (see PFT, A-a).

aA Abampere.

A1A Alpha-I-antitrypsin (= A1AT; á1AT).

A-1's & A-2's Very small arteries in the brain.

A-1 & A-2 pulleys Slings for tendons in the hand.

A&A Aid and attendance (payment - VA.); Anesthesia and Analgesia (journal); Arthroscopy and arthrotomy; Awake and aware.

AIIA Angiotension II/2 antagonist (Type AT1) (see SARB).

10AA Mixture of 10 aminoacids.

AAA Abdominal aortic aneurysm/ aneurysmectomy; Acetoacetic acid (= Acetone carboxylic/ Acetylacetic/ Diacetic acid); Acne-associated arthritis; Acquired aplastic anemia; Acute angina(l)/ anxiety/ asthma(tic) attack; Adenine-adenine-adenine (three consecutive adenine bases); Adenylyl adenylyl adenoxine; Advances in Automated Analysis (journal); Agonist-antagonist analgesic (see OAAA); Alpha/ Anti adrenergic agent (see AA; AABA; ABA); Amalgam; Ambulance Association of America; American Academy of Allergy/ Anatomists/ Audiology; American Aging/ Anthropology/ Arbitration Association; American Association of Anatomists; Androgenic anabolic agent; Aneurysm of ascending aorta; Anti-allergic action; Anti-allergic/ anemic /anginal/ angiogenesis/ angiogenic/ anxiety/ arrhythmic/ arthritic agent (see AAM); Anti-amebic antibody; Anti-androgen(ic) action/ivity; Antibiotic anticancer agent (e.g. Bleomycin, Dactinomycin, Daunorubicin, and Mitomycin) (= AAA or Antineoplastic antibiotic); Antigen-extracted, autolyzed, allogeneic (bone/ bone regeneration); Aortic arch atheroma; Area Agency on Aging; Aromatic amino acid; Arterioarterial anastomosis; Atomic absorption analysis.

aaa amalgam.

αAA α-adrenergic activity/ agent (see AAA; AABA; ABA)/ antagonist; **α**-adrenoceptor/ adrenoreceptor antagonist (Doxazosin, Indoramin, Phentolamine, Phenoxybenzamine, Prazosin, Tetrazosin).

α1AA Alpha-1 adrenergic activity/ antagonist.

A-2 AA Alpha-2 adrenergic agonist (= AARA).

AAAA Acute abdominal aortic aneurysm (see ITP).

AAAAI American Academy of Allergy, Asthma and Immunology.

AAACRR American Association of Academic

Chief Radiology Residents.

AAAD Aromatic amino acid decarboxylase.

AAAE Amino acid activating enzyme.

AAAHE American Association for the Advancement of Health Education.

AAAI American Academy of Allergy and Immunology.

AAALAC American Association for Accredition of Laboratory Animal Care.

AAAM American Association for Automotive Medicine.

AAAMQ American Association for Automative Medicine Quarterly.

AAAN American Academy of Applied Nutrition.

AAAS American Academy of Arts and Sciences; American Association for the Advancement of Science.

AAAT Antimicrosomal antithyroid antibody titer.

AAATCM American Academy of Air Traffic Control Medicine.

AAB Acute alcoholic binge; Adenoameloblastoma; African-American baby; Alpha-adrenergic blocker (see AABA); Alzheimer-afflicted brain; American Association of Bioanalysts (= AABA); Aminoazobenzene; Anterior Achilles bursitis (= Albert's disease); Autoantibody (= AAb; AENAA; ANA; ATG; ATP; GADA; IAA; ICA; ISMG; etc.); Average absolute bioavailability.

Aab Autoantibody (see AAB).

AABA Alpha-adrenergic blocking agent (= AAB); Alpha aminobutyric acid; American Association of Bioanalysts (see AAB).

AABB American Association of Blood Banks.

AABC Alkylating agent-based chemotherapy; Association for the Advancement of Blind Children.

AABCC Alertness (consciousness), airway, breathing, circulation, cervical spine.

AABD Aid to the Aged, Blind, and Disabled.

αABE Alpha-adrenergic blocking effect.

AABEVM Association of American Boards of Examiners in Veterinary Medicine.

AABGA American Association of Botanical Gardens and Arboreta.

AABS Automobile accident, broadside.

AABT Association for Advancement of the Behavioral Therapies.

AAC Acanthoma adenoides cysticum (see EAC); Acinar/ Acinic/ Acinous adenocarcinoma (see ACAC); Acute abdominal condition; Adequate asthma control; Anaplastic astrocytoma (= Glioma multiforme) (see GBM); Anti-aging compound (= AAF); Antibiotic-associated pseudomembraneous colitis; Antigen-antibody complex (= IC - Immune complex); Antimicrobial agent-associated/-induced colitis; Antimicrobial Agents and Chemotherapy (medical journal); Approach-approach conflict (a conflict caused by the need to choose between two or more things that are wanted); Approach-avoidance conflict (a conflict caused by something that is both wanted and not wanted); Argentaffin cell (see ECC); Articulatio acromioclavicularis (see SCJ); Association of Analytical Chemists; Augmentative and alternative communication; Avoidance-avoidance conflict (see Conflict).

AACA Acylaminocephalosporanic acid; Additive anticonvulsant activity; American Association of Certified Allergists.

AACC American Association for Clinical Chemistry/ of Clinical Chemists; Association for the Aid of Crippled Children.

AACCN American Association of Critical-Care Nurses.

AACCP American Association of Colleges of Chiropody-Podiatry.

AACE American Association for Cancer Education; American Association of Clinical Endocrinologists.

AACG Acute angle closure glaucoma.

AACHP American Association for Comprehensive Health Planning.

AACIA American Association of Clinical Immunology and Allergy.

AACLSA American Association of Clinical Laboratory Supervisors and Administrators.

AAcLV Avian acute leukemia virus (=AclV).

AACM American Academy of Compensation Medicine.

AACMS American Association of Councils of Medical Staffs.

AACN American Association of Colleges of

Nursing.

AACO American Association of Certified Orthoptists.

AACOMAS American Association of Colleges of Osteopathic Medicine Application Service.

AACP Alcohol Abuse Control Program (USN); American Academy of Cerebral Palsy; American Academy of Child Psychiatry; American Academy of Clinical Psychiatry; American Association of Colleges of Pharmacy; American Association of Colleges of Podiatry; American Association of Correctional Psychologists.

AACPDM American Academy for Cerebral Palsy and Developmental Medicine.

AACPJ American Academy of Child Psychiatry Journal.

AACPM American Association of Colleges of Podiatric Medicine.

AACPR American Association of Cleft Palate Rehabilitation.

AACPS American Association of Clinic Physicians and Surgeons.

AACR American Association for Cancer Research.

AACS American Academy of Clinical Sexologists; American Academy of Cosmetic Surgery.

AACSH Adrenal androgen corticotropic stimulating hormone.

AACT American Academy of Clinical Toxicology.

AACU American Association of Clinical Urologists.

AAD Acid-ash diet; Acute agitated delirium; Acute abdominal distress/ disturbance; Acute aortic dissection (see AAAA; IRAD; ITP); Acyanotic congenital defect; Adhesive absorbent dressing; Adult celiac/ chronic (see FOAD; FPT) disease; Alloxazine adenine dinucleotide (= FAD; FADN; Flavine a.d.); Alpha-1-antitrypsin deficiency; American Academy of Dentists/ Dermatology; Amino acid deficiency/ disorder; Anti- addiction/ anginal/ angiogenesis/ angiogenic/ anxiety/ arrhythmic/ arthritic/ asthma drug (see AAM); Antibiotic-associated diarrhea; Anticancer diet (recommended by the ACS, NAS and NCI; includes reduction in fatty foods, adequate intake of high-fiber foods, foods rich in vitamin A and C, and vegetables such as broccoli, cabbage, and cauliflower, and limits to the intake of alcohol and salt-cured, smoked or nitrate-cured foods, etc.); Antiviral amantadine derivative (e.g. Tromantadine); Aromatic acid decarboxylase; Association of American Dentists; Atlanto-axial dislocation; Auto-antibody development/ disorder.

AAdA Aminoadipic acid.

AADC Amino acid decarboxylase.

AADD Adult attention deficit disorder (see ADHD).

AADE American Association of Dental Editors/ Examiners; American Association of Diabetes Educators.

AADEBB American Association of Dental Examiners Board Bulletin.

AADGP American Academy of Dental Group Practice.

AADN American Association of Doctors' Nurses.

A-aDN$_2$ Alveolar-arterial nitrogen partial pressure/ tension difference.

A-aDO$_2$ Alveolar-arterial oxygen tension difference (see PFT).

AADP American Academy of Denture Prosthetics; Amyloid A-degrading protease.

AADPA American Academy of Dental Practice Administration.

AADR American Academy of Dental Radiology; American Association for Dental Research.

AADS American Academy of Dermatologic Surgery (Atlanta); American Association of Dental Schools.

AAE Active assistive exercise; Acute allergic encephalitis; American Association of Endodontists; Annuloaortic ectasia; Anti-allergic/ arrhythmic/ asthmatic effect; Anti-androgen effect (such as gynecomastia) of a drug (e.g. cimetidine).

AAEC Australian Atomic Energy Commission.

AAEE American Academy of Environmental Engineers; American Association for Electromyography and Electrodiagnosis.

AAEH Association to Advance Ethical Hypnosis.

AAEM American Academy of Environmental Medicine.

AAETS American Academy of Experts in Traumatic Stress.

AA ex Active assistive exercise.

A/AEX Active assistive exercise (= AA ex).

AAF Academic Aid Fund; Acetic acid-alcohol-formalin (mixture - a fixing fluid); Acetyl-amino-fluorine (a carcinogen); Acute adrenal failure; Acute atrial fibrillation; Allylamine antifungal (e.g. Terbinafine); Anti-aging formula (see AAC); Anti-angiogenesis factor; Army Air Force; Ascorbic acid factor (a corticotropin in ACTH).

AAFA Asthma and Allergy Foundation of America.

AAFB Acid and alcohol fast bacilli.

AAFD American Academy of Family Doctors.

AAFGH Al-Anon Family Group Headquarters.

AAFM American Association of Feed Microscopists.

AAFMC American Association of Foundations for Medical Care.

AAFMG American Association of Foreign Medical Graduates.

AAFP American Academy of Family Physicians (formerly AAGP).

AAFPRS American Academy of Facial, Plastic, and Reconstructive Surgery.

AAFS American Association for Forensic Science; Association for the Advancement of Family Stability; Atomic absorption flame spectrometer; Australian Academy of Forensic Sciences.

AAG Abdominal angiogram/graph(y); Acute absolute glaucoma; Adenylyl adenylyl guanosine; Allergic angiitis and granulomatosis; Alopecia androgenetica; Alpha-1-acid glycoprotein; Alveolar arterial gradient; Anti-angiogenesis/ genetic (drug used in cancer therapy such as combrestatin and endostatin); Auto-antigen.

AAGA Anti-angiogenesis agent (= AS - Angiostatin; AGI - Angiogenesis inhibitor; ES - Endostatin) (see AAGT).

AAGBI Association of Anaesthetists of Great Britain and Ireland.

AAGD Anti-angiogenesis drug (see AAGA).

AAGL American Association of Gynecological Laparoscopists.

AAGN Acute active glomerulonephritis.

AAGP Alpha-amino-guanidino-propionic acid; American Academy of General Practice (now AAFP); American Academy of General Practitioners (now AAFP); American Association for Geriatric Psychiatry.

AAGPC Alkylacyl glycerophosphatidylcholine.

AAGS American Association of Genitourinary Surgeons (= AAGUS).

AAGT Anti-angiogenic therapy (blood-vessel growth inhibition therapy, used in cancer) (see AG; AAGA; AGB; AGI; AS; ES; TNP-470).

AAGUS See AAGS.

AAH Acute alcoholic hepatitis; Amino acid homoeostasis; Analgesic abuse headache; "Anti-aging" hormone(s) - associated suggestively with enhancing energy, building muscle mass, increasing sexual drive, improving sleep, and preventing jet lag (such as DHEA - Dehydroepiandrosterone, Estrogen, hGH - Human growth hormone, Melatonin - the pineal gland hormone, and Testosterone, etc.).

AAHA American Animal Hospital Association; American Association of Hospital Accountants.

AAHAJ American Animal Hospital Association Journal.

AAHC American Association of Hospital Consultants; Association for Academic Health Centers.

AAHD American Academy of the History of Dentistry; American Association of Hospital Dentists.

AAHDC American Association of Hospital Dental Chiefs.

AAHE Association for the Advancement of Health Education.

AAHPER American Association for Health, Physical Education, and Recreation.

AAHM American Association of the History of Medicine.

AAHP American Association of Health Plans; American Association for Hospital Planning/

Podiatrists; American Association for Humanistic Psychology; Army artificial heart pump.

AAHPA American Association of Hospital Purchasing Agents.

AAHPER American Academy/ Alliance for Health, Physical Education and Recreation.

AAHPhA American Animal Health Pharmaceutical Association.

AAHS American Association for Hand Surgery.

AAI Accrued analyzed information; Acute adrenal insufficiency; Acute alcohol intoxication (see AEI); Acute alveolar injury; Adolescent Alienation Index; American Association of Immunologists; American Audio Institute; Arteria alveolaris inferior (L.) (see IAA); Artificially acquired immunity (e.g. by vaccination); Atrial inhibited (pacemaker).

AAIA Antigen/ antibody interaction.

AAIAN Association for the Advancement of Instruction about Alcohol and Narcotics.

AAIB Alpha-1-aminoisobutyrate; American Association of Instructors of the Blind.

AAID Acquired autoimmune disease/ disorder; American Academy of Implant Dentistry; American Association of Implant Dentures; American Association of Industrial Dentists.

AAIN American Association of Industrial Nurses.

AAIP American Association of Indian Physicians.

AAIT American Association for Inhalation Therapy.

AAJ Absent ankle jerk; Amphidiarthrodial joint (a hinge joint, allowing movement in one plane only, such as the temporomandibular joint); Atlanto-axial joint.

AAK Allo-activated killer.

AAL Anterior atlanto axial/ occipital ligament; Anterior axillary line; Aortic arch lesion; Available arch length (the length or space in a dental arch that is available for all the natural teeth).

AALAS American Association for/ of Laboratory Animal Science.

AALIPS Arthur Adaptation of the Leiter International Performance Scale.

AALL American Association for Labor Legislation.

AAM Acute alcoholic myopathy; Acute aseptic meningitis; American Academy of Microbiology; Aminoacid metabolism/ mixture; Anterior atlantooccipital membrane; Anti-aging medicine; Anti-anginal/ angiogenesis/ angiogenic/ anxiety/arthritic medication (= AAA; AAD; AAT); Arachidonic acid metabolism (with production of prostaglandins) (see AAPP); Azole antimycotic.

AAMA American Academy/ Association of Medical Administrators/ Assistants.

AAMBP Association of American Book Publishers.

AAMC American Association of Marriage Counselors; American Association of Medical Clinics; Association of American Medical Colleges.

AAMCB Association of American Medical Colleges Bulletin.

AAMCH American Association for Maternal and Child Health.

AAMCOMA Association of American Medical Colleges' Office of Minority Affairs.

AAMD American Academy of Medical Directors; American Association on Mental Deficiency.

AAME Acetylarginine methyl ester.

AAMFC American Association of Marriage and Family Counselors.

AAMFT American Association for Marriage and Family Therapy.

AAMI Association for the Advancement of Medical Instrumentation; Association of Allergists for Mycological Investigations.

AAMIH American Association for Maternal and Infant Health.

AAMIJ Association for the Advancement of Medical Instrumentation Journal (now MIJ).

AAMMC American Association of Medical Milk Commissions/ers.

AAMP American Academy of Maxillofacial Prosthetics; American Academy of Medical Prevention.

AAMR Age-adjusted mortality rate; American Academy of Mental Retardation.

AAMRL American Association of Medical

Record Librarians.
AAMRS Automated ambulatory medical record system.
AAMS Acute aseptic meningitis syndrome.
AAMSE American Association of Medical Society Executives.
AAMSI American Association for Medical Systems and Informatics.
AAMT American Association for Medical Transcription.
AAMVA American Association of Motor Vehicle Administrations.
AAN AIDS-associated nephropathy; Alpha-amino nitrogen; American Academy of Neurology/ Nursing/ Nutrition; American Association of Neuropathologists; Amino acid nitrogen; Analgesic abuse/ associated nephropathy; Attending's admission notes.
AANA American Association of Nurse Anesthetists.
AANAJ American Association of Nurse Anesthetists Journal.
AANM American Association of Nurse-Midwives.
AANN American Association of Neurosurgical/ Neuroscience Nurses.
AANNT American Association of Nephrology Nurses and Technicians.
AANPI American Association of Nurses Practicing Independently.
AANS American Academy of Neurosurgical Surgery; American Association of Neurological Surgeons; American Association of Neurosurgical Surgeons.
AAO Academy of Applied Osteopathy; Acute arterial occlusion (by embolus, thrombus, etc.); American Academy of Ophthalmology/ Optometry/ Osteopathy/ Otolaryngology; American Association of Ophthalmologists/y/ Orthodontists; Amino acid output/ oxidase; Awake, alert and oriented.
A-aO_2 Alveolar-arterial oxygen gradients/ tension.
AAO x 3 Awake and oriented to time, place, and person.
AAOC American Association of Osteopathic Colleges; Antacid of choice.
AAOD Agonist-antagonist opioid drug (see AAA; OAAA).
AAofA Ambulance Association of America.
AAOG American Association of Obstetrics and Gynecologists.
AAO-HNS American Acadamy of Otolaryngology - Head and Neck Surgery.
AAOM American Academy of Occupational Medicine; American Academy of Oral Medicine.
AAOME American Association of Osteopathic Medical Examiners.
AAOMS American Association of Oral and Maxillofacial Surgeons.
AAON American Association of Orthodontists Newsletter (now Orthodontic Bulletin).
AAOO American Academy of Ophthalmology and Otolaryngology.
AAOOT American Academy of Ophthalmology and Otolaryngology Transactions.
AAOP American Academy of Oral Pathology.
AAOPS American Association of Oral and Plastic Surgery.
AAOS American Academy/ Association of Orthopedic Surgeons.
AAP Accelerated aging phenotype (DNA aging); Acid aspiration prophylaxis; Acute alcoholic pancreatitis; Air at atmospheric pressure; American Academy of Pediatrics/ Pedodontics/ Periodontics/tology/ Psychoanalysis/ Psychotherapists; American Association of Pathologists; Aminoacidopathy; Amino acid peptide; Anti-angiogenic property (e.g. of fumagillol); Anti-androgenic property; Anti-apoptotic factor (such as G-CSF & GM-CSF); Anti-apoptosis; Assessment adjustment pass; Association of Academic Physiatrists; Association for the Advancement of Psychoanalysis/ Psychology/ Psychotherapy; Association of American Physicians/ Publishers; Autoantibody production.
37 AAP 37 amino acid peptide (= Amylin, previously known as DAP or Diabetes-associated peptide).
AAPA American Academy/ Association of Pathologist/ Physician Assistants.
AAPB American Association of Pathologists and Bacteriologists.
AAPC Antibiotic-associated pseudo-membra-

nous colitis.

AAPCO Association of American Pesticide Control Officials.

$AAPCO_2$; (A-a)PCO_2 Alveolo-arterial carbon dioxide tension difference.

AAPF Anti-arteriosclerosis polysaccharide factor.

AAPHD American Association of Public Health Dentists.

AAPHP American Association of Public Health Physicians.

AAPL American Academy of Psychiatry and the Law.

AAPLB American Academy of Psychiatry and the Law Bulletin.

AAP-LOG American Association of Pro-Life Obstetricians and Gynecologists.

AAPM American Academy of Pain Medicine; American Association of Physicists in Medicine.

AAPMC Antibiotic-associated pseudo-membranous colitis.

AAPMR; AAPM&R American Academy/ Association of Physical Medicine and Rehabilitation.

$AaPO_2$; (A-a)PO_2 Alveolo-arterial oxygen tension difference (see PFT).

AAPP Arachidonic acid/prostaglandin pathway (pivoted in diabetes-induced neural tube defects and other congenital malformations) (Obstetrics).

AAPPP American Association of Planned Parenthood Physicians.

AAPRP Acute ascending polyradiculopathy.

AAPRS American Association of Plastic and Reconstructive Surgery.

AAPS American Association of Physicians and Surgeons; American Association of Plastic Surgeons; Arizona Articulation Proficiency Scale; Asian Association of Pediatric Surgeons; Association of American Physicians and Surgeons.

AAPSC American Association of Psychiatric Services for Children.

AAPSCN American Association of Psychiatric Services for Children Newsletter.

AAPSRO American Association of Professional Standards Review Organizations.

AAR Active avoidance reaction; Acute adaptive response; Acute allergic reaction; Acute allograft rejection; Acute articular rheumatism; Against all risks; Alliance for Aging Research; Alpha adrenergic receptor (see αAR); Anamnestic antibody response; Angioma arteriale racemosum; Antigen-antibody/ antiglobulin reaction; Australian antigen radioimmunoassay.

αAR Alpha-adrenergic receptor (= Alpha receptor; AAR or Alpha-adrenegic receptor).

AARA Alpha adrenergic receptor agonist (see A-2 AA); Anti-acetylcholine receptor antibody.

AARD Altanto-axial rheumatoid disease.

AARE Automobile accident, rear end.

AARF Age-adjusted risk factor.

AARNN Alberta Association of Registered Nurses Newsletter (Canada).

AAROM Active assertive range of motion.

Aaron's sign Pain and soreness between the navel and the right hip bone (MacBurney's point), during an attack of appendicitis.

AARP American Association of Retired People/ Persons.

AARS American Association of Railway Surgeons.

AART Academy of Assisted Reproductive Technology (LA); American Archives of Rehabilitation Therapy (journal); American Association of Radiologic Technology; American Association for Rehabilitation/ Respiratory Therapy.

AAS Academy of Applied Science; Acid aspiration syndrome; Air-abrasion system (dentistry); Alcoholic abstinence syndrome; Alveolar air space; Ambient air standard (the highest amount permitted by the Federal authorities in the US of any air pollutant, such as lead, nitrogen dioxide, sodium hydroxide, sulfuric dioxide, etc.); American Academy of Sanitarians; American Analgesia Society; Aminoacid sequence; Anabolic-androgenic steroid; Androgenic-anabolic steroid; Aneurysm of atrial septum; Anthrax antiserum; Anti-aging substance (e.g. melatonin); Antigen-antibody system; Aortic arch syndrome; Associate in Applied Science; Atlanto-axial/axis sublaxation; Atomic absorption spectrophotometry/roscopy; Atypical absence seizure; Axoaxonic synapse (junction or synapse of the axon of one neuron with the dendrites of another).

AASA American Association of Surgery/ Surgical Assistants.

AASCRN Amino acid screen.

AASD American Academy of Stress Disorders.

AASEC American Association of Sex Educators and Counselors.

AASECT American Association of Sex Educators, Counselors and Therapists.

aa seq amino acid sequence.

AASH Adrenal androgen stimulating hormone; American Association for the Study of Headache.

AASJ American Analgesia Society Journal.

AASLD American Association for the Study of Liver Diseases.

AASM Airtight aerosol saving manifold (jet nebulizer).

AASND American Association for the Study of Neoplastic Diseases.

AASP Acute atrophic spinal paralysis; American Association of Senior Physicians; Ascending-aorta synchronized pulsation.

AAST American Association for the Surgery of Trauma; Anabolic androgenic steroid therapy.

AASS American Association for Social Security.

AAT Aachen Aphasia Test; Academic Aptitude Test; Acardiac acephalic twin (Obstetrics); Acute abdominal tympany; Acute air trapping; Alanine aminotransferase (see ALT; GPT; SGPT); Alkylating agent therapy; Alpha-1-antitrypsin; American Academy of Toxicology; American Association of Trauma; Anti-aging (see AAH)/ anginal/ angiogenesis/ angiogenic/ anxiety/ arthritic therapy/ treatment (see AAM); Anti-asthma therapy/ treatment; Antibody absorption test (as in syphilis); Atrial triggered (pacemaker); Auditory apperception test; Automatic atrial tachycardia; Aspartate aminotransferase (see ASP-AT; AST; SGOT).

A1AT; α1AT Alpha-I-antitrypsin (= A1A).

AATCC American Association of Textile Chemists and Colorists.

AATG Acardiac-acephalus twin gestation (Obstetrics).

AATR Appropriate antibacterial therapeutic regimen.

AATS American Association of Thoracic Surgeons/ Surgery.

AAU Acute anterior uveitis; Amateur Athletic Union; Amino acid uptake.

AAUP American Association of University Professors.

AAV Adeno-associated virus; Adenovirus-associated virus; Adequate alveolar ventilation; Adolescent acne vulgaris; AIDS-associated virus (see ARV); Artificially assisted vision.

AAVA Artery-artery vascular anastomoses/mosis (between fetuses) (Obstetrics).

AAVMC Association of American Veterinary Medical Colleges.

AAVP American Association of Veterinary Parasitologists; Association of American Volunteer Physicians.

AAVS American Anti-Vivisection Society.

AAVV Accumulated alveolar ventilatory volume.

AAW Acute alcohol withdrawal; Anterior aortic wall.

AAWH American Association for World Health.

AAWHN American Association for World Health News (journal).

AAZPA American Association of Zoological Parks and Aquariums.

AAZV American Association of Zoo Veterinarians.

AB Abdominal; Able-bodied; A blood type (ABO system); Abnormal; Abortion (= Ab; ab; ABORT; Abort; abort); Ace bandage; Active bilaterally; Aid to the Blind; Alcian blue; American Board; Analytical Biochemistry (journal); Antibiotic; Antibody; Antigen binding; Apex beat; Archives of Biochemistry (journal); Asbestos body; Assisted breach (a technique in which a baby being born feet or buttock first is permitted to be born spontaneously as far as its navel, and is then fully extracted by the attending midwife or physician) (= PBE or Partial breech extraction); Asthmatic bronchitis; Axiobuccal; Bachelor of Arts (L. Artium Baccalaureus); Blood group AB; Roswell Park Memorial Institute code for experimental substances.

Ab Abortion (see AB); Antibody (= ab; aby).

aB Azure B; Trimethyl derivative of thionine.

ab abortion (see AB); about; antibody (see Ab); away from/ from - prefix (L.).

Aβ Beta-amyloid (peptide) - a 'metalloprotein' which binds to metals such as copper, iron, and zinc; responsible for amyloid plaques in Alzheimer's disease (= APP).

A/B Acid/base (ratio); Apnea/bradycardia.

A>B Air greater than bone (conduction).

A&B Apnea and bradycardia.

A2B2 Hemoglobin p.

3AB 3-aminobenzamide.

AB 100 Bis (ethyleneimido)phosphorourethane - a cytotoxic agent.

AB 103 Benzodepa (= Benzcarbimine; NSC 37096) - an antineoplastic agent; has been used in the treatment of advanced bronchogenic carcinoma.

AB 132 Meturedepa (= Dimethylurethimine; NSC 51325) - an antineoplastic agent Has been given with radiotherapy in the treatment of bronchogenic carcinoma.

ABA Abbot Bichromatic Analyzer; Abscissic acid; Absolute bioavailability; Adrenergic blocking agent (= AAA or Antiadrenergic agent); Alcohol-Benzocaine-Anesthetic (or Compound Benzocaine Injection - BPC, containing a sterile solution of Benzyl Alcohol, Benzocaine, and the Anesthetic Ether in arachis oil); Alkaline buffering agent; Allergic broncho-pulmonary aspergillosis; American Bar/ Burn Association; American Board of Anesthesiologists/y; Antibacterial activity/ agent; Antibacterial agent; Antigen-binding affinity; Applied Behavioral Analysis.

AbA Atom-by-atom.

Abadie's sign A twitch of the eyelid sometimes seen with a hyperactive thyroid gland.

ABAI American Board of Allergy and Immunology.

ABA_m Mean absolute bioavailability (= MABA).

AbAP Antibody-against-panel (assays).

ABAS American Board of Abdominal Surgeons.

ABB Abnormal breast biopsy; Acid-base balance; Albright-Butler-Bloomberg (syndrome); American Board of Bioanalysis; Archives of Biochemistry and Biophysics (journal); Artificial breeding box (insects).

ABBA Antiquarian Booksellers Association of America.

Abbe flap Lip-switch flap for repair of unilateral and bilateral cleft lip deformities.

ABBI Advanced breast biopsy instrumentation.

AbBI Antibody-bound insulin.

ABBQ Acquired Immunodeficiency Syndrome Beliefs and Behavior Questionnaire.

Abbr; Abbrev Abbreviated/ion.

ABC Absolute band/ basophil count; Absolute bone conduction; Acid balance control; Aconite, belladonna, chloroform (linament); Advanced bladder/ bone/ brain/ breast cancer/ carcinoma; Airway, breathing, and circulation; Alternative birth center; Alum, blood, and charcoal (purification and deodorizing method); Alum, blood, and clay (sludge deodorizing method); American Biology Council; American Blood Commission (HEW); Aneurysmal bone cyst; Annales de Biologie Clinique (Fr journal); Antibacterial chemotherapy; Antigen-binding capacity; Apnea, bradycardia, cyanosis; Artificial beta cells; Aspiration biopsy cytology; Assessment of basic competency; Atomic, biological, chemical (warfare - see CBR); Axiobuccocervical; Breathing and blood circulation (formerly CPR, now ARC); Check for open airway; (Potassium) acetate bicarbonate (urate).

A&BC Air and bone conduction.

ABCAST American Breast Cancer Adjuvant Study Group.

ABCC American Board of Clinical Chemistry; Atomic Bomb Casualty Commission (AEC, now RERF).

ABCD Screening tests for: 1) Breathing and

blood circulation (= ARC; CPR): **A** Airway (check for open airway) - **B** Breathing (check) - **C** Circulation (bloodcheck) - **D** Definitive (initiate definitive therapy); 2) Congenital defects: **A** Affected family - **B** Bilirubin level - **C** Congenital rubella syndrome - **D** Defects of the ear, nose, or throat; 3) Mole changes in melanoma: **A** Asymmetry - **B** Border irregularity - **C** Color (non-uniform pigmentation) - **D** Diameter (more than 6 cm/ sudden increase in size).

ABCDE Botulism toxin/ toxoid pentavalent.

ABCE American Board of Clinical Engineering.

ABCH American Board of Clinical Hypnosis.

ABCIL Antibody-mediated cell-dependent immunolympholysis (system).

ABCL American Birth Control League (now PPFA).

ABCN American Board of Clinical Neuropsychology.

ABCOP American Board for Certification in Orthotics and Prosthetics, Inc.

ABCP Association of Blind Chartered Physiotherapists.

ABCRS American Board of Colon and Rectal Surgery.

ABCS American Board of Counseling Services.

ABCs For controlling CAD or Coronary artery disease. **A**spirin and ACE inhibitors. **B**lood pressure control and **B**eta-blockers. **C**holesterol control and glu**C**ose.

ABCT Automated blood chemistry test(s) (see SMA ...analyzer).

ABC warfare Atomic, biological, chemical warfare (see ABC).

ABD Abdomen; Acid-base disorder/ disturbance; Acute bleeding disorder; Acute bloody diarrhea; Acute/ Anoxic brain damage; Adolescent brain development; Adrenergic-blocking drug (see GABD; PABD); After bronchodilator; Aged, blind, and disabled; Aggressive behavioral disturbance; All but dissertation; American Board of Dermatology; Antibody-based drug; Autologous blood donation; Average body dose.

α, β, δ, θ alpha, beta, delta, theta-electromagnetic waves (see Symbols - 5).

ABDCT Atrial bolus dynamic computer tomography.

Abd. Hyst Abdominal hysterectomy (operation/ gynecology).

Abdom/abdom Abdomen/inal (see Abd/abd).

ABDPH American Board of Dental Public Health.

ABE Acute bacterial endocarditis/ exacerbation; Adult basic education; American Board of Endodontics; Antibacterial effect; Botulism equine trivalent antitoxin.

Abd; abd Abdomen/inal (= abdom); Abduct/ion/or.

ABEA American Broncho-Esophageal Association.

ABEM American Board of Emergency Medicine; Annals of Biochemistry and Experimental Medicine (journal).

ABEP American Board of Examiners in Psychotherapy; Auditory brainstem-evoked potentials.

ABEPH American Board of Examiners in Psychological Hypnosis.

ABEPP American Board of Examiners in Professional Psychology.

aber aberrant.

ABESPA American Board of Examiners in Speech Pathology and Audiology.

A-beta Beta amyloid protein (degenerates into fibrils, neurofibrillary tangles and plaques, in Alzheimer's disease).

ab ext From externally (L. ab externo).

ABF Ameloblastic fibroma; Antiberiberi factor (= Thiamine HCl) (see Vitamins - B1); Aortobifemoral.

ABFP American Board of Family Practice.

ABG Abnormal brain growth (as in autistic children see SMC); Aortoiliac bypass graft; Arterial blood gases (laboratory/ blood gas); Autogenous bone graft; Axiobuccogingival.

ABH Ameloblastic hemangioma; Hexachlorocyclohexane.

ABHP American Board of Health Physics.

ABHs "America's Best Hospitals".

ABI American Baking Institute; Ankle/brachial index; Atherothrombotic brain infarct/ion; Autograft-bone interface (see

BAJ).

ABIC Adaptive Behavior Inventory for Children.

ABID Antibody identification.

A-bile Bile from the common duct.

ABIM American Board of Internal Medicine.

ABIMCE American Board of Internal Medicine certifying examination.

AbioCor The first fully implantable artificial heart (constructed in 2001 by Abiomed, US) (= FIAH).

AbIT Antibody instructive theory (that each contact with an antigen causes the body to make a new antibody).

ABJS Association of Bone and Joint Surgeons (US).

ABK Antibacterial-keratolytic (topical, such as 2% Salicylic acid in 70% Alcohol) (= ASK); Aphakic bullous keratopathy.

ABL α-β-Lipoproteinemia; Accelerated bone loss; African Burkitt's lymphoma; Albight-Butler Lightwood (syndrome); Allograft-bound lymphocytes; Alpha-beta-lipoproteinemia; Amobarbital level; Angioblastic lymphadenopathy; Anticipated/ Average blood loss; Antigen-binding lymphocyte; Army Biological Laboratories/tory; Automated biological laboratory; Axiobuccolingual.

ABLAM American Board of Laboratory Animal Medicine.

ABLB Alternate binaural loudness balance (test).

ABLP Abetalipoproteinemia (a rare inherited fat disorder, with low or absent betalipoproteins which carry cholesterol in the blood stream) (= BKS).

ABLR American Burkitt Lymphoma Registry.

ABM Acid-base metabolism; Adjusted body mass; Allogeneic/ Aplastic bone marrow; Alveolar basement membrane; American Board of Microbiology; Angioblastic meningioma; Appendicular bone mass (Orthopedics); Autologous bone marrow.

ABMC Amino-benzyloxy-methyl cellulose.

ABMDR American Bone Marrow Donor Registry.

ABMI Autologous bone marrow implant.

ABMLS Accrediting Bureau of Medical Laboratory Schools (AMT).

ABMM American Board of Medical Management.

A/B Mods Apnea/bradycardia moderate stimulation.

ABMS Advisory Board for Medical Specialties; American Board of Medical Specialists/ties.

A/B MS Apnea/bradycardia mild stimulation.

ABMT Allogeneic/ Autologous bone-marrow transplant(ation).

ABMTR Autologous Bone and Marrow Transplant Registry (of North America).

ABN American Board of Nutrition; Aseptic bone necrosis; Association of British Neurologists.

AbN Antibody nitrogen.

ABN; Abn; abn Abnormal/ity/ities (= Abnor).

ABNM American Board of Nuclear Medicine.

ABNMP Alpha-benzyl-N-methyl phenethylamine.

Abnor Abnormal (see ABN; Abn; abn).

ABNP American Board of Neurology and Psychiatry.

ABNS American Board of Neurological Surgery.

ABO Abortion; Absent bed occupancy; Acute bronchial obstruction; Alveolar bone osteoclast (Orthopedics); American Board of Ophthalmology/ Opticianry/ Orthodontics/ists/ Otolaryngology; Blood group system of antigens.

ABOB Moroxydine hydrochloride - a biguanide derivative used formerly in the treatment of viral infections, but with doubtful value.

ABOE American Board of Ophthalmic Examinations.

ABOG American Board of Obstetrics and Gynecology.

ABO-HD ABO hemolytic disease.

ABOHN American Board for Occupational Health Nurses.

A-Bomb A cigarette prepared from a mixture of marijuana and heroin (see Cannabis; Diamorph HCl).

ABOMS American Board of Oral and Maxillofacial Surgery.

ABOP American Board of Oral Pathology.

Abor; Abort Abortion (= Ab).

Abortion A spontaneous or deliberate termination of pregnancy which includes Habitual, Infected, Septic, Threatened, or Voluntary abortion.

ABOS American Bibliography/ Board of Orthopedic Surgery; American Board of Oral Surgery; American Board of Orthopaedic Surgeons (US).

ABP Acute back pain; Adaptive balance profile; Alcohol brain pathology; Ambulatory blood pressure; American Board of Pathology/ Pediatrics/ Pedodontics/ Periodontology/ Proctology/ Prosthodontics/(ists); American Business Press; Aminobiphosphonate (= Alendronate) - a specific inhibitor of osteoclast-mediated bone resorption (in PMO - Postmenopausal osteoporosis); Amyloid beta protein (found in the brains of people with Alzheimer's disease); Androgen/ Antigen-binding protein; Antibacterial peptide (found in leeches); Arterial blood pressure; Autograft bone paste (Orthopedics); Avidin-biotin peroxidase.

ABPA Allergic bronchopulmonary aspergillosis.

ABPC American Board of Pediatric Cardiology; Antibody-producing cell.

ABPD American Board of Podiatric Dermatology.

ABPE Acute bovine pulmonary edema.

ABPI Ankle Brachial Pressure Index (an indicator of PAD - Peripheral arterial disease); Association of the British Pharmaceutical Industry

ABPLA American Board of Professional Liability Attorneys.

ABPM Ambulatory blood pressure monitoring; American Board of Preventive Medicine.

ABPMR American Board of Physical Medicine and Rehabilitation.

ABPN American Board of Psychiatry and Neurology.

ABPP American Board of Professional Psychology.

ABPS American Board of Plastic Surgery; American Board for Psychological Services, Inc.

ABR Abortus Bang Ring probe (test); BABR); Advances in Brain Research (journal); American Board of Radiology; Aortic body reflex (a normal chemical reaction in the body due to a decrease in blood oxygen, causing faster breathing to build up oxygen supplies); Auditory brainstem response; Average blood replacement.

A Br Agglutination test for brucellosis.

Abr; Abras Abrasion(s).

ABRA American Blood Resources Association.

Abram lens Abraham lens, a Goldmann fundus lens which has been coated with an antireflective compound and a small 66-D powered button bonded excentrically on the surface; used as a contact lens in laser surgery.

ABRET American Board of Registration of Electroencephalographic Technologists.

ABRMT Ames bacterial reverse mutation test.

ABRT Ames bacterial reversion test (see ABRMT).

ABS Abdominal surgery; Acid-base state/ status (see ABA; ABB; ABD); Acrylonitrile-butadiene-styrene (= Acryzonitrile-b-s) - a copolymer; Acute bacterial sinusitis/ synovitis; Acute brain syndrome; Adaptive Behavior Scale; Admitting blood sugar; Adult bovine serum; Aging brain syndrome; Alkylbenzene sulfonate (= Alkylbenzyl s.); Allograft bone supplement; Aloin-belladonna-strychnine (a laxative); Ameloblastic sarcoma; American Board of Surgery; American Biological Society; Amniotic band sequence/syndrome; Amphoric breath sound (as is heard with a stethoscope in pneumothorax); Animal Behavior Society; Antibacterial spectrum; Antibody system (of immunity) - antibodies produced by B cells (see HIS); Anti-B serum; Antibodies (= Abs); Antley-Bixier syndrome; Arterial blood sample; Arterial bypass surgery; Artificial blood substitute (a synthetic blood substitute called Hemopure or Oxygent, based on the chemical Perflubron, and used on deep water divers to absorb nitrogen bubbles in their blood due to rapid resurfacing, with the painful and sometimes fatal condition, called the bends) (= SBS); At

Abs Absorbance; Absorption (see absorp); Antibodies (see ABS); Auer bodies (Red-staining rods found in myeloblasts of leukemia patients) (see ARs - Auer rods).
abs Absent (L. absente)/ away from; Absolute; Absorb.
ABSA American Biological Safety Association.
Absc Abscess, Abscissa (L. abscissus; abscindo) - tearing off/ cutting off.
abs conf Absolute configuration.
Ab (score) Abstract (score) (psychology).
ABSe Ascending bladder septum.
abs feb In the absence of fever/ fever being absent/ while fever is absent (L. absente febre).
absorp Absorption (= Abs).
ABSR Auditory brain stem response.
AbSR Abnormal skin reflex.
A/B SS Apnea/bradycardia self-stimulation.
AbST Antibody specific theory (of production of specific antibodies to antigens) (= CTS - Clinical selection theory).
Abst; Abstr Abstract.
ABT Accessory bypass tract (or pathway, as in WPW - Wolff-Parkinson-White and LGN - Lown-Ganong-Levine syndromes); Air-borne transmission (of disease); Allogeneic blood transfusion; Aminopyrine breath test; Autologous blood transfusion/ bone transplant(ation).
Abt About.
ABT-378 Lopinavir (an antiviral, protease inhibitor drug).
ABTA American Brain Tumor Assocation.
ABTS American Board of Thoracic Surgery.
ABU American Board of Urology; Asymptomatic bacteriuria.
ABV Acceptable baseline value(s); Actinomycin D-bleomycin-vincristine; Alternobaric vertigo; Arthropod-borne virus; Asymptomatic bacterial vaginosis; Average baseline value.
ABVD Adriamycin, bleomycin, vinblastine, and dacarbazine.
ABW Actual/ Average body weight.
ABx Antibiotics.
ABY Acid bismuth yeast (agar/ medium).
Aby Antibody (= Ab).
AC Abdominal circumference/ compression; Absorption coefficient; Abuse case; Acetate; Acetylcholine; Acetyl-cysteine; Acidified complement; Acinetobacter calcoaceticus; Acromioclavicular; Acta Chirurgica (journal); Acta Cytologica (journal); Activated charcoal; Active-controlled (study) (see ACS); Acupuncture clinic; Acute; Acute cholecystitis; Adaptive control; Adenocarcinoma; Adenylate cyclase; Adherent cell; Adrenal cortex; Adrenocorticoid; Adult and Child (journal); Advertising Council; Affinity chromatography; Air chamber; Air changes; Air conditioning; Air conduction (hearing test); Alcoholic cirrhosis; Alternating current; Alveolar crest; Ambulatory care; Amniocentesis (at 16-18 weeks' gestation, second trimester); Amplitude of convergence (also called Fusional amplitude - Vergence ability); Analog computer; Analytical Chemistry (journal); Anchored catheter (see A/C); Anesthesia circuit; Angewandte Chemie (journal); Angiocellular; Anodal closure; Ante cibum (L. before meals); Antecubital; Anterior chamber (eye examination); Anterior column; Anterior commissure; Antibiotic concentrate; Anticoagulant; Anticomplement/ary; Anticonvulsant (e.g. phenytoin) (see PDA); Anti-inflammatory/ Antiphlogistic corticoid; Aortic closure; Aortocoronary; Arm circumference; Arterialized capillary; Ascending colon; Assist control (see A/C); Atriocaratid; Auricular-carotid (interval); Autocorrelation; Axiocervical; Before meals (L. ante cibum).
Ac Accelerator (e.g. Ac globulin); Acetate; Acetyl; Acryl group; Actinium (atomic no. 89 - see Elements); Arabinosyl cytosine (= aC).
aC Abcoulomb; Arabinosyl cytosine (see Ac); Monomethyl thionine (basic dye).
ac Acceleration; Acid; Acute; Alternating current; Ante cibum (L. before meals); Antecubital; Anterior chamber; Axiocervical; Before meals (L. ante cibum).
A-C Adult-versus-child; Air-conditioned; Aortocoronary (bypass); Atriocarotid; Auriculocarotid.
A/C Albumin/coagulin (ratio); 5-Amino-4-imidazolicarboxamide; Anchored catheter (=

AC); Anterior chamber (of eye); Assist control (= AC).

5-AC Azacitidine.

AC 601 Buramate (=2-Hydroxyethyl N-benzylcarbamate) - an anticoagulant and tranquilizer used in the treatment of convulsive disorders in children.

ACA Abnormal coronary artery; Acinar cell adenoma (see PACA); Acrodermatitis chronica atrophicans; Acromioclavicular arthritis/ articulation (see ACJ); Acute cerebellar ataxia; Acyclovir (see ACV); Adenine-cytosine-adenine; Adenocarcinoma; Adequate clinical assessment; Adrenoceptor antagonist (**α,β**); Adult child of an alcoholic; American Chiropractic Association; Aminocaproic acid; American College of Allergists/ Anesthesiologists/ Angiology/ Apothecaries; American Council on Alcoholism; American Crystallographic Association; Aminocaproic/ Aminocephalosporanic acid; Ammonia, copper, and acetate; Amyotrophic choreoacanthocytosis; Anterior cerebral artery; Anterior communicating aneurysm/ artery; Anticancer agent (see CSACA); Anticardiolipin/ Anticentromere/ Anticollagen/ Anticycloplasmic antibody; Anticholinergic action/ agent (such as Atropine, Benzhexol, Ipratropium bromide {N-isopropyl noratropine}, Orphenadrine, Papaverine, Procyclidine, Stramonium, etc.) (= ACD); Anticoagulant/ convulsant action/ activity; Anticomplement activity; Antimetabolite cytotoxic agent (see AMCA); Apparent cardiac arrest; Automated computer analysis; Automatic Clinical Analyzer.

AC/A Accommodative convergence/ accommodation (ratio).

ACAAI American College of Allergy, Asthma and Immunology.

ACABCC Airway clearance, Assisted breathing, Chest compression (CPR) (see CPP; MPP; MtM; PRFCC).

ACAC Acinic cell adenocarcinoma (= AAC); Activated charcoal artificial cell.

AcAc Acetoacetate.

ACACN American Council of Applied Clinical Nutrition.

ACAD Asymptomatic coronary artery disease.

Acad Academy.

ACAG Anticancer gene.

A-CAH Autoimmune chronic active hepatitis.

ACAJC American Chiropractic Association Journal of Chiropractic.

ACAO Acyl coenzyme A oxidase.

ACAP Acetaminophen; American Council on Alcohol Problems.

A cap ad cal From head to heel (L. a capite ad calcem) - in describing symptoms.

ACAS Asymptomatic carotid-artery stenosis (cardioembolic stenosis, lacunar stenosis, etc.; Asymptomatic Carotid Atherosclerosis Study (US).

ACAST Advisory Committee on the Application of Science and Technology.

ACAT Automated computerized axial tomography.

ACB Additional clinical benifit; Adrenoceptor blocker (see ACBA); Airman, Classification Battery (psychology); Alberta Cancer Board (Canada); Alveolar-capillary block; Annals of Clinical Biochemistry (journal); Antibody-coated bacteria; Aortocoronary bypass (saphenous vein); Arterialized capillary blood; Asymptomatic carotid bruit.

acb before breakfast.

ACBA Adrenoceptor blocking agent (see SACBA; AABA).

AC/BC Air conduction/bone conduction (time ratio).

ACBE Air contrast barium enema.

ACBG Aortocoronary bypass graft; Autogenous cortical bone graft (Orthopedics).

ACBS Advisory Committee of Borderline Substances.

ACC Accommodation; Acetyl coenzyme A carboxylase; Acetylsalicylic acid, caffeine, codeine (proprietary drug); Acinic cell carcinoma; Acute care center; Acute (spinal) cord compression; Adenoid cystic carcinoma; Administrative control center; Adrenal chromaffin cell; Adrenocortical carcinoma; Alveolar cell carcinoma; Ambulatory care center; American College of Cardiology/ Chemosurgery; Anodal closure clonus/ contraction (= ACCI; AnCC); Anode closing current (= AnCC) - electrotherapy; Anterior cingulate cortex (brain); Anticoagulant clinic;

Antitoxin-containing cell; Aplasia cutis congenita; Arm cylinder cast (made of plaster of Paris or fiberglass, to keep the arm rigid from the wrist to above the elbow); Arthropod cell culture (medium); Articular chondrocalcinosis; Artificial classification cavity (Dentistry) - any tooth decay or cavity that may be classified in one of six groups: Class I. Cavities linked to structural tooth defects such as pits and fissures; Class II. Cavities in the sides of premolars and molars; Class III. Cavities in the sides of canines and incisors, not interfering with the edge of the tooth; Class IV. Cavities in the sides of canines and molars requiring restoration of the tooth edge; Class V. Cavities, except pit cavities, near the gum; Class VI. Cavities on the edges and cusp tips of the teeth; Aspirin-containing compound; Associated clinical condition; Autologous cultured chondrocyte.

Acc Acceleration (see Accel); Accident; Accommodation (= Accom) - eye examination; Adenoid cystic carcinoma (see ACE).

acc Acceleration; Accelerator; Accident; Accommodation; According (to).

ACCA American Clinical and Climatological Association; American Credit Card Association.

ACCC Association of Committee Cancer Centers.

ACCEL American College of Cardiology Extended Learning.

Accel Acceleration (= Ace).

ACCEPT Alcoholism Center Coordinating Education Prevention and Treatment.

ACCESS Ambulatory Care Clinic Effectiveness Systems Study; American College of Cardiology Extended Study Services; Amgen Cancer & Chemotherapy Educational Support System (an information program for women receiving chemotherapy for breast cancer - US).

ACCH Association for the Care of Children's Health.

AcCh Acetylcholine (= ACh).

AcChR Acetylcholine receptor.

AcCHS Acetylcholinesterase.

ACCI Action Committee of Childhood Immunization.

Accid Accident.

Acc insuff Accommodation insufficiency.

ACCI Anodal closure clonus (see ACC) - electrotherapy.

ACCME Accreditation Council for/ Advisory Committee on Continuing Medical Education (AMA).

AcCoA Acetyl coenzyme A.

Accom Accommodation (see Acc).

Accord According(ly).

ACCP American College of Chest Physicians; American College of Clinical Pharmacology.

ACCPB American College of Chest Physicians Bulletin.

ACCR Amylase creatinine clearance ratio.

ACCS American College of Chest Surgeons.

Accu-Chek Blood glucose meter with digital read-out for diabetic patients to examine their own blood glucose; reads Chemstrip blood glucose.

Accum Accumulation.

Accur Accurately; most carefully (L. accuratissime).

ACD Absolute cardiac dullness; Absolute claudication distance; Acid, citrate, dextrose (see A.C.D.) - Strumia's solution, an anticoagulant for blood samples and preservative for donor blood; Acta Radiologica Diagnosis (journal); Actinium emanation (chemical symbol for); Actinomycin D; Active claudication distance; Acute cardiac/ cerebral/ coronary damage/ disease; Adrenal cortex deficiency; Adult celiac disease; Advanced care directive; Aerosol conservation device; Alcoholic cerebellar degeneration; Allergic contact dermatitis; American College of Dentists; Anglokeratoma corporis diffusum (universale) - Fabry's syndrome; Anterior chamber/ chest diameter; Anticancer drug (see CSACA); Anticholinergic drug (see ACA); Anticlotting/ convulsant drug; Anticoagulant, citrase, dextrose (see A.C.D.); Area of cardiac dullness; Arnold-Chiari deformity; Articular cartilage damage; Australasian College of Dermatologists; Automatic computing densitometer; Awareness context of death; Citric acid, trisodium citrate, dextrose (see A.C.D.); Dactinomycin; Trisodium, citrate, dextrose (see A.C.D.).

A.C.D. Anticoagulant and citrate dextrose solution (= ACD; A.C.D. sol) - a sterile solution of sodium citrate, citric acid, and dextrose in Water for Injection. Used as an anticoagulant and preservative for donor blood. Also known by the name Strumia's solution.

Ac̄D Alive with disease.

AC-DC Bisexual (homosexual and heterosexual).

AC/DC Alternating current/ (or) Direct current.

ACDI Agricultural Cooperative Development, International.

ACDJ American College of Dentists Journal.

ACDQ Association des Chirurgiens Dentistes du Québec.

ACDs Anticonvulsant drugs.

ACDSJ Anglo-Continental Dental Society Journal (UK).

A.C.D. sol Anticoagulant and citrate dextrose solution (see A.C.D.).

ACDT Anticonvulsant-drug therapy.

ACDUTRA Active Duty for Training (for personnel assigned to naval research dental units).

ACE Acetonitrile; Acetylcholinesterase (= AchE) - an enzyme responsible for cholinergic neurotransmission; see E 2020; Acute cerebral encephalopathy; Acute coronary event; Adrenal cortical extract; Adrenocortical extract; Adrenocorticoid effect; Adverse circulatory event; Adverse clinical event; Alcohol, chloroform, ether (anesthetic mixture); 6-allyl-8b-carboxy-ergoline (a metabolite of cabergoline, used in the treatment of Parkinson's disease); American College of Epidemiology; American Council of/on Education; Angiotensin converting enzyme; Anticholinergic/ coagulant/ convulsive effect; Anticholinesterase; Association for Childbirth Education; Association of Conservation Engineers.

ACe Adriamycin and cyclophosphamide (combination therapy).

Ace Marijuana cigarette (obsolete) - see Cannabis.

ace acentric; acetone (= Acet).

ACEA Angiotensin converting enzyme antagonist (= AT1RA; AT2RA).

ACEAHPS Advisory Committee on Education for the Allied Health Professions and Services (AMA).

ACED Anhidrotic congenital ectodermal dysplasia.

ACEDS Angiotensin-converting enzyme dysfunction syndrome.

ACEE Acetylcholine esterase enzyme (see ACE).

ACEH Acid cholesterol ester hydrolase.

ACEI Angiotensin-converting enzyme inhibitor.

ACEMBP Annual Conference on Engineering in Medicine and Biology Proceedings.

ACEP American College of Emergency Physicians.

ACEPUAEMS American College of Emergency Physicians and the University Association for Emergency Medical Services.

ACERP American College of Emergency Room Physicians.

AcEst Acetyl esterase.

Acet Acetone (= ace); Vinegar (L. acetum).

acetab Acetabular/um.

acetyl-CoA Acetyl coenzyme A.

ACF Accessory clinical finding(s); Acute care facility; Acute circulatory failure (cardiac shock) (see CGS; HTS); Acute clinical filariasis; Additional contributory factor; Adrenoceptor/ cortical function; Anterior cervical fusion; Area correction factor; Asthmatic Children's Foundation.

ACFDN Association of Canadian Faculties of Dentistry Newsletter.

ACFEM L'Association canadienne des fabricants d'équipement médical (CAMMD).

ACFMR Accreditation Council for Facilities for the Mentally Retarded.

ACFO American College of Foot Orthopedists.

ACFON American College of Foot Orthopedists Newsletter.

ACFS American College of Foot Surgeons.

ACG Accelerator globulin; American College of Gastroenterology; Angiocardiogram/graphy; Angle-closure glaucoma; Aortocoronary graft; Apexcardiogram (procedure/ cardiology).

AcG; Ac-G; Ac-g Accelerator globulin - see Factor V.

ACGE American College of Gastroenterology.

ACGEHA Accrediting Commission on Graduate Education for Hospital Administration.

ACGIH American Conference of Governmental Industrial Hygienists.

ACGME Accreditation Council on Graduate Medical Education (program).

ACGP American College of General Practitioners.

ACGPOMS American College of General Practitioners in Osteopathic Medicine and Surgery.

ACGS Aerospace Cartographic and Geodetic Service.

ACGT Advisory Committee on Genetic Testing (DoH, UK); Antibody-coated grid technique.

A,C,G,T Alanine, Cytosine, Guanine, and Thymine - the four chemical (aminoacid) bases or gene sequences making up the DNA. These bases are arranged in pairs, "A" bonding with "T", and "C" with "G", forming the steps of the DNA's double helix. Humans have 3 billion chemical letter steps of base pairs, positioned in 23 pairs of chromosomes. On them are 50,000 to 100,000 genes, an average gene possessing 30,000 to 60,000 base pairs or gene sequences.

ACH Accident Case Histories (SFPC bulletin); Acetaldehyde; Acetylcholine (see ACh); Achalasia; Active chronic hepatitis; Acute-care hospital; Adrenal cortical hormone (see Hormones); Aftercoming head; Aluminium chlorhydroxide (antiperspirant); Amyotrophic cerebellar hypoplasia; Arm girth, chest depth, height, or hip width (see ACH nutritional index).

Ach; Ach Acetylcholine (= ACH; Ach).

ACHA American College Health Association; American College of Hospital Administrators.

AChA Anterior choroidal artery.

ACHC Association of Community Health Councils (England and Wales).

AChE Acetylcholinesterase.

AchE-I Acetylcholinesterase inhibitor (= E 2020) (see ACE).

ACHEMA Exhibition of Chemical Apparatus (German: Ausstellung für Chemisches Apparatewesen).

ACH index Arm girth, chest depth, hip width index (of nutrition).

ACHOO Autosomal dominant compelling helio-ophthalmic outburst (syndrome).

ACHP L'Association Canadienne d'Hygiène Publique (CPHA).

AChR Acetylcholine receptor.

AC/hr Air changes per hour.

AChRAb Acetylcholine receptor antibody.

AChRP Acetylcholine receptor protein.

AchS; AchS Associate of the Society of Chiropodists.

AC&HS Before meals and at bed time (L. ante cibum & hora somni).

ACI Acoustic comfort index; Acute cardiac insufficiency; Acute coronary infarction/ insufficiency; Adenylate cyclase inhibitor; Adrenocortical insufficiency; Aftercare instructions; Angiotensin convertase inhibition; Anticholinesterase inhibitor; Anticlonus index; Autologous chondrocyte implant(ation).

ACID Arithmetic, Coding, Information, and Digit Span.

Acid LSD-25 (see LSD).

Acid phos Acid phosphatase (see Acid p'tase) - laboratory/ chemistry.

Acid p'tase Acid phosphatase (= ACP; AC-PH; Ac phos; Ac p'tase; AP) - laboratory/ chemistry.

ACIF Against/anti complement immunofluorescence (test for).

ACIL American Council of Independent Laboratories.

ACIOL Anterior chamber intraocular lens (= ACL).

ACIOLI Anterior chamber intraocular lens implant (= ACLI).

ACIP Acute canine idiopathic polyneuropathy; Advisory Committee on Immunization Practices (USPHS) - see CD.

ACIR Automotive Crash Injury Research.

ACIS Adenocarcinoma in situ (abnormal gland tissue that may become cancerous, as in the colon and endometrium).

ACJ Acromioclavicular joint (see SCJ).

AcK Francium (Actinium K).

ACL Achievement Check List; Acromegaloid features, cutis verticis gyrata, (corneal) leucoma (syndrome); Acute childhood leukemia; Air conditioner lung (= Humidifier lung, a type of pneumonitis); Amaurosis congenita of Leber (see LCA); Anterior chamber lens (see ACIOL); Anterior cruciate ligament.

ACl Aspiryl chloride.

ACLA American Clinical Laboratory Association; Amide-compound local anesthetic (such as Bupivacaine, Dibucaine, Etiodocaine, Lidocaine, Mepivacaine, Prilocaine).

ACLC Assessment of Children's Language Comprehension.

ACLD Association for Children with Learning Difficulties/ Disabilities.

ACLI American Council on Life Insurance; Anterior chamber lens implant (see ACIOLI).

ACLM American College of Legal Medicine.

ACLPS Academy of Clinical Laboratory Physicians and Scientists.

ACLS Advanced cardiac life support; American Council of Learned Societies; Annals of Clinical Laboratory Science.

ACLSS Advanced Cardiac Life Support Subcommittee (AHA).

ACLTCF Accreditation Council for Long-Term Care Facilities (JCAH).

ACLU American Civil Liberties Union.

AclV (Avian) acute leukemia virus (see AAcLV)..

ACM Abnormal cell metabolism; Acute/ Alcoholic cardiomyopathy; Acute cerebrospinal meningitis; Adhesive copolymeric matrix (used in wound dressings); Adriamycin, cyclophosphamide, methotrexate; Albumin-calcium-magnesium; All-cause mortality; Alveolar capillary membrane; Anticardiac myosin; Anticholinergic medication; Anticonvulsant medication; Appropriate contraceptive measure; Arnold-Chiari malformation; Association for Computing Machinery.

ACMB Advisory Council of Medical Boards.

ACMC Association of Canadian Medical Colleges.

ACME Advisory Council on Medical Education; Aphakic cystoid macular edema; Automated Classification of Medical Entities.

ACMF Arachnoid cyst of the middle fossa.

ACMG American College of Medical Genetics.

ACMH American College of Medical Hypnosis.

ACMI American Cystoscope Makers Inc.

ACML Atypical chronic myeloid leukemia.

ACMP Alveolar-capillary membrane permeability.

ACMR Advisory Committee on Medical Research (WHO).

ACMS Advisory Committee on Medical Science; American Chinese Medical Society; American Council of Medical Staffs.

ACMT American College of Medical Technologists; Artificial circus movement tachycardia.

ACMV Assist-controlled mechanical ventilation.

ACMVAT Anticytomegalovirus antibody test.

ACMW American Committee on Maternal Welfare.

ACN Acute conditioned neurosis; American College of Neuropsychiatrists/ Nutrition; Anterior crural/ cutaneous nerve.

ACn Air conduction (in the presence of bone conduction noise).

ACNB American College of Neuropsychiatrists Bulletin.

ACNHA American College of Nursing Home Administrators.

ACNM American College of Nuclear Medicine; American College of Nurse-Midwives.

ACNP American College of Neuropsychopharmacology; American College of Nuclear Physicians.

ACO Acute coronary occlusion; Alert, cooperative, and oriented; Ambulatory-care organization; American College of Orgonomy; American Council of Otolaryngology; Anodal closing/sure odor; Anticholinergic overdose ("Red as a beet, blind as a bat, dry as a bone, mad as a hatter and hotter than hell!") (= ACT).

ACoA Adult children of alcoholics; Anterior communicating artery.

ACOB Association Canadienne des Optométristes Bulletin.
ACOG American College of Obstetricians and Gynecologists.
ACOGN American College of Obstetricians and Gynecologists Newsletter.
ACOGTB American College of Obstetricians and Gynecologists Technical Bulletin.
ACOHA American College of Osteopathic Hospital Administrators.
ACO-HNS American Council of Otolaryngology - Head and Neck Surgery.
ACOI American College of Osteopathic Internists.
ACOM American College of Occupational Medicine.
ACOMA Adriamycin, Cyclophosphamide, Oncovin, Methotrexate and arabinosyl Cytosine (Chemotherapy).
ACOMS American College of Oral and Maxillofacial Surgeons.
ACOOG American College of Osteopathic Obstetricians and Gynecologist.
ACOP American College of Osteopathic Pediatricians.
A-COPP Adriamycin-Cytoxan, Oncovin, Prednisone, Procarbazine (in the treatment of neoplastic disease).
ACORDE A Consortium On Restorative Dentistry Education.
ACORN Automated Coder Of The Report Narrative.
ACOS American College of Osteopathic Surgeons.
ACOSN American College of Osteopathic Surgeons News.
Acou- prefix meaning hear (Gr. akous).
Acous Acoustic(s)/cal.
ACP Abnormal cell proliferation; Accessory conduction pathway; Acetyl-carrier protein; Acid phosphatase (see Acid p'tase); Active-control patient; Acute cor pulmonale; Acyl carrier protein; Adenomatous colon polyp; Adrenal cortisol production; Adult competent patient; Ambulatory constipated population; American College of Pathologists/ Pharmacists/ Physicians/ Prosthodontists/ Psychiatrists; AMSA, Chlorambucil and pred-Care Panel; Anodal closing picture; Anticancer protein; Antichole-cystokinin peptide; Aspirin, caffeine, phenacetin (proprietary drug); Association Canadienne des Physiciens; Association for Child Psychiatrists; Association of Clinical Pathologists (UK); Association of Correctional Psychologists; Asthma Control Program; Ataxic/ Athetoid cerebral palsy.
AcP Acupuncture (see AP).
ACPA Acute cardiopulmonary arrest; American Chronic Pain Association; American Cleft Palate Association; Anticytoplasmic antibodies.
ACPAP Advisory Committee on Physician's Assistant Programs.
ACPC Aminocyclopentane carboxylic (acid).
ACPE American College of Physician Executives; American Council on Pharmaceutical Education.
ACPEF American Cleft Palate Educational Foundation.
AC-PH; Ac phos Acid phosphatase (see Acid p'tase).
ACPM Acute-care patient monitoring; American College of Preventive Medicine.
ACPMR American College of Physical Medicine and Rehabilitation.
ACPP Adrenocorticopolypeptide.
ACPP PF Acid phosphatase prostatic fluid.
ACPS Acrocephalopolysyndactyly.
Ac p'tase Acid phosphatase (see Acid p'tase).
ACq Air conduction in quiet.
ACR Abnormally contracting region; Absolute catabolic rate; Accounts of Chemical Research (journal); Acriflavine; Active-Controlled Response (see ACRRI); Adenomatosis of colon and rectum; Adrenocortical reserve; Albumin : creatinine ratio (urinary) (in mg/mmol, geometric mean tolerance factors); Allergic cross reaction; American College of Radiologists/ Radiology/ Rheumatology; Americans for Children's Relief; Annals of Clinical Research (journal); Anticonstipation regimen; Axillary count rate.
Acr Acrylic.
Acr- prefix meaning extremity or peak (Gr.

ACRB American College of Radiology Bulletin.

ACRC AIDS Clinical Research Center.

ACRF Acute cardiorespiratory failure, Advanced chronic renal failure; Ambulatory care research facility.

ACRM American College of Rehabilitation Medicine; American Congress of/on Rehabilitation Medicine.

ACRMD Association for Children with Retarded Mental Devolopment.

ACRRI Active-controlled response Responder Index.

ACS Abortion counseling service(s); Acetabular Cup System (see OI/OP); Acetylstrophanthidin; Acrocallosal syndrome; Acrocephalosyndactylism (= Apert's syndrome); Acrocephalosyndactyly; Acromioclavicular separation; Acta Chemica Scandinavica (journal); Active-controlled study; Acute calcinic synovitis (of the knee joint); Acute chest/ cholinergic/ coronary syndrome; Acute confusional state; Alcon Closure System; Adrenal catecholamine secretion; Adrenocortical steroid; Adrenocortical steroidogenesis; Advance Closure Systems (Calif) (use of radio waves as adhesives in replacing stitches or staples); Ambulatory care services; American Cancer Society; American Chemical Society; American College of Surgeons/ Surgery; Ankylosed cervical segment/ spine; Anodal closing sound; Anterior chamber shallowing (eye); Antireticular cytotoxic serum; Aperture current setting; Appropriate clinical standard(s); Arterial cleansing system (IV chelation therapy); Association of Clinical Scientists.

acs before supper.

ACSA Adenylate cyclase-stimulating activity.

ACSB Ambulatory Care Statistics Branch (NCHS); American College of Surgeons Bulletin.

ACSE Association of Component Society Executives.

ACSH American Council on Science and Health.

ACSJMC American Chemical Society Journal of Medicinal Chemistry.

ACSM American College of Sports Medicine.

(A-CS)O_2 Myocardial oxygen extraction.

ACSP Adenylate cyclase-stimulating protein; Advisory Council on Scientific Policy.

ACSS Acute caretaker stress syndrome.

ACSV Aortocaronary saphenous vein.

ACSVBG Aortocoronary saphenous vein bypass graft.

ACSW Academy/ Association of Certified Social Workers.

ACT Abdominal computerized tomogram/graph(y); Achievement through Counseling and Treatment; Actinomycin; Activated cephalin/ clotting/ coagulation time; Adjuvant chemotherapy; Adrenal cortical tissue/ tumor; Advanced Cell Technology (Biotechnical concern); Advanced Coronary Treatment; Alkylating cytotoxic (e.g. Carboplatin; Cyclophosphamide); Allergen challenge test; Alternative/ anticancer therapy/ treatment; Anagen (growth phase) → Catagen (acute follicular regression or transitional phase) → Telogen (resting or shedding phase) - 3 phases of the hair growth cycle; American College Testing (Program) (see ACTP); Anterocolic transposition; Anticholinergic toxidrome (see ACO; TD); Antichymotrypsin; Anticoagulant/ Anticonvulsant therapy; Anxiety control training; Appropriate corticosteroid therapy/ treatment; Assisted conception technique; Atropine coma therapy.

Act Actinomycin; Active/vity (= Activ).

ACTA American Corrective Therapy Association; Automatic computerized transverse axial (tomographic scanner - see CAT; CT).

ACTAS Automatic computerized transverse axial scanner (see ACTA).

ACTC; ActC; Act-C Actinomycin C.

ACTD Adrenocorticotropic deficiency.

ACTD; ActD; Act-D Actinomycin D (cosmogen/ dactinomycin).

ACTe Anodal closure tetanus.

Act Ex Active exercise.

ACTG AIDS Clinical Treatment/ Trial Group.

ACTH Adrenal corticotropic hormone (= Adrenocorticotropic hormone) - see Hormones.

ACTH 1-24 b-1-24-corticotropin.
ACTH-LI Adrenocorticotropin-like immunoreactivity.
ACTH/MSH (basophils) Adrenocorticotropic hormone/ melanocytic-stimulating hormone (basophils) (see Hormones).
ACTH-RF Adrenocorticotropic hormone releasing factor.
Actin- prefix meaning ray or radius (Gr. aktis).
ACTION American Council To Improve Our Neighbourhoods (a former name for an independent Federal agency).
Activ Active/vity (see Act).
ACTJ American Corrective Therapy Journal.
ACTN Adrenocorticotropin (see Hormones).
ACTP Adrenocorticotropic/pin polypeptide (see Hormones); American College Testing Program.
ACTR Adrenocorticotropic reserve.
ACTS Acute cervical traumatic sprain/ syndrome; Anti-Cancer Treatment Status; Auditory Comprehension Test for Sentences.
ACTSEB Anterior chamber tube shunt encircling band.
ACU Acquired cold urticaria; Acute care/ coronary unit; Agar colony forming unit; Ambulatory care unit.
Acu- prefix meaning hear (Gr. akous).
Acup Acupuncture.
ACV Acute cardiovascular disease (see ACVD); Acute/Allergic conjunctivitis vernalis; Acyclovir (an antiviral drug); Anterior cardiac vein; Atrial/ carotid/ ventricular.
A/CV Assisted/Controlled ventilation.
ACVB Aortocoronary venous bypass.
ACVD Acquired color vision deficiency; Acute/ Alcoholic/ Atherosclerotic cardiovascular disease.
ACVT American College of Veterinary Toxicologists.
ACW Anterior chest wall; Arterial circle of Willis.
Ac/w A cetone/water (mixture).
AD Absorbed/ Analgesic/ Arthritic dose; Accident department/ dispensary; Acetate dialysis; Achievement drive; Acid/ Alkaline diuresis; Active/ Adjuvant/ Adult/ Aleutian disease; Acute dermatomyositis; Addict(ion); Adenoid(al) degeneration (agent/ virus); Adhesive disc; Admitting diagnosis; Adrenostenedione; Advanced directive; Aerosol deposition; Affective disorder; After discharge; Aid to disabled; Alcohol dehydrogenase; Alcoholic dementia; Aldehyde dehydrogenase (see ADG); Allergic/ Atopic diathesis; Allodynia (pain generated by minor stimulation of the skin); Alternating days; Alveolar diffusion; Alveolar duct; Alzheimer's dementia/ disease (cerebral sclerosis, with memory lapses, confusion, and slow dementia); American Druggist (journal); Analog-to-digital; Anno Domini (L.) - in the year of the Lord i.e. the Christian era (used in dates); Anodal duration; Ante diem (L.) - before the day; Anterior division; Antigenic determinant; Aortic dissection; Appropriate disability; Archives of Dermatology (journal); Associate Degree; Atopic dermatitis; Atrium dexter (L.) - right atrium; Attentional disturbance; Auris dextra (L.) - right ear; Autonomic dysreflexia; Autosomal dominant; Average deviation/ duration; Axiodistal; Axis deviation; Axonal degeneration; Diphenylchlorarsine; Donor recovery time (see A/D); Drug addict (see DA); Right atrium (L. atrium dexter); Right ear (L. auris dextra).
Ad; ad Add/ Add up to (= add) (L. adde)/ Let them be added (L. addantur)/ Let there be added (L. addetur)/ To (L.); Adenovirus; Adrenal; Anisotropic disk; Axiodistal; Right ear (L. auris dextra) - see AD.
ad- prefix meaning to or up to (L.).
A&D Admission and discharge; Alcohol and drug(s); Ascending and descending; Vitamins A and D.
ADA Adenosine deaminase (see ADase); American Dental/ Dermatological/ Diabetes/tic/ Dietetic Association; Americans with Disabilities Act; Anterior descending artery; Antideoxyribonucleic acid antibody; Antidepressant action; Antidepressive agent; Antidiabetic/ diarrheal agent (= ADD); Antidopaminergic activity; Approved dietary allowance; Aspiration drug abuse (e.g. cocaine snorting; glue sniffing); Australian Dental Association.

ADAA American Dental Assistants' Association; Anxiety Disorders Association of America.

ADA diet American Diabetic Association diet.

ADADS Assistant Director Army Dental Service.

ADAF Alcoholism and Drug Addiction Foundation (Toronto, Canada); American Diabetes Association Forecast (journal).

ADAJ American Dental Association Journal.

ADAM Amniotic deformity, adhesion, mutilation (syndrome).

ADAMHA Alcohol Drug Abuse and Mental Health Administration (HEW).

ADAN American Dental Association News.

ADAP AIDS Drug Assistance Program; Alzheimer's disease associated protein; American Dental Assistant's Program; Assistant Director of Army Psychiatry.

ADARC Aaron Diamond AIDS Research Center (NYC).

ADARF Alcoholism and Drug Addiction Research Foundation (Ontario, Canada).

ADAS Alzheimer's Disease Assessment Scale.

ADA-SCID Adenosine deaminase - severe combined immune deficiency (a rare genetic disease).

ADAS-COG ADAS (cognitive portion of).

ADase Adenosine deaminase (= ADA; ADD).

ADAU Adolescent drug abuse unit.

ADAV&RS Assistant Director Army Veterinary and Remount Services.

ADB Abdominal-diaphragmatic breathing; Accidental death benefit; Anti DNase B.

ADC Acute dilated cardiomyopathy; Affective/ Anxiety disorder(s) clinic; Aid to dependent children; AIDS Dementia Complex; Albumin, dextrose, catalase (media); Alzheimer's Disease Center (UCLA); Ambulance design criteria; Analog-to-digital converter; Androgen-dependent cancer (e.g. of the prostate); Anodal duration contraction; Antidromic conduction (of a nerve impulse in a direction contrary to the normal i.e. backwards); Archives of Diseases in Childhood (BMA journal); Arrested dental caries; Arterial dilatation catheter (= Gruntzig balloon catheter - used in iliac artery dilatation); L'Association Dentaire Canadienne (CDA); Average daily census; Axiodistocervical.

AdC Adenylate cyclase; Adrenal cortex.

ADCC Acute disorder of cerebral circulation; Adult day care center; Antibody-dependent cell-mediated/ cellular cytotoxicity.

Ad Com Administration committee.

ADCP Adenosine deaminase complexing protein.

ADCS Ahumada del Castillo syndrome (absence of menstruation in non-pregnant females, sometimes associated with a pituitary gland tumor and the presence of breast milk); Alzheimer's Disease Cooperative Study; Argonz del Castillo syndrome.

ADD Accidental death and dismemberment (insurance); Adduction; Adenosine deaminase deficiency (see ADase; PSPE); Adult degenerative disease; Antibody deficiency disease; Antidepressive/ diabetic/ diarrheal drug (see ADA); Attention deficit disorder; Autosomal dominant disease/ disorder; Average daily dose.

add Add (L. adde) (see Ad/ad); Addition; Adduction/tor; Let them be added (L. addantur) (see Ad/ad); Let there be added (L. addetur) (see Ad/ad).

add c trit Add with triturition (L. adde cum tritu).

ADDD Adenosine deaminase deficiency disease (see ADD; PSPE).

adde (L.) add.

Ad def an To the point of fainting (L. ad defectionem animi).

Ad deliq To fainting (L. ad deliquium).

Addend To be added (L. addendus).

ADDH Attention deficit disorder with hyperactivity (see ADHD)..

ADD/HA Attention deficit disorder/hyperactivity (see ADHD).

Addict Addiction/tive.

ADDL Association of Drug Detection Laboratories.

Addn Addition.

ADDP Adolescent Drug Depending Program; Apollo Double-Diaphragm Pump.

Add poll Adductor pollicis.

ADDS American Digestive Disease Society; American Diopter and Decibel Society.

ADDU Alcohol and drug dependence unit.
ADE Accumulated dose equivalent (an estimate of the maximum safe dose of radiation over a life-time); Acneform drug eruption; Acrodermatitis enteropathica (an autosomal recessive, hypotrichosis with alopecia, diarrhea, acral and periorificial dermatitis, and failure to thrive); Acute disseminated encephalitis/ encephalomyelitis (see ADEM); Adverse drug effect/ event; AIDS-defining event(s); American (Medical Association) Drug Evaluation; Antibody-dependent enhancement; Apparent digestible energy.
Ade Adenine.
AdeCbl Adenosyl cobalamine.
ADEE Age-dependent epileptic encephalopathy.
Ad effect Until effective/tual (L. ad effectum).
ADEK Fat-soluble vitamins A, D, E and K.
ADEM Acute disseminated encephalomyelitis.
aden- prefix meaning gland (Gr. aden).
Adenoca Adenocarcinoma.
Adeq Adequate.
ADF Audio-Digest Foundation (CMA).
Ad feb Fever being present (L. adstante febre).
ADFN Albinism-deafness syndrome.
ADFR Activate (bone metabolism with phosphorus to stimulate parathroid activity - 4 days) → Depress (osteoclasts with a diphosphonate such as alendronate or etidronate - 14 days) → Free period (with calcium and Vit D - 12 weeks) → Repeat (the cycle - A → D → F at least 12 times) - a cyclic phosphate/ diphosphonate/ calcium sequence in the treatment of osteoporosis.
ADFU Agar diffusion for fungus.
ADG Aldehyde dehydrogenase (= AD); Atrial diastolic gallop; Axiodistogingival.
ADGID Angiodysplastic gastrointestinal disease.
Ad gr. acid; Ad grat. acid To an agreeable acidity or sourness (L. ad gratum aciditatem).
Ad gr. gust; Ad grat. gust To an agreeable taste (L. ad gratum gustum).
ADH Academy of Dentistry for the Handicapped; Acquired dislocation of the hip; Adhesion; Adrenalin-heparin (complex); Alcohol dehydrogenase; Antidiabetic hormone - the insulins (see Hormones); Antidiuretic hormone i.e. vasopressin (see Hormones); Arginine dihydrolase.
Adh Adhesion/sive; Antidiabetic/ Antidiuretic hormone (see ADH).
ADHA American Dental Hygienists' Association; American Drug and Hospital Association.
ADHD Antidiuretic hormone disorder; Attention-deficit-hyperactivity/ve disorder.
Adhib Administer/ apply/ take/ to be administered (L. adhibendus).
ADHR Antidiuretic-hormone-resistant (diabetes).
ADI Absolute Doppler index; Academy of Dentistry International; Acceptable/ Allowable daily intake; Acute dangerous/ depressive/ dyspeptic illness; Adverse drug interaction; Alcohol/ Aldehyde dehydrogenase inhibitor (e.g. Disulfiram, Fomepizole, etc.); American Documentation Institute (Library of Congress); American Drug Index; Artificial diverticulum of the ileum; Atlasdens interval; Autosomal dominant inheritance (genetic disease); Axiodistoincisal.
ADIM Audio-Digest of Internal Medicine.
ad int In the meantime/ meanwhile (L. ad interim).
adip- prefix meaning fat (L. adeps).
ADJ Amelodentinal junction (see DEJ); Australian Dental Journal (Australian Dental Association).
adj adjacent; adjective; adjoining; adjunct; adjuvant.
ADK Adenosine kinase; Adirondack Mountain Club.
ADKC Atopic dermatitis with kerato-conjunctivitis.
ADL Activities of daily living; Adrenoleukodystrophy (Lorenzo's disease); Amsterdam Depression List; Arthur D Little, Inc.; Acute disc lesion.
ADLC Antibody-dependent lymphocyte-mediated cytotoxicity.
Ad lib As desired/ at pleasure (L. ad libitum).
ADLMA American Dental Library and Museum Association.

ADM Abductor digiti minimi; Adequate/ Appropriate dietary management; Administrative medicine; Adriamycin hydrochloride (= Doxorubicin HCl) - a cytotoxic agent; Aggravated diabetes mellitus.

Adm; adm Administrate/tion/tor; Admission/mit(ted); Apply (L. admove).

AdM Administrative medicine; Adrenal medulla.

ADMA American Drug Manufacturers Association; Aran-Duchenne muscular atrophy (see PSMA).

Ad man. med Deliver to the physician (L. ad manus medici).

Adm Dr Admitting doctor.

ADME Absorption, Distribution, Metabolism and Elimination (of a drug).

Admin Administer/tration (see Adm; adm).

Admov Add/ apply/ let it be applied/ let there be added/ let there be applied (L. admove, admoveatur).

Adm Ph Admitting physician.

ADMR Average daily metabolic rate.

ADMS Assistant Director of Medical Services.

ADMX Adrenal medullectomy.

ADN Antideoxyribonuclease; Aortic depressor nerve; Associate Degree in Nursing; Deoxyribonucleic acid (proprietary name in France) - see DNA.

Ad naus To the extent/ point of producing nausea (L. ad nauseam).

ADN-B Antideoxyribonuclease B.

Ad neut To neutralization (L. ad neutralizandum).

ADO Adenosine; Adolescent medicine; Association of Dispensing Opticians (UK); Audio-Digest Otorhinolaryngology (journal); Axiodistoocclusal.

Ado Adenosine.

Ad-OAP Doxorubicin (Adriamycin), vincristine (Oncovin), cytarabine (cytosine Arabinoside), and prednisone.

ADOD Arthrodentosteodysplasia.

AdoDABA Adenosyldiaminobutyric acid.

ADOG Audio-Digest Obstetrics-Gynecology (ADF).

AdoHcy S-Adenosylhomocysteine.

adol adolescent.

AdoMet S-Adenosylmethionine.

Adonis complex Male body obsession (see MBO).

Adox Oxidized adenosine.

ADP Additional diagnostic procedure; Adenopathy; Adenosine diphosphate; Administrative psychiatry; Alveolar distending pressure (the pressure difference between the pulmonary alveoli and the intrapleural space); Amino-diphenyl (a carcinogen); Antidepressant poison(ing); Antidiabetic principle - the insulins (see Hormones); Appropriate/ Approved diagnostic procedure; Approved drug product; Area diastolic pressure; Arterial demand pacing; Atrial premature depolarization; Audio-Digest Pediatrics/ Psychiatry (journals); Automatic data processing; Automatic dual programmed; Acute disc prolapse.

AdP Adductor pollicis.

Ad part. dol To the painful parts (L. ad partes dolentes).

Ad part. dolent See Ad part. dol.

ADPase Adenosine diphosphatase.

AD pattern Arterial deficiency pattern.

ADPD Autosomal dominant Parkinson's disease (see parkin gene).

ADPI Alzheimer's Disease Prevention Initiative.

ADPKD Autosomal dominant polycystic kidney disease.

ADPL Average daily patient load.

Ad pond. om To the weight of the whole (L. ad pondus omnium).

ADPR Adenosine diphosphate ribose.

ADPS Antideformity positioning and splinting (Orthopedics).

ADQ Abductor digite quinte.

Adq Adequate.

ADR Accepted Dental Remedies (published by the American Dental Association); Accepted dental remedy; Acute dystonic reaction; Adjusted death rate; Adrenodoxin reductase; Adverse drug reaction - Type A (Augmented), Type B (Bizarre); Airway dilation reflex; Alzheimer's Disease Research (program - AHAF); Appropriate dosage regimen; Arrested development of righting response; Assigned daily range;

Asymmetrical ('eccentric') dose regimen; Ataxia-deafness-retardation (syndrome); Autonomic dysreflexia; Doxorubicin (Adriamycin) (see ADM).

Adr; adr Adrenal; Adrenalectomy; Adrenalin(e); Adriamycin.

Ad rat As reasonable (L. ad rationem).

ADRBR Adrenergic beta-receptor.

ADRC Alzheimer's Disease Research Center.

ADRDA Alzheimer's Disease and Related Disorders Association.

Adria Adriamycin (see ADM).

ADRN Associated Degree Registered Nurse.

ADRV Adult rotavirus.

ADS Active drug substance; Acute death/ diarrheal syndrome; Acute disseminated strongyloidiasis; Alcohol Dependence Scale; Alcohol dependence syndrome; Alternative delivery system; Alveolar dead space; American Dental Society; Anatomical dead space; Anonymous donor's sperm; Anterior dislocation of the shoulder; Anterior drawer sign (see DS; PDS; PDT); Antibody deficiency syndrome; Antidiphtheritic serum (= Diphtheria antitoxin); Antidiuretic substance (= ADH; Antidiuretic hormone) (see Hormones); Archives of Dermatology and Syphilogy; Army Dental Service; Audio-Digest Surgery (journal); Automatic Development System (Blue Shield); Axodendritic synapse (Obstetrics).

ADSA American Dairy Science Association; American Dental Society of Anesthesiology.

ADSAPI Accentuated decrease in systemic arterial pressure during inspiration.

Ad sat To saturation (L. ad saturandum).

ADSS Axodendrosomatic synapse (junction or synapse of the axon of one neuron with the dendrites plus cell body of another).

Adst. feb When/ while fever is present (L. adstante febre).

ADSU Ambulatory diagnostic surgery unit.

ADT Accepted Dental Therapeutics; Adenosine triphosphate; Admission, discharge, transfer; Agar-gel diffusion test; Alternate-day therapy/ treatment; Androgen-dependent tumor; Anodal duration tetanus; Anticipate discharge tomorrow; Antidepressant/sion/sive therapy; 'Antidoping' test(s) (e.g. to athletes, suspected drug users, traffic violators, etc.); Any desired thing/ anything desired/ anything you desire or like/ "any damn thing" (a placebo prescription); Alzheimer's-type dementia; Auditory Discrimination Test; Automated dithionate test.

ADTA American Dance Therapy Association; American Dental Trade Association.

ADTe Anodal duration tetanus (Tetanic contraction).

A-DTIC Doxorubicin (Adriamycin) and dacarbazine (DTIC).

ADTP Adolescent Day Treatment Program.

ADU Active duodenal ulcer; Allen-Doisy unit; Acute duodenal ulcer.

Ad us According to custom (L. ad usum).

Ad us. ext For external application/ use (L. ad usum externum).

ADV Adenovirus; Adventia; Aleutian disease virus; Arterio deep venous (see A/DV).

A/DV Arterio/deep venous (= ADV).

Adv; adv Adenovirus (see ADV); Adverse to/ against (L. adversum); Advertisement.

ADV-4 Adenovirus (type 4).

ADV-7 Adenovirus (type 7).

Ad 2 vic At two times/ for two doses (L. ad duas vices).

ADVIRC Autosomal dominant vitreo-retinochoroidopathy.

Ad virus Adenovirus.

ADVOCAP Advocate Community Action Committee.

ADW Assault with deadly weapon; Avoirdupois weight (the English system of weights, in which there are 7,000 grains, 256 drams, or 16 ounces to 1 pound. One ounce equals 28.35 grams and one pound equals 453.59 grams).

A5 D5 W Alcohol 5%, dextrose 5%, in water.

ADWS Acute drug-withdrawal syndrome.

ADX Adrenal-ectomized.

AE Above elbow (amputation); Accident and emergency (department); Acrodermatitis enteropathica; Acta Endocrinologica (Denmark journal); Activation energy; Adult erythrocyte; Adverse event(s)/ experience(s); After-effect; Agarose electrophoresis; Air embolism/ entry; Alcoholic embryopathy;

Alveolar Echinococcosis; Aminoethyl; Angioneurotic edema; Anoxic encephalopathy; Anti-epileptic; Antitoxin unit (German Antitoxin-Einheit); Apoenzyme; Aryepiglottic; Atherosclerotic encephalopathy; Atomic emmision; Atopic eczema; Avian encephalomyelitis; Energy of activation.

A-E Dow Chemical Co. code for experimental substances.

A+E Accident and Emergency (Department/ Ward); Analysis and evaluation.

AEA Above elbow amputation; Acute exacerbated/tory asthma/ attack; Alcohol, ether, acetone (mixture); Alkaline Elution Assay (= Ames in vitro assay in rat hepatoctes, for mutagenicity of a drug) (see CAA); Anti-epileptic activity/ agent; Apocrine membrane antigen; Atomic Energy Authority (UK).

AEA sol Alcohol-ether-acetone solution.

AEB Acute erythroblastopenia; As evidenced by; Avian erythroblastosis.

AEC Allergic eye condition; Ankyloblepharon, ectodermal defects, and cleft lip (syndrome); At earliest convenience; Atomic Energy of Canada Ltd. (see AECL); Atomic Energy Commission (now defunct).

AECB Acute exacerbation of chronic bronchitis.

AECCC American-European Concensus Conference Committee.

AECD Allergic eczematous contact dermatitis.

AECG Abdominal electrocardiograph.

AECL Atomic Energy of Canada Limited (= AEC; EACL).

AECM Albert Einstein College of Medicine (New York).

AED Accident and Emergency department; Acute endothelial dysfunction; Anhidrotic ectodermal dysplasia (see CST - Christ ST); Anorexic and Eating Disturbances (Symposium, NY, May 2001); Anti- emetic/ epileptic/ estrogen drug; Antihidrotic ectodermal dysplasia; Automated external defibrillator; Average effective dosage/ dose.

AEDP Automated external defibrillator pacemaker.

AEDT Anti-epileptic drug therapy/ treatment.

AEE Anti-emetic effect; Antiepileptic effect/ efficacy; Atomic Energy Establishment (UK).

AEEU Admission entrance and evaluation unit.

AEF Allogenic-effect factor; American Epilepsy Foundation; Amyloid enhancing factor.

AEG Air encephalogram/graphy (procedure/ neurology); Apolipoprotein E genotyping (e.g. in Alzheimer's disease); Atrial electrogram.

Aeg The patient (L. aeger; aegra).

AEGIS Aid for the Elderly in Government Institutions.

AEH Adynamia episodica hereditaria (a rare inherited defect seen in infants, also called HPP or Hyperkalemic periodic paralysis); Antiembolism hose (elastic stockings worn to prevent clotting or thromboembolic defects); Anti-estrogen hormone; Archives of Environmental Health.

AEHA Army Environmental Hygiene Agency.

AEI Acute ethanol intoxication (Alcohol, C2H5OH) (= AAI) - Degree I: Well-being: talkativeness, revelry, subjective elevation of the psyche; Degree II: Inebriation: slurred speech, emotional instability, incoordination, loss of sensory perception; Degree III: Intoxication: blurred vision, loss of sensory perception, muscular incoordination, ataxia, slow reaction time, slurred speech; Degree IV: Severe intoxication: severe ataxia, blurred or double vision, coma, convulsions; Degree V: Very severe intoxication: coma, hyporeflexia, hypothermia, respiratory depression, poor airway protection; Adequate electolyte intake; American Enterprise Institute; Arbitrary evolution index; Atrial emptying index.

AEIPPR American Enterprise Institute for Public Policy Research.

AEM Accident and emergency medicine (UK); Ambulatory electrocardiographic monitoring; Analytical electron microscopy; Annals of Emergency Medicine (journal); Anti-epileptic medication; Avian encephalomyelitis.

AEMB Alliance for Engineering in Medicine and Biology.

AEMIS Aerospace and Environmental Medicine Information System.

AEN Aseptic epiphyseal necrosis.
AENAA Anti-extractable nuclear antigen antibody (see AAB).
A2 England English influenza epidemic (1972).
AEO Abbe-Estlander operation (mouth skin-graft procedure).
AEOS Alopecia-Epilepsy-Oligophrenia syndrome (Epilepsy, severe mental retardation - an ectodermal dysplasia) (= MS - Moynihan syndrome).
AEP Acute edematous pancreatitis; Acute ethanol poisoning; Adjudicated endpoint (see CEAC); Advanced ectopic pregnancy; Adverse event/ experience profile; Ambulant elderly patient; 2-Aminoethylphosphonic acid; Artificial endocrine pancreas; Auditory (brain-stem and cortical) evoked potential; Average evoked potential.
AEPR Acute extra-pyramidal reaction.
AEPs Average evoked potentials.
AEq Age equivalent.
Aeq; aeq Equal (L. aequales).
AEQI Agricultural Environmental Quality Institute (BARC-USDA).
AER Abduction/ external rotation; Acoustic/ Auditory/ Average evoked response; Acute exertional rhabdomyolysis; Advances in Enzyme Regulation (journal); Agranular endoplasmic reticulum; Albumin/ Aldosterone excretion rate; Anion exchange resin (cholestyramine); Apical ectodermal ridge; Averaged electroencephalic response.
aer- prefix meaning air (Gr. aer).
AERD Atheroembolic renal disease.
AERE Atomic Energy Research Establishment (UK).
AERJ American Educational Research Journal.
Aer M Aerosol mask.
Aero Aerobacter - a genus of microorganisms of the family Enterobacteriaceae; e.g. A. aerogenes (= Aero. aerogenes; Bacillus lactis a.; Enterobacter a.) - causes urinary tract and other infections in man.
Aeron Aeronautics.
AERP Antegrade/ Atrial effective refractory period.
AERPAP Antegrade effective refractory period accessory pathway.
Aer T Aerosol tent.
AES Abnormal electric signal (heart); Acetone-extracted serum; Acute ethmoidal sinusitis; Adult Emergency Service; American Electroencephalographic/ Encephalographic/ Endocrine /Endodontic/ Endoscopic/ Entomological/Epidemiological/ Epidermological/ Epilepsy/ Eugenics Society; Anterior esophageal sensor; Anti-embolic stockings; Anti-eosinophil sera; Antral ethmoidal sphenoidectomy; Aortic ejection sound; Auger electron spectroscopy; Auto-erythrocyte sensitization.
Aes Adverse events/ experiences.
AESOP Automated Endoscopic System for Optimal Positioning (an electro-mechanical arm for positioning an endoscope).
AEST Aeromedical evacuation support team; American Entomological Society Transactions.
aeste- prefix meaning feel or perceive (Gr. aisthe-).
AET Absorption-equivalent thickness; Acute ethanol toxicity; S-(2-aminoethyl) isothiouronium bromide; Anti-emetic/ Anti-estrogen therapy/ treatment; Atrial ectopic tachycardia.
Aet; aet Aetiology (= Aetiol; Etiol; Etiliogy); Age (L. aetas)/ Of age (L. aetatis) (= Aetat).
Aetat Aged/ Of age (see Aet; aet).
Aetiol Etiology (Brit. aetiology) (see Aet; aet).
AEV Avian erythroblastosis virus.
AF Abnormal frequency; Acid-fast; Adult female; Afebrile; Aflatoxin; Air Force; Albumin-free (see Tuberculin); Albumose-free; Aldehyde fuchsin; Amaurosis fugax; Aminophylline; Amniotic fluid; Angiogenesis factor; Annulus fibrosus (of the intervertebral disc); Anteflexion; Anterior fontanelle; Antibody-forming; Antifibrinogen; Antifog; Aortic flow; Aortofemoral; Armed Forces; Arthritis Foundation; Artificial feeding; Ascitic fluid; Atomic fluorescence; Atrial fibrillation/ flutter (= Af; AFib; AFl); Atrial fusion; Attenuation factor; Attributable fraction; Audio frequency; Audiology Foundation; Auricular fibrillation/ flutter.
Af Atrial flutter (see AF).
af Audio frequency (see AF).

aF Abfarad.
af- alternate spelling of prefix ad.
A-F (tuberculin) Albumin-free (tuberculin) (see Tuberculin).
AFA Acromegaloid facial appearance; Advanced first aid; Alcohol-formaldehyde-acetic acid (fixative); Allergy Foundation of America; American Forestry Association; Antifungal activity/ agent.
AFACA Associate Fellow of the American College of Allergists (= AFACAL).
AFACAL See AFACA.
AF/Afl Atrial fibrillation/Atrial flutter (see AF).
AFAR American Foundation for Aging Research.
AFARA Arthritis Foundation's American Rheumatism Association.
AFB Acid-fast bacillus (tuberculosis) (laboratory/ bacteriology); Aflatoxin B; Air fluidized bed; American foulbrood; American Foundation for the Blind; Aortofemoral bypass; Aspirated foreign body.
AFB1 Aflatoxin B1.
AFBG Aortofemoral bypass graft.
AFBN American Foundation for the Blind Newsletter.
AFBP Anhydrous free base peptide.
AFC Adult foster care; Air-filled cushions; Amniotic fluid complement (C3) - a marker of intra-amniotic infection; Antibody-forming cell(s); Automatic frequency control.
AFCI Acute focal cerebral ischemia.
AFCR American Federation/ Foundation for Clinical Research.
AFD Accelerated freeze drying; Acute febrile disease (see AFI); Acute fetal distress; Air flow direction; Alcohol-free diet; Antifungal drug (see AFA; AFP); Axial flow device (artificial heart).
AFDA American Food and Drug Administration (see FDA).
AFDC Aid to Families with Dependent Children (program).
AFDC-FC Aid to Families with Dependent Children - Foster Care.
AFDCO Aid For Dependent Children's Organization.
AFDH American Fund for Dental Health.
AFDW Ash-free dry weight.
AFE Adenofibroma edematode(s); Amniotic fluid embolism.
AFEB Armed Forces Epidemiological Board.
afeb afebrile.
AFF Atrial filling fraction.
Aff; aff Afferent; Affinity/ Having an affinity with but not identical with (L. affinis).
AFG Aflatoxin G; Alfa fetoglobulin (liver test); Amniotic fluid glucose; Average fibular graft (Orthopedics).
AFGE American Federation of Government Employees.
AFGP Antifreeze glycoprotein.
AFH American Foundation for Homeopathy; Angiofollicular hyperplasia; Anterior facial height; Atopic family history.
AFHPSP Armed Forces Health Professions Scholarship Program.
AFI Acute febrile illness; Adequate/ Ample fluid intake; Amaurotic familial/ family idiocy; Amniotic fluid index; Amniotic fluid infection (see Amnionitis); Artificially-fed infant.
AFib Atrial/ Auricular fibrillation (see AF).
AFIP Armed Forces Institute of Pathology.
AFIPS American Federation of Information Processing Societies.
AFIS Amniotic fluid infection syndrome.
AFL American Federation of Labor; Antifatty liver (related to a factor in pancreatic tissue); Artificial limb; Atrial flutter (see AF).
AFl Atrial flutter (see AF).
AFL/CIO American Federation of Labor and Congress of Industrial Organizations.
AFLD Alcoholic fatty liver disease.
AFLNH Angiofollicular lymph node hyperplasia.
AFLP Acute fatty liver of pregnancy.
AFM Acute fulminant myocarditis; Aflatoxin M; Air-Flow meter (see PFT); Air Force Manual; Anal-finger-mouth (transmission of infection, as in *Enterobius* vermicularis infestation); Android fat mass (see TFM); Archives of Family Medicine; Atomic force microscope.
AFMCH American Foundation for Maternal and Child Health.
AFMD Armed Forces Medical Department.

AFMJ Armed Forces Medical Journal.

AFML Armed Forces Medical Library.

AFN Afunctional neutrophil.

AFNA American Federation for Negro Affairs.

AFNC Air Force Nurse Corps.

AFND Acute febrile neutrophilic dermatosis.

AFNSW Asthma Foundation of New South Wales.

AFO Acid-fast organism; Ankle-foot orthrosis; Annual flu outbreak.

AFOCC Asian Federation of Organizations for Cancer Research and Control.

AFOS American Foundation of Oncologic Societies.

AFOSR Air Force Office of Scientific Research (US).

AFP Acute facial palsy/ paralysis; Acute febrile polyneuritis (see AIP; GBS); Acute fulminating pneumonitis; Alpha-fetoprotein - a respiratory carrier (raised in anencephaly, spina bifida, Down's syndrome, etc.) (laboratory/ chemistry); American Family Physician (journal); Anterior faucial pillar; Antifungal powder; Antifungal preparations (such as the Allylamine antifungal, Terbinafine; the Aslylamine antifungal, Naftifine; the antifungal Antibiotic, Griseofulvine; Butenafine; Ciclopiroxolamine; the Imidazole derivative antifungals, Bifonazole, Clotrimazole, Econazole, Isoconazole, Ketoconazole, and Miconazole; the Keratolytic antifungals, Benzoic acid and Salicylic acid; Nystatin; the Polyene antibiotic, Amphotericin B; Tolnaftate; the Triazole antifungals, Fluconazole and Itraconazole; Undecylenic acid; etc.) (see AFA; AFD); Atypical facial pain; Archives Françaises de Pédiatrie (French journal); Axial flow pump (see PBD; PBH).

AfP Affiliate physician.

aFP Alpha-fetoprotein.

AFPD American Federation of Physicians and Dentists.

AfPh Affiliate physician.

AFPP Acute fibropurulent pneumonia.

αFPT Alpha feto-protein (blood) test (for Hepatitis B infection).

AFQ Aflatoxin Q.

AFQT Armed Forces Qualification Test.

AFR Adequate follicular response; Allergic food reaction (= FAR); Aqueous flare response; Ascorbic free radical.

AFRAX Autism-fragile X (syndrome).

AFRD Acute febrile respiratory disease.

AFRI Acute febrile respiratory illness.

AFRRI Armed Forces Radiobiology Research Institute.

AFS Absolute fixed stiffness (of prosthetic device - orthopedics) (see MFS; MIS); Acquired/ adult Fanconi syndrome; Acute frontal sinusitis; Allergic fungal sinusitis; American Fertility/ Fracture Society; American Field Service; Amniotic fluid sampling; Annual flu shot; Antifibroblast serum; Awakening from sleep.

AFSAM Air Force School of Aerospace Medicine.

AFSC Allied Forces Sports Council; American Friends Service Committee.

AFSCI American Foundation for the Science of Creative Intelligence (TM).

AFSP Acute fibrinoserous pneumonia; American Foundation for Suicide Prevention.

AFT Aflatoxin; Albumose-free tuberculin (see Tuberculin); Agglutination-flocculation test; Antifungal therapy/ treatment; Auditory fatigue test(s).

Aft After.

AFTA American Family Therapy Association; Autonomously functioning nodule.

AFTC Apparent free testosterone concentration.

AFTN Autonomously functioning thyroid nodule.

AFU Air flow unit.

AFUD American Foundation for Urologic Disease Inc.

AFV Air flow velocity; Amniotic fluid volume.

AFVSS Afebrile, vital signs stable.

AFX Air-fluid exchange.

AG Abbot Laboratories code for experimental substances; Abdominal girth; Agarose; Aminogluthethimide; Aminoglycoside; Analytical grade; Angiogenesis (a process of capillary proliferation by which a malignant tumor stimulates its own growth) (see

AAGT); Anion gap; Antigen; Antiglobulin; Antigravity; Aphakic glaucoma; Atrial gallop; Attached gingiva; Axiogingival; Azurophilic granule(s).

A/G Albumin/globulin (ratio).

Ag Antigen; Silver (L. argentum) - atomic no. 47 (see Elements).

ag- alternate spelling of prefix ad-.

AGA Accelerated growth area (embryology); Acute gonococcal/ gouty arthritis; Galactosidase A (= Agalsidase alfa) - a product of generic engineering technology as a human cell line, and used by infusion in the treatment of Fabry Disease or other inherited metabolic diseases, as long-term enzyme replacement therapy (see FD); Allergic granulomatosis and angiitis; American Gas/ Gastroenterological/ Genetic(s)/ Geriatric(s)/ Glaucoma/ Goiter Association; Aminoglycoside antibiotic (e.g. Framycetin, Gentamycin, Kanamycin, Paromomycin, Streptomycin, Tobramycin, etc.); Androgenetic alopecia; Anion gap acidosis; Antagavinistic activity (at 5H2, D1, D2, H1 and alpha nerve receptors); Anterograde amnesia; Antigalactose/ Antiglomerular antibody; Antigonadotrophic activity; Antigout agent; Anti-IgG autoantibody; Appropriate for/ Average gestational age.

AgAb complex Antigen-antibody complex or molecule.

AGADP Agarosehexane-adenosine diphosphate.

AGAMP Agarosehexane-adenosine monophosphate.

AGATP Agarosehexane-adenosine triphosphate.

AGB Abnormal genital bleeding; Angiogenesis blocker (angiostatin, endostatin, etc. - see AGI).

AGBAD Alexander Graham Bell Association for the Deaf.

AGBM Antiglomerular basement membrane.

AGC Absolute granulocyte count; Automatic gain control.

AgCl Silver chloride.

AgCN Silver cyanide.

AGCT Antiglobulin consumption test; Army General Classification Test.

AGD Academy of General Dentistry; Active/ Acute gut disease/ disorder; Agar/ agarose gel diffusion (method); Adiposogenital dystrophy (= AGS; Frolich's syndrome); Age-related disease; Angular growth deformity (e.g. at knee) (Orthopedics); Antigalactic drug.

AGDD Agar gel double diffusion.

AGDJ Academy of General Dentistry Journal.

AGE Acrylamide gel; Acute gastroenteritis; Adequate glycemic control; Advanced glycation end(product) (Glycated product/ protein); Agarose gel electrophoresis; Anesthetic group equipment (MET-sol); Angle of greatest extension.

AGEA American Gastro-Enterological Association.

AGED Automated general experimental device.

Agent Orange A deadly defoliant, whose most toxic element, dioxin, has been linked with birth defects and chloracne in humans, and cancer in animals. Used by US forces in the Viet Nam war. Also known as Herbicide Orange, it consists of a 50:50 combination of 2 herbicides: 2,5-D and 2,4,5-T, the latter containing Dioxin.

Agent X A viroid, virus-like agent, also known as kuru agent or scrapie agent, believed to be the cause of certain diseases of man and animals such as: BSE - Bovine spongiform encephalopathy (also known as Mad Cow disease; thought to be caused by rogue proteins called prions, which eat away at cow brains, eventually killing the cows). CJD - Creutzfeldt-Jacob disease (human equivalent of BSE). Kuru - a deadly disease found among one cannibal tribal population of New Guinea. Scrapie - a similar, brain-destroying disease of sheep, and TME - Transmissible mink encephalopathy, a similar disease found in minks.

AGEPC Acetyl glyceryl ether phosphorylcholine.

AGEPT Agarose gel electrophoretic test (done on cerebrospinal fluid to demonstrate oligoconal banding).

AGF Adrenal growth factor; Angle of greatest flexion; Autologous growth factor.

Ag. feb When/ while the fever increases/ is

coming on (= Aggred feb) - L. aggrediente febre.

AGG Agammaglobulinemia; Aggravated (= Agg; agg).

Agg; agg Agglommeration (see Agglom); Agglutination (see Agglut); Aggravate(d)/tion (see AGG); Aggregate/tion (see Aggreg).

Aggl Agglomeration (see Agglom); Agglutination/ted (see Agglut).

Agglom Agglomeration (= Agg; agg; Aggl).

Agglut Agglutination/ted (= Agg; agg; Aggl).

Aggrav Aggravate(d)/tion (see AGG).

Aggred. feb While the fever increases/ is coming on (see Ag. feb).

Aggreg Aggregate/tion (= Agg; agg) - (in botanical names) including two or more species which resemble each other closely.

AGGS Antigas gangrene serum.

AGGT Angiogenesis gene therapy.

AGH Asthenia gravis hypophyseogenea (see Asthenia).

AGI Alan Guttmacher Institute (PPFA); Angiogenesis inhibitor (= AAGA; AGB; AS; ES) (see AAGT); Ascending genital infection.

AgI Silver iodide.

AGII Acute gastrointestinal illness.

Agit Agitate/tion; Shake/ stir (L. agita) (medical orders/ prescriptions).

Agit ante sum Shake before taking (L. agita ante sumendum).

Agit vas Shake the vial/ the vial being shaken (L. agitato vase).

AGJ Anterior gastrojejunostomy.

AGL Acute granulocytic leukemia; Agglutination; Aminoglutethimide.

A GLACTO-LK Alpha galactoside leukocytes.

AGM Adnexal gestational mass; Anterograde memory (= Senile memory); Antigout medication/cine; Antigravity muscle(s) (the muscles that keep joints or other body parts in proper position by opposing the effects of gravity on the body, e.g. the jaw muscles that automatically raise the lower jaw and keep the mouth closed).

AGMIAPQ Association des Gardes-Malades et Infirmiers Auxiliaires de la Province de Québec.

AGMK African green monkey kidney (cell) (= AGMkK).

AGMkK African green monkey kidney (cell) (see AGMK).

AGN Acute glomerulonephritis; Agnosia; Antegonial notch (a depression or low place present at the corner of the lower jaw).

VIII_{AGN} Factor VIII antigen.

agn Agnosia (see AGN).

AGNAD Agarosehexane-nicotinamide adenine dinucleotide.

$AgNO_3$ Silver nitrate.

AgNOR Silver-staining nucleolar organizer region.

Ag_2O Silver oxide.

-agogue suffix meaning leading or inducing (Gr. agogos).

Agonist A ligand which produces an appropriate response when it binds to its receptor (e.g. histamine is an agonist at histamine receptors) (see Ligand).

AGOS American Gynecological and Obstetrical Society.

AGP Acid glycoprotein; Agar gel precipitation; Anogenital pruritus; Antigerminal pole (that pole of an ovum at which the greater amount of food yolk is deposited) (= Vegetal pole); Archives of General Psychiatry (journal).

AGPA American Group Practice/ Psychotherapy Association.

AGPI Agar-gel precipitin inhibition.

AGPOLY (I) Agarose polyriboinosinic acid.

AGPT Agar-gel precipitation test.

AGR Aniridia, genitourinary abnormalities, and mental retardation; Anticipatory goal response; Asialoglycoprotein receptor.

-agra suffix meaning catching or seizure (Gr. agra).

A/G ratio Albumin/ globulin ratio (laboratory/ chemistry).

AGRF American Geriatrics Research Foundation.

Agri; Agric Agriculture.

AGRIS Agricultural Information System (FAO).

AGS Adiposogenital syndrome (see AGD); Adrenogenital syndrome; Alternating gradient synchrotron; Amelogenesis imperfecta (an inherited defect in which the teeth are brown in color, either due to severe lack of calcium or poor growth of the enamel (= HEB or Hereditary brown enamel; HEH or Hereditary enamel hypoplasia); Amenorrhea-galactorrhea syndrome; American Geriatric(s)/ Gerontological/ Gynecological Society; Artificial-gut system; Audiogenic seizures; Automated gene sequencer.

AGs Aminoglycosides (Bacterial agents which inhibit production of messenger and transfer RNA, thus interrupting bacterial synthesis. They include amikacin, gentamycin, kanamycin, neomycin, netilmicin, streptomycin and tobramycin).

Ag_2S Silver sulfide.

AgSD Silver sulfadiazine.

AGSM Acta Genetica et Statistica Medica (journal - now HH).

Ag_2SO_4 Silver sulfate.

AGT Abnormal/ Abnormality of glucose tolerance; Activitity group therapy; Acute generalized tuberculosis; Angiogenesis therapy (injections into heart muscle, etc.); Antiglobulin test; Autogenic therapy (a mental-health therapy [MHT] based on the concept that natural brain forces are capable of removing disturbing influences).

agt agent.

A,G,T,C Adenine, guanine, thymine, and cytosine-nucleotides, forming 64 possible three-way combinations, in the building of cellular gene aminoacids. "Triplet" repeats or Trinucleotide repeats of defective genes, occur in genetic diseases such as: CAG in Huntington's chorea - on chromosome 4 and in Spinocerebellar ataxia - on chromosome 6; CGG in Fragile X syndrome - on chromosome X; CTG in Myotonic dystrophy, etc. The average chromosome holds 120 million nucleotides.

AGTH Adrenoglomerulotropic hormone.

AGTr Adrenoglomerulotropin.

AGTT Abnormal glucose tolerance test.

AGU Active/ Acute gastric ulcer.

AGV Aniline gentian violet.

AH Abdominal hysterectomy; Absorptive hypercalciuria; Accidental hyperthermia; Acetohexamide; Acid hydrolysis; Acta Haematologica (journal); Active Handicapped (journal); Acute hepatitis; Adaptive hormones: secreted during adaptation to unusual circumstances (see Hormones); Adrenal hyperplasia; Adult home; After hyperpolarization; Agnathiaholoprosencephaly; Alcohol(ic) hallucinosis; Alcoholic hepatitis; Allen and Hanbury's code for experimental substances; Amenorrhea and hirsutism; Amenorrhea-hyperprolactinemia; Aminohippurate; Androgenic hormones: the masculinization hormones, androsterone and testosterone (see Hormones); Animal Health (journal); Anterior/ Arcuate hypothalmus; Antihistamine; Antihyaluronidase; Anxiety hysteria; Army Hospital; Arterial hypertension; Artificial heart; Ascites hepatoma; Assisted hatching (puncture of the outer membrane or shell of the embryo, to aid implantation in the uterus); Asteroid hyalosis (see VAH); Astigmatic hypermetropia; Ataxic hemiparesis; Atrium His (atrionodal-bundle interval); Autonomic hyperreflexia; Axillary hair; Conduction time -see A-H (interval/ time); Hypermetropic astigmatism (see Ah; ah).

aH Abhenry.

Ah; ah Hypermetropic astigmatism (= AH).

A/H Amenorrhea/ hyperprolactinemia.

A+H Accident & Health (policy).

A*h Ampere hour.

A-H (interval/ time) Conduction time through the Atrio-ventricular node (A-V node), from the atrium to the Bundle of His (= AH).

a.h. Every other hour (L. alternis horis).

AHA Acetohydroxamic acid - a specific inhibitor of urease. Its use has been suggested in the treatment of hepatic coma; Acquired/ acute hemolytic anemia; Adipic hydrazide agarose; Alpha hydroxy acid; American Health/ Heart/ Hospital/ Humane/ Humanist Association; Anterior hypothalamic area; Antiheart/ antihistone antibody; Antihyperglycemic activity; Antihypertensive agent (see AHD); Area Health Authority; Arthritis-hives-angioedema (syndrome); Aspartyl-hydroxamic acid - a specific inhibitor of urease(used as in Acetohydroxamic acid); Associate, Institute of Hospital Administrators; Autoimmune hemolytic anemia.

AHAb Antihypocretin antibody (= AOAb) (see HR2G).

AHAF American Health Assistance Foundation.

AHAM Association of Home Appliance Manufacturers.

"aha" reaction A sudden idea that occurs, especially during deep thought (Psychology).

AHAT Amebiasis hemagglutination titer.

AHA (T) Area Health Authority (Teaching).

AHB Alkyl-4-hydroxybenzoate (a paraben); Alpha-hydroxybutyric (acid); Antegrade heart block; Available hospital bed.

α-HBDH Alpha-HBDH (see HBDH).

AHBuBP 4-amino-1-hydroxybutylidene-1,1-biphosphonate (a drug utilized in the treatment of menopausal osteoporosis).

AHC Academic health care; Academic Health Center; Acute hemorrhagic conjunctivitis/ cystitis; Acute hypertensive crisis; Ad Hoc Committee; American Health Congress; Antihemophilic factor C; Anterior horn cell.

AHCA American Health Care Association.

AHCD Anterior horn cell disease/ disorder/ dysfunction; Antihypercholesterolemic drug (e.g. clofibrate, colestipol, etc.) (see ALD).

AHCF Antihemophilic C factor (see Factor XI).

AHCO Accreditation of Health Care Organizations.

AHCPR Agency for Health Care Policy and Research.

AHCS American Health Care System (1999) (NEJM).

AHCy Adenosyl homocysteine.

AHD Acquired hepatocerebral degeneration; Acute hepatic diathesis/ disease/ disorder; Acute/ Adult/ Arteriosclerotic/ Atherosclerotic heart disease; Adequate historical data; Anti hemorrhagic/ histamine drug; Antihyaluronidase; Antihypertensive diuretic/ drug; Arteriohepatic dysplasia; Autoimmune hemolytic disease.

AHDMS Automated hospital data management system.

AHDP Azacycloheptane diphosphonate.

AHE Acute haemorrhagic encephalomyelitis; Acute hepatic encephalopathy; Acute hypoglycemic episode; Alcoholic hepatic encephalopathy (see HEA); Antihypertensive effect/ efficacy.

AHEA American Home Economics Association; Area health education activity.

AHEC Area Health Education Center(s) (HEW).

AHEL Army Human Engineering Laboratories.

AHES Artificial heart energy system.

AHF Acquired hemostatic failure; Acute heart/ hepatic failure; American Health/ Hepatic Foundation; American Hospital Formulary; Antihemolytic factor (see Factor VIII); Antihemophiliac/lic factor (see Factor VIII); Argentinian hemorrhagic fever (caused by the Junin virus, an arenavirus and transmitted by the small South American rodent, *Calomys* musculinus); Artificial Heart Fund (UK); Associated Health Foundation.

AHFS American Hospital Formulary Service (ASHP).

AHG Acta Hepato-Gastroenterologica (journal); Acute hemorrhagic gastritis; Aggregated/ Antihemolytic/ Antihemophilic/ Antihuman globulin (see Factor VIII); Annals of Human Genetics (journal).

AHGC Antihuman globulin consumption.

AHGG Aggregated human/ Antihuman gamma globulin; Acquired hypogammaglobulinemia.

AHGS Acute herpetic gingival stomatitis.

AHH Adrenal androgenic hyperfunction; Alpha-hydrazine analogue of histidine; Anosmia and hypogonadotropic hypogonadism (syndrome); Aryl Hydrocarbon hydroxylase (an enzyme that changes cancer-causing chemicals in tobacco smoke and in polluted air, into active cancer-causing agents within the lungs); Association for Holistic Health; Asymptomatic hypotonic hyponatremia (see PAH).

AHI Active hostility index; Animal Health Institute; Apnea-hypopnea index (in SDB - Sleep-disordered breathing); Apnea-plus-hypopnea index; Arizona Heart Institute; Artificial hip implant.

AHIG Antihuman immunoglobulin.

AHIP Assisted Health Insurance Plan.

AHIS Automated hospital information system.
AHJ Acromiohumeral joint; American Heart Journal; Artificial hip joint.
AHL Active hair loss (see FHL; MAHL; MPHL; PHL; SHL; VHL); Anagen hairloss (see ACT); Apparent half-life.
AHLE Acute hemorrhagic leukoencephalitis.
AHLG Antihuman lymphocte globulin.
AHLS Antihuman-lymphocyte serum.
AHM Allied health manpower; Ambulatory Holter monitor; Antihypertensive medication.
AHMA American Holistic Medicine Association; Antiheart muscle auto-antibody.
AHMC Association of Hospital Management Committee(s).
AHME Association for Hospital Medical Education.
AHMP Asthma home management plan.
AHN Acute hepatic necrosis; Adenomatous hyperplastic nodule; Army/ Assistant Head Nurse.
A(H5N1) Avian influenza virus (bearing H - Hemagglutinin and N - Neuraminidase surface protein molecules in its genes).
AHNC Anterior horn nerve cell (= AHC).
AHO Acute hematogenous osteomyelitis; Albright's hereditary osteodystrophy.
AHP Acute hallucinatory paranoia; Acute hemorrhagic pancreatitis; Adenohypophysis (see LCH); Adrenal hypoplasia; After hyperpolarization; Air at high pressure (i.e under hyperbaric conditions); Allied health personnel; Allied Health Professions; Ambulatory hypertensive patient; Angiohemophilia (= VWD; vWD; or von Willebrand's disease); Artificial Heart Program; Assistant House Physician; Associated Health Professions (Division of) (HRD); Athletic/ Asthenic habitus, pyknic (Gr. pyknos = thick); Automatic hardware programmed.
AHPA American Health Planning Association.
AHPAT Allied Health Professions Admissions Test.
17 AHPC 17-Alpha-hydroxyprogesterone caproate.
AHPE Accreditation of Health Professions Education (San Francisco).
AHPO (area) Anterior hypothalmic pre-optic (area).
AHPPT Allied Health Professions Personnel Training (Act).
AHR Abdominal hernia repair; Abnormal heart rhythm (arrhythmia); Acute hypersensitivity reaction (e.g. anaphylaxis, angioedema, bronchospasm, urticaria, etc.); A.H. Robins Co. code for experimental substances; Antihyaluronidase reaction; Association for Health Records; Autonomic hyperreflexia.
AHR 85 Methocarbamol (= 2-Hydroxy-3-O-methoxyphenoxypropyl carbamate); a centrally acting muscle relaxant, used for the relief of muscle spasm, and as an adjunct to physiotherapy, in the treatment of myositis, spondylitis, bursitis, and arthritis.
AHR 438 Metaxalone (= 2-Oxo-5-[3,5,xylyloxymethyl]oxazolidine) - a centrally acting muscle relaxant, of limited value in the treatment of chronic spastic states such as multiple sclerosis, and degenerative disease of the central nervous system.
AHR 504 Glycopyrronium bromide (= Glycopyrrolate) - a peripheral parasympatholytic, used in the symptomatic treatment of peptic ulcer and other gastro-intestinal disorders.
AHR 619 Doxapram hydrochloride - an analeptic, used as a post-operative respiratory stimulant, as well as in the treatment of respiratory distress conditions such as emphysema.
AHR 857 Sulfamethoxydiazine (= Sulfametin; Sulfametorinum) - a sulfonamide drug, rapidly absorbed and slowly excreted.
AHRA American Hospital Radiology Administration.
a/H ratio Ratio of A-wave to the total excursion during systole.
AHRC Association for the Help of Retarded Children.
AHRF Acute hypoxemic respiratory failure; American Hearing Research Foundation.
AHS Academy of Health Sciences; Adaptive hand skills; Adie-Holmes syndrome (= Adie's pupil; Toxic pupil; Weill's syndrome); Adult Health Study; African horse sickness; Alveolar hypoventilation syndrome; American Hearing Society (now NAHSA); American Horticultural/ Hospital/ Humane

Society; Anaphylactic hypersensitivity; Antihuman serum; Assistant house surgeon; Athletic heart syndrome (= Athlete's heart).

AHSC American Hospital Supply Corp.; Army Health Services Command.

AHSDF Area health service development fund.

AHSN Assembly of Hospital Schools of Nursing.

AHSR Association for Health Services Research.

AHT Abnormal hair texture; Aggregation half time; Ameba/ Amebiasis hemagglutination titer; Antihyaluronidase titer/ titration (enzyme); Antihypertensive therapy/ treatment; Apathetic hyperthyroidism; Augmented histamine test; Autoantibodies to human thyroglobulin; Autogenous hamster tumor.

AHTA Antihypertensive agent (= AHTD).

AHTD Antihypertensive drug (see AHTA).

AHTG Antihuman thymocytic globulin.

AHTP Antihuman thymocytic plasma.

AHTS Antihuman thymus serum.

AHU Acute hemolytic uremic (syndrome); Arginine, hypoxanthine, and uracil; Asymptomatic hyperuricemia.

AHuG Aggregated human IgG.

AHV Artificial heart valve (see CGP; CLP); Avian herpes virus.

AHW Active hairy wart.

AI Accidental injury; Accidentally incurred; Adenine and inosine; Adiposity/ Aggregation/ Allergy/ Anxiety/ Articulation/ Atherogenic index; Advances in Immunology (journal); Adynamic ileus; Alcohol intake; Alginine infusion(s); Allergy and immunology; Allergy Information (journal); Ambulatatory induced; Amnesty International (political prisoners); Anal intercourse; Anaphylatoxin inactivator; Angiogenesis inhibitor; Angiotensin I; Aortic incompetence/ insufficiency; Aorto-iliac; Apical impulse; Artificial insemination/ intelligence; Atrial insuffiency; Autoimmune/nity; Auto-infection; Axioincisal.

aI Active ingredient; Mixture of azure A and azure B.

A-I Antero-inferior.

A&I Allergy and immunology.

AIA Acute invasive aspergillosis; Adults with Incapacity Act (Scotland, 2000); Allergy Information Association; Allyliso-propylacetamide; Amylase inhibitor activity; Anti-idiotype/ Anti-immunoglobulin/ Anti-insulin antibody; Anti-infective/ influenza agent; Anti-inflammatory action/ activity/ agent; Aspirin-induced allergy/ asthma; Automated image analysis.

AI-Ab Anti-insulin antibody (= AIA).

AIAP Allantoidoangiopagus (see OAP - Omphaloangiopagus).

AIAR Arthroscopic intraarticular repair (of the meniscus - knee joint) (Orthopedics).

AIB Active internal bleeding; Aminoisobutyrate (see AIBA); Avian infectious bronchitis.

AIBA Amino-isobutyric acid.

AIBCS American Intersociety Board of Certification of Sanitarians.

AIBF Anterior interbody fusion.

AIBL Angioimmunoblastic lymphadenopathy (see AIL).

AIBS American Institute of Biological Sciences; Antigen-induced bronchospasm.

AIC Ambulatory Infusion Center; American Institute of Chemists; 5-Aminoimidazole-4-carboxamide (a metabolite of the antineoplastic drug, temozolomide); Association des Infirmières Canadiennes.

AIC# Acute intracapsular fracture (see AICF).

A-IC Average integrated concentration.

AICA Anterior inferior cerebellar artery; Anterior inferior communicating artery; Association Internationale de Computation Analogue (Fr.) - International Association for Analog Computation.

AI-CAH Autoimmune-type chronic active hepatitis.

AICAR Amino-imidazole-carboxamide ribonucleotide.

AICB Artificial-intelligence cognitive being (see AS - Asperger syndrome).

AICC Acute ischemic cardiac complication(s).

AICD Automatic implantable cardioverter defibrillator.

AICDD Activation-induced cytidine deaminase deficiency (= AID).

AICE Angiotensin I converting enzyme.

AICF Acute intracapsular fracture (of the femoral neck) (see AIC#); Autoimmune complement fixation.

AIChE American Institute of Chemical Engineers.

AICJ Anaesthesia and Intensive Care Journal.

AICO Association of Institutes of Clinical Oncology (Italy).

AICR American Institute for Cancer Research.

AID Absolute iron deficiency; Activation-induced (cytidine deaminase) deficiency (see AICDD); Active/ Acute inflammatory disease; Acquired immune deficiency (see AIDS); Acute infectious diarrhea/ disease; Acute ionization detector; Advanced inoperable disease (see LAID); Agency for International Development; America-India Dispensary; Antibiotic-induced diarrhea; Anti-impotence/ infective/ inflammatory dose/ drug; Antiinitiator drug (a substance that may cause cancer, or be used to prevent it if given before exposure to a carcinogen); Approval for individual diagnosis; Argon ionization detector; Artificial impregnation - donor (= heterologous impregnation/ insemination); Artifial insemination by donor (heterologous insemination); Autoimmune deficiency/ diabetes/ disease/ disorder; Automatic implantable defibrillator; Automatic infiltration detector; Automatic injection device; Average interocular difference.

AIDC Autoimmune Disease Center.

AIDKS Acquired immune deficiency (syndrome) with Kaposi's sarcoma.

AIDP Acute inflammatory demyelinating polyradiculopathy.

AIDS Acquired immune deficiency syndrome caused by the AIDS virus (ARV; HIV; HTLV-3; LAV; LAV/HTLV III) (LAV/HTLV III = Lymphadenopathy associated virus/ Human T cell lymphotropic virus III) (see HTLV III & HIV or Human immunodeficiency virus); AIDS - older name, GRID or Gay-related immune/immuno deficiency (syndrome) (see HTLV-3; HTLV-III; LAV). There is a growing arsenal of biological inhibitor drugs used against HIV (see II; PI; RTI).

AIDS cocktail See II (Integrase inhibitors); RTI (Reverse transferase inhibitors).

AIDS DRUGS Clinical trials of acquired immunodeficiency drugs (MEDLARS data base).

AIDS-KS Acquired immune defiency syndrome with Kaposi's sarcoma.

AIDSLINE On-line information on acquired immunodeficiency syndrome (MEDLARS data base).

AIDS-RKS AIDS-Related Kaposi's Sarcoma (= AIDS-KS).

AIDSTRIALS Clinical trials of acquired immunodeficiency syndrome drugs (MEDLARS data base).

AIDT Academic-industry drug trial.

AIE Acute inclusion-body encephalitis; Acute infectious encephalitis; Acute infective endocarditis/ enterocolitis; Anti-inflammatory effect; Autoimmune endocrinopathies/hy.

AIEC Advanced ion exchange cellulose.

AIEEE Annals of the Institute of Electrical and Electronics Engineers.

AIEP Amount of insulin extractable from the pancreas.

AIF Anemia-inducing/ Anti-inflammatory/ Anti-invasion factor; Anti-insulin factor (adrenal glands, epinephrine, immunological factors, etc.); Aorticiliac-femoral; Atomic Industrial Forum (Inc).

AIFD Acute intrapartum fetal distress.

A2IFN Alpha 2 - interferon.

AIFNAb Anti-interferon antibody.

AIFT Alpha interferon therapy.

AIG Anti-immunoglobulin; Aorto-iliac graft (for AAA - Abdominal aortic aneurysm).

AIGE Acute infantile gastroenteritis.

AIH Acute idiosyncratic hepatitis; American Institute of Homeopathy/ Hypnosis; Artificial impregnation - husband (= homologous impregnation/ insemination); Artificial insemination by husband (homologous insemination); Autoimmune hepatitis/ hypothyroidism (= AIHT).

AIHA Acute idiopathic hemolytic anemia; American Industrial Hygiene Association; Autoimmune hemolytic anemia (see AHA).

AIHAJ Aerican Industrial Hygiene Association Journal.

AIHC American Industrial Health

Conference.

AIHD Acquired immune hemolytic disease; Acute idiopathic hepatic disease.

AIHJ American Institute of Homeopathy/ Hypnosis journal.

AIHOM Archives of Industrial Hygiene and Occupational Medicine (journal).

AIHT Autoimmune hypothyroidism (see AIH).

AII Acute intestinal infection; Alcohol-induced impairment.

AIIA Angiotensin II antagonist (Type AT1) (see SARB).

AIIE American Institute of Industrial Engineers.

AIIMS All-India Institute of Medical Sciences (= AIMS).

AIIRA Angiotensin-II (AT1) receptor antagonist (such as Candesartan, Irbesartan, Losartan, Valsartan, etc.).

AIIS Acute inflammatory infective stage; Anterior inferior iliac spine.

AIIT Amiodarone-iodine-induced thyrotoxicosis.

AIJR Accelerated idiojunctional rhythm (= AIR).

AIKC Autoimmune Killer cell (e.g. in the pancreas, destroyed by TNF or Tumor necrosis factor).

AIL Acute infectious lymphocytosis; Angiocentric immunoproliferative lesion; Angioimmunoblastic lymphadenopathy; Anti-itch lotion.

AILD Alcohol-induced liver disease; Alveolar interstitial lung disease; Angioimmunoblastic lymphadenopathy with dysproteinemia; Autoimmune lung disease.

AIM Abridged Index Medicus; Academy - International, of Medicine; Action for Independent Maturity (AARP - NRTA); Annals of Internal Medicine (journal); Anti-inflammatory mechanism; Anti-infective/ inflammatory medication/ medicine; Archives of Internal Medicine (journal); Artificial intelligence in medicine (see SUMEX-AIM); Autoimmune myocarditis.

AIMC American Institute of Medical Climatology.

AIMD Abnormal involuntary movement disorder.

AIMS Abnormal involuntary movement scale; All-India Institute of Medical Sciences (see AIIMS); Arthritis Impact Measurement Scales.

AIN Acute interstitial nephritis; American Institute of Nutrition; Anal intraepithelial neoplasia; Anterior interosseous nerve; Association of Interpretive Naturalists.

AINA American Indian Nurses Association; Automated immunoephelometric assay.

AINP Anterior interosseous nerve palsy.

AINS Anti-inflammatory non-steroidal.

A Insuf Aortic insufficiency.

AIO Acute intestinal obstruction.

AION Anterior ischemic optic neuropathy.

AIP Acute idiopathic pericarditis; Acute idiopathic polyneuritis (= AFP or Acute febrile polyneuritis; GBS or Guillain-Barré syndrome); Acute infectious polyneuritis; Acute intermittent porphyria; Acute iron poisoning; Aerosolized iloprost (a prostaglandin analogue used by inhalation in the treatment of PPH or Primary pulmonary hypertension); Alcohol-induced impairment (e.g. in performance); Aldosterone-induced protein; Allergic interstitial pneumonitis (= Allergic alveolitis; DHP or Diffuse hypersensitivity pneumonia; EAP or Extrinsic allergic pneumonia); Ambulatory infusion pump (for hyperalimentation, chemotherapy, etc.); American Institute of Physics/ Planning; American Institute for Psychoanalysis; Anatuberculin, Petragnani's integral; Angiogenesis inhibitor protein (angiostatin); Annual Implementation Plan; Anti-inflammatory properties/ty; Autoimmune pathogen(esis)/ process; Automated immunoprecipitation; Average intravascular pressure.

AIPE Acute interstitial pulmonary emphysema.

AIPFP Acute idiopathic peripheral facial (nerve) palsy.

AIPM Alternative infusion preparation method.

AIPS American Institute of Pathologic Science.

AIR Abdominal inguinal ring; Accelerated idiojunctional rhythm (see AIJR); Accelerated idioventricular rhythm (see AIVR); Active inflammatory response; Acute infusion/ inflammatory reaction; Aminoimidazole ribonucleotide; American Institute for Research; Anergic immunoregulatory (protein receptors such as CD45RA and CD45RO); Australasian Institute of Radiography; Autoimmune reaction/ response; Average impairment rating.

AIRA Anti-insulin receptor antibody.

Aircast braces Ankle brace, ankle training brace, armband brace, knee brace, leg brace, and walking brace.

AIRE Acute Infarction Ramipril Efficacy (Study).

AIRF Alterations in respiratory function.

AIRS Amphetamine Interview Rating Scale.

AIS Abbreviated Injury Scale/ Score; Alternate/ Alternative infusion site; Amniotic infection syndrome; Analytical Instrument Specialties Co.; Androgen insensitivity syndrome; Anterior interosseous (nerve) syndrome; Anti-insulin serum; Asiatic intestinal schistosomiasis (caused by the worm *Schistosoma* japonicum); Autoimmune sequence/ syndrome; Autonomic instability syndrome (with cardiac dysrhythmia, diaphoresis, irregular blood pressure, tachycardia, etc.) (see NMS).

AISA Acquired idiopathic sideroblastic anemia.

AISI American Iron and Steel Institute.

AIS/ISS Abbreviated Injury Scale/ Injury Severity Score.

AIS/MR Alternative Intermediate Services for the Mentally Retarded.

AIT Acute intensive treatment; Adoptive/ Allergen immunotherapy; Agglutination inhibition test; Aging-intervention therapy; Anti-infective/ inflammatory/ ischemic therapy/ treatment; Aseptic injection technique; Autoimmune thrombocytopenia/ thyroiditis.

AITED Autoimmune thyroid eye disease (= ATED).

AITP Acute/ Autoimmune idiopathic thrombocytopenic purpura.

AITT Arginine/ Augmented insulin tolerance test.

AIU Absolute iodine uptake; Antigen-inducing unit.

AIUM American Institute of Ultrasound in Medicine.

AIUR Autoimmune uveoretinitis.

AIV Avian influenza virus.

AIVR Accelerated idioventricular rhythm.

AIVV Anterior informal vertebral vein.

AIWC Acutely inflamed weeping condition (skin).

AJ The American Journal; Ankle jerk (see A/J).

A/J Ankle jerk (= AJ).

aj Before breakfast (L. ante jentaculum).

AJA American Jewish Appeal; American Journal of Acupuncture/ Anatomy/ Audiology (see JSLHR); Australian Journal of Audiology.

AJAC Audiology, the Journal of Auditory Communication (ISA).

AJAT American Journal of Art Therapy.

AJBS American Journal of Biological Sciences.

AJC American Joint Committee; American Journal of Cancer/ Cardiology.

AJCCS American Joint Committee for Cancer Staging.

AJCD American Journal of Clinical Dermatology.

AJCH American Journal of Clinical Hypnosis (ASCH).

AJCM American Journal of Chinese Medicine.

AJCN American Journal of Clinical Nutrition.

AJCP American Journal of Clinical Pathology.

AJD Advanced joint destruction/ disease; Australasian Journal of Dermatology (formerly Australian Journal of Dermatology).

AJDC American Joint Distribution Committee; American Journal of Diseases of Children.

AJDD American Journal of Digestive Diseases.

AJDDN American Journal of Digestive Diseases and Nutrition.

AJE American Journal of Epidemiology.

AJEBMS Australian Journal of Experimental Biology and Medical Science.

AJEEGT American Journal of

Electroencephalographic (EEG) Technology.

AJFS Australian Journal of Forensic Sciences (AAFS).

AJG American Journal of Gastroenterology.

AJH American Journal of Hematology/ Hygiene/ Hypertension; Apophysial joint arthritis.

AJHG American Journal of Human Genetics.

AJHP American Journal of Hospital Pharmacy (AHSP).

AJIC American Journal of Infection Control.

AJIVT American Journal of Intravenous (IV) Therapy.

AJM American Journal of Medicine.

AJMD American Journal of Mental Deficiency.

AJMS African Journal of Medical Sciences; American Journal of the Medical Sciences.

AJMT American Journal of Medical Technology (ASMT).

AJN American Journal of Neuroradiology/ Nursing (ANA).

AJO American Journal of Ophthalmology/ Optometry (AOA)/ Orthodontics (AAO)/ Orthopsychiatry (AOA).

AJOG American Journal of Obstetrics and Gynecology.

AJOPO American Journal of Optometry and Physiological Optics (AAO).

AJOT American Journal of Occupational Therapy.

AJP American Journal of Pathology/ Pharmacy/ Physics/ Physiology/ Proctology/ Psychiatry (APA)/ Psychotherapy (AAP); Australasian Journal of Pharmacy.

AJPH American Journal of Public Health (APHA).

AJPHNH American Journal of Public Health and the Nation's Health (now AJPH).

AJPM American Journal of Physical/ Podiatric Medicine.

AJR Abnormal jugular reflex; Accelerated junctional rhythm.

AJRCCM American Journal of Respiratory and Clinical Care Medicine.

AJRGS Audio Journal Review: General Surgery.

AJRRTNM American Journal of Roentgenology, Radium Therapy and Nuclear Medicine (ARRS).

AJS Acute joint syndrome; American Journal of Surgery.

AJSGVD American Journal of Syphilis, Gonorrhea, and Venereal Diseases (formerly AJSN).

AJSM American Journal of Sports Medicine.

AJSN American Journal of Syphilis and Neurology (now AJSGVD).

AJTCR American Journal of Therapeutics and Clinical Reports (Cases and Comments).

AJTMH American Journal of Tropical Medicine and Hygiene.

AJVR American Journal of Veterinary Research (AVMA).

AK Above knee - signifying amputation, operation, or Plaster of Paris application; Acetate/ Adenosine/ Adenylate kinase (AKA); Actinic keratosis; Artificial kidney.

A/K; ak Above knee.

A→K Ankle to knee.

AKA Above knee amputation (= AK; AK amp.); Adenylate kinase (= AK); Alcoholic ketoacidosis; All known allergies; Also known as; Anti-Kell antibody (= RCA - Red cell antibody); Antikeratin antibody.

A/K/A Personian coefficient.

AK amp Above knee amputation (see AKA).

AKC Angiokeratoma circumscriptum (a rare skin defect in which bumps and pimples appear in small patches on the legs and on the trunk); Associate King's College (London).

AKCD Angiokeratoma corporis diffusum (= FD - Fabry's disease).

AKD Advanced kidney disease (see ARD).

AKE Acrokeratoelastoidosis.

AKF Acute kidney failure (see ARF); American Kidney Fund; American Korean Foundation.

A/kg Amperes per kilogram.

Akinesia (= Akinesis). 1. An abnormal state of physical and mental activity with absence or poverty of movement due to inability to move the muscles. 2. The temporary paralysis of a muscle or group of muscles by the injection of a local anesthetic such as Amethocaine, Benzocaine, Lignocaine, Procaine, etc. Akinesia algera - paralysis or voluntary abstinence of movement often seen in neuras-

thenic states, or by the intense pain associated with muscular movements such as Mobius/ Moebius syndrome (congenital bilateral paralysis of the facial and oculomotor muscles, with periodic migraine (Apraxia algera) - Paul Julius Mobius, German neurologist [1853 - 1907]).
Akinesia amnestica. - loss of motor power due to disuse.
Crossed akinesia - motor paralysis on the side opposite the lesion.
O'Brien akinesia - paralysis of the orbicularis oculi muscle with the injection of a local anesthetic (into the orbital branch of the 7th. [Facial] nerve).
Reflex akinesia - loss of reflex movement.

AKP Alkaline phophatase (see Alk. p'tase); Artificial Kidney Program.

AKR Aldoketoreductase.

AKS Alcoholic Korsakoff syndrome; Arthroscopic knee surgery; Auditory and kinesthetic sensation(s) (see Aks; aks).

Aks; aks Auditory and kinesthetic sensation(s) (= AKS).

AL Absolute latency; Acinar lumen; Acute leukemia; Adaptation level; Albumin; Alcoholism; Alignment (mark/ cardiography); Allergy (index); American Laboratory (journal); Amyloidosis; Antihuman lymphocytic (globulin); Argon laser; Arterial line; Avian leukosis; Axial length; Axillary loop; Axiolingual; Left ear (L. auris laeva).

Al Allantoic; Allergic/gy; Aluminium (atomic no. 13) (see Elements).

al (Ethyl) alcohol (ethanol); Left ear (= AL).

A-L Antero-lateral.

Al 0361 Hydroxyphenamate (= Oxyfenamate; P301; 2-Hydroxy-2-phenylbutyl carbamate) - a sedative used in the treatment of anxiety and tension states.

ALA Alanine (see Ala); Amebic liver abscess; American Laryngological/ Leukemia/ Library/ Lung Association; Aminolevulinic acid; Antileukemia agent (= ALD); Apolipoprotein A; Atropine-like action; Axillary lymphadenopathy; Axiolabial (see A La); Axiolabiolingual (see A La L); Asymmetrical lobar atrophy (see PD - Pick's disease).

αLA Alpha-lactalbumin (a protein present in breast milk) (= alpha-lac) (see HAMLET); Alpha-lipoic acid.

ALa; A. La Axiolabial (= ALA).

Ala Alanine (= ALA).

ALA-AT Alanine-aminotransferase (erythrocyte).

ALAB American Lung Association Bulletin.

ALAb Antilatent/lytic antibody.

AL-Ab Antilymphocyte antiantibody.

ALAC Antibiotic-loaded acrylic cement; Artificial limb and appliance center.

ALAD Abnormal left axis deviation; Aminolevulinic acid dehydrase/ dehydrogenase (= ALaD; ALA-D).

ALaD; ALA-D Aminolevulinic acid dehydrase/ dehydrogenase (see ALAD).

ALADO Latin American Association of Orthodontics.

ALAG Axiolabiogingival (= ALaG; A. La. G.).

ALaG; A. La. G Axiolabiogingival (see ALAG).

ALAL Axiolabiolingual (see A. La. L.).

ALaL; A. La. L Axiolabiolingual (= ALA; ALAL).

Al-Anon Alcoholics Anonymous (A world-wide group better known as AA).

AlaP; ala-P Alafosfalin.

ALARA As low as reasonably achievable (radiation exposure).

ALARM Adjustable leg and ankle repositioning mechanism.

ALAS American Lapidus Airfloat System (Lapidus bed - for control and treatment of decubitus ulcers; Aminolevulinic acid synthetase..

ALAT Alanine aminotransferase (= Alanine transaminase) (see SGPT).

Alateen A world-wide group giving health and guidance to children of alcoholics (see AA; Al-Anon).

ALB Albumin (see Alb); Apolipoprotein B; Avian lymphoblastosis.

Alb Albumin (= ALB); White (L. albus).

alb- prefix meaning white (L. albus).

ALBC Albumin clearance.

ALB/GLOB Albumin/globulin (ratio).

ALBP Acute low back pain; Afterload blood

pressure (the pressure against which the left ventricle ejects the blood during systole).

Albus (L.) White.

ALC Absolute lymphocytic count; Activated liquid cephaloplastin; Acute lethal catatonia; Alcohol (see Alc; EtOH); Adverse laboratory change(s); Allogenic lymphocytic cytotoxicity; Alternate level of care; Alternative Lifestyle Checklist; Amoeba-less life cycle; Apical lung cancer/ carcinoma (= PT - Pancoast's tumor); Approximate lethal concentration; Avian leukosis complex; Axiolinguocervical.

Alc Alcohol (= ALC; Alcoh) (see EtOH); Alcoholic/lism (= Alcoh).

ALCA Anomalous left coronary artery.

ALCAPA Anomalous origin of left coronary artery from pulmonary artery.

ALCAR Phosphoribosyl-5-amino-imidazole-carboxamide.

Alcar Acetyl-L-carnitine (an 'antiaging' nutrient, anti-oxidant, and dietary supplement).

ALCEQ Adolescent Life Change Event Questionnaire.

Alcoh Alcohol(ic)/lism (see Alc).

ALCOR Appalachian Leaders and Community Outreach.

AlcR; alcR Alcohol rub.

Al Cr Aluminium crown.

ALD Active/ Acute/ Advanced liver disease; Adrenoleukodystrophy - a fatal genetic disorder caused by excessive VLCFAs in the blood (see VLCFA); Alcoholic liver disease; Aldolase; Anterior latissimus dorsi; Antileprotic drug (used to treat leprosy); Antileukemia drug (see ALA); Antilipidemic diet/ drug (= AHCD); Appraisal of Language Disturbance; Appropriate loading dose; Approximate lethal dose; Arch length deficiency (the difference in a dental arch between the length needed for all the natural teeth and the natural space available); Average lethal dose - the average dose of the drug or organism (in culture) which will kill a particular species of animal.

Ald Aldolase (see ALS).

ALDF American Lyme Disease Foundation.

ALDH Aldehyde dehydrogenase.

Aldo; ALDOST Aldosterone.

ALE Adverse laboratory experience(s) (see LAE); Allowable limits of error.

ALEC Artificial lung-expanding compound.

ALEP Atypical lymphoepitheloid (cell) proliferation.

Aleppo boil A skin disease caused by *Leishmania* tropica (also called Cutaneous leishmaniasis, Delhi boil, Old World leishmaniasis, Oriental sore, Tropical sore).

ALERT All-Africa Leprosy and Rehabilitation Center.

ALF Abnormal liver function; Acute liver failure; Altered laboratory finding(s); American Leprosy/ Liver Foundation.

ALFT Abnormal liver function test.

ALG Antihuman lymphocytic globulin; Antilymphocyte/tic globulin; Axiolinguogingival.

alg Allergy.

alg- prefix meaning pain (Gr. algos).

ALGB Acute leukemia group B.

-algia suffix meaning pain (Gr. algos).

ALGOL A computer programming language (ALGOrithmic Oriented Language).

ALH Angiolymphoid hyperplasia; Anterior lobe hormone; Anterior lobe of the hypophysis.

ALHE Angiolymphoid hyperplasia with eosinophilia.

ALI Active/ Acute liver inflammation; Active/ Acute lung infection/ inflammation/ injury; Air-liquid interface (in the pulmonary alveolus); Annual limit of intake; Anterior lens implant; Argon laser iridotomy.

ALIMD Association of Life Insurance Medical Directors.

ALIMDA Association of Life Insurance Medical Directors of America.

ALIP Abnormal localized immature (myeloid) precursor.

ALK; Alk Alkaline; Alkylating.

ALK ISO Alkaline (phosphatase) isoenzymes.

ALK-P; Alk. phos Alkaline phosphatase (see Alk. p'tase).

Alk. p'tase Alkaline phosphatase (= AKP; ALK-P; Alk. phos; ALP; AlPase) - orthophosphoric monoester phosphohydrase.

ALL Acute lymphoblastic/ lymphocytic leukemia; Anterior longitudinal ligament;

Attempted limb lengthening (by osteotomy, physeal distraction or separation, etc.) (Orthopedics).

all Allergic/gy.

all- prefix meaning other or different (Gr. allos).

ALLA Acute lymphoctic leukemia antigen.

ALLO Atypical Legionella-like organism.

ALLHAT Antihypertensive and Lipid Lowering treatment to prevent Heart Attack Trial.

ALM Acral lentigenous melanoma; Adenoleiomyofibroma; Aerial lentiginous melanoma; Alpha loop maneuver (performed when difficulty is encountered during colonoscopy, if the advancing colonoscope fails to negotiate the "alpha loop" of the colon at the junction of the sigmoid and descending colon; this is accomplished under fluoroscopic guidance); Alveolar living material; American Leprosy Missions.

ALMA Adoptee's Liberty Movement Association.

ALME Acetyl-lysine methyl ester.

ALMI Anterior lateral myocardial infarct.

ALMV Anterior leaflet of the mitral valve.

ALN Adaptive learning network; Allylnitrile; Anterior lymph node; Axillary lymph node.

ALNRC American Legion National Rehabilitation Committee.

ALO Average lymphocyte output; Axiolinguo-occlusal.

Al_2O_3 Aluminium oxide (= ALOX).

$Al(OH)_3$ Aluminium hydroxide.

ALOP Appropriate level of protection.

ALOS Average length of stay.

ALOSH Appalachian Laboratory for Occupational Safety and Health.

ALOX Aluminium oxide (see Al_2O_3).

ALP Acute leukemia protocol; Acute lupus pericarditis; Alkali-labile pepsin; Alkaline phosphatase (see Alk. p'tase); Alupent; Alveolar proteinosis; Anterior lobe of pituitary; Antilymphocyte/tic plasma; Apolipoprotein; Argon laser photocoagulation.

ALPA Air Line Pilots Association.

AlPase Alkaline phosphatase (see Alk. p'tase).

ALPC Argon laser photocoagulator (used in diabetic retinopathy).

ALPHA Area-wide and Local Planning for Health Action.

alpha See α. Greek letter alpha; Angular acceleration; first (carbon atom next to the carbon atom bearing the active group in organic compounds); optical rotation; probability of type I error; solublity coefficient.

alpha-lac Alpha-lactalbumin (see αLA; HAMLET).

alpha2-AP Alpha 2-antiplasmin.

alpha-GLUC Alpha-glucosidase.

alpha2M Alpha2-macroglobulin.

ALPS Angiolymphoproliferative syndrome; Aphasia Language Performance Scale.

ALPZ Alprazolam.

ALR Advances in Lipid Research (journal).

Alr Allergenic.

ALRI Acute lower respiratory infection; Anterolateral rotatory instability.

ALROS American Laryngological, Rhinological, and Otological Society (Triological Society).

ALS Abdominal laparoscopic surgery; Absence-like seizure (epilepsy); Academic life science(s); Acute lateral sclerosis; Advanced Life Support (system); Afferent loop syndrome; Aldolase (= Ald); Amyotrophic lateral sclerosis (= Lou Gehrig's disease); Anaphylactic-like shock (syndrome); Angiographic lumen stenosis (in CAD); Angiotensin-like substance; Anterolateral sclerosis; Anticipated life span; Antilymphatic/ Antilymphocyte serum; Assembly of Life Sciences (NRC); Average life span; Azar lid speculum (ophthalmology).

ALSD Advanced-life support device (on aircraft, such as the automated external defibrillator); Alzheimer's-like senile dementia.

ALS-PD Amyotrophic lateral sclerosis-parkinsonism-dementia (complex).

ALT Abnormal lab(oratory) test; Activated liquid thromboplastin; Alanine transaminase (= Alanine aminotransferase - formerly GPT or Glutamic-pyruvic transaminase; also SGPT); Antero-lateral thigh (see VLM or Vastus lateralis muscle); Antileukemic therapy; Argon laser therapy/ trabeculoplasty; Average length of time; Avian laryngo-tracheitis.

AlT Aluminium tartrate (= Alt; alt).

Alt; alt Alternate/tive; Altitude; Aluminium tartrate (see AlT).

2 alt Argon laser trabeculoplasty; Every other day (see Alt dieb).

ALT/AST Alanine/Aspartate aminotransaminase (= GPT/GOT; SGPT/SGOT).

ALTB Acute larngo-tracheo-bronchitis.

ALTC Antileukotriene compound.

Alt dieb Alternate days/ every other day (L. alternis diebus) (= 2 alt).

ALTE Apparant life-threatening event.

ALTEE Acetyl-L-tyrosine ethyl ester.

Alt h; Alt hor Alternate hours/ every other hour (L. alternis horis).

Alt noc Alternate nights/ every other night (L. alternis nocta/te).

ALTS Acute lumbar traumatic sprain/ syndrome.

ALU Arithmetic and logic unit (computer).

ALV Abelson leukemia virus; Adeno-like virus; Alveolar/lus; Apical lordotic view (X-ray taken with the patient leaning backward at an angle of about 45 degrees); Ascending lumbar vein; Avian leukosis virus.

Alv Alveolar/lus (= ALV).

A/LV Apex cardiography.

ALVAD Abdominal left ventricular assist device.

Alv adst When constipated/ when the bowels are constipated (L. alvo adstricta).

Alv deject Alvine dejections/ discharge from the bowels (L. alvi dejectiones).

alve- prefix meaning cavity, channel or trough (L. alveus).

ALV M Alveolar mucosa.

ALVs Abnormal laboratory values (see ALT).

ALVT Aortic and left ventricular tunnel.

alv vent Alveolar ventilation.

Alvx Alveolectomy.

ALW Arch-loop-whorl (fingerprint).

ALWMI Anterolateral wall myocardial infarct (ion).

AM Academy of Medicine (Canada); Acta Medica (journal); Actomyosin; Actomysin; Acute myelofibrosis; Addictions Magazine; Adolescent Medicine (journal); Adult male/ monocyte; Aerospace Medicine (journal); Air meatography (lumbar puncture); Akinetic mutism; Alternative medicine (see CM); Alveolar macrophage/ mucosa; Amacrine cell; Amalgam; Ambulatory; American Medicine (journal); Amethopterin; Ametropia; Ametropia and meterangle; Ammeter; Amperemeter; Ampicillin; Amplitude modulation; Amyl; Amylase; Anovular menstruation; Applied Microbiology (journal); Arithmetic mean; Arousal mechanism; Articular manipulation; Aviation medicine; Axiomesial; Before death (L. ante mortem); Before noon/ in the morning/ morning (L. ante meridianus/ meridiem); Extracellular space; Master of Arts (= MA) (L. Artium Magister); Medial amygdaloid nucleus; Meter angle; Mixed/ myopic astigmatism; Prehemodialysis.

Am American (see Amer); Americium (atomic no. 95, see Elements); Amethropterin (= AM); Amyl (group) (= am); Amnion.

am amyl (see Am); as in AM. e.g. ametropia, amplitude, meter-angle, mixed/ myopic astigmatism, etc.

A/m Amperes per meter.

A-M Antero-medial.

A-m² Ampere-square meter.

α2M α2-macroglobulin (a plasma protein).

AMA Acute metabolic acidosis/ alkalosis; Acute migraine attack; Aerospace Medical Association; Against medical advice; American Management/ Mathematical/ Medical Association; Ames mutation assay; Antimalarial agent (= AMD); Antimeasles/ mitochondrial/ myocardial/ myosin/ mumps/ mycoplasma antibody; Antimetabolite agent (it interferes with the making of DNA, and is used in cancer therapy (= ANA; AND); Antimicrobial action/ activity (see AME); Antimicrobial/ migraine/ mitotic/ motility/ muscarinic/ mutagenic agent (see AMD); Antimuscarinic action (decrease in detrusor pressure in the urinary bladder); Antimycobacterial/cotic agent (isoniazid, rifabutin, rifampicin, etc.) (see AFA); Antithyroid microsomal antibody; Apothecaries of Medieval Allemagne; Audiometric analysis (for auditory acuity); Austin Moore arthroplasty (see AMP);

Australian Medical Association.
AMAA Aviation Medical Assistance Act (1998) (US).
AMA-AMPAC American Medical Association - American Medical Political Action Committee.
AMACD American Medical Association Council on Drugs.
AMAD Morning admission.
AMA-DE American Medical Association - Drug Evaluation.
AMAEI American Management Associations Extension Institute.
AMAERF American Medical Association Education and Research Foundation.
AMAG Adrenal medullary autograft.
AMAJ American Medical Association Journal.
AMAL Aero-Medical Acceleration Laboratory.
Amal Amalgam (see Amalg); Amobarbital.
Amalg Amalgam (= Amalg) (tooth filling).
AMA-MRP American Medical Association - Medical Retirement Plan.
AMAN American Medical Association (AMA) News - now American Medical News (AMN).
AMAP As much as possible.
AMA-SRF American Medical Association - Sears Roebuck Foundation (community medical assistance).
AMAT Antimalignant antibody test.
A-MAT Amorphous material.
AMATAB Antimicrosomal antithyroid antibody (titer - found in Sjogren's syndrome).
AMAU American Medical Association Update (journal).
AMB Active major bleeding; Ambivalent group; Ambulate/tory (see Ambul); Amphotericin B; Anomalous muscle bundle; Avian myeloblastosis.
Amb; amb Ambient; Ambiguous (see Ambig); Ambulance/ate/ation/atory (see Ambul).
Ambig Ambiguous (= Amb).
AMBL Acute megakaryoblastic leukemia.
Amblyopia ('amblys' - Modern L., derived from Gr. = dull + 'o~ps' = eye) - Dimness of/ reduced vision, or early amaurosis in an eye that appears to be normal and has no detectable ocular organic lesion, such as:
Alcoholic amblyopia (or Amplyopia alcoholica) - Impairment of vision due to alcohol poisoning (see Toxic amblyopia).
Arsenic amblyopia - Visual disturbance due to arsenic poisoning (see Toxic amblyopia).
Astigmatic amblyopia - due to imperfect development of retinal vision.
Color amblyopia - Impairment of color vision due to toxins, etc. (see Toxic amblyopia).
Amblyopia crapulosa = Alcoholic amblyopia.
Crossed amblyopia - Amblyopia affecting one eye, with ipsilateral hemianesthesia.
Amblyopia cruciata = Crossed amblyopia.
Amblyopia ex anopsia - Suppression of vision due to chronic illness.
Hysterical amblyopia - Amblyopia associated with hysteria.
Nocturnal amblyopia - Dimness of vision at night.
Postmarital amblyopia - Amblyopia caused by excessive sexual activity.
Quinine amblyopia - Disturbed vision due to anemia of the retina, following large doses of quinine (see Toxic amblyopia).
Reflex amblyopia - Amblyopia resulting from peripheral irritation.
Suppression amblyopia - Amblyopia caused by subconscious inhibition or repression of vision.
Tobacco amblyopia - Impairment of vision caused by excessive smoking (active/ passive inhalation of nicotine) (see Toxic amblyopia).
Toxic amblyopia - Amblyopia due to poisoning by toxins i) chemicals, such as Alcohol, Arsenic, Nicotine (tobacco), Quinine, etc., as well as ii) infections (bacterial, viral, etc.).
Uremic amblyopia - Visual disturbances sometimes seen in ESRD/ Uremic attacks.
Ambul Ambulance/ate/ation/atory (= AMB; Amb; amb).
AMC Abnormal mental condition; Academic medical center; Acetylmethyl carbinol; Acute medical care/ crisis; Acute metabolic crisis (Hypoglycemia, ketoacidosis, etc); Adjusted mean change(s); Amebic meningo-encephalitis; Animal Medical Center; Antibody-mediated cytotoxicity; Antimalaria campaign;

Antimicrobial compound; Appalachian Mountain Club; Arm muscle circumference; Army Medical Corps; Arthrogryposis multiplex congenita; Association Médicale Canadienne; Atypical mononuclear cell; Autologous marrow cell; Automated mixture control; Axiomesiocervical.

AMCA American Medical Curling Association; Aminomethylcyclohexane carbonic acid; Antimetabolite cytotoxic agent (= ACA).

AM-CAP American Medical-Computer Assistance Program.

AMCAS American Medical College Application Service.

AMCC Advanced metastatic colorectal cancer.

AMCHA Tranexamic acid (= Aminomethylcyclohexane-carboxylic acid; Trans-4-[aminomethyl]cyclohexane carbolic acid).

AMCJ Association Médicale Canadienne Journal.

AMCN Anteromedial caudate nucleus.

AMCR Amylase to creatinine ratio.

AMCs Additional marker chromosomes.

AMD Above-mentioned disorder; Acid maltase deficiency; Aclometasone diproprionate (a topical steroid); Acromandibular dysplasia; Actinomycin D; Active/ Acute myocardial damage; Adjusted mean difference (between two therapies); Adrenomedullary dysfunction/ dysplasia; Adrenomyelodystrophy; Advances in Metabolic Disorders (books); Aerospace Medical Division (US Air Force); Age-related macular degeneration; Aleutian mink disease; Alpha-methyldopa; Ancient medical dictum; Antimalarial/ mutagenic/ mycotic drug (see AMA); Antimitotic drug; Antimotility drug (i.e. for diarrhea); Antimuscarinic drug (a drug that causes the "flight or fight" response with HTN, hypoptyalism and tachycardia) (= AMA); Appropriate maintenance dosage/ dose; Arbitrary medical decision; Association for Macular Diseases; Axiomesiodistal.

AMDA Airline Medical Directors' Association.

AMDGF Alveolar macrophage-derived growth factor.

Am Doc American doctor.

AMDR Association of Medical Device Reprocessors (US).

AMDS Association of Military Dental Surgeons.

AMDST Antimicrobial disk susceptibility test (NCCLS).

AME Acute manic episode; Adenomyoepithelioma (= ACC or Adenoid cystic/ Adenocystic carcinoma, Cribriform carcinoma, Cylindroma, Cylindromatous carcinoma); Adverse metabolic effect(s); Amphotericin methyl ester; Ankle-motion exercise(s); Antimicrobial effect (= AMA); Antimitotic effect; Aseptic meningoencephalitis; Aviation Medical Examiner.

AMEA American Medical Electroencephalographic Association (see AMEEGA).

AMEAE Acute monophasic experimental autoimmune encephalomyelitis.

AMEDS Army Medical Service.

AMEE Association for Medical Education in Europe.

AMEEGA American Medical Electroencephalographic Association (= AMEA).

AMEGL; AMegL Acute megakaryoblastic leukemia.

AMEL Aero-Medical Equipment Laboratory.

Amer American (= Am).

AMES Air medical evacuation system.

Ameslan American Sign Language (for the deaf).

AMet Adenosyl-L-methionine.

AMF Adenomyofibroma; Adrenomedullary function; American Menopause Foundation; American mountain fever (see CTF); Anthropometric factor (Gr. anthropos = man; metron = measure); Antimetastatic/ Antimuscle factor; Autocrine motility factor.

AmFAR American Foundation for AIDS Research.

AMG Acoustic myography; Americal Medical Graduate; Aminoglycoside; Amyloglucosidase; Antimacrophage globulin; Axiomesiogingival.

A2MG Alpha-2-macroglobulin.

AMGA American Medical Golf Association.

AMGP Association of Medical Group Psychoanalysts.

AMGT Adenovirus-mediated p53 gene transfer (in the treatment of advanced lung cancer - NSCLC).

AMH Adrenal medullary/ Adrenomedullary hormones (see Hormones); Adrenomedullary hypofunction; Antimüllerian hormone; Archives of Medical Hydrology (journal); Automated medical history; Mixed astigmatism with myopia predominating (see Amh).

Amh Mixed astigmatism with myopia predominating (= AMH).

AMHA Association of Mental Health Administrators.

AMHAI Association for Mental Health Aid to Israel.

AMHF American Mental Health Foundation.

AMHP Austin Moore hip prosthesis.

AMHT Automated multiphasic health testing.

AMI Abnormal maternal immunization; Acquired monosaccharide intolerance; Acute meningeal irritation; Acute myocardial infarction/ ischemia; Advocates for Medical Information (a student organization); American Meat Institute; American Medical International; Amitriptyline; Anterior myocardial infarction; Assistance Médicale Internationale (Canadian journal); Association of Medical Illustrators; Atypical mycobacterial infection; Atheltic Motivation Inventory; Axiomesioincisal.

AMIA American Medical Informatics Association.

Amies Amyl nitrite (capsules - see Amyl nitrite).

AMIKA Amikacin sulfate.

AMI-P Acute myocardial infarction and pericarditis.

AMIS Aspirin Myocardial Infarction Study (NIH).

Amish Member of a Mennonite sect.

AMJA American Medical Joggers Association.

AMKL Acute megakaryoblastic leukemia.

AML Acute monocytic/ myeloblastic/ myelocytic/ myelogenous/ myeloid leukemia; Acute mucosal lesion; Anatomic medullary locking; Anterior mitral leaflet; Argon Microsurgical Laser; Automated Medical/ Multitest Laboratories/ry; Trademark (Orthopedic Implants).

AMLB test Alternate Monaural Loudness Balance test.

AMLC Adherent macrophage-like cell; Autologous mixed lymphocte culture.

AMLFC Association des Médecins de Langue Française du Canada.

AMLR Autologous mixed lymphocyte reaction.

AMLS Antimouse lymphocyte serum.

AMLSGA Acute myeloblastic leukemia surface glycoprotein antigen.

AMM Agnogenic myeloid metaplasia; Ammonia (see Ammon); Anterior mediastinal mass (see AMT); "Antimissile missile" (e.g. Anti-IgE therapy in allergic disease); Army Medical Museum; Antibody to murine (cardiac) myosin; World Medical Association (French: Association Médicale Mondiale).

Amm Ammonia (see Ammon).

AMMA American-Mexican Medical Association.

AMMAJ American-Mexican Medical Association Journal.

AMML Acute monomyelogenous/ myelomonocytic leukemia.

AMMoL Acute myelomonoblastic leukemia.

Ammon Ammonia (= AMM; Amm).

AMN Acne miliaris necrotica; Acriflavine mononucleotide (= Riboflavine phosphate); Acute muscle necrosis Adrenomyeloneuropathy; Alloxazine mononucleotide; American Medical News (formerly AMAH); Aminonucleoside (see AMNS); Anterior median nucleus; Anterior mediastinal neoplasm/ node.

Amnesia Lack of memory, esp. inability to remember past experiences.
Antegrade amnesia - for events occurring after the responsible episode.
Auditory amnesia - word deafness.
Broca's amnesia - inability to remember spoken words.
Hysteric amnesia - amnesia associated with extreme hysteric anxiety, excitability, emotional conflict, or neurosis.
Infantile amnesia - the normal or usual inabil-

ity of recalling events of early childhood.
Lacunar amnesia - loss of memory only for certain isolated events.
Localized amnesia - amnesia for events associated with a certain incident, place, or time.
Olfactory amnesia - loss of the sense of smell.
Patchy amnesia - lacunar amnesia.
Posthypnotic amnesia - amnesia under the influence of hypnotic suggestion or directed forgetfulness.
Posttraumatic amnesia - loss of memory due to head injury or other trauma.
Retroactive amnesia - amnesia for events taking place before the trauma or disease causing it.
Retrograde amnesia - retroactive amnesia.
Tactile amnesia - inability to recognize objects or to appreciate their form by touching or feeling them, i.e. Astereognosis.
Tropic amnesia - loss of memory affecting white people in the tropics, such as 'coast memory', which is very prevalent on the west coast of Africa.
Tropical amnesia - tropic amnesia.
Verbal amnesia - loss of memory for words.
Visual amnesia - word blindness.

AMNH American Museum of Natural History.

amnio amniocentesis.

Amnionitis. Infection of the amniotic fluid (see Chorioamnionitis; Funisitis; Villitis) (= AFI).

AMNS American Medical News Service; Aminonucleoside (= AMN); Arthromyoneuropathy syndrome.

AMN SC Amniotic (fluid) scan.

AMO Aerobic/ Anaerobic micro-organism; Laser (ophthalmology); Assistant medical officer; Axiomesio-occlusal.

amo Amorphous (see Amorph).

A-MODE Time/amplitude modulation.

AMoL; AMOL Acute monoblastic/ monocytic leukemia.

Amorph; Amor Amorphous (= amo; Amor).

AMOX; Amox Amoxicillin trihydrate (= Amox).

AMP Accelerated mental process(es); Accepted medical practice; Acid mucopolysaccaride/ saccharide (see AMPS); Adenosine monophosphate (= Adenosine-3,5'-monophosphate; APM; Muscle adenylic acid; Phosphentacide) - see CAMP; cAMP - a nucleotide constituent of animal cells, being concerned with the storage and release of energy. Has been used as a vasodilator in angina pectoris and also in the treatment of multiple sclerosis and porphyria - see Vitamins B8; Age-matched patient; Alternative medical practice/titioner (such as Acupuncture, Aroma therapy, Chiropractic/axis, Energy healing, Homeopathy, Massage therapy, Meditation, Naturotherapy, Osteopathy, Reflexology, Reiki, Shiatsu, Syntology, etc.); Aminomethylpropanol; Ammonium molybdophosphate; Amphetamine; Ampicillin (on culture and sensitivity reports); Ampoule; Ampul; Amputation/tee (see Amp); Androgenomimetic progestogen; Antimicrobial preservative; Austin Moore prosthesis (for replacement of femoral head) (Orth); Average mean pressure.

Amp Amperage/re; Amplification/fy; Ampoula/le (see Ampul); Amputation/utee (= AMP).

AMPA American Medical Publishers Association; Amino-3-hydroxy-5-methylisoxazole-4-propionic acid.

AMPAC American Medical Political Action Committee (AMA).

AMP-c Cyclic adenosine monophosphate.

AMPD Amino-methyl-propanediol.

AMPE Acute massive pulmonary embolism (= MPE).

AMPH Amphetamine (see Amphet).

Amph Amphoric.

Amph- prefix meaning both or doubly (Gr. amphi).

Amphet Amphetamine(s) - a cerebral stimulant increasing mental activity and physical energy, with relief of fatigue. It averts sleep in narcolepsy, and oculogyric crises in postencephalitic parkinsonism. Repeated use causes severe addiction (= Benzylmethyl carbinamine). Other names are: Bam; Benny; Benz; Benzedrine; Black beauty (biphetamine); Brain tickler (amphetamine pill); Brownie; BZ (Dimethoxymethyl-amphetamine); Cartwheel (amphetamine tablet); Chalk (amphetamine tablet); Copilot (dexedrine tablet); Crank; Crossroad (amphetamine tablet); Crys (methamphetamine); Crystal (any soluble amphetamine, desoxyn, or methedrine); DAS (Dextroamphetamine sulfate); Dephadren (Dexamphetamine sulfate tablet); Dex (Dexedrine); Dexamed (Dexamphetamine sulfate tablet); Dexamphetamine sulfate; Dexedrine (Dexamphetamine sulfate); dexie (Dexedrine tablet [Dexamyl/ Drinamyl] - proprietary tablets containing 5 mg dexamphetamine sulfate and 32 mg amylobarbitone); DOET (= Dimethoxy-ethyl amphetamine; 2,5-Dimethoxy-4-ethyl amphetamine); doll; DOM (= Dimethoxymethyl amphetamine; 2,5-Dimethoxymethyl-amphetamine; BZ; STP); Ecstasy (see MDMA); Football (diphetamine pill); Forward (amphetamine) pill); Heart (Dexedrine heart-shaped tablet); IT-290 (Indole analog of amphetamine); Leaper (amphetamine tablet); Lid popper (amphetamine tablet); MDMA (= Ecstasy; 3,4-methylenedioxymethamphetamine; 3-methylfentanyl) - the so-called synthetic heroin drug, a derivative of Oil of Sassafras or Oil of Nutmeg; ME (= Methamphetamine hydrochloride) - a hallucinogen; Meth (Methedrine); MMDA (= Methoxy-methyl-ene-dioxy-amphetamine; trimethoxy-amphetamine); Orange (dexedrine tablet); Speed (Methamphetamine); Splash; STP (Methyl-dimethoxy-methylphenethylamine); Ten A (10-milligram amphetamine tablet); Thruster (amphetamine pill); Upper (amphetamine pill); Ups (amphetamine pill); Water (Methamphetamine); White (amphetamine/ benzedrine pill).

Amp/hr; amp-hr Ampere-hour; Amperes per hour.

Ampl Large (L. amplus).

A-M pr Austin-Moore prosthesis.

AMPRCA Antibody-mediated pure cell aplasia (as in reaction to therapy with epoetin alfa - rHuEPO).

AMPS Abnormal mucopolysacchariduria; Acid mucopolysaccaride/ saccharide (= AMP); Assembly of Mathematical and Physical Sciences (NRC).

AMP scale/ system Assessment of the severity of psychiatric symptoms (German: Arbeitsgemeinschaft für Methodik und Dokumentation in der Psychiatrie).

AMPT Alpha-methylparatyrosine.

AMP therapy Atropine metaraminol pyridine aldoximes therapy.

Ampul Ampule/Ampoule (= Amp) (L. ampulla).

AMR Alternating motion reflex(es); Annual morbidity/ mortality rate; Antibody-mediated response; Arthroscopic meniscus repair (Knee joint) (Orthopedics).

AMRA American Medical Record Association.

AMRC Academy of Medical Royal Colleges (UK).

AMRDC Army Medical Research and Development Command; Association of Medical Rehabilitation Directors and Coordinators.

AMRI Anteromedial rotatory instability.

AMRIID Army Medical Research Institute of Infectious Diseases (see USAMRIID).

AMRL Aerospace Medical Research Laboratories/tory.

AMRNL Army Medical Research and Nutrition Laboratory.

AMRS Adrenal Metabolic Research Society; Automated medical record system.

AMS Academy of Medical Sciences (Moscow); Accelerator mass spectrometry; Acta Medica Scandinavica (journal); Activated mouse serum; Acute maxillary sinusitis; Acute mountain sickness; Adenomyosarcoma (e.g. Wilms' tumor); Adequate medical supervision; Aggravated in military service; Agricultural Marketing Service; Allen-Masters syndrome (see MAS; UJC); Altered mental status; American Mathematical/ Meteorological/ Microbiological/ Microchemical/ Microscopical Society; Amount of a substance (see ams); Amylase; Angiomyosarcoma; Anticipated mean/ median survival; Antimacrophage serum; Antimicrobial serum (= Antiserum; Immune serum); Antimyosin scintography; Arkansas

Medical Society; Army Medical Service; Aseptic meningitis syndrome; Association of Medical Students; Association of Military Surgeons; Atypical measles syndrome; Audiometric screening; Auditory memory span; Automated multiphasic screening; Average(d) mean score; Awkward motor skill(s) (as in Asperger syndrome - see GS; MRP; ORB; PDD; SMC).

ams Amount of a substance (= AMS).

AMSA Acridinylamine methanesulfon-m-anisidide; American Medical Society on Alcoholism; American Medical Student(s) Association; Amsacrine.

AMSAB American Medical Students' Association of Bologna (Italy).

AMSC Army Medical Specialist Corps.

AMSD Acute musculoskeletal disorder.

AMSH Alpha melanocytic-stimulating hormone - a new treatment for arthritis (see Hormones).

AMSIT Portion of the mental state examination: **A** - appearance, **M** - mood, **S** - sensorium, **I** - intelligence, **T** - thought process.

AMSRDC Army Medical Service Research and Development Command.

AMSS Albright-McCune-Sternberg syndrome (with very early puberty in females) (= Albright's syndrome; OFD or Osteitis fibrosa disseminata).

AMST Antimicrobial susceptibility test.

AMSUS Association of Military Surgeons of the United States.

AMT Active malignant tumor; Acute miliary tuberculosis; Adrenal medullary tissue/ tumor (= PCC - Pheochromocytoma); Allogeneic marrow transplant (see HABMT); Alpha-methyltyrosine; Ambulance medical technician; American Medical Technologist(s); Amethopterin; Amitriptyline; Amphetamine(s); Anterior mediastinal tumor (e.g. thymoma, lymphoma, endocrine tumor, germ-cell tumor, etc.) (= AMM); Antimicrobial therapy; Anxiety management training; Appropriate medical therapy/ treatment.

Amt Amount.

AMTA American Massage and Therapy Association; American Medical Tennis Association; American Music Therapy Association.

AMTD Antibody-mediated tissue damage.

AMTJ American Medical Technologists Journal.

AMU Army Medical Unit; Atomic mass unit (see Amu).

Amu Atomic mass unit (dalton) (= AMU; Dal).

AmuLV Abelson/ Amphotrophic murine leukemia virus.

AMV Assisted mechanical ventilation; Avian myeloblastosis virus (reverse transcriptase).

Am. VD American Venereal Disease (Association).

AMVER Automated Mutual Assistance Vessel Rescue Center (Coast Guard).

AMVI Acute mesenteric vascular insufficiency.

AMVL; aMVL Anterior mitral valve leaflet.

AMWA American Medical Women's/ Writers' Association.

AMWAJ American Medical Women's Association Journal.

AMWS American Men and Women of Science (book).

AMX Amoxicillin.

AMY; Amy Amyl nitrite (vial of) - see Amyl nitrite; Amylase.

amyl- prefix meaning starch (Gr. amulos).

Amyl nitrite Amyl NO_2 (= Amies; Amy; Amylis Nitris; Amylium Nitrosum; AN; Azotite d'Amyle; Christmas tree [Dexamyl capsule]; Isoamyl Nitrite; Nitrito de amylo; Pentanoli Nitris; Poppers [Amyl nitrite or Butyl nitrite]; Rush [Amyl nitrite/ Butyl nitrite]; Snapper). When inhaled, causes severe vasodilatation and flushing of the face, the head and neck perspire, and the heart-beat is accelerated. The action is short and usually lasts only 2 to 3 minutes. Used in the treatment of attacks of angina of effort by producing instant coronary vasodilatation. Also much abused in its use by drug addicts, because of the flushing and vasodilating action.

AN Acanthosis nigricans; Acne neonatorum; Acoustic neuroma; Adult, normal; Ala nasi; American Nurse (ANA journal); Amyl nitrite;

Anesthesiology; Aneurysm; Anisometropia (see An); Annals of Neurology; Anode; Anorexia nervosa; Antenatal; Anterior; Antineuraminidase (antibody); Anxiety neurosis; Archives of Neurology (ANA); Aseptic necrosis; Associate Nurse/ in Nursing; Atmosphere normal; Atrionodal; Auditory neuropathy; Autonomic neuropathy; Avascular necrosis; Axonal neuropathy.

An Actinon; Anisometropia (= AN) - eyes requiring different refractive corrections; Anode/dal; Normal atmosphere (see A/~ N).

an aneurysm.

A/N Acid/neutral; As needed.

A/~ N; A/~ n Normal atmosphere (= An).

an- prefix meaning absent/ no/ not (Latin); positive/ up (Greek).

ANA Acetylneuraminic acid; Acoustic Neuroma Archive (journal); American Narcolepsy/ Neurological/ Nurses' Association; Anesthesia/thetic (see Anesth); Angioneurotic anuria; Antibody to nuclear antigens; Antineoplastic agent (see CSACA); Antineoplastic antibiotic (see AAA or Antibiotic anticancer agent); Antineutrophil antibody; Antinuclear antibody (laboratory/ serology); Antinuclear autoantibody (see AAB); Aspartyl naphthylamide; Atypical neuroleptic agent.

Ana Anaesthesia (journal); Anaesthetist (journal); Anesthesia/thetic (see Anesth); Of each/ equal parts (= aa) (see ana-).

ana- combining form meaning of each, up, or positive (Gr.) (= Ana).

ANAb Antinuclear antibody (see ANA).

Anachem Association of Analytical Chemists.

ANACP American Nurses' Association Careers Program.

ANAD Anorexia nervosa with associated disorders.

ANADG Antinicotine amide dinucleotide glycohydrolase.

ANAE Alpha-naphthyl acetate esterase.

Anaes; Anaesth Anaesthesia/thetic (see Anesth).

ANAG Acute narrow angle glaucoma.

ANAL; Anal Analgesia/ic; Analysis/yses/ytic; The Analyst (journal).

Anal Psychol Analytical psychology.

ANALYZ (program) Automatic syntactic analysis (program).

ANAMH Australian National Association for Mental Health.

ANAP Agglutination negative, absorption positive (reaction).

Anaphylaxis Gr. ana- = excess; phylaxis = protection. An exaggerated, unusual, or severe allergic response to a foreign substance or antigen. Also called Antigen-antibody reaction, Hypersusceptibility, or Protein sensitization. Known as the Theobald-Smith phenomenon in guinea pigs.

Acquired anaphylaxis - produced by administration of a foreign protein.

Active anaphylaxis - the anaphylactic state produced in an animal by the injection of a foreign protein.

Aggregate anaphylaxis - a severe allergy caused by injecting a foreign substance (antigen).

Antiserum anaphylaxis = Passive anaphylaxis.

Chronic anaphylaxis = Enteritis anaphylactica, a laboratory condition in sensitized dogs, characterized by chronic hemorrhagic inflammation of both legs and small intestine, following a second dose of an anaphylactogen (Charles Robert Rickets, French physiologist).

Cutaneous anaphylaxis - an allergic skin reaction.

Cytotoxic anaphylaxis - anaphylaxis caused by chemical compounds or other cytotoxins.

Heterologous anaphylaxis - a passive anaphylaxis caused by transfering serum from an animal of a different species (see Passive anaphylaxis).

Homologous anaphylaxis - a passive anaphylaxis induced by the transference of serum from an animal of the same species (see Passive anaphylaxis).

Indirect anaphylaxis - anaphylaxis induced by one's own protein modified in some way.

Inverse anaphylaxis - an anaphylactic shock produced by a single IV injection of a heterogenetic antibody (Forssman).

Passive anaphylaxis - anaphylaxis occurring in a normal person as a result of an injection

of serum from a previously sensitized individual (e.g. Heterologous anaphylaxis; Homologous anaphylaxis).
Psychic anaphylaxis - an attack of neurosis due to early psychic trauma.
Reverse anaphylaxis - anaphylaxis due to the injection of antigen following the injection of antiserum.

ANAR Appropriate neutralizing antibody response.

ANAS Anastomosis (see Anast); Auditory nerve activating substance.

Anast Anastomosis (= ANAS).

Anat Anatomical/mist/my.

ANB Adrenergic neurone blocker (e.g. bethanidine); Anorexia nervosa with bulimia; Aseptic/ Avascular necrosis of bone (= Caisson disease or Decompression sickness syndrome); "As needed" basis; Autonomous bladder (= Flaccid bladder) (see UBD); Avascular necrosis of bone.

ANBD Adrenergic neurone blocking drug (see ANB).

ANC Absolute neutrophil count; Acid/ Antigen neutralizing capacity; Adequate nursing care; Antenatal care/ clinic; Archinephric canal (see PND); Army Nurse Corps.

ANCA Anthracene-9-carboxylic acid; Antineutrophil cytoplasmic antibody.

AnCC; ANCC Anodal closure contraction (= ANCC).

ANCD Alcoholic-nutritional cerebellar degeneration (also called CCD or Cerebellar cortical degeneration).

anch anchored.

ANCM Association of New Chinese Medicine.

ANCOVA Analysis of covariance.

ancyl- prefix meaning crooked or looped (Gr. agkulos).

AND Adolescent nutritional disorder; Algoneurodystrophy; Antenatal diagnosis/ disease/ disorder (= PND); Anterior nasal discharge; Antineoplastic drug (see CSACA); Archinephric duct (see PND); Autonomy drive.

ANDA Abbreviated New Drug Application.

ANDD Algoneurodystrophic disorder (= Sudeck's disease).

ANDI Acquired nephrogenic diabetes insipidus.

andr- prefix meaning man (Gr. andros).

ANDRO; Andro Androsterone.

Andro 4-Androstenediol; Androstenedione.

ANDTE; AnDTe Anodal duration tetanus.

ANE Angioneurotic edema (= AE; Quincke's disease; Toxic edema); Antineoplastic effect.

Anes Anesthesia/thetic (see Anesth); Anesthesiology (journal).

ANESR Apparent norepinephrine secretion rate.

Anesth Anaesthesia/thetic; Anesthesia/thetic (= ANA; Ana; Anaes; Anaesth; Anes).

Aneurysm A bulging of the wall of a blood vessel, usually caused by atherosclerosis or hypertension, but sometimes due to injury, infection, or an inherited weakness in the vessel wall (artery or vein).
Abdominal aneurism - an aneurysm of the abdominal aorta.
Ampullary aneurism - Sacculated aneurysm.
Aneurysma anastomotica - aneurysm by anastomosis, with dilatation of several arteries, forming a pulsating subcutaneous tumor.
Aortic aneurism - aneurysm of the aorta.
Arteriovenous aneurism - an aneurysm (i) caused by the simultaneous rupture of an artery into a neighboring vein, as in Aneurysmal varix or Rodrigues's aneurysm, or (ii) rupture into two veins, as in Park's aneurysm, or (iii) caused by the blood flowing directly into such a vein by a connecting sac, as in Varicose aneurysm (= Pott's aneurism).
Axial aneurism - an aneurysm in which the entire circumference of the vessel is dilated.
Axillary aneurism - an aneurysm of the axillary artery.
Bacterial aneurism = Mycotic aneurysm.
Bérard's aneurism - an arteriovenous aneurysm in the tissues around a vein or outside an injured vein (see Arteriovenous aneurism).
Berry aneurism - a small saccular or sacculated aneurysm of the cerebral artery (see Sacculated aneurism).
Bone aneurism - a pulsating vascular bone tumor (= Osteoid aneurism).

Branching aneurism - a Cirsoid aneurysm (see Racemose aneurism).
Cardiac aneurism - an aneurysm caused by dilatation/ weakening of a portion of the myocardial (heart) wall, as following MI (= Mural aneurism).
Cerebral aneurism - a ballooning of an artery in the brain (cerebrum) (see also Berry aneurism).
Circumscribed aneurism = True aneurysm.
Cirsoid aneurism - a Branching aneurysm (see Racemose aneurism).
Compound aneurism - an aneurysm in which some of the coats are ruptured and others merely dilated (= Mixed aneurism).
Consecutive aneurism = False aneurysm.
Crisp's aneurism - aneurysm of the Splenic artery (see Serpentine aneurism).
Cylindroid aneurism - the uniform dilatation of a considerable part of an (= Tubular aneurism).
Cystogenic aneurism - an aneurysm resulting from the rupture of a cyst into an artery.
Diffuse aneurism = False aneurysm (see).
Dissecting aneurism - one in which the blood 'dissects' or is forced between the coats of an artery, as in Dissecting Aorta, Shekelton's aneurism, etc.
Ectatic aneurism - one formed by arterial distension without rupture of the coats or walls of the artery.
Embolic aneurism - an aneurysm caused by embolism.
Embolomycotic aneurism - an aneurysm caused by embolism from some fungal, mycotic, or vegetative heart condition.
Endogenous aneurism - an aneursym associated with disease of the blood vessel wall (= Spontaneous aneurism).
Erosive aneurism - an aortic aneurysm caused by the extension of heart valve disease, resulting in ulcerative endocarditis and destruction of the intima.
Exogenous aneurism - an aneurysm caused by injury to the vessel wall (= Traumatic aneurism).
External aneurism - an aneurysm not situated in a body cavity.
False aneurism - one in which all the vessel coats are ruptured and the blood is retained by the surrounding tissues (= Consecutive aneurism; Diffuse aneurism; Spurious aneurism).
Fusiform aneurism - a spindle-shaped arterial dilatation (= Richet's aneurism).
Hernial aneurism - an aneurysm in which the inner coat herniates or projects through the outer.
Innominate aneurism - aneurysm of the brachiocephalic trunk.
Internal aneurism - an aneurysm situated within any of the body cavities.
Intracranial aneurism - an aneurysm within the cranium.
Intramural aneurism - one in which the blood remains within the arterial wall.
Lateral aneurism - an aneurysm which projects from one side of an artery.
Medical aneurism - a deep-seated aneurysm not accessible by surgery (such as Thoracic aneurism).
Miliary aneurism - an aneurysm of a minute artery or capillary (such as: Intracranial aneurism).
Mixed aneurism = Compound aneurysm.
Mural aneurism - an aneurysm of the heart wall (e.g. Cardiac aneurism).
Mycotic aneurism - an aneurysm produced by growth of microorganisms in the vessel wall (= Bacterial aneurism).
Orbital aneurism - an aneurysm found within the orbit of the eye. Osteoid aneurism = Bone aneurysm (see). Park's aneurism - an arteriovenous aneurysm in which the arterial dilatation communicates with two veins (see Arteriovenous aneurism ii).
Pelvic aneurism - an aneurysm found within the pelvis.
Phantom aneurism - a condition in which the patient complains of severe throbbing in the region of the palpable aorta (= Aortismus abdominalis; Students' aneurysm).
Pott's aneurism - an Aneurysmal varix or Varicose aneursym (see Arteriovenous aneurysm iii.).
Racemose aneurism - an aneurysm in which the blood vessels become dilated, lengthened, and tortuous (= Branching aneurism; Cirsoid

aneurism).
Rasmussen's aneurism - a dilatation of a terminal artery in a tuberculous cavity (lung), its rupture causing hemorrhage in the late (3rd) stage of the disease (TBC).
Renal aneurism = Gull's renal epistaxis (a disease of middle adult life, marked by renal hemorrhage, but with no known lesion. Also called Angioneurotic hematuria, Essential renal hematuria, and Renal hemophilia).
Richet's aneurism = Fusiform aneurysm.
Rodrigues's aneurism - a varicose aneurysm with the sac lying contiguous to the artery (see Arteriovenous aneurism i.).
Sacculated aneurism - a saclike arterial dilatation which opens by a small opening, with the said artery (= Ampullary aneurism; Berry aneurism).
Secondary aneurism - one that recurs after apparent cure.
Serpentine aneurism - an elongated, varicose, so-called senile condition of arteries such as the iliac, splenic (e.g. Crisp's aneurism), and temporal arteries.
Shekelton's aneurism - a dissecting aneurysm (see Dissecting aneurism).
Silent aneurism- an aneurysm not felt or seen (i.e. producing no signs or symptoms).
Spongy aneurism - an angioma.
Spontaneous aneurism = Endogenous aneurysm.
Spurious aneurism = False aneurysm.
Students' aneurism = Phantom aneurysm.
Surgical aneurism - one that can be treated by a surgical operation.
Thoracic aneurism - an aneurysm situated within the thorax (see Medical aneurism).
Traction aneurism - an aneurysm produced by traction on the aorta by an incompletely atrophied ductus arteriosus.
Traumatic aneurism - an aneurysm caused by injury (see Exogenous aneurism).
True aneurism - an aneurysm in which the sac is formed by the arterial walls of which, one at least is unbroken (= Circumscribed aneurism).
Tubular aneurism = Cylindroid aneurysm.
Valvular aneurism - an aneurysm formed between the layers of a heart valve.
Varicose aneurism - an aneurysm in which the artery communicates with a contiguous vein by means of an intervening sac (see Arteriovenous aneurism iii.).
Venous aneurism - aneurysm of a vein.
Ventricular aneurism - aneurysmal dilatation of a heart ventricle.
Verminous aneurism - an aneurysm containing hematozoa.
Worm aneurism - aneurysm in horses caused by the larvae of the parasitic nematode worm, *Strongylus* equinus.

AnEx; an ex Anodal/de excitation.

ANF Abnormal/ Absent nerve function; Acoustic neurofibroma (= Acoustic neurilemmoma/ neurinoma/ neuroma); Alpha-naphthoflavone; American Nurses' Foundation; Antineuritic/ Antinuclear factor(s) (laboratory/ serology); Atrial natriuretic factor.

A(NF)M Acute (non-fulminant) myocarditis.

ANG; Ang Acute necrotizing gingivitis (= Trench mouth; Vincent's angina); Angiogram/graphy (see Angio); Angiotension; Angle e.g. Ang of scapula; Anglican Church of Canada member; Angular.

Angel dust Phencyclidine and marijuana mixture (see Cannabis).

Angels' trumpets The long flowers of some species of the *Datura* plant, infused into 'teas' and often associated with drug abuse (see 'Jimson weed').

Ang GR Angiotensin generation rate.

angi- combining form meaning vessel (Gr. aggeion).

Angio Angiogram/graphy (= ANG; Ang) (procedure/ cardiovascular); Angiologica (journal).

Ang pect Angina pectoris.

ANH Antineoplastic hormone; Artificial nutrition and hydration.

Anh; anh Anhydrous.

ANHA American Nursing Home Association (now HCA - Health Care Association).

ANHE Acute necrotizing hemorrhagic encephalopathy (= AHLE).

ANHI Fatty acid mixture A of National Heart Institute.

ANHS Alaska Native Health Service.

ANI Absolute nutrient intake; Acquired neurological injury; Acute nerve irritation.

ANIA Automated nephelometric immunoassay.

ANIF Antinuclear immunofluorescence.

ANIS Anorexia Nervosa Inventory for Selfrating.

Aniso Anisocytosis (of red blood cells).

aniso- prefix meaning unequal or dissimilar.

ANIT Alpha-naphthyl-isothiocyanate.

ANJ Australian Nurses' Journal (RANF).

Ank Ankle.

ankyl- prefix meaning crooked or looped (Gr. agkylos).

ANL Acute non-lymphoblastic leukemia; Argonne National Laboratory.

ANLI Antibody-negative with latent infection.

ANLL Acute non-lymphoblastic/phocytic leukemia.

ANM Acne necrotica miliaris; Assistant nurse midwife.

Ann Annals (journal); Annual.

Ann fib Annulus fibrosus.

Annot Annotation.

ANO Acute narcotic overdosage.

AnOC; ANOC Anodal opening contraction (= ANOC; AOC).

ANOCL Anodal opening clonus.

Anon Anonymous.

ANOVA; ANOV Analysis of variance (= ANOV; AOV).

ANP Acute necrotizing pancreatitis; A-norprogesterone; Archives of Neurology and Psychiatry (journal); Atrial natriuretic peptide; Autonomic neuropathy.

ANP 235 Meclofenoxate hydrochloride (= Centrophenoxine/ Clophenoxate/ Meclofenoxane HCl); Proprietary name: Lucidril. A stimulant of the central nervous system, used in the treatment of depression, mental confusion, anorexia neonatorum, and delirium tremens.

ANPO Alpha-naphthyl-phenyl-oxazole (scintillator).

A-NPP Absorbed normal pooled plasma.

ANR Autonomic reflex.

ANRC American National Red Cross.

ANRL Antihypertensive neutral renomedullary lipid(s).

ANS Academy of Natural Sciences; Acanthion; Acta Neurologica Scandinavica (journal); American National Standard; American Neurotology/ Nuclear/ Nutrition Society; 8-Anilino-l-naphthalene sulfonic acid - it releases thyroxine (T4) from endogenous thyroxine-binding globulin (TBG); Anterior nasal spine; Antineutrophilic serum; Antirat neutrophil serum; Aqueous nasal spray; Army Nursing Service; Arterionephrosclerosis; Associate in Nursing Science; Autonomic nervous system.

Ans Anserine.

ans answer.

ANSC Adult neural stem cell; American National Standards Committee.

ANSCII American National Standard Code for Information Interchange.

ANSI American National Standards Institute (formerly ASI; USASI).

ANSS American Nature Study Society.

ANSU Aphthous non-specific ulcer.

ANSWER Algorithm for non-synchronized waveform error reduction.

ANT Acoustic noise test; Adenine nucleotide translocator (in dialated cardiomyopathy); 2-Amino-5-nitro-thiazol (Enheptin); Anterior (see ant); Antidote; Antineoplastic therapy; Attenuated neuromuscular transmission (as in DMD - Duchenne's muscular dystrophy) (see DNT).

Ant Antenna; Anterior (see ant); Antimycin.

ant Anterior (= ANT; Ant) (front of/ front of body).

ant- prefix meaning against (Gr. anti).

AntA Antimycin A.

Antag Antagonist(ic).

Antagonist (= Antag) A ligand which prevents the effects of an agonist (e.g. cimetidine is an antagonist of the action of histamine at one subtype of histamine receptors - H2) (see Agonist; Ligand).

Ant. ax. line Anterior axillary line.

Ant. cib Before meals (L. ante cibum).

ante- (L.) prefix meaning before.

Anthrop Anthropology.

Anthropom Anthropometry.

anti- (Gr.) prefix meaning against or opposed to.

ANTI A:AGT Anti blood group A antiglobulin test.

Antibioto 1600 Aminosidin sulfate (= Amminosidin sulfate; Crestomycin sulfate; FI 5853). The sulfate of an antimicrobial substance produced by the growth of Streptomyces chrestomyceticus. Has been shown to be chemically and physically identical with paromomycin (produced by growth of Streptomyces rimosus forma paromomycinus). Used in the treatment of intestinal and hepatic amebiasis, lambliasis, and acute bacillary dysentery.

Antibodies anti-B core: positive sign for acute hepatitis; anti-Kell: red cell antibody; anti-Kidd; anti-Lutheran; antimicrosomal antithyroid: found in Sjogren's syndrome; antimitochondrial; antismooth muscle: found in sera of patients with chronic active hepatitis.

Anti bx Antibiotic.

anti DNP Antidesoxyribonucleoprotein.

anti GBM Antiglomerular basement membrane.

anti HBc Hepatitis B core antibody.

anti HBe Antibody to Hepatitis B early antigen.

anti HBs Hepatitis B surface antibody.

anti-I Cold autoantibody.

anti NP Antinucleoprotein.

anti-PNM Ab Antiperipheral nerve myelin antibody.

Antiq Antiquity.

Ant. jentac Before breakfast (L. ante jentaculum).

Ant. pit Anterior lobe of pituitary.

ANTR Apparent net transfer rate.

antr- Prefix meaning cavern (Gr. antron).

Ant. sag D Anterior sagittal diameter.

Ant. sup Anterior superior.

Ant. sup spine Anterior superior (iliac) spine/ spine (of ilium) (= ASS).

ANTU Alpha-naphthyl-thiourea (rat poison/ rodenticide).

ANuA Antinuclear antibody.

ANUG Acute necrotizing ulcerative gingivitis.

ANV Antineuritic vitamin (= Thiamine HCl) (see Vitamins - B1); Avian nephritis virus.

ANW Above-normal weight (Obs./ Pediatrics).

Anx Anxiety/ious.

ANYAS Annals of the New York Academy of Sciences (journal).

ANZAC Australian and New Zealand Army Corps.

ANZCP Australian and New Zealand College of Psychiatrists.

ANZJOG Australian and New Zealand Journal of Obstetrics and Gynecology.

ANZJP Australian and New Zealand Journal of Psychiatry (ANZCP).

ANZJS Australian and New Zealand Journal of Surgery (RACS).

ANZSNM Australian and New Zealand Society of Nuclear Medicine.

AO Abdominal aorta; Achievement orientation; Acid output; Acridine orange (test); American Optical (Company/ Corporation); Angle Orthodontist (AOREF journal); Ankle orthosis; Annals of Ophthalmology (ASCO journal); Anodal/ Aortic opening; Anterior oblique; Aorta (see Ao); Applied Optics (journal); Archives of Ophthalmology/ Otolaryngology (journal); Association of Osteosynthesis; Atomic orbital (countour); Atrioventricular opening (i.e of the AV valves); Auriculoventricular-valve opening; Average optical (density); Axio-occlusal; Plate or screw (orthopedics).

Ao Aorta (= AO); Aortic root.

a/o account of.

A&O; A/O Alert and oriented.

A&O x 3 Awake and oriented to person, place, and time.

A&O x 4 Awake and oriented to person, place, time, and date.

AOA Administration on Aging; Alpha Omega Alpha; American Ontoanalytic/ Optometric/ Orthopedic/ Orthopsychiatric/ Osteopathic Association; Antiobesity (= AOD)/ Anti-osteoarthritic/ oxidant agent; Argentine Odontological Association; Atrophic osteoarthritis; Australian Optometrical Association.

AoA Academy of Aphasia; Administration on Aging (OHD).

AOAA Amino-oxyacetic acid.

AOAb Anti-orexin antibody (see AHAb; HR2G).

AOAC Association of Official Agricultural (now called, Analytical) Chemists.
AOAJ American Optometric Association Journal.
AOAN American Optometric Association News.
AOAO American Osteopathic Academy of Orthopedics.
AOAP As often as possible.
AOAS American Osteopathic Academy of Sclerotherapy.
AOB Accessory olfactory bulb; Adjustable orthodontic band (Dentistry); Alcohol on breath; Archives of Oral Biology (UK journal).
AOBA American Osteopathic Board of Anesthesiology (AOA).
AOBD American Osteopathic Board of Dermatology (AOA).
AOBI Adult-onset brain impairment.
AOBIM American Osteopathic Board of Internal Medicine (AOA).
AOBNP American Osteopathic Board of Neurology and Psychiatry (AOA).
AOBOG American Osteopathic Board of Obstetrics and Gynecology (AOA).
AOBOO American Osteopathic Board of Ophthalmology and Otorhinolaryngology (AOA).
AOB Path American Osteopathic Board of Pathology (AOA).
AOB Ped American Osteopathic Board of Pediatrics (AOA).
AOB Proc American Osteopathic Board of Proctology (AOA).
AOBR American Osteopathic Board of Radiology (AOA).
AOBRM American Osteopathic Board of Rehabilitation Medicine (AOA).
AOBS Acute organic brain syndrome; American Osteopathic Board of Surgery (AOA).
AOC Abridged ocular chart; Advanced ovarian cancer/ carcinoma; Agent of choice (see DOC); American Orthoptic Council; Amyloxycarbonyl; Anodal opening contraction (see AnOC); Antacid of choice; Apparent oral clearance (of a drug) (see CL/F); Area of concern.
AOCA American Osteopathic College of Anesthesiologists.
AOCD American Osteopathic College of Dermatology; Anemia of chronic disease.
AOCl Anodal opening clonus.
AOCPA American Osteopathic College of Pathologists.
AOCPR American Osteopathic College of Proctology.
AOCR American Osteopathic College of Radiology/ Rheumatology.
AOCRE American Osteopathic College of Rehabilitation.
AOCS American Oil Chemists' Society.
AOD Academy of Operative Dentistry; Academy of Oral Dynamics; Acridine-orange diagnosis (see AO technique); Accidental/ Acute overdosage/ se; Acute organ dysfunction Adult onset diabetes (see AODM); Alleged onset date; Anti-obesity drug (see AOA); Arterial occlusive disease; Assistant Officer-of-the-Day.
AODA Alcohol and other drug abuse.
AODM Adolescent offsping of diabetic mother; Adult onset diabetes mellitus (= AOD) (Type II diabetes).
AODME Academy of Osteopathic Directors of Medical Education.
AODP Alcohol and other drug problems.
AOF Anti-oncogenic factor.
AOFS Adult-onset Fanconi syndrome; American Orthopedic Foot Society.
AOG Angle-closure glaucoma (acute g) (see CAG).
AOH Annals of Occupational Hygiene; Anti-obesity hormone (Leptin).
AOHA American Osteopathic Hospital Association.
AOI Association for Osteosynthesis Institute.
ao-il aorta-iliac.
AOIVM Angiographically ocult intracranial vascular malformation.
AOJ Atlantooccipital joint.
AOL Acro-osteolysis; Apical odontoid ligament (connecting the spine to the skull); Archives of Otolaryngology (AMA journal) (see AO).
AOM Academy of Occupational Medicine; Acute otitis media; Alternatives of manage-

ment; Ancillary obstetric maneuver(s); Ascending oblique muscle (see OIA); Azoxymethane; Master of Obstetric Art(s).

AOMA American Occupational Medical Association.

AOMP; AoMP Aortic mean pressure.

AoN All-or-none (drug effects/ response).

AoNL All-or-none law (a principle in physiology).

AOO Anodal opening odor; Atrial synchronous (competitive, fixed-rate) (pacemaker).

AOOD Acute oral overdose.

AOP Academy of Orthomolecular Psychiatry; Acetoxy pregnenolone; Adverse outcome(s) of pregnancy; Anodal opening picture; Aortic pressure.

AOPA Aircraft Owners and Pilots Association; American Orthotic and Prosthetic(s) Association.

AOPCP Methylene-adenosine diphosphate.

AOPCPOP Methylene-adenosine triphosphate (= AOPOPCP).

AOPOPCP See AOPCPOP.

AOPW; AoPW Aortic posterior wall.

AOQ Age-old question.

AOR Acute organ rejection; Adjusted odds ratio; Alvarado Orthopedic Research (instruments); Auditory oculogyric reflex.

AOREF Angle Orthodontists Research and Education Foundation.

AORGS Alvarado Orthopedic Research Guide System (a system of guides and instruments used in total knee replacement).

AORL Annals of Otology, Rhinology, and Laryngology (journal).

AORN Association of Operating Room Nurses.

AORNJ Association of Operating Room Nurses Journal.

AORT Association of Operating Room Technicians.

AORTF American Organization for Rehabilitation through Training (ORT) Federation.

Aort regurg Aortic regurgitation (A. incompetence).

Aort sten Aortic stenosis.

AO-RV Aorta - right ventricle.

AOS Acro-osteolysis syndrome (see ADOD; CHS); Adams-Oliver syndrome (birth defects with incomplete formation of limbs such as deficiency of phalangeal bones and syndactylism, scaly defects with scarring alopecia - aplasia cutis/ autosomal dominant, congenital hypotrichosis); Algebraic operating system (calculator); American Ophthalmological Society; American Otological Society (see A.Ot.S); Anodal opening sound; Anterior (o)esophageal sensor.

A2-os Aortic second heart sound, opening snap.

AOSD Adult onset Still's disease.

AOSSM American Orthopedic Society for Sports Medicine.

AOT Accessory optic tract; Add-on therapy/ trial; Anodal opening tetanus (see AOTe); Association of Occupational Therapists (UK); Average operating time.

AOTA American Occupational Therapy Association.

AOTAN American Occupational Therapy Association Newsletter (now OT).

AOTD Acute oral toxic dose.

AOTe Anodal opening tetanus (= AOT).

AO technique Acridine orange technique (for cancer cells) (see AOD).

AO test See AO technique.

A.Ot.S American Otological Society (= AOS).

AOU American Ornithologist's Union; Apparent oxygen utilization.

AOV Analysis of variances (see ANOVA); Anti-oxidant vitamin (A, C and E); Aortic valve (see AoV).

AoV Aortic valve (= AOV).

AOW Acute opoid withdrawal.

AOWL Average obligatory water loss(es).

AP Abdominal perineal; Academy of Periodontology; Accessory pathway; Acid phoshphatase (see Acid p'tase); Acinar parenchyma; Acta Paedopsychiatrica (IACPAP journal); Action potential; Active pepsin; Acupuncture (= AcP); Acute pancreatitis/ phase/ pneumonia/ proliferative; Adenomatous polyposis; Adolescent psychiatry; Agarose plate; Alkaline phosphatase (see Alk. p'tase); Alkaline/ Allergic potential; Alum precipitated (with reference to vaccines); American Patient/ Psychologist (journals); Aminopeptidase; Aminopurine; Ammonium persulfate; Ampicillin; Amyloid P-component; Anesthesia Progress (ADSA journal); Angina pectoris; Antepartum (obstetrics); Anterior pituitary (gland); Anterior/ posterior (see A/P); Anterior-posterior/ Anteroposterior (see A-P); Antidromic potential; Antipyrine; Antral peristalsis; Aortic pressure; Aorto-pulmonary; Apical pulse; Apoptosis (an orderly self-destruction of cells); Apothecary; Appendectomy; Appendicitis; Appendix; Apurinic acid; Archives of Pathology/ Pediatrics (journals); Area postrema; Arithmetic progression; Arterial pressure; Artificial pneumothorax; Aspiration pneumonia; Assessment and plans; Associated Press; Association period; Atherosclerotic plaque; Atrial pacing; Atrioventricular pathway; Attending physician; Axiopulpal; Before dinner/ meals (see ap); Before parturition (L. ante partum); Doxorubicin (Adriamycin) and cisplatin (platinum compound); Position on X-ray table.

A-P Analytic-psychological psychiatrist; Anterior-posterior (= AP); Anteroposterior (= AP).

A/P Anterior/posterior (= AP); Ascites/plasma (ratio).

Ap Apex.

ap Attachment point; Before dinner/ meals (= AP) - L. ante prandial/ium.

A&P Active and present; Anatomy and physiology; Anterior and posterior; Apothecaries and Physicians (Guild of); Assessment and plans; Auscultation and palpation/ percussion.

3-AP 3-Acetylpyridine.

A2>P2 Aortic second sound is louder than the pulmonary second sound.

A2<P2 Aortic second sound is less (loud) than the pulmonary second sound.

AP 43 Amolanone hydrochloride - has been used for local anesthesia of the lower urinary tract.

APA Acidophilic adenoma (= Eosinophilic adenoma of the pituitary, causing gigantism or acromegaly); Action potential amplitude; Active pituitary adenoma; Acute periarthritis; Acute pyogenic arthritis; Addisonian pernicious anemia; Aggressive prevention action; Aldosterone-producing adenoma; Alkaline phosphatase activity; All purpose antiseptic; Ambulatory Pediatric Association; American Pancreatic/ Patients/ Pharmaceutical/ Pharmacopoeial/ Physiotherapy/ Podiatric/try/ Polygraph/ Psychiatric/ Psychoanalytic/ Psychological/ Psychopathological/ Psychotherapy Association; Aminopenicillinacic acid; Anaplastic astrocytoma (a malignant glioma); Antipernicious anemia (factor); Antiphospholipid antibody; Antiplatelet activity/ agent/ antibody; Antiprotoplasmatic agent (an agent that damages the living substance or protoplasm of a cell); Antipruritic/ pyretic agent (see APD); Antipruritic agent; Antipsychotic action/ activity/ agent (see APD); Aplastic anemia; Ascending pharyngeal artery; Assistance Payments Administration (SRS); Atriopulmonary anastomosis; Australian Paediatric Association.

6-APA 6-Aminopenicillanic acid.

APAA American Physicians Art Association.

APAAP Alkaline phosphatase-anti-alkaline phosphatase (labeling).

APAB Antiphospholipid antibody.

APAC Anaplastic astrocytoma.

APACHE Acute Physiology, Age and Chronic Health Evaluation (severity-of-illness index); Astral Program for the Advancement of Continuing Health Education.

APAD Atherosclerotic peripheral arterial disease.

APAF Antipernicious anemia factor (= Cyanocobalamin; Extrinsic factor; LLD factor or *Lactobacillus* lactis Dorner factor; Vitamin B12).

APAJ American Podiatric/ Psychoanalytic Association Journal.

APAM Alternating pressure air mattress; Archives of Pediatrics and Adolescent Medicine.

APAN Ambulatory Pediatric Association Newsletter.

APAP Acetylparaminophenol.

APAS; APAbS Antiphospholipid antibody syndrome.

APB Abductor pollicis brevis; Active pathological bleeding (a hemostatic disorder such as BPU - Bleeding peptic ulcer or ICB, Intracranial bleeding, etc.); Antipyretic bath; Atrial/ auricular premature beat(s).

APBI Association of British Pharmaceutical Industry.

APBSCT Autologous peripheral-blood stem-cell transplant(ation).

APC Academic Progress Charts; Acetylsalicylic acid, phenacetin, caffeine (tablets); Activated protein C; Active peptic ulceration; Acute pulmonary coccidioidomycosis (Valley fever); Adenoidal-pharyngeal-conjunctival (virus); Adenomatous polyposis coli; Advanced Personal Computer; Advanced prostatic cancer/ carcinoma; Advances in Protein Chemistry (books); All-purpose capsule; Anisopoikilocytosis; Antepartum care; Antigen-presenting cell; Antiphlogistic corticoid; Aperture current; Apneustic center; Appropriate palliative care; Aspirin, phenacetin, caffeine (tablets/ mixture); Atrial/ auricular premature contraction(s); Average peak concentration (of a drug).

ApC Adenylyl phosphate cytidine.

APCA Accident Prevention Control Agency; Air Pollution Control Association; Antiparietal cell antibody.

APCB Air Pollution Control Board (APCA).

APCC; APC-C; APC&C Aspirin, phenacetin, and caffeine with codeine (= APC&C).

APCD Acquired prothrombin complex deficiency (syndrome); Adult polycystic (kidney) disease (see APCKD).

APCF Acute pharyngoconjunctival fever.

APCG Apex cardiogram; Atypical plasma cholinesterase gene.

APCKD Adult/ Adult-type polycystic kidney disease (= APCD).

APC virus Adenoidal-pharyngeal-conjunctival virus.

APD Achondroplastic dwarf (see FAP); Acid/ Active/ Acute peptic disease (see APUD); Action potential duration; Acute panic disorder (recurrent unexpected attack of acute anxiety, peaking within ten minutes, and characterized by palpitations, chest pains, sweating, chills or hot flushes, trembling, shortness of breath or choking, lightheadedness or feeling of unreality, and fear of losing control or dying) (see CFR, FFF, GAD, PD, PTSD); Acute paralytic disease; Acute paranoid disorder (a psychological condition with false beliefs of being persecuted); Acute/ Adult polycystic disease (see PKD); Afferent pupillary defect; Aggravated Parkinson's disease; Alzheimer's presenile dementia; Ambulatory peritoneal dialysis; Aminohydroxypropylidene diphosphate; Anteroposterior diameter (see A-PD); Antiparasitic/ parkinsonian/ platelet/ pyretic (= APA)/ pruritic/ psychotic drug; Antiperistaltic drug (i. Narcotics, such as diphenoxylate, loperamide, paregoric, etc. ii. Anticholinergic drugs such as atropine, dicyclomine, papaverine, etc.); Antisocial personality disorder; Association of Professors of Dermatology; Atrial premature depolarization; Autoimmune progesterone dermatitis; Automated peritoneal dialysis; Avalanche photodetector.

A-PD Antero-posterior diameter (= APD).

APD 50 per cent Action potential duration at 50% repolarization.

APD 100 per cent Action potential duration at full repolarization.

APDA American Parkinson Disease Association Inc.

APDC Ammonium pyrrolidine dithiocarisamate; Anxiety and Panic Disorder Clinic.

APDER Anterior-posterior dual energy radiography.

APDI Adult Personal Data Inventory.

APDIC Arizona Poison and Drug Information Center.

APDP Adult and Pediatric Dialysis Program (UCLA).

APDT American Practitioner and Digest of Treatment.

APE Acetone powder extract; Acute polioencephalitis; Acute psychotic episode; Acute pulmonary edema/ embolism; Adapted physical educator; Airway pressure excursion; Aminophylline, phenobarbital, ephedrine; Anesthetic-proof equipment (= MET-501; SPE); Anterior pituitary extract (see

Hormones - APH); Anthropometric examination; Antiproliferative/ Antiprolactinemic/ Antiprotease effect; Antipsychotic efficacy (of a drug); Arthroplasty of elbow (Ewald); Asthma of physical effort; Avian pneumoencephalitis.

APECED Autoimmune polyendocrinopathy-candidosis-ectodermal dystrophy.

APEX Advance purchase excursion.

APF Acidulated phosphate-fluoride; Adenoid punch forceps (Meltzer - Otolaryngology); Advance prognostic feature(s); Amaurosis partialis fugax (see STPB); American Physicians Fellowship (for the Israel Medical Association); American Psychological Foundation; Anabolism-promoting factor; Animal protein factor; Antiperinuclear factor; Aortopulmonary fenestration (see CCA); Australian Pharmaceutical Formulary; Axoplasmic flow (the continuous pulsing movement of the cytoplasm between the cell body of a neuron and the nerve cell extension or axon).

APFS Antepartum fetal surveillance (e.g. in pregnant diabetic patients).

APG Acid-precipitated globulin; Air plethysmograph(y); American Physicians Guild; Aminopropyl glass; Animal pituitary gonadotropin; Anterior pituitary gland; Antral-predominant gastritis (in DUD) - affects the neuroendocrine cells responsible for the secretion of gastrin, which in turn increases the basal and postprandial output of acid from the gastric corpus (see ASC; ASG; BAO; EAS; GAO; GAS; HAG; PPO); Apgar (score) (see APGAR); Autogenous periosteal graft.

ApG Adenylyl phosphate guanosine.

APGA American Personnel and Guidance Association.

APGAR American Pediatric Gross Assessment Record.

APGBI Association of Physicians of Great Britain and Ireland.

APGL Alkaline phosphatase activity of the granular leukocytes.

AP gland Anterior pituitary gland.

APGO Association of Professors in Gynecology and Obstetrics.

APH Acetylphenylhydrazine; Adult psychiatric hospital; Alcohol-positive history; Alternative pathway hemolysis; Aminoglycoside phosphotransferase; Antepartum hemorrhage (obstetrics); Anterior pituitary hormones (see Hormones); Association of Private Hospitals.

Aph Aphasia.

-aph (Gr.) suffix meaning touch.

APHA American Protestant Hospital Association; American Public Health Association.

APhA American Pharmaceutical Association.

APHAB Abbreviated Profile of Hearing Aid Benefit (inventory).

APHAS Automated Patient History Acquisition System.

APHB American Printing House for the Blind.

APHIS Animal and Plant Health Inspection Service (USDA).

APHP Antipseudomonas human plasma.

API Acid-pump inhibitor (see PPI); Acute pelvic/ pulmonary infection; Acute pulmonary insufficiency; Alkaline protease inhibitor; Analytical Profile Index; Ankle/ Arm/ Arterial pressure index; Artificial passive immunization; Atmospheric pressure ionization (for mass spectroscopy); Autonomy Preference Index.

APIC Association for Practitioners in Infection Control.

APID Acute pelvic inflammatory disease.

APIE Assessment, plan, implementation, and evaluation.

APIM (Fr.) Association Professionnelle Internationale dès Médecins (an international body).

APIP Additional personal injury protection.

APIVR Artificial-pacemaker-induced ventricular rhythm.

APJ Australian Paediatric Journal (APA).

APKD Adult-onset polycystic kidney disease.

APL Abductor pollicis longus; Accelerated painless labor; Acute premyelocytic leukemia; Acute promyelocytic leukemia Animal placenta lactogen; Anterior pituitary-like (substance or hormone) (see Hormones - HCG); Human chorionic gonadotropin (a commercial product); Programming language computer.

APL; aPL Antiphospholipid (see APS).

AP&L; A-P&L Anterior-posterior and lateral (views - X-ray/ chest).

APLA AIDS Project Los Angeles; Antiphospholipid antibody.

APLAb Antiphospholipid antibody (see APS).

APLH Anterior pituitary-like hormone (see Hormones - HCG).

APLM Archives of Pathology and Laboratory Medicine (now Arch. Path).

APLS Anterior pituitary-like substance (see Hormones - HCG); Antiphospholipid syndrome (see APS).

APLUB Association of Learned University Professionals of Brazil.

APM Academy of Parapsychology and Medicine; Academy of Physical/ Psychosomatic Medicine; Acid precipitable material (xerosin); Acute pain management; Acute pulmonary mycosis; Adenosine 3',5'-monophosphate (see AMP); Alternating (air) pressure mattress; Allo/ Auto plastic maneuver; Anteroposterior movement; Anterior poliomyelitis (affecting the anterior horn cells of the spinal cord) (see SPM); Antipsychotic medication/cine (such as the phenothiazines, pimozide, sertindole, etc.) (see APD); Archives of Physical Medicine; Aspartame; Association of Professors of Medicine.

APM-12 Alum-precipitated streptococcal type 12M protein.

APMA American Podiatric Medical Association.

APMB Association for Psychoanalytic Medicine Bulletin.

APME Aspartyl-phenylalanine methyl ester (a sweetening agent); Association of Plastics Manufacturers in Europe.

APMR Archives of Physical Medicine and Rehabilitation (journal); Association for Physical and Mental Rehabilitation.

APN Accessory phrenic nerve; Acetylcholine-producing neuron; Acute polyneuropathy; Aetiopathogenetic nuance(s) (see EPN); Average peak noise.

Apnea I. The transient cessation of automatic breathing, such as: Cardiac apnea - abnormal, short-term absence of breathing, as in Cheyne-Stokes respiration:

Central sleep apnea - (CSA), a condition in which a person stops breathing during sleep due to reduced output from the central nervous system; maybe associated with a brain tumor, polio, or other causes (= OSA or Obstructive sleep apnea).

Deglutition apnea - the normal absence of breathing during swallowing, due to the temporary arrest of the activity of the respiratory nerve center.

Apnea neonatorum - disturbance of the respiratory mechanism in an infant, occurring shortly after birth (see Periodic apnea of the newborn [PAN]).

Obstructive sleep apnea (OSA) - see Central sleep apnea (CSA).

Periodic apnea of the newborn - a normal condition in the full-term, newborn child, with rapid breathing followed by a brief period in which breathing stops (= Apnea neonatorum).

Primary apnea - a total lack of breathing, common after birth in the newborn baby, who may not breathe until the blood carbon dioxide reaches a certain level.

Reflex apnea - an unwilled cessation of respiration caused by irritating, harmful vapors or gases.

Secondary apnea - an abnormal condition in which breathing has stopped after apparent recovery (see Secondary asphyxia).

Traumatic apnea - arrest of respiration as a result of sudden or severe compression of the thorax and/ or upper abdomen (= Traumatic asphyxia).

II. Asphyxia (apnea - negative + Gr. sphix - pulse) - Suffocation due to severe lack of oxygen or anoxia:

Blue apnea = Asphyxia livida.

Apnea carbonica - suffocation from inhalation of coal gas, carbon monoxide, or water gas.

Apnea cyanotica = Asphyxia livida.

Fetal apnea - asphyxia in utero due to premature placental separation, causing interference with blood circulation in the fetus.

Apnea livida - asphyxia due to lack of blood

oxygen, with blue or cyanotic change in skin color (= Blue asphyxia; Asphyxia cyanotica).
Local apnea - with intermittent attacks of pallor or cyanosis of the extremities, as in Raynaud's disease.
Apnea neonatorum - imperfect breathing in newborn infants (see Apnea neonatorum; Periodic apnea of the newborn).
Apnea pallida - asphyxia with skin pallor, weak pulse, and abolition of the reflexes (= White asphyxia).
Apnea reticularis - also called Livedo annularis or Livedo racemosa, a peripheral condition characterized by a reddish-blue, netlike mottling of the skin of the extremities.
Secondary apnea - asphyxia recurring after apparent recovery from suffocation (= Secondary apnea).
Traumatic apnea - arrest of respiration as a result of trauma (see Traumatic apnea).
White apnea = Asphyxia pallida.

APNPS Sulfanitran.

APNS Asymptomatic Pulmonary Nodule Study.

APO Abductor pollicis obliquous; Acquired pendular oscillation; Acute paracetamol overdose; Acute pulmonary edema; Adriamycin, prednisone, oncovine (vincristine) (chemotherapy); Adverse pregnancy outcome (fetal death, large-for-gestational age fetus, toxemia of pregnancy, etc.) (Obstetrics); Aphoxide; Apolipoprotein; Apomorphine; Apoprotein triethylene-phosphoramide.

Apo; apo Apolipoprotein, Apomorphine, Apoprotein (= APO).

apo- (Gr.) prefix meaning away from or detached.

apoA-1 Major apoprotein of high-density lipoproteins.

apoB Apoprotein B (of low-density lipoproteins).

apoC Apolipoprotein C (see apoC-III).

apoC-III Major apoprotein of very low-density lipoproteins.

APOE Apolipoprotein E (allele) - ε2, ε3 and ε4 (present in Alzheimer's disease) (= apoE).

apoE Apolipoprotein E.

APOM Association of Occupational Medicine.

Ap. Op Applied Optics (journal).

APORF Acute postoperative renal failure.

Apoth Apothecary.

APP Acute phase protein; Allergy-provoking protein; Alternating-pressure pad; Aluminium hydroxide, papaverine hydrochloride, phenobarbitone (proprietary stomach powder/ tablets); Aluminium-polyethylene pouch (for blister packs, tablets, etc.); Alum-precipitated pyridine; American Professional Pharmacist (journal); Aminopyrazolopyrimidine; Amyloid peptide precursor; Amyloid precursor protein; Antero-posterior phlebogram/aph; Antiplatelet plasma; Antiproliferative properties/ty; Anxiety prone personality; Aphonia paranoica (loss of speech functions with no underlying physical cause, as in some forms of mental illness); Aqeous procaine penicillin; Automated physiologic profile; Avian pancreatic polypeptide; Aviation Psychology Program.

App; app Apparatus (see Appar); Apparent (see Appar); Appendectomy (see Appy); Appendix (see Append); Appetite (see Appet); Appliance (see Appl); Applicand (see Applic); Application (see Applic); Applied (see Appl); Apply (see Appl); Appointment (see Appt); Appreciate (see Apprec); Approximate(ly) (see Approx).

APPA American Professional Practice Association; American Psychopathological Association.

Appar (= App; app) Apparatus; Apparent.

Append (= App; app) Appendectomy; Appendix.

Appestab Appetite center (in the hypothalamus).

Appet (= App; app) Appetite.

APPG Aqueous procaine penicillin G.

Appl (= App; app) Appliance; Applicand (see Applic); Application (see Applic); Applied; Apply.

Applan Flattened (L. applanatus).

Applic (= App; app.) L. applicandus - Applicand (= To be applied); Application.

APPP Association of Planned Parenthood Physicians; Australian Polyp Prevention Project.

Appr; appr Appreciate (see Apprec);

Approximate(ly) (see Approx).

APPRE Alum-precipitated pyridine ragweed extract.

Apprec; apprec (= App; app; Appr) Appreciate(d).

Approx; approx (= App; app; Appr) Approximate(ly).

APPSS AutoPap Primary Screening System (see TPPT).

APPT Activated partial prothrombin time.

Appt (= App; app) Appointment.

Appx Appendix.

Appy (= App; app) Appendectomy.

APQC Air Products Quick Connect.

APR Abdominoperineal resection; Absolute proximal reabsorption; Acute phase reactant; Acute-phase reaction (as in myocardial damage/ necrosis); Allergic perennial rhinitis; All-purpose replacement (e.g. prosthesis); Amebic prevalence rate; Anatomic porous replacement (see OI/OP); Anterior pituitary reaction; Antiretroviral Pregnancy Registry; Association of Patient Representatives.

Apr April.

Ap Rad Applied Radiology.

Aprax Apraxia. Inability to perform simple, purposeful, or routine acts or movements, especially to make proper use of an object:
Akinetic apraxia - inability to carry out a quick or spontaneous movement without thinking.
Apraxia Algera = Akinesia algera (see Akinesia).
Amnestic apraxia - inability to perform a movement on command due to the inability to remember the command itself.
Cortical apraxia = Motor apraxia.
Ideational apraxia - Failure to understand the use of an object (see Sensory apraxia).
Ideokinetic apraxia - a form of apraxia in which simple movements can be executed, but not complicated ones, due to an interruption between the ideation center and the center for limb control (= Ideomotor apraxia; Limb-kinetic apraxia; Transcortical apraxia).
Ideomotor apraxia = Ideokinetic apraxia.
Innervation apraxia = Motor apraxia.
Liepmann's apraxia - inability to perform coordinated limb movements despite the fact that there is no actual paralysis.
Limb-kinetic apraxia = Ideokinetic apraxia.
Motor apraxia - inability to use an object or perform a task needing a certain arm or leg muscle (= Cortical apraxia; Innervation apraxia).
Sensory apraxia - inability to use an object properly, due to lack of perception of its proper nature and purpose (= Ideational apraxia).
Apraxia of speech - inability to speak understandably due to loss of control of the speech muscles, caused by brain damage.
Transcortical apraxia = Ideokinetic apraxia.

A&P repair; A-P repair Anterior and posterior/ Anterior-posterior colporrhaphy or repair (operation/ gynecology).

APRL American Prosthetic(s) Research Laboratory (US Army).

Apro Aprobarbital (see Barb).

AProL Acute promyelocytic leukemia.

APRP Acidic proline-rich protein; Acute phase reactant protein.

APRPD Antero-posterior renal pelvic diameter (increased by 4 mm or more in fetal hydronephrosis) (Obstetrics).

A.Pr.S American Proctologic Society.

APRT Adenine phosphoribosyl transferase (the adenine salvage enzyme).

APRTase Ampyrophosphoryl transferase.

APS Academy of Pharmaceutical Sciences; Acta Physiologica Scandinavica (journal); Acute painful shoulder (syndrome) (see ASB; AST); Adenosine phosphosulfate; Adolescent/ Adult parasuicide; Adult Psychiatric Service; Advance pathologic stage; Ambulatory Patient Severity (Index); American Pain/ Paraplegia/ Pediatric/ Philosophical/ Physical/ Physiological/ Proctologic/ Prostate/ Prosthodontic/ Psychiatric/ Psychological/ Psychosomatic Society; Aminopolystyrene; Anionic polysaccharide; Antepartum surveillance (see DUAV); Antiphospholipid syndrome (=APLS); Antiplasmacyte; Anxietas presenilis (a state of extreme anxiety linked with the change of life); Association of Pediatric Surgeons; Atriopulmonic sulcus; Attending physician's statement; Autoimmune polyglan-

dular syndrome; Automated patient system.
APSA American Pediatric Surgical Association.
APSAC Acylated plasminogen streptokinase activator complex (= Anistreplase).
APSD Alzheimer's presenile dementia; Aortopulmonary septal defect.
APSGN Acute poststreptococcal glomerulonephritis.
APSQ Abbreviated Parent Symptom Questionnaire.
APSS Association for the Psychophysiological Study of Sleep.
APT Acid perfusion test (Bernstein - Esophageal motility studies); Acupuncture/ Antipsychotic therapy/ treatment; Adjunctive psychotherapy (including music, occupational, physical, and recreational therapy); All-patients-treated (analysis); Alum-precipitated toxoid; Aminophenyl-thioether; Antiplatelet/ pseudomonal therapy; Archives of Physical Therapy; Atrial pacing time; Autogeneic patellar tendon (grafted in reconstruction of the Anterior cruciate ligament) (see LKP).
APTA American Physical Therapy Association.
APTD Aid to Permanently and Totally Disabled.
APTI Active-passive tetanus immunization (see CAPI).
APTIC Air Pollution Technical Information Center (EPA).
APTT Activated partial thromboplastin time (laboratory/ coagulation).
aPTT See APTT.
A-PTX Adenomectomy.
ApU Adenylyl phosphate uridine.
APUA Alliance for the Prudent Use of Antibiotics.
APUD Acid/ Active/ Acute peptic ulcer disease (= APD); Amine precursor uptake and decarboxylation (cells).
APUH Antepartum uterine hemorrhage (= AUH).
APV Abnormal posterior vector.
APVC Anomalous pulmonary venous connection.
APVR Aortic pulmonary valve replacement.
APVS Absent pulmonary valve syndrome (see SAPVS).
APW Alkaline peptone water; Asymptomatic pregnant woman/women.
APWA American Public Welfare Association.
AQ Accomplishment/ Achievement/ Aphasia quotient; Any quantity.
Aq Aqueous (= Aqu); Water (L. aqua).
Aq ad Add water (L. aquam ad).
Aq astr Frozen water (L. aqua astricta).
Aq bull Boiling water (L. aqua bulliens).
AQC Automatic quench compensation.
Aq cal Warm water (L. aqua calida).
Aq comm; Aq com Common water (= Aq com) (L. aqua communis).
Aq conct Concentrated water (L. aqua concentrata).
Aq dest Distilled water (L. aqua destillata).
Aq ferv Hot water (L. aqua fervens).
Aq fluv River water (L. aqua fluvialis).
Aq font Spring water (L. aqua fontalis).
Aq frig Cold water (L. aqua frigida).
AQL Acceptance quantity level.
AQLQ Asthma Quality of Life Questionnaire.
Aq mar Sea water (L. aqua marina).
Aq menth pip Peppermint water (L. aqua menthae piperitae).
Aq niv Snow water (L. aqua nivalis).
Aq pluv Rain water (L. aqua pluvialis).
Aq pur Pure water (L. aqua pura).
AQRS Mean vector of ventricular activation (on the electrocardiogram).
AQS Additional qualifying symptoms.
Aq tep Tepid water (L. aqua tepida).
AQTS Acquired QT syndrome (see Q-T).
Aqu Aqueous (see Aq).
AR Achievement ratio; Acta Radiologica (journal); Actinic reticuloid (syndrome); Active renin/ resistance (exercise); Adherence ratio; Admitting room; Adverse reaction; Age-corrected survival rate; Agonal rhythm (see CAR); Airway resistance; Alarm reaction (stress); Alcohol related; Aldose reductase (an enzyme); Alkali reserve; Allergen-reagin; Allergic rhinitis; Alloy restoration; Aloud rehearsal; Amplitude ratio; Analytic(al) reagent; Androgen receptor; 'Antabuse' reaction (dizziness, flushing and palpitations in response to alcohol ingestion); Anterior root; Aortic regurgitation/ root; Apical radial

(pulse); Apical rate; Applied Radiology (journal); Arcuate nucleus; Argyll Robertson (pupil); Aromatase; Arsphenamine (see Ars); Arthritis and Rheumatism (ILAR journal - see A&R); Articulare (craniometric point); Artificial/ Assisted respiration; Assisted reproduction (see ART); At rest/ risk; Atrial rate; Atrophic rhinitis (of swine); Augmented Reality; Aural rehabilitation; Australasian Radiology (RACR journal); Automated reagin; Autoradiography; Autorefractor; Autosomal recessive; Code for experimental substances (Stanlabs Inc).

Ar Argon (atomic no. 18) - see Elements; Articulare.

ar aromatic.

A/R; A-R Apical/radial (pulse).

A&R Adenoidectomy with radium; Advised and released; Arthritis and rheumatism (= AR) (ILAR journal).

5AR 5-alpha-reductase.

ARA Academy of Rehabilitative Audiometry; Acetylcholine-receptor antibody/ antigen (see SARAA); Acetylene reduction activity; Active rheumatoid arthritis; Acute respiratory ailment; Acute rheumatic/toid arthritis; ADP (Adenosine diphophate) - receptor antagonist (e.g. clopidogrel); Adrenoceptor antagonist (see β-ARA); Aluminium-related anemia; American Rheumatism/ Rheumatology Association; Angiotensin II-receptor antagonist (AT1 receptor subtype); Antirachitic activity/ agent; Antireceptor/ reticulin/ rubella antibody; Antiresorptive agent (used in the treatment of osteoporosis); Antirheumatic agent (= ARD); Aortic root angiogram; Arabinose (see Ara; ara); Arachidonic acid; Associate of the Royal Academy; Autosomal recessive agammaglobulinemia (see PIDD).

Ara; ara Arabinose (= ARA).

ARAA Acetylcholine-receptor-antibody assay (see SARAA).

ARA-A; Ara-A; ara-A Adenine arabinoside (= Ara-A; ara-A; Vidarabine).

Ara= A 9-B-D-arabinofuranosyladenine.

ARA-AC Fazarabine.

ARA-C; Ara-C Arabinosyl cytosine (= Ara-C; Cytarabine; Cytosine arabinoside) - a cytotoxic drug used in the treatment of acute leukemia.

arachn- prefix meaning spider (Gr. arachne).

ARAMIS American Rheumatism Association Medical Information System.

ARAR Acute renal allograft rejection.

ARAS Anti-rotation arm sling (Orthopedics); Ascending reticular activating system.

ARASCO Arachidonic acid - (rich) single-cell oil (dietary fat in infant formula).

ara-U Arabinosyluracil.

ARB Accrediting Review Board (NAACLS); Adrenergic receptor binder; Age-related bruising (see ARSC); Angiotensin II-receptor blockade/ker (see ARA; SARB) (such as candesartan cilexetil, irbesartan, losartan, and valsartan) (see ARA); Animal Resources Branch (NIH); Annual Review of Biochemistry (journal); Antibiotic-resistant bacteria/ium; Any reliable brand (medical orders/ prescriptions).

arb Arbitrary (unit).

ARBA Acetylcholine-receptor-binding antibody (highly specific for myasthenia gravis) (see ARA; SARAA); Adrenergic-receptor-blocking agent (β 1-selective, Cardioselective, etc.).

ARBD Alcohol-related birth defect(s); Aluminium-related bone disease.

ARBOR Arthropod-borne (virus) (= Arbovirus).

Arbovirus See ARBOR.

ARBOW Artificial rupture of bag of water.

Arb u Arbitrary unit.

ARC Absorption rate constant (of a drug taken up by the body in a set amount of time); Accelerating rate calorimetry; Accessory root canal (a side-branch of the pulp canal in a tooth); Active renin concentration; Adjuvant radiotherapy and chemotherapy (for neoplastic disease) (= RCC); Age-related cataract (see REACT)/ change; Agriculture Research Center (USDA)/ Council (UK); AIDS-related complex/ condition (see AIDS); Alcohol-related crime; Amberlite resin column (used in determining iron-binding capacity); American Red Cross; Ames research Center (NASA); Anomalous retinal correspondence; Anorectal cancer/ carcinoma; Antigen reactive cell; Appalachian

Regional Commission; Arcuate; Arthritis and Rheumatism Council (UK); Arthritis Rehabilitation Center; Assessment Referral Committee; Association of Rehabilitation Centers; Association for Retarded Children/ Citizens; Asthma Research Council (UK); Atherosclerosis Risk in Communities (project - WHO); Average response computer; Check for open airway; Respiration and blood circulation (see CPR).

ARCA Acquired red cell aplasia; American Rehabilitation Counseling Assocation.

ARCBS Americal Red Cross Blood Services.

Arch Archives.

arch- prefix meaning beginning or origin (Gr. arche).

Arch Intern Med Archives of Internal Medicine (see AIM).

Arch Path Archives of Pathology (see APLM).

Archaeol Archaeology/Archeology.

Archit Architecture.

ARCI Addiction Research Center Inventory.

ARC-NMs AIDS-related complex - Neurological manifestations (cerebral toxoplasmosis, cryptococcal meningitis, cytomegalovirus or CMV retinitis, dementia, primary and metastatic brain lymphoma, progressive multi-focal leucoencephalopathy, etc.) (see AIDS).

Arco Arcology.

ARCR Arthritis and Rheumatism Council for Research (UK).

ARCS Achievement Rewards for College Scientists (Foundation); Associate/ Association of the Royal College of Science.

ARCSE Associate of the Royal College of Surgeons of England.

ARD Absolute reaction of degeneration; Acid-reducing drug; Acid reflux disease (see GERD); Acid-related disease/ disorder/ dyspepsia (e.g. DUD; GERD; GUD; PUD; etc.); Active/Acute/ Advanced renal disease/ disorder/ dysfunction (e.g. acidosis, anuria, elevated serum creatinine, etc.); Acute radiation disease; Acute/ Adult/ Allergic/ Atopic respiratory disease; Advanced renal disease (= AKD); Age-related damage (e.g. of mitochondria, etc.)/ difference/ disease/ disorder; Annals of the Rheumatic Diseases (ILAR journal, UK); Anorectal disease/ disorder/ dressing; Antibiotic/ Antimicrobial removal device; Antirheumatic drug (see ARA); Arthritis-related disease (e.g. scleroderma); Aphakic retinal detachment; Arthritis and rheumatic diseases; Autosomal recessive deficiency/ disorder (as in Gaucher's disease) (see ART; HLE).

ARDC Air Research and Development Command.

ARDL Adelberg Research and Development Laboratories.

ARDS Acute/ Adult respiratory distress syndrome (also called Congestive atelectasis; Pump, Shock, or Wet lung).

ARDSN Acute Respiratory Distress Syndrome Network (NIH).

ARE Acute radiation episode; Acute rejection episode (following organ transplant); Active-resistive exercises; Adverse renal effect (of drugs); Age-related effect; AIDS-related encephalitis; Annual rectal examination; Annual Review of Entomology (books); Antigen-receptor episome; Aqueous ragweed extract.

AREDS Age-related Eye Disease Study (NEI) (see AMD).

AREDYLD Acrorenal (field defect), ectodermal dysplasia, lipoatrophic diabetes (syndrome).

ARES Antireticulo-endothelial serum.

ARF Abnormal renal function; Acute renal/ respiratory failure; Acute rheumatic fever; Addiction Research Foundation (Canada); American Rehabilitation Foundation; Annual retention fee (GMC; UK); Antibiotic-resistant fever (= ARP); Area resource file; Arthritis and Rheumatism Foundation; Associated risk factor.

ARFC Active rosette-forming T-cell(s); Autologous rosette-forming cell(s).

ARFPD Autosomal recessive familial Parkinson's disease (see parkin gene).

ARG Annual Review of Genetics (books); Antigen-receptor gene; Autosomal recessive gene.

Arg Arginine; Autoradiography; Silver (atomic no. 47) (L. argentum) (see Elements -

Silver).

arg silver (see Arg).

ARH Appalachian Regional Hospitals.

ARHP American Hospital in Poland; Association of Reproductive Health Professionals.

ARI Acid regular insulin (see Insulin); Acute renal/ respiratory illness/ infection/ inflammation/ insufficiency; Aderoside reuptake inhibitor (e.g. Dipyridamole); Advanced renal insufficiency (see ESRD); Airway reactivity index; Aldose reductase inhibitor; Anxiety reaction, intense; Artificial retina(l) implant (in the subretinal space); Autosomal recessive inheritance (non-dominant inheritance) (see ASI).

ARIA Automated radioimmunoassay.

ARIC Atherosclerosis Risk in Communities (study); Associate/tion of the Royal Institute of Chemistry.

ARID Autosomal recessive immunodeficiency (see SCID).

ARIDD Autosomal recessive immunodeficiency disease/ disorder (see SCID).

AR/IR Active/inactive renin (ratio).

ARISE Appointment Registration Information System and Evaluation.

ARIT American Registry of Inhalation Therapists.

Ar Kr Argon-krypton (laser).

ARL Acute regional lymphadenitis; Applied Research Laboratories; Average remaining lifetime.

ARLD Alcohol-related liver disease.

ARLL American Right to Life League.

ARM Active range of movement (of a joint); Adregernic receptor material; Aerosol rebreathing method; American reimplantation Mission (to China); Anorectal manometry; Antibiotic-resistant microbe; Anxiety reaction, mild; Appropriate rescue medication; Armenian (hamster); Artificial rupture of the membranes; Atomic resolution microscopy.

ARMA American Records and Management Association; Autoregressive moving average.

ArMA Arizona Medical Association.

ARMC Annual Reports in Medicinal Chemistry (books).

ARMD Age-related macular degeneration; Alzheimer's related mitochondrial dysfunction.

ARMH Academy of Religion and Mental Health.

ARMS Adverse Reaction Monitoring System; Alveolar rhabdomyosarcoma; Amplification refractory mutation system.

ARMT Ames reverse mutation test (for mutagenesis).

Army disease Morphine (see PAPAVER).

ARN Acute renal/ retinal necrosis; Arcuate nucleus; Association of Rehabilitation Nurses.

ARNC Age-related nuclear cataract. ARO. Asthma-related outcome.

ARNM Applied Radiology and Nuclear Medicine (journal).

ARNMD Association for Research in Nervous and Mental Disease(s).

ARNP Acute radial nerve palsy; Advanced Registered Nurse Practitioner.

ARO After receipt of order; Antibiotic-resistant organism; Army Research Office (US); Associate/tion for Research in Ophthalmology.

AROA Autosomal recessive ocular albinism.

AROM Active range of motion; Artificial rupture of membranes.

arom aromatic.

AROS Annual Report On Stress (Hans Selye).

ARP Absolute refractory period; Activity-related pain; Acute relapse phase; Advanced research project(s); Advances in Radiological Protection (journal); Alcohol rehabilitation program; Alcohol-related problem(s) (hepatic cirrhosis, etc.); Alpha redistribution phase; American Registry of Pathologists/ Pathology; Animal Resource Program; Annual Review of Physiology (serial); Antibiotic-resistant pathogen/ plague/ problem/ pyrexia (see ARF); Appetite-regulating protein (e.g. Leptin); Argyll Robertson pupil (= AR); Assay reference plasma; Assimilation regulatory protein; At risk period; Automaticity recovery phase.

ARPA Advanced Research Projects Agency (DoD).

ARPD Autosomal recessive Parkinson's disease (see ARFPD).

ARPES Angular resolved photoelectron spectroscopy.

ARPKD Autosomal recessive polycystic kidney disease.

ARPP Annual Review of Plant Physiology (books).

ARPPRN Nadide.

ARPS Australian Radiation Protection Society.

ARPT American Registry of Physical Therapists.

ARR Acute renal rejection (posttransplant); Age-related risk; Alzheimer's Research Review (journal - ADR); Antiretroviral regimen (see PIBCT; RTI); Aortic root replacement.

Arr; arr Arrest(ed); Arrival/ve(d).

ARRC Associate/tion of the Royal Red Cross.

ARRD American Review of Respiratory Disease (Am. Thoracic S. journal).

Arrhy Arrhythmia.

ARRS American Roentgen Ray Society.

ARRT American Registered Respiratory Therapist; American Registry of Radiologic Technologists.

ARS Acid reactive substance (see TBARS); Acquiescence response scale; Acute radiation sickness; Acute relapse stage; Acyclovir-resistant (viral) strain (such as, of CMG, HHV, HIV, RSV, VZV, etc.); Adult Reye's syndrome; Agricultural Research Service (USDA); Alizarin red S; American Radium/ Rhinologic Society; Animal reproduction study; Antirabic/ies serum; Arsphenamine (see Ars); Arylsulfatase; At-risk status; Autonomously replicating sequence.

ARs Auer rods (found in patients with acute granulocytic leukemia) (see ABs).

Ars Arsphenamine (= AR; ARS).

ARSA American Reye's Syndrome Association.

ARSACS Autosomal recessive spastic ataxia of Charlevoix-Saguenay.

ARSC Age-related skin change(s) - Lowered moisture retention and oil production with dry, itchy and scaly skin, less manufacture of collagen causing thinness and more fragile skin, deterioration of the quality of elastin with crisscrossing and wrinkling, increase in broken capillaries, spider veins, age spots (lipofucsin) and bruising of the thinner skin, making them more obvious with age, and gradual breakdown of the immune system and weakening of the skin's natural protecting mechanisms with greater vulnerability to cosmetic and medical problems such as new growths; Associate of the Royal Society of Chemistry.

AR-SCID Autosomal recessive severe combined immunodeficiency (see ARID; ARIDD).

ARSM Acute respiratory system malfunction; American Review of Soviet Medicine.

ARSPH Associate of the Royal Society for the Promotion of Health (UK).

ART Absolute retention time; Accredited Record Technician; Achilles (tendon) reflex test; Acoustic reflex test/ threshold(s); Active resistance training; Adequate/ Appropriate replacement therapy; Adjuvant radiotherapy; Aggressive-radical therapy (Psychiatry); Algebraic reconstruction technique (for an image); Allogenic renal transplant; American Review of Tuberculosis; Antirejection therapy; Antireperfusion (see ERT)/ resorptive (in osteoporosis)/ retroviral therapy (see ARVT); Arterial/ery; Assisted Reproductive Technique/nology (see SART); Assisted reproductive therapy/ treatment; Automated reagin test; Automaticity recovery time; Autosomal recessive trait (see ARD)/ transmission (of disease, such as Parkinson's disease, etc.).

Art; art Arterial/ery; Article; Articulation (see Artic); Artificial (see Artif).

arter- prefix meaning artery (Gr. arteria).

Arteriosonde 1010 To measure blood pressure in the newborn.

ART gene Antirepressor transactivating gene - a regulatory gene of the AIDS virus (HIV-1) genome, that promotes viral mRNA translation.

Arth Arthritis.

Artic Articulated/tion (= Art).

artic- prefix meaning joint (L. articulus).

Artif Artificial (= art).

art insem artifial insemination.

ARTPB Acta Radiologica: Therapy, Physics,

Biology (journal).

ARTS Audio response time-shared.

Art T Art therapy.

ARU Atherosclerosis Research Unit.

ARV AIDS related virus/ retrovirus (see HTLV III); Anterior right ventricle; Antiretroviral (HIV therapy); Avian retrovirus.

ARVA Antiretroviral agent.

ARVD Antiretroviral drug (see ARVM).

ARVL Age-related vision loss (see ARMD).

ARVM Antiretroviral medication (= ARVD; ARVR; ARVT).

ARVO Association for Research in Vision and Ophthalmology.

ARVR Antiretroviral regimen (see ARVM).

ARVT Antiretroviral therapy.

ARWY; Arwy Airway.

ARXT American Registry of X-ray Technologists.

AS Abdominal Surgery (ASAS journal); Absence seizure (see PMS); Abstinence syndrome (= WS - Withdrawal syndrome); Acetylstrophanthidin; Acidified serum; Acoustic schwannoma/ stimulation; Activated/ve sleep; Active sarcoidosis; Adams-Stokes disease; Advances in Surgery (journal); Aesculapian Society (Canada); Age spot (see LF - Lipofuscin); Alport/ Angelman/ Anovulatory syndrome; Alveolar sac; American Scientist (journal); American Surgeon (SESC journal); Amyloid substance; Anal sphincter; Androsterone sulfate; Angiostatin (an anti-angiogenesis compound, such as TNP-470) (= AAGA; AGB; AGI) (see AAGT); Ankylosing spondylitis; Annals of Surgery (ASA journal); Answering service (doctors on call); Antigenic shift (of viruses); Antiserum; Antisocial; Antistreptolysin; Antral spasm; Anxiety state; Aortic sound/ stenosis; Aqueous solution/ suspension; Archives of Surgery (AMA journal); Arteriosclerosis (see ASC); Artificial sweetener; Ascendance- submission (see A-S); Ascending aorta; Aseptic meningitis; Asperger syndrome (a mild form of autism, marked by awkwardness, impaired social ability and a predilection for unappreciated soliloquies); Assisted suicide; Astigmatism (see Ast); Asymmetric; Atherosclerosis (see ASC); Atrial septectomy/ septum/ stenosis; Atropine sulfate; Audiogenic seizure; AutoSuture; Left ear (see as); Sickle cell trait.

A.S. Auto Suture: A.S curet. A.S EEA: instrument for end-to-end anastomosis, and skin and fascia stapler. A.S GIA stapler: for gastrointestinal anastomosis. A.S Surgiclip: for vascular surgery. A.S TA 50 staple gun: originally used for thoracoabdominal surgery, but generally used for transection and resection of intestine.

As Arsenic (atomic no. 33) (see Elements - Arsenic); Astigmatism (see Ast); Asymptomatic.

as Left ear (= AS) - L. auris sinistra.

aS Absiemens.

A (s) Asplenia syndrome.

as- alternate spelling of prefix ad-.

A*s Ampere second.

A-S Anterior-superior; Ascendance-submission (= AS).

^{A}s Very small curve on impedance audiogram.

A x s Ampere per second.

AS 18908 Sulfalene (= Sulfamethopyrazine; Sulfamethoxypyrazine; Sulphalene) - a long-acting sulfonamide with a serum "half-life" of more than 48 hours.

ASA Acetylsalicylic acid (aspirin); Acetylsalicylic acid, acetophentidin, caffeine (a proprietary drug); Active systemic anaphylaxix; Acoustical Society of America; Acute severe asthma; Acute surgical abdomen; Adams-Stokes attack (= A-S attack); Addiction Services Agency; American Schizophrenic/ Stroke/ Surgical Association; American Society of Anesthesiologists; American Standards Association (now ANSI); Amino-salicylic acid; Aminosuccinic acid (= Asp or Aspartic acid); Anterior spinal artery; Antibody-to-surface antigen; Antiseborrheic agent; Antiseizure activity (see ACA); Antiserum anaphylaxis (= Serum anaphylaxis); Antistreptococcal antibody (= ADN); Argininosuccinic acid (see ASAS); Argininosuccinic acidemia (an inherited metabolic disorder); Argininosuccinic aciduria (an autosomal, recessive hypotrichosis nodosa with mental retardation, seizures, ataxia, brittle nails and recurrent vomiting); Arthroscopic acromioplasty/ assessment; Arylsulfatase-A; Aspirinsensitive asthma; Associate of the Society of Actuaries; Association for the Study of Abortion; Auditory system assessment; Australian Society of Anaesthetists; Autism Society of America.

ASA I Healthy patient with localized pathological process.

ASA II A patient with mild to moderate systemic disease.

ASA III A patient with severe systemic disease limiting activity, but not incapacitating.

ASA IV A patient with incapacitating systemic disease.

ASA V Moribund patient not expected to live.

ASAA Acquired severe aplastic anemia; American Sleep Apnea Association.

ASAAD American Society for Analgesia and Anesthesia in Dentistry; American Society for the Advancement of Anesthesia in Dentistry.

ASAC Acidified serum-acidified complement.

ASACL American Society of Anesthesiologists Classification (ASA I-V)

ASAE American Society of Agricultural Engineers.

ASAGAD American Society for the Advancement of General Anesthesia in Dentistry.

ASAH Aneurysmal subarachnoid hemorrhage (= ASH); Antiobiotic sterilized aortic (valve) homograft.

ASAHP American Society of Allied Health Professions (formerly Association of Schools of Allied Health Professions).

AS/AI Aortic stenosis/ aortic insufficiency.

ASAIO American Society for Artificial Internal Organs.

ASAP Alcohol Safety Action Program; American Society for Adolescent Psychology; Anti-oxidant Supplementation in Atherosclerosis Prevention (study); Aspirin-sensitive asthmatic patient (see ASA); As soon as possible.

ASAPN American Society for Adolescent Psychiatry Newsletter.

ASAPS American Society for Aesthetic Plastic Surgery.

ASAS American Society of Abdominal Surgeons/ Surgery; Arginosuccinate synthetase (= ASA synthetase).

ASAT Aspartate aminotransferase.

ASA triad Asthma, nasal polyps, and aspirin-induced wheezing.

A-S attack Adams-Stokes attack (see ASA).

ASB Acute subacromial bursitis (see APS); Agalsidase beta (a recombinant form of galactosidase A, produced by recombinant DNA technology, using mammalian CHO or Chinese Hamster Ovary cell culture); American Society of Bacteriologists/gy; Anencephaly and spina bifida (syndrome); Anatomic snuffbox (a small, cup-like low space at the back of the hand, near the wrist); Anesthesia standby; Antisocial behavior; Anxiety Scale for the Blind; Appropriate social behavior (absent in autism or mind-blindness) (see MBS; PDD); Archives of Sexual Behavior; Asymptomatic bacteriuria/teruria.

asb apostib (unit for light density).

ASBC American Society of Biologic(al) Chemists.

ASBD Antisocial behavior disorder (see ASPD).

ASBP American Society of Bariatric Physicians.

ASBS American Society of Breast Surgeons.

ASBV Avocado sunblotch viroid.

ASC Acetylsulphanilyl chloride; Acid-secreting cell (in the glands of the gastric corpus or body of the stomach) (see APG; GAS); Aerosol storage chamber; Adult stem cell; Allergic skin condition; Altered/ Alternate state of consciousness; Ambulatory surgical center; American Society of Cybernetics/ Cytology; American Standard Code (information exchange); American Sterilizer Co.; Anterior subcapsular cataract; Antigen-sensitive cell; Antimony sulfur colloid; Antiseptic skin cleanser; Arteriosclerosis/otic (= AS; ATS); Ascending (see Asc); Ascorbate; Ascorbic acid; Asthma symptom check-list; Atherosclerosis (see Athsc); Atypical squamous cell (on Pap cervical smear).

Asc Anterior subcapsular; Ascending (= ASC).

ASCA American Speech Correction

Association; Anabolic Steroids Control Act (1990 - US); Anti Saccharomyces cytoplasmic antibody.

ASCAD Atherosclerotic coronary artery disease.

A-scan An ultrasound procedure which records the size and shape of the eye, and is used to help determine the focusing or optical power of the intraocular lens.

ASCAo Ascending aorta.

ASCB American Society for Cell Biology.

ASCC American Society for the Control of Cancer (= ASCCG).

ASCCG See ASCC.

ASCD Arcing-spring contraceptive diaphragm (a flexible-disk, contraceptive, intrauterine device [IUD], especially used in women with cystocele, rectocele, or uterine prolapse) (see CSCD; FSCD; CDF; Contraceptives).

ASCE American Society of Childbirth Educators/ Civil Engineers.

ASCH American Society of Clinical Hypnosis/ Hypnotists.

ASCI American Society for Clinical Investigation.

ASCII American Standard Code for Information Interchange.

ASCLT American Society of Clinical Laboratory Technicians.

ASCM American Society for Chinese Medicine.

ASCMS American Society of Contemporary Medicine and Surgery.

ASCN American Society of Clinical Nutrition.

ASCO American Society of Clinical Oncology; American Society of/ for Contemporary Ophthalmology; Association of Schools and Colleges of Optometry.

ASCP American Society of Clinical Pathologists/Consultant Pharmacists.

ASCPC American Society of Clinical Pharmacology and Chemotherapy.

ASCPT American Society for Clinical Pharmacology and Therapeutics.

ASCR American Society of Chiropodical Roentgenology.

Ascr Ascribed to (L. ascriptum).

ASCRS American Society of Colon and Rectal Surgeons.

ASCS Agricultural Stabilization and Conservation Service (USDA).

ASCT Allogeneic/ Autologous stem cell transplantation.

ASCUS Atypical squamous cells of undetermined significance (Pap smear).

ASCVD Arterio/ Atherosclerotic cardiovascular/ cerebrovascular disease.

ASD Acute schizophrenic/niform/ stress disorder; Acute skin/ stress disease/ disorder; Adolescent/ Adult Spectrum (of HIV) Disease (project); Advanced stage disease; Albers-Schonberg disease (with an overall increase in bone density caused by faulty bone resorption, resulting from a lack of osteoclasts. Also known as Osteopetrosis, Osteosclerosis fragilis, and Marble or Ivory bones); Aldosterone secretion defect; Alzheimer senile dementia; American Surgical Dealer (journal); Antisecretory/ Appetite suppressant/essing drug; Antiseizure drug (see AE - Anti-epileptic; AED); Antiseptic drug/ dressing; Antisiphon device; Application site disorder (e.g. cellulitis, contact dermatitis, injection site reaction, etc.); Arthroscopic debridement/ decompression (of the rotator cuff in shoulder surgery)/ diagnosis; Atherosclerotic disease; Arthritis syphilitica deformans; Arthroscopic subacromial decompression; Atrial septal defect; Atypical somatoform disorder; Autism/ Autistic spectrum disorder; Autosomal defect/ disease/ disorder (see ASI).

ASD2 Atrial septal defect - secundum type.

ASDA American Sleep Disorders Association; American Stundent Dental Association.

ASDAN American Student Dental Association Newsletter (ADA journal).

ASDC American Society of Dentistry for Children; Anxiety and Stress Disorders Clinic (Ohio State University, US); Association of Sleep Disorders Centers; Autosomal dominant condition.

ASDH Acute subdural hematoma.

ASDI Automatic selective dissemination of information.

ASDR Age-standardized death rate; American Society of Dental Radiographers.

ASDS American Society for Dermatologic

Surgery.

ASE Acute septic endocarditis; Acute stress erosion/ event; Adverse side effect; American Society for Electrotherapy; Arthroscopic evaluation/ examination; Autologous (normal) skin extracts; Axilla, shoulder, elbow (bandage).

ASEB American Society for Experimental Biology.

ASEE American Society for Engineering Education.

ASEEGT American Society of Electroencephalographic Technologists (= ASET).

ASEP American Society for Experimental Pathology.

ASET American Society for Extracorporal Technology; American Society of Electroencephalographic Technologists (see ASEEGT).

ASF Abnormal sexual function; Added safety factor; African swine fever; Aniline, sulfur, formaldehyde - a synthetic resin compound (microscopy); Anterior spinal fusion (Orthopedics).

ASFR Age-specific fertility rate.

ASFT Ammonium sulfate flocculation test (see LFT iv).

ASG Acid-secreting gland (in the stomach corpus) (see APG; GAS); Acute simple glaucoma; Advanced cell group; American Society for/ of Genetics; Anatomical Society of Germany; Anterior segment of globe (eye); Antiseptic gauze; Army Surgeon General.

ASGB See ASGBI.

ASGBI Anatomical Society/ Association of Surgeons of Great Britain and Ireland (= ASGB).

ASGDJ American Society for Geriatric Dentistry Journal.

ASGE American Society for Gastrointestinal Endoscopy.

AS/GP Antiserum, guinea pig.

ASGTP American Society for Group Therapy and Psychodrama.

ASH Action on Smoking and Health (society/ journal); Adrenal stimulating hormone (see ACTH); Adrenal stress hormone (= Cortisol; HSH); Adrenoglomerulotropin; Aldosterone-stimulating hormone; Alkylosing spinal hyperostosis; American Society for/ of Hematology/ Hypertension; Aneurysmal subarachnoid hemorrhage (see ASAH); Antistreptococcal hyaluronidase; Asymmetrical septal hypertrophy.

AsH Hypermetropic astigmatism.

A&Sh Arm and shoulder.

ASHA American School Health Association; American Social Health Association (VD); American Speech and Hearing Association; Antistreptohyaluronidase.

ASHBM Associate Scottish Hospital Bureau of Management.

ASHCSP American Society for Hospital Central Service Personnel.

ASHCVD Atherosclerotic hypertensive cardiovascular disease.

ASHD Arteriosclerotic/ Atrioseptal heart disease.

ASHE American Society for Hospital Engineers (A Hosp. A).

ASHET American Society for Health Manpower Education and Training.

ASHG American Society for Human Genetics.

ASHI Association for the Study of Human Infertility.

ASHN Acute sclerosing hyaline necrosis.

ASHNS American Society for Head and Neck Surgery.

AS/Ho Antiserum, horse.

ASHP American Society for Hospital Planning/ of Hospital Pharmacists.

ASHPA American Society for Hospital Personnel Administration.

ASHPRD American Society for Hospital Public Relations Directors.

ASHRAE American Society of Heating, Refrigerating and Air-conditioning Engineers.

ASHSP American Society of Health-System Pharmacists.

ASHT American Society of Hand Therapists.

ASH (test) Antistreptococcal hyaluronidase (test).

ASI Active specific immunotherapy (see ASIT); Addiction severity index; American Statistical Index; Animal-source insulin; Anxiety staus inventory; Arthroscopic screw installation; Autosomal inheritance (= ADI; ARI).

ASIA American Spinal Injury Association.

ASIF Association for the Study of Internal Fixation.

ASII American Science/ Society Information Institute.

ASIM American Society of Internal Medicine.

ASIS American Society for Information Sciences; Anterior superior iliac spine.

ASIT Active specific immunotherapy (= ASI).

ASK Abnormally scanning key (SMAC); Antiseptic-keratolytic (see ABK); Antistreptokinase.

ASL Active/ Adult sex life; Acute spleno medullary/ myelogenous leukemia (see ASML); American sign language; Antistreptolysin (titer); Argininosuccinate lyase; Atherosclerotic lesion; Atmospheric Sciences Laboratory (US Army).

ASLHA American Speech, Language, and Hearing Association (see ASHA).

ASLIB Association of Special Libraries and Information Bureaux.

ASLM American Society of Law and Medicine.

ASLMS American Society for Lasers in Medicine and Surgery.

ASLO Antistreptolysin-O (titer) (= ASL-O; ASO; ASOT; AST; ASTO) (laboratory/ serology).

ASL-O See ASLO.

ASLT Antistreptolysin test.

ASM Additional/ Appropriate supportive measure(s) (see AST); Airway smooth muscle; American Society for Metals/ for Microbiology/ of Mammologists; Anterior scalenus muscle; Antiseizure medication.

AsM Myopic astigmatism.

ASMA Aerospace Medical Association; Alaska State Medical Association; Ames Salmonella/ microsome Mutagenesis Assay (for DNA modifying activity); Antismooth muscle antibody; Antistriated muscle antibody (present in thymoma and myasthenia gravis).

ASMBED Association of State Medical Board Executive Directors.

ASMC Arterial smooth muscle cell.

ASMD Atonic sclerotic muscle dystrophy.

ASME American Society of Mechanical Engineers; Association for the Study of Medical Education (London).

ASMI Anteroseptal myocardial infarct.

As/Mk Antiserum, monkey.

ASML Acute spleno medullary/ myelogenous leukemia (= ASL).

ASMPA Armed Services Medical Procurement Agency.

ASMR Age-standardized mortality ratio.

ASMS Acute skeletal muscle spasm.

ASMT American Society for Medical Technologists/gy.

ASN Adiponecrosis subcutanea neonatorum (also called Pseudosclerema, Subcutaneous fat necrosis); Alkali-soluble nitrogen; American Society of Nephrology; American Society for Neurochemistry; Arteriosclerotic nephritis; Asparagine (see Asn); Associate in Nursing; Average sample number.

Asn Asparagine (= ASN; Aspg; AspN; Aspn).

ASNDT American Society for Non-Destructive Testing.

ASNL American Standard National Language.

ASNS American Society for Nutritional Sciences.

ASO Aldicarb sulfoxide; Allele-specific oligonucleoside; American Society of Orthodontists; Antistreptolysin-O (see ASLO); Arteriosclerosis obliterans; Automatic step over (chromatography); Automatic stop order.

AS_2O_3 Arsenic trioxide.

ASOOA American Society of Ophthalmologic and Otolaryngological Allergy.

ASOS American Society of Oral Surgeons.

ASOT Antistreptolysin-O test/ titer (see ASLO).

ASP Abnormal spinal posture; Accidental self-poisoning; Acute suppurative parotitis; Acute symmetric polyarthritis; Additional (= SSP)/ Arthroscopic surgical procedure; African swine pox; Aged substrate plasma; Age-specific prevalence (e.g. of autoimmune diseases); Alcoholic skin preparation; Alkalistable pepsin; American Society of Parasitologists/gy; Anastomotic substitution pathway(s); Ankle systolic pressure (see

DPA; PTA); Ankylosing spondylitis; Anorectal malformation, sacral bony abnormality and presacral mass; Antisocial personality; Antiviral Substances Program (NIAID); Aortic/ Area systolic pressure; Application-site pain/ pruritis; Arteriosclerotic parkinsonism (an association of cerebral arteriosclerosis with idiopathic parkinsonism); Asparaginase (see Asp); L-Aspartic acid (see Asp); Aspirin-sensitive patient; Atherosclerotic plaque; Australian Society for Parasitology; Automatic software programmed.

Asp Asparaginase; L-Aspartic acid (= ASP).

asp aspartate; aspartic acid; aspiration.

ASPA American Society of Physician Analysts/ Podiatric Assistants.

ASPAT Antistreptoccal polysaccharide test.

ASP-AT Aspartate aminotransferase (erythrocyte) (= AST).

ASPC Antishock pelvic clamp.

ASPD American Society for/ of Preventive Dentistry; Antisocial personality disorder (= ASP; SPD).

ASPDJ American Society for Preventive Dentistry Journal.

ASPDM American Society of Psychosomatic Dentistry and Medicine.

ASPDMJ American Society of Psychosomatic Dentistry and Medicine Journal.

ASPEN American Society for Parenteral and Enteral Nutrition.

ASPET American Society for Pharmacology and Experimental Therapeutics.

ASPG Antispleen globulin.

Aspg Asparagine (see Asn).

ASPH Association of Schools of Public Health.

Asphyxia Suffocation (see Apnea II).

ASPI Audio speech perception index.

ASPIRE Advanced Surgical Planning Interactive Research Environment (a computer software program in vascular surgery at the Stanford Medical School, US).

ASPM American Society of Paramedics; Aided speech perception measure(s).

AspN; Aspn Asparagine (see Asn).

ASPO American Society for Psychoprophylaxis in Obstetrics; American Society of Preventive Oncology.

ASPP Association for Sane Psychiatric Practices.

ASPRS American Society of Plastic and Reconstructive Surgeons.

ASPS Advanced sleep phase syndrome; American Society of Plastic Surgeons (see ASPRS).

ASPVD Atherosclerotic peripheral vascular disease.

ASQ Abbreviated Symptom Questionnaire; Anxiety Scale Questionnaire.

ASQC American Society for Quality Control.

ASR Abortion Surveillance Report (USPHS); Acute synovial rupture; Additional systemic reaction(s) (e.g. to Penicillin, such as: abdominal distension, candidiasis, chest pain, chills, dysuria, edema, epistaxis, erythema, facial swelling, fatigue, flatulence, glossitis, headache, itching, malaise, mucosal bleeding, nausea, substernal pain, tightness in throat, urine retention and vomiting); Air-sea rescue; Aldosterone secretion rate; Allergic seasonal rhinitis; Allergic skin rash/ reaction; Antisocial reaction (see ASPD); Antistreptolysin reaction; Application site reaction (see LSR); Artificial silicon retina; Atrial septal resection; Authentic Science Research (NYAS).

ASRA Ames *Salmonella* reversion assay.

AS/Rab Antiserum, rabbit.

ASRC Accident Services Review Committee (of Great Britain and Ireland).

ASRM Adenosarcorhabdomyoma; American Society for Reproductive Medicine.

ASRPP American Society for Research in Psychosomatic Problems.

ASRT American Society of Radiologic Technologists.

ASS Aarskog-Scott syndrome; Acute serum sickness; Acute spinal stenosis; Adams-Stokes syndrome (see AS; HB; SAS); Adrenal stress syndrome/ system; Adult schizophrenia syndrome; Advice to stop smoking; African sleeping sickness (a parasitic disease caused by protozoal organisms, one of them *Trypanosoma* cruzi, and carried to humans by the bite of bloodsucking insects such as the reduviid bug *Panstrongylus*) (also

ASS — Apgar scoring system

	0	1	2
Heart rate	Absent	Slow (below 100 beats/min)	Over 100 beats/min
Respiratory effort	Absent	Slow or irregular	Good crying
Muscle tone	Limp	Some flexion of extremities	Active motion
Response to catheter in nostril (tested after oropharynx is clear)	No response	Grimace	Cough or sneeze
Color	Blue or pale	Body pink, extremities blue	Completely pink

called African/ Brazilian/ Cruz/ South American trypanosomiasis, Carcotrypanosis, Chagas'/ Chagas-Cruz disease, Thyroiditis parasitaria); Allergen skin sensitization; Ankylosed spinal segment; Anosigmoidoscopy; Anterior superior spine (of ilium) (see Ant sup spine); Apgar scoring system (= IEB - Infant evaluation at birth) (see table); Arthroscopic surgery; Axosomatic synapse (Obstetrics).

Ass Assessment.

ass associated (see Assoc).

ASSA Aminopterin-like syndrome sine aminopterin; American Society for the Study of Allergy; Association of Surgeons of South Africa.

Assby Assembly.

ASSC Acute splenic sequestration crisis.

ASSE American Society of Safety Engineers.

ASSH American Society for Study/ Surgery of the Hand.

ASSI Accurate Surgical and Scientific Instruments.

ASSIM Assimilate/tion.

Assn Association (see Assoc).

ASSO American Society for the Study of Orthodontics; Australasian Society for the Study of Obesity.

Assoc Associate(d)/tion (= ass; Assn; Assocd).

Assocd Associated (with) (see Assoc).

ASSOJ American Society for the Study of Orthodontics Journal.

ASSR Adult situation stress reaction.

Asst Assistant.

AST Acid suppressive therapy/ treatment; Acute supraspinatus tendinitis (see APS); Acute symptomatic therapy/ treatment (such as acetaminophen [paracetamol, "Tylenol", et al.], acetylsalicylic acid [aspirin], codeine, ergotamine, metaclopramide, etc.); Adhesive skin traction; Aggressive supportive/ symptomatic therapy; Allergy serum transfer; Anabolic/ Androgenic steroid therapy (see AAST); Angiotensin sensitivity test; Anterior spinothalamic tract; Antibiotic sensitivity/ susceptibility test; Antibody specific theory (concerning the growth of antibodies) (= CST - Clonal selection theory); Antisense therapy; Antisocial tendency; Antistreptolysin titer (see ASLO); Aphasia Screening Test (Reitan - psychological test); Appropriate supportive therapy/ treatment; Arthroscopic technique. Aspartate aminotransferase (see ASP-AT) - also known as aspartate transaminase, (formerly GOT; SGOT); Assisted reproductive therapy/ treatment; Association of Medical Technologists; Astemizole; Astigmatism (see Ast); Atlantic standard time; Atrial stimulation; Audiometry sweep test; Autoserous therapy/ treatment.

Ast Astigmatism (= AS; As; AST; Astig).

ASTA Antistaphylolysin.

ASTEC Association of Science Technology Centers; Australian Science and Technology Council.

A sten Aortic stenosis.

Asth Asthenia; Asthenopia; Asthma.

Asthenia 1. Lack or loss of strength or energy; weakness; debility; 2. Lack of dynamic force in the personality.
Asthenia gravis hypophyseogenea (AGH) - a pituitary cachexia marked by emaciation, anorexia, amenorrhea, constipation, hypothermia, hypotonia, and hypoglycemia.
Myalgic asthenia - asthenia with muscular pains and general fatigue.
Neurocirculatory asthenia (NCA) - a psychosomatic syndrome characterized by various symptoms such as breathlessness, palpitation, chest pain in the region of the precordium, giddiness, and a sense of fatigue, etc. Also called Soldier's heart, Effort syndrome, IHS or Irritable heart syndrome, DAH or Disordered action of the heart, Anxiety neurosis, Cardiac neurosis, DCS or DaCosta's syndrome, and Neurasthenia.
Periodic asthenia - periodically returning attacks of severe asthenia.
Asthenia pigmentosa = Addison's disease, with partial or complete failure of the adrenal glands.
Tropical anhidrotic asthenia - a condition caused by almost complete, generalized anhidrosis, usually in high temperature conditions, and characterized by drowsiness with headache and vertigo, inability to concentrate, anorexia, and a tendency to overfatigability and irritability, etc.
Asthenia universalis (Stiller's theory, Budapest) - Visceroptosis with associated neurasthenia, gastrointestinal atony, and vasomotor weakness.

ASTHO Association of State and Territorial Health Officers/cials.

ASTI Antispasticity index.

Astig Astigmatism (see Ast).

ASTM American Society for Testing and Materials/ of Tropical Medicine.

ASTMH American Society of Tropical Medicine and Hygiene.

ASTMS Association of Scientific, Technical, and Management/ Managerial Staffs (UK).

ASTO Antistreptolysin-O (titer) (see ASLO).

as tol as tolerated.

ASTPHLD Association of State and Territorial Public Health Laboratory Directors.

ASTPP Academy's Science and Technology Policy Program.

ASTR American Society of Therapeutic Radiologists.

Astron Astronomy.

ASTRUP pH and pCO_2 gases done on baby.

ASTS American Society of Transplant Surgeons.

ASTZ (test) Antistreptozyme (test).

ASU Acute stroke unit; Ambulatory surgical unit.

A (sulf) Arylsulfatase.

ASUTS American Society of Ultrasound Technical Specialists.

ASV Anodic stripping voltammetry (a chemical process used to detect trace metals); Antiscorbutic vitamin (= Ascorbic acid) (see Vitamins - C); Antisiphon valve; Antisnake venom; Arterio superficial venous (see A/SV); Avian sarcoma virus.

A/SV Arterio/superficial venous (= ASV).

ASVCPB American Society of Veterinary Clinical Pathologists Bulletin.

ASVD Arteriosclerotic vessel disease; Atherosclerotic vascular disease.

ASVO American Society of Veterinary Ophthalmology.

ASVPP American Society of Veterinary Physiologists and Pharmacologists.

ASW Anteroseptal wall (heart); Artificial seawater.

ASWG Accomodation Strategy Working Group (GMC, UK).

Asx Asparagine and/or aspartic acid (amino acid that gives aspartic acid after hydrolysis); Asymptomatic.

asym asymmetric(al)/ry.

ASZ American Society of Zoologists.

AT Abdominal tympany; Academic Therapy

(journal); Achard-Thiers (syndrome); Achievement test; Achilles tendon; Activity therapist/py; Adaptive thermogenesis; Adenine and thymine (see AT type); Adenine-thyronine; Adipose tissue; Adjunctive therapy; Air temperature; Allergy treatment; Alt tuberculin (German: Old Tuberculin); Aminotransferase; Anaerobic threshold; Anaphylotoxin; Angiotensin (a peptide hormone derived from the protein precursor angiotensinogen, by the sequential actions of proteolytic enzymes, including catalysis by the angiotensin-converting enzyme - ACE) (see ATG); Anterior tibia; Antithrombin; Antitrypsin; Antral transplantation; Applantation tonometry; Applied Therapeutics (journal); Art therapy; Ataxia telangiectasia (see A-T); Atlas Chemical code for experimental substances; Atmosphere; Atraumatic; Atresia, tricuspid; Atrial tachycardia; Atropine; Attenuate/ation; Axonal terminal; Old Tuberculin (German: Alt tuberculin).

AT; αT α-tocopherol (= Vitamin E).

A-T Ataxia-telangiectasia (a complex syndrome of combined immunodeficiency associated with neurologic, endocrinologic, hepatic and cutaneous abnormalities, with increased susceptibility to cancer. The defective mutant gene, ATM resides on chromosome 11q22.3 and encodes a phosphatidylinositol 3-kinase-like protein enzyme) (see HCID; OCT; PCA; RBSPD; TAGVHD).

At Acidity, total; Astatine (atomic no. 85) (see Elements); Atrial/ium.

at airtight; atom (ic).

at- alternate spelling of prefix ad-.

AT I Angiotensin I.

AT II Angiotensin II.

AT III Angiotensin III; Antithrombin III.

AT 7 Hexachlorophene.

AT 10 Dihydrotachysterol (= DHT; Dichysterol) - an analogue of vitamin D, closely related chemically to calciferol. Used in correcting the hypocalcemia of hypoparathyroidism, and in the treatment of acute, chronic, and latent forms of parathroid tetany; also in vitamin D-resistant rickets and osteomalacia.

ATA Abnormal threshold adaptation; Air Transport Association (US); Alimentary toxic aleukia; American Thyroid/ Tinnitus Association; Aminotriazole; Anterior tibial artery; Antithrombotic action/ agent; Antithymic/ Antitumor(al) activity; Antithyroglobulin/ Antithyroid/ Antitoxoplasma antibody; Antitumor agent; Associate Technical Aid; Atmosphere absolute (see At A); Atransferrinemic anemia (see ATFA); Aurintricarboxylic acid (industrial dye).

At A Atmosphere absolute (pressure unit) (= ATA).

ATAA Antitumor alkylating agent.

ATAT Antitoxoplasma antibody test.

ATB Antibiotic (see AB; Ant bx); At the time of the bomb(ing) (i.e A-bomb on Hiroshima); Atrial tachycardia with block.

ATBC Alpha-Tocopherol, Beta-Carotene (Lung Cancer Prevention Study) (NCI).

ATBCCPS Alpha-Tocopherol, Beta Carotene Cancer Prevention Study (see ATBC).

ATC Activated thymus cell; Air traffic controller; Alcoholism therapy class (es) (see ATU); Alcoholism treatment center (see ATU); Alloimmune thrombocytopenia; Antitumor compound (see ANA; CSACA); Appropriate terminal care; Autoreactive T-cell; Around the clock.

ATCase Aspartate carbamoyl-transferase.

ATCC American Type Culture Collection (cell depository).

ATCS Anterior tibial compartment syndrome.

ATD Adjusted treatment difference; Aid to the totally disabled; Allograft-transmitted disease (= ATI); Alzheimer-type dementia; Androstatrienedione; Anthropomorphic test dummy; Antithermic (see APD - Antipyretic drug)/ Antithyroid/ Antitubercular/ Antitussive drug; Antithrombin deficiency; Antithrombotic/ tumor drug; Aqueous tear deficiency; Asphyxiating thoracic dystrophy; Autoimmune thyroid disease; Autotome drill (Neurosurgery) (see OTD).

AtD Analogue-to-digital (converter).

atd angle (a,t,d) triradius angle.

ATDC Association of Thalidomide Damaged Children.

ATG — Angiotensinogen

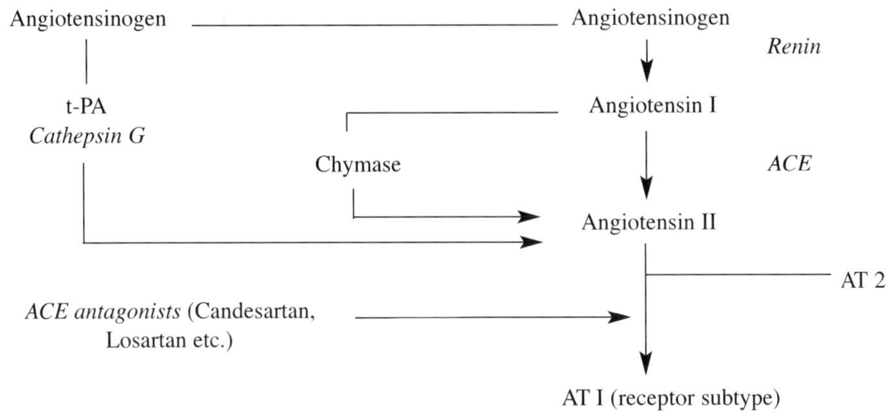

ATDT Antithyroid drug therapy/ treatment.

ATE Acute toxic encephalopathy; Adequate therapeutic effect; Adipose tissue extract; Arterial/ Athero-thromboembolism; Autologous tumor extract; Automatic test equipment.

ATEA Arterial thromboembolic accident (see ATED).

ATED Arterial thromboembolic disease (e.g. CVA, MI, etc.); Autoimmune thyroid eye disease (see AITED).

ATEE N-acetyl-1-tyrosine-ethyl ester.

ATEM Analytic transmission electron microscopy.

Aten Atenolol.

ATEP Arterial thrombo-embolic process.

ATER Arterial thromboembolic/ism risk (see ATEA; ATED).

ATF Abnormal thyroid/ tubal (obstetrics & gynecology) function; African tick fever (a relapsing fever caused by various strains of the *Borrelia* spirochete, esp. B. duttonii, and also called West African relapsing fever as well as Famine, Recurrent, Spirillum or Tick fever); Alcohol, Tobacco, and Firearms (Bureau of); Aminotransferase; Ascites tumor fluid; Asthma Task Force; Axis traction forceps (deWeese).

ATFA Atransferrinemic anemia (= ATA).

At fib Atrial fibrillation (see Atr fib).

AT III FUN Antithrombin III functional.

ATG Active treatment group; Adenine-thymidine-guanine (antihuman) thymocyte globulin; Angiotensinogen (see Scheme); Antithrombocyte globulin; Antithymocyte globulin; Antithyroglobulin (see AAB); Aspirin-treated group.

ATGAM Antithymocyte gamma-globulin.

ATGC Adenosine, Thymine, Guanine and Cytosine (chemical aminoacid building blocks, arranged in three-letter 'words' along the length of the DNA molecule) (see AT/GC).

AT/GC Adenine-thymine/guanine-cytosine (ratio).

ATH Acetyl-tyrosine hydrazide; Allergic-type hypersensitivity (reaction).

ATh Associate in Therapy.

ATHC Allotetra-hydrocortisol.

ATHR Angina threshold heart rate.

Athsc Atherosclerosis (see ASC).

ATI Abdominal trauma index; Active/Antitetanus immunization; Acute traumatic injury; Allograft-transmitted infection (see ATD); Alpha-trypsin inhibitor; American Tobacco Institute; Attitude(s) toward integration.

ATL Achilles tendon lengthening; Adult T-cell

leukemia; Aminotransferase level; Anterior tricuspid leaflet; Antitension line; Atypical lymphocyte (see AtL).

AtL Atypical lymphocyte (= ATL).

ATLA Adult T-cell leukemia (virus-associated) antigen; Association of Trial Lawyers of America.

ATLAS An electronic digital computer.

ATLL Adult T-cell leukemia/ lymphoma.

ATLS Acute tumor lysis syndrome; Advanced Trauma Life Support (Program).

ATLV Adult T-cell leukemia virus.

ATM Abnormal tumor myelin; Acute transverse myelitis/ myelopathy; Ataxia telangictasia mutation (a mutant protein); Atmosphere/ric (see atmos); Automatic teller machine (bank).

atm atmosphere/ric (see atmos); Standard atmosphere.

ATMA Advanced Technology Management Association; Antithyroid (plasma) membrane antibody.

At ma Atrial milliamp.

atmos atmosphere/ric (= ATM; atm).

ATMP Annals of Tropical Medicine and Parasitology.

ATN Acute tubular necrosis; Anterior tibial node (leg lymph-node); Augmented transition network.

ATNC Atraumatic normocephalic.

aTNM Autopsy staging of cancer.

at no atomic number (see Z).

ATNR Asymmetrical tonic neck reflex.

ATO Affected target organ.

ATP Abnormal tear production; Active treatment period; Acute toxic phenomena/menon; Addiction treatment program; Adenosine triphosphate (= Adenosine 5'-triphosphate; Adenylpyrophosphoric acid; Triphosadenine) - a nucleotide constituent of animal cells concerned with the storage and release of energy; Adult Treatment Panel (see NCEP-ATP); Alphagenic training progression; Altered taste perception; Ambient temperature and pressure; Ampullary tubal pregnancy (ectopic); Antithyroid peroxidase (see AAB); Atlas of Tumor Pathology (ARP); Authorization to purchase; Autoimmune Thrombocytopenic purpura; Autologous Transfusion Program; Autotopagnosia (the inability to recognize or locate the various parts of the body because of organic brain damage. Also called BIA or Body-image agnosia; BSD or Body-scheme disorder).

A-TP Adsorbed test plasma.

AT-P Antitrypsin-Pittsburgh.

AtP Attending physician.

AT-PAS Aldehyde-thionine-periodic acid Schiff (test).

ATPase Adenine triphosphatase.

ATPD Ambient temperature and pressure, dry (see PFT).

ATPM Association of Teachers of Preventive Medicine.

ATP-2Na Adenosine triphosphate disodium.

ATPS Ambient temperature and pressure, saturated (with water vapour) (see PFT).

ATR Achilles tendon reflex; Adverse tissue reaction/ response; Allergic/ Anaphylactic/ Anaphylactoid-type reaction (including chest tightness, dyspnoea, faintness, fever, flushing, nausea, pruritus, rash, [hypotensive] shock, sweating, tachycardia, urticaria, etc.); Antibacterial/ Appropriate therapeutic regimen (see AATR); Attenuated total reflection; Audio-tape replay.

atr atrial; atrophy.

AT1RA Angiotensin I receptor antagonist (Candesartan, Losartan, etc.) (see ACEA).

AT2RA Angiotensin II receptor antagonist (see ACEA).

AT1RB AT1 or Angiotensin II receptor blocker (see ARA, ARB).

Atr fib Atrial fibrillation (= At fib).

ATRO; Atrop Atropine.

ATS Achard-Thiers syndrome; Acid test solution; Active/ Anionic tubular secretion (kidneys); Acute toxicity studies/dy; Alpha-D-tocopherol acid succinate; American Temperance/ Therapeutic/ Thermographic/ Thoracic/ Trauma/ Trudeau Society; Ankylosed thoracic spine (as in Rheumatoid spondylitis); Annals of Thoracic Surgery (STS journal); Antirat thymocyte/ Antithymocyte serum; Antitetanic/nus serum (tetanus antitoxin); Anxiety tension state; Applications technology satellite (NASA); Arteriosclerosis (see ASC); Artificial tobacco substitutes; Atherothrombotic stroke; Automatic test system; Autotransfusion service/ system.

ATS-6 Applications/ Applied Technology Satellite-Six.

ATSA Antitopiosomerase (II anticancer) agent.

ATSD Adult-type stable diabetes/tic (type II DM).

ATSDR Agency for Toxic Substances and Disease Registry.

ATS-F Applications/ Applied Technology Satellite-F.

ATT African tick typhus (an infection caused by *Rickettsia* microorganisms and transmitted by ixodial ticks); Alpha-tocopherol therapy; Antithyroid/ tumor therapy; Arginine tolerance test; Aspirin tolerance time.

Att; att attend/ance/ding; attitude.

AT&T American Telephone and Telegraph Co.

atto- Symbol: A; a. Metric prefix for 10^{-18}.

Attrib Attributive(ly).

AT type Adenine and thymine type (with reference to pentosenucleic acids).

ATU Alcoholism treatment unit (= ATC).

ATV Abelson transformed virus; All-terrain vehicle; Avian tumor virus.

At vol Atomic volume (= AV).

At wt Atomic weight (= AW).

ATx Adult thymectomy.

atyp atypical.

ATZ Atazanavir (a PI anti-HIV drug - Bristol-Myers Squibb); Atypical transformation zone.

AU Absorbance/ Allergenic unit; Ad usum (L. - according to custom); Alopecia universalis (an inherited condition associated with mutation of both copies of the gene on chromosome 8, resulting in total baldness, with no body hair, eyelashes, or eye-brows); Angstrom unit (= A.) - 10^{-10} meter; Antitoxin unit (e.g. diphteria AU); Arbitrary unit; Australia (antigen); Azauridine; Both ears together (= au) (L. aures unitas); Each ear (= au) (L. auris uterque).

Au Australia (antigen) (see AU); Gold (L. aurum) - Z = 79 (see Elements - Gold).

au See AU.

^{198}Au; Au-198 Gold-198 (= Au-198) - Radioactive gold (nuclear medicine/ radioactive isotope).

AUA Acquired uterine anomaly (e.g. fibroids); American Urological Association; Anti-ulcer agent.

Au a Auberger blood group.

Au Ag Australia antigen.

Au antigen Australian hepatitis antigen.

AUB Abnormal uterine bleeding; American University of Beirut.

AUC Area under the plasma concentration time curve within a dose time interval (see AUC).

AUCC Association of Universities and Colleges of Canada.

$AuCl_3$ Gold chloride.

Auct Of authors (L. auctorium).

AUD Arthritis of unknown diagnosis.

Aud Auditory.

AUD COMP Auditory comprehension.

Audiol Audiologie/ Audiology (journal, see AJAC).

Audiometry The testing of the sense of hearing, such as:
Cortical audiometry - measures the brain's response to pure tones.
Impedence audiometry - testing the middle ear by measuring muscle responses to sound with a probe inserted in the auditory canal.
Localization audiometry - measurement of the patient's ability to locate the source of a sound.
Pure tone audiometry - determines the patient's ability to hear sound frequencies ranging usually from 125 to 8,000 hertz (Hz), in order to test if the hearing loss is caused by problems in the middle ear, the inner ear or the auditory nerve.
Speech audiometry - tests the ability to repeat certain words.

AUDRI Automated drug identification system (California Institute of Technology).

Aud-vis Audiovisual.

AUE Active unresisted exercise(s).

Auer bodies/ rods In granulocytic leukemia a few of the myeloblasts may contain one or more bodies or rods that stain red.

Aufranc Mold for cup arthroplasty.

AUFS Absorbance units full scale.

AUG Acute ulcerative gingivitis; Adenosine-uracil-guanine (a specific start codon in the mRNA molecule, which determines the point of initiation of peptide chain synthesis) (see Codon; mRNA); Adenylyl uridylyl guanosine (initiation codon).
Aug Auger/ to increase (L. augere); August.
AUGH Acute upper gastrointestinal hemorrhage.
AUGIB Acute upper gastrointestinal bleeding.
AUGID Active ulcerative gastrointestinal disease.
AUGII Acute upper gastro-intestinal illness.
AUH American University Hospital (Beirut); Antepartum uterine hemorrhage (see APUH).
Au-HAA Australia-hepatitis associated antigen.
AUI Alcohol Use Inventory.
AUL Acute undifferentiated leukemia.
AUN Acute urate nephropathy.
AUO Adequate urinary/ urine output; Amyloid of unknown origin.
AuP Australian antigen protein.
AUPHA Association of University Programs in Health/ Hospital Administration.
AUPO Association of University Professors of Ophthalmology.
AUR Acute urinary retention; Association of University Radiologists.
aur auricle/cular.
aur- prefix meaning ear (L. auris).
AURA Atacand (Candesartan cilexetil) Under Real-Life Aspects (trial).
AURE Alliance of UK Regulators on Europe.
Aur fib; Aur fibr Auricular fibrillation.
Auric Auricle/cular.
AURPO Association of University Radiation Protection Officers (UK).
AUS Acute urethral syndrome.
Ausc; aus Ausultation.
AuSH; AuSh Australian serum hepatitis (antigen).
Aust. P Austrian Pharmacopoeia (Österreichisches Arzneibuch).
Austral Australian.
Aut Autopsy.
aut autistic.
Auto Automedica (journal).
auto- prefix meaning self.
Autolet A home device to check blood sugar in diabetics.
Auto-PEEP Self-controlled positive end-expiratory pressure.
Autoplot Used in eye examination.
AUU Adenylyl uridylyl uridine.
Aux Auxillary.
aux- prefix meaning increase (Gr. auxo).
AV Acne vulgaris; Adenovirus; Adrenal virilism; Adriamycin and vincristine; Air velocity; Allergic vasculitis; Anteroventral; Anteversed/sion; Anticipatory vomiting; Antivirin; Aortic valve (see A-V); Arenavirus (a genus of viruses usually carried to humans by mouth or skin contact with the waste matter of wild rodents, causing illnesses in various geographic areas such as in Argentine [AHF or Argentine hemorrhagic fever], in Bolivia [BHF or Bolivian hemorrhagic fever], and in Liberia, Nigeria, and Sierra Leone [LF or Lassa fever]); Arteriovenous (see A-V); Artificial/ Assisted ventilation; Astrovirus; Atomic volume (see At vol); Atrioventricular (see A-V); Atrophic vaginitis; Audiovisual/ Auditory visual (aids) (see A-V); Augmented vector; Auriculoventricular (see A-V); Average (see Av; av); Aviation medicine; Avoirdupois (= avdp) (see Av; av); Avulsion.
Av; av Air velocity; Average (= AV; Avg); Avoirdupois (= AV; Avdp; avdp); Avulsion.
aV abvolt.
A-V (= AV) Aortic valve; Arteriovenous; Atrioventricular; Audiovisual/ Auditory visual (aids); Auriculoventricular; A-variant (carbohydrate).
A/V Ampere/volt; Arteriovenous.
AVA Activity vector analysis; Antiviral activity/ antibody; Antiviral agent (= AVD); Aortic valve atresia; Arbovirus arthropathy; Arteriovenous anastomosis/ angioma (e.g. of the brain - an inborn tumor); Australian Veterinary Association.
AV/AF Anteverted/anteflexed.
AVB Abnormal vaginal bleeding; Atrioventricular block (= A-V block)/ bundle (= Av b; A-V b; Bundle of His).
AVC Aberrant ventricular conduction; Academy of Veterinary Cardiology; Allantoid vaginal cream; Antiviral chemotherapy;

Association of Vitamin Chemists; Associative visual cortex; Atrioventricular canal (= A-V canal); Atrioventricular conduction (see AVCS); Automatic volume control.

AVCB Atrioventricular conduction block.

AVCS Atrioventricular conduction system.

AVD Antiviral drug (see AVA); Aortic valvular disease; Apparent volume of distribution; Army Veterinary Department; Assisted vaginal delivery; Atrioventricular dissociation.

AVDA American Venereal Disease Association; Arterial vasodilator activity.

$AVDO_2$ Arteriovenous oxygen content/ saturation difference (= $[A\text{-}V]O_2$).

AVDP Asparaginase, vincristine, daunorubicin, and prednisone; Average diastolic pressure.

Avdp; avdp Avoirdupois (see Av; av).

AVE Acute vascular emergency; Acute viral encephalitis; Adolescent vertebral epiphysitis (= Juvenile kyphosis or Scheuermann's disease); Antiviral effect; Aortic valve echocardiogram.

ave; aver average.

A-Ve Atrioventricular extrasystole.

AVENS Audiovisual Education in Neurosurgery.

AVF Acute visual failure; Anterior vaginal fornix; Antiviral factor; Apolipoprotein vulnerability factor (a specific gene on chromosome 19); Arteriovenous fistula; Augmented (V) unipolar lead (VF), on the left foot (leg) - on the electrocardiogram (Left leg vs left arm + right arm V - i.e. Arioventricular - Foot).

aVF Augmented unipolar limb lead - left leg (see AVF).

AVG Autologous vein graft.

Avg Average (see Av; av).

AVGs Ambulatory visit groups.

AVH Acute viral hepatitis; Ankylosing vertebral hyperostosis (see DISH).

AVHD Acquired valvular heart disease.

AVI Air velocity index; Arbovirus infection; Association of Veterinary Inspectors.

AVID Angiography vs. Intravascular Ultrasound-Directed (Stent Placement).

AVJ Atrioventricular junction; Australian Veterinary Journal (AVA).

AVJR Atrioventricular junction rhythm.

AVJRe Atrioventricular junctional reentrant.

AVL Augmented (V) unipolar lead (VL), on the left wrist (arm) - on the electrocardiogram (Left arm vs left leg + right arm = Atrioventricular - Left).

aVL Augmented unipolar limb lead - left arm (see AVL).

AVLINE Audiovisual On-Line (Data base) (NLM: National Library of Medicine).

AVLT Auditory-Verbal Learning Test.

AVM American Veterans Movement; Arteriovenous/ Atrioventricular malformation; Automated Ventilation Module; Aviation medicine.

AVMA Action for Victims of Medical Accidents (GMC, UK); American Veterinary Medical Association.

AVMAJ American Veterinary Medical Association Journal.

A-V Miniclinic Portable unit used to test pacemaker functions.

AVN Acute vasomotor nephropathy; Arteriovenous nicking; Atrioventricular/ Auriculoventricular nodal conduction or node (= A-VN); Avascular necrosis.

AVN; AV nicking A blood vessel abnormality seen on the retina, when a vein is pressed together by an artery crossing it (arteriovenous nicking). The vein appears "nicked" because of narrowing or spasm, as a result of Hypertension, Arteriosclerosis, and other blood vesel disorders affecting the eye.

A-VN See AVN.

AVNA Atrioventricular nodal ablation.

AVNB Atrioventricular nodal block (see AVND).

AVND Atrioventricular nodal disease; Atrioventricular node dysfunction.

AVNF Atrioventricular nodal function.

AVNFH Avascular necrosis of the femoral head.

AVNFRP Atrioventricular node functional refractory period.

AVNR Atrioventricular nodal reentry.

AVNRT AV Nodal reentry tachycardia.

AVO Atrioventricular opening.

Avo-; avo- 10^{-24}. (prefix for) Symb. A (see A: Avo-).

$(A\text{-}V)O_2$ See $AVDO_2$.

Avoc Avocation.

AVP Abnormal vasopressin; Actinomycin-vincristine-Platinol; Altered visual perception; Ambulatory venous pressure; Ankylosing vertebral hyperostosis; Antiviral properties/ty/ protein; Aortic valve prosthesis; Aqueous/ Arginine vasopressin (hormone) plasma (see Hormones); Arginine vasopressin; Arteriovenous passage time.

AVR Accelerated venticular rhythm; Advances in Virus Research (annual book); American Veterinary Review (journal); Antiviral regulator; Aortic-valve regurgitation/ replacement; Augmented (V) unipolar lead (VR), on the right arm (wrist) - on the electrocardiogram (Right arm vs left leg + left arm = Atrioventricular - right).

aVR Augmented unipolar limb lead - right arm (see AVR).

AVRI Acute viral respiratory infection.

AVRP Atrioventricular refractory period.

AVRT Atrioventricular reciprocating/ reentrant tachycardia.

AVRTI Acute viral respiratory tract illness/ infection.

AVS Acanthoma verrucosa seborrheica (= Seborrheic keratosis/ wart); Antiviral state (primed A-V state of cells); Aortic valve stenosis/ surgery; Arteriovenous shunt; Atrioventricular synchrony (physiologic or atrial pacing, with atrial or dual-chamber pacemaker - as opposed to ventricular pacing); Association for Voluntary Sterilization; Atrioventricular septum; Auditory vocal sequencing; Auriculoventriculostomy (a surgical procedure directing the cerebrospinal fluid [CSF] into the blood circulation as in the treatment of hydrocephalus; also called VAS - Ventriculo-atrial shunt or Ventriculoatriostomy); Aversive stimulus (see AVT).

AVSD Atrioventricular septal defect.

AVSL Auditory vocal sequencing with language.

AVSPI Audiovisual speech perception index.

AVSS Afebrile, vital signs stable.

AVS (test) Auditory Vocal Sequencing (test).

AVSV Aortic valve stroke volume.

A-VSV Allport-Vernon Study of Values.

AVT Acute venous thrombosis; Allen vision test; Antiviral therapy; Arginine vasotonin; Asymptomatic ventricular tachycardia; Atrioventricular/ Atypical ventricular tachycardia; Aversion therapy (a form of behavior therapy in which drugs, punishment, unpleasant or painful stimulation such as electric shock, are used to stop undesirable behavior. Also called Aversive conditioning); Aviation Medicine Technician.

AVV Antiviral vaccine; Ascending vertical vein (Obstetrics); Atrioventricular valve.

Av3V Anteroventral third ventricle.

AVZ Avascular zone.

AW Abdominal wall; Able to work; Abnormal wave; Above waist; Abrupt/ Alcohol withdrawel; Alveolar/ Anterior wall; Asthma Wellfarer (AFNSW journal); Atomic warfare; Atomic weight (see At wt).

aw airway; water activity.

A/W Able to work; Alive and well (= A & W).

A&W Alive and well.

AWA Animal Welfare Act (of 1970).

awa as well as.

AWARE Addiction Workers Alerted to Rehabilitation and Education.

A waves Atrial contraction waves.

AWBM Alveolar wall basement membrane.

AWC Arterial-wall calcification.

AWCL Antegrade Wenckebach cycle length.

AWD Aortic-wall disease.

AWDW Assault with a deadly weapon.

AWF Adrenal weight factor (a corticotropin in ACTH).

AWG American Wire Guage (same as Brown and Sharpe - see B&S).

AWI Anterior wall infarction (see AWMI); Average weekly intake (of alcohol).

AWDA Americans With Disabilities Act.

AWM Average weight maintenance.

AWMI Anterior wall myocardial infarction (= AWI).

AWMS Annals of Western Medicine and Surgery.

AWO Airway obstruction.

AWOL Absent without leave.

AWP Airway pressure; Average of the wholesale prices.

AWR Acute withdrawal reaction(s) (see

AWS).
AWRA American Water Resources Association.
AWRS Anti-whole rabbit serum.
AWRU Active wrist rotation unit.
AWS Acute withdrawal syndrome; Alcohol withdrawel syndrome.
AWTA Aniridia-Wilms' tumor association.
Awu; awu Atomic weight unit.
Ax; ax Axial; Axilla; Axillary; Axis; Axon; Coalescence of small rounded pneumoconiotic opacities (radiograph symbol).
ax- prefix meaning axis (Gr. axon).
Axa Antithrombotic activity.
AXD Axial skeletal defect.
AXF Advanced x-ray facility.
AXG Adult xanthogranuloma.
ax grad axial gradient.
AXL Axillary lymphoscintigraphy.
AXM Acetoxycyclo-hexamine (a catecholamine).
axon- prefix meaning axis (Gr. axon).
AXR Abdominal X-ray.
AXS Acute xerostoma (in head and neck cancer).
AXT Alternating exotropia.
AXV Antixerophthalmic vitamin (= Retinol) (see Vitamins - A).
AY Ayerst Laboratories code for experimental substances.
Ay Yellow (mouse).
AY 5710 Magaldrate (= Hydrated Magnesium Aluminate; Monalium Hydrate) - an antacid.
AY 64043 Propranolol hydrochloride (ICI 45,520) - a blocking agent acting on the adrenergic beta-receptors, reducing or preventing sympathetic nerve stimulation. Used in the treatment of cardiac arrhythmias, acute coronary insufficiency and angina pectoris, and also in the relief of essential hypertension.
AYA Acute yellow atrophy.
AYF Antiyeast factor.
AYP Autolysed yeast protein.
AYV Aster yellow virus
AZ Alzheimer's (disease); Automatic zero.
Az Azote (French: azote - old name for nitrogen).
A-Z Ascheim-Zondek (test for pregnancy) (= AZPT; AZT).
AZA Azathioprine.
5 AZA Azacitidine.
AzC Azacytosine.
AzG; Azg; azg Azaguanine.
A-ZH Ascheim-Zondek hormone (see Hormones - LH v).
AZJP Anatomic zero joint position (the starting point of the natural movement of a joint).
AZM Active zone material (the macromolecular scaffold massed in the cytoplasm of nerve endings); Adoral zone of membranellae (in protozoans).
AZO; azo chemical group -N=N-.
AZPT Ascheim-Zondek pregnancy test (see A-Z).
AZQ Diaziquone.
AZR Alizarin.
AZS Azoospermatism/ermia (absence or lack of spermatozoa in the semen).
AZT Ascheim-Zondek test (see A-Z); Azidothymidine (= BW A509U; Compound S; 3'-azido-3'deoxythymidine; Zidovudine - now known as) - A tentative drug used in the treatment of AIDS (Acquired immune deficiency syndrome).
AZT-TP 3'-azido-3'-deoxythymidine triphosphate.
AZU Azauracil.
AzUR See 6-AzUR.
6-AzUR Azauridine (= 6-Azauridine; NSC 32074) - A cytotoxic agent, which by inhibiting enzymic action, interferes with pyrimidine biosynthesis and retards the formation of cell nucleic acids. Has been used in the treatment of acute leukemias in adults.

B

B Asparagine and/or Aspartic acid; Bacillus; Bacterium; Balneum (L.) bath; Balsam, e.g. B. of Peru (= Peruvian b) - a resin combined with oil; Bands; Barometric; Base (of a prism - in chemical formulas); Basophil(ic) (WBC count); Bath (L. balaneum); Baumé scale (= B scale for expressing the specific gravity of fluids); Behavior; Bel; Benoist scale (= B scale for expressing the hardness of roentgen rays); Benzoate; Beta; Bhang (Marijuana - see Cannabis); Bicuspid; Bilateral; Bilis (L.) bile, e.g. B. bovina or ox-bile); Black; Blanc (Fr. - white); Blood; Blood type (B) of the ABO system; Bloody; Blue; Body (in psychology); Boils at; Bolton point; Bolus (L./Gr.) - a lump, e.g. B. alba or kaolin; Bone marrow-derived (B cell or lymphocyte); Born; Boron (Z = 5) (see Elements - Boron); Both; Bound; Bovine; Boy; Brachium (L./Gr. brachion - arm/ arm-like process or structure) (e.g. B. cerebri); Break; Bregma; Bronchial/hitis/hus; Brother; Brucella; Bruit; Buccal; Bucky (film in cassette in Potter-Bucky diaphragm); Bulb (L. bulbus/ Gr. bolbos), e.g. B. of urethra or Bulbus penis); Bulbus, e.g. B. aortae (Bulb of aorta); Bulla (= a bladder or bubble), e.g. B. fornicis (= B. of fornix; corpus mamillare; mamillary body); Bundle, e.g. B. of His (= Atrioventricular b.); Bursa cells (of thymus or lymph nodes); Bypass; Corticosterone; Gauss (unit of magnetic flux density or induction); Kelco Co. code for experimental substances; Magnetic field; Sand bath (L. balneum arenae) - see Bal ar; Supramentale (point); Vitamin B group (see Vitamins - B).

b barn; base; bis (L.) twice/ two times; boils at (°C/°F); born; computer bit; supramentale (point).

β beta - the second letter of the Greek alphabet - an anomer of a carbohydrate; buffer capacity; in chemistry referring to the carbon atom in organic compounds - a carbon atom separated from a carboxyl by one other carbon atom in aliphatic compounds; a constituent of a plasma protein fraction; a probability of Type II error; a substituent group of a steroid that projects above the plane of the ring; a symbol designating second.

B-1, B-2 craniotome attachment sizes (used with the Midas Rex drill in neurosurgery).

1-ß Power of statistical test.

B0 Constant magnetic field in nuclear magnetic resonance.

B1 Radiofrequency magnetic field in nuclear magnetic resonance; Thiamine (see Vitamins - B1).

B2 Riboflavine (see Vitamins - B2).

B3 Nicotinamide; Pantothenic acid (see Vitamins - B3).

B4 Before; Bilateral bundle branch block (BBBB).

B5 A growth factor in rats (see Vitamins - B5).

B6 Pyridoxine (see Vitamins - B6).

B7 Biotin (see Vitamins - B7).

B8 Adenosine phosphate (see Vitamins - B8).

B10 Folic acid-type compound (see Vitamins - B10).

B11 same as in B10 (see Vitamins - B11).

B12 Cyanocobalamin (see Vitamins - B12).

B14 Anti-oncogenic vitamin (see Vitamins - B14).

B15 Pangamic acid (see Vitamins - B15).

B 436 Prenylamine lactate (= B436 base; Hoechst 12512) - a coronary vasodilator, said to be of value in the prophylaxis of angina pectoris.

B 518 Cyclophosphamide (= Cyclophospham) - an alkylating agent used in the treatment of malignant diseases such as Hodgkin's disease, lymphosarcoma, multiple myeloma, etc. It has also been used as an immunosuppressive agent in prolonging the survival of homografts, as in kidney transplantation, and in severe cases of rheumatoid polyarthritis.

B 663 A Chloro-isopropyliminophenazine compound (= G 30320) - has been used experimentally in the treatment of leprosy, mycobacterial ulceration, and tuberculosis.

B 1459 Corn Sugar Gum (= Polysaccharide B 1459; Xantham Gum; NRLL B1459) - A polysaccharide gum produced from dextrose by bacterial fermentation with Xanthomonas campestris. A soft bulky powder with a yeast-like color and odor. A hydrophilic colloid, compatible with alcohols, sugars, and high concentrations of electrolytes.

BA Bachelor of Arts; Backache (see B/A); Bacterial agglutination; Balneum arenae (L.) sand bath - see Bal ar; Basilar/ Brachial artery; Basion (craniometric point); Benzyladenine; Benzyl alcohol; Best amplitude; Beta-methasone acetate; Bilateral asymmetrical; Bile/ Boric acid; Biliary atresia; Bioengineering Abstracts (EI journal); Bioavailability (= BAA); Biological Abstracts (journal); Biological activity; Blocking antibody; Blood agar (culture medium); Blood alcohol; Blue acid (LSD - 25) - see LSD; Bone age; Bourns assist; Bovine albumin; Bowel anastomosis; Brain abscess; Brain atrophy (see CA); Breathing apparatus; Bronchial asthma; Buccoaxial; Buffered acetone.

B/A Backache (= BA).

B>A Bone (conduction) greater than air (conduction) to sound.

B&A Brisk and active.

Ba Barium (Z = 56) - see Elements - Barium; Barium enema; Basion (see ba).

ba basion (= BA; Ba) - craniometric point.

ba- prefix meaning go, walk or stand (Gr. baino).

βA Beta-amyloid (see Aβ).

Ba-29837 Desferrioxamine hydrochloride (= Deferoxamine HCl; DFM HCl; DFOM HCl; Desferrioxamine B HCl) (see Ba-33112).

Ba-33112 Desferrioxamine Mesylate (= Deferoxamine Mesylate; Desferrioxamine B Mesylate; DFM Mesylate; DFOM Mesylate) - An iron chelating agent; given by injection it increases the excretion of iron; given by mouth it renders non-toxic any iron remaining in the alimentary tract.

BAA Below-ankle amputation (Syme); Benzoyl arginine amide; Beta-agonist activity; Bioavailability (see BA); Binding-antibody assay (standard assay, and specific for myasthenia gravis) (see SARAA); Blocking-antibody assay (measures the blocking of bungarotoxin-binding to the acetylcholine receptor) (see SARAA); Branched amino acid.

βAA Beta-adrenergic agonist/ antagonist; β-adrenoceptor/ adrenoreceptor agonist (see β-ARA; BARA)/ antagonist (Adrenaline, Fenoterol, Formoterol, Isoetharine, Isoprenalinc, Orciprenaline, Pirbuterol, Rimiterol, Riproterol, Terbutaline) (= SMD - Sympathomimetic drug).

BAAS British Association for the Advancement of Science.

BaaW Body as a whole.

BAB Beta-adrenergic blocker (see BABA); Blood agar base; Body (current) activated (circuit) breaker.

βAB β-adrenergic blocker.

BAb Blocking antibody.

Bab Babinski (reflex); Baboon.

BABA Beta-adrenergic blocking agent (= BAB); Beta-aminoisobutyric acid.

BABD Beta-adrenoceptor blocking drug.

BABI Blastomere analysis before implantation.

BabK Baboon kidney.

Ba bolus Barium swallow (see Ba swallow).

BABR Bile acid-binding resin (e.g. cholestryamine, colestipol).

Baby Marijuana (see Cannabis).

BAC Back-action condenser (a dental instrument for compacting filling material or amalgams); Bacterial adherent colony; Bacterial antigen complex; Benzalkonium chloride; Bioactive concentration; Biological active component; Biological applications of computers; Blood alcohol concentration; Bovine albumin crystallized; British Association of Chemists; Bronchoalveolar cells; Buccoaxiocervical.

Bac; bac Bacillus; Bacillus; Bacillary.

BACCUP Belarussian Aid for Children, Cardiff Undergraduate Programme (Wales, UK).

bacill- prefix meaning rod (L. bacillus).

$BaCl_2$ Barium chloride.

BACOD Bleomycin, Adriamycin, Cytoxan, Oncovin and Dexamethasone (Decadron) (Chemotherapy).

BACON Bleomycin, Adriamycin (doxorubicin), CCNU (lomustine), Oncovin (vincristine), and Nitrogen mustard (mechlorethamine or mustine).

BACOP Bleomycin, Adriamycin (doxorubicin), Cyclophosphamide, Oncovin (vincristine), and Prednisone.
BACS Bulletin of the American College of Surgeons.
Bact; bact Bacteria(l); Bacteriology (see Bacteriol); Bacterium; Bacterium.
bacter- prefix meaning rod (Gr. bakterion).
Bacteriol Bacteriology (= Bact).
BAD Biological aerosol detection; Bipolar affective disorder; Brachial artery diameter; British Association of Dermatologists/gy.
Baden silastic rod Fixation of finger.
Badger's triangle Area just below the medial malleolus.
BADS Biodegradable antibiotic delivery system; British Association of Dermatology and Syphilology.
BAE Bovine aortic endothelium; Bronchial artery embolization.
BaE Barium enema (X-ray/ colon) (= Ba; BaEn; Ba enem).
BAEC Bovine aortic endothelial cells.
BAEE Benzoyl arginine ethyl ester.
BaEn Barium enema (see Ba E).
Ba enem Barium enema (see Ba E).
BAEP Brainstem auditory evoked potential.
BAER Brainstem auditory evoked response.
BAEs Buerger-Allen exercises (postural exercises for peripheral vascular disease).
BAF Bacterial adherence factor.
Baffes' operation Operation on the aortic valve.
BAG Beta amyloid gene (present in Alzheimer's disease); Buccoaxiogingival.
BAGECO Bacterial Genetics and Ecology (Symposium).
BAGG Bruton's agammaglobulinemia (an inherited illness); Buffered azide glucose glycerol (broth).
Bah Baha'i member (religious faith).
Bahnson clamp Used in vascular surgery.
BAHS Butoctamide hydrogen succinate.
BAI Basilar artery insufficiency; Beta-aminoisobutyrate; Bronchial asthma of infancy (see ISB).
BAIB Beta-aminoisobutyric (acid).
BAIF Bile acid independent flow.
BAIS Basilar artery insufficiency syndrome.
BAIT Bacterial automated identification technique.
BAJ Bone-autograft junction (Orthopedics) (= ABI).
BAL Blood alcohol level; Breath alcohol level (g/dl) (see BAS); British anti-Lewisite (= Dimercaprol; 2,3-dimercaptopropanol) - a war gas; Bronchoalveolar lavage (cell, technique).
Bal Balance (journal); Balance(d) (= bal); Balsam (see Bals); Bath (L. balneum).
bal balance (see Bal).
Bala Beta-alanine.
Bal ar; Bal aren; Bal arenae Sand bath (= B; BA; Bal aren; Bal arenae) - L. balneum arenae.
BALB Binaural alternate loudness balance.
BALF Bronchoalveolar lavage fluid.
ball- prefix meaning throw (Gr. ballo).
Bal mar Salt or sea-water bath (L. balneum maris).
BALs Biologically active lipids (leukotrienes, platelet activating factor - PAF, prostaglandins, thromboxanes, etc.) - released by phospholipid hydrolysis, as a result of activation of the enzyme phospholipase A2 (PLA2), with subsequent initiation of the inflammatory process, viz. vasodilatation, increased capillary permeability, edema formation, recruitment of circulating cells and ultimately, tissue damage (see HMs; PMsI).
Bals; bals Balsam (= Bal).
Bal sin Mustard bath (L. balneum sinapis).
BALT Bronchoalveolar lavage technique; Bronchus-associated lymphoid tissue.
Bal vap Steam or vapour bath (L. balneum vaporis).
BAM Basilar artery migraine; Basophil-associated mononuclear; Bilaminar amniotic membrane (Obstetrics); Brachial artery mean (pressure); Buccal administration of medication/cine.
BaM Barium meal.
Bam Benzamide (amphetamine pill) - see Amphet.
βAM Beta-agonist medication (see βAT).
Bamboo spine Ankylosing spondylitis (see MSD).
BAME Benzoylarginine methyl ester.

BAMM British Association of Manipulative Medicine.
BAMT Benign adrenal medullary tumor.
BAN British Approved Name; British Association of Neurologists.
BANA Bridge anticoagulant neutralizing agent.
Bands Banded neutrophils (on white blood cell counts).
Bang Heroin (see Diamorph HCl).
BANS Back, arm, neck, and scalp.
BAO Bachelor of the Art of Obstetrics; Basal acid output; Basilar artery occlusion; Brachial artery output; British Association of Otolaryngologists.
BAO/MAO Basal acid output/Maximum acid output (ratio).
BAOT British Association of Occupational Therapists.
BAP Bacterial/ Bone-specific alkaline phosphatase; Behavior Activity Profile; Beta-amyloid peptide; Beta-amyloid plaque(s)/ protein (found in the brains of Alzheimer's disease patients); Blood-agar plate; Bovine albumin in phosphate buffer; Brachial artery pressure.
BaP Benzo-alpha-pyrene.
Bap Baptist.
BAPA Benzol-dl, arginine, p,nitro-analide.
BAPhysMed British Association of Physical Medicine.
BAPI Barley alkaline protease inhibitor.
BAPN Beta-aminoproprionitrile (fumarate).
BAPS Biomechanical ankle platform system; Bovine albumin phosphate saline; British Association of Paediatric/ Plastic Surgeons.
BAPT British Association of Physical Training.
BAPV Bovine alimentary papilloma virus.
BAQ Brain-age quotient.
BAQD-10 Dequalinium chloride.
BAR Balfour abdominal retractor; Bariatrics; Barometer(tric) - see Bar; Beta-adrenergic receptor; Biphasic absorption release (of drugs - in a dual-release manner).
Bar Barometer(tric) (= BAR; bar); Marijuana (see Cannabis).
bar barometric (see Bar).
bar- prefix meaning weight (Gr. baros).
β-ARA; BARA . Beta-adrenoceptor/ adrenoreceptor antagonist (Acebutolol, Atenolol, Betaxolol, Bisoprolol, Labetalol, Metoprolol, Nadolol, Oxyprenolol, Penbutolol, Pindolol, Practolol, Propranolol, Sotalol, Timolol) (= βAA).
Barb; barb Barbiturate; Barbituric. Other names are: Apro (aprobarbital); Blockbuster; Blue (numorphan or amytal); Bluebird (sodium amytal capsule); Blue heaven (amytal capsule); Bomber (barbiturate cigarette); Brain tickler (barbiturate pill); Compound 25,398 (methohexitone sodium); Courage (barbiturate pill); DEBA (Diethylbarbituric acid); Dexamyl (as in Dexie); Dexie (proprietary tablet containing 5 mg dexamphetamine sulfate and 32 mg amylobarbitone) - known also as Dexamyl or Drinamyl; Dial (allobarbital); Doll; Downer; GB or Goofball (Barbiturate pill); Gorilla (Barbiturate pill); Idiot (Barbiturate pill); King-Kong (Barbiturate or other sedative pill); Mexican red (sodium secobarbital); NB (Nitrous oxide barbiturate); Nebbie, Nemish, Nemmie, Nimby (Nembutal capsules i.e. Pentobarbitone); Wild Geronimo (barbiturate dissolved in an alcoholic drink); Yellow or Yellow jacket (nembutal capsule).
BARC Beltsville Agricultural Research Center (USDA); Bhabha Atomic Research Centre (India).
BARI Bypass Angioplasty Revascularization Intervention.
BARL Baylor Auditory Research Laboratory (Texas Medical Center).
BARN Bilateral acute retinal necrosis.
BARP British Association of Radiology and Physiotherapy.
BARR British Association of Rheumatology and Rehabilitation.
BARS Brachial artery reactivity study.
BART Blood-activated recalcification time.
BAS Balloon atrial septostomy; Basilar artery stenosis (with cerebral infarction); Basophil(s) (= Bas; Baso) white blood count; Battalion aid station; Benzyl analog(ue) of serotonin; Benzyl anti-serotonin; Beta-adrenergic stimulation; Bile-acid sequestrant (e.g. cholestyramine); Biological air sampler; Boric acid solution; Breast augmentation

surgery; Breath alcohol sensor (see BAL); British Anatomical/ Antivivisection Society; Bulletin of the Atomic Scientists (journal).

BaS Ball-and-socket (joint, e.g. the hip joint) (Orthopedics); Barium swallow.

Bas; bas Basilar; Basophil/ Basophilic/ Basophils (see BAS).

β2-AS β2-adrenergic stimulant (= β2-agonist).

BASA Beta-adrenergic stimulating agent; Bile-acid sequestering agent (see BAS); Boston Assessment of Severe Aphasia.

BASCT Benign adrenal subcapsular cell tumor.

BASE B27-arthritis-sacroiliitis-extra-articular features (syndrome).

BASH Body acceleration synchronous with heart rate.

BASHP Bulletin of the American Society of Hospital Pharmacists.

BASIC Beginner's All-Purpose Symbolic Introduction Code (a computer programming language).

BASJ Ball-and-socket joint (a spheroid joint such as the hip joint) (see MAJ).

BASK Basket (cell).

Baso; baso Basophil (see BAS).

$BaSO_4$ Barium sulfate.

BASO STIP Basophilic stippling.

Ba swallow Barium swallow or Ba bolus (see BaS) (X-ray/ esophagus).

BAT Basic aid training; Best available technology; Binet age test (the mental age of a person, especially a child, as determined by the Binet-Simon tests. The Binet or mental age corresponding to: "profoundly retarded" is 1 to 2 years of age; "severely retarded" is 3 to 7 years of age; "mildly retarded" is 8 to 12 years of age); Blunt abdominal trauma (see BAW); Brain attack team (neurology); Breast/ Brown adipose tissue; Bronchoalveolar tumor (see MFBAT); Tropine benzylate.

βAT Beta-agonist therapy (for bronchial asthma) (= βAM).

BATF Bureau of Alcohol, Tobacco, and Firearms (Treasury Dept.).

BATs Beta amyloid tangles (see BAG).

batt battery.

BAU British Association Unit.

BAUS British Association of Urological Surgeons.

BAV Bicuspid aortic valve; Bunyamwera arbovirus (one of a group of ABVs or Arthropod-borne viruses that infect humans, and are carried by mosquitoes from rodent hosts, causing California encephalitis, Rift valley fever, and other diseases).

BAVCP Bilateral abductor vocal cord paralysis.

BAVFO Bradycardia after arteriovenous fistula occlusion.

BAVMP Brain Aneurysm and Vascular Malformation Program (UCLA Medical Center).

BAVP Balloon aortic valvuloplasty.

BAW Blunt abdominal wound (= BAT); Bronchoalveolar washing.

BAX Baxter Laboratories code for experimental substances.

BAYa 1040 Nifedipine (= MW 343). A dihydropyridine derivative. A calcium antagonist and coronary dilator, used in the treatment of cardiac arrhythmias and angina pectoris.

Bayer 205 Suramin (= Fourneau 309; Germanin; Moranyl; Naganin; Naganol; Sodium Suramin; Suraminum Natricum). A naphthalene-trisulphonic acid compound, used in the treatment of early trypanosomiasis. It is ineffective in the advanced disease affecting the central nervous system as it does not penetrate the blood-barrier into the cerebrospinal fluid.

Bayer 1362 Butaperazine (= Riker 595). A phenothiazine derivative. An antipsychotic tranquillizing agent used in the treatment of chronic schizophrenia.

Bayer 2353 Niclosamide. A tenicide active against most tapeworms, including Taenia saginata (beef tapeworm), Taenia solium (pork tapeworm), Diphyllobothrium latum (fish tapeworm), and Hymenolepis nana (dwarf tapeworm).

Bayer 3231 Triaziquone. - A benzoquinone cytotoxic agent, acting on proliferating cells by alkylating the nucleic acids of the chromosomes. Used in the palliative treatment of neoplastic diseases, particularly those of lymphoid and hemopoietic tissues such as

Hodgkin's disease, lymphosarcoma, etc.

Bayer 5360 Metronidazole (= RP 8823). A trichomonacidal agent used in the oral treatment of Trichomonas vaginalis infections of the female genito-urinary tract in males and females.

Bayer 8169 Demeton (= E 1059; Systox). A mixture of Demeton-O and Demeton-S (phosphorothionate drugs). An organophosphorus insecticide.

Bayer 17147 Azinophos-methyl (= DBD; Gusathion; Guthion). An organophosphorus insecticide.

Bayer 21/199 Coumaphos (= Asuntol; Co-Ral). An organophosphorus insecticide.

Bayer 29493 Fenthion (= Baytex; Entex; S 1752; Tiguvon). An organophosphorus insecticide.

Bayer B 186 Chlophedianol hydrochloride (= Clofedanol HCl; SL 501). A centrally-acting cough suppressant with a mild local anesthetic action.

Bayer L 13/59 Trichlorphon (= Chlorophos; Dipterex; Metriphonate; Nevugon; Tugon). An organophosphorus compound used as an agricultural insecticide and a veterinary anthelmintic.

BAZ Boric acid, adrenaline solution, zinc sulfate solution (eye-drops).

BB Baby boy; Backboard; Bad breath; Battling the Breeze (Emph. Anon. (journal); Bed bath/ board; Before bed/ breakfast; Beta blockade/ blocker; BioBreeding (rat); Blanket bath; Blood bank/ buffer; Blow bottle; Blue bloaters (emphysema); Body belt/ burden (radionuclides); Both bones (regarding fractures - see bb); Bowel and bladder (see B&B); Brain/ Breast biopsy; Brain CPK isoenzyme (see CPK-1); Breakthrough bleeding; Brush border; Buffer base; Bundle branch; Bureau of Biologics (FDA); Isoenzyme of creatine kinase containing two B subunits (see CPK-1); Potassium sorbate (see BB powder).

bb Bolton point; both bones (= BB).

B/B Backward bending; Bowel and bladder (see B&B).

B&B Bowel and bladder (= BB; B/B).

Bb-12 A strain of the probiotic microbe, *Bifidobacterium*; used in treatment of infantile diarrhea (see PB - Probiotic).

BBA Bad Breath Anonymous; Behavioral Biology Abstracts (journal); Beta blocking activity/ agent; Biochimica et Biophysica Acta (journal); Born before arrival.

BBAD Biologically based anxiety disorder (see BBMI).

BBB Basic building block(s) (in peptides, genes, etc.); Better Business Bureau; Blood-borne bacteria/ium; Blood-brain barrier; Blood buffer base; Buccal Barr bodies; Bundle branch block; Component (a filixic acid c.).

BbB Breath-to-breath (minute ventilation, etc.).

BBBB Bilateral bundle branch block (see B4).

BBC Bad brain chemistry; Bowel biopsy capsule (= Carey/ Crosby capsule); Brain-body connection; Brain Bio Center; Bromobenzylcyanide (a war gas).

BBD Before bronchodilator; Benign breast disease; Benzylamino-nitro-benz-oxadiazole; Biologically based data; Bisbiguanide disinfectant (such as Chlorhexidine, etc.); Blockbuster drug (e.g. Fluoxetine ["Prozac"], etc.); Blood-bank donor; Brittle bone disease (= Osteoporosis); Broad beta disease (hereditary type of HLP - Hyperlipoproteinemia); 'Bubble boy' disorder (in children with ADA - adenosine deaminase deficiency).

BBDCB Blood-borne disease-causing bacterium.

BBDCP Blood-borne disease-causing parasite.

BBDCV Blood-borne disease-causing virus.

BBE Bacteroides bile esculin (agar); Bee body extract (Bee antigen vaccine).

BBEP Brush border endopeptidase.

BBF Biting basket forceps (Wolf - arthroscopy); Brain/ Bronchial blood flow; Breakbone fever (with severe muscle and joint pain) (= Aden/ Bouquet/ Dandy/ Dengue/ Solar fever) - a viral infection transferred to humans by the AEDES mosquito.

BBG Baby-boom generation (of the late nineteen forties).

BBI Blood-borne infection; Bowman-Birk (soybean) inhibitor.

B-bile Bile from the gall-bladder.

BBIUI Blood-borne intrauterine infection.
BBL Bastard bipolar lead Bird; breeder's lung (see PBD).
BB leprosy Borderline leprosy.
BBM Banked breast milk; Biochemical bone marker (see BCBM); Biologically based model; Blood based metabolism; Bone-building mechanism; Brush border membrane.
BBMC Bone-bone marrow consortium (Orthopedics).
BBMI Biologically based mental illness (= BBAD).
BBMT Blood Bank Medical Technologist (ASCP).
BBMV Brush border membrane vesicle.
BBN Broad band noise.
B-bomb Benzedrine inhaler.
BBOT Butyl-benzoxazolyl thiopene (scintillator).
BBP Baseline blood pressure; Basic biochemical pathway; Behaviorally-based program; Blood-borne pathogen (such as Hepatitis virus, HIV, etc.).
BBPAL Big big prolactin.
BBPC Blood-borne progenitor cell (associated with rHuEPO or Epoetin therapy in MCMM and PPMM) (see MCMM; PPMM).
BB powder Potassium sorbate (= BB).
BBPS Build and blood pressure study.
BBR Bainbridge reflex (reflex acceleration of the heart beat, resulting from stimulation of the wall of the left atrium due to increased pressure in, or increased distension of the large somatic veins, such as by large amounts of intravenous fluids).
BBRC Biochemical and Biophysical Research Communications (journal).
BBRS Burks' Behavior Rating Scale.
BBS Bardet-Biedl syndrome (an inherited disorder due to a Mendelian recessive trait, characterized by a variable phenotype with defects in vision, plydactyly, obesity, and learning difficulties); Basal blood sampling (e.g. glucose, C-peptide, etc); Bashful bladder syndrome; Battered baby syndrome (= BCS); Benign breast syndrome; Bilateral breath sounds; Bombesin; British Births Survey; Broad-bean syndrome (= Favism) (see G6PD); Bronchial breath sound; Brown bowel syndrome (gastrointestinal ceroidosis, with brown ceroid deposition on the gastrointestinal tract, associated with Vitamin E malabsorption).
BBT Basal body temperature; Benign bone/ brain tumor; Biceps brachii tendon; Blood bank technologist; Bloodborne transmission (of infection); 'Blunder-buss' therapy.
BBTMFP Basal body temperature method of family planning (see NFPM).
BB to MM Belly button to medial malleolus.
BB unit Berga-Broida unit.
BBV Blood-borne virus; Brain blood vessel; British-Bee-Venom (propietary drug).
BB/W BioBreeding/Worcester (rat).
BBx Breast biopsy.
BC Baby Care (journal); Bachelor of Surgery (L. Baccalaureus Chirurgiae); Back care; Bactericidal concentration; Baker's cyst; Balance of competence; Banjo curet (Obstetrics and Gynecology); Basal/ Basket cell; Battle casualty; Bed and chair (see B&C); Before Christ; Bicarbonate; Biliary colic; Biomedical Communications (journal); Biotin carboxylase; Bipolar cell; Birth/ Bourn control; Blastic crisis; Blood Cells (journal); Blood center/ count/ culture; Blood cholesterol (see LFT iv); Blood/ British Council; Blue Cross (plan); Board certified; Bone conduction (hearing test); Boundary conduction; Brachiocephalic; Bradycardia; Breast cancer; Bronchial carcinoma/ challenge; Buccal cartilage; Buccocervical; Buffy coat; Bureau of the Census.
B&C Board and care; Bed and chair (rest) (= BC); Biopsy and curettage (operation/ gynecology); Breathed and cried.
B/C Because; Bed to chair (patient); Blood urea nitrogen/ creatinine (ratio).
b/c benefit/cost (ratio).
B1C (= C3) Serum complement (globulin).
BC 48 Demecarium bromide. A miotic drug used in the treatment of certain types of glaucoma by local instillation into the conjunctival sac.
BC 51 Cholinesterase inhibitor.
BC 105 Pizotyline.
BCA Background-corrected absorbance; Bacterial cell assay (in vitro assay or Ames

test); Bactericidal agent (lethal); Balloon catheter angioplasty; Basal cell acanthoma (see BCP)/ adenoma/ atypia; Base Case Analysis; Benefit-cost analysis; Benign colonic amebiasis; Biochemical abnormalities/ty; Blood color analyzer; Blue Cross Association; Body composition assessment; Boric acid, cocaine hydrochloride, adrenaline solution (eye-drops); Brachiocephalic arteritis (= Martorell's syndrome, Pulseless disease, Reversed coarctation, Takayasu's arteritis); Brachiocephalic artery; Branchial cleft anomaly; Breast cancer antigen; Bronchoconstricting activity; Buffy Coat Analysis (a quantitative blood count examination).

BCAA Branched chain-enriched amino acid.

BCAT Brachiocephalic arterial trunk.

B cat Branhamella catarrhalis.

B-CAVe Bleomycin, CCNU (lomustine), Adriamycin (doxorubicin), and Velbe (vinblastine).

BCAZ Boric acid, chlorbutol, adrenaline, zinc sulfate solution (eye-drops).

BCB Benign chondroblastoma (Orthopedics); Blood-cerebrospinal (fluid) barrier; Brilliant cresyl blue.

BC/BC Fraction of serum complement.

BCBM Biochemical bone marker (= BBM).

BCBR Bilateral carotid body resection.

BC/BS Blue Cross/Blue Shield (plan).

BCC Basal cell carcinoma (= BCE or Basal cell epithelioma, Basaloma, Basiloma, Basiloma terebrans, CBC or Carcinoma basocellulare, HMC or Hair matrix carcinoma, Rodent ulcer); Baseline clinical characteristic(s); Basosqamous cell carcinoma (see BSCC); Biliary cholesterol concentration; Bipolar cord coagulation (Obstetrics); Brain/Breast-cancer care/ cell; Breast Care Center; Birth Control Clinic.

bcc body-centered-cubic.

BCCa Basal cell carcinoma (see BCC).

BCCG British Co-operative Clinical Group.

BCCI British Columbia Cancer Institute.

BCCP Biotin carboxyl-carrier protein.

BCD Basal cell dysplasia; Binary-coded decimal; Bleeding colonic diverticulosis (see CDH); Bleomycin, cyclophosphamide, dactinomycin; Bone cell differentiation (see BCP; BCR); Blood cell destruction; Bone collagen degradation (Urinary markers of BCD are hydroxyproline, deoxypyridinoline, cross-linked N-telopeptides of type I collagen, etc.); Brain cell damage/ death/ decay/ dysfunction; Breast cancer detection/ diagnosis; Bryan cervical disc (artificial polyurethane spinal disc).

BCDDP Breast Cancer Detection Demonstration Project.

BCDF B-cell differentiation factor.

BCDL Brachmann-Cornelia de Lange (syndrome).

BCDS Blue Cross Data Service.

BCDSP Boston Collaborative Drug Surveillance Program.

BCE Basal cell epithelioma; Benigh childhood epilepsy; Bubble chamber equipment.

BCEDP Breast and Cervical Cancer Early Detection Program (SFMS). Also known as: Breast Care Early Detection Program (SFMS; TSRI).

B-cell Bone marrow(-derived) cell - lymphocyte (see B lymphocyte).

BCF Basket cutting forceps; Basophil chemotactic factor; Bio-concentration factor; Biosynthesis coagulation factor; Blood clotting/ coagulation factor (see Factor); Breast cyst fluid; Bronchial collateral flow (network of lung tissue capillaries).

BCFA Birth Control Federation of America (now PPFA).

BCFo Occluded bone conduction with frontal placement.

BCFP Board-certified family physician; Breast cyst fluid protein.

BCFRS Benign congenital focal Rolandic seizure (= BFNE).

BCFu (= BCM). Unoccluded bone conduction with mastoid placement.

BCG Bacille Calmette-Guérin (TB vaccine); Ballistocardiogram/aphy (procedure/ cardiology); Bicolor guaiac (test); Bromcresol/syl green (albumin indicator/ reagent).

BCGF B-cell growth factor.

BCG test Bicolor guaiac test.

BCH Basal cell hyperplasia; Basic clinical history; Benzolhexachloride; Boston

Children's/ City Hospital.

BCh Bachelor of Surgery (= B Chir) - L. baccalaureus chirurgiae.

B-chain cystometrogram Urography.

BChD Bachelor of Dental Surgery (= BDS) - L. baccalaureus dentalis chirurgiae.

B Chir Bachelor of Surgery (see BCh).

Bchl; bChl Bacterial chlorophyll.

BCHS Bureau of Community Health Services (HEW; Health Services Administration).

BCI Biventricular cardiac insufficiency.

BCIC Birth Control Investigation Committee.

BCJ British Chiropody Journal (now British Journal of Chiropody).

BCKA Branched-chain keto acid(uria).

BCKD Branched-chain alpha-keto acid dehydrogenase.

BCL Basic cycle length; Breast-conserving lumpectomy.

βCL Beta-cell lymphoma.

β-HCG Beta-Human chorionic gonadotropin (pregnancy test) (see Hormones - HCG).

BCLA Board of Certified Laboratory Assistants.

BCLL B-cell chronic lymphocytic leukemia.

BCLP Bilateral cleft of lip and palate.

BCLS Basic cardiac life support.

BCM Biochemical marker; Birth control medication; Blood chemistry/ concentration monitor(ing); Blood-clotting mechanism (effects); Body cell mass; Bone conduction with mastoid (placement) - see BCFu; Mannomustine hydrochloride (= Mannitol Mustard). A cytotoxic agent used in the palliative treatment of certain neoplastic diseases, particularly those of lymphoid and hemopoietic tissues, e.g. Hodgkin's disease, lymphosarcoma, etc.; Bovine cervical mucus; Bursal chrondromatosis (Orthopedics).

BCME Bis-chloromethyl ether (a carcinogen).

BCMN Bureau Central de Mesures Nucléaires (Fr.) (= Central Bureau for Nuclear Measurements - part of Euratom).

BCN Basal cell nevus; Bilateral cortical necrosis; Blue Care Network (Michigan, US).

BCNP Board Certified Nuclear Pharmacist.

BCNS Basal cell nevus syndrome.

BCNU Carmustine (= Bischloroethyl-nitrosurea; 1,3-bis-{2-chloroethyl}-1-nitrosourea; Bischloronitrosourea; NSC 409962). A cytotoxic drug used in the treatment of brain tumors and Hodgkin's disease.

BCO Bilateral cryptorchidism; Biliary cholesterol output; Bipolar cord occlusion (Obstetrics); Board-certified ophthalmologist.

BCO_2 Bound carbon dioxide.

BCOG Board-certified obstetrician/ gynecologist.

BCOP BCNU (carmustine), cyclophosphamide, vincristine, procarbazine. A combination treatment used in certain neoplastic diseases.

BCP Basal cell papilloma (= BCA or Basal cell acanthoma, Seborrheic keratosis, Seborrheic wart); Basic calcium phosphate; BCNU (carmustine), cyclophosphamide, and prednisone; Birth control pill; Bladder control problem; Blood cell processor/ profile; Blue Cross Plan; Bone cell proliferation (see BCD; BCR); Breast cancer patient; Bromcresol/syl purple.

B-CP B-cell precursor.

BCPD; BCP-D Bromcresol/syl purple deoxylate/ desoxycholate (culture medium).

BCPT Breast Cancer Prevention Trial (NCI).

BCPV Bovine cutaneous papilloma virus.

BCR Baseline-controlled study (see MCBCS); B-cell reactivity/ receptor; Beryllium Case Registry; Birth control regimen; Board-certified radiologist; Bone cell replication (see BCD; BCP); Brain cell regeneration; Brain corticosteroid receptor (see BSCR); Breast cancer research/ risk; Bromocriptine.

BCR; bcr Breakpoint cluster region.

BCRA Breast Cancer Risk Assessment (test).

BCRC Baltimore Cancer Research Center (NCI).

BCRD B-cell receptor deficiency (see IgD); British Council for Rehabilitation of the Disabled.

BCRE Beta-Carotene and Retinol Efficacy (Trial) (NCI).

BCRx Birth control drug.

BCS Baseline-controlled study (see MCBCS); Battered child syndrome; Biochemical study; Biracial community study; Blood cell separator; Breast cancer screening/ specialist/ surgery/ survivor; Breast Carcinoma Study;

Breast-conserving surgery; British Cardiac Society; Budd-Chiari syndrome.

BCSI Breast cancer screening indicator.

BCSR Board-certified skeletal radiologist; Brain corticosteroid receptor (= BCR).

BCSS Bone-cell-stimulating substance (Orthopedics).

BCST Breast cancer screening test (mammography).

BCT Base channel threshold; Blood coagulation test(s) (see Factor): Bleeding time (BT) (min) / Fibrinogen (= Plasma thromboplastin factor I - PTAH) (g/L); Partial thromboplastin time (PTT) (sec) / Platelets (x 10,000,000,000 l); Procoagulant factor VIII (= Antihemophilic factor - AHF) / Prothrombin time (sec) / Thrombin time (% of control); Brachiocephalic trunk (= Brachiocephalic artery; Innominate artery); Branched-chain (amino acid) transferase; Buffy coat transfusion (see GCT).

B + CT Bleeding plus clotting time.

BCTF Breast Cancer Task Force (NCI).

BCtg Bovine chymotrypsinogen.

BCTP Breast cancer transplant program.

BCtr Bovine chymotrypsin.

BCU Basic chemical unit (base-pair in the DNA gene); Bicornate uterus; Burn care unit.

B-curve Finding in impedance audiogram; a completely flat "curve" or pattern.

BCV Bicuspid valve (= Left atrioventricular or Mitral valve); Brachiocephalic vein (or Innominate vein).

BCVP BCNU (carmustine), Cyclophosphamide, Vinblastine, Procarbazine.

BCVPP BCNU (Carmustine), Cyclophosphamide, Vinblastine, Procarbazine and Prednisone (Chemotherapy).

BCW Bacterial cell wall; Biological and chemical warfare.

BCYE Buffered charcoal-yeast extract (agar).

BD Band (neutrophil); Barbital-dependent; Barbiturate dependence; Base deficit; Base of prism down; Basophilic degeneration; Batten's/ Behcet's/ Byler's disease; Behavior(al)/ Briquet disorder; Belladonna; Benzoylated DEAE; Bicarbonate dialysis; Bile duct; Binocular deprivation; Bipolar disorder (= BPD); Birth date/ defect; Black death; Blastodisc; Block design (psychological test); Blood donor; Blue diaper (syndrome); Borderline dull; Bornholm disease (a viral myositis in adults); Bottle/ Bronchial drainage; Bound; Brain damage/ dead/ death; Bronchodilation/tor; Buccodistal; Bureau of Drugs (FDA); Twice a day (L. bis die) (see bd; Bis in die).

B-D Becton-Dickinson.

B&D Bondage and discipline.

Bd Board; Buoyant density; Diastolic blood pressure.

bd band; bundle; twice a day (L. bis die) (= BD; Bis in die).

BDA Balloon dilation angioplasty; Benzodiazepine antagonist (see BDZA); British Dental/ Dermatological/ Diabetes(tic)/ Dietetic Association.

BDAC Bureau of Drug Abuse Control (FDA).

BDAE Boston Diagnostic Aphasia Examination.

BDAS Biomedical Data Acquisition System.

BDB Bis-diazotized-benzidine.

BDBS Bonnet-Déchaume-Blanc syndrome.

BDC Bazex-Dupré-Christol (syndrome); Biodegradable carrier (for antibiotics, etc.); Blood Donor Center; Breast diagnostic center; Bureau of Domestic Commerce; Burn-dressing change.

BDC-OH Bis-dimethylamino-diphenyl carbinol.

BDD Body dysmorphic disorder (a deep or grim fixation on some flaw in one's appearance) (see OCD; OCI).

BDE Bile duct examination/ exploration; Bronchodilating effect; Bulletin of Dental Education (AADS journal).

BDentSci Bachelor of Dental Science (Dublin).

BDF Biopsy drill forceps (Palmer - Obstetrics and Gynecology); Bipolar diathermy forceps (Autosuture); Black divorced female; Bulldog forceps (used in surgery).

BDG Buccal developmental groove; Buffered desoxycholate glucose (broth).

BDGF Bone-derived growth factor (see BCSS).

BDH British Drug House code for experimental substances; Bubble-diffusion humidifier.

BDH 1298 Megestrol acetate (= SC 10363). A synthetic sex hormone with pronounced progestational properties and an inhibitor of ovulation.

BDH 1921 Melengestrol acetate. A synthetic sex hormone with pronounced progestational properties, but more potent than progesterone. It produces prolonged remission in advanced inoperable endometrial carcinoma.

BDI Beck's Diagnostic Inventory (developed by A.T.Beck in the 1970s as a diagnostic and therapeutic tool for the treatment of childhood mental disorders) (see DSM; DSM III); Birth Defect Institute (New York State Health Department); Bureau of Disability Insurance (SSA).

BDI SF Beck Depression Index - Short Form.

BDJ British Dental Journal (British Dental Association).

BDL Below detectable limits; Bile duct ligation.

BDLS Brachmann-de Lange syndrome.

BDM Becker's muscular dystrophy; Black divorced male.

BDNF; BDNGF Brain-derived nerve-growth factor.

BDOO Bureau of District Office Operations (SSA).

B-DOPA Bleomycin, Dacarbazine, Oncovin (vincristine), Prednisone, and Adriamycin (doxorubicin).

BDP Beclomethasone dipropionate; Beginning diastolic pressure; Benzodiazepine; Bilateral diaphragmatic paralysis; Bone derivative preparation (Orthopedics); Brain-damaged patient/ person; Bronchopulmonary displasia.

BDPRA Benzodiazepine receptor antagonist (see BRA).

BDR Background diabetic retinopathy; Bronchodilator response.

BDS Bachelor of Dental Surgery (see BChD); Biological detection system; Blessed Dementia Scale (see MMSE); Bone-density study.

bds to be taken twice a day (L. bid in die summendus).

BDSc Bachelor of Dental Science.

BDT Bronchodilation/tor therapy.

BDU Brick dust urine (containing uric acid precipitates).

BDUR Bromodeoxyuridine.

BDW Buffered distilled water.

Bdw Wild bird species.

Bdy wt Body weight.

BDZ Benzodiazepine(s) (= BDP) - an Anxiolytic group of drugs, including Alprozalam, Bromazepam, Brotizolam, Carbamazepine, Chlordiazepoxide, Clobazam, Clonazepam, Clorazepate, Clozapine (Di BDP), Diazepam, Flunitrazepam, Ketazolam, Lorazepam, Medazepam, Nitrazepam, Nordiazepam, Olazapine (Thieno BDP), Oxazepam, Oxcarbazepine and Triazolam.

BDZA Benzodiazepine antagonist (= BDA).

BDZR Benzodiazepine receptor.

BDZRA Benzodiazepine receptor antagonist (see BRA).

BDZS Benzodiazepine screen (see UDS).

BE Bacillary emulsion (Ger. bacillen e.) (see Tuberculin - BE); Bacterial endocarditis; Barium enema (X-ray/ colon); Barrett's esophagus; Base excess (plasma bicarbonate); Below elbow (see B/E); Bile esculin (test); Binding energy (electron-volts); Biomedical Electronics (journal); Biomedical Engineering (journal); Bovine enteritis; Brain edema; Brain encephalitogen; Bread equivalent; Breast examination; Broncho-esophagology; Bunionectomy (Podiatry): Akin, Austin, Barker, cap, closing ABD wedge, crescentic, Drato, Hohmann, Jones, Keller, lapidus, Logracino, Mayo, Mitchell, McBride, opening ABD wedge (Trethawain), ORD (off-set reverse dome), Peabody, Reverdin, Silver bunionectomies.

Be Beryllium (Z = 4) (see Elements - Beryllium).

Bé Baumé scale (Specific gravity s).

B/E Below-elbow (= BE - amputation/ fracture/ operation).

B↑E Both upper extremities.

B↓E Both lower extremities.

B&E Brisk and equal.

BE 419 Ioglycamic acid. An X-ray contrast medium given intravenously for the radiographic examination of the biliary tract.

BEA Below-elbow amputation; Bioelectrical activity; Blood ethyl alcohol; British Epilepsy Association; Bromoethylamine.

Be a Becker antigen (blood group).

BEAM Behavioral, Emotional, Academic and Medical (therapy); Brain electrical activity mapping/ monitoring.

BEAMOS Beam-accessed metal-oxide semiconductor.

BEAP Bronchiectasis, eosinophilia, asthma, pneumonia.

BEAR Biological effects of atomic radiation.

BEARC Biological Effects of Atomic Radiation Committee (NAS-NRC).

Beast LSD-25 (see LSD).

BEB Benign essential blepharospasm.

BEBM-USSR Bulletin of Experimental Biology and Medicine of the USSR.

BEC Background of equivalent concentration (spectroscopy); Bacterial endocarditis; Blood ethanol concentration (= BAC; BEA) (see AEI); Bromo-ergocryptine; Buccal epithelial cell (= OAC); Bureau of Employees' Compensation.

BECEC Board of Examiners for Clinical Engineering Certification.

BECF Blood/ Brain extracellular fluid.

BECOS Benign Epilepsy of Childhood with Occipital Spikes.

Becquerel One nuclear disintegration per second (= 2.7 x 1/1,000,000,000,000 curie).

Bedt Bedtime.

BEE Basal energy expenditure; Bi-exponential elimination (of a drug).

Bee Marijuana (see Cannabis).

BEEC Biomedical Engineering Education Committee (ASEE).

BEF Best excitatory freqencies; Bronchoesophageal fistula.

Bef Before.

BEG Benge eating disorder.

Beg; beg Begin(ning).

Beh; beh Behavior/ral/rism.

Beh Sp Behavior specialist.

BEI Back-scattered electron imaging; Balanced electrolyte intake; Biological Exposure Indexes; Biomedical Engineering and Instrumentation (Branch) (see BEIB); Butanol-extractable iodine (thyroid test).

BEIB Biomedical Engineering and Instrumental Branch (NIH).

BEIR Biological Effects of Ionizing Radiation (NAS report).

BEK Bi-exponential kinetic (distribution/ elimination of a drug); Bovine embryonic kidney (cells).

BEL Blood ethanol level; Bovine embryonic lung.

BELIR Beta-endorphin-like immuno-reactivity.

Bel; bel Well; good (L. bene).

Belg. P Belgian Pharmacopoeia (Pharmacopée Belge).

BEM Biochemical efficacy marker; Buccal epithelial mucosa (= BES).

BENAR Blood eosinophilic non-allergic rhinitis.

Benny Benzedrine pill (see Amphet).

Benz; benz Benzedrine (see Amphet); Benzene; Benzidine; Benzoate.

BEP Basic element of performance; Bleomycin, etoposide, and cisplatin (platinum compound); Brain/ Brainstem evoked potential.

B-EP ß-endorphin.

BEPTI (X+Y+Z) Malaria incidence factors - an expression used in malaria epidemiology. These five factors are: B - Bionomics, E - Environment, P - Plasmodium, T - Treatment, and I - Immunity, with: X - Human carrier, Y - Mosquito vector, and Z - Human victim.

BER Basic electrical rhythm.

BERA Brainstem evoked response audiometry.

Bernie Cocaine (see Erythroxylum).

BES Balanced electrolyte solution; Bioequivalence/lent study; Biological Engineering Society (British); British Engineering System (of units); Buccal epithelial surface (see BEM).

BESI Balloon-expandable-stent implant(ation).

BESJ British Endodontic Society Journal.

BESM Bovine embryonic skeletal muscle.

BESP Bovine embryonic spleen (cells).

Bé specific gravity scale Baumé specific gravity scale.

BEST Battery energy storage test; Bombay

Electric Supply Tramway; Breast examination (through) simultaneous temperature (evaluation).

BET Bacillen emulsion tuberculin (see Tuberculin); Bacterial endotoxin; Benign epithelial/ essential tremor; Bicycle exercise test; Brunauer-Emmett-Teller (surface area method/ test).

3 beta-HSD 3-beta-p-hydroxysteroid dehydrogenase.

BETE Tropine benzylate.

BEV Baboon endogenous virus; Bleeding esophageal varix; Billion electron volts (see BeV).

BeV; Bev; beV; bev; BEV Billion (109) electron volts - now GEV (see GeV).

bev beverage.

BEVA British Equine Veterinary Association.

BEWT Bureau of East-West Trade.

BF Backlash feelings; Bentonite flocculation (test) - see BFT; Bile/ Blood flow; Biofeedback (see BFB); Black female (see B/F); Blastogenic factor; Blister fluid; Body fat; Bouillon filtrate (Fr. bouillon filtré); Bouillon filtrate tuberculin or Denys' tuberculin, a culture medium for tubercle bacilli (see Tuberculin - BF); Bound free (see B/F); Boyfriend; Breakfast fed; Breast feeding; Buffered; Burning feet (syndrome); Bureau of Foods (FDA); Butter fat.

bf bouillon filtrate (tuberculin) - see BF.

B/F Black female (= BF); Bound free (antigen ratio) (= BF).

BF# Butterfly fracture (a bone break in which two cracks form a triangle) (= BFF).

B3F Band 3 cytoplasmic fragment.

BFA Baby for adoption; Bifemoral arteriogram; Brassfounder's ague (see MFV).

BFB Bifidobacteria/rium (found in breast milk); Biofeedback/ Biological feedback (= BF); Bottle-/ Breast-fed baby (see BFI); Bronchial foreign body; Butterfly bandage.

BFC Benign febrile convulsion; Biceps flexor cubiti (= Biceps; Biceps brachii).

BFD Bucco-facial dyskinesia.

BFDI Bronchodilation following deep inspiration.

BFEC Benign focal epilepsy of childhood.

BFE Blood flow energy.

BFF Base-forming food (a food that makes urine less acid, such as fruits, vegetables, and dairy products); Butterfly fracture (see BF#).

BFGF Basic fibroblast growth factor.

BFH Benign familial hematuria.

BFI Bismuth-formic-iodide (compound) - a proprietary antiseptic dusting powder; Breast-fed infant (= BFB; HMFI).

BFL Bird fancier's lung; Borjeson-Forssman-Lehmann (syndrome); Breast firm and lactating; Bulk forming laxative (see Lax; lax).

BFLS Borjeson-Forssman-Lehmann syndrome.

BFM Blood flow meter; Breast-feeding mother.

BFMIRA British Food Manufacturing Industries Research Association.

BFNE Benign focal nocturnal epilepsy (see BCFRS).

BFO Balanced/ Ball-bearing forearm orthosis; Best-frequency oscillator; Blood-forming organ; Breast-fed offspring.

BFP Bacterial food poisoning; Biologic/cal/cally false positive/vity (test/ting), e.g. in serological tests for syphilis (see BFPSTS); Bipolar femoral prosthesis (Orthopedics); Bisferious pulse (an arterial pulse with two separate peaks, the second slightly stronger than the first) (see DCP); Brain Fingerprinting; Buccal fat pad (sucking pad, in infants).

BFP; bFP; βFP Beta fetoprotein (a protein found in fetal liver and in some adults with liver disease. It is identical with normal liver ferritin).

BFPO Dimefox (= DIFO; Pestox 14; Tetramethylphosphorodiamidic floride). An organophosphorus insecticide.

BFPR Biologic/cal/cally false positive reaction.

BFPSTS Bilogic/cal/cally false positive serological test for syphilis.

BFR Biologic false-positive reactor; Biologic false reaction; Bird-face retrognathism (an abnormal profile with an undeveloped lower jaw); Blood flow rate/ response; Bone formation rate; Buffered Ringer's (solution) - see BFR sol.

B frag Bacillus fragilis.

BFRI Boston Federation of Residents and Interns.

BFR sol Buffered Ringer's solution (for infusion).

BFS Bedford finger stall; Blood fasting sugar (see FBS); Bronchofibroscopy (see FOB - Fiberoptic bronchoscopy); Burning feet syndrome.

BFT Bendroflumethiazide (diuretic and antihypertensive drug); Benign familial tremor; Bentonite flocculation test (for rheumatic factor); Biceps femoris tendon; Biofeedback training; Bouillon filtrate tuberculin (see Tuberculin - BFT).

BFTI Bone-fibrous-tissue interface (Orthopedics).

BFU Burst-forming unit (see HGF).

BFU-E; BFU Burst-forming unit, erythroid (cell) - see HGF.

BFU-ME Burst-forming unit, myeloid/ erythroid - see HGF.

BFV Blood-flow velocity; Bovine feces virus.

BFW Behavior following wakefulness; Bilateral facial weakness; Breast-feeding woman/ women.

BG Baby girl; Basal ganglion; Basic gastrin; Behavior Genetics (journal); Bender Gestalt (test); Beta-galactosidase; Beta-glucuronidase; Bicolor guaiac (test); Birbeck granule; Blood glucose (laboratory/ chemistry) (see BGlu); Bone graft (operation/ orthopedics); Bordet-Gengou bacillus (see B-G); Brilliant green; Buccogingival; Bypass graft.

Bg beige (mouse).

B-G Bender-Gestalt (test) (= BG); Bordet-Gengou (agar/ bacillus/ phenomenon).

BGA Biogenic amine (such as norepinephrine, acetylcholine, & dopamine); Blood gas analysis (arterial); Blue-green algae; British Geriatric(s) Association.

BGAg Blood group antigen.

B-GAL B-galactosyl (grouping).

B-GALACTO Beta galactosidase.

BGAV Blue-green algae virus.

BGC Basal ganglion calcification; Blood glucose concentration (see BGL; BSL)/ control; Blood group class; Bronchogenic carcinoma/ cyst.

BGCA Bronchogenic carcinoma.

BGCT Benign granulosa/lotheca cell tumor.

BGD Blood-gas determination (analysis of the acid-base balance or pH of the blood); Blood group degradation.

BGDC Bartholin gland duct cyst.

BGE Butyl glycidyl ether.

BGF Blood growth factor.

BGG Bovine gamma-globulin.

BGGRA British Gelatine and Glue Research Association.

BGH Bovine growth hormone (= bGH) (see Hormones - BGH; GH).

bGH Bovine growth hormone (see BGH).

BGJ BGJ culture medium, modified by Fitton Jackson (see BGJ); Biggers Gwatkin Judah (culture medium).

BGL Biogenetic law (see RCT - Recapitulation theory); Blood glucose level.

BGLB Brilliant green lactose broth.

BGlu Blood glucose (= BG).

BGM Bacterial gene mutation; Blood glucose monitor(ing); Bordet-Gengou medium; Green monkey kidney cells.

BGMV Bean golden mosaic virus.

BGP Bermuda grass pollen; Beta-glycerophosphatase; Bigeminal pulse (or Bigeminy); Bone GLA protein; Bone-grafting procedure; Butyl glycolyl-butyl phthalate.

BGR Background radiation (naturally occurring radiation given off by elements in the soil, ground waters, and building materials; also by radioactive substances in the body, especially potassium 40 [40K], plus cosmic rays from outer space, the average individual being exposed each year to 44 millirad [mrad] of cosmic radiation, 44 mrad from the environment, and 18 mrad from naturally occurring internal radioactive sources - a total of some 106 mrads); Bone graft reconstruction (Orthopedics); Brain-growth regulator(s) incoded in genes, as in VIPs or Vaso-active intestinal peptides).

B/G ratio Length of basal layer/ length of granular layer ratio (thyroid).

BGS Bacterial growth substratum; Balance, gait, and station; Beta-galactosidase (= Lactase); Blood group substance; Bone graft substitute; British Geriatrics Society;

Buccoglossal syndrome.

BGSA Blood granulocyte-specific activity.

BGSM Blood glucose self-monitoring (= GSM) in IDDM.

BGT Background therapy; Blood-gas tension.

B-G test Bordet-Gengou test.

BGTT Borderline glucose tolerance test.

BGU Benign gastric ulcer; Biochemical Genetics Unit.

BH Base hospital; Benzalkonium and heparin; Bill of health; Birth history; Bishop-Harman (instruments); Board of Health; Bolton-Hunter (reagent); Borderline hypertensive; Both hands; Brain hormone; Breath holding; Bronchial hyper-reactivity; Bryan high titer; Bulletin of Hygiene (journal); Bundle of His.

BH# Buttonhole fracture (any broken bone caused by a bullet) (= BHF)

B3H Corticosterone - 1,2-3H.

BH4 Tetrahydrobiopterin.

BHA Beta-hydroxyisovaleric aciduria (see BHIA); Bound hepatitis antibody; Butylated hydroxyanisole. An antioxidant for oils and fats, used for their preservation in pharmaceutical practice; also for the preservation of vitamin oil concentrates.

Bhang Marijuana (see Cannabis).

BHAT Beta-blocker Heart Attack Trial (US).

BHB Basic Hospital Benefits (program); Beta-hydroxybutyrate; Buttonhole bypass (see MIDCAB).

bHb Bovine hemoglobin.

BHBA Beta-hydroxybutyric acid.

BHC Basic health care; Benign hereditary chorea; Benzene hexachloride (= HCH - Hexachlorocyclohexane) - A chlorinated insecticide and scabicide; Breast Health Center (USC); Braxton Hicks contraction(s) (irregular tightening of the pregnant uterus that begins during the first 3 months of pregnancy. Also called Braxton Hicks sign or False labor); Brunnstrom hemiplegia classification.

BHCDA Bureau of Health Care Delivery and Assistance.

BHD BCNU (= carmustine), hydroxyurea, and dacarbazine; Bird-headed dwarfism (distinctive bird-like facies, with beaked nose, micrognathia and low-set ears, dwarfism and microcephaly and premature, greying, abnormal hair - probably an autosomal recessive, congenital hypotrichosis) (= PAS; SS - Seckel's syndrome); Bulletin of the History of Dentistry (AAHD journal).

BHE Bureau of Health Education.

BHET Bicycle heart exercise test (Ergometer).

B-HEXOS-A-LK Beta hexosaminidase A leukocyte(s).

BHF Bolivian hemorrhagic fever (caused by the Machupo virus, an arena virus and transmitted by the Bolivian mouse, *Calomys* callosus); Bone-holding forceps (= LJC); British Heart Foundation; Buttonhole fracture (see BH#).

BHHC Bunker Hill Health Center.

BHHCC Bureau of Health and Hospital Careers Counseling.

BHI Biological Homeopathic Industries; Biosynthetic human insulin; Blues Health Insurance; Brain-heart infusion (agar/ broth); British Humanities Index; Bureau of Health Insurance (HEW).

BHIA Beta-hydroxyisovaleric aciduria (an inherited metabolic disease caused by the lack of an enzyme needed to process the amino acid leucine) (see MSUD); Brain-heart infusion agar.

BHI-ac Brain heart infusion (broth) with acetone.

BHIB Brain-heart/ Beef-heart infusion broth.

BHIBA Brain-heart infusion blood agar.

BHIRS Brain-heart infusion and rabbit serum.

BHIS Beef heart infusion supplemented (with broth or agar).

BHJ British Heart Journal (BCS); British Homeopathic Journal.

BHK Baby hamster kidney (cells); Type-B Hong Kong (influenza virus).

BHL Bilateral hilar lymphadenopathy; Biological half-life (= MHL) (see Half-life).

BHM Blackett-Healy method (of positioning a patient for X-raying of the shoulder area); Bone histomorphometry (see QHM); Bulletin of the History of Medicine; Bureau of Health Manpower (HEW).

BHME Bureau of Health Manpower Education (NIH, now defunct).

BHN Bephenium hydroxynaphthoate; Bridging hepatic necrosis; Brinell hardness number.

BHOLN Bulletin of the Health Organization, League of Nations (defunct journal).

B Hormone Melanin-stimulating hormone (see Hormones - MSH ii).

BHP Basic health profile; Behavioral health professional; Benign hyperplasia; Blood hydrostatic pressure; Bureau of Health Professions (NIH).

BH_2PO_4 One equivalent of base (B), combined with the phosphate radical.

B_2HPO_4 Two equivalents of base (B_2), combined with the phosphate radical.

BHPRD Bureau of Health Planning and Resources Development.

BHR Basal heart rate; Benign hypertrophic prostatitis; Bronchial hyperreactivity.

B-HR Bolton-Hunter Reagent (^{125}I).

BHRA Bureau of Health Resources Administration (HEW).

BHRD Bureau of Health Resources Development (HEW).

BHS Bachelor of Health Sciences; Basic health services; Beating-heart surgery; Behavioral Health Services; Beta-hemolytic streptococcus; Bicap Hemostatic Source (cautery unit used with the endoscope); Braxton Hicks sign (see BHC); Breast health services; Breath-holding spell; British Hypertension Society; Bronchial hypersecretion (as in bronchiectasis); Bureau of Health Services.

BHSR Bureau of Health Services Research.

BHT Benign hepatic tumor (= BLT); Beta-hydroxytheophylline; Black "hairy" tongue; Breath hydrogen test; Brinnell hardness test (for surface hardness of materials use in dentistry); Bucket-handle tear (longitudinal tear in the knee cartilage or meniscus); Butylated hydroxytoluene - An antioxidant for oils and fats, no longer recommended for use in food products because of its possible hazard to health.

BHTD Bureau of Hygiene and Tropical Diseases (UK).

BHTN Benign hypertension.

BHTT Bennet hand tool test (used in occupational therapy and job-aptitude testing to measure hand function, coordination, and speed of performance).

BHU Basic health unit.

BHV Bovine herpes virus; Braxton Hicks version (a maneuver used to turn the fetus from an undesirable position to one that promotes delivery); Butterfly heart valve (Gott).

BH/VH Body hematocrit/venous hematocrit (ratio).

BHyg Bachelor of Hygiene.

BI Background interval; Bacterial/icidal/iological index; Base-in (prism) (Base of prism in); Basilar impression; Behavioral imagery (see VMBR); Billroth I (operation); Biological indicator; Bodily/dy/ Bone injury; Bovine insulin (see Insulin - BI); Bowel impaction; Brain injured/ry; Broder's index (a classification of the degree of malignancy of tumors, based on histologic features); Brookings Institution; Burn index.

Bi Bismuth (Z = 83) (see Elements - Bismuth).

bi- combining form meaning life (Gr. bios); prefix meaning two or twice (L. bi).

BIA Bioimpedance analyzer; Biolectric impedance analysis; Bioimmunoassay; Body-image agnosia (see ATP); Braille Institute of America; Bureau of Indian Affairs (USA - Dept. of Interior).

Bi a Bile antigen (blood group).

BIAC Bioinstrumentation Advisory Council.

BIB Biliointestinal bypass; Brought in by.

Bib; bib Drink (L. bibe) - medication order.

Biblio; biblio Bibliography.

BIBRA British Industrial Biological Research Association.

B-IBS B-immunoblastic sarcoma.

BIC Blood isotope clearance; Brain Imaging/ Injury Center; Bureau of International Commerce.

Bic Biceps.

BICAO Bilateral internal carotid artery occlusion.

Bicarb; bicarb Bicarbonate (= $NaHCO_3$ - sodium bicarbonate).

BICH Benign intracranial hypertension (= BIH; Meningeal hydrops; PTC or Pseudotumor cerebri).

BiCNU Carmustine (a cytotoxic drug - see BCNU).
BICROS Bilateral contralateral/ crossing routing of signals.
BID Bacterial infectious diarrhea; Bibliographic information and documentation; Bipolar-induced disorder; Brought in dead (see DOA).
bid Twice a day/ Twice daily (L. bis in die) (see Bis in die).
BIDA British International Doctors Association (2002, formerly ODA) (GMC, UK)
BIDLB Block in posteroinferior division of left branch.
BIDS Biological Integrated Detection System; Brittle hair, intellectual impairment, decreased fertility, and short stature (syndrome).
Bif Bifocal(s).
BIG 6 Analysis of 6 serum components.
Big Chief Mescaline (see Mesc).
big D LSD-25 (see LSD).
BIGGY Bismuth glycine glucose yeast.
BIH Benign intracranial hypertension; Bilateral inguinal hernia; British Institute of Homeopathy; Bureau International de l'Heure.
BIHCC. Bayer Institute for Health Care Communications (US).
BIHM Bulletin of the Institute of the History of Medicine.
bihor during two hours (L. bihorium).
BII Basel Institute for Immunology; Billroth II (operation); Biphasic insulin injection (see Insulin - BII); Butanol-insoluble iodine.
Bi Isch Between ischial tuberosities.
BIL Basal insulin level; Bilirubin (see Bili); Brother-in-law.
Bil Bile (L. bilis); Bilirubin (see Bili).
bil bilateral (see bilat).
bil- prefix meaning bile (L. bilis).
BIL/ALB Bilirubin/albumin (rate/tio).
Bilat; bilat Bilateral (= bil).
BILAT SLC Bilateral short leg case.
BILAT SXO Bilateral salpingo-oophorectomy.
BILG Boston Interhospital Liver Group.
Bili; bili Bilirubin (= BIL; Bil; Bilirub).
Bili-c; bili-c Conjugated bilirubin.
Bilirub; bilirub Bilirubin (see Bili).
Bilis Bile (L.), e.g. B. bovina = ox-bile.
BIM Brain imaging machine.
BIMA Bilateral internal mammary artery.
BIMC Beth Israel Medical Center.
BIN Twice nightly (see bin).
bin Twice a night/ Twice nightly (= BIN) (L. bis in nocte/tus).
Bind Binding.
Biochem Biochemistry (journal).
biochem biochemical/istry.
Biochemie (journal).
$(BiO)_2CO_2$ Bismuth subcarbonate.
BIOD Bony interorbital/ intraorbital distance.
Bio-des Diethylstilbestrol (proprietary/ trade name).
bioeng bioengineering.
BIOETHICSLINE Bioethical Information On-Line.
BIOF Biofeedback.
Biofizika (journal).
Biokh Biokhimiya (biochemistry journal translated from Russian).
Biol; biol Biological/gy.
bioLH Bio-assay of luteinizing hormone.
Biophys; biophys Biophysics/cal.
Biopoly Biopolymers (journal).
Biopsy The removal of a small piece of living tissue for microscopic examination in order to establish a diagnosis or follow the course of a disease. Kinds of biopsy include:
Aspiration biopsy = Needle biopsy (see).
Fractitional biopsy - histologic study of only fragments of tissue which have been removed for this purpose.
Needle biopsy - Biopsy of material obtained by aspiration through a needle.
Punch biopsy - Biopsy of material obtained by a punch into the tissue.
Sponge biopsy - Biopsy obtained by rubbing a sponge of suitable material over the lesion and examining it as a routine specimen.
Sternal biopsy - Biopsy of the sternal bone marrow obtained by puncture.
Surface biopsy - Examination under the microscope of cells obtained by scraping the surface of suspected lesions.
Surgical biopsy - Biopsy of material obtained

by surgical excision.
Total biopsy - Histologic examination of a growth removed in its entirety.

Biorheology (journal).

BIOS British Intelligencc Objective Subcommittee.

BIOSEM Biological scanning electron microscope.

Bios I Inositol (= hexahydroxycyclohexane). Belongs to the Vitamin B complex group.

Bios II Biotin (identical with Vitamin H and coenzyme R). Belongs to the Vitamin B complex group (see Vitamins - H).

BIOSIS BioScience Information Service.

BIP Bacterial intravenous protein; Benign idiopathic pericarditis (= Dressler's syndrome; Postinfarction syndrome); Bezafibrate Infarction Prevention (Study); Biparietal (diameter of skull); Bismuth Iodoform Paraffin; Blue Cross interim payment; Brief infertility period; Bromo-imidazolyl propionic acid monohydrate.

BIPD; bipd Biparietal diameter.

BIPLED Bilateral, independent, periodic, lateralized, epileptiform discharge.

BIPM Bureau International des Poids et Mesures (Fr.: International Bureau of Weights and Measures).

BIPP Bismuth Iodoform Paraffin/ Petrolatum Paste.

BIQ 16 Hedaquinium chloride (= Hexadecamethylenebis-isoquinolinium chloride). An antibacterial and antifungal agent, used in the treatment of tinea pedis and other fungous infections.

BIR Basal insulin requirement; Basic incidence rate; British Institute of Radiology.

BIREME Biblioteca Regional de Medícina (Brazil).

BIRK Rabbit kidney cells.

Birth The act or process of being born, as in:
Breech birth - in which the baby is born feet, knees, or buttocks first.
Cross birth - labor with the fetus lying in the transverse position in the womb.
Dead birth = Stillbirth (see).
Head birth - Head-presenting birth.
Live birth - in which the body exhibits any sign of life, such as breathing, heart beat, umbilical cord pulsation, or muscle movement.
Multiple birth - the birth of two or more babies produced in the same gestation period.
Post-term birth - birth of a post-term or postmature baby.
Premature birth - birth of a premature infant.
Stillbirth - birth of a fetus which during or before delivery, has lost all signs of antenatal life, heartbeat, movement, etc. (= Dead birth).

BIS Body's immune system; Bone cement implantation syndrome; Brain-imaging studies/dy; Brain Information Service (UCLA); Building illness syndrome; Sodium bicarbonate and invert sugar.

bis (L.) twice.

bis- prefix meaning two/ twice (L. bis).

BIS-GMA Bisphenol-A and glycidyl methacrylate (see GMA).

Bis ind Twice a day/ Twice daily (see Bis in die).

Bis in 7d Twice a week. (= biw); twice in 7 days (L. bis in septum diebus).

Bis in die (L.) Twice a day/ Twice daily (= BD; bd; bid; Bis ind).

BISp; BISP Between ischial spines (pelvic measurement).

bisp bispinous diameter (see Bisp diam).

Bisp diam Bispinous diameter (= bisp) (pelvic measurement).

BIST British Institute of Surgical Technicians, Inc.

BIT Biological/ Brain-imaging technique/test (see CAT; CT; MRI; NIT; PET); Bitrochanteric (between great/ greater trochanters).

bit binary digit.

BITP Benzisothiazole piperazine.

BITU Benzyl thiourea.

BIU Barrier isolation unit; Basic intelligence unit.

BIV Bolus intravenous (injection); Bovine immunodeficiency virus.

BIV → FIV → SIV → HIV Mutation evolution of the immunodefiency virus from cattle → cat → monkey → human.

biw Twice a week (L., Eng. bis in week) (see Bis in 7d).

BIZ-PLT Bizarre platelets.

BJ Bence Jones (protein/ proteinuria); Biceps jerk; Bielschowsky-Jansky (syndrome); Biochemical/ Biophysics Journal; Bone and joint (see B&J).

B-J Bezold-Jarisch (reflex) - bradycardia and hypotension from enhanced vagal activity (as occurs sometimes in Myocardial Infarction, etc.).

B&J Bone(s) and joint(s) (= BJ).

BJA British Journal of Addiction/ Anaesthesia/ Audiology.

BJC British Journal of Cancer/ Chiropody.

BJCP British Journal of Clinical Practice/ Pharmacology.

BJD British Journal of Dermatology.

BJDC British Journal of Diseases of the Chest; British Journal of Disorders of Communication.

BJDR Baby Jane Doe regulations (established in 1984 by the USHHSD. Also called Baby Doe rules) (see USHHSD).

BJE Bone and joint/ Bones, joints, and examination.

BJEP British Journal of Experimental Pathology.

BJH British Journal of Haematology.

BJHM British Journal of Hospital Medicine.

BJIM British Journal of Industrial Medicine.

BJM Benign juvenile melanoma (= CMC or Compound melanocytoma; SCN or Spindle cell nevus; Spitz nevus); Bones, joints, and muscles.

BJME British Journal of Medical Education.

BJMH British Journal of Medical Hypnotism.

BJMP British Journal of Medical Psychology.

BJMS British Journal of Mental Subnormality (BSSMS).

BJN British Journal of Nutrition.

BJO British Journal of Ophthalmology/ Orthodontics (BSSO).

BJOS British Journal of Oral Surgery.

BJP Bence-Jones protein/ proteinuria; British Journal of Pharmacology/ Psychiatry (RCP); British Journal of Psychology.

BJPMIH British Journal of Physical Medicine and Industrial Hygiene.

BJPO British Journal of Physiological Optics (BOA).

BJ protein Bence-Jones protein (= BJP).

BJPS British Journal of Plastic Surgery.

BJPSM British Journal of Preventive and Social Medicine.

BJR British Journal of Radiology (BIR).

BJRL Bone & Joint Research Laboratory (DVAMC).

BJS British Journal of Surgery (ASGBI).

BJT British Journal of Tuberculosis.

BJU British Journal of Urology.

BJVD British Journal of Venereal Disease.

BK Below knee (with reference to amputation stump, fracture, or Plaster of Paris application) (see BKA); Bovine kidney (cells); Bradykinin; Bullous keratopathy.

Bk Berkelium (Z = 97) (see Elements - Berkelium).

B/K Bladder/kidney.

B-K Initials of two patients after whom a multiple cutaneous nevus (mole) was named.

bk back.

BKA Below-knee amputation (= BK; BK amp).

BK-A Basophil kallikrein of anaphylaxis.

BK amp Below-knee amputation (see BKA).

BKC Blepharo-keratoconjunctivitis.

Bkf; bkf; Bkfst; bkfst; Bkft; bkft Breakfast.

Bkg Background.

BKS Barrel knot suture (see Sut); Bassen-Kornzweig syndrome (see ABLP); Beekeeper serum.

BKTT Below knee to toe.

BKU Back up.

BKV Bovine kidney virus (see HPV).

BK virus Bovine kidney virus (see HPV).

BKVN BK virus nephropathy (see HPV).

BKWP Below knee walking plaster.

BL Barré-Lieou (syndrome); Basal lamina; Baseline; Baseline latency; Before lunch; Bessey-Lowry (method/ unit); Biocontainment laboratory; Bioluminescence; Black light; Bland; Blast cell(s); Bleeding; Blind loop; Blood level/ loss; Bone marrow lymphocyte; Borderline lepromatous; Bronchial lavage; Buccolingual; Burkitt's lymphoma.

B-L Buschke-Loewenstein (syndrome) (= GCA - Giant condyloma acuminata).

Bl Black; Bladder; Blood.

bl bath (L. balneum); black; bleeding; blood;

blue.

B-l Bursa-equivalent lymphocyte.

B&L Bausch and Lomb, Inc.

BL 139 Aminopentamide sulfate (= Dimevamide sulfate; Valemeramide sulfate). An anticholinergic drug, used as an antispasmodic in the symptomatic treatment of gastric and duodenal ulcer, and in other visceral conditions for which atropine is indicated.

BL 700B Ambutonium bromide (= R 100). A drug having peripheral anticholinergic actions similar to those of atropine; used in the treatment of peptic ulcer, and to reduce hypermotility of the gastro-intestinal tract.

BLA Benign lymphadenopathy (see GGCH); Beta-lactam antibiotics; Biologic assay (= Bioassay); Biological activity.

black beauty biphetamine capsule (see Amphet).

black pill opium (see Papaver).

black Russian hashish (see Cannabis).

black stuff opium (see Papaver).

β-lactam antibiotics Bactericidal agents which inhibit cell wall synthesis in bacteria, such as the penicillins, cephalosporins and monobactams (aztreonam, etc.).

BLAD Borderline left axis deviation.

blad bladder.

Blanc (Fr.) White, e.g. Blanc fixe or Barium sulfate.

blanco heroin (see Diamorph HCl).

-blast- combining form meaning an object in an early stage of growth (Gr. blastos).

BLAT Blind Learning Aptitude Test.

BLB Baker-Lima-Baker (mask); Bessey-Lowry-Brock (method/ unit); Black light bulb; Bone-ligament-bone (complex) (Orthopedics); Boothby-Lovelace-Bulbulian (oxygen mask); Bulb (syringe).

BLBK Blood bank.

BL = BS Bilateral equal breath sounds.

BlC Base-line characteristic(s); Blood culture (= bl cult) (laboratory/ bacteriology).

BLCL Burkitt's lymphoma cell line.

bl cult Blood culture (see BlC).

BLD Basal liquefactive degeneration; Benign lymphoepithelial disease; Bilineage differentiation; Bitrochanteric lipodystrophy (common in women); Black lung disease (anthracosis, asbestosis, pneumoconiosis, silicosis, etc); Bullous lung disease.

Bld; bld Blood.

bldg bleeding.

bld tm bleeding time.

BLE Baseline endoscopy; Both lower extremities.

BLE; βLE Beta-lactamase enzyme.

BLEL Benign lympho-epithelial lesion.

BLEO Bleomycin (see Blm).

-blep- combining form meaning look/ see (Gr. blepo).

Bleph; bleph Blepharitis.

blephar- combining form meaning eyelid (Gr. blepharon).

BLESS Bath, laxative, enema, shampoo, and shower.

BLF Baseline fracture; British Lung Foundation; Bubble lattice file.

BLFD Buccolinguofacial dyskinesia.

BLG Beta-lactoglobulin.

BLH; BLHTN Baseline hypertension.

BL-H Bristol Laboratories code for experimental substances.

blH Biologically active luteinizing hormone.

BLHS Base-line hypertension status.

BLI Base-line information; Benign lymphocytic infiltration; Bombesin-like immunoreactivity.

BLI, βLI Beta-lactamase inhibitor.

BLIP Brookhaven Linac isotope producer.

Blk; blk Black.

BLL Base-line level; Below lower limit; Bilateral lower lobe.

BLLD British Lending Library Division.

BL leprosy Borderline-lepromatous leprosy.

BLM Baseline morbidity/ mortality; Bilayer lipid membrane; Bimolecular liquid membrane; Bleomycin (see Blm); Borderline myocarditis; Buccolinguomasticatory.

Blm Bleomycin (= Blenoxane; BLEO; BLM).

BLMT Buccolinguomasticatory triad (of uncontrollable head, jaw, lip, & tongue movements seen in tardive dyskinesia).

BLN Beta-lactamase negative (= Penicillinase negative) (= Positive culture for microorganisms resistant to Penicillin drugs); Bronchial lymph node.

BLNK B-cell linker (adapter/ mutant protein).

Blntd Balantidium. A genus of Protozoa, e.g. Blntd. coli.
BLOBS; Bl obs; bl obs Bladder observation/ obstruction.
block opium (see Papaver).
blockbuster Barbiturate pill (see Barb).
blond hash hashish/ marijuana (see Cannabis).
Blood (journal of hematology).
BLOT British Library of Tape (Recordings).
BLP Balloon-like protusion (e.g. in a blood vessel, as in brain aneurysm); Beta-lipoprotein; Biologic psychiatry.
Bl P; bl p Blood pressure (see B/P).
BLP 413 Diphenicillin sodium (= SKF 12141; Sodium 2-Biphenylylpenicillin). A semi-synthetic penicillin compound with a specific range of antibacterial activity, particularly affecting staphylococci.
B-LPH Beta-lipoprotein hormone.
B-LPN Beta-lipotropin.
BLPO Beta-lactamase-producing organism.
bl pr blood pressure (see BP).
BLQ Both lower quadrants.
BLRA British Leprosy Relief Association.
BLROA British Laryngological, Rhinological, and Otological Association.
BLS Bacteria-laden stool (in Colon diverticulitis, Peritonitis, etc.); Bare lymphocyte syndrome; Basic life support (CPR); Blind loop syndrome; Blood and lymphatic system; Blood sugar (see BlS); Bloom syndrome (see BlS); Borderline schizophrenia (also called Latent schizophrenia, PNS or Pseudoneurotic schizophrenia, PPS or Pseudopsychopathic schizophrenia); Bureau of Labor Statistics.
BlS Blood sugar (= BLS); Bloom syndrome (= BLS).
BLSA Baltimore Longitudinal Study on Aging.
BLSD Bovine lumpy skin disease.
BLSP Basic life support procedure.
BLT Benign liver tumor (see BHT); Bleeding time (see Blx); Blood-lead test; Blood-clot lysis time; Blood test/ type/ typing (see BlT).
BlT Bleeding time (= BLx); Blood test/ type/ typing (= BLT).
Bl time Bleeding time (see Blx).
BLU; B-LU Bessey-Lowry unit.
Blue Amytal/ Numorphan (see Barb).
Blue acid LSD-25 (see LSD).
Bluebird Sodium amytal capsule (see Barb).
Blue heaven Amytal capsule (see Barb).
BLV Base-line value/ volume; Blood viscosity/ volume (see BlV); Bovine leukemia virus.
BlV Blood viscosity/ volume (= BLV).
BLVB Baylor Left Ventricular Bypass (device).
BLVL Baseline virus load.
BLVR Biliverdin reductase.
Blx Bleeding time (= BLT; BlT; Bl time).
B lymphocyte (= B cell). Bone marrow-derived lyphocyte (a potential synthesizer of immunoglobulins).
BM Bachelor of Medicine (= BMed; MB); Balneum maris (L.) - sea-water bath (see bm); Barotitis media (or 'airplane ears') - caused by pressure differential in the middle ear during flight; Basal medium/ metabolism; Basement/ Basilar membrane; Behavior modification; Betamethasone; Biomass; Biomedical; Biomedical Medicine (journal); Black male (see B/M); Body/ Buccal mass; Boehringer Mannheim (test); Bohr magneton; Bone marrow; Bowel movement; Breast milk; British Medicine (journal); Buccal margin (see MB); Buccomesial; Bureau of Medicine (FDA).
bm Salt-water/ Sea-water bath (= BM) (L. balneum maris).
B/M Black male (= BM).
B2M; ß2M Beta-2-microglobulin.
BMA Bacterial mutation assay (Ames test); Bavarian Medical Association (Fed. Rep. of Germany); BioMonitoring Applications, Inc.; Bone marrow arrest/ aspirate; British Medical Association.
BmA Brugia malayi adult (antigen).
BMAP Biventricular microaxial pump (= BMP); Bone marrow acid phosphatase.
BMB Biomedical belt; Biomolecular barrier (protecting the brain); Bone marrow biopsy; Bone mineral balance; British Medical Bulletin.
BMBL Benign monoclonal B cell lymphocytosis.
BMC Benign mesenchymoma; Blood mononuclear cell; B-mode contrast

(Echocardiogram); Boehringer Mannheim Corporation; Bone marrow cell; Bone mineral content; Brain Mapping Center (Ahmanson-Lovelace, UCLA).

BMD Basophilic myocardial degeneration; Becker's muscular dystrophy; Benign mammary disease/ disorder; Boehringer Mannheim Diagnostics; Bone marrow damage/ density/ depression/ disease/ disorder/ donor/ dysplasia; Bone mineral density; Boston Medical Center; Bovine mucosal disease; Bureau of Medical Devices (EHD; HPB).

BMDC Bangladesh Medical and Dental Council; Biomedical Documentation Center.

BMDDP Bureau of Medical Devices and Diagnostic Products (FDA).

BME Basal medium, Eagle's (culture medium); Biomedical engineering; Bis (N-maleimidomethyl) ether; Biundulant meningoencephalitis; Bone marrow exam(ination); Brief maximal effort.

BMED Biomedical engineering device (used in the treatment of SCI).

BMed Bachelor of Medicine (see BM).

BMedBiol Bachelor of Medical Biology.

BMedSci Bachelor of Medical Science.

BMEI Biomedical Engineering and Instrumentation Branch (NIH).

BMES Biomedical Engineering Society.

BMET Biomedical electronic/ engineering/ equipment technician.

BMF Black married female; Bone marrow failure/ fibrosis/ function; Bovine milk fat.

BMG Benign monoclonal gammopathy; Bone-marrow graft(ing).

BMH British Ministry of Health.

BMHR Basal metabolic heart rate.

BMI Bio-Medical Insight (journal); Biomedical instrumentation; Body-mass index (= Weight in kg/height^2 in meters); Body-mind interaction.

BMic Bachelor of Microbiology.

BMJ Bones, muscles, joints; Breast milk jaundice; British Medical Journal (BMA).

Bmk; bmk Birthmark.

BML Bell-Magendie law (an axiom stating that the inner nerves of the spinal cord control muscular movement and the external nerves control the senses (= Bell's law; Magendie's law); Biomolecular level; Bone marrow lymphocytosis; Bone mineral loss.

BMLH Businessman's lunchtime high; Dimethyl tryptamine (see DMT).

BMLS Billowing mitral leaflet syndrome.

BMM Black married male; Bone micrometastases/sis; Boundary maintenance mechanism(s) (behavior and practices that keep out members of one group from the customs and values of another).

BMMD Body mass measurement device.

BMMP Benign mucous membrane pemphigoid/gus.

BMN Bone marrow necrosis; Breast malignant neoplasm.

BMNC Blood mononuclear cell.

BMOC Brinster's medium for ovum culture.

BMod; Bmod Behavior modification (therapy).

B-mode Brightness modulation.

BMP Barometric pressure (= Atmospheric pressure - the pressure of the weight of the atmosphere, at sea level approx. 14.7 pounds per sq. inch and at 30,000 feet above sea level, only 4.3 pounds per square inch); Behavior management plan; Benign mastopathy; Bimanual palpation; Biomechanical properties/perty (Orthopedics) (see BMS; CBS); Biventricular microaxial pump (see BMAP); Bone morphogenetic protein; Brain-mapping project.

BMPAL Bureau of Medical Practitioner Affairs Limited (UK).

BMPase Bone morphogenetic proteinase.

BMPI Bronchial mucous proteinase inhibitor.

BMPRSC Biomedical Pattern Recognition Subcommittee (IEEE Computer Society).

BMQA Board of Medical Quality Assurance.

BMR Basal metabolic rate; Best motor response; Bibliography of Medical Reviews (contained in Index Medicus of NLM); Biomedical research; Bone marrow recipient; Bone mass reserve; Buttock-meter reading (Orthopedics).

BMRC Biomedical research community; British Medical Research Council.

BMS Bachelor of Medical Science(s); Betamethasone; Biomechanical study (of

Knowles pins and other prosthetic devices) (see CBS); Biomedical monitoring system; Biomedical science; Bleomycin sulfate; Bone marrow sarcoma/ suppression; Bottle-mouth syndrome (see NBC or Nursing-bottle caries); Buccal-mucosa scraping; Bureau of Medical Services; Bureau of Medicine and Surgery (US Navy); Burning mouth syndrome.

BMSA British Medical Students Association.

BMSB Bis-methylstyryl benzene (scintillator).

BMSC Bone marrow stem cell.

BMSF Bristol-Myers Squibb Foundation.

BMSH Beta melanocyte-stimulating hormone (= B hormone) (see Hormones - MSH).

BMSJ British Medical and Surgical Journal (now NEJM); British Medical Students Journal.

BMSSVD British Medical Society for the Study of Venereal Diseases.

BMST Bruce maximal/mum stress test.

BMT Bachelor of Medical Technology; Basement membrane thickening; Behavioral modification technique; Behavior modification therapy; Benign mesenchymal tumor; Bilateral myringotomy and tubes; Bone marrow transplant(ation)/ toxicity; Bronchomotor tone.

BMTP Bone marrow transplant patient.

BMTT Bilateral myringotomy with tympanic tubes.

BMTU Bone marrow transplant unit.

BMU Basic metabolic unit; Basic multicellular unit.

BMV Bioprosthetic mitral valve.

BMW Bulbar muscle weakness.

BMZ Basement membrane zone.

BN Bedside Nurse (journal); Behavioral Neuropsychiatry (journal); Biology of the Neonate (journal); Biomedical News (journal); Bladder neck; Brain News (journal); Brachial neuralgia (= NAT); Branchial/ Bronchial neuritis; Bronchial node; Brown Norway (rat); Bulimia nervosa; Bulimic neurosis; Bulletin on Narcotics (US).

BNA Basle Nomina Anatomica (Basel anatomical nomenclature); Beta-naphthylamine (an organic compound used in aniline dyes and a cause of bladder cancer in humans).

BNC Baseline neutrophil count; Bladder neck contracture.

BNCDS British National Child Develepmont Study.

BNCT Boron neutron capture therapy.

BND Barely noticeable difference; Bulletin of Narcotic Drugs (now Bulletin on Narcotics); 'Bullneck' diphtheria (fulminant form of diphtheria).

BNDD Bureau of Narcotics and Dangerous Drugs (now DEA).

BNEd Bachelor of Nursing Education.

BNF British National Formulary; British Nutrition Foundation.

BNFC Bulletin of the National Formulary Committee.

BNFL British Nuclear Fuels Ltd.

BNIH Bulletin of the National Institutes of Health (formerly, HLB).

BNIST Bureau National d'Information Scientifique (Fr.: National Bureau of Scientific Information).

BNL Brookhaven National Laboratory (Upton, New York).

BNLC Benign nocturnal leg cramps (= NLC; NLMC).

BNMC Bethesda Naval Medical Center.

BNO Bladder-neck obstruction; Bowels not opened.

BNP Benign neoplasm; Blocked nasal passage(s); B-type natriuretic peptide (such as Nesiritide, a recombinant therapy for CHF or Congestive heart failure).

BNPA Binasal pharyngeal airway.

BNR Bladder neck retraction.

BNS Behavioral neuroscientist; Benign nephrosclerosis.

BNSc Bachelor of Nursing Science.

BNST Bed nucleus of the Stria terminalis (situated in front and just below the thalamus and above the Amygdala, at the base of the brain: it is the emotional core of the brain triggering the fear response, and when activated it perpuates it, with continuation of unease and anxiety).

BNT Barrier nursing technique; Bionanotechnology; Boston Naming Test; Brain neurotransmitter.

BNW Below-normal weight (Obs./Pediatrics).

BNYVV Beet necrotic yellow vein virus.
BO Bachelor of Osteopathy; Bad odor; Base (of prism) out; Behavior objective; Belladonna and opium (see B&O); Body odor; Bolton (see Bo); Bowel obstruction; Bowel(s) open; Bucco-occlusal.
Bo Bohemium. Former name of the element, now called Rhenium (Re). Z = 75 (see Elements - Rhenium); Bolton (craniometric point) (= BO; BP); Bowel(s) (see bo).
bo bowel(s) (= Bo).
B&O Belladonna and opium (= BO) (medical orders/ prescriptions).
BOA Behavior observation audiometry; Born on arrival; Born out of asepsis; British Optical/ Orthopaedic Association; Butoxyacetanilide.
BoA Bursa of Achilles.
BoaS Beads-on-a-string (sign = CWS/ Obs/Gyn).
BOB Ball on back; Benign osteoblastoma; Bureau of Biologics (FDA).
BOBA Beta-oxybutyric acid.
BOC Blood oxygen capacity; Bone organ culture (Orthopedics); Bureau of Census; Butyloxycarbazate/bonyl.
BoCarAl Boric acid, carbolic acid (phenol), alum.
BOCES Boards of Cooperative Educational Services.
BOD Bilateral orbital decompression; Biochemical/ Biological oxygen demand; Board of Directors; Bodansky (unit) (see Bod); Bureau of Drugs.
Bod Bodansky (unit) (= BOD).
BOE Bilateral otitis externa.
BOEA Ethyl biscoumacetate (= Bis-oxy-coumarin-ethylacetate; Ethyldicoumarol; Neodicumarin). An anticoagulant drug, more rapidly absorbed and excreted than dicoumarol. Maximum therapeutic effect is obtained within 24 hours, and the prothombin time usually returns to normal within 48 hours.
BOF Binocular fixation.
BOF; BO# Blow-out fracture (a broken bone beneath the eyeball caused by a blow that suddenly increases intra-ocular pressure).
BoF Ball of (the) foot.
BOH Board Of Health.
BoH Bundle of His.
BOHB; ßOHB D-beta-hydroxybutyrate.
6B-OH-F 6B, 11B, 170C, 21, tetrahydroxypregn-4-3,20-dioxide.
BOI Bone-osteoid interface (Orthopedics).
Boil Boiling.
BOJ Benign obstructive jaundice.
Bol; bol Bolus or large pill (L. bolus).
bol- combining form meaning throw (Gr.).
BOL-148 d-2-bromolysergic acid (see LSD).
BOLD Bleomycin, Oncovin, Lomustine, Dacarbazine.
Bolivian marching powder Cocaine (see Erythroxylum).
BOM Bilateral otitis media; Biological oxygen monitor; Bureau of Medicine (FDA).
BOMA Bilateral otitis media, acute.
Bomber A barbiturate or a marijuana cigarette (see Barb; Cannabis).
BOMS Bulletin de l'Organisation Mondiale de la Santé (= BWHO or Bulletin of the World Health Organization).
Bonita Milk sugar used to dilute heroin (see Diamorph HCl).
BOO Bladder outlet obstruction.
Boo Marijuana (see Cannabis).
BOOP Bronchiolitis obliterans-organizing pneumonia.
BOP Binocular parallax (a major factor in depth perception; also called SSP or Stereoscopic parallax); Biocompatible osteoconductive polymer; Bipolar operational power (supply); Buffalo orphan prototype (virus).
BOR Basal optic root; Before time of operation; Benevolent over-reaction; Board of Registry (ASCP, formerly RMT); Bowels open regularly; Branchio-oto-renal (syndrome).
BORR Blood oxygen release rate.
Bos (L.) Cow, e.g. B. sinicus - Schistosomiasis in cattle.
BOSH Bureau of Occupational Safety and Health (ECA).
BoSM Bolivian squirrel monkey.
BOSS Bureau of State Security.
BOT Binovular/ Biovular twins (see DZT); Butorphanol tartrate (a narcotic given before

and during surgery).
BOT; BoT Base of tongue; Botulinum toxin.
Bot Botanical/ny.
bot bottle.
Botox Botulinum toxin.
BOU Branchio-oto-ureteral (syndrome).
Bouncing powder Cocaine (see Erythroxylum).
BOV Binocular vision; Brown oil of Vitriol (= Sulfuric acid).
BOW Bag of waters (amniotic sac).
Boy Heroin (see Diamorph HCl).
BP Bachelor of Pharmacy (see BPharm); Back pain/ pressure; Barometric pressure; Basic protein; Bathroom privileges (= BPR); Bed pan (see bp); Before the present; Behavior pattern; Bell's/ Bulbar palsy; Benzoyl peroxide; Benzpyrine (= benzapyrine/zopyrine - a carcinogen); Benzyl penicillin; Beta-protein; Bichromatic photometry; Biochemical Pharmacology (journal); Biological parent; Biological Psychiatry (SPB journal); Biotic potential; Biparietal (diameter of head - see BPD); Biphenyl; Bipolar; Birthplace; Blood pressure (see B/P); Body phlethysmography; Boiling point (see bp); Bolton point (see Bo); Borderline personality; British Petroleum; British Pharmacopoeia (see BPh); Bronchopleural; Bubonic plague (caused by *Yersinia* pestis, of the family of gram-negative bacteria, *Enterobacteriaceae*); Buccopulpal; Bulletin of Pharmacy (journal); Bullous pemphigus; Butylphenol; Bypass (operation/ cardiovascular).
bp base pair (of double-stranded DNA); bed pan (= BP); boiling point (= BP).
B/P Blood pressure (= Bl P; bl p; BP).
BP I Bipolar (affective disorder), type I.
BPA Back Pain Association (UK); Basophilic adenoma; Benign pancreatic adenoma; Biological Photographic Association; Blood pressure assembly; Bovine plasma albumin; Brachial plexus anesthesia; British Paediatric Association; Bronchopulmonary aspergillosis; Burst-promoting activity.
BPAA Biphenylacetic acid (an active metabolite of the NSAID agent, Fenbufen).
BPAC Blood Products Advisory Committee (FDA).
BPAEC Bovine pulmonary artery endothelial cell.
BPAN Black Psychiatrists of America Newsletter.
BPAR Biopsy-proven acute rejection.
BPAS Benzamido-salicylic acid sodium (salt).
BPB Biliopancreatic bypass; Bipolar pacemaker battery; Bromophenol/Bromphenol blue.
BPBD Butylphenyl-biphenyl-oxadiazole (scintillator).
BPC Basis pedunculi cerebri (a part of the brain consisting of nerve fibers that descend from the cerebral cortex to form the nerve bundles of the pons) (= Crus cerebri); Behavior Problem Checklist; Bile phospholipid concentration; Blood pressure check/ control/ cuff; Bonded-phase chromatography; British Pharmaceutical Codex (PSGB)/ Conference; British Pharmacopoeia Commission.
BPD Benzoporphyrin derivative (a light-sensitive compound); Biliopancreatic disease/ disorder/ diversion; Biopsy-proved disease; Biparietal diameter (of head) (= BP); Bipolar disorder (see BD); Blood pressure decrease; Borderline personality disorder; Bowen's precancerous dermatosis (see IEC); Branch pulmonary displasia; Bronchopulmonary disease/ displasia.
BPd Diastolic blood pressure.
BPDE Broparodioestrol.
BPDE-I Benzo(a)pyrene dihydrodiol epoxide - I (a substance found in tobacco smoke that causes cancer).
BPE Bacterial phosphatidylethanolamine; Benign prostate enlargement (see BPH); Blood pressure elevation.
BPEC Benign partial epilepsy of children; Bipolar electrocardiogram.
BPEI Blepharophimosis-ptosis-epicanthus inversus.
BPEIS Blepharophimosis-ptosis-epicanthus inversus syndrome.
BPF Bone peg fixation (= CBPF); Bradykinin-potentiating factor; Bronchopleural/ pulmonary fistula; Burst-promoting factor.
BPG Benzathine penicillin G; Bipolar pulse

generator (pacemaker); Blood pressure gauge; Body plethysmograph(y); Bypass graft.

BPH Bachelor of Public Health; Benign prostatic hyperplasia/ hypertrophy.

BPh British Pharmacopoeia (= BP; PhB); Buccopharyngeal.

BpH Blood pH (hydrogen ion concentration or acidity/ alkalinity of the blood).

Bph Bacteriopheophytin.

BPHA Bureau for Population and Humanitarian Assistance (AID).

BPharm Bachelor of Pharmacy (= BP).

BPHEng Bachelor of Public Health Engineering.

BPHMD Benign pseudohypertrophic muscular dystrophy (= BMD or Becker's muscular dystrophy).

BPHN Bachelor of Public Health Nursing.

BPI Basic Personality Inventory; Beef-pork insulin; Biparental inheritance (= Amphigonous inheritance; Duplex inheritance); Blood pressure increase; Brachial plexus injury; Brief Pain Inventory (a validated pain measurement scale); British Pharmaceutical Industry.

bpi bits per inch (magnetic tape).

BPI-71-1 High-protein rice.

BPL Basophilic leukemia; Benign proliferative lesion; Benzylpenicilloyl-polylysine; Beta-propiolactone (= B-propiolactone; ß-propiolactone; Propiolactone) - a powerful disinfectant used mainly for the gaseous sterilization of pharmaceutical and surgical materials. Recently reported to be a carcinogen; Blood pressure level; Brachial plexus lesion.

BPLA Blood pressure, left arm; Blood-pressure-lowering activity.

BP 120/80 LA/LAr/lar Blood pressure 120 (systolic), 80 (diastolic), left arm reclining/ recumbent.

BPLE Blood pressure lowering effect (of drugs).

BPM Beats per minute (see bpm); Biperidyl/ Bipiperidyl mustard; Biphasic manner; Blood pressure monitor(ing); Brain pacemaker (= DBS or Deep-brain stimulator); Breaths per minute (see bpm); Brompheniramine maleate; Bulbar poliomyelitis (including the medulla and the brain stem).

bpm beats per minute (= BPM) (heart/ pulse rate); breaths per minute (= BPM) (respiration rate).

BPMC Banstead Place Mobility Center (UK).

BPMF British Postgraduate Medical Federation.

BPMS Blood plasma measuring system.

BPN Bacitracin, polymyxin B, neomycin sulfate; Brachial plexus neuropathy/ neurapraxia.

BPO Basal pepsin output; Benzyl penicilloyl; Benzoyl peroxide.

BPO-FLYS Benzyl penicilloyl-formyl-lysine.

BPP Biophysical profile; Bipolar programmable pacemaker (Cardiology); Blister-pack pill; Bovine pancreatic polypeptide; Brachial plexus paralysis (as in Erb-Duchenne paralysis or Erb's palsy); Bradykinin potentiating peptide.

BP&P Blood pressure and pulse.

BPPC Biopsy-proven prostate/atic cancer.

BPPN Benign paroxysmal positioning nystagmus.

BPPP Bilateral pedal pulses present.

BPPS Biophysical profile scoring.

BPPV Benign paroxysmal positional vertigo; Bovine paragenital papilloma virus.

BPQ Berne pain questionnaire.

BPR Bilirubin/ Blood production rate (= BRP); Blood per rectum; Blood pressure recorder/ reduction/ response; Brachial plexus repair (Orthopedics).

BPRA Blood pressure, right arm.

BPRS Behavior Psychiatric Rating Scale (= PAS; PRS); Brief Psychiatric Rating/ Reacting Scale.

BPS Bacterial protein synthesis; Bard-Pic syndrome (characterized by progressive jaundice, enlarged gallbladder, and deterioration associated with advanced pancreatic cancer); Barré's pyramidal sign (the inability of the hemiplegic to remain in a flexed position); Basophilic stippling; Beats/ Bits/ Breaths per second; Behavioral Pharmacological Society; Bilateral partial salpingectomy; Biophysical profile scoring; Biophysical score (test for fetal well-being in diabetic pregnancies) (see NRNST); Bovine papular stomatitis; Brain protein solvent; Brief Placement Scale;

British Pharmacological/ Psychoanalytical Society; Bureau of Product Safety (FDA); Bypass surgery.

BPs Systolic blood pressure.

BPSA Bronchopulmonary segmental artery.

BPSD Bronchopulmonary segmental drainage.

BPSP Biopsychosocial phenomenon.

BPsTh Bachelor of Psychotherapy.

BPT Bacteriophage typing; Benign paroxysmal torticollis; Bombay phenotype (a rare genetic trait involving the ABC blood groups; first reported in Bombay, British India); Brief psychotherapy.

BPTI Basic pancreatic/ polyvalent trypsin inhibitor.

BPU Bleeding peptic ulcer(ation).

BPV Benign paroxysmal/ positional vertigo; Bioprosthetic valve; Bovine papilloma virus.

BP(Vet) British Pharmacopoeia (Veterinary).

Bq Becquerel.

BQA Bureau of Quality Assurance (HEW).

BQC Dibromoquinone-chlorimide (= 2,6-dibromoquinone-chlorimide solution). An amebicide, bactericide, and fungicidal agent.

BQT Benedict's qualitative test (for sugar in the urine) (= Benedict's method).

BR Bacteriological Review (journal); Barrier reared (experimental animals); Baseline recovery; Bathroom; Bed/ Bowel rest; Bedside rounds; Benzing retrograde; Bibliography of Reproduction (journal); Bilirubin; Bills receivable; Biologic response; Biological Reviews/ Rhythms (journals); Birth/ Breathing rate; Blink reflex; Boiling range (see br); Botanical Review (joural); Brain Research (journal); Branch (see br); Branchial (see br); British Revision (of BNA, with reference to anatomical nomenclature); Bronchial/chitis/chus (see Br); Brucella (see Br); Brucellosis (see Br); Bulimorexia (binge eating, then vomiting); By report.

Br Breath (see br); Breech; Bregma; Bridge (dental); British (= Brit); Bromide; Bromine (Z = 35) (see Elements - Bromine); Bronchial/chitis/chus (= BR); Broncho- (e.g. Br pn or Br pneumonia); Brown; Brucella (= BR; Bruc) - a genus of small, gram-negative, coccobacilli of the family Brucellaceae); Brucellosis; Plasma unconjugated bilirubin concentration.

br boiling range (= BR); brachial (= Brach); branch (= BR); branchial (= BR); breath (= Br); brother (= Bro; bro).

BRA Bailey rib approximator (General and Thoracic Surgery); Benzodiazepine receptor antagonist (e.g. Flumazenil) (= BDPRA; BDZRA); Beta-resorcylic acid; Bilateral renal agenesis; Bone regeneration ability; Bone-resorbing activity; Brain-reactive antibody.

Bra Brain.

BRAC Basic rest and activity cycle.

Brach Brachial (see br).

brachi- prefix meaning arm (Gr. brachion).

brachy- prefix meaning short (Gr. brachus).

Brady; brady Bradycardia.

brady- prefix meaning slow (Gr. bradus).

Brain (UK journal).

Brain tickler Barbiturate or amphetamine pill (see Barb; Amphet).

BRAO Branch retinal artery occlusion.

BRAP Burst of rapid atrial pacing.

BrAP Brachial artery pressure.

BRAT Bananas, rice (cereal), applesauce, and toast; Baylor rapid autologous transfusion (system).

BRATT Bananas, rice, applesauce, tea and toast.

Braz. P Brazilian Pharmacopoeia (Farmacopeia dos Estados Unidos do Brasil).

BRB Biomedical Research Branch (NIDA); Blood-retinal barrier; Bright red blood; Bronchoreversibility.

β2RB β2-receptor blockade/ blocker.

BRBC Bovine red blood cell.

BRBN Blue rubber bleb nevus.

BRBNS Blue rubber bleb nevus syndrome.

BRBPR Bright red blood per rectum (= BRBR).

BRBR Bright red blood per rectum (see BRBPR).

BRbx Breast biopsy.

BRC Balance-related cue; Blood-related cancer (e.g. leukemias, lymphomas, myelomas, etc.); Bone-resorbing cell (i.e. Osteoclast).

Brc Bromocriptine.

BRCA 1 Breast Cancer 1 (gene).

BRCA 2 Breast Cancer 2 (gene).

BRCM Below right costal margin.

BRCPS Biological Reviews, Cambridge Philosophical Society.
BRCS British Red Cross Society.
BRD Bilirubin direct; Bladder retraining drill; Bovine respiratory disease; Bulletin on Respiratory Diseases (journal).
Brd Bird.
BRDU; BrdU; BrdUrd Bromodeoxyuridine (= 5-bromodeoxyuridine).
"4-7-8" Breath A yogic relaxing breath exercise for overcoming anxiety disorders (this involves inhaling through the nose for 4 seconds, holding the breath for 7 seconds, and exhaling through the mouth for another 8 seconds).
brevis (L.) short.
BRF Behavioral/ Biggest risk factor(s); Bone-resorbing factor; Brain Research Foundation, Inc. (University of Chicago).
BRH Benign recurrent hematuria; Bureau of Radiological Health (FDA).
Brhp Bronchophony.
BRHS British Regional Heart Study.
BRI Bacterial respiratory infection; Behavior Research Institute; Bio-Research Index; Brachial reactivity index; Brain Research Institute (UCLA); Bristol Royal Infirmary (UK); British Royal Infirmary.
BRIC Benign recurrent intrahepatic cholestasis.
BRIME Brief repetitive isometric maximal exercise.
Brit Britain/tish (see Br).
BRJ Brachial radialis jerk.
BRKF; Brkf; BRKT Breakfast.
BRL Beecham Research Laboratories (UK firm).
BRL 152 Phenethicillin potassium (= P 152; Penicillin B; Potassium α-phenoxyethylpenicillin). A penicillin derivative antibiotic.
BRL 284 Propicillin potassium (= PA 248; Potassium α-phenoxypropylpenicillin). A penicillin derivative antibiotic.
BRL 1241 Methicillin sodium (= P 35; X 1497; Dimethyoxyphenicillin sodium; Dimethoxyphenyl penicillin sodium). A penicillin derivative antibiotic.
BRL 1341 Ampicillin (= P 50; {D[-]-α-Aminobenzyl}penicillin). A penicillin derivative antibiotic.
BRL 1400 Oxacillin sodium (= P 12; {5-Methyl-3-phenyl-4-isoxazolyl}penicillin sodium). A penicillin derivative antibiotic.
BRL 1621 Cloxacillin sodium (= P 25; Sodium 3-O-chlorophenyl-5-methyl-4-isoxazolyl-penicillin monohydrate). A penicillin derivative antibiotic.
BRL 1702 Dicloxacillin sodium (= R 13423; Sodium 6-3{3-[2,6-dichlorophenyl]-5-methylisoxazole-4-carboxyamido}penicillinate). A penicillin derivative antibiotic.
BRM Bacterial reverse mutation; Biological response modifier (a substance which boosts the body's immune system, such as interferon and various cytokines); Birth-related morbidity/ mortality; Biuret reactive material; Bone regenerative matrix; Bone-replacement mechanism.
BRMP Bilateral reduction mammoplasty.
BRMT Board of Registry of Medical Technologists.
BRN Board of Registered Nursing.
brn brown.
BRO Bone-resorbing osteoclast; Bronchoscopy (see Bronch).
Bro; bro Bronchoscopy (see Bronch); Brother (see br).
brom bromide.
brom- combining form meaning stench (Gr. bromos).
Bron Bronchoscopy (see Bronch).
Bronch Bronchi/hial/hoscopy/hus (= BR; Br; BRO; Bro; bro; Bron).
bronch- prefix referring to bronchus or windpipe (Gr. brogchos).
Brother Heroin (see Diamorph HCl).
Brown Heroin (see Diamorph HCl).
Brownie Amphetamine (see Amphet).
Brown stuff Opium (see Papaver).
BRP Bacterial receptor protein; Balance-related problem; Bathroom privileges (see BP); Bed-ridden patient/ person; Bilirubin/ Blood production (rate) (see BPR); Biomedical Research Panel; Bone remodeling process; Brain Research Publications; Brief reactive psychosis; Bronchophony (see Brph).
Brph Bronchophony (= BRP).
BrPM Breath(s) per minute.

BRR Baroceptor reflex response; Block-replace regimen (in medical treatment) (see SFHD); Body righting reflex; Brachioradialis reflex (see DTR); Breathing reserve ratio.
BR RAO Branch retinal artery occlusion.
BRS Battered root syndrome; Behavior(al) Rating Scale (for Dementia); Bibliographic Retrieval Services; Biofeedback Research Society; Bladder repair/ replacement surgery; Breast reduction surgery; British Roentgen Society; Buffered Ringer's solution.
BRSH British Royal Society of Health.
BRSI Bureau of Retirement and Survivors Insurance (SSA).
BRSM British Royal Society of Medicine.
BrSM Brazilian squirrel monkey.
BrSo; Br sounds Breath sounds.
BRT Bilirubin, total; Brook reaction test.
BRTA Bureau of Resource and Trade Assistance.
Brth; brth Breath.
BRU Bone remodeling unit.
BRU; BrU Bromide urine.
BrU Bromouracil.
Bruc *Brucella* (see Br).
bruit de canon French: "canon sound" - A type of heart sound or murmur.
BRVO Branch retinal vein occlusion.
BRW Brown-Robert-Wells (stereotactic system).
BRX Bulletin RX (journal).
bry- combining form meaning full of life (Gr. bryo).
BS Bachelor of Science (see BSc)/ Surgery (see ChB); Bacillus subtilis; Balloon septostomy; Bartter/ Behcet/ Bloom syndrome; Barb staple (Orthopedics); Base strap; Beauty shop/ sleep; Bedside; Before sleep/ supper; Bennett seal; Benzyl salicylate; Bilateral symmetrical; Bile salt; Binet-Simon (test) (see B-S); Biological sciences; Biometric/ Biophysical Society; Bismuth sulfate/fite; Boerhaave's syndrome (spontaneous rupture of the esophagus); Blood sugar; Blue Shield (plan); Borderline schizophrenia; Bowel/ Breath sound(s); Breaking strength; British Standard; Buffered saline; Bureau of Standards/ Statistics; Bypass surgery.
Bs Systolic blood pressure.
bs bedside; bowel sound; breath sound.
B-S Binet-Simon (= BS). Intelligence test.
B&S Bartholin's and Skene's (glands); Brown and Sharp (sutures); Brown and Sharpe (standard wire guage - same as AWG).
b X s brother and sister (inbreeding).
BS 572 Cyclandelate. A peripheral vasodilator used in the treatment of vascular disorders due to arterial spasm, such as acrocyanosis, chilblains, erythrocyanosis, and Raynaud's disease.
BS 5930 Orphenadrine hydrochloride (= Mephenamine HCl). It has an inhibitory effect on cerebral motor areas, resembling the central effect of atropine. Used in the symptomatic treatment of rigidity in paralysis agitans, and other cases of Parkinsonism; also to reduce the extra-pyramidal side-effects of neuroleptic drugs, such as the phenothiazines.
BS 6987 Deptropine citrate (= Dibenzheptropine citrate). Has the properties and uses of the antihistamine drugs. It is much more potent than promethazine hydrochloride, and has marked anticholinergic and antiserotonin properties.
BSA Bacteriostatic agent (inhibitory); Benzenesulfonic acid; Biofeedback Society of America; Bismuth sulfate/fite agar; Bis-trimethylsilyl-acetamide; Blind Service Association; Blue Shield Association; Body surface area; Botanical Society of America; Bovine serum albumin (see bsa); Bowel sounds active; Boy Scouts of America; Breakseal ampoule; Broad-spectrum antibiotherapy/otic; Bronchosecretolytic action (see BSL).
bsa bovine serum albumin (= BSA).
B2SA Beta 2 stimulating agent.
BSAB Balthazar Scales of Adaptive Behavior.
BSABA Broad spectrum antibacterial agent.
BSAEP Brain stem auditory evoked potential (EEG).
BSAG Bristol Social Adjustment Guides.
BSAM Basic sequential access method.
BSAP Bone-specific alkaline phosphatase; Brief short-action potential; Brief, small, abundant potentials.
BSAVA British Small Animal Veterinary Association.

BSB Bedside bag; Body surface burned; Brookhaven Symposia in Biology.

BS = BL Breath sounds equal bilaterally.

BSC Basophilic stippling of (red blood) cells; Bedside care/ commode; Bench scale calorimeter; Bennet's small corpuscle(s) (transparent cell[s] found sometimes in the fluid of ovarian cysts) (= Drysdale's corpuscle); Best supportive care; Bilateral stereotactic cingulotomy (see LSS); Bile salt concentration; Biological Stain Commission; Biomedical Science Corps; Blood sugar control; Burn scar contracture.

BSc Bachelor of Science (= BS; SB; ScB).

BSC-1; BS-C-1 Cercopithecus monkey kidney cells.

BSCABB Bulletin of the South Central Association of Blood Banks.

B scale (see B) Baumé scale; Benoist scale.

BSCB Bulletin de la Société Chimie Biologique (Fr.) - Bulletin of the Biochemical Society.

BSCC Basosquamous cell carcinoma (= BCC); Biotechnology Science Coordinating Committee; British Society for Clinical Cytology.

BSCEP Brain stem and cortical evoked potential (see AEP; BSEP).

BSCP Bovine spinal cord protein.

BSCS Biological Sciences Curriculum Study (NSF).

BSD Baby soft diet; Bacterial sputum density; Bedside drainage; Body-scheme disorder (see ATP); Brain stem death/ disease/ disorder; Breath sounds diminished; Brill-Symmer's disease (see GFL; GFLA); Bronchospastic disease/ disorder (see OLD; OPD).

BSDLB Block in anterosuperior division of left branch.

BSE Bachelor of Science in Engineering; Backscattered electron (imaging) (see BSEI); Bacteriologic sputum examination; Bad side effect(s); Behavior summarized evaluation; Bilateral(ly) symmetrical and equal; Bovine spongiform encephalopathy (see Agent X); Brain stem encephalitis; Breast self-examination.

BSEI Backscattered electron image/ imaging (analysis/ technique).

BSEP Brain stem evoked potential.

BSepF Black separated female.

BSepM Black separated male.

BSER Brain stem evoked response (audiometry).

BSF Back scatter factor (X-rays); Black single female; Bradford solid/ split frame; Bromsulfalein; Bromsulfein; Bureau of Sport Fisheries and Wildlife (Dept of Interior, now FWS); Busulfan (= BUS).

BSG Brain stem glioma; Branchio-skeleto-genital (syndrome); British Society of Gastroenterology.

BSGA Beta Streptococcus group A.

BSGH; BSGh Biosynthetic growth hormone.

BSGT "Be Safe. Get Tested" (HIV/AIDS campaign, US).

BSH Brain-stem herniation.

BSHR Baseline fetal heart rate.

BSI Bacterial skin infection; Behavior Status Inventory; Body substance isolation; Borderline Syndrome Index; Bound serum iron; Brainstem injury; British Society of Immunology; British Standards Institution; Bromosuccinimide.

BSID Bayley Scale of Infant Development.

BSIF Bile salt independent fraction.

BSJR Bureau of Standards Journal of Research.

BSL Benign symmetric lipomatosis; Bio-Science Laboratories; Bisexual libido; Blood sugar level; Broad-spectrum light; Bronchosecretolytic (such as acetylcysteine, bromhexine, carbocysteine, and streptokinase-streptodornase enzymes).

BSL 1,2,3, etc. Biosafety level 1,2,3, etc. (Lab) (CDC).

BSM Bachelor of Science in Medicine; Bedside manner; Behavior/ Body systems model; Bile salt metabolism; Black single male; Bronchial smooth muscle.

BSMJ British Medical Students' Journal.

BSMT Board of Schools of Medical Technology.

BSN Bachelor of Science in Nursing; Benign skin neoplasia (= SBN); Bone scan negative; Bowel sounds normal.

BSNA Bowel sounds normal and active.

BSNE Bachelor of Science in Nursing

Education.

BSNT Breast soft and non-tender.

BSO Bean-shaped organelle (such as a mitochondrion); Bilateral sagittal osteotomy (operation/ orthopedics); Bilateral salpingo-oophorectomy (operation/ gynecology); British School of Osteopathy; Buthionine sulfoximine (a chemotherapeutic anti-cancer drug).

BSOM Bilateral serous otitis media.

BSP Biosynthesis pathway; Brachial systolic pressure; Breast screening procedure/programme; Broad spectrum penicillin (see BSA); Bromsulphalein (sodium) (= Bromsulphophthalein Sodium; SBP; Sulfobromophthal Sod; Sulphobromophthalein Sodium) - Used for testing the functional capacity of the liver, particularly of its reticuloendothelial cells (see LFT iv).

BSp Bronchospasm.

BSPA Bowel sounds present and active.

BSPh Bachelor of Science in Pharmacy.

BSPM Body surface potential mapping.

BSQ Behavior Style Questionnaire.

BSR Basal skin resistance (compare GSR); Basic science research; Blood sedimentation rate (see ESR); Bowel sounds regular; Brain stem response (see ABSR); Brain stimulation reinforcement; British Society of Rheumatology.

BSRA British Society for Research on Ageing.

BSRP Basic Science Research Program.

BSS Bachelor of Sanitary Science; Backache-sciatica syndrome; Bacteriostatic saline/ sodium chloride/ solution; Balanced salt solution; Balloon septostomy (= Rashkind procedure); Bedside scale; Bernard-Soulier syndrome (see B-SS); Bismuth subsalicylate; Black silk suture; Blood-stained sputum; Brain stem syndrome; Breast-saving surgery (chemotherapy before surgery for breast cancer); Bridging spinal syndesmophyte(s) (seen in EA; ERA); Brown-Séquard syndrome; Buffered saline/ salt solution; Buffered single substrate; Buffered sterile solution.

B-SS Bernard-Soulier syndrome (= BSS).

BSSE Bile salt-stimulated esterase.

BSSG Sitogluside.

BSSI Bureau of Supplemental Security Income (SSA).

BSSL Bile salt-stimulated lipase.

BSSMS British Society for the Study of Mental Subnormality.

BSSO British Society of the Study of Orthodontics.

BSSS Benign sporadic sleep spikes.

BST Bacteria screening test; Bedside testing; Bile solubility test (used to differentiate between pneumococcal/ streptococcal infection); Biochemical Society Transactions (UK journal); Blood serologic(al) test (for syphilis) (see STS); Brain scan technology; Brain stem tumor; Brief stimulus therapy (psychology); Brown-Sequard's treatment (= Organotherapy).

BSTFA Bis-(trimethylsilyl)trifluoroacetamide.

BSTs Binet-Simon tests (see BAT).

BSU Bartholin, Skene, urethral (glands); Basic structural unit; British standard unit.

BSV Batten-Spielmyer-Vogt (syndrome); Binocular single vision.

BSW Bachelor of Social Work; Bloodsucking worm (such as the European medicinal leech, *Hirudo* medicinalis).

BT Bacillus thuringiensis (pesticide); Base of tongue; Bedtime; Bentiromide test (for pancreatic insufficiency); Bentonite test (for rheumatoid arthritis and trichinosis); Biological therapy; Biomedical Therapy (journal); Biotachometer; Bitemporal (diameter of head); Bitrochanteric; Bituberous; Bladder/ Brain/ Breast tumor; Bleeding time (laboratory/ coagulation); Blood transfusion/ type/ping; Blue tetrazolium (a histological stain); Blue tongue; Body temperature; Borderline tuberculoid; Bovine turbinate (cells); Brachytherapy (radioactive seed implants in prostate cancer); Brain theory; Breath test (for DWI).

Bt *Bacillus* thuringiensis (a microorganism which, combined with genetically engineered corn, is transformed into a transgenic seed used as a pesticide).

B-T Blalock-Taussig (shunt).

76-BT National Fire Protection Association safety tests.

BTA Benzoyl-tyrosine amide (= N-benzoyl-L-tyrosine amide); Blood Transfusion Association; British Tuberculosis Association.

BtA Balloon-to-artery (ratio) (Angiography); Biological Terrain Assessment (with the aid of enhanced software, graphs and visual biofeedback tools).

B12TAM Vitamin B12 tannate aluminium monostearate. A long-acting vitamin B12 suspension, prepared in sesame oil for intramuscular injections.

BTB Breakthrough bleeding; Bromthymol blue (an indicator).

BtB Bench-to-bedside (medical research); Blood-to-blood (spread of infection); Breath-to-breath (variations in minute ventilation, etc.).

BTBL Bromthymol blue lactose.

BTBV Beat to beat variability.

BTC Basal/ Body temperature chart; Benign thrombocytosis (= STC or Secondary thrombocytosis); Benzalkonium chloride; Biliary tract cancer; Bioptome tip catheter (designed to obtain samples of the cardiac endocardial lining); Bladder tumor check; Blood trough concentration; Bone Tumor Center (Univ. of Bologna, Bologna, Italy); By the clock; Organon Laboratories code for experimental substances.

BtCk Battery check.

BTD Bedtime dose; Biliary tract disease; Bitter tasting drug; Blood Type Diet (now criticized and refuted).

BTDS Benzoylthiamine disulfide.

BTE Behind-the-ear (hearing aid); Blood-tissue exchange; Bovine thymus extract; Tropine benzylate.

BTF Biduotertian fever (a form of malaria); Biotransformation; Blastic transformation (late stage in bone cancer); Blenderized tube feeding; Bowtie filter (in radiology).

BTFS Breast tumor frozen section.

BTG Beta-thromboglobulin (= ß-TG).

ß-TG Beta-thromboglobulin (see BTG).

BTg Bovine trypsinogen.

BTGH Ben Taub General Hospital (Texas Medical Center).

BThU British thermal unit (see BTU).

BTI Beef tapeworm infection (caused by the tapeworm TAENIA saginata); Biotechnology industry.

BTI; βTI Beta-thalassemia intermedia.

BTIN Balkan tubulointerstitial nephritis.

BTK; Btk Bruton tyrosine kinase (gene) (a mutant protein).

Btk Buttock.

BTL Bell Telephone Laboratories; Bergonie-Tréboneau law (concerning tissue-cell sensitivity in X-ray therapy); Bilateral tubal ligation (operation/ gynecology).

BT leprosy Borderline-tuberculoid leprosy.

BTLS Basic trauma life support.

BTM Benign tertian malaria; Biothesiometer (for determining sex sensation threshold).

BTMD Batten-Turner muscular dystrophy (syndrome).

BTMMD Bayley Test of Mental and Motor Development.

BTMSA Bis-trimethylsilacetylene.

BTP Biliary tract pain; Biotransformation pathway; Blalock-Taussig procedure (heart surgery); Blood-typing protein; Body temperature & pressure; Breakthrough pain; Bronchial tree penetration (of antibiotics, etc.).

BTPABA N-Benzoyl-L-tyrosyl-p-aminobenzoic acid.

BTPD Body temperature and pressure (ambient pressure in prevailing atmosphere), dry (Pulmonary function test reports - see PFT).

BTPS Body temperature, pressure (ambient pressure in prevailing atmosphere), and saturation (with water vapor/ gas) (Pulmonary function test reports - see PFT).

BTR Bezold-type reflex; Biceps tendon reflex; Bladder tumor recheck; Body temperature regulation.

BTr Bovine trypsin.

BTRL Bartlett Tree Research Laboratories.

BTS Bithionol sulfoxide; Blood transfusion service; Blue toe syndrome; Bradycardia-tachycardia syndrome; Brain Tissue Scanner (a novel microscopic camera, capable of picking up details as tiny as 1/100,000 of an inch or 0.254 μ, smaller than an individual neuron); British Thoracic Society.

BtS "Back to Sleep" (campaign fostered by the NIH to prevent SIDS or Sudden infant death syndrome in babies).

BTSH; bTSH Bovine thyroid stimulating hormone (see Hormones - TSH).

BTT Batrachotoxinin; Bismuth triple therapy (in *Helicobacter* pylori gastritis) - a combination of colloidal bismuth with the antibiotic amoxycillin or tetracycline, and metronidazole or tinidazole 3 times daily for 2 weeks (see ODT; OTT).

BTU; Btu British thermal unit (= BThU).

BTV Basal tidal volume; Blue tongue virus.

BTW Beef tapeworm (= *Taenia* saginata).

BTX Benzene, toluene, xylene; Brevetoxin.

BTX-B Brevetoxin-B.

BTZ Benzothiazepine.

BU Babson/ Bethesda/ Bodansky/ Burn unit; Base of prism up; Below umbilicus; Blood urea; Bromouracil.

Bu Butyl.

bu bullae (radiograph symbol); bushel.

BUA Blood uric acid; Broadband ultrasonic attenuation.

BUC Blood urea concentration.

Buc; Bucc Buccal.

bucc- combining form meaning cheek (L. bucca).

BuChE Butyrylcholinesterase.

BUD Budesonide.

Bud Buddhist.

BUDD Bureau of Devices and Diagnostics (FDA).

BUDR Bromodeoxyuracil; Bromodeoxyuridine (= 5-bromo,2-deoxyuridine; Bromouridine; BUDU).

BUDS Bilateral upper dorsal sympathectomy.

BUDU Bromo-deoxyuridine (see BUDR).

BUE Both upper extremities.

BUF Buffalo (rat).

BUFA Baby up for adoption.

BUG Buccal ganglion; Bulbourethral gland (also called Cowper's gland).

BUI Brain uptake index.

BUL Benign uterine leiomyoma; Bulbar (palsy).

BULIT Bulimia test.

BULL Buccal or upper lingual of lower.

Bull Bulletin.

bull let it boil (L. bulliat).

BuMed Bureau of Medicine and Surgery (USN).

BuMines Bureau of Mines (Department of the Interior).

BUMP Behavioral Regression or Upset in Hospitalized Medical Patients (scale).

BUN Blood urea nitrogen (= UN) (laboratory/ chemistry - see KFT).

Bun Bunion.

bun br bundle branch.

BUN/CR Blood urea nitrogen/creatine ratio.

BUO Bleeding/ Bruising of undetermined origin.

βUP β-ureido-propionase.

BUPA British United Provident Association.

BUQ Both upper quadrants.

BUR Back-up rate (ventilator); Bilateral ureteral occlusion.

Bur Bureau.

Burd Burdick (suction).

Burese Cocaine (see Erythroxylum).

Burns (ISBI journal).

BUS Bartholin's, urethral and Skene's (glands); Bonnevie-Ullrich syndrome (a chromosome disorder marked by the absence of one X chromosome - better known as Turner's syndrome or Monosomy X); Busulfan (see BSF).

BUSAMD Bulletin of the United States Army Medical Department.

bush Marijuana (see Cannabis).

BUSM Boston University School of Medicine.

BUT Bipolar union transistor.

But; but Butter (L. butyrum); Butyrate/ric.

BUTI Butirosin (sulfate).

Button Peyote.

BV Bacitracin V; Bacterial vaginitis/ vaginosis; Basilic vein; Biological value/ valve; Blood vessel/ volume; Blurred vision (see PMA); Borna virus (see BVI); Bronchovesicular (breath sounds); Vapor bath (see bv).

bv Balneum vaporis (L.) - Steam/ Vapor bath (= BV).

BVA Ball-valve action (the opening and closing of a hole by a buoyant, ball-shaped mass acting as a valve, such as can occur with kidney stones, gall stones, and blood clots); British Veterans/ Veterinary Association.

BVAD Biventricular assist device.
BVC Bivalve cast; British Veterinary Codex (see BVetC).
BVD Bovine viral diarrhea; Vincristine; BCNU (Carmustine), Vincristine and Dacarbazine (Chemotherapy); Blood/ Brain vessel damage; Blood vessel disorder; Blood volume deficiency (= Hypovolemia); Bronchial venous drainage.
BVDT Brief vestibular disorientation test.
BVDU Bromovinyldeoxyuridine.
BVE Binocular visual efficiency; Blood vessel endothelium; Blood volume expander; Borna virus encephalitis (causes encephalitis in horses; suspected by some scientists of being associated with mental illness in humans, such as schizophrenia, depression, and bipolar disorder).
BVetC British Veterinary Codex (= BVC).
BVF Baseline vertebral fracture.
BVH Biventricular hypertrophy (heart).
BVI Blood vessel invasion; Borna virus infection (a psychiatric illness).
BVJ British Veterinary Journal.
BVL Bilateral vas ligation (operation/ genitourinary).
BVM Bronchovascular markings; Bureau of Veterinary Medicine (FDA).
BVMGT Bender Visual-Motor Gestalt Test (= BVMOT).
BVMOT Bender Visual-Motor (Gestalt Test) (see BVMGT).
BVMS Bachelor of Veterinary Medicine and Science.
BVMT Bacterial reverse mutation test (Ames).
BVO Branch vein occlusion.
BVOP BCNU (= Carmustine), vincristine, vinblastine, procarbazine. A combination treatment used in certain neoplastic diseases.
BVP Bacterial vaginosis/ vulvovaginosis pathogen - (1) common pathogens such as *Chlamydia* trachomatis, *Neisseria* gonorrhoeae, etc. or (2) potential pathogens such as *Gardnerella* vaginalis, *Mobiluncus* mulieris, *Mycoplasma* hominis, *Peptostreptococcus* spp., etc. (see NBVP); Blood vessel prosthesis; Blood volume pulse; Bonhoeffer-Van der Pol model; Burst of ventricular pacing.
BVR Baboon virus replication; Biphasic ventilatory reaction/ response.
BvR; bvr Benefit-versus-risk (drug balance).
BVRT Benton Visual Retention Test.
BVS Blanked ventricular sense; Blood vessel surgery.
BVSc Bachelor of Veterinary Science.
BVT Basal vagal tone.
BVU Bromoisovalerylurea (= Bromisovalum).
BVV Bovine vaginitis virus.
BVW Blood-vessel wall.
BW Bacteriological warfare; Bedwetting; Below waist/ weight; Biological warfare/ weapon; Birth weight (see BWt); Bite-wing (radiograph); Bladder washout; Blood Wassermann (reaction - see WR; STS); Body water/ weight (see bw); Brain wave; Burroughs Wellcome Research Institute code for experimental substances.
B&W Black and white (milk of magnesia and cascara extract).
bw body water/ weight (= BW).
BW 50-63 Pyrimethamine (= RP 4753). A synthetic diaminopyrimidine anti-malarial drug affecting the nucleo-protein metabolism of the parasites by interference in the folic-folinic acid systems during nuclear division. Used chiefly as a suppressant in the eradication of malaria.
BW 61-32 Stilbazium iodide. An anthelmintic reported to be effective against roundworms, threadworms, and whipworms.
BW 56-158 Allopurinol (= HPP - Hydroxy-pyrazolo-pyrimidine). It reduces the production of uric acid by inhibiting xanthine oxidase; used in the treatment of gout, and in the reduction of hyperuricemia from other causes, such as anti-neoplastic drugs.
BW 57-233 Lucanthone hydrochloride (= Lucanth. hydrochlor; NSC 14574). Used in the treatment of schistosomiasis.
BW 57322 Azathioprine. Acytotoxic agent, converted slowly into mercaptopurine in the body. Used chiefly as an immunosuppressive agent for the survival of renal transplants, and in the treatment of acute and chronic leukemia.
BWA Bed wetter admission; Bioweapons agency (see BWR).

BW A509U see AZT.
BWB Body-weight basis.
BWC Blood warming coil (a device made of coiled plastic tubing, used for warming blood before transfusion) (see EBW).
BWCS Bagged white cell study.
BWD Bacillary white diarrhea (in chicks); Biphasic (low-energy) waveform defibrillation (see RBV; TBS; TVD).
BWE Bioweapons engineer (see BWR).
BWF Backward failure (congestive heart failure developing when the right ventricle cannot empty, causing the blood to back up in the pulmonary veins and the lungs, thus resulting in pulmonary edema); Bite-wing film (a type of dental X-ray film that has a central tab or wing); Blackwater fever (with dark red or black urine as seen in chronic falciparum malaria).
BWFI Bacteriostatic water for injection.
BWG Body weight gain.
BWH Bureau of Water Hygiene.
BWHO Bulletin of the World Health Organization (BOMS).
BWI Bi-weekly interval.
BWidF Black widowed female.
BWidM Black widowed male.
BWL Body weight loss.
BWM Bulletin of War Medicine.
BWN Brooker-Wills nail (see IIN) (Orthopedics).
BWR Biological weapons research (for spread of anthrax, plague, smallpox, etc.); Body weight ratio; Boiling-water reactor.
BWS Battered woman/ wife syndrome; Beckwith-Wiedemann syndrome; Brain wave synchronizer.
BWSA Black widow spider antivenin.
BWST Black widow spider toxin.
BWSV Black widow spider venom.
BWt Birth weight (= BW).
BWYV Beet western yellow virus.
BX; Bx; bx Bacitracin X; Biopsy.
BX BS Blue Cross and Blue Shield.
Bx factor Para-aminobenzoic acid.
BXM B cell crossmatch.
BXO Balanitis xerotica obliterans.
BYDV Barley yellow dwarf virus.
BYE Barile-Yaguchi-Eveland (culture medium).
byte a sequence of bits (computer).
BZ Benzodiazepine (see BZD); Benzene (see Bz); Benzoyl (see Bzl); Biochemische Zeitschrift (Ger. journal, now EJB); Dimethyoxymethylamphetamine (same as DOM; STP) (see DOM).
Bz Benzene (= BZ); Benzodiazepine (see BZD); Benzoyl (see Bzl).
BZ 55 Carbutamide (= Glybutamide; U 6987). A sulfonylurea, formerly used in the oral treatment of diabetes mellitus; an extremely toxic drug, now superceded by other safer anti-diabetic agents.
BZD Benzodiazepine (= BZ; Bz; BZDZ); Brill-Zinsser disease (associated with and following louse-borne typhus) (see LBT).
BZDZ Benzodiazepine (see BZD).
BZE Benzoyl ecgonine (see UDS).
Bzl Benzoyl (= BZ; Bz).
BZQ Benzquinamide.
BZS Bannayan-Zonana syndrome.

C

C About (L. circa); Approximate (L. circa); Bruised (L. contusus); Caffeine; Calcitonin-forming (cell); Calculus; Calor (L.) heat, e.g. C. febrilis - the heat of fever; Calorie (Large); Campylobacter; Candida; Candle; Canine (tooth); Cannabis (see Cannabis); Capacitance; Carbasus (L.) (Gr. karpasos) - Cotton (an old name for cotton or lint, e.g. C. absorbens = absorbent guaze; Carbo (L.) charcoal, e.g. C. activatus - activated charcoal; Carbohydrate (diet order); Carbon (Z = 6) - see Elements - Carbon; Cardiac; Cardiovascular (disease); Carrier; Cast; Cathodal; Cathode; Catholic (Roman) - see Cath; Caucasian; Cell; Celsius (= Cel; Centigrade) - thermometer scale; Centi- (10^{-2}), e.g. cg (centigram) = 10^{-2} gram; Centigrade (L. celcius) - above; Central; Central electrode placement in electroencephalography; Centrometric or constitutive heterochromatic chromosome (banding); Centum (L.) one hundred; Cerebrospinal (fluid) - see CSF; Certified; Cervical; Cesarian (section); Charas - marijuana (see Cannabis); Chest; Chest (precordial lead in electrocardiography - see CF 1); Chicken; Child; Chlamydia; Chloramphenicol (on culture and sensitivity reports) - see CAP; Cholesterol; Circa (L.) about (= c; ca; cir; circ) - approximate date, figure, etc.; Clark II - diphenylcyanoarsine (a war gas); Class; Clearance (in kidney function tests); Clearance rate; Clonus (= clonic muscular contraction); Clostridium; Closure; Clubbing; Coarse (with reference to bacterial colonies); Cocaine (see Erythroxylum); Codeine; Coefficient; Colon; Color; Color (response - Rorschach); Color (sense); Colored (guinea pig); Complement (a constituent of all normal plasma, consisting of an activatable system of 11 plasma proteins reacting with one another in the form of 9 components [C1-C9] in a set sequence, and thus being capable of leading to the destruction of antibody-bearing cells, e.g. anti-C globulin); Complete; Complex; Compliance (pulmonary artery); Component; Compound (L. compositus); Concentration, e.g. Hydrogen ion c (= hydrogen exponent or pH), Ionic c (gram atoms of ion per unit volume), MCc (limiting living population density of microorganisms possible in any fluid culture medium), etc.; Concretion (calculus, abnormal union, hardening or solidifying process); Concussion; Conditioned/ning; Conduction; Condyle; Congius (L.) gallon - a measure of volume; Constant (= c; const); Consultation; Contact, e.g. direct c (in communicable diseases), occlusal c (in dentistry); Contract; Contraction/ture; Control (with reference to a group in an experiment); Conventionally reared (experimental animal); Convergence; Correct; Correspondence (the condition of being in agreement or conformity); Cortex; Costa (L.) rib; Coulomb; Cryptococcus; Crystalline (enzyme); Cubic; Cubitus; Cum (L.) with; Cup; Curie (= c; cu) - a unit of radioactivity; Cyanosis; Cycle; Cylinder, e.g. Eye examination, Urinary c (a urinary cast); Cysteine; Cytidine; Cytochrome; Cytosine; Gallon (L. congius) (= Cong; gal); Horn (L. cornu); Hundred (L. centum); Large calorie; Molar heat capacity; Rh gene (allelic form); Rib (L. costa); Squibb, ER & Sons code for experimental substances; Vitamin C; With (L. cum).

c about, approximate(ly) (L. circa); allelic form of Rh gene; calorie (small); candle; canine (tooth - deciduous); capacity; carat; centi- (prefix for 1/100); centum (L.) one hundred; century; cibus (L.) meal; circa (L.) about, approximate(ly) (= cir; circ); coenzyme - an organic dialyzable thermostable compound with which an apoenzyme must unite in order to function: cI - diphosphopyridine nucleotide, cII - triphosphopyridine nucleotide (= cW), cA - pantothenic acid, cR - biotin, cW - Warburg's enzyme (= cII; triphosphopyridine nucleotide); complementary (strand); concentration; constant (see C Constant); contact; copyright; count(s); cubic; cum (L.) with; cup; curie (see C Curie); cycle/lic; meal (L. cibus); specific heat capacity; speed of light; with (L. cum).

°C degree Celcius (= Centigrade) (see C; Cel).

C' Complement.
c' coefficient of portage.
c̄ with (L. cum) (= c).
C(0) Estimated concentration of a drug at the time of injection.
C1 First Cervical nerve/ vertebra; First rib (L costa); Cytochrome 1; First component of complement.
C1; C'1 Activated first component of complement (in man).
C2 Second cervical nerve, cervical vertebra, component of complement, etc.
CI First Cranial nerve.
CII Second cranial nerve, etc.
$\underline{C}_2$ Second rib; Cytochrome 2, etc.
$\bar{C}2$; C'2 Activated second component of complement (in man), etc.
C3 Collins' solution; Cytochrome 3; Third rib.
C3 (population) population that is mentally or physically deficient.
$\bar{C}3$; C'3 Activated third component of complement (same as B1C globulin).
C-4 Cyclotrimethylene trinitramine (a plastic explosive).
C-6 Hexamethonium (Vegolysin).
C10, C-10 Dexamethonium iodide (= Dexameth Iod; Dexamethonium biiodatum) - a depolarizing muscle relaxant, used to obtain muscular relaxation during surgical operations.
C11; C-11 A radioisotope of carbon with a half-life of 20 minutes.
C-14; ^{14}C Radioactive carbon (isotope) (= Carbon-14).
C-56 Hexachlorocyclopentadiene.
^{137}C Radioactive caesium/cesium (= ^{137}Cs) (see Elements - Caesium).
295 C51 Tripolidine hydrochloride (a potent antihistamine).
311 C 90 Zolmitriptan - an oral 5-hydroxytryptamine (5HT) IB/ID receptor agonist, used in the treatment of migraine.
373 C57 Bretylium tosylate. A hypotensive agent which acts by selectively blocking the peripheral adrenergic or sympathetic nerves, preventing the release of adrenaline and noradrenaline at the nerve endings.
467 C60 Bethanidine sulfate (= N-Benzyl-N'N"-dimethylguanidine hemisulfate). A hypotensive agent, chemically related to bretylium and guanethidine, and acting by blocking impulses in the peripheral sympathetic nerves. Used in the treatment of severe hypertension.
C 1428 Cyclarbamate. A muscle relaxant and tranquilizer.
C 5581 Phenyltoloxamine citrate (= Phenyltolyloxamine citrate; PRN - an isomer of diphenhydramine and an antihistamine drug).
C 11925 Phanquone (= Phenanthrolinquone; Pheninquone; 4,7-Phenanthroline-5,6-quinone). An anti-amebic and antibacterial agent, active against both intestinal and extra-intestinal amebiasis.
C 17922 Sulphaphenazole (= Sulfaphenazole; Sulphophenylpyrazol). A sulphonamide derivative and bacteriostatic.
CA Anterior commissure (L. commissura anterior); Bromobenzyl cyanide; Calcium antagonist; California (rabbit); Cancer; Cancer antigen; Candida albicans; Caproic/ Cholic/ Citric acid; Carbonic anhydrase; Carcinogenesis Abstracts (NCI + SIS journal); Carcinoma; Cardiac aneurysm/ arrest/ arrhythmia; Carotid/ Celiac/ Coronary artery; Cast; Catecholamine(rgic) (Central); Cathode; Caucasian adult; Celiac axis; Cellulose/ Cortisone acetate; Centrifugal analyzer; Cerebral abscess/ angiography/ aqueduct/ arteritis/ atrophy; Cervicoaxial; Chemical Abstracts (ACS journal); Chemotactic activity; Child abuse; Chloroamphetamine; Chromosomal aberration/ abnormality; Chronic alcoholic/ism/ anovulation; Chronological/ Conceptional age; Clinical Allergy/ Anesthesia (journals); Clinical associate; Clotting assay; Coagglutination; Coarctation of the aorta; Cocaine Anonymous; Coefficient of absorption; Cold agglutinin (test); Colloid/ Common antigen; Compressed air; Conditioned abstinence; Condylomata acuminata; Coronary angioplasty; Corpora alata/ amylacea; Corpus albicans; Coucil Accepted (AMA); Cortical atrophy (brain); Cranial arteritis (= GCA or Giant cell arteritis); Cricoid arch; Croup-associated (virus); Cytosine arabinoside; Cytotoxic anti-

bodies/dy.

C_A See C alb.

Ca Calcium (Z = 20) - chemical symbol (see Elements - Calcium); Cancer; Candida albicans; Carcinoma; Cathodal/de.

ca about/ approximate (L. circa); cancer; candle; carcinoma; circa (L.) - about, approximate (with reference to time).

C&A Clinitest and Acetest (urine test/ diabetes).

CA-2 Second colloid antigen.

CA 15-3; CA 19-9; CA-50 Tumor marker antigens (see CA-125).

CA-125 Tumor marker antigen (Radioimmunoassay test: uses a monoclonal antibody to monitor the course of epithelial ovarian carcinoma).

CAA Canadian Association of Anatomists; Cardiac anti-arrhythmic (e.g. quinidine) (see PDA); Carotid arterial atherosclerosis; Carotid audiofrequency analysis; Carotid/ Cerebral artery aneurysm; Centrally acting agent(s) (such as alcohol, hypnotics, sedatives, tranquilizers, etc.); Cerebral amyloid angiopathy; Chromosomal/some Aberration Assay (in vitro assay in Chinese hamster ovary [CHO] cells/ in vivo assay in mice - for mutagenicity of a drug) (= CAT); Chronic alcohol abuse; Circulating anodic antigen; Clean Air Act (1970); Community Action Agency; Computer-aided/ assisted analysis; Computer-assisted assessment; Computer augmented accounting; Constitutional aplastic anemia; Coronary artery aneurysm/ atherosclerosis (see CAS); Crystalline amino acids; Cyanoacrylate adhesive (used in prosthetic devices); Cytosolic autoantigen; Cytotoxic anticancer agent (= CAD).

Caa 40 Isoxsuprine hydrochloride (= Compound 5029; Phenoxyisopropyl-norsuprifen). A vasodilator acting directly on the muscle wall of the arteries. Used in the treatment of peripheral vascular disease associated with arterosclerosis, causing intermittent claudication and thromboangiitis obliterans.

CAAS Coronary artery atherosclerosis (see CAS).

CAAT Computer-assisted axial tomography (see CAT).

CAB California Association of Bioanalysts; Captive air bubble; Catheter-associated bacteruria; Cellulose acetate butyrate; Cerebellar angioblastoma; Circumscribed abscess of bone (= Brodie's abscess); Civil Aeronautics Board; Coronary artery blockage/ bypass (graft - see CABG).

CABA Coronary artery balloon angioplasty (see MRP).

"cabbage" A nickname for coronary bypass (see CABG).

Caballo Heroin (see Diamorph HCl).

CABAS Computerized Automated Blood Analysis System.

CABD Combined/ Compensated acid-base disorder/ disturbance.

CABG Coronary artery bypass graft(ing) (= CAB).

CABGS Coronary artery bypass graft surgery.

CaBI Calcium bone index.

CABO Computer-assisted bypass operation.

CABP Coronary artery bypass.

CABS Cognitive behavioral-analysis system (of psychotherapy); Coronary artery bypass surgery.

CABT Combined antibacterial therapy.

CAC Cardiac-accelerator center; Cardiac arrest code; Carotid arterial circulation; Carotid artery clamp; Carotid/ Cerebral/ Coronary -artery calcification; Circulating anticoagulant; Codex Alimentarius Commission (WHO); Commonly associated condition(s); Consecutive amenorrheic cycle(s).

cac- prefix meaning bad, ill, or abnormal (also kak-, Greek: kakos) (e.g. cacesthesia, cacosmia, etc.).

CaC_2 Calcium carbide.

Ca-ca Counterfeit heroin (see Diamorph HCl).

CaCC Cathodal/de closing/sure contraction (= CCC).

CAC/CIC Chronic active/inactive cirrhosis.

CACHP Charleston Area Comprehensive Health Planning (Agency).

CACI Computer-assisted continuous infusion.

$CaCl_2$ Calcium chloride.

$Ca(ClO_3)$ Calcium chlorate.

CaCl(OCl) Chlorinated lime.

CACMLE Colorado Association for

Continuing Medical Laboratory Education.

caco- A combining form meaning bad, ill, etc. (see cac-).

$CaCO_3$ Calcium carbonate.

CaC_2O_4 Calcium oxalate.

CACP Cardiac accessory conduction pathway; Cisplatin.

CACT Central anticholinergic toxicity (= CAT).

CaCTe Cathodal closure tetanus.

Cactus Peyote. A drug obtained from the Mexican cactus, Anhalonium or Lophophora. Used by the natives to produce a state of intoxication marked by feelings of ecstasy (see Lophophora; Mesc).

CaCV Calicivirus.

CACX, CaCX, CaCx Carcinoma/ Cancer of the (uterine) cervix.

CAD Cadaver(ic) (see cad); Calcific aortic disease; Carbolic acid derivative (e.g. Sodium valproate/ Valproic acid); Carotid-artery disease/ dissection; Center for Advanced Dentistry (Fullerton, California); Centrally-acting drug; Chronic airways disease; Chronic autoimmune disorder (see CAID); Clinical anxiety disorder; Cold agglutitin disease; Complete/ Conventional axillary dissection (for axillary breast cancer metastasis - see SLNM; SLNs; SNR); Compressed air disease; Computer-aided/assisted design/ diagnosis/ disease; Concurrently administered drug (= CAM); Congenital abduction deficiency; Coronary artery disease (obstructive); Current arrhythmic disorder; Cystic arachnoidal diverticula/lum (Orthopedics); Cytotoxic anticancer drug (see CAA).

Cad; cad Cadaver(ic) (= CAD).

CADC Committee on Ambulance Design Criteria (NAS-NRC).

CADD Committeee on Alcoholism and Drug Dependence (AMA).

Cadence (ASMT journal).

CADL Communicative Abilities in Daily Living.

CADM Congenital autoimmune diabetes mellitus.

CADTe Cathodal-duration tetanus.

CaDTPA Calcium trisodium pentetate (= Calcium trisodium diethylene-triamine-pentaacetate).

CAE Caprine arthritis-encephalitis; Cellulose acetate electrophoresis; Clinical adverse experience; Clinically/ Common adverse event(s); Compressed air experience (see ANB; CAD); Contingent after-effects; Coronary artery embolism; Cyclophosphamide, Adriamycin (doxorubicin), and Etoposide.

CaE Calcium excretion; Cause and effect (relationship); Chicken-and-egg (issue/ problem/ question).

CAEC Cardiac Arrhythmia Evaluation Center; Cytokine-activated epithelial cell.

CaEDTA Calcium disodium edathamil (= Calcium disodium edetate; $CANA_2EDTA$; $CaNa_2EDTA$) - Calcium disodium ethylene diamine tetraacetate.

CAEE Cytokine-activated epithelial cell.

CAEP Cortical auditory evoked potential.

caerul dark blue-green (L. caeruleus).

CAEV Caprine arthritis-encephalitis virus.

CAF CD8 antiviral factor (a WBC protein which checks the progress of diseases such as AIDS); Cell adhesion factor; Chest auscultatory finding(s); Chloramphenicol (see CAP); Chronic adrenal failure; Chronic atrial fibrillation; Citric acid fermentation; Cross-action forceps; Cyclophosphamide, Adriamycin (doxorubicin), and Fluorouracil.

Caf; caf Caffeine.

CaF_2 Calcium fluoride.

café-au-lait French: light brown spots on the skin.

CAFOR Conference on Association Functions, Organization and Relationships.

CAFP California Academy of Family Physicians.

CAFT Clinitron air fluidized therapy.

CAG Cardioangiogram/graph(y); Carotid/ Cerebral angiogram/graph(y); Cholangiogram/raphy; Chronic atrophic gastritis; Closed angle glaucoma; Continuous ambulatory gamma globulin (infusion); Coronary angiography; Cytosine-adenine-guanine (nucleotide sequence in DNA).

CaG Calcium gluconate.

CAGE Cut down, annoyed by criticism, guilty about drinking, eye-opener drinks (a test for alcoholism).

CAH Center on Aging and Health; Chronic active/ aggressive hepatitis; Combined atrial hypertrophy; Compromised adult height; Congenital adrenal hyperplasia; Cyanacetic acid hydrazide (= Cyacetazide; Cyanacetic acid hydrazine; Cyanoacetohydrazide).

CAHD Coronary arteriosclerotic/ atherosclerotic heart disease.

CAHEA Committee on Allied Health Education and Accreditation.

CaH_2O_2 Calcium hydroxide.

CAHPS Council on Allied Health Professions and Services.

CAHS Central alveolar hypoventilation syndrome.

CAHV Central alveolar hypoventilation (see CAHS).

CAI Carbonic anhydrase inhibitor (Diuretics such as Acetazolamide, Brimonidine, Brinzolamide, Dorzolamide, etc.); Carboxy amino imidazole (an anti-cancer drug); Cardiac arrest intervention; Cellular autoimmunity; Central auditory imperception; Civil Aeromedical Institute; Complete androgen insensitivity; Computer-administered/ aided/ assisted instruction; Confused artificial insemination.

Ca i Capsula interna (thalamus).

CAIA Clinical adverse interaction.

CAID Chronic autoimmune disorder (= CAD); Convention of American Instructors of the Deaf.

CAIP Community-acquired infectious pneumonia (= CAP).

CAIS Complete androgen insensitivity syndrome.

CAL Café au lait; Calcium test (dentistry); Calculated average life; Calories; Carotid/ Cerebral/ Coronary-artery lesion; Chronic airflow limitation; Computer-assisted learning; Coracoacromial ligament.

Cal Calcium (see Calc); Caliber (= cal); Callus; Calorie - large (= 1000 cal; diet order).

cal caliber (see Cal); calorie - small.

C_{alb} Albumin clearance (see KFT).

Calc Calcium (= Cal).

calc calculate/tion.

calc- prefix meaning stone or heel (L. calx, calcis).

calCd calculated.

-calcemia suffix meaning calcium.

calcif calcification.

cal ct calorie count.

CALD Chronic active liver disease.

calef make warm (L. calefac); warm(ed) (L. calefactus).

CALGB Cancer and leukemia group B.

CALH Chronic active lupoid hepatitis.

cALL Common null cell acute lymphocytic leukemia.

cALLA; cALLa Common acute lymphoblastic/ocytic leukemia antigen.

CALM Café-au-lait macules; Candesartan And Lisinopril Microalbuminuria (study in diabetic hypertensive patients with the ARB drug, Candesartan and the ACE inhibitor, Lisonipril).

calor- prefix meaning heat (L.).

CALS Café-au-lait spot(s) - as in Albright-McCune-Sternberg syndrome (= Albright's syndrome, Osteitis fibrosa disseminata), Neurofibromatosis (= Multiple neuroma, Neuromatosis, von Recklinghausen's disease), & in Normal people.

Cal Tech California Institute of Technology.

CAM Calf aortic microsome; Canadian Association of Manufacturers; Caucasian adult male; Cell-associating molecule; Cellular adhesion molecule (see ICAM-1; LFA-1); Center for Athletic Medicine (USC); Children's Antispasmodic Mixture (trade name); Chloramphenicol (see CAP); Choreoathetoid movement(s); Chorioallantoic membrane; Chorioamniotic membrane(s); Circulating adhesion molecule (soluble E-selecten, sICAM; and sVCAM); Committee on Acute Medicine (Am Soc Anesth); Complementary and alternative medicine (see AMP); Computer-aided manufacturing; Computer-aided/assisted myelography; Computerized axial myography; Concurrently administered medicine (see CAD); Contralateral axillary metastasis.

C_{am} Amylase clearance (laboratory/ chemistry).

CAMAC Computer assisted/ automated mea-

surement and control.
CAM-AQI Amodiaquin.
CAMC Canadian Association of Medical Clinics.
CAMEO Cancer Management and Education Optimization (Program).
CAMF Cyclophosphamide, Adriamycin, methotrexate, fluorouracil.
CAMH Center of Addiction and Mental Health (Univ. of Toronto, Canada).
CAMHDD Commonwealth Association for Mental Handicap and Developmental Disabilities.
CAMI Civil Aviation Medicine Institute.
CAMLT California Association of Medical Laboratory Technologists.
CAMMD Canadian Association of Manufacturers of Medical Devices (ACFEM).
CAMO Chief Administrative Medical Officer.
CAMP Childhood Asthma Management Program (research group/ study); Christie-Atkins-Munch-Peterson (test); Computer-assisted medical procedure (see CAP; CARS); Computer-assisted menu planning; Concentration of adenosine monophosphate; Cyclic adenosine monophosphate (see cAMP); Cyclophosphamide, Adriamycin, methotrexate, and procarbazine.
cAMP Cyclic adenosine-3',5'-monophosphate (= CAMP; cyclin AMP).
CAMPF Clinton P. Anderson Meson Physics Facility (Los Alamos).
Campl heaping spoonful (L. cochleare amplum).
CAMR Canadian Association for the Mentally Retarded.
CAMRL Canadian Association of Medical Record Librarians.
CAMS Computer-assisted monitoring system.
CaMV Cauliflower mosaic virus.
CAN Cord around neck; "Cure Autism Now" (activist group, US); Current Articles on Neoplasia (journal); Cyclosporine-associated nephropathy/ toxicity.
Can Canada/dian (= Canad); Cancer (also: journal); Candida (see Candida); Cannabis (see Cannabis).
can morphine (see Papaver).
CA/N Child abuse and neglect.
CANA Circulating antineuronal antibody.
Canad Canada/dian (see Can).
Canad. F Canadian Formulary (1949).
Canadian black Marijuana (see Cannabis).
$CANA_2EDTA$; $CaNa_2EDTA$ Calcium disodium edathamil (see CaEDTA; EDTA).
canc cancelled.
Canceled stick Marijuana cigarette (see Cannabis).
Cancer (ACS journal).
Cancerline Computer data base; on-line cancer bibliography (NLM).
CANCERLIT Cancer Literature.
CANCERPROJ Cancer Research Projects.
cancr- prefix meaning crab or cancer (L. cancer) (see carcin-).
Candida (= Can). A genus of yeast-like fungi producing mycelia, of the family Cryptococcaceae. Other names for this genus are: Cryptococcus; Endomyces; Monilia; Myocandida; Mycotoruloides; Oidium; Parasaccharomyces; Saccharomyces; Syringospora; Torula; Torulopsis; and Zymonema, e.g. Candida albicans (= CA; Can albicans) - causes candidiasis or thrush in man.
Candle (Brit. Epilepsy Assoc. journal).
CANDLES Children of Auschwitz Nazis' Deadly Laboratory Experiments Survivors.
Cannabis (= Can). A genus of plants of the Hemp and Hop family, Cannabinaceae, e.g. C. sativa. The Hemp plant, an erect annual with deeply palmate-lobed leaves. It originated in central Asia but has been cultivated for centuries in eastern countries for the narcotic resin it contains. The dried flowering tops yield the resin Cannabinone, containing the active principles, Cannabinol (CBN) & Tetrahydrocannabinol (THC), psychoactive hallucinating drugs causing euphoria, mental confusion, and motor excitement. The initial phase of inebriation is succeeded by irritability and somnelescence, and after some hours by a comatose sleep. Cannabis is variously known by some 100 or more names, as: A-Bomb (a cigarette prepared from a mixture of marijuana and heroin); Ace (cigarette - now obsolete); Angel dust (a mixture of cannabis

with phencyclidine); Baby; Bar; Bee; Bhang; Black Russian; Blond Hashish; Bomber (m. cigarette); Boo; Bush; Can; Canadian black; Canamo indiano; Cancelled stick (m. cigarette); Cannabis Indica; Chanore Indien; Charas; CS; Dagga; Duby; Dynamite (concentrated m.); Finger (hashish; marijuana); Gangster (m.); Ganga (m.); Gold (concentrated m.); Grass; Green; Grefa; Greta; Grifa (m. cigarette); Gruner Turke; Guaza; Gunga; Hanfkraut; Haschischol; Hash; Hashish; Hay; Hemp; Herb; Indian hay; Indian hemp; J (m. cigarette); Jay (m. cigarette or joint); Joint (m. cigarette); Juanita; Kick stick (m. cig.); Kief (cannabis); Kif (cannabis); Killer weed (potent m.); Kilter; Lebanese (hashish); Loco; Macon (cannabis); Majoon (candy containing hashish or cannabis); Mariahuana; Mariajuana; Marihuana; Marijuana; Mary Ann; Mary Jane; Mexican brown; Mexican green; Mj (Mary Jane/m.); MJ (Mary Jane/m.); Moon (hashish/ peyote); Moota; Mota; Mu; Muggle (m. cig.); Muta; Number (m. cig.); Oil (hashish extract high in THC - tetrahydrocannabinol); Panama; Panama Red; Pin (m. cig.); Pot; Rag (ragweed - dilute m.); Ragweed (dilute m.); Red (Panama red/m.); Reefer (m. cig.); Root (m. cig.); Rope; Roter Libanese; Schwarzer Afghane; Sinsemilla (a seedless marijuana species, produced through intensive cultivation of only the female plant - Spanish American); Snop; Stick (m. twig); Sweet Lucy; Tea; Texas tea; THC (tetrahydrocannabinol - a major active ingredient of marijuana); Thumb (m. cig.); TJ (m. purchased in Tijuana, Mexico); Twist; Weed; Wheat; Yerba; Z purple (m. grown in Zacatecas, Mexico).

Can Nur Canadian Nurse (journal).

CANP Calcium-activated neutral protease.

CANS Central auditory nervous system.

CAO Canadian Association of Optometrists; Cardioactive outcome; Chronic airflow/ airway obstruction; Chronic aluminium overload; Coronary artery obstruction/ occlusion.

CaO Calcium oxide.

CAOB Canadian Association of Optometrists Bulletin.

CaOC Cathodal opening clonus/ contraction (= CaOCl; COC; COCl; KOC; KOCl).

CaOCl Cathodal opening clonus (see CaOC).

CA_{O2}-CV_{O2} Calculated arterio-venous oxygen difference.

CAOD Coronary artery occlusive disease.

$Ca(OH)_2$ Calcium hydroxide.

CAOM Chronic adhesive otitis media.

CAOT Canadian Association of Occupational Therapists; Controlled add-on trial.

CaOTe Cathodal opening tetanus (= COTe).

CAP Camptodactyly-arthropathy-pericarditis (syndrome); Canadian Association of Pathologists/ Physicists; Capreomycin; Caproyl; Capsular arthroplasty (Orthopedics); Capsule; Captopril; Carbolic acid poisoning (as in hydroxybenzene, oxybenzene, phenol, phenylic acid poisoning, etc.); Cardiac arrest program; Catabolite gene-activator protein; Cell-adhesion protein (e.g. collagen, fibronectin, integrins, etc.) - produced by stimulation with TGF-β - Transforming growth factor-β, of fibroblasts and other cells. Likewise the production of ECMP - Extracellular-matrix protein) (see TGF-β); Cell attachment protein; Cellular acetate propionate; Cellulose acetate phthalate (used as an enteric-coating material for tablets and capsules); Central apical part; Chloramphenicol (= C; CAF; CAM; Ch; CHL; Chl; CM; CMC; CMP); Chloroacetophenone; Chronic alcoholic pancreatitis; Chronic ankle pain; College of American Pathologists; Community Action Program; Community-acquired pneumonia; Complement-activated plasma; Compound action potential; Computer-assisted procedure (see CARS); Contact-allergenic (sensitizing) potential (= CSP); Coronary angioplasty (= CA); Coronary angioplasty procedure; Cup arthroplasty (see OI/OP); Coupled atrial tracing; Cyclic AMP-binding protein; Cyclophosphamide, Adriamycin, and Platino (cisplatin); Cystine aminopeptidase; Let him take (see Cap).

CaP Cancer of the prostate.

Cap; cap Capacity; Capsule (L. capsula) (see caps); Let him/ the patient take (L. capiat) (= CAP; Cpt).

Ca/P Calcium to phosphorus ratio.

CAPA Cancer-associated polypeptide antigen.
CAPB Central auditory processing battery.
CAPD Chronic/ Continuous ambulatory peritoneal dialysis.
CAPE Caffeic acid phenethyl ester; Coalition of American Public Employees.
CAPERS Computer Assisted Psychiatric Evaluation and Review System.
CAPHLD California Association of Public Health Laboratory Directors.
CAPhO Canadian Association of Pharmacy in Oncology.
CAPI Combined active-passive immunization (e.g. against tetanus) (= APTI; PAI).
capiend to be taken (L. capiendus).
capit- prefix meaning head (L. caput).
CAPM Chinese Academy of Preventive Medicine.
cap moll soft capsule (L. capsula mollis).
CAPMR Canadian Association of Physical Medicine and Rehabilitation.
CAPNA Columbia Advanced Practice Nurse Associates (NY).
CAPO Computer aid to physician's office.
$Ca_3(PO_4)_2$ Tribasic calcium phosphate.
CAPP Concerted Action Polyposis Prevention (Study, EURope).
CAPPS Council for the Advancement of the Psychological Professions and Sciences; Current and Past Psychopathology Scale.
cap quant vult Let the patient take/ To be taken as much as he/one wants to (L. capiat quantum vult).
CAPRCA Chronic, acquired, pure red cell aplasia.
CAPRI Cardiopulmonary Research Institute.
CAPS Coronary Atherosclerosis Prevention Study (see WOSCOPS).
caps capsule (L. capsula) (= Cap; cap; capsul).
caps- combining form meaning container (L. capsa).
capsul capsule (see caps).
CAPTA Child Abuse Prevention and Treatment Act (1974).
CAPYA Child and adolescent psychoanalysis.
CAR Canadian Association of Radiologists; Cancer-associated retinopathy; Cardiac agonal rhythm (an idioventricular rhythm, pertaining to or seemingly the "agony of death", at fewer than 30 heart-beats per minute); Cardiac ambulation routine; Chronic articular rheumatism; Common adverse reaction; Computer-assisted research; Conditioned avoidance response; Crossed adductor response (knee jerk).
Car; car Carcinogen; Carotid.
CARA Chronic aspecific respiratory ailment.
CARB Carbohydrate (see Carb; carb).
Carb; carb Carbenicillin disodium (= CB; CBC; CBCN); Carbohydrate (= CARB; Carbo; carbo); Carbonate.
Carbo; carbo Carbohydrate (see Carb; carb).
carb carbonate noncarboxylate anion (= CNCA).
carb- prefix meaning coal or carbon (L. carbo).
carbam carbamate carboxylate anion (= CCA).
CARC Canadian Arctic Resources Committee.
carcin- prefix meaning crab or cancer (Gr. karkinos) (see cancr-).
CARD Cardiac automatic resuscitative device.
Card; card Cardiac; Cardiology (see Cardiol; cardiol).
card- combining form meaning heart (Gr. kardia).
Card insuff Cardiac insufficiency.
Cardiol; cardiol Cardiology (= Card; card).
CARE Cholesterol and Recurrent Events (Study/ Trial); Clinical AIDS Research and Education (see CCARE); Community Action to Reach the Elderly; Computerized adult and records evaluation (system); Cooperative for American Relief Everywhere (formerly Cooperative for American Remittances to Europe).
CARED Concerned Americans for a Responsible Exit with Dignity.
CARET Beta-Carotene and Retinol Efficacy Trial (NCI).
CARF Commission on Accredition and/of Rehabilitation Facilities.
CARIH Children's Asthma Research Institute and Hospital (University of Colorado, Denver, US).
CARJ Canadian Association of Radiologists Journal.

Carn Carnosine.
CARS Childhood Autism Rating Scale; Children's Affective Rating Scale; Coherent anti-Stokes Raman scattering; Computer-assisted robotic system (see CAMP; CAP; RAHO; RAOR; RAS; RSD; RSE; RSS).
cart cartilage.
Cartwheel Amphetamine tablet (see Amphet).
cary- combining form meaning nut, kernel, or nucleus (Gr. karyon).
CAS Calcarine sulcus; Calcific aortic stenosis; Canadian Anaesthetists' Society; Cancer Attitude Survey; Carbohydrate-active steroid; Cardiac adjustment scale; Cardiac surgery; Carotid artery stenosis; Carotid/ Cerebral/ Coronary atherosclerosis (= CAA; CAAS); Carotid/ Coronary arterial/ery stenosis/stenting/ surgery; Celite-activated normal serum; Center for Alcohol Studies; Central axial skeleton (Orthopedics); Ceramic acetabular socket (Hip joint arthroplasty); Cerebral arteriosclerosis/ atherosclerosis; Chemical Abstract(s) Service; Children's Aid Society; Chronic arteriosclerosis; Chronic asthma studies/dy; Cold agglutinin syndrome; Community-acquired sinusitis; Complex absence seizure; Comprehensive appraisal scheme (GMC, UK); Compressed air system; Computer-assisted surgery; Confusion-ataxia syndrome; Congenital alcoholic syndrome; Control adjustment strap; Conventional acoustic stethoscope (see FES); Coronary artery spasm; Council of Academic Societies; Council on Atmospheric Sciences; Czechoslovak Academy of Science.
Cas Casualty.
cas castrate/ted/tion.
CASA Cardiac Arrest Survival Act (US); Computer-aided/assisted self assessment/ sperm analysis/yzer; Computer-assisted semen analysis.
Casc Cascara (= CASCARA sagrada)
CASH Commission for Administrative Services in Hospitals; Cortico-adrenal stimulating hormone; Cruciform anterior spinal hyperextension.
CASHD Coronary arteriosclerotic heart disease.
CASI Cognitive Abilities Screening Instrument.
CASIT Center for Advanced Surgical and Interventional Technology (UCLA).
CASMD Congenital atonic sclerotic muscular dystrophy.
$CaSO_4$ Calcium sulfate.
CASP Child Analytic Study Program.
CASPR Central Application Services for Podiatric Residencies (ETS).
CAS-REGN Chemical Abstracts Service Registry Number.
CASRT Corrected adjusted sinus (node) recovery time.
CASS Computer-aided sleep system; Coronary Artery Surgery Study.
CASSIS Classification and Search Support Information System (Patent Office).
CAST Cardiac Arrhythmia Suppression Trial; Children of Alcoholism Screening Test; Clearinghouse Announcements in Science and Technology; Council for Agricultural Science and Technology.
CASU Centro de Accion Social Universitaria.
CASW Council for the Advancement of Science Writing.
CAT California Achievement Test; Capillary agglutination test; Cardiovascular analog trainer; Catalase (see CAT'ase); Cataract (= cat); Catecholamine; Cerebral/ Coronary artery thrombosis/bus; Central anticholinergic toxicity (see CACT); Children's Apperception Test; Chloramphenicol acetyltransferase; Chlormerodrin accumulation test; Choline acetyltransferase (= Choline-o-acetyl transferase); Chopra's antimony test (for Kala-Azar); Chromosome aberration test (see CAA); Chronic abdominal tympany; Cochran-Armitage test (for trend in adverse event data or drug reaction); Cognitive Abilities Test; Cold agglutination test; College Ability Test; Computer-aided/-assisted technology; Computed/ Computer-assisted/ Computerized abdominal tomography; Computer/ Computer-assisted/ Computerized axial tomography (= CAAT; CATS; CAT scan; CT; CTAT; CTS; CT scan; X-ray scan); Computer of average transients (EEG); Concomitant antibiotic therapy.
Cat Heroin (see Diamorph HCl).

cat catalysis/st; cataract (see CAT).
CaT Total serum calcium (see Ca-Tot).
cat-; cata- prefix meaning down, negative (Gr. kata).
CA/TA Cortical area/total area (ratio).
CAT'ase Catalase.
CATCH Child and Adolescent Trial for Cardiovascular Health; Community Actions to Control High Pressure.
Catch 22 A No-win situation where there are no options, with a "heads-I-win, tails-you-lose" alternative.
Cath; cath Cathartic (L. catharticus); Catheter(ize); Cathode; Catholic (= C).
Catheter A hollow, flexible, tubular device for insertion into body cavities, canals, passageways or vessels, to permit injection or withdrawal of fluids or to keep a passage open. Kinds of catheters include:
Acorn-tipped catheter - a flexible hollow tube with an acorn-shaped tip, often used in urology.
Balloon-tip catheter - a catheter with an inflatable sac around one end, the sac being inflated with air or sterile water after insertion, in order to secure the catheter in the correct position. The Foley and Swan-Ganz catheters are of this type.
Bicoudate catheter - a twice-bent Mercier's catheter (= Catheter bicoudé).
Bioptome-tip catheter - designed to obtain samples of the endocardium).
Bozeman-Fritsch catheter - a double-current uterine catheter (= Bozeman's/ Fritsch's catheters).
Bozeman's catheter = Bozeman-Fritsch catheter (see).
Catheter bicoudé = Bicoudate catheter (see).
Catheter coudé - an Elbowed catheter (see).
Catheter à demeure. - a catheter that is held in position in the urethra.
de Pezzer catheter - a self-retaining catheter with a bulbous extremity (= Pezzer's catheter).
Elbowed catheter - a catheter with a sharp bend near the beak, used principally in cases of enlarged prostate.
Eustachian catheter - an instrument for extending the eustachian tube and for treating diseases of the middle ear (= Itard's catheter).
Faucial catheter - an Eustachian catheter used through the fauces.
Female catheter - a short catheter for passage through the female urethra.
Flexible catheter = Néaton's catheter (see).
Foley catheter - a Balloon-tip catheter inserted into the urinary bladder.
Fritsch's catheter = Bozeman-Fritsch catheter (see).
Gouley's catheter - a solid, curved, steel instrument grooved on its inferior surface for easy passage over a guide through a urethral stricture.
Indwelling catheter - a catheter held in position in the urethra.
Intrauterine catheter - a catheter introduced within the uterus through the cervical canal.
Itard's catheter - a variety of Eustachian catheter (see).
Lobster-tail catheter - a catheter with three joints at the tip.
Mercier's catheter - a flexible catheter elbowed at the end; used in patients with enlarged prostate.
Nélaton's catheter - a catheter of soft India rubber (= Flexible or Soft catheters).
Pezzer's catheter = de Pezzer catheter (see).
Phillips' catheter - a urethral catheter with a woven filiform guide.
Prostatic catheter - a catheter having a short angular tip for passing an enlarged prostate.
Railway catheter - a straight elastic tube with an open end, introduced with a filiform guide in cases of stricture.
Schrötter's catheter - a hard-rubber catheter of various calibers, used for dilating laryngeal strictures.
Self-retaining catheter - a catheter so constructed as to be retained at will and used in drainage of the urinary bladder (e.g. Skene's catheter).
Skene's catheter - a strong glass Self-retaining catheter (see), used in the female urinary bladder.
Soft catheter = Nélaton's catheter (see).
Squire's catheter - a Vertebrated catheter (see).
Swan-Ganz catheter - a Balloon-tip catheter

used in measuring the pressure in the pulmonary artery.
Two-way catheter - a catheter used in irrigation.
Vertebrated catheter - a catheter fitted together in small sections so as to make it more flexible (e.g. Squire's catheter).
Whistle-tip catheter - a catheter with a terminal opening plus a lateral one.
Winged catheter - a catheter with two projections on the end, in order to retain it in the urinary bladder.

CATLINE Catalog On-Line (on-line bibliography data for all books and serials catalogued at the National Library of Medicine since 1965).

Ca-Tot Total serum calcium (= CaT).

CATRS Cocaine Abuse Treatment and Research Service.

CATS Canadian American Ticlopidine Study; CAT scan (see CAT).

CAT-S Children's Apperception Test, Supplemental.

CAT scan Computed axial tomography scan (see CAT).

CATT Card agglutination test (for *Trypanosoma* brucei gambiense infection i.e. Gambian trypanosomiasis or 'sleeping sickness').

CATT; CaTT Calcium tolerance test.

CATV; CaTV Cable television.

CAU Chronic anterior uveitis.

Cau; Cauc Caucasion.

Caud; caud Caudad; Caudal.

caud- prefix meaning tail (L. cauda).

Cauf Unfilterable calcium.

Caut; caut Cauterization/ze.

CAV Chronic acne vulgaris (= Acne indurata); Computer-aided ventilation; Congenital absence of vagina; Congenital adrenal virilism; Constant angular velocity; Coronary artery vasoconstriction (see CAVC; CAVS)/ vasodilatation/lation (see CAVD)/ vasospasm (see CAVS); Croup-associated virus; Cyclophosphamide, (cytosine) arabinoside, vincristine.

Cav; cav Cavity.

cav- combining form meaning hollow (L. cavus).

CAVB Complete atrioventricular block.

CAVC Common atrioventricular canal; Coronary artery vasoconstriction.

CAVD Complete atrioventricular dissociation; Completion, Arithmetic problems, Vocabulary, following Direction (Direction-following) (test) (in psychology, a battery of four intelligence tests); Coronary artery vasodilatation.

CAVE Contra-indications due to allergy or vasomotor episodes.

CAVe CNU (Lomustine), Adriamycin and Vinblastine (Chemotherapy).

C(ave); Cave; C(avg); Cavg Average plasma concentration.

CAVH Continuous arteriovenous hemofiltration.

CAVHD Continuous arteriovenous hemodialysis.

CA virus Croup-associated virus (see CAV).

CAVLT Children's Auditory Verbal Learning Test.

CAVO Common atrioventricular orifice.

CAVP College Audio-Visual Presentation.

CAV-P-VP Cyclophosphamide, Adriamycin (doxorubicin), Vincristine, Platino (cisplatin), and Etoposide VP (podophyllotoxin derivative).

CAVS Conformance Assessment to Voluntary Standards; Coronary artery vasospasm (= CAV).

CAVU Continuous arteriovenous ultrafiltration.

CAW Central airways; Commission on Atomic Weights (IUPAC).

C_{aw} Airway conductance.

CB Bachelor of Surgery (L. chirurgiae baccalaureus); Calcium blocker; Cancer Bulletin (journal); Carbenicillin (see Carb) (on culture and sensitivity reports); Carbobenzoxy; Carotid body; Census Bureau (Department of Commerce); Cephalic blade (forceps used in delivery); Cesarean birth; Chest - Back; Chester Beatty Research Institute and Allen & Hanburys code for experimental substances; Children's Bureau (OCD); Child's Brain (ISPN journal); Chirurgiae Baccalaureus (L) - Bachelor of Surgery; Chlorambucil (see CB 1348); Chocolate blood (agar); Chromatin body; Chronic bronchitis; Chronobiology; Ciba Pharmaceutical Co; Circumflex branch; Citizen's band (radio); Clinical Biochemistry (Canada journal); Code blue; Color blind; Coltsfoot Bronchials (proprietary drug); Compensated base; Conference Board; Coracobrachial; Culture of bladder (through cystoscope); Doriden pill (= Glutethimide; Alpha-phenyl-α-ethyl-glutaric acid imide - Ciba - a hypnotic drug).

Cb Columbium (Z = 41), former name for the chemical element Niobium (Nb) (see Elements - Niobium).

C&B Chair and bed (rest); Crown and bridge.

CB 1 Chest lead, with indifferent electrode on subject's back (ECG).

CB 11 Phenadoxone hydrochloride. An analgesic with a slight hypnotic action.

CB 154 2 bromo-alpha-ergocryptine.

CB 1348 Chlorambucil (= CB). A nitrogen mustard derivative and cytotoxic agent which acts by damaging dividing cells, by fragmentation of their nuclear chromosomes. Used in the treatment of follicular lymphoma, lymphocytic lymphoma, and other related neoplastic diseases.

CB 1678 Propiomazine maleate (= Propiomazine hydrogen maleate). A depressant of the central nervous system; is used by mouth as a sedative, tranquillizer, or hypnotic.

CB 2041 Busulphan (= Busulfan; GT 41; Myelosan; Tetramethylene dimethanesulfonate; 1,4-Di[methanesulphonyloxy]butane). A cytotoxic agent having a selective depressant action on bone marrow. In small doses it depresses granulocytopoiesis and to a lesser extent thrombocytopoiesis, but has little effect on lymphocytes. Because of its selective action busulphan is particularly useful in the treatment of chronic myeloid leukemia.

CB 3025 Melphalan (= NSC 8806; PAM; Phenylalanine nitrogen mustard; Sarcolysinum). An antineoplastic agent used in the treatment of multiple myeloma by systemic administration, and malignant melanomas by isolated perfusion technique.

CB 8019 Carisoprodol (= N-Isopropylmeprobamate). A muscle relaxant and analgesic used in the relief of pain associated with acute muscle spasm, such as low back pain, stiff neck, fractures, dislocations and sprains, etc.

CB 8053 Thiamphenicol (= Dextrosulphenidol; Thiophenicol; Tiophenicol; Win 5063-2). A broad-spectrum antibiotic, whose action resembles that of chloramophenicol.

CBA Calcium-based antacid; Carcinoma bearing animal; Chemical-Biological Activities (file); Chemical Bond Approach (project in general chemistry); Child-bearing age; Chronic bronchitis and asthma; Complete bone attachment (Orthopedics); Congenital berry aneurysm (intracranial a); Cosmetic breast augmentation (Cosm. surgery); Cost-benefit analysis.

CBA 93626 Clonixin.

CBAB Complement-binding antibody.

CBADAA Certifying Board of the American Dental Assistants Association.

CBAI Computer-based anatomical imagery.

CBAS Cognitive behavior(al)-analysis system (of psychotherapy).

CBAT Coag/ Coulter battery.

CBB Cancer Biochemistry-Biophysics (UK journal); Coomassie brilliant blue (stain); Cord blood bank(ing) (umbilical cord).

CBC Calcium-based ceramics/ composites (in bone reconstruction); Carbenicillin (see Carb); Carcinoma basocellulare (see BCC); Case by case (basis); Cavernous body of the clitoris (or Corpus cavernosum in the female); Cellular blood component; Child-behavior characteristics; Complete blood cell count (= cbc); Complete blood count (= cbc).

cbc See CBC.

CBCG Cooperative Breast Cancer Group.

CBCL Child Behavior Checklist.

CBCL/2-3 Child Behavior Checklist for ages 2-3.

CBCN Carbenicillin (see Carb).

CBCS; CBCs Complete blood counts.

CBCT Cisplatin-based chemotherapy; Community-based clinical trial; Consumer-bank communication terminal (same as RSU).

CBCTR Cooperative Breast Cancer Tissue Resource (NCI, US).

CBD Carotid body denervation; Cash before delivery; Cat-bite disease (see CBF); Childhood behavior disturbance(s) (ADD; ADHD; SLD); Chronic bronchopulmonary disease (see CBPD; COPD); Closed bladder drainage; 'Clotbusting' device/ drug (e.g. Balloon angioplasty; the 'Xpeedior 100' intra-arterial catheter which blasts blood clots with jets of saline [Possis Medical, Minneapolis, USA]; etc.); Commerce Business Daily (journal); Common bile duct; Congenital (urinary) bladder diverticulum; Congenital bleeding disorder.

CBDC Chronic bullous disease of children.

CBDE Common bile duct exploration.

CBDF Cord Blood Donor Foundation.

CBE Center for Bioethics; Center for Biomedical Ethics; Chronic bronchitis with emphysema (see COPD); Clinical breast examination; Communities for a Better Environment; Council of Biology Editors; Current Bibliography of Epidemiology (journal).

CBET Certified biochemical equipment technician.

CBF Capillary/ Collateral/ Coronary/ Cortical blood flow; Cat-bite fever (= CBD) (see CSD; CSF - Cat-scratch fever); Cerebral blood flow (= CF); Childbed fever (= Puerperal fever/ septicemia) (= CF); Ciliary beat frequency; Clinical blood flowmeter; Continuous blood flow (as in the artificial heart, the Jarvik 2000 assist device).

CBFS Cerebral blood flow studies/dy.

CBFV Cerebral blood flow velocity.

CBG Cancellous bone graft(ing); Capillary blood gases/ glucose; Center for Biomedicine & Genetics (US) - a research-based facility of the COH institute (see COH); Copper-balance gene (which prevents excess accumulation of dietary copper in the liver. An abnormal, autosomal, recessive gene fails to do so, resulting in excessive hepatic copper concentration, as is found in Wilson's disease); Coronary bypass graft; Cortico-steroid-binding globulin (transcortin); Cortisol-binding globulin.

CBGv Corticosteroid-binding globulin variant.

CBH Chronic benign hepatitis; Common bundle of His (heart); Cutaneous basophilic hypersensitivity.

CBHL Center for Bioethics and Health Law (Univ. of Utrecht, Holland).

CBHP Community Breast Health Project.

CBI Carpal bone injury (Orthopedics); Chronic bacterial infection; Chronic brain injury; Close-binding-intimate; Continuous bladder irrigation.

CBIL; CBil Conjugated bilirubin.

CBIR Cell-based immune response (see CMIR; CMS).

CBL Caffeine, belladonna, luminal (proprietary tablet); Chronic blood loss (= cbl); Circulating blood lymphocyte(s); Cord blood leukocyte(s).

Cbl Cobalamin.

cbl chronic blood loss (see CBL).

CBM Capillary basement membrane.

CBMMP Chronic benign mucous membrane pemphigus.

CBMT Capillary basement membrane thickness.

CBN Cannabinol (see Cannabis); Central benign neoplasm; Chronic benign neutropenia; Commission on Biochemical/ Biological Nomenclature (IUPAC-IUB); Community-based nurse; Complete(ly) balanced nutrition.

CBNS Center for the Biology of Natural Systems.

CBO Congenital bowel obstruction; Congressional Budget Office.

CBOC Completion of bed occupancy care.

CBP Caged-ball prosthesis (an artificial heart valve made up of a plastic ball in a metal cage); Calcium/ Carbohydrate/ Cobalamin-binding protein; Cavernous body of the penis (or Corpus cavernosum in the male); Child-bearing potential; Chlorobiphenyl; Chronic back/ benign pain; Chronic bacterial prostatitis; Chronic belly pain; Cognitive/ Complex behavior performance; Collagen breakdown product(s); Community-based physician; Comparative Biochemistry and Physiology (journal); Controlled blood pressure; Cord-blood program; Cyclical breast pain.

CBPA Competitive protein-binding assay.
CBPC Community-based primary care.
CBPD Chronic bronchopulmonary disease (see COPD).
CBPF Cortical bone peg fixation (see BPF).
CBPS Coronary bypass surgery.
CBR Carotid bodies resected; Carotid body reflex (see ABR); Center for Blood Research; Chemical, biological, and radiological (warfare) (see ABC); Chemically-bound residue; Chronic bed rest; Commercial breeder reactor; Cord Blood Registry; Cosmetic breast reduction (Cosm. surgery); Complete bed rest; Cost-benefit ratio; Crude birth rate.
C_{Br} Hepatic bilirubin clearance (see LFT iv).
CBRS Culture-bound reactive syndrome (psychiatry).
CBRU Computer-Based Resource Unit(s).
CBS Cardiac bypass surgery (see "cabbage"; CABG; CABS); Cervicobrachial syndrome; Chronic brain syndrome (= Chr Br Syn); Colloidal bismuth subnitrate; Communication behavior scale; Community-based study; Comparative biomechanical study (of fractures); Computer-based scanner; Conjugated bile salts; Coronary bypass surgery (see CABG; OHCBS); Cruveilhier-Baumgarten syndrome; Culture-bound syndrome; Cystathionine beta-synthase.
CBSP Common bedside surgical procedure(s).
CBT Carotid body tumor; Chronic behavior(al) technique; 'Clotbuster' therapy; Cognitive behavior(al) therapy; Computed/ Computerized body tomography; Congenital brain tumor; Cord blood transplant(ation); Core body temperature.
CbT Covariate-by-treatment (interaction).
CBU Chronic bleeding ulcer (peptic).
CBV Capillary blood (cell) velocity; Catheter balloon valvuloplasty; Central/ Cerebral/ Circulating/ Corrected/ Cortical blood volume; Cerebral/ Coronary blood vessel; Coxsackie B virus.
CBVD Cerebrovascular disease (see CVD).
CBW Chemical-biological warfare; Critical band width (of noise).
CBX Computer-based examination.
CBZ; CBz Carbamazepine (see G 32883) - An anticonvulsant; Carbenzoxy chloride.
CC Calcaneal-cuboid; Calcium cyclamate; Cancer Cyotology (PACCS journal); Cardiac catheterization/ compression (resuscitation)/ contusion/ cycle; Cardiovascular clinic; Case coordinator; Cathodal closing (see KC); Cell culture; Central compartment; Cereal Chemistry (journal); Cerebral commissure/ concussion/ cortex; Cerebral compression/ contusion/ cry; Chamber of Commerce; Chest circumference; Chief complaint; Cholecalciferol; Cholinergic crisis; Chondrocalcinosis; Choriocarcinoma (see CCA); Chronic complainant/ainer/aint; Circuit course; Circular chromatography; Circulatory collapse; Classical conditioning; Clean catch (of urine); Clindamycin (on culture and sensitivity reports); Clinic(al) Center (NIH); Clinical Chemistry (journal); Clinical course; Clomiphene citrate; Closed cup; Closing capacity; Coefficient of correlation; Collateral coronary; Colony count; Colorectal cancer; Columnar cell(s); Commission certified (with reference to stains); Common cold; Compound cathartic; Compression constant; Computer calculated; Congenital cardiopathy/ cataract; Consumption/tive coagulopath(y); Contrast cystogram; Conversion complete; Coracoclavicular; Cord compression (umbilical); Coronary collaterals; Corpora cardiaca (endocrinology); Corpus callosum/ cavernosum; Costochondral; Coulter counter; Craniocervical; Creatinine clearance (see Ccr; KFT); Critical care/ condition; Cronkhite-Canada (syndrome); Crus cerebri; Cubic centimeter (see cc); Current complaint; Current Contents (journal); With correction (see cc).
Cc Concave (= cc).
cc centuries; concave (see Cc); corrected; cubic centimeter (= CC, ccm, cu cm, ml, 10^{-3} l); with correction (= CC) (ophthalmology).
C_c Creatinine clearance (see C_{cr}; KFT).
C-C Convexo-concave.
C&C Cold and clammy.
CC 914 Thiocarbasone.
CC 1037 Thioarsenate.
CCA Calcium channel antagonist(s) (see CCB); Calcium-containing antacid; Canadian Chiropractic Association; Cancer-causing agent; Carbamate carboxylate anion (see car-

bam); Cardiac conduction abnormality; Careful clinical assessment; Case- crossover analysis; Cephalin cholesterol antigen; Chick cell agglutination (unit); Chimpanzee coryza agent (= RSV - Respiratory syncytial virus); Chondrocalcinosis articularis (Orthopedics); Choriocarcinoma (= CC); Chronic cocaine addict; Circulating cathodic antigen; Circumflex coronary artery; Citizens for Clean Air; Clinica Chimica Acta (journal); Combined contraceptive agent; Common carotid artery; Concentrated/ Critical care area; Congenital cardiac anomaly - any defect(s) of the heart or great blood vessels existing from birth. These include: AS - Aortic/ Atrial stenosis. ASD - Atrial septal/ Atrioseptal defect. CA - Coarctation of the aorta. ECD - Endocardial cushion defect. PDA - Patent ductus arteriosus. PS - Pulmonary/nic stenosis. TA - Tricuspid atresia. Tet F; TF - Tetralogy of Fallot. TGV - Transportation of the great vessels. VS - Valvular stenosis. VSD - Ventricular septal defect; Congenital contractural arachnodactyly; Constitutional chromosome abnormality; Cytidyl cytidyl adenyl (see C-C-A).

C-C-A Cytidyl cytidyl adenyl (= CCA).

CCAHS Consumer Commission on the Accreditation of Health Services (NYC).

CCAP Capsule cartilage articular preservation.

CCARE Center for Clinical AIDS Research and Education (UCLA).

CCAT Chick cell agglutination test; Conglutinating complement absorption test (for the serological diagnosis of glanders).

CCAVB Congenital complete atrioventricular block (see CCHB).

CCB Calcium channel blocker(s); Closed-chest bypass (see CCBHBO; CDRS).

CCBB Clinical-center blood bank.

CCBHBO Closed-chest, beating heart, bypass operation.

CCBV Central circulating blood volume.

CCC A normal cat cell strain; Cancer Care Center; Cancer causes control; Care-cure coordination; Cathodal closing/sure contraction (= CaCC; KCC; KSC); Cathode closing current (electrotherapy); Central counteradaptive change; Certificate of Clinical Competence; Child care clinic; Child Care Center; Chronic calculous cholecystitis; Chronic cardiac complication (e.g. cardiomyopathy); Chronic catarrhal colitis; Chronic (spinal) cord compression; Cisplatin-containing chemotherapy (in lung cancer) (= CCR); Citrated calcium carbimide/ cyanamide; Civilian Conservation Corps; Clear-cut consensus; Columbia Clinical Classification; Commission on Clinical Chemistry; Commodity Credit Corporation; Common cold cure and Tonic (proprietary drug); Comprehensive care clinic; Comprehensive Cancer Center (NCI); Concomitant clinical condition; Consecutive case conference; Continuing community care; Cooperating Clinics Committee (ARA); Copyright Clearance Center, Inc. (US); Coronary collateral circulation; Council on Clinical Cardiology; County Community Consortium; Crafoord coarctation clamp; Crile crushing clamp (artery forceps); Critical Care Clinic; Critical care complex; Current Concepts in Cancer (journal); Cylindrical confronting cisternae; Cytidylyl cytidylyl cytosine.

CC&C Colony count and culture.

CCCA Commission on Critical Choices for America.

CCC-A Certificate of Clinical Competence in Audiology.

CCCC Centrifugal countercurrent chromatography; Citizens' Committee for the Conquest of Cancer; Comprehensive Cancer Care Conference (Washington, DC).

CCCD Complex congenital cardiac disease/ disorder; Current Citations on Communication Disorders (journal).

cccDNA Convalently closed circular deoxyribonucleic acid.

CCCE Certification Commission for Clinical Engineering.

CCCl Cathodal/de closure clonus.

CCCM Chest and Critical Care Medicine.

CCCP Carbonyl cyanide m-chlorophenylhydrazone; Current Contents: Clinical Practice (journal).

CCCPC Cancer: Cause, Control and Possible Cure (ACS).

CCCR Closed chest cardiac resuscitation.
CCCS Comparator-controlled clinical study; Condom catheter collecting system.
CCC-SP Certificate of Clinical Competence in Speech-Language Pathology.
CCCT Closed craniocerebral trauma.
CCCU Comprehensive cardiac/ cardiovascular care unit.
CCD Calibration curve data; Cancer/ Complete cell death; Carbonate compensation depth; Cardiac conduction defect/ disorder/ dysrhythmia; Catheterization and Cardiovascular Diagnosis (journal); Central core disease; Cerebellar cortical degeneration (see ANCD); Chagas-Cruz disease (see ASS); Charge-coupled device; Childhood celiac disease; Chronic cardiac disease; Chronic cerebral/ chest disease; Coded Classification of Disease (RCGP); Committee on the Care of the Diabetic; Complement component deficiency; Complex carbohydrate diet; Complex coronary disease; Congenital cardiac disorder; Congenital chloride diarrhea; Conventional corticosteroid dosage/ dose (regime); Coronary circulatory disturbance; Countercurrent distribution; Cumulative cardiotoxic dose; Cytocidal drug.
CCDA Chenodeoxycholic acid.
CCDC Canadian Communicable Disease Center.
CCDEP Central Clinical Drug Evaluation Program.
CCDM Commonwealth Congress on Diarrhea and Malnutrition (Darwin, Australia).
CCDN Central Council for District Nursing.
ccDNA Closed circle deoxyribonucleic acid.
CCDS Color-coded Doppler system (see CFDS); Coronary catheter dilating system.
CCE Carboline carboxylic acid ester; Chamois contagious ecthyma; Chronic constitutional eczema; Clear-cell endothelioma; Clinical Cardiac Electrophysiology; Clubbing, cyanosis, and edema; Countercurrent electrophoresis.
CCEI Crown-Crisp Experimental Index.
CCEPM Center for Continuing Education in Podiatric Medicine.
CCF Cancer coagulation factor; Carbohydrate-containing food; Cardiolipin complement fixation; Carotid-cavernous fistula; Centrifuged culture fluid; Cephalin-cholesterol flocculation (see CCFT); Chronic clinical filariasis; Cleveland Clinic Foundation; Compound comminuted fracture; Congenital clubfoot (Orthopedics); Congestive cardiac failure (see CHF); Crystal-induced chemotactic factor.
CCFA Cefotoxin-cycloserine fructose agar; Center for Craniofacial Anomalies (University of Illinois).
CCFAS Compact colony-forming active substance.
CCFE Cyclophosphamide, cisplatin, fluorouracil, and estramustine.
CCFF Canadian Cystic Fibrosis Foundation.
CCFMG Cooperating Committee on Foreign Medical Graduates.
CCFS Center for Child and Family Studies.
CCFT Cephalin-cholesterol flocculation test (Hanger's test) (= CCF) (see LFT iv).
CCG Cancer-cell growth; Cardiocairograph (X-rays of the heart made at any point in its cycle); Cholecystogram, cholecystography; Conventional care group.
CCGC Capillary column gas chromotography.
CCH C-cell hyperplasia; Central control hypothesis; Chronic care hospital; Chronic cholestatic hepatitis; Chronic cluster headache (see CTTH); Cork County Hospital (Chicago, USA).
CCHA Canadian Council on Hospital Accreditation.
CCHB Congenital complete heart block (fetal) (see CCAVB, MAPLS).
CCHD Committee to Combat Huntington's Disease (Inc.); Cyanotic congenital heart disease.
CCHE Central Council for Health Education.
CCHF Chronic congestive heart failure; Congo/ Crimean hemorrhagic fever (caused by a nairovirus of the Bunyaviridae group and transmitted by ticks, principally *Hyalomma* sp).
CCHMS Central Committee for Hospital Medical Services.
CCHP Consumer Choice Health Plan.
CCHPA California Council for Health Plan Alternatives.

CCHRT Continuous-combined hormone replacement therapy (estrogen with progestin).
CCHS Congenital central hypoventilation syndrome.
CCI Calcium-channel inhibitor (see CCB); Center for Clinical Immunology (Stanford Univ., US) (see CIC); Chronic cardiac/ coronary insufficiency; Coexisting current illness; Corrected count increment; Cross Cancer Institute (Edmonton, Canada).
CCJ Costochondral joint/ junction.
CCK Cholecystokinin (in Choliangiography; with secretion, a main mediator of hormonal regulation; a gut hormone which mediates impulses from the digestive tract and helps produce satiety) (see Hormones - CCK).
CCK-8 Cholecystokinin octapeptide (see CCK-OP).
CCK-GB Cholecystokinin cholecystography.
CCKLI Cholecystokinin-like immunoreactivity.
CCK-OP Cholecystokinin octapeptide (= CCK-8).
CCK-PZ Cholecystokinin-pancreozymin (see PZ-CCK).
CCL Carcinoma/ Certified cell line; Cardiac catheterization laboratory; Charcot-Leyden crystal; Coronary catheter line (a torquable, eccentric laser catheter); Cortical cell loss; Critical carbohydrate level; Critical condition list.
CCl_4 Carbon tetrachloride.
CCl_3CHO Chloral.
$CCl_3CH(OH)_2$ Chloral hydrate.
CCLE Chronic cutaneous lupus erythematosus.
CCLI Composite clinical and laboratory index.
CCM Calcium-containing medication; California College of Medicine; Candesartan cilexetil monotherapy (for HTN); Careful clinical monitoring; Cerebrocostomandibular (syndrome) (see CCMS); Clinical Care Medicine (journal); Congestive cardiomyopathy; Continuous cardiac monitoring Craniocervical malformation; Critical care medicine; Cryptococcal meningitis; Cyclophosphamide, CCNU (= CeeNu; lomustine), and methotrexate.
c cm; cm^3 cubic centimeter (see cc); cubic centimeter(s) per minute.
CCMA Certified Color Manufacturers Association.
CCMC Committee on the Cost(s) of Medical Care.
CCMD Critical Care Medicine Department (Clinical Center, NIH).
CCME Center for Clinical Medical Ethics; Coordinating Council on Medical Education (AMA).
CCMG Charing Cross Medical Gazette (UK journal).
CCMR Cross-cultural medical research.
CCMS Cerebrecostomandibular syndrome (= CCM); Clean catch midstream (see CCMSU); Clinical care management system; Committee on Challenges of Modern Society; Congress of County Medical Societies.
CCMSU Clean catch midstream urine (= CCMS; CCMU) (procedure/ urine culture; see KFT).
CCMT Catechol-o-methyltransferase.
CCMU Clean catch midstream urine (see CCMSU); Critical care medical unit.
CCN Caudal central nucleus; Coronary/ Critical care nursing.
CCNSC Cancer Chemotherapy National Service Center.
CCNU Chlorethyl cyclohexyl nitrosurea (= Chlorethyl cyclohexyl nitrous urea; Lomustine; N-(2-chloroethyl)-N'-cyclohexyl-N-nitrosourea) - a cytotoxic drug used in the treatment of brain tumors and Hodgkin's disease; Cyclophosphamide, Methotrexate and Lomustine (small cell carcinoma) [Methotrexate, Doxorubicin, Cyclophosphamide and Lomustine (non-oat cell carcinoma)] Procarbazine, Vincristine, Cyclophosphamide and Lomustine (3 Chemotherapy combinations); Lomustine (= CeeNU; CNU; LO).
CCO Comprehensive care organization; Cytochrome C oxidase.
C-collar Cervical collar.
CCOM Chicago College of Osteopathic Medicine.
CCOT Cervical compression overloading test.

CCP Cancer control program (NCI); Cancer Cure Program; Carrier control point (NWN - National Warning Network for nuclear attack - UK); Chronic calcifying pancreatitis; Ciliocytophthoria; Comprehensive cancer program; Contemporary clinical practice; Contraceptive pill/ precaution/ protection; Co-operative Cardiovascular Project; Critical care physician; Cytidine cyclic phosphate.

CCPA Committee on Chemistry and Public Affairs (ACS); Consumer Credit Protection Act.

CCPD Continuous cycling/ cyclical peritoneal dialysis.

CCPDS Centralized Cancer Patient Data System.

CCPR Crypt cell production rate.

CCR Cancer Chemotherapy Reports (NCI journal); Cardiac catheterization recovery; Cell cycle regulation/tor; Center for Cancer Research (MIT); Central chemoreceptor(s) (located at the base of the brain) (= MCR); Cerebro-colic reflex (Defecation reflex initiated in the conscious brain - on awakening, through motivation, visual and other stimuli, etc.) (see GCR); Cisplatin-containing regimen (see CCC); Closed-cell rubber/ rubber foam (used in orthopedics); Commission on Civil Rights; Common research center (Euratom); Complete continuous/ Continuous complete remission; Critical Care Research (Laboratory in southern California).

C_{cr} Creatinine clearance (= CC; Ccr; CCT; Cl_c) (see KFT_{cr}).

CCRA Comprehensive cancer risk assessment (a vital part of the COH Cancer Center) (see COH); Computer-controlled robotic arm (Robotic surgery).

CCRC Continuing care residential community.

CCRCB Closed-chest robotic coronary bypass (see CCB; CCBHBO; CDRS).

CCRF Children's Cancer Research Foundation; Central Cancer Registry of Puerto Rico.

CCRIS Chemical Carcinogenesis Research Information System.

CCRMP California Committee for Regional Medical Programs.

CCRN Critical Care Registered Nurse.

CCRS A seven-transmembrane protein, chemokine (virus) receptor.

CCRT Concomitant chemoradiotherapy (for cancer).

CCRU Critical care recovery unit.

CCS Canadian Cancer/ Cardiovascular Society; Cardiac conduction system; Case-control/ crossover study; Casualty clearing station; Cat-cry syndrome (a rare, inherited defect seen at birth with a kitten-like cry, low weight, small head, "moon-face", wide-set eyes with strabismus, and low-set misshaped ears. Also called CDCS or Cri-du-chat syndrome and C5pS or Chromosome 5p-syndrome); Causal connecting statement(s); Cell cycle specific; Central chondrosarcoma (= ECS); Central cord syndrome (as in myelopathy of spinal cord); Child Care Services (UCLA); Cholecystosonography; Chronic cerebellar stimulation; Chronic compartment syndrome; Cloudy cornea syndrome; Colon cancer syndrome; Committee on Chemical Safety (ACS); Complex clinical state; Concentration camp syndrome; Constant current source; Controlled clinical study; Costoclavicular syndrome; Crippled Children Services; Critical carotid stenosis (i.e. >70%); Cronkite-Canada syndrome (diarrhea, weakness, weight loss, diffuse hair loss and nail dystrophy); Cryoconservation of sperm.

CCSCS Central cervical spinal cord syndrome.

CCSE Cognitive Capacity Screening Examination.

CCSG Children's Cancer Study Group.

CCSP Central canal of the spinal cord.

CCST Certificate of Completion of Specialist Training.

CCT Calcitrol; Carotid compression tomography; Cancer/ Cytotoxic chemotherapy (see CST); Cardiac conducting tissue; Cardiac/ Central conduction time; Cathodal/de closing/sure tetanus (= CCTe; KCT; KST); Cephacetrile; Cerebro-cranial trauma; Chocolate-coated/covered tablet; Chronic corticosteroid therapy; Closed cerebral trauma; Coated compressed/ Compressed coated tablet; Combination chemotherapy;

Combined cortical thickness; Complex clinical state; Composite cyclic therapy; Computerized cranial tomography; Congenitally corrected transposition (of the great vessels); Controlled clinical trial; Controlled cord traction; Conventional cancer therapy/ treatment (such as chemotherapy, radiation therapy or surgery); Conventional chemotherapy; Coronary care team; Cranial computed tomography; Creatinine clearance test (see C_{cr}; KFT); Crude coal tar; Cyclocarbothiamine.

CCTA Cancer chemotherapeutic agent.

CCTe Cathodal closure tetanus (see CCT).

CCTG Coccidioidomycosis Cooperative Treatment Group.

CCTGA Congenitally corrected transposition of the great arteries.

CCT in PET Crude coal tar in petroleum.

CCTP Coronary care training program/ project.

CCTRT Combined chemotherapy and radiotherapy (= CTRT).

CCTV Closed-circuit television.

CCTVS Council on Cardio-Thoracic and Vascular Surgery (AHA).

CCU Cardiac/ Cardiovascular/ Continuing/ Coronary/ Critical Care Unit; Cellular calcium uptake; Cherry-Crandall unit; Common Cold Unit; Community care unit.

CCUA Clean catch urinanalysis.

CCUP Colpocystourethropexy.

CCV Channel catfish virus; Conductivity cell volume; Congenital calcaneo-valgus (= Pes calcaneo-valgus congenitus [L]); Congenital coxa vara (Orthopedics); Custom cancer vaccine.

CCVCC Consonant, consonant, vowel, consonant, consonant (utterance).

CCVD Chronic cerebrovascular disease; Congenital cardiovascular disorder.

CCVM Congenital cardiovascular malformation.

CCW Chest wall compliance; Childcare worker; Counterclockwise.

CCX Complications.

CD Cadaver donor (transplantations); Caesarean/ Cesarean/ Cesarian/ Complicated delivery/red (obstetrics); Canadian Doctor (journal); Canine distemper/ dose; Carbohydrate dehydratase; Carbon dioxide; Cardiac diameter/ disease/ dullness/ dysrythmia; Cardiovascular/ Castleman's/ Celiac/ Childhood/ Communicable/ Contagious/ Crohn's disease; Cardiovascular Disease (journal); Carrel-Dakin (fluid); Cathodal duration (= KD); Caudad; Caudal (see Cd); Cell dissociation; Cell/ Cerebellar/ Cerebral degeneration/ dysfunction; Certificate of deposit (bank); Cervical dystonia; Cervicodorsal; Chagas' disease (a Latin American form of trypanosomiasis, named after Carlos Chaga who identified the sickle-shaped, protozoan parasite *Trypanosoma* cruzi, previously discovered by Dr. Oswaldo Cruz in Central Brazil, as the transmitter of this disease by the feces of reduviid or triatomid bugs, also known as conenose or "kissing" bugs, of the family *Reduviidae*; these parasites burrow into the heart muscle and other organs, causing divers illnesses such as congestive cardiomyopathy of Chagas' disease); Character/ Communication/ Conduct(ion)/ Convulsive disorder; Chemical dependency; Chemist and Druggist (journal); Child Development (journal); Chronic Disease (journal); Circular dichroism; Civil defence; Clinical Dentistry (journal); Clinical diagnosis (see OSCD); Cluster of differentiation (an antigen molecule on the surface of T cell lymphocytes: CD3 molecules act as antigen receptors, CD4 molecules recognize class II antigens, CD8 molecules recognize class I antigens, including viral antigen and so on); Coccygeal (see Cd); Colla dexter (L.) - with the right hand; Collagen disease/ disorder; Combination drug; Common duct; Completely denatured; Conjugate diameter (L. conjugata diagonalis) - diagonal diameter of the pelvic inlet; Consanguineous donor; Contact dermatitis; Continuous drainage; Control diet; Conventional dialysis; Convulsive/ Curative dose; Corneal dystrophy; Cot death; Cotrel-Dubousset (rod); Crib death (see SIDS); Crossed diagonal; Cushing's disease (see CS); Cutdown; Cystic duct; Cytarabine and daunorubicin.

Cd Cadmium (Z = 48) - see Elements -

Cadmium; Caudal (= CD; cd); Caudatum (thalamus); Coccygeal (= CD) (with reference to vertebrae; in vertebral numbers); Color-denial (Rorschach); Condylion.

cd candela (L) - candle. A unit of intensity of light (luminous intensity; new candle); caudal (see Cd).

C/D; C/d; c/d Cigarettes per day; Cup to disc ratio.

C&D Curettage and desiccation; Cystoscopy and dilatation/ dilation (procedure/urology).

CD3 An antigen molecule which acts as an antigen receptor (see CD).

CD4 HIV helper cell count; Lymphocytes/ Protein receptors (involved in the function of other immune cells).

CD8 HIV suppressor count; Lymphocytes/ Protein receptors (the killer cells and suppressor cells of the immune system); White blood cells of the human immune system.

CD 10 The common acute lymphoblastic antigen.

CD 45 The common leukocyte, surface protein antigen (see CLSP).

CD_{50} Median curative dose (i.e. that which abolishes symptoms in 50% of test subjects).

CD 68 Chlordane (= Chlordan; Octachlor; Octa-Klor; Toxichlor; Velsicol 1068). A methanoindane chlorinated insecticide.

^{115}Cd Radioactive cadmium.

CD 154 T-cell surface molecule (see TCSM).

Cd 412 Peruvoside.

CDA Canadian Dental/ Diabetic Association; Certified Dental Assistant; Chenodeoxycholate/ cholic acid (see CDCA); Ciliary dyskinesia activity; Complement-dependent antibody (activity); Completely denatured alcohol; Concomitant drug administration; Congenital dyserythropoietic anemia; Corticosteroid-dependent aspergillosis.

2-CdA 2-Chlorodeoxyadenosine (= Cladribine). A powerful new, anti-lymphocyte, anti-cancer drug, used in the treatment of hairy cell leukemia, multiple sclerosis, and other auto-immune diseases (see DCF).

CDAA Chloro-diallylacetamide (a herbicide).

CDAD *Clostridium* difficile-associated disease (the most severe form of which is PMS - pseudomembranous colitis).

CDAI Crohn's Disease Activity Index.

CDAJ Canadian Dental Association Journal.

CDAK Cordis Dow Artificial Kidney.

CDAPCA Comprehension Drug Abuse Prevention and Control Act.

CDB Colonic diverticular bleeding (see CDH).

C&DB Cough and deep breath.

CDBT Chewable-dispersible buffered tablet (see CDT; CT).

CDC Calculated date/ day of confinement; Cancer detection/ diagnosis center; Capillary diffusion capacity; Carboplatin, doxorubicin, and cyclophosphamide; Cardiac diagnostic center; Cell division cycle; Centers for Disease Control (USPHS, Atlanta); Chenodeoxycholate/ cholic acid (see CDCA); Child Development Center; Child development clinic; Chronic disease care; *Clostridium* difficile colitis (see ClDC); Communicable Disease Center (PHS, Atlanta); Community Development Corporation; Complement-dependent cytotoxicity; Cycloheptaamylose-dansyl chloride.

CD-C Controlled drinker-control.

CDCA Chenodeoxycholate/ deoxycholic acid (= CDA; CDC); Choledochocaval anastomosis.

CDCC Child day-care center.

CDCP Centers for Disease Control and Prevention (see CDC); Council on Dental Care Programs (ADA).

CDCS Cri-du-chat syndrome (see CCS).

CDD Cardiodepressant drug (procainamide, quinidine, etc.); Catecholamine-depleting drug (e.g. reserpine); Centre for Digestive Diseases (Leeds, UK); Cerebral degenerative disease (e.g. ataxic telangiectasia, juvenile Huntington's disease, lysosomal enzyme deficiency, Wilson's disease); Certificate of disability for discharge; Choledochoduodenostomy; Chronic degenerative/ disabling disease; Chronic depressive disorder; Chronic disabling dermatosis; Chronic disc degeneration; Clot-dissolving drug (= CDM); Continuous daily dosing.

CDDP Cis-diaminedichloroplatinum.

CDE Canine distemper encephalitis; Central dopaminergic effect; Certified Diabetes

Educator; Chlordiazepoxide (see CDX); Common duct exploration; Coronary disease event(s); Council on Dental Education (ADA).

C,D,E Three Rh genes.

c,d,e three allelic forms of Rh genes.

CDEB Chemical Defence Establishment in Britain.

CDER Center for Drug Evaluation and Research (FDA).

CDF Cardiac dysfunction; Cartilage derived factor (Orthopedics); Children's Defence Fund; Chondrodystrophia foetalis; Contiguous-disk file (computer); Contraceptive diaphragm fitting (see Contraceptives).

CDG Cancer detection guideline(s); Central developmental groove.

CDGP Constitutional delay of growth and puberty.

cDGS Complete form of DiGeorge's syndrome.

CDH Canadian Dental Hygienist (CDHA journal); Central dislocation of the hip (Orthopedics); Ceramide dihexoside; Cervical disc herniation; Chronic daily headache; Chronic disease hospital; Colonic diverticular hemorrhage (= BCD; CDB; RDB); Congenital diaphragmatic hernia; Congenital dislocation/ dysplasia of the hip.

CDHA Canadian Dental Hygienists Association.

CDI Carbonyl-diimidazole; Central/ Chronic/ Cranial diabetes insipidus; Children's Depression Inventory; Choriodecidual infection (see Chorioamnionitis); Clinical Drug Investigation (journal, Auckland, New Zealand).

C_{Di} Concentration of dialysate.

CDILD Chronic diffuse interstitial lung disease.

CDK Climatic droplet keratopathy; Cyclin-dependent kinase (see Cdk 5).

Cdk 5; CDK 5 Cyclin-dependent kinase 5 (the enzyme responsible for neurofibrillary tangle formation by altering the structure of the tangles' main component, the protein tau in Alzheimer's disease) (see AD, CDK, ICH, NFT, NTF, THP).

CDKI Cyclin-dependent kinase inhibitor (= p27).

CDL Chlordeoxylincomycin/ Chlorodeoxylincomycin; Curriculum Development Laboratory (TERC).

CDLE Chronic discoid lupus erythematosus.

CDLS Cornelia de Lange syndrome.

CDM Cancer detection method (such as CEA, PSA, TMT, etc.); Chemically-defined medium; Chronic Disease Management (journal, now CD); Clinical decision making; Clinical diabetes mellitus; Cloth-dissolving medicine (see CDD).

CDMD Council on Dental Materials and Devices.

CDN Clindamycin.

CDNA; cDNA Circular/ Complementary deoxyribonucleic acid.

CDNB 1-chloro-2,4-dinitrobenzene.

CDNHW Canadian Department of National Health and Welfare.

CDOS Cervicodorsal outlet syndrome (Orthopedics).

CDP Center for Diabetes in Pregnancy (Obstetrics); Central disc prolapse; Cervical discogenic pain; Child Development Program; Chondrodysplasia punctata (Ichthyosis, stippled calcification of epiphyses, saddle nose, congenital cataracts, dwarfism - an autosomal and sex-linked/ X-L dominant, congenital hypotrichosis) (= CHS); Chronic destructive periodontitis; Chronic Disease Program (USPHS); Collagenase-digestible protein; Communicable Diseases Program (WHO); Congenital dislocation of the patella; Constant/ Continuous distending pressure; Coronary drug project (NHLI); Cytidine/ Cytosine diphosphate.

CDPC Cytidine diphosphate choline.

CDPs Common digestive problems.

CDPX X-linked chondrodysplasia punctata.

CDQ Chronic Disease Quarterly (journal); Corrected development quotient.

CDR Calcium-dependent regulator; Clinical Dementia Rating; Clinical dose range; Clinical drug research; Complement decay rate; Computerized digital radiography; Continuous daily regimen; Continuous disability review; Council on Dental Research

(ADA); Cup/ disk ratio; Crude Death Rate (deaths per thousand per month) (Public Health).

CDRF Canadian Dental Research Foundation.

CDR(H) Cup-to-disc ratio (horizontal).

CDRS Children's Depression Rating Scale; Computer-driven robotics system (used in heart surgery; called "Zeus" - see CCBHBO).

CDRT Committee on Diagnostic Reading Test.

CDR(V) Cup-to-disc ratio (vertical).

CDS Cardiovascular surgery; Catechol-3,5-disulfonate; Caudal dysplasia syndrome; Cervical disc syndrome; Chemical Data Systems, Inc.; Child development service(s); Choriodecidual space; Christian Dental Society; Chromatography data system; Chronic disease state(s); Comprehensive discharge summary; Computer densitometer system; Cumulative duration of survival.

cds cul-de-sac (Fr. culs-de-sac = [lit] bottom of a sack) - 1. A passage or position with only one outlet; 2. A situation from which there is no escape.

CDSC Communicable Diseases Surveillance Center (London).

CDSM Committee on Dental and Surgical Materials.

CDSPQ College of Dental Surgeons of the Province of Quebec.

cd-sr candela-steradian.

CDSS Clinical decision support system.

CDT Carbon dioxide therapy; Cathodal/de duration tetanus (see CDTe); Certified Dental Technician; Chewable-dispersible tablet (see CDBT); Chronic drug therapy; Clinical drug trial; Cloning-derived therapy/ treatment (see TCT); Clostridium difficile toxin; Combined diphtheria tetanus (vaccine); Complex drug therapy; Comprehensive diagnostic treatment; Concentration-dependent toxicity (e.g. amino/ cardiac glycosides, cytotoxic agents, psychoactive drugs, etc.); Council on Dental Therapeutics (ADA).

CDTA Cyclohexylene dinitrilo-tetraacetic acid.

CDTe Cathodal/de duration tetanus (= CDT; KDT).

CDTS Clinical-Drug-Trial System.

CDU Chemical dependency unit; Cumulative dose unit.

CDUD Compulsive/ dependent use of drugs (see CUD; EUD; RUD).

CDV Canine distemper virus.

CDW Contaminated drinking water.

CDX Chlordiazepoxide (= CDE; CDZ). A benzodiazepine tranquillizer.

Cdyn; C_{dyn} Dynamic compliance (lung).

CDZ Chlordiazepoxide (see CDX); Conduction delay zone.

CE California encephalitis; Cardiac enlargement; Cardioesophageal; Catamenial epilepsy; Cataract extraction; Cauda equina (terminal nerve filaments of the spinal cord) (see FT); Cell/ Crude extract; Central episiotomy; Centriole; Cephaloridine; Cerebral edema/ embolism; Chemical energy; Chick embryo; Childbirth Education (ASPO journal); Chloroform ether; Cholesterol ester(s); Chorioepithelioma; Chromatoelectrophoresis; Ciliated/ Columnar epithelium; Clinical Endocrinology (UK journal); Clinical engineer/ examination; Commission exhibit; Community/ Continuing education; Conjugated estrogen(s); Constant error; Contractile element (of skelettal muscle); Contrast echography; Conversion electron; Converting enzyme; Cytopathic effect.

CE; C/E; C-E Cost-effective.

Ce Cerium (Z= 58) (see Elements - Cerium); Center median (thalamus).

C-E Chloroform-ether (anesthesia mixture).

C/E Church of England; Collagen/ elastin (ratio).

C&E Consultation and examination; Cough and exercise; Curettage and electrodesiccation.

^{58}Ce Radioactive cerium.

C1E1 C1 and E1 esterase inhibitor.

CEA Carcinoembryonic antigen (test); Cardiac electrical activity; Carotid endarterectomy; Cat's eye amaurosis (blindness in one eye in which a bright reflexion from the pupil is seen - caused by a swelling or cancerous tumor); Central edge angle. Formed with one arm taken vertically from the head of the femur and the other from this point (i.e. the femoral head), to the upper edge of the acetabulum; Childbirth Education Association; Cholesterol-esterifying activity; Commission à l'Énergie Atomique (France); Cost-effectiveness analysis; Council of Economic Advisors; Crystalline egg albumin.

CEAC Clinical Endpoint Adjudication Committee (see AEP; PEP; SEP).

CEAR Congress of the European Association of Radiology.

CEARP Continuing Education Approval and Recognition Program.

CEASD Conference of Executives of American Schools for the Deaf.

CEAT Carcinoembryonic antigen test (Roche); Chronic ectopic atrial tachycardia.

CEBD Controlled extrahepatic biliary damage.

CEBP Cancer Epidemiology Biomarkers Prevention (Study/ Trial).

cEBV Chronic Epstein-Barr virus (infection).

CEC Cauda equina compression (e.g. in Paget's disease) (see CECS); Chick embryo cell (culture medium); Ciliated epithelial cell; Clinical Endpoints Committee; Clinical ethics committee; Council for Exceptional Children.

CeC Carcinoma en cuirasse (a rare cancer developing along with advance breast cancer, or cancer of the rectum).

cec- prefix meaning blind (L. caecus) (e.g. cecum, cecal vision, etc.).

CECC Clinical Engineering Certification Commission; Committee on Emergency Cardiac Care (AHA).

CECH Center for the Enhancement of the Capabilities of the Handicapped (FIRL).

CECOS Center for the Study and Conservation of Sperm (Fr. Centre pour l'Étude et Conservation du Sperme).

CECS Cauda equina compression syndrome (Orthopedics).

CECT Contrast-enhanced computed tomography.

CED Chondroectodermal dysplasia (Acromegalic dwarfism, 50% congenital heart disease and oligodontia - attachment of upper lip to gingiva - an autosomal recessive dysplasia) (= EVC - Ellis van Crefeld's); Chronic endothelial dysfunction.

CEDC Community Economic Development Corporation.

CEE California equine encephalitis (= STE); Central European encephalitis; Chick embryo extract.

CEEA Curved end-to-end anastomosis (stapler).

CEEB College Entrance Examination Board.

CEEG Clinical Electroencephalography (journal); Computer-analyzed electroencephalography.

CeeNU Lomustine (see CCNU; LO).

CEES Center for Energy and Environmental Studies (Princeton Univ, NJ).

CEEV Central European encephalitis virus.

CEF Centrifugation extractable fluid; Chick embryo fibroblast; Constant electric field; Coronary endothelial function.

CEFIC Centre Européen des Fédérations de l'Industrie Chimique (Fr.) (European Center of Federations of the Chemical Industry).

CEFMG Council on Education for Foreign Medical Graduates.

CEFP Continuing Education for the Family Physician (journal).

CEG Chronic erosive gastritis.

CEH Cholesterol ester hydrolase.

CEHC Calf embryonic heart cell.

CEI Carbapenem enzyme inhibitor; Cauda equina injury; Center for Economic Information (UN); Character education inquiry; Clinical and Experimental Immunology (journal); Committee on Environmental Improvement (ACS); Committee for Environmental Information; Continuous extravascular infusion; Converting enzyme inhibitor.

CEID Calibrated electronic infusion device; Crossed electroimmunodiffusion.

CEJ Cement-enamel junction.

CEK Chick embryo kidney.

CEL Cardiac exercise laboratory; Cholesterol-enriched lipoprotein (see CETRL).

Cel Celluloid (see Cell; cell); Celsius (= C; Cels; cent; Centigrade degree) (thermometer scale).

cel A unit of velocity (1 cm/sec).

cel- prefix meaning hollow (Gr. koilos).

-cele suffix meaning tumor, swelling, or herniation (Gr. kele).

Cell (journal).
Cell; cell Celluloid (= Cel) (dentistry).
cell- combining form meaning room or cell (L. cella).
CELO Chicken embryonal lethal orphan (virus).
Cels Celsius (see Cel).
CEM Composite efficacy measure; Computerized electroencephalographic map; Conventional transmission electron microscope (= CTEM); Cutting-edge medicine.
CEMS Committee on Emergency Medical Services (AMA and NAS-NRC).
CEN Center for Nuclear Energy Studies (Belgian - Centre d'Études de l'Énergie Nucléaire); Center for Nuclear Studies (Fr. Centre d'Études Nucléaires); Certificate for Emergency Nursing; Comité Europeen de Normalisation (standards); Continuous emergency/ enteral nutrition.
cen central (= cent); centromere.
cen- prefix meaning common (Gr. koinos).
C&EN Chemical and Engineering News (ACS).
ceno- prefix meaning empty (Gr. kenos).
CENP Centromere protein.
cent centigrade (see Cel); centimeter (see cm); central (see cen).
cent- prefix meaning hundred (L. centum).
-cente suffix meaning puncture (Gr. kentes).
centi- metric prefix for 1/100.
CENU Chloroethylnitrosourea (anti-cancer agent, e.g. in gliomas).
CEO Chick embryo origin; Chief Executive Officer; Chronic exogenous osteomyelitis; Clinically evident ophthalmopathy (in Graves' disease); Conjugated equine oestrogen.
CEOP Chronic progressive external ophthalmoplegia.
CEOT Calcifying epithelial odontogenic tumor.
CEP Capsule endoscopy procedure (the capsule used contains a powerful package of diagnostic tools, including a color camera, four light sources, a radio transmitter and batteries; the casing is watertight and acid-resistant, and the capsule relies on peristalsis to push it through the digestive tract, as it records two images per second, providing more than 50,000 images to aid diagnosis); Cardiac electrophysiology; Chronic effusive pericarditis; Chronic eosinophilic pneumonia; Chronic/ Congenital erythropoietic porphyria; Clinical end point; Cognitive evoked potential; Common effect parameter; Continuing education program; Cortical evoked potential (EEG); Counter-/ Countercurrent-/ Counterimmuno-electrophoresis.
CEPA Chloroethane phosphoric acid.
CEPH Cephalic; Cephalosporin.
Ceph; ceph Cephalin; Cephalometry.
Ceph 87/4 Cephaloridine (= Compound 40,602). A broad-spectrum bactericidal antibiotic (see Compound 40,602).
cephal- prefix meaning head (= kephal-) (Gr. kephale).
CEPH FLOC; Ceph Floc Cephalin flocculation (test).
CEPP Clinical and Experimental Pharmacology and Physiology (joural).
cept- combining form meaning take or receive (L. capio).
CEQ Council on Environmental Quality.
CER Ceramide (see Cer); Conditioned emotional response; Control(led) electrical rhythm; Cortical evoked response; Cost effective ratio; Cumulative event rate (Kaplan-Meier); Cutting-edge research.
Cer Ceramide (= CER).
cer- combining form meaning wax (L. cera; Gr. keros).
CE&R Central episiotomy and repair.
CERA Cortical evoked response audiometry.
cerat cerate (wax or fat ointment) (L. ceratum).
cerat- combining form meaning horn (Gr. keras; keratos).
CERCLA Comprehensive Environmental Response, Compensation, and Liability Act.
CERD Chronic end-stage renal disease.
cerebr- prefix meaning cerebrum (L).
CERES Consumers for Ethics in Research (UK).
CERN Centre Européen pour la Recherche Nucléaire (French; Geneva) - European Center for Nuclear Research.
Cert; cert Certificate/fied.

CERULO Ceruloplasmin.
cerv cervical/vix.
Cervic-; cervic- prefix meaning neck (L. cervix; cervicis).
CES California Epilepsy Society; Capital Expenditures and Services (controls - NHI); Cardiac electrical stability; Cardioembolic stroke; Cat's eye syndrome; Cauda equina syndrome; Central Excitatory Scale; Central excitatory state; Chronic electrophysiological study; Cognitive environmental stimulation; Conditioned escape response; Conjugated estrogenic substance(s); Cooperative Extension Service; Cutting-edge scientist/ service(s).
CESD Cholesterol ester storage disease; Chronic environmental stress disorder.
CES-D Center for Epidemiological Studies - Depression.
CET Capital expenditure threshold; Clinical efficacy/ experience trial; Concentration-effect-toxicity (of a drug); Concurrent estrogen therapy; Congenital eyelid tetrad; Corrected effective temperature; Cost-effective therapy; Cutting-edge.
CETA Comprehensive Employment and Training Act.
CETC Chick embryo tissue culture.
CETE Central European tick-borne encephalitis.
CETI Communication with Extraterrestrial Intelligence.
CETIS Centre Europe̒en de Traitement de l'Information Scientifique (Fr.) (European Center for Processing Scientific Information) (part of Euratom).
CETRL Cholesterol-enriched triglyceride-rich lipoprotein.
CEU Congenital ectropion uveae; Continuing education unit.
CEV California encephalitis virus; *Citrus* exocortis viroid; Coxsackie enterovirus; Cyclophosphamide, etoposide, and vincristine.
CEX Clinical evaluation exercise.
CEZ Cefazolin.
CF Calcium leucovorin; Calf blood flow; Calibration/ Chemotactic/ Clotting/ Colicin/ Colonization/ Coupling factor; Canadian Formulary (CPA); Cancer-/ Carrier-free; Caput forceps (for delivering head of baby); Carbofuchsin; Carbol-fuchsin; Carbon filtered; Cardiac failure; Carotid foramen; Carworth Farms; Cascade filtration; Case file; Caucasian female; Centrifugal force; Cephalothin (on culture and sensitivity reports); Characteristic frequency; Chemotherapy Foundation; Chest and left leg (ECG lead) (see CF 1); Chiari-Frommel (syndrome); Chick fibroblast; Chikungunya/ Childbed (see CBF) fever; Children's Formula; Chorion frondosum (placenta); Christmas factor (see Factor IX); Cisplatin and fluorouracil; Citrovorum factor (= Calcium folinate/ Folinic acid/ leucovorin); Clotting factor (= AT III - Antithrombin III); Collagen fibril; Collected fluid; Colony forming; Color and form (response - Rorschach); Complement factor (one of the accessory factors in the six major components of the immune system); Complement fixation (test); Complement-fixing (see C'F); Computed fluoroscopy; Conservation Foundation; Constant/ Cough frequency; Contractile force; Coronary flow (see CBF); Count fingers (eye examination); Counting finger; Cubic feet (of gas); Cycling fibroblast; Cystic fibrosis; Cystic Fibrosis (journal).
Cf Californium (Z = 98) (see Elements - Californium).
cf centrifugal force; compare (bring together, confer, refer to) (L. confer; confero).
C'F Complement-fixing (= CF).
c/f colored female.
CF 1 Chest lead with indifferent electrode on left leg (ECG) (= C; CF).
CFA Cancer fighting agent; Colonization factor antigen; Colony-forming assay; Common femoral artery; Complement-fixing activity/ antibody; Complete Freund adjunct/juvant; Configuration frequency analysis; Congenital facial abnormality; Consumer Foundation of America; Continuous flow analysis; Cryptogenic fibrosing alveolitis.
CFAC Complement-fixing antibody consumption.
C-factor; C-fact Cleverness factor (psychology test).

CFB Central fibrous body; Corneal foreign body.
CFBS Canadian Federation of Biological Societies.
CFBSS Chronic failed back surgery syndrome.
CFC Capillary filtration coefficient; Cardiofaciocutaneous (syndrome) - a minor hypotrichosis with sporadic inheritance, patchy scalp alopecia, psychomotor and growth retardation, and cardiac abnormalities; Cervical fibronectin concentration (see PMP; VFC); Chemical feed computer; Chlorinated Fluoro-Carbon(s); Chlorofluorocarbon(s); Clotting-factor cascade/ concentrate (see CF); Colony-forming capacity/ cell; Combined Federal Campaign; Continuous flow centrifugation; Craniofacial Clinic (UCLA).
CFC_{12} Fluorocarbon 12.
CFC_{13} Fluorocarbon 13.
CFCs Chlorofluorocarbons.
CFD Canadian Food Directorate; Cancer-fighting drug; Cephalofacial deformity; Cerebellar/ Cerebral function disease/ disorder; Chronic fibrotic/ filarial disease; Class F diabetes (= DN, DNP - Diabetic nephropathy); Craniofacial defect/ deformity; Craniofacial dysostosis.
CFDA Canadian Food and Drug Act.
CFDD Canadian Food and Drug Directorate.
CFDE Canadian Fund for Dental Education.
CFDS Color-flow Doppler system (see CCDS); Craniofacial dyssynostosis.
CFDSQ Canadian Forces Dental Services Quarterly (journal).
CFF Critical flicker fusion (test/ threshold) (used as an index of sedation and drug-induced drowsiness) (= cff); Critical flicker/ fusion frequency (= cff); Cystic fibrosis factor; Cystic Fibrosis Foundation.
CFF; CF# Complex femoral fracture.
cff Critical flicker fusion (see CFF); Critical fusion frequency (see CFF).
CFFA Cystic fibrosis factor activity.
CFFT Critical Flicker Fusion Threshold.
CFG Cancer-fighting gene.
CFH Council on Family Health.
cfh cubic feet per hour.
CFHb Cell-free hemoglobin.
CFI Chemotactic factor inactivator; Chronic fungal infection(s); Color flow image/ imaging (Ultrasound); Complement fixation inhibition (test); Cost, freight, and insurance.
CFICA Complement fixing islet-cell antibody.
CFIDS Chronic fatigue immune dysfunction syndrome (see CFS; ICL).
CFL Calcaneo-fibular ligament; Cisplatin, fluorouracil, and leucovorin calcium; Cosmetic face-lift (Cosm. surgery).
CFM Chlorofluoromethane (a fluorocarbon); Close-fitting mask; Corometric fetal monitor (see CMS); Craniofacial microsomia; Cubic feet per minute (see cfm); Cyclophosphamide, fluorouracil, and citoxantrone.
cfm cubic feet per minute.
CFMA Council For Medical Affairs.
CFMG Commission of Foreign Medical Graduates.
CFN Council on Foods and Nutrition (AMA).
CFND Craniofrontonasal dysostosis.
CFNS Chills, fever, and night sweats; Craniofrontonasal syndrome.
CFP Canadian Family Physician (journal); Cancer-fighting properties/ty; Cancer-free polyp; Carbol-fuchsin paint (contains boric acid, phenol, resorcinol, fuchsin, acetone, and alcohol in water. Used to treat fungus infections of the skin. Also called Castellani's paint); Cardiac filling pressure; Chronic false-positive (test); Clinical Fellowship Program; College of Family Physicians (Canada); Committee on Food Protection (FNB of NRC); Complication-free recovery; Craniofacial reconstruction; Cyclophosphamide, fluorouracil, prednisone; Cystic fibrosis of the pancreas; Cystic fibrosis protein.
CFPP Craniofacial pattern profile.
CFPR Canadian Familial Polyposis Registry.
CFPT Cyclophosphamide, fluorouracil, prednisone, and tamoxifen.
CFQ Carboxyfluoroquinolone(s) (Quinolone group of antibiotics such as Ciprofloxacin, Levofloxacin, Moxifloxacin, Nalidixic acid, Ofloxacin, and Perfloxacin) (Especially effective against *Enterobacteriaceae* and *Pseudomonas*); Cystic Fibrosis Quaterly

(journal).

CFR Capillary filtration rate; Case-fatality rate/ ratio; Center for Futures Research; Citrovorum-factor rescue; Classic fear response (with activation of the amygdala, thalamus, locus ceruleus, and hippocampus of the brain, resulting in sweaty palms, rapid heartbeat, increased blood pressure, and a burst of adrenaline) (see APD, FFF, GAD, PD, PTSD); Code of Federal Regulations; Complement-fixation reaction (see CFT); Correct fast reaction; Cyclic flow reduction.

CFRF Cystic Fibrosis Research Foundation.

CFS Cancer family syndrome; Carbol-fuchsin solution (= Castellani's paint) (see CFP); Center for Food Safety (USDA); Chiari-Frommel syndrome; Child and Family Services; Chronic fatigue syndrome (see CFIDS; ICL); Circumferential fiber shortening; Continuous flushing system; Craniofacial stenosis; Crush fracture syndrome; Culture fluid supernatant; Cystic Fibrosis Society.

cfs; cf/s cubic feet per second.

CFSE Crystal field stabilization energy.

CFSG Charge-free spacer gel.

CFSQE Center for Food Safety and Quality Enhancement (Univ of Georgia).

CFSR Circumferential fiber shortening rate.

CFSS Chronic Fatigue Syndrome Society.

CFSTI Clearinghouse for Federal Scientific and Technical Information (later NTIS - see NTIS).

CFT Carbon-13 and Fourier transform (nuclear magnetic resonance spectroscopy); Cardiac function test(s): Blood volume % of body weight - Cardiac output L/min./sq.m body surface area - Cardiac pressure mm Hg - Right atrium - mean pressure - Right ventricle (systolic, diastolic pressure) - Pulmonary artery (systolic, diastolic, mean pressure) - Circulation time (arm to tongue) sec - Venous pressure mm water; Cardiolipin flocculation test; Clinical full time; Closed functional treatment (of fractures) (Orthopedics); Complement-fixation test (= CFR; CF test); Complement-fixing (antibody) titer; Cystic fibrosis therapy.

CF test Complement fixation test (see CFT).

CF 1TL Colonoscope (C = colon; F = flexible; 1 = single channel; T = treatment; L = long).

CFTR Cystic fibrosis transmembrane (conductance) regulator.

CFU Clinical follow-up (see LFU); Colony-forming unit (see HGF); Color-forming unit.

CFU-C Colony-forming unit - culture (see HGF).

CFU-E Colony-forming unit - erythrocyte (Erythroid cell CFU - see HGF).

CFU-Eo; CFU-Eos Colony-forming unit - eosinophil (see HGF).

CFU-F Colony-forming unit - fibroblastoid (see HGF).

CFU-GEMM Colony-forming unit - granulocyte/ erythrocyte/ monocyte/ megakaryocyte (see HGF).

CFU-GM Colony-forming unit - granulocyte macrophage; CFU granulocyte/ macrophage (see HGF).

CFU-L Colony-forming unit - lymphoid (see HGF).

CFU-M; CFU-Meg Colony-forming unit - megakaryocyte (see HGF).

CFU-NM Colony-forming unit - neutrophil/ monocyte (see HGF).

CFU-S Colony-forming unit - spleen (see HGF).

CFV Continuous flow ventilation.

CFW Carworth Farms (mouse), Webster strain.

CFWM Cancer-free white mouse.

CFX Cefoxitin; Circumflex coronary artery.

CFZ Capillary free zone.

CFZC Continuous-flow zonal centrifugation.

CG Cardiography; Cardiogreen (= iodocyanine green) - a dye; Center of gravity (= cg); Central gray (region of brain); Chloasma gravidarum (skin discoloration occurring in pregnancy) (= CU); Choking gas (phosgene); Cholecystogram; Chorea gravidarum; Choriogenic gnynecomastia; Chorionic gonadotropin (see Hormones - CG; HCG); Chromogranin; Chronic glomerulonephritis; Cingulate gyrus; Colloidal gold; Contact guarding; Control group; Controlled gavage; Cyroglobulin; Phosgene (choking gas).

cg center of gravity (see CG); centigram (= cgm; 10^{-2} gram); chemoglobulin; coccygeal.

C_G Glucose clearance rate (= K_G) (see KFT_G - C).

CG-1 Carbimazole (= CGI).

CGA Catabolite gene activator; Compressed Gas Associations Inc.; Cryoglobulinaemia; Crystallographic analysis (of kidney stones); Cytogenetic abnormalities/ty/ analysis (see CGF).

C-GAP Cancer Genome Anatomy Project.

CGAS Children's Global Assessment Scale.

CGB Chronic gastrointestinal (tract) bleeding; Chronic gonadotropin, beta-unit.

CGC Carcinoma gigantocellulare (see GCC); Child guidance center; Colloidal gold curve; Computer-generated copy (of the brain, etc.).

CGD Career grade doctor (NHS, UK); Chromosomal gonadal dysgenesis; Chronic granulomatous disease (formerly FGD); Cytogenetic damage/ disease/ disorder.

CGDE Contact glow discharge electrolysis.

CGE Computer-guided electrode.

CGEB Center for Genetic Engineering and Biotechnology (Havana, Cuba).

CGF Cellular growth factor; Cockroft-Gault formula (140 - age) X body wt (kg) X K/serum creatinine (1/2mol/l). K = constant (1.25 for men and 1.03 for women) - for calculation of Creatinine clearance, Glomerulation filtration rate, etc.; Cytogenetic finding (in bone marrow, etc.) (see CGA).

CGFH Congenital fibrous histiocytoma.

CGFNS Commission on Graduates of Foreign Nursing Schools.

CGFT Colloidal gold flocculation test (see LFT iv).

CGH Cervicogenic headache; Chorionic gonadotropic hormone (see Hormones - CGH; HCG).

CGI Carbimazole (see CG-1); Chronic granulomatous inflammation; Clinical Global Impression (scale); Computer-generated imagery.

CGIAR Consultative Group on International Agricultural Research.

CGIC Clinician's global impression of change.

CGKD Complex glycerol kinase deficiency.

CGL Cephaloglycin; Chorionic gonadotropin level (see SCG); Chronic granulocytic leukemia.

C Gl Carrier glucose.

c gl correction with glasses.

CGM Central gray matter (spinal cord); Continuous glucose monitoring.

cgm centigram (see cg).

CGMMV Cucumber green mottle mosaic virus.

CGMP See cGMP.

cGMP Cyclic guanosine monophosphate (= CGMP; Cyclic 3'5'-gm; GMP).

CGN Chronic glomerulonephritis.

CGNB Composite ganglioneuroblastoma.

CG/OQ Cerebral glucose/oxygen quotient.

CGP Carbenzoxy-glycyl-phenylalanine (= N-carbenzoxy-glycyl-L-phenylalanine); Carcinogenic potential; Choline glycerophosphatide; Chorionic growth hormone prolactin (see Hormones - GH); Circulating granulocyte pool; Clastogenic potential; College of General Practice (Canada).

CGPM Conférence Générale des Poids et Mesures (1960) - France (General Conference of Weights and Measures).

CGR Center for Genome Research (Univ. of Edinburgh).

CGRP Calcitonin gene-related peptide.

CGS Carcinogenetic/genicity study; Cardiogenic shock; Catgut suture; Centimeter-gram-second (see cgs); Chromic gut suture; Cytogenetic study.

CGs Cancer genes (HER-2 genes, Oncogenes, Adenovirus-p53 genes, TSG [Tumor suppressor genes], Antisense genes, Anti-telomerase genes, Anti-angiogenic drugs such as angiostatin, endostatin, and vasculostatin).

cgs centimeter-gram-second (system of units) (= CGS).

cg/s centigrams per second.

CGSR Co-ordinating Group on Standards for Registration (GMC, UK).

CGT Cancer gene therapy (see HGT; SGT); Carbenzoxy-glutamyl-tyrosine (= N-carbenzoxy-α-glutamyl-L-tyrosine); Chorionic gonadotropin (see Hormones - HCG); Clinical gene therapy; Cyclodextrin glucanotransferase.

CGTH Chorionic gonadotropic hormone (see

Hormones - HCG).

CGTT Cortisone glucose tolerance test (diabetes detection - laboratory/ chemistry).

CGU Cerebral glucose uptake (see CMRG).

cGy Centigray (1 rad).

CH Case history; Catabolic hormone(s) - e.g. catecholamines, cortisol, glucagon, growth hormone, etc); Chediak-Higashi/ Conradi-Hunermann (syndrome); Chiasma; Chinese hamster; Chloral hydrate; Cholestatic hepatitis (see CJ); Cholesterol (see Chol); Christchurch chromosome (see Ch'); Chromaffin hormones (see Hormones - CH i); Chronic hepatitis (= CHH)/ hypertension; Classic hepatitis (viral); Cluster headache; Cochlear hydrops (a clinical variant of Meniere's disease); Common hepatic (duct); Communicating hydrocele; Community Health; Complement, hemolytic (see CH50); Completely healed; Compulsory hospitalization; Congenital hypothyroidism; Continuous heparin (infusion); Convalescent hospital; Conversion hysteria; Cortical hormone (see Hormones - CH ii); Crown-heel (length of body/ fetus); Cycloheximide; Cystic hygroma; Wheelchair.

ch chest (= Ch); chief (= Ch); child (= Ch); chronic (= Ch).

Ch Chapter; Check; Chest (see ch); Chido (antibody); Chief (see ch); Child (see ch); Chloramphenicol (see CAP); Choline; Christchurch (chromosome/ syndrome - see Ch'); Chromosome; Chronic (see ch).

cH Hydrogen ion concentration (see cH^+).

C_H Constant domain of H chain; Hydrogen ion concentration (see cH^+).

cH^+ Hydrogen ion concentration (= cH; C_H).

Ch' Christ-church chromosome/ syndrome (= CH; Ch).

C&H Coarse and harsh (breathing); Cocaine and heroin (see Erythroxylum; Diamorph HCl).

$(CH_2)_2$ Ethylene.

(CH_3) Methyl group.

CH_4 Methane.

C_2H_2 Acetylene.

C_6H_6 Benzene.

CH50; C'H50 Complement, hemolytic (50% hemolyzing dose of complement) (total serum).

CHA California/ Canadian/ Catholic Hospital Association; Capillary hemangioma (= Hemangioma simplex; Strawberry mark); Catholic Health Association; Cavernous hemangioma (= Angioma cavernosum; Cavernoma); Chest and Heart Association (UK); Child health associate; Children's health advocate; Chinese hamster; Chronic hemolytic anemia; Common hepatic artery; Congenital hemolytic anemia; Congenital hypoplasia of adrenal (glands); Congenital hypoplastic anemia; Continuously heated aerosol; Cyclohexyladenosine; Cyclohexylamine.

ChA Choline acetylase.

CHAART Center for Health Applications of Aerospace Related Technologies.

CHABA Committee on Hearing and Bio-Accoustics (Armed Forces - National Research Council).

ChAC; ChAc Choline acetyltransferase (see ChAT).

CHAD Control (and treatment) of Hypertension, Atherosclerosis, and Diabetes; Cyclophosphamide, Hexamethylmelamine, Adriamycin (Doxorubicin), (and cisplatin).

chaero- prefix meaning rejoice (Gr. chairein) (= chairo-; chero-).

CHAI Continuous hepatic artery infusion.

CHAIR Consortium on HIV/AIDS Interregional Research (Kaiser Permanente, Pasadena, California.

chairo- See chaero-.

chalk amphetamine tablet (see Amphet).

$C_6H_9AlO_6$ Aluminium acetate {the solution, also containing $Al_2(SO_4)_3$ or Aluminium sulfate plus $CaCO_3$ or Calcium carbonate, is known as Burrow's solution, used as a skin cream and antiseptic).

CHAM Consistent, hierarchical, arbitrary, and monothetic (method used to classify psychiatric states or conditions.

CHAMOCA Cyclophosphamide, Hydroxyurea, Actinomycin D (dactinomycin), Methotrexate, Oncovin (vincristine), Calcium folinate (leucovorin), and Adriamycin (doxorubicin).

CHAMP Certified Hospital Admission

Monitoring Program; Children's Hospital Automated Medical Program; Commonwealth Hospital Admissions Monitoring Program (Massachusetts).

CHAMPUS Civilian Health and Medical Program of the Uniformed Services.

CHAMPVA Civilian Health and Medical Program - Veterans Administration.

chancr- prefix meaning crab or cancer (L.).

CHANDS Curly hair - ankyloblepharon - nail dysplasia syndrome.

Chang C Chang conjunctiva (cells).

Chang L Chang liver (cells).

CHAOS Cambridge Heart Antioxidant Study.

CHAP Certified Hospital Admission Program (California); Child health associate practitioner; Children's Health Assurance Program (New York); Community Health Accreditation Program; Corporate Headquarters Alcoholism Program; Cyclophosphamide, Hexamethylmelamine, Adriamycin (doxorubicin), and Platinum compd (cisplatin).

chap chapter.

CHARGE Coloboma, heart disease, atresia choanae, retarded growth and retarded development (and/or CNS anomalies), genital hypoplasia, and ear anomalies and/or deafness (syndrome).

C_{HARLEM} Non S sickling hemoglobin.

Charles Cocaine (see Erythroxylum).

Chart Paper(s) (L. charta; chartulae).

Chart bib Blotting paper (L. charta bibula).

Chart cerat Waxed paper (L. charta cerata).

CHAS Center for Health Administration Studies.

Chase Chondroitin lyase.

CHAT Checklist for Autism in Toddlers.

ChAT Choline acetyltransferase (= ChAC; ChAc).

CHB Chronic hepatitis B; Complete/ Congenital heart block.

CHb Carbanino-hemoglobin.

ChB Bachelor of Surgery (L. chirurgiae baccalaureus) (= BS).

CHBHA Congenital Heinz body hemolytic anemia.

CHBM Chinese hamster bone marrow (used for in vivo micronucleus test for chromosomal aberrations).

ChbMet Cyanomethemoglobin (a form of hemoglobin formed during nitrite therapy for cyanide poisoning (= HbCMet).

CHBPR Council for High Blood Pressure Research.

C_2H_5Br Ethyl bromide.

CHC Capitated health care; Childhood cancer; Community Health Center/ Computing/ Council; Coordinate home care; Cultured human cell.

CH_3CCNU Semustine.

CHCF California HealthCare Foundation (COH).

C_2H_5CHO Acetone (see CH_3COCH_3).

$CH_3CHOHCOOH$ Lactic acid (= $C_3H_6O_3$).

$CHCl_3$ Chloroform.

$C_2H_4Cl_2$ Ethylene chloride.

C_2H_5Cl Ethyl chloride.

$C_2HCl_3(OH)_2$ Chloral hydrate.

CH_3COCH_3 Acetone (=C_2H_5CHO; C_3H_6O).

$C_2H_5CO_2NH_2$ Ethyl carbamate.

$(CH_3CO)_2O$ Acetic anhydride.

CH_3COOH Acetic acid (= $C_2H_4O_2$).

C_4H_9COOH Valerianic acid (=$C_5H_{10}O_2$).

C_6H_5COOH Benzoic acid (=$C_7H_6O_2$).

CHCP Comprehensive/ Correctional Health Care Program (SSA); Coordinated Home Care Program; County health care plan.

CHCs Chlorinated hydrocarbons (see VSA).

CHCVD Chronic hypertensive cardiovascular disease.

CHD Center/ Chronic hemodialysis; Chediak-Higashi/ Childhood disease; Chinese herbal drug; Chronic heart/ hepatic disease; Chronic heavy drinker; Common hepatic duct; Congenital heart damage/ defect(s); Congenital/ Congestive/ Coronary/ Cyanotic heart disease; Congenital hip dislocation; Constitutional hepatic dysfunction.

ChD Doctor of Surgery (L. chirurgiae doctor) (= DS; DSur).

Chd Child.

CHDC California Health Data Corporation.

CHDD Continuous high daily dosage/ dose.

C-HDL Alpha-lioprotein (high density).

CHDM Comprehensive hospital drug monitoring; Coronary heart disease mortality.

CHDP Child Health and Disability Prevention

(Program).
CHE Cholinesterase (see ChE); Chronic hepatic encephalopathy.
ChE Chemical engineer; Cholinesterase (= CHE; Che; CHS).
Che Cholinesterase (see ChE).
che a gene involved in chemotaxis.
CHEC Community Hypertension Evaluation Clinic.
CHEF Chinese hamster embryo fibroblast.
cheil- prefix meaning lip (Gr. cheilos).
cheir- combining form meaning hand (Gr. cheir).
Chem; chem Chemistry; Chemical; Chemotherapy.
Chem ID Chemical Identification.
CHEMLINE Chemical (Dictionary) On-Line (i.e. Chemical information retrieval service NLM).
Chemo Chemotherapy (journal).
ChemoRx Chemotherapy.
CHEMRAWN Chemical research applied to world needs (IUPAC).
CHEMTREC Chemical Transportation Emergency Center.
Ch Eng Church of England (member).
Cheno Chenodeoxycholic acid.
chero- prefix meaning rejoice (see chaero-).
CHERSS Continuous high-amplitude EEG rhythmical synchronous slowing.
CHES Community Health Educatonal Services (Albany, New York).
CHESS Community Health and Environmental Surveillance System (EPA).
Chest (ACCP journal).
CHF Canadian Heart Foundation; Chick embryo fibroblast; Chronic/ Clinical heart failure; Congenital hepatic fibrosis; Congestive heart failure (= CCF); Crimean hemorrhagic fever; Cyclophosphamide, Hexamethylmelamine and 5-Fluorouracil (Chemotherapy).
CHFC Carnegie Hero Fund Commission.
CHFD Controlled high flux dialysis.
CHFV Combined high-frequency ventilation.
CHG Community Health Group.
chg change(d).
CHH Cartilage-hair hypoplasia (autosomal recessive disease) (fine, light-colored, silky and sparse hair, dwarfism, metaphyseal dysostosis, and susceptibility to infections - an autosomal recessive, congenital hypotrichosis); Chronic hepatitis (see CH); Country House and Hospital (Hollywood, California).
CH_3H_4GLU Methyltetrahydrofolate.
CHI Catastrophic health insurance (for severe or long-term illness or injury); Closed head injury; Chronic hepatic impairment/ insufficiency; Commission for Health Improvement (NHS, Brit); Creatinine-height index.
chi chimera.
CHI_3 Iodoform.
C_2H_5I Ethyl iodide.
Chi-A Chimpanzee leukocyte antigen.
Chick Heroin (see Diamorph HCl).
Chief LSD-25 (see LSD).
CHILD Congenital hemidysplasia with icthyosiform erythroderma and limb defects (syndrome).
Chil. P Chilean Pharmacopoeia (Farmacopea Chilena).
CHIME Coloboma, heart anomaly, icthyosis, mental retardation, and ear abnormality.
Chimia (Swiss journal).
Chin Chinese.
CHINA Chronic infectious neurotropic agent.
Chinese white Concentrated heroin (see Diamorph HCl).
Chin. P Chinese Pharmacopoeia.
CHIP Catastrophic (see CHIPS)/ Comprehensive Health Insurance Plan; County Health Improvement Program; Curb Heroin in Plants (United Auto Workers' factory program); Iproplatin.
CHIPASAT Children's Paced Auditory Serial Addition Task.
CHIPS Catastrophic health insurance plans.
chir- combining form meaning hand (Gr. cheir).
Chir Doct; Chir Doc Doctor of Surgery (L. chirurgiae doctor).
Chiro Chirogram (journal).
Chirop Chiropodist (journal).
chirurg surgical (L. chirurgicalis).
Chix Chickenpox (see Chpx).
Chk Check.
CHL Childhood hearing loss; Chinese hamster lung; Chlorambucil; Chloramphenicol

(see CAP); Chloroquine (see CQ); Chlorpromazine (see CPZ); Cochlear hearing loss.

Chl Chloramphenicol (see CAP); Chloroform; Chlorophyll; Chloroquine (see CQ); Chlorpromazine (see CPZ); Cholesterol (see Chol).

CHLA Childrens Hospital Los Angeles; Cyclohexyl linoleic acid.

Chlb Chlorobutanol.

CHLCA Chinese hamster (in vitro) lung cell assay (for chromosomal abberations).

CHLD Chronic hypoxic lung disease.

chlor chloride.

chlor- combining form meaning green (Gr. chloros).

Chloral hydrate JJ; Joy juice; Knockout drops (liquid chloral); Mickey Finn; Torpedo; and other names.

CHM College of Human Medicine; Community health medic; Compound heterozygous mutation (gene); Coronary heart morbidity/ mortality; Council on Health Manpower.

ChM Master of Surgery (L. chirurgiae magister).

Chm Chairman.

CHMA Comprehensive Health Manpower Act (1971).

CHMAb Campath-1H monoclonal antibody (directed against T cells in MS).

CHMC Children's Hospital Medical Center (Boston); City of Hope Medical Center (Duarte, California).

CHMD Clinical hyaline membrane disease.

CHMS Council of Heads of Medical Schools (UK).

CHMTA Comprehensive Health Manpower Training Act.

CHN Carbon, hydrogen, and nitrogen (elemental analysis of); Child Neurology (journal); Children's Hospital Notes (journal); Chinese (hamster); Chinese-herb nephropathy (a serotonin nephropathy caused by Aristolochic acid present in the Chinese herb *Aristolochia* fangchi, and resulting in the apoptosis of the tubular cells of the kidneys in this disease. The incidence of urothelial carcinoma in such patients has been attributed to the continued ingestion of this medicinal herb); Community health nurse.

Chng Change.

$C_6H_5NH_2$ Aniline.

CHNMC Children's Hospital National Medical Center (Washington, DC).

$C_3H_5(NO_3)_3$ Glyceryl trinitrate (nitroglycerine).

$C_5H_4N_4O_3$ Uric acid.

$C_5H_{11}NO_2$ Amyl nitrite.

C_8H_9NO Acetanilid.

$C_9H_9NO_3$ Hippuric acid.

$C_6H_2(NO_2)_3OH$ Trinitrophenol (picric acid).

CHO Carbohydrate; Carbohydrate exchange (in dietary regimes); Chinese hamster ovary; Chorea.

Cho Cholesterol (see Chol); Choline (= Chol).

(CHO-) Aldo-group.

CH_2O Formaldehyde; Water clearance.

CH_2O_2 Formic acid (see HCOOH).

CH_4O Methy alcohol (see CH_3OH).

$C_2H_2O_4$ Oxalic acid (see HOOCCOOH).

$C_2H_4O_2$ Acetic acid (see CH_3COOH).

$(C_2H_5)_2O$ Ether (ethyl ether) (= $C_4H_{10}O$).

C_2H_6O Ethyl alcohol (see C_2H_5OH).

C_3H_6O Acetone (see CH_3COCH_3).

$C_3H_6O_3$ Lactic acid (see $CH_3CHOHCOOH$).

$C_3H_8O_3$ Glycerin - see $C_3H_5(OH)_3$.

$C_4H_6O_2$ Crotonic acid.

$C_4H_6O_6$ Tartaric acid - see $(CHOHCOOH)_2$.

$C_4H_8O_2$ Butyric acid (isobutyric acid).

$C_4H_{10}O$ Ether (ethyl ether) - see $(C_2H_5)_2O$.

$C_5H_{10}O_2$ Valerianic acid (see C_4H_9COOH).

$C_5H_{12}O$ Amyl alcohol (see $C_5H_{11}OH$).

C_6H_6O Phenol (carbolic acid) (see C_6H_5OH).

$C_6H_8O_7$ Citric acid - see $COOHC(OH)(CH_2COOH)_2$.

$(C_6H_{10}O_5)_n$ Starch.

$C_6H_{12}O_6$ Dextrose (d-glucose).

$C_7H_4O_7$ Meconic acid.

$C_7H_6O_2$ Benzoic acid (see C_6H_5COOH).

$C_7H_6O_3$ Salicylic acid (see $C_6H_4OHCOOH$).

$C_7H_6O_5$ Gallic acid.

$C_{12}H_{22}O_{11}$ Cane sugar (sucrose).

$C_{14}H_{10}O_9$ Tannic acid.

$C_{15}H_{10}O_4$ Chrysophanic acid.

$C_{17}H_{14}O_4S$ Rofecoxib (an inhibitor of prostaglandin synthesis, via inhibition of COX-2/ Cyclooxygenase-2, and used in the treatment of osteoarthritis).

$C_{17}H_{21}NO_4$ Cocaine (see Erythroxylum).

$C_{18}H_{34}O_2$ Oleic acid.

$C_{18}H_{36}O_2$ Stearic acid.

Choc Chocolate.

CHOCAA Chinese Hamster Ovary Chromosome Aberration Assay.

CH_3OH Methyl alcohol (=CH_4O; MeOH).

C_2H_5OH Ethyl alcohol (=C_2H_6O; EtOH).

$C_3H_5(OH)_3$ Glycerin (= $C_3H_8O_3$).

$C_5H_{11}OH$ Amyl alcohol (=$C_5H_{12}O$).

C_6H_5OH Phenol (carbolic acid) (=C_6H_6O).

$(CHOHCOOH)_2$ Tartaric acid (=$C_4H_6O_6$).

$C_6H_4OHCOOH$ Salicylic acid (= $C_7H_6O_3$).

CHOL Cholesterol (see Chol).

Chol Cholesterol (= CH;Chl; Cho; CHOL); Choline (see Cho).

chol- prefix or suffix meaning bile (Gr. chole).

c̄ hold withhold.

cholecyst prefix meaning gallbladder.

Chol est Cholesterol ester(s).

chondr- prefix meaning cartilage (Gr. chondros).

CHOP Cyclophosphamide, hydroxydaunomycin (doxorubicin), Oncovin (vincristine), and prednisone (program).

CHOP-BLEO Cyclophosphamide, Hydroxydaunomycin (Doxorubicin), Oncovin (Vincristine), Prednisone and Bleomycin (Chemotherapy).

CHOR Cyclophosphamide, Hydroxydaunomycin (Doxorubicin), Oncovin (Vincristine) and radiation (Chemotherapy with Radiation).

chord- combining form meaning string or cord (Gr. chorde).

chord chirurg surgical suture (L. chorda chirurgicalis).

chori- combining form meaning protective fetal membrane (Gr. chorion).

Chorioamnionitis Infection of the fetal membranes (see Amnionitis; Funisitis; Villitis) (= CDI).

CHP Capillary hydrostatic pressure; Capitated health plan; Charcoal hemoperfusion; Chemical Hygiene Plan; Child psychiatry (see ChP); 6-Chloro-17-α-hydroxypregna-1,4,6-triene-3,20 dione; Chronic health problem; Coalition for Health Planning (HRD); Common human pattern; Comprehensive Health Planning (Division of, - HRD); Coordinating hospital physician; Cup hip prosthesis (see OI/OP); Cutaneous hepatic porphyria.

ChP Chairperson; Chest physician; Child psychiatry (= CHP).

CHPA Comprehensive Health Planning Act.

CHPC Center for High Performance Computing (Univ. of Utah, USA).

CHPP Comprehensive health planning program.

CHPS Comprehensive Health and Planning Services (Act).

CHPV Cervical human papilloma virus (= HPV).

Chpx Chickenpox.

CHQ Chloroquinol.

CHR Cercarien hullen reaction; Cerebrohepatorenal (syndrome); Clinical Hypertension Research (Uppsala, Sweden) (see SCOPE); Community health representative.

CHr Candle-hour (see c hr).

Chr Chromatography; Chromobacterium (e.g. Chr amythistinum); Chronic (see chron).

chr chromosome; chronic (see chron).

c hr Candle-hour (= CHr).

c-hr curie-hour. A unit of dose equivalent to that obtained by exposure for one hour to radioactive material disintegrating at the rate of 3.70 x 10^{10} atoms per second.

ChRBC Chicken red blood cell.

Chr Br Syn Chicken brain syndrome (see CBS).

CHRIS Cancer Hazards Ranking and Information System; Chemical Hazards Response Information System (USCG).

Christmas tree Dexamyl capsule (see Amyl nitrite).

chro- combining form meaning color (Gr. chros).

Chromo Chromosome (journal).

Chromosome 22 The Philadelphia chromosome.

Chron Chronological.

chron chronic (= Chr; chr).

CHRP College of Health Related Professions.

CHRPE Congenital hypertrophy of the retinal

pigment epithelium.

CHRS Cerebrohepatorenal syndrome; Committee on Human Rights of Scientists (NYAS); Congenital hereditary retinoschisis.

CHS Canadian Hemophilia Society; Center for Human Sexuality; Central hypoventilation syndrome; Chediak-Higashi syndrome; Chemical hypersensitivity syndrome (see MCS); Cheney-Hadju syndrome (see ADOD; AOS); Cholinesterase (see ChE); Chondroitin sulfate; Colloidal hydrated silica (an excipient); Community Health Services/ Survey; Comprehensive (Program for Elective) Surgery (see CPES); Compression hip screw; Congenital hypoventilation syndrome; Conradi-Hunerman syndrome (see CDP); Contact hypersensitivity.

ChSci Christian Science (member).

CHSD Children's Health Services Division.

CHSO Total hemolytic serum C activity.

CHSPQ Cattell High School Personality Questionnaire.

CHSR Cellular hypersensitivity reaction (see CMIR; Type IV HS).

CHSS Comprehensive (HEW)/ Cooperative Health Statistics System.

CHT Cerebellar hemisphere tumor; Colonoscopic hemostatic therapy; Combined hormone therapy; Congenital hypotrichosis (see HDA); Contralateral head turning; Cosmetic hair transplant (Cosm. surgery).

ChTg Chymotrypsinogen.

ChTK Chicken thymidine kinase.

CHTN Compensated/ Controlled hypertension.

CHTZ Chlorothiazide (see CTZ).

CHU Closed head unit.

"Church-spire" A coined phrase indicating a high, spiked peak in the serum electrophoresis.

CHV Canine herpes virus; Centigrade heat unit; Chief Health Visitor (NHS, UK).

CHW Community Health Work.

chy- combining form meaning pour (Gr. cheo; chy).

CI Cardiac index (l/min/m^2) = Cardiac output/ body surface area (CO/BSA); Cardiac/ Convergence/ Coronary insufficiency; Cell immunity inhibition; Cell(ular) immunity; Cellular Immunology (journal); Cephalic/ Chemotactic/ Chemotherapeutic/ Clonus/ Color/ Contamination/ Cytotoxic index; Cerebral infarction/ ischemia; Cesium/ Cochlear implant; Chain-initiating; Chemical ionization; Chromatid interchange; Chronic infection/ insomnia; Chronically infected; Clinical investigation/tor; Clomipramine; Coefficient of intelligence; Colloidal iron; Commitee on Injuries (AAOS); Complete iridectomy; Confidence interval; Continued insomnia; Continuous infusion; Contra-indication (see C/I); Corrected (count) increment; Crystalline insulin; Cumulative incidence; Parke, Davis & Co code for experimental substances.

Ci Curie (a unit of radioactivity - 3.70 x 10^{10} disintegrations or atoms/second.

C/I Contra-indication.

CI 395 Phencyclidine hydrochloride. A potent analgesic and anesthetic, which is said not to cause depression of cardiovascular and respiratory functions. Has been used in the treatment of psychoneurosis and in obsessional illness. Also known by the slang name, Elephant.

CI 416 Triclofenol piperazine (= Piperazine trichlorophenate; Piperazine Trichlorphate). An anthelmintic active against roundworms and hookworms.

CI 427 Prodilidine hydrochloride (see A-1981-12).

CI 440 Flufenamic acid (= INF 1837). An anthranilic acid derivative and an anti-inflammatory agent, used in the treatment of articular rheumatism.

CI 473 Mefenamic acid (= INF 3355; N-2,3-Xylylanthranilic acid). An anti-inflammatory analgesic used in the treatment of osteoarthritis and other arthroses.

CI 501 Cycloguanil embonate (= Cycloguanil pamoate). An active metabolite of proguanil; has been tried out in the prophylaxis of malaria.

CI 581 Ketamine hydrochloride. A cyclohexanone derivative; a potent analgesic and anesthetic, with actions similar to those of phencyclidine (see CI 395).

CI 642 Ambutyrosin.

CIA Central Intelligence Agency; Chemiluminescent immunoassay; Chemotherapy-induced anemia; Chemotrypsin inhibitor activity; Chronic idiopathic anhidrosis; Collagen-induced arthritis; Collegium Internationale Allergologicum (Switzerland); Colony-inhibiting activity; Congenital intestinal aganglionosis.

C'IA Complement immune adherence (serum).

CIAA Competitive insulin autoantibodies.

CIAE Clinically important adverse experience.

CIAED Collagen-induced autoimmune ear disease.

CIAG CAMAC Industry Applications Group (see CAMAC).

CIAI Complicated intra-abdominal infection.

CIAP Climatic Impact Assessment Program (DOT).

CIAT International Center of Tropical Agriculture (Colombia).

CIB Carnation Instant Breakfast; Crying-induced bronchospasm; Cytomegalic inclusion bodies; International Council for Building Research Studies and Documentation; Cytoplasmic inclusion bodies/ body (found in some viruses).

cib Food, meal (L. cibus).

Ciba Name of Swiss chemical and pharmaceutical firm (Chemical Industries of Basel).

CIBD Chronic inflammatory bowel disease.

CIBHA Congenital inclusion-body hemolytic anemia.

CIBI Clinician Interview Based Impression.

CIBIC Clinician's Interview Based Impression of Change.

CIBIS Cardiac Insufficiency Bisoprolol Study (-II).

CIBP Chronic intractable benign pain.

CIBPS Chronic intractable benign pain syndrome.

CIC Cardiac Imaging Center (NY); Cardiac intensive care; Cardioinhibitor center; Chronically infected cell (as in AIDS); Circulating immune complex; Clinical immunology center (see CCI); Clinical Interventions Catalogue (Pharmacy software program, used to document pharmaceutical services); Combined induction/tive chemotherapy (see CICT); Completely-in-the-canal (ear instrument/ hearing aid/ shell); Concomitant inhaled corticosteroid; Constant initial concentration; Consumer Information Center (GSA); Coronary intensive care; Crisis intervention center/ clinic.

CICA Cervical internal carotid artery.

CICD Center to Improve Care of the Dying (George Washington University, Washington, DC).

CICE Combined intracapsular cataract extraction.

CICNRD Committee for International Coordination of National Research in Dermography.

CICP Chloropropham (see CIIPC).

CICS Customer information control system.

CICT Combined induction/tive chemotherapy (= CIC).

CICU Cardiac intensive/ Cardiovascular inpatient/ Coronary intensive care unit.

CID Cardiac iron deposits; Cellular immunodeficiency; Center for Infectious Diseases; Central Institute for the Deaf; Cervical immobilization device; Chick infective dose; Childhood infectious disease; Chronic inflammatory disease (e.g. Rheumatoid arthritis); Clinical Infectious Diseases (journal); Combined immunodeficiency disease (= SCID); Congenital immune/no deficiency; Cytomegalic inclusion disease; Information and Documentation Center (Euratom).

CiD Choice in Dying (Washington, DC).

-cid suffix meaning cut or kill (L. caedo) (= -cide).

CID$_{50}$ Callus inhibition dose (dose producing a specified inhibition of callus formation).

CIDBMCPCT Clinic-initiated, double-blind, multicenter, placebo-controlled trial.

CIDCOM Council for Interdisciplinary Communication in Medicine.

-cide See -cid.

CIDEP Chemically induced dynamic electron polarization.

CIDF Congress of the International Diabetes Federation.

CIDNP Chemically induced dynamic nuclear polarization.

CIDP Chronic idiopathic polyradiculopathy; Chronic inflammatory demyelinating polyradiculoneuropathy (= CIP-D).

CIDS Cellular immunity deficiency syndrome; Circular intensity differential scattering; Continuous insulin delivery system.

CIE Cellulose ion exchange; Counter immunoelectrophoresis (= Counter immunoelectrosmophoresis; Counter-current immunoelectrophoresis; CIEP) - of the cerebrospinal fluid, against specific antisera in detection of the degradation products of bacteria; Crossed immunoelectrophoresis.

CIEA Continuous infusion epidermal analgesia/ anesthesia.

CIEBM Committee on the Interplay of Engineering with Biology and Medicine (NAE).

CIEM Counter immunoelectrophoric method (see CIE).

CIEP Council on International Economic Policy; Counter immunoelectrophoresis (see CIE).

CIES Council for International Exchange of Scholars (ACE).

CIF Cloning inhibiting/tory factor; Cost, insurance, and freight (included in price).

CIFC Council for the Investigation of Fertility Control.

CIG Cold-insoluble globulin; Complement inhibitor gene.

CIG; Cig; cig Cigarette(s).

CIg Intracytoplasmic immunoglobulin.

cigM Cytoplasmic immunoglobulin M.

CIGMB Conférence International du Génie Médical et Biologique (ICMBE).

CIGN Center for Image-Guided Neurosurgery (Cleveland, Ohio).

CIH Carbohydrate-induced hyperglyceridemia; Certificate of/in Industrial Health; Children in hospital.

CIHD Chronic ischemic heart disease.

CIHDM Committee for the Improvement of Hereditary Disease Management.

CIHP Coalition of Independent Health Professionals.

ci-hr curie-hour.

CIHS California Institute for Health Systems (COH); Central infantile hypotonic syndrome.

CII Cancer Immunology and Immunotherapy (journal); Carnegie Interest Inventory; Chronic intestinal inflammation (e.g. Crohn's regional ileitis; Inflammatory Bowel Disease, etc.); Clinically insignificant increase; Computerized internal imaging.

CIIA Common internal iliac artery.

CIIP Clinical Immunology and Immunopathology (journal); Chronic idiopathic intestinal pseudo-obstruction.

CIIPC Chloropropham (= Chlorpropham; CICP; CIPC; Isopropyl N-m-chlorophenylcarbamate).

CIIT Chemical Industry Institute of Toxicology.

cili- combining form meaning eyelid (L. cilium).

CIM Chronic intestinal malfunction; Cimetidine; Cortically induced movement; Crystal impedence meter; Cumulated Index Medicus.

Ci/ml Curies per milliliter.

CIMMYT Centro Internacional de Mejoramiento de Maize y Trigo (Sp.) (International Maize and Wheat Improvement Center, El Batan, Mexico) (= IMWIC).

CIMS Chemical ionization mass spectrometry.

CIN Central inhibition; Cerebriform intradermal nevus; Cervical intra-epithelial neoplasia; Chronic interstitial nephritis.

C_{in} Insulin/ Inulin clearance.

CIN1; CIN I Cervical intraepithelial neoplasia, grade 1 (mild dysplasia).

CIN2; CIN II Cervical intraepithelial neoplasia, grade 2 (moderate-severe dysplasia).

CIN3; CIN III Cervical intraepithelial neoplasia, grade 3 (severe dysplasia and carcinoma in situ).

CINCA Chronic infantile neurological cutaneous and auricular (syndrome).

CINE Chemotherapy-induced nausea and emesis; Cineangiogram.

cine- prefix meaning move (Gr. kineo).

C1 INH Inhibitor of first complement of component.

CINJ Cancer Institute of New Jersey.

CIO Chronic iron overload.

CIOMS Council for International

Organizations of Medical Sciences (WHO).

CIOS Center for International Occupational Safety (= CIS).

CIP Cardiac Injury Panel; Cellular immunocompetence profile; Chronic idiopathic polyradiculoneuropathy; Chronic intestinal pseudo-obstruction; Clinical incubation period; Clinical Investigator Program (VA); Collection de l'Institut Pasteur; Critically ill/ injured patient/ patient/ person; Cystic intestinal pneumaosis; International Potato Center (Peru).

CIPA Collagen-induced platelet aggregation.

CIPC Chloropropham (see CIIPC).

CIPD Chronic inflammatory demyelinating polyradiculoneuropathy (see CIDP); Chronic intermittent peritoneal dialysis.

CIP-D Chronic inflammatory polyneuropathy - demyelinating (see CIDP).

CIPF Chronic interstitial pneumonitis and fibrosis (see CIP-F); Clinical illness promoting factor.

-cipient suffix meaning take or receive (L. capio).

CIPN Chronic idiopathic/ inflammatory polyneuropathy.

CIPP Committee on Injury and Poison Prevention (AAP).

CIPSO Chronic intestinal pseudo-obstruction.

CIR Cardiac index at rest; Cellular immune reaction (to viruses such as HIV); Cellular/ Chronic immune response; Cerebral infarction; Committee of Interns and Residents (New York State).

Cir; cir; Circ; circ Circa (L.) - about (see c); Circle; Circuit; Circular (see circul); Circulating/tion/tory (see circul); Circumcised/cision (see circum); Circumference (see circum).

CIRA Chromatographic infrared analyzer.

Circa; circa about (see C; c; ca; Cir; cir; Circ; circ).

Circ & sens Circulation and sensation.

CIRC artery Circumflex coronary artery.

Circul Circulation (AHA journal).

circul (= Cir; cir; Circ; circ) Circular; Circulating/tion/tory.

circum (= Cir; cir; Circ; circ) Circumcised/cision/ference.

circum- prefix meaning around (L. circum).

CIRF Chronic interstitial renal fibrosis.

CIRM Centro-Internazionale Radio-Medico.

CIRS Committee for Rotation of Surgeons-in-training; Cumulative Illness Rating Scale.

CIS Cancer-in-situ (=see IEC; PIC, which see); Carcinoma in situ (also called Cancer in situ, IEC or IECa - Intraepithelial carcinoma, PIC or PICa - Preinvasive carcinoma); Carotid insufficiency syndrome; Catheter-induced spasm; Cellular/ Compromised immune system; Center for International (Occupational) Safety (see CIOS); Central inhibitory state; Chemical/ Clinical/ Congressional Information Service; Childhood immunization schedule; Chronic impingement syndrome (shoulder) (see SIS); Clean intact skin; Clinical information system; Color Imaging System; Complete immunization schedule; Cytotoxic immunosuppressant.

CI-S Calculus index, simplified.

CiS Cingulate sulcus.

-cis combining form meaning cut or kill (L. caedo).

CISC Clean intermittent self-catheterization.

CISCA Cisplatin, cyclophosphamide, and Adriamycin (doxorubicin).

CISD Critical Incident Stress Debriefing.

cis-DPP Cisplatin.

CISM Conseil International Sport Militaire (International Military Sports Council).

CISP Chronic intractable shoulder pain.

CIT California Institute of Technology; Casoni's intradermal test (for Echinococcus infection); Citrate (see cit); Clinic-initiated trial (see CIDBMCPCT); Cold-ischemia time; Combined intermittent therapy; Computer-imaging technology; Conjugated-immunoglobulin technique. Conventional immunosuppressive/ insulin therapy.

cit; Cit citrate (= CIT; Cit).

Citat Citation (AMA forensics journal).

cit disp; cito disp Dispense quickly (L. cito dispensetur).

Citn Citrulline.

CIU Chronic idiopathic urticaria.

CIUC Copper intrauterine contraceptive (device) (see CIUCD).

CIUCD Copper intrauterine contraceptive device.
CIUP Coordinator of Improvement of University-level Personnel.
CIVI Continuous intravenous infusion.
CIVII Continuous intravenous insulin infusion.
CIVS Continuous intravenous sedation.
CIWAAS Clinical Institute Withdrawal Assessment of Alcohol Scale (Canada) (see ADAF).
CIXA Constant infusion excretory urogram.
CJ Cholestatic jaundice (see CH); Clinical Journal; Conjunctivitis.
CJA Chronic juvenile arthritis (= SD - Still's disease)/ arthrodesis.
C-Jakob Creutzfeldt-Jakob (disease) (see CJD).
CJB Canadian Journal of Biochemistry.
CJC Cancer Journal for Clinicians (ACS journal).
CJCM Canadian Journal of Comparative Medicine.
CJCMVS Canadian Journal of Comparative Medicine and Veterinary Science (now CJCM).
CJD Creutzfeldt-Jakob disease (the human equivalent of MCD or Mad Cow Disease) (= C-Jakob; CJS) - named after Hans Gerhard Creutzfeldt and Alfons Jacob, the two German neuropsychiatrists who first isolated this disease in 1920. A spongiform degenerative encephalopathy, resulting in ataxia, loss of memory, dementia and death. Since 1984, suspected of being caused by slow-virus infection through tissue transplants, or contaminated injections of hGH (human growth hormone) used in cases of pituitary dwarfism (see Agent X).
CJGC Canadian Journal of Genetics and Cytology.
CJI *Campylobacter* jejuni infection.
CJM Canadian Journal of Microbiology.
CJMT Canadian Journal of Medical Technology (CSLT).
CJNS Canadian Journal of Neurological Sciences.
CJO Canadian Journal of Ophthalmology (COS)/ Optometry (CAO)/ Otolaryngology (COS).
CJOT Canadian Journal of Occupational Therapy.
CJP Cholestatic jaundice of pregnancy.
CJPH Canadian Journal of Public Health (CPHA).
CJPN Canadian Journal of Psychiatric Nursing (PNAC).
CJPP Canadian Journal of Physiology and Pharmacology.
CJR Canadian Journal of Research.
CJRRNM Canadian Journal of Radiography, Radiotherapy, and Nuclear Medicine (CSRT).
CJS Canadian Journal of Surgery; Creutzfeldt-Jakob syndrome (see CJD).
CJT Conjugated twins (such as Siamese twins). These are Monozygotic twins, equally developed twin fetuses produced from the same egg (see MZT).
CK Calf/ Chicken kidney; Cholecystokinin; Choline kinase; Conductive keratoplasty (radiofrequency waves used in eye surgery); Contralateral knee; Creatine kinase (see CPK); Cyanogen chloride (war gas); Cytokinin.
Ck; ck Check(ed).
C_k Renal clearance (= C_r) (see KFT - C_k; C_r).
CK-BB Creatine kinase - BB band.
CKC Cold-knife conization.
CKD Congenital kidney disease/ disorder.
CKF Chronic kidney failure (see CRF, ESRD).
CKG Cardiokymography.
CKI Chronic knee instability (Orthopedics).
CK-ISO Creatine kinase isoenzyme.
CK-MB Creatine kinase - methyl bromide.
CK-MM Creatine kinase - MM band.
Ckn Chicken.
CK-PZ Cholecystokonin-pancreozymin.
CKR Chemokine receptor; Cytokine reaction/ receptor/ response.
CKS Classic form of Kaposi's sarcoma.
CKT Cadaveric kidney transplant; Cardiokinetic therapy/ treatment.
CKW Clockwise.
CL Cancer Letter (journal); Capillary lumen; Cardiolipin; Cell line; Centralis lateralis; Chemiluminescence; Chest and left arm (ECG lead/ connection); Cholelithiasis;

Cholesterol-lecithin (test); Chronic leukemia; Cirrhosis of the liver; Clavicle (= clav); Clear liquid; Clearance; Cleft lip; Clinical laboratory; Clomipramine; Clostridium (= Cl); Colistin (on culture and sensitivity reports) (= Cl); Complex loading; Confidence level/ limit; Contact lens; Corpus luteum; Cricoid lamina; Criterion level; Critical list; Cross-linked; Cutis laxa; Cutter and Lederle Laboratories code for experimental substances; Cycle length; Cytotoxic lymphocyte.

C_L Constant domain of L chain; Lung compliance (see PFT - C_L)

Cl Chloride (laboratory/ chemistry); Chlorine (Z = 17) (see Elements - Chlorine); Claustrum (thalamus); Clavicle; Clear (= cl); Clindamycin (see CLM); Clinic (see Clin); Clostridium (see CL); Closure (of an electric current); Colistin (see CL); Total clearance.

cl centiliter (= 1/100 liter; 10^{-2} liter; 10 cc; 10 ml); clarified; clean; clear (see Cl); cleft; clinic (see Clin); clinical; clonus; clotting; cloudy (see cldy).

CL 1 Chest lead, with indifferent electrode on left arm (ECG).

CL 13,900 Puromycin (= L 3128; P 638). An antibiotic produced by the growth of Streptomyces albo-niger. Has been used in the treatment of African sleeping sickness and amebic dysentery.

CLA Certified Laboratory Assistant (ASCP); Cervicolinguoaxial; Cholesterol-lowering agent; Clarithromycin (an antibiotic) (see RBT); Clinical laboratory assistant; Community living arrangements; Conjugated linoleic acid; Contralateral local anesthesia; Cyclic lysine anhydride.

Cla Clarithromycin.

CLAC Clinical Laboratory Association of California.

ClAc; Clac Chloracetyl.

CLAD Cystine lactose electrolyte deficient (agar).

CLAH Congenital lipoid adrenal hyperplasia.

CLam Cervical laminectomy.

CLAO Contact Lens Association of Ophthalmologists.

Clap (the) Gonorrhea.

CLAPA Cleft Lip and Palate Association (UK).

CLAPSRO California - Los Angeles Professional Standards Review Organization (PSRO).

Clark II Diphenylcyanoarsine = $(C_6H_5)_2AsCN$ - a war gas.

CLAS Cholesterol Lowering Atherosclerosis Study; Clinical laboratory automation system; Congenital localized absence of skin.

clas- combining form meaning break (Gr. klao, klas).

CLASB Citizen's League Against the Sonic Boom.

CLASP Committee on Laboratory Standards and Practices.

CLASS Clinical Anatomy Study System.

Class; class; Classif; classif Classification.

clav clavicle (see CL).

CLB Capeline bandage (a caplike bandage wrapped to look like a cap, used to protect the head, shoulder, or the stump of a limb. Also called Hippocrates' bandage); Chlorambucil; Current Literature of Blood (journal); Curvilinear body.

CLBBB Complete left bundle branch block.

CLBP Chronic low back pain.

CLBSE Chlorobenzene-sulfenic acid.

CLBSI Chlorobenzene-sulfinic acid.

CLBSO Chlorobenzene-sulfonic acid.

CLC Cancerous lymphoma cell; Charcot-Leyden crystal; Choledocholithiasis (= Biliary calculus; Gallstones); Clerc-Levy-Critesco (syndrome); Cork leather and celastic (orthotic); Corpus luteum cyst.

Cl_3CCHO Chloral.

CL/CP Cleft lip/cleft palate.

Cl_{Cr} Creatinine clearance (ml/min) (see KFT - C_{Cr}).

CLD Cadaveric liver donor; Cephaloridine; Cholesterol-lowering drug; Chronic liver/ lung/ lymphoproliferative disease; Chronic Lyme disease (see TBI); Congenital limb deficiency; Corpus luteum deficiency; Coumarin-like drug (anticoagulant).Crystal ligand field.

ClDC *Clostridium* difficile colitis (assoc. with PMC - Pseudomembranous colitis) (= CDC).

CLDH Choline dehydrogenase.

CLDL Cadaveric liver donor list.

cldy cloudy (= cl).
CLE Centrilobular emphysema; Continuous lumbar epidural (anesthesia); Cutaneous lupus erythematosus; Cytologic evidence.
CLEA Conference on Laser Engineering and Applications.
CLED Cystine-lactose-electrolyte-deficient (agar).
CLEOS Conference on Laser and Electro-Optical Systems.
CLEX Cephalexin.
CLF Cardiolipin fluorescent (antibody); Cholesterol-lecithin flocculation; Contact lens fatigue.
CL/F Mean plasma clearance.
CLGB Cancer and Leukemia Group B (see ECOG).
CLH Chronic lobular hepatitis; Contralateral hemisphere (brain); Corpus luteum hormone(s) i.e. progesterone (see Hormones - LH iv); Cutaneous lymphoid hyperplasia.
CLI Chronic Lyme infection; Corpus luteum insufficiency; Cost-of-living index.
CLIA Clinical Laboratories Improvement Act (1967).
CLIF Chemistry Linac irradiation facility (BNL); Cloning inhibitory factor; Crithidia luciliae immunofluorescence.
Clin; clin Clinic(al) (= Cl; cl).
clin- combining form meaning bend, incline, lay/ lie down (Gr. klino).
ClinC Clinical conference.
Clini Clinitest.
Clinician (journal).
Clinics (journal).
Clin path Clinical pathology.
Clin proc Clinical procedure.
CLINPROT Clinical (Cancer) Protocols.
Clin Radiol Clinical Radiology (UK journal).
CLIP Corticotropin-like intermediate lobe peptide.
CLip Cerebral lipidosis.
CLJ Contact Lens Journal (UK).
Clk Clock.
CLL Cholesterol-lowering lipid; Chronic lymphatic/ lymphocytic leukemia; Cow lung lavage.
CLLE Columnar-lined lower esophagus.
Cl liq Clear liquid.
CLM Cholesterol-lowering medication; Clindamycin (= Cl; CM).
CLMA Clinical Laboratory Management Association.
CLML Clinical/ Current List of Medical Literature.
CLMV Cauliflower mosaic virus.
CLN Cervical lymph node.
CLNR Cleft lip-nasal revision.
CLO Chronic lymphatic obstruction; Cod liver oil.
CLO; Clo Close.
clo "clothing" - a unit of thermal insulation.
CLOF Clofibrate.
CLON Clonidine.
Clon Clone; Clonorchis.
Clostr Clostridium.
Clothespin graft See H graft.
Clox Cloxacillin.
CLP Caged-lens prosthesis (an artificial heart valve made up of a plastic disk in a metal cage); Chymotrypsin-like pepsin; Cleft lip with cleft palate; Clinical laboratory parameter; Cross-legged position (Orthopedics); Cross-linked polyethylene; Cycle length-paced.
CL(P) Cleft lip without cleft palate.
ClP Clinical Pathology.
CL&P Cleft lip and (cleft) palate (= CLP).
Cl Pal Cleft palate.
CLPC Childhood Lead Poisoning Control (Program - CDC).
Clq A complement component.
CLR Cerebellar ataxia; Chloride test (dentistry); Cleft lip repair (Plastic surgery); Comparative leukemia research; Cysteinyl leukotriene receptor (see CysLT1, 2); Cytogenetics Laboratory Report (chromosome studies on newborn).
CLr Renal clearance.
CLr_m Mean renal clearance.
CLRO Community leave for reorientation.
CLRP&D Council on Long-Range Planning and Development.
CLS Capillary-leak syndrome (causing pulmonary edema); Cardiac life support; Cholesterol-lowering statin (see CLSD); Clinical Laboratory Scientist (journal); Closed-loop system (for IPT or Insulin pump

therapy); Coffin-Lowry syndrome; Confused-language syndrome; Contralateral side (e.g. of the head); Cornelia de Lange syndrome; Cosmetic liposuction; Cystitis like syndrome.

CLs̄ Subunit of human complement.

CLSD Cholesterol-lowering statin drug (= CLS).

CLSE Calf lung surfactant extract.

CLSH Corpus luteum stimulating hormone (see Hormones - CLSH).

CLSL Chronic lymphosarcoma (cell) leukemia.

CLSP Center for Law and Social Policy; Common Leukocyte Surface Protein (= CD 45).

CLT Cancerous lung tumor (see BGC; BGCA); Certified/ Clinical Laboratory Technician; Chemiluminescence technique; Cholesterol-lowering therapy; Chronic lymphocytic thyroiditis; Clinical laboratory technology/ test(ing); Clot-lysis/ Clotting time; *Crithidia* lucillae test (DNA antibody test) (*Crithidia* = a genus of Zoomast Protozoans); Cysteinyl leukotriene(s) (LTC4, LTD4, LTE4) - potent inflammatory eicosanoids or humoral mediators, released from mast cells, eosinophils, etc. (see HMs - Humoral Mediators).

CL_{TB} Total body clearance.

Cl time Clotting time (laboratory/ coagulation).

CLT(NCA) Certified Laboratory Technician (certified by the) National Certification Agency (for Medical Laboratory Personnel).

ClTP Chlorothiophenol.

CLU Cerebral lactate uptake (see CMRL).

clus- combining form meaning shut (L. claudo; clusus).

CLV Cassava latent virus; Complete loss of vision (= CVL); Constant linear velocity.

CL VOID Clean voided (specimen) - viz. of urine.

CLW Contact lens wearer.

clysis hypodermoclysis (procedure/ fluid infusion).

-clysis suffix meaning injection (Gr. klysis).

CLZ Clozapine.

CM California mastitis (test); California/ Clinical/ Computer Medicine (journals); Calmodulin; Capreomycin; Carboxymethyl; Carcinomatous myopathy (see ELPS); Cardiac monitor/ muscle; Cardiomyopathy; Carpo-metacarpal; Caucasian male; Causa mortis (L.) - cause of death; Cell membrane; Center of mass; Cerebellar/ Cerebral malformation; Cerebral malaria/ mantle; Certified Midwife; Cervical mucosa/cus; Chick-Martin (coefficient); Chloramphenicol (see CAP); Chloroquine-mepacrine; Chondromalacia; Chopped meat (medium); Circular muscle; Circulating monocyte; Circumferential measurement; Clindamycin (see CLM); Clinical medicine/ microbiology/ modification; Coccidioidal meningitis; Cochlear microphonic (response); Common migraine; Complementary medicine (see AM); Complete/ Conditioned/ Contrast/ Culture medium; Complication(s); Congenital malformation; Congestive myocardiopathy; Continuous murmur; Conus medullaris; Conventional mores; Copulatory mechanism; Costal margin; Cow's milk; Culture media/ium; Current medication; Cybernetic Medicine (ISCM journal); Cystic mesothelioma; Cytometry; Cytoplasmic membrane; Master of/in Surgery (L. chirurgiae magister); Narrow-diameter endosseous screw implant (Fr. crête manche); Of sound mind (L. compos mentis); Tomorrow morning (L. cras mane) (see cm).

Cm Curium (Z = 96) (see Elements - Curium); Maximum compliance.

cM centi-morgan.

cm centimeter (= 10^{-2} meter; 10^{-2} m; cent); costal margin; cras mane (L) - tomorrow morning (= CM).

C_m Maximum clearance (with reference to UCl test - see KFT).

C/M Counts per minute.

C&M Cocaine and Morphine (mixture) (see Ertythoxylum; Papaver).

cm^{-1} reciprocal centimeter or kayser (unit of wave number).

cm^2 square centimeter.

cm^3 cubic centimeter (see cc).

CMA California/ Canadian/ Chilean/ Chinese Medical Association; Carbohydrate Metabolism Abstracts (journal); Centrally mediated action; Certified Medical Assistant (AAMA); Chemical Manufacturers Association; Chimeric monoclonal antibody (such as Trastuzumab or Traztuzumab [Herceptin TM], used in the treatment of HER2-positive breast cancer - see HER2; HumAB4D5-8); Chronic metabolic acidosis; Community Medical Alliance (HMO); Compound myopic astigmatism; Cow's milk allergy; Cultured macrophages; Current Medicine for Attorneys (journal); Cytokine-mediated activation (of fibroblasts, etc.).

CMAA California Medical Assistants Association.

CMAAO Confederation of Medical Associations in Asia and Oceania.

CMAF Centrifuged microaggregate filter.

CMAIR Cell-mediated autoimmune response.

CMAJ Canadian Medical Association Journal (JAMC).

CMAP Compound motor/ muscle action potential; Current Medical Abstracts for Practitioners.

CMAS Continuous motor activity syndrome (= IS or Isaac's s).

Cmax; C_{max} Maximum/ Peak plasma/ serum level/ concentration (of any drug, i.e. in ng/ml).

CMB Carbolic methylene blue; Central Midwives' Board; Chloromercuribenzoate; Cross-matched blood.

CMBBT Cervical mucous basal body temperature.

CMBES Canadian Medical and Biological Engineering Society (SCGMB).

CMBF Cow milk-based formula (see CMDF).

CMC Calcium-mediated contraction; Cancer-modified cell; Carboxymethyl cellulose; Carcinoma mucocellulare (or Krukenberg's tumor) (a metastatic tumor of the ovary); Cardiac muscle cell; Care management consulting/ counselling; Care management continuity (see CMCt); Carpometacarpal; Cell-mediated cytolysis/ cytotoxicity; Center for Medical Consumers (NYC); Cerebellomedullary cistern; Chloramphenicol (see CAP); Chronic mucocutaneous candidiasis/idosis (see CMCC); City/ Community/ Cornell Medical Center; Coexisting medical condition; Combined multiple chemotherapy (see CMCT); Conventional medical care (see CMSs); Critical micellar concentration; Cyclophosphamide, Methotrexate and CeeNu (Lomustine) (Chemotherapy - high dose/ standard dose).

CMCC Chronic mucocutaneous candidiasis (= CMC).

CMCN Community medical center nurse.

CMCT Combined multiple chemotherapy (= CMC); Controlled multicenter trial.

CMCt Care management continuity across settings (= CMC).

CMD Cartilage matrix deficiency; Childhood/ Congenital muscular dystrophy; Chronic/ Continued/ Continuous maintenance dose; Chronic metabolic disease (e.g. Diabetes mellitus, etc.); Chronic myeloproliferate/ Cytomegalic disease; Clinically manifest disease; Comparative mean dose; Confirmed metastatic disease; Congenital myotonic dystrophy; Continuous microinfusion device; Contralateral mediastinal disease (metastatic cancer, lung); Conventional medical doctor (see CMSs); Count, median diameter (of particles); County medical director; Cranio-mandibular disorder; Current Medical Dialog (journal).

CMDA Concomitant multiple-dose administration.

CMDF Cow milk-derived formula (for infants) (= CMBF; CMF).

CMD-FT Congenital muscular dystrophy - Fukuyama type (a common genetic disorder, especially in Japan, where gene mutation on chromosome 6 that encodes a protein fukutin, causes defects in neurone growth during brain development as well as progressive muscle degeneration. The mutation is apparantly caused by a so-called retro-transposon, a roving snippet of genetic information copied into the chromosome about 2,000 to 2,500 years ago.

CMDL Clinical Molecular Diagnostic Laboratory (COH).

CMDMCS Chloromethyl-dimethyl-chlorosilane.

CMDP Cis-2-methoxycarbonyl-1-methylvinyl-dimethyl phosphate (=

Mevinphos; Phosdrin; OS 2046). An organophosphorous insecticide.

CMDTB Cyanomethyl-dithio-benzoate.

CME Carolina Medical Electronics; Cervical mediastinal exploration; Cholinomimetic effect; Commission/ Council on Medical Education (AMA); Comprehensive/ Continuous medical examination; Continuing/ Continuous medical education; Crude marijuana extract; Cystoid macular edema.

CMEH Council of Medical Education and Hospitals (AMA).

CMER Current medical evidence of record.

CMF Cacium-magnesium free; Catabolite modular factor; Chondromyxoid fibroma; Christian Medical Fellowship; Cold mitten fraction; Cortical magnification factor; Cow milk formula (see CMDF); Craniomandibulofacial; Cyclophosphamide, methotrexate/ methrotrexame, and 5-fluorouracil (combination chemotherapy for breast cancer).

CMFP Calendar method of family planning (= Rhythm method) (see NFPM; Cyclophosphamide, methotrexate, fluorouracil, and prednisone.

CMFT Cardiolipin microflocculation test.

CMF-TX Cyclophosphamide, Methotrexate, 5-Fluorouracil and Tamoxifen (Chemotherapy).

CMFV Cyclophosphamide, methotrexate, fluorouracil, and vincristine.

CMFVP Cyclophosphamide, methotrexate, fluorouracil, vincristine, and prednisone.

CMG California/ Community Medical Group; Canine/ Congenital myasthenia gravis; Center for Molecular Genetics; Chopped meat glucose (agar/ broth/ medium); Cystometrogram/aphy.

CMGH Cleveland Metropolitan General Hospital.

CMGM Center for Molecular and Genetic Medicine.

CMGN Chronic membranous glomerulonephritis.

CMGS Chopped meat-glucose-starch (medium).

CMGT Chromosome-mediated gene transfer.

CMgT Choline magnesium trisilicate (= CMT).

CMH Canada's Mental Health (journal); Cephalexin monophosphate (a cephalosporin antibiotic); City of Memphis Hospital (Memphis, Tennessee); Combined (mixed) hyperlipidemia (Fredrickson Types IIa and IIb); Complete medical history; Congenital malformation of heart.

CMHC Community Mental Health Center; Community Mental Health Centers (Act of 1963).

CMHD Community Mental Health Department.

CMHJ Community Mental Health Journal.

CMH&MRC Community Mental Health and Mental Retardation Center.

CMHN Community Mental Health Nurse.

cmH_2O centimeters of water.

CMHP Carboxymethyl hydroxypropyl.

CMHS Community mental-health services.

CMHT Clinical manifestation of hyperthyroidism (see GHT; SHT); Cochran -Mantel-Haenszel test (for categorical variables, in psychiatry).

CMI Carbohydrate metabolism index; Care management integration; Cell/ Cellular-mediated immune (response - see CMIR); Cell-mediated immunity; Cell multiplication inhibition; Centers for Medical Innovations; Chronic mesenteric ischemia; Chronic mycoplasmal infection (some somatiform disorders such as CFS, FMS, GWI, GWS, PTSD and PTSS are caused by it) (see SFDs); Circulating microemboli index; Colonic motility index; Commonwealth Mycological Institute; Comprehensive medical insurance; Computer-managed instruction; Conventional medical imaging (X rays); Cornell Medical Index/ Inventory.

CMID Cytomegalic inclusion disease.

cmil centimilliliter (= centimil; 10^{-5} liter; 10^{-2} ml; 10^{-2} cc).

CMIM Cardiac myosin-induced myocarditis.

C/Min; c/min Counts/ Cycles per minute (see cpm).

Cminss Steady-state trough concentration (of a drug) (in µg/ml).

CMIR Cell/ Cellular-mediated immune

response (= CMI).
CMIT Current Medical Information and Terminology.
CMJ Canadian Medical Journal; Carpometacarpal joint.
CMK Chloromethyl ketone; Congenital multicystic kidney.
CML Cardinal movements of labor (of the baby, through the pelvis during labor); Cell-mediated lymphocytotoxicity/ lympholysis/ lysis; Chronic myelocytic/ myelogenous/ myeloid leukemia; Current-mode logic.
CMM Cell-mediated mutagenesis; Chemoreceptor-mediated mechanism (= CRMM); Chinese Materia Medica; Close medical monitoring; Colored married male; Costimulatory molecule (CD 28, CD 80, CD 86, etc.); Cross-modality matching; Cutaneous malignant melanoma.
cmm cubic millimeter (see cu mm).
CMMaL Chronic myelomacrocytic leukemia (= CMML).
CMMB Catholic Medical Mission Board (New York City).
CMME Chloromethyl methyl ether (a carcinogen).
CMMHCS Center for Mindfulness in Medicine, Health Care and Society (anti-stress program, Univ. of Massachusetts, USA).
CMML Chronic myelomacrocytic leukemia (see CMMaL); Chronic myelomonocytic leukemia (see CMMoL).
CMMoL Chronic myelomonocytic leukemia (= CMML).
CMMS Columbia Mental Maturity Scale.
CMN Caudal mediastinal node; Congenital malignant neoplasm; Congenital mesoblastic nephroma; Cystic medial necrosis (of the aorta).
CMNA Complement-mediated neutrophil activation.
CMN-AA Cystic medial necrosis of the ascending aorta.
CMO Cardiac minute output; Card made out; Chief Medical Officer; Cell-mediated oxidation; Cetyl myristoleate; Comfort measures only; Common main objective (stereomicroscope); Corticosterone methyloxidase.
cMO centimorgan.
CMOL Chronic monocytic leukemia.
CMOP Cyclophosphamide-MOPP (see MOPP).
CMOPP Cyclophosphamide, Mustine, Oncovin, Procarbazine and rednisone (Chemotherapy) (see MOPP).
CMOS Complementary metal-oxide semiconductor.
CMP Carbon monoxide poisoning (see CO P); Cardiomyopathy; Cervical mucus penetration; Chloramphenicol (see CAP); Chondromalacia patellae; Cognitive and Motor Performance; Competitive/ Comprehensive medical plan; Cow's milk protein; Crook measuring prosthesis (Otolaryngology); Custom-made prosthesis; Cytidine monophosphate.
CMPA Canadian Medical Protective Association.
CMPB Chlordiazepoxide hydrochloride (= 7-Chloro-2-methylamino-5-phenyl-3H-1,4-benzodiazepine-4-oxide hydrochloride; Libraxin [trade name]; Librium [trade name]; Methaminodiazepoxide; Ro 5-0690). A benzodiazepine tranquillizing drug.
CMPC Caldwell-Moloy pelvic classification (a system for classifying the structure of the bony pelvis of the female, to predict her ability to give birth normally). Categories include:
Android pelvis - heart-shaped opening, with thick and heavy bones, typical of the male, but also found in women. Difficult childbirth.
Anthropoid pelvis - oval opening, and antero-posterior diameter much greater than the transverse. Normal childbirth.
Gynecoid pelvis - nearly round opening, typical in women. Ideal for childbirth.
Platypelloid pelvis - round inlet, but the back section is made shorter due to its flat and heavy border. Found in about 3% of women. Vaginal birth is not often possible in this type of pelvis.
CMPD Chronic myeloproliferative disorder.
CMPGN Chronic membranoproliferative glomerulonephritis.
CMPI Cow's milk protein intolerance.
cmps centimeters per second.
CMPT Cervical mucus penetration test.

CMQ Catholic Medical Quarterly (journal); Cook-Medley Questionnaire (psychological test for assessment of hostility).

CMR Carbon-13 magnetic resonance (spectroscopy); Cell-mediated response (see CMIR); Cerebral metabolic rate; Certified/ Chronic/ Continued mental retardation; Certified medical representative; Chief medical resident; Cholinergic muscarinic receptor; Common mode rejection; Competitive (non-depolarizing) muscle relaxant (see NDMR); Crude mortality ratio.

CMR 807 Trichlormethiazide. A chlorothiazide diuretic with a greater potency and duration of action than chlorothiazide.

CMRG Cerebral metabolic rate of glucose (= CGU; CMRglu; CMRgluc).

CMRglu; CMRgluc See CMRG.

CMRI Children's Medical Relief International.

CMRL Cerebral metabolic rate of lactate (= CLU; CMRlactate).

CMRlactate See CMRL.

CMRNG Chromosomally-mediated resistant Neisseria gonorrhoeae.

CMRO; $CMRO_2$ Cerebral metabolic rate of oxygen (= COU).

CMRR Common mode rejection ratio.

CMRT Certified Medical Records Technician.

CMS Camptomelic syndrome (or Camptomelia, an inherited defect in which one or more limbs are bent or permanently curved); Candidate of Medical Sciences; Cell-mediated system (of immunity) - associated with the action of killer T cells (see HIS); Cervical mediastinoscopy; Changed mental status; Christian Medical Society; Chronic malabsorption/ myelodysplastic syndrome; Chronic mononucleosis syndrome (see PVFS); Chromosome modification site; Circulation, motion, and senation; Clofibrate-induced muscular syndrome; Close medical supervision; Clyde Mood Scale; Color, motion, sensation; Colorado Medical Society; Complement-mediated solubility; Complementary Medicine Services; Congenital myasthenic syndrome(s); Connecticut Medical Service; Consolidated Medical Systems; Cornmeal-soy (flour); Corn-milk, soybean (powdered milk/ high-protein food mixture); Corometrics Medical System (device for fetal monitoring); Council on Medical Service/ Staffs (AMA); County medical society; Cumulative myelosuppression.

cms take/ to be taken tomorrow morning (L. cras mane sumendus).

cm/s; cm/sec centimeters per second.

cm/s^2; cm/sec^2 centimeters per second per second.

CMSA Coal Mine Safety Act.

CMSH Center for Male Sexual Health (Albany, NY).

CMSI Commission on Medical Services and Insurance (ACR).

CMSJ Christian Medical Society Journal.

CMSS Center for Marital and Sexual Studies; Circulation, motor ability, senation, and swelling; Cooperative Medical Service System; Council of Medical Speciality Societies.

CMSs Conventional medical services (see CMC, CMD).

CMSUA Clean midstream urinanalysis.

CMSUE Change in Mental Status of Unknown Etiology.

CMT California mastitis test; Cancer multistep therapy; Carbon monoxide toxicity (see CO T); Cardiolipin microflocculation test (for syphilis - see STS); Catechol methyltransferase; Cervical motion tenderness; Charcot-Marie-Tooth (atrophy/ disease/ syndrome) (= CMTA; CMTD; CMTS); Choline magnesium trisilicate (see CMgT); Circus movement tachycardia; Combined modality therapy (as for cancer - surgery, radiotherapy and chemotherapy); Congenital muscular torticollis (Orthopedics); Continued maintenance therapy/ treatment; Continuous memory test; Contrast medium technique; Council on Medical Television; Cricomyotomy; Current Medical Terminology (AMA publication); Cutis marmorata telangiectasia.

CMTA Charcot-Marie-Tooth atrophy (see CMT).

CMTC Cutis marmorata telangiectatica congenita.

CMTD Cell-mediated tissue damage;

Charcot-Marie-Tooth disease (see CMT).

CMTS Charcot-Marie-Tooth syndrome (see CMT).

CMU Chlorophenyldimethylurea; Complex motor unit; Colonic mucosal ulceration.

CMUA Continuous motor unit activity.

CMULP Carboxylate-modified uniform latex particle.

CMV Cisplatin, methotrexate, and vinblastine; Constant/ Controlled mandatory volume; Continuous mandatory ventilation; Controlled/ Conventional mechanical ventilation; Cool mist vaporizer; Cucumber mosaic virus; Cytomegalovirus (= HCMV).

CMV-IGIV; CMV-IgIV Cytomegalovirus immune globulin intravenous.

CMV-MN Cytomegalovirus mononucleosis.

CMVS Culture midvoid specimen.

CMX Cefmenoxime.

CN Cahiers du Nursing (Canadian journal); Canadian Nurse (CNA journal); Cancer News (journal); Cardiovascular Nursing (AHA journal); Catholic Nurse (NGEW journal); Caudate/ Cochlear nucleus; Cellulose nitrate; Charge nurse; Child nutrition; Chloroacetophenone (a war gas); Clinical nurse/sing; Colon neurosis (see IBS); Compensation neurosis; Congenital nephrosis/ nystagmus; Cranial nerve; Crigler-Najjar (syndrome); Cyanide; Cyanogen (see Cn); Cyanogen radical; Cyanosis neonatorum; Parke, Davis & Co code for experimental substances; Tomorrow night (L. cras nocte) (see cn).

Cn Colistin; Cyanide; Cyanogen (= CN).

cn calcification (in small pneumoconiotic opacities) (radiograph symbol); cras nocte (L) - tomorrow night (= CN).

C_n Color-naming (Rorschach).

C/N Calorie-Nitrogen (ratio) - i.e. the quantitative relationship in the diet between calories and nitrogen (= protein/6.25); Carbon/Nitrogen (ratio); Carrier/ Contrast Noise (ratio).

CN- Cyanide ion.

CN I-XII Cranial nerves 1-12.

CN 1115 Quinocide hydrochloride (= Chinocide; Win 10,448). A methoxyquinoline structural isomer of primaquine, widely used in Russia in the treatment and prophylaxis of vivax malaria. A well tolerated anti-malarial drug.

CNA Calcium nutrient agar; Canadian Nuclear/ Nurses' Association; Chart not available.

CNAF Chronic non-valvular atrial fibrillation.

CNAG Chronic narrow angle glaucoma.

CNAP Compound nerve action potential.

CNB Central nervous blockade; Core needle biopsy (see SCNB); Cutting needle biopsy.

CNC Clinical nursing conference.

CNCA Carbonate noncarboxylate anion (see carb).

CNCACG Chronic non-congestive angle-closure glaucoma.

CNCbl Cyanocobalamin.

CNCMH Canadian National Committee for Mental Hygeine.

CND Canned; Cannot determine; Cranial nerve damage.

CNDC Chronic non-specific diarrhea of childhood; Chronic non-suppurative destructive cholangitis.

CNDI Congenital nephrogenic diabetes insipidus.

CNE Chronic nervous exhaustion; Concentric needle electrode; Cortical norepinephrine.

C'3NeF C3 (complement component) nephritic factor.

CNegP Continuous negative pressure (see CNP).

CNES Chronic nervous exhaustion syndrome.

CNF Chromosomally normal fetus (Obstetrics); Chronic nodular fibrositis; Congenital nephrotic syndrome of the Finnish (type); Cyclophosphamide, Novatrone (mitoxantrone), and fluoro-uracil.

CNH Central neurogenic hyperpnea; Community Nursing Home.

CNHD Congenital non-spherocytic hemolytic disease.

CNHI Committee for National Health Insurance.

CNI Center of nuclear image; Chronic nerve irritation.

CNIC Centre National de l'Information Chimique (France).

CNK Cortical necrosis of the kidneys.

CNL Cardiolipin natural lecithin; Chronic neutrophilic leukemia; Cranial nerve lesion.
CNM Certified-Nurse Midwife; Computerized nuclear morphometry; Congenital neonatal malaria.
CNMDD Chronic non-psychotic major depressive disorder.
CNMRF Children Nationwide Medical Research Foundation (US).
CNMS Cooperative Neonatal Meningitis Study.
CNMT Certified Nuclear Medicine Technologist.
CNN Cable News Network; Cephanone; Congenital nevocytic nevus.
CNND Committee on Nursing in National Defence (ANA).
CNO Chief of Naval Operations (USN).
CNOH Cyanic acid (= HNCO).
CNOR Certified Nurse, Operating Room.
CNP Chinese National Pharmacopoeia; Chronic neck/ neuropathic pain; Clinical nursing procedure; Community nurse practitioner; Community nutrition program; Continuous negative pressure (= CNegP); Cortical neuropeptide(s) - include GHRIF or Growth hormone release inhibiting factor (= Somastatin; Somatostatin), CRF or Corticotrophin releasing factor, VIP or Vasoactive intestinal polypeptide, CCK or Cholecystokinin, NT or Neurotensin, and Substance P; Cranial nerve palsy; 2',3'-cyclic nucleotide 3'-phosphodiesterase.
CNPA Chronic necrotizing pulmonary aspergillosis.
CNPase 2'3'-cyclic nucleotide 3'-phosphohydrolase.
CNPC Chronic non-productive cough.
CNPV Continuous negative pressure ventilation.
CNR Civil nursing reserve.
CNRC Conseil National de Recherches Canada (National Research Council of Canada).
CNRD Clinical Notes on Respiratory Diseases (ATS journal).
CNRN Certified Neurosurgical Registered Nurse.
CNRS Centre National de la Recherche Scientifique (National Scientific Research Center, France).
CNRT Corrected (sinus) node recovery time.
CNS Central nervous system; Clinical nurse specialist; Clinical nursing skill; Coagulase-negative staphyloccoci; Cognitive Neuroscience Society; Committee on Nomenclature and Statistics (American Psychiatric Association); Congenital nephrotic syndrome; Congress of Neurological Surgeons/ery; Sulfocyanate; Take tomorrow night (see cns).
cns take/ to be taken tomorrow night (L. cras nocte sumendus) (= CNS).
CNSD Central nervous system depressant (such as alcohol, barbiturates, and other hypnotics, etc.); Central nervous system disorder/ dysfunction (Acute psychosis, Drugs, Hemorrhage, Inflammatory & demyelinating diseases, Mass lesions, Stroke, Trauma, etc.).
CNSF Compromised nervous system function.
CNSHA Congenital non-spherocytic hemolytic anemia.
CNSL; CNS-L Central nervous system leukemia.
CNSLD Chronic non-specific lung disease.
CNSR Clinical neuroscientific research.
CNSS Central nervous system stimulant (such as amphetamines, caffeine, etc. Also called Analeptic); Central nervous system/ CNS syndrome (caused by a massive whole-body dosage of radiation).
CNST Central nervous system tumor (of the brain or spinal cord).
CNT Clinical nursing technique; Could not test.
CNTBI Chronic non-tuberculous bronchial infection.
cntd continued.
CNU Cartridge-Needle Unit; Clinical non-union (bone fracture, grafting, osteotomy, etc.); Lomustine (see CCNU; LO).
CNV Choroidal neovascularization; Contingent negative variation; Cutaneous necrotizing vasculitis.
CO Carbon monoxide; Cardiac output (liters per minute; l/min); Castor oil; Casualty officer; Centric occlusion; Cervical orthosis; Cervico-axial; Check out (see C/O; c/o);

Cholesterol/ Choline oxidase; Cocaine (see Erythroxylum); Coccygeal; Coenzyme (see Co); Community organization (degree - MSW); Community organizer; Complains of (see C/O; c/o); Compound(ed) (see Co); Compulsive overeating; Control; Corneal opacity; Court order; Cross over (genetics - drug study); Cutoff.

Co Cobalt (Z = 27) (see Elements - Cobalt); Coenzyme (= CO); Company; Compound(ed)/ Compounded of/ A compound (L. compositus) (= CO; co; Comp; Compd); Concrete (score) (psychology).

co abnormal cardiac size or shape (radiograph symbol); compound(ed) (see Co).

C/O; c/o (= CO) Care of/ In care of; Check out; Complains of.

co- prefix meaning with or together (L. con).

C=O Keto group.

CO-1 Cardiac output at one minute; Coenzyme-1 (see Co-I; Co-1).

CO I; CO 1; Co I; Co 1 Coenzyme I (see Co-I; Co-1).

Co-I; Co-1 Coenzyme I/ Coenzyme-1 (= CO I; CO 1; Co I; Co 1; CO- I; CO-1; Diphosphopyridine nucleotide; DPN; NAD; Nadide; Nicotinamide adenosine dinucleotide; Nicotinamide adenine dinucleotide).

CO II; CO-II; CO 2; CO-2; Co II; Co 2 Coenzyme II (see Co-II; Co-2).

Co-II; Co-2 Coenzyme II/ Coenzyme-2 (= CO II; CO 2; Co II; Co 2; CO-II; CO-2; TPN; Triphosphopyridine nucleotide).

CO_2 Carbon dioxide.

CO_3 Carbonate.

^{57}Co; ^{56}Co Radioisotopes of cobalt.

^{60}Co; Co-60 Radioactive cobalt (nuclear medicine).

COA Canadian Ophthalmological/ Orthopaedic Association; Cervico-oculo-acusticus syndrome; Chondro-osteoarthritis; Condition on admission; Cyclic oral administration.

CoA Coarctation of the aorta; Coenzyme A; Coferment A.

COAD Chronic obstructive airway (see COLD)/ arterial disease.

COAG Chronic open angle glaucoma.

Coag; coag Coagulase (on bacteriological reports; Coagulate/ted/tion.

COAGSC Coagulation screen.

Coag time Coagulation time.

COAP Cytotoxan (cyclophosphamide), Oncovin (vincristine), Ara-C (arabinosyl cytosine), and Prednisone. A combination of four drugs used in chemotherapy in the treatment of acute leukemia.

CoASH Acetyl coenzyme (uncombined coenzyme A).

CoA-SPC Coenzyme A-synthetizing protein complex.

COAT Children's Orientation and Amnesia Test.

COB Chronic obstructive bronchitis; Circumscribed (= Osteoid osteoma)/ Cortical osteoblastoma; Cisplatin, Oncovin (vincristine), and bleomycin; Coordination of benefits.

coban cohesive bandage.

COBD Chronic obstructive bronchopulmonary disease (see COBPD; COLD; COPD).

COBE Committee on Board Establishment (ACEP).

COb/Gyn Contemporary Ob/Gyn (journal).

COBOL Common business-oriented language (computer).

COBPD Chronic obstructive bronchopulmonary disease (see COPD).

COBRA Consolidated Omnibus Budget Reconciliation Act (Health insurance coverage).

COBS Caesarian-obtained barrier-sustained (i.e. animals delivered by caesarian section into a germ-free environment); Chronic organic brain syndrome.

COBT Chronic obstruction of the biliary tract.

COC Cardiac output computer; Cathodal opening clonus/ contraction (see CaOC); Cleveland open cup (flash point test); Coccygeal (see Coc); Combination (type)/ Combined oral contraceptive; Community-oriented care.

Coc Coccygeal (= COC).

Cocaine See Erythroxylum.

cocc- combining form meaning pill or seed (Gr. kokkos).

COCCIO Coccideimycosis.

coch; cochl; cochleat A spoonful/ by spoonfuls (L. cochlear, cochleare, cochleatum).

coch/cochl amp A heaped/ping spoonful (L. cochleare amplum).

coch/cochl infant A teaspoonful (L. cochleare infantis) (see coch/cochl parve).

coch/cochl mag A large spoonful or tablespoonful (L. cochleare magnum) - about 14 ml.

coch/cochl med A desertspoonful (L. cochleare medium) - about 7 ml (= coch/cochl mod).

coch/cochl min A small spoonful or teaspoonful (L. cochleare mininimum) (see coch/cochl parve).

coch/cochl mod A dessertspoonful (L. cochleare modicum) (see coch/cochl med).

coch/cochl parv A teaspoonful (L. cochleare parvum) - about 4 ml (= coch/cochl infant/min; c parve).

COCI Consortium on Chemical Information.

COCl Cathodal opening clonus (see CaOC).

COCM Congestive cardiomyopathy.

CO_2 comb Carbon dioxide combining power (laboratory/ blood gas).

CO_2 cont Carbon dioxide content (laboratory/ blood gas).

CO_2CP Carbon dioxide plasma concentration.

coct boiling (L. coctio).

COD Cash on delivery; Cause of death; Chemical oxygen demand; Chondro-osseous dysplasia; Chondro-osteo-dystrophy (Orthopedics); Chronic/ Continued/ Continuous overdosage/se; Codeine (see Cod; cod); Condition on discharge; Coronary occlusive disease; Council of Deans; Cytosine arabinoside, Oncovin (vincristine), and Daunorubicin.

Cod; cod Codeine (= COD; Schoolboy).

CODAP Client Oriented Data Acqusition Process (NIAAA).

CODATA Committee on Data for Science and Technology.

CODEN Six-letter code which identifies all serial publications (ASTM).

COD-MD Cerebro-ocular dysplasia-muscular dystrophy (syndrome).

CODO Codocytes.

Codon A gene base nucleotide coding, with one or more other codons for a particular amino acid in the genetic code.

Cod SO_4 Codeine sulfate.

CODye Cardiac output (estimation) by dye (dilution technique).

COE Council on Oceanic Engineering (IEEE); Cyclooctene.

Coeff; coeff Coefficient.

coel prefix meaning hollow (Gr. koilos).

COEPS Cortically originating extra-pyramidal symptoms.

COESH Center for Occupational and Environmental Safety and Health (Stanford University).

COF Cutoff frequency.

CoF Cobra (venom) factor; Cofactor.

COFAL Complement-fixation test for avian leucosis virus.

COFS Cerebro-oculo-facial-skeletal (syndrome).

COG Central Oncology Group; Clinical Obstetrics and Gynecology (journal); Cognitive (function tests).

CoG Center of gravity.

Cog; cog Cognition/tive (function/ impairment/ performance/ score/ unit).

Cogito, ergo sum L. - "I think, therefore I am". French philosopher and scientist René Descartes (1596-1650), in his famous Discourse on Method for Rightly Conducting One's Reason and for Seeking Truth in the Sciences (1637).

CoGME Council on Graduate Medical Education.

COGO Cognition.

COGTT Cortisone/ Cortisone-primed oral glucose tolerance test.

COH Carbohydrate; City of Hope (US Institute in basic scientific research, genetic & molecular medicine, cancer research center, Southern California) (see CBG); Coefficient of haze (soiling index); Controlled ovarian hyperstimulation (see COHS).

COHb Carboxyhemoglobin (= Carbon monoxide hemoglobin; COHgb) (laboratory/ chemistry).

COHgb See COHb.

COHLA Spanish-Latin American

Odontological Congress.
COHR Center for Oral Health Research.
COHS Carrear Opportunities in the Health Sciences; Controlled ovarian hyperstimulation (e.g. with FSH).
COHSE Confederation of Health Service Employees.
COI Cellular oxidative injury; Central Obesity Index; Community onset infection.
COIF Congenital onychodysplasia of the index finger.
Coke Coca-Cola; Cocaine (see Erythroxylum).
Col Cola (L.) - strain; Colicin; Collagen (see Coll); Collateral (see Collat); Collect(ion/ive/ively) (see Collect); College (see Coll); Colloidal (see Coll); Colony (on culture reports); Color(ed); Column; Cortisol; Strain (L. cola).
col- prefix meaning: i) lower intestine (Gr. kolon). ii) with or together (L. con).
colat strained (L. colatus) (= colen; colet).
COLD Chronic obstructive lung disease (= COAD; COPD; CORD; ROAD).
COLD A Cold agglutinin titer.
colen let them be strained (L. colentur) (see colat).
colet let it be strained (L. coletur).
Coli Colistine (sulfate).
Coll Collagen (= Col); Collateral (see Collat); Collect(ion/ive/ively) (see Collect); College (= Col); Colloidal(= Col); Eyewash (see Collyr); Mouth wash (see Collut); Nose wash (see Collun).
Collat Collateral (= Col; Coll.)
Collect Collection/ive/ively (= Col; Coll).
Collun Nose wash (L. collunarium) (= Coll).
Collut Mouth wash (L. collutorium) (= Coll).
Coll vol Collective volume.
Collyr Eyewash (L. collyrium) (= Coll).
col/ml colonies per milliliter.
colon- prefix meaning lower intestine (Gr. kolon).
Color; color Colorimetry; Let it be colored (L. coloretur).
colp colporrhaphy.
colp- prefix meaning hollow or vagina (Gr. kolpos) (= kolp-).
COM *Candida* (hematogenous) (see HCO)/ Chronic osteomyelitis; Caput ossis metacarpalis; Chronic otitis media; Chronic over-medication; College of Osteopathic Medicine; Computer output microfiche/ film; Cyclophosphamide, Oncovin, and Methotrexate.
com comminuted; commitment.
com- prefix meaning together or with (L. con) (see con-).
Comb; comb Combination; Combine(d); Combining.
COMC Carboxymethylcellulose.
comf comfortable.
COMLA Cyclophosphamide, Oncovin (vincristine), methotrexate, leucovorin (l. calcium), and Ara-C (cytarabine).
Comm Commission; Committee.
comm; commun communicable.
commun dis communicable disease.
COMP Complicate(d)/tion (see Comp); Cyclophosphamide, Oncovin (vincristine), methotrexate, and prednisone.
Comp; comp Comparative; Compare; Compensate; Compensated (heart disease); Compensation (case); Compete/tition (= Compet); Complaint (= Compl); Complete(d)/tion (= Compl); Complicate(d)/tion (= Compl; Complic); Compose; Composition (= Compn); Compound(ed) (see Co); Comprehension/sive (care); Compress(ion) (= Compr); Computer.
Comp Care; Comp care Comprehensive Care (i.e. Comprehensive Health Care Program of the Children's Hospital, Washington, DC).
Comp case Compensation case.
Compd; compd Compound(ed) (see Co).
Compd S Compound S (see Compound S).
Compendex Computerized Engineering Index (EI).
Compet Compete/tition (see Comp).
Compl; compl (see Comp) Complaint; Complete(d)/tion; Complicate(d)/tion.
Complic Complicate(d)/tion (see Comp).
Compn; compn Composition (see Comp).
compos mentis Latin: of sound mind.
Compound 269 Endrin. A dimethanonaphthalene chlorinated insecticide.
Compound 711 Isodrin. A dimethanonaphtha-

lene chlorinated insecticide.

Compound 933 F Piperoxan hydrochloride (= Piperoxane HCl; Benzodioxane HCl; F 933; Fourneau 933). An adrenergic blocking drug which has been used to differentiate hypertension due to a phaeochromocytoma (chromaffin tumor) or to paragangliomas from other forms of hypertension. Also as an antidote for overdoses of adrenaline and noradrenaline in surgical emergencies. Piperoxan has largely been replaced by the use of phentolamine mesylate.

Compound 1003 Guanoxan sulfate. A guanidine sulfate derivative and hypotensive agent thought to act by blocking the release of adrenaline and noradrenaline from post-ganglionic nerves, and possibly also by its effect on the central nervous system. Used in the treatment of severe hypertension.

Compound 1029 Guanoclor sulfate. A guanidine sulfate derivative and hypotensive agent, thought to act by adrenergic blockade, and also by inhibition of the enzyme dopamine â-oxidase, thereby blocking the conversion of dopamine to noradrenaline. Used in the treatment of severe hypertension.

Compound 1080 Sodium fluoroacetate (= Sodium Monofluoroacetate). A highly effective rodenticide, but must be used with great caution because of its toxicity to other animals and to man.

Compound 1081 Fluoroacetamide. Used as a rodenticide; highly toxic. In Britain its use is restricted to the destruction of rats in ships and in sewers.

Compound 4047 Malathion (= Carbofos; Malathon). An organophosphorus insecticide, active both as a stomach and as a contact poison for controlling lice, and against mosquitoes ans houseflies.

Compound 5029 Isoxsuprine hydrochloride (see Caa 40).

Compound 25,398 Methohexitone sodium (= Sodium methohexital; Enallynymalnatrium). A very short-acting barbiturate which has similar actions and uses to thiopentone sodium. It is given intravenously for the induction of general anesthesia or as the sole anesthetic for minor operative procedures which do not require muscular relaxation (see Barb).

Compound 29,275 Capreomycin (= Capromycin). An antimicrobial polypeptide produced by the growth of Streptomyces capreolus. Given by intramuscular injection, in conjunction with other drugs, in the treatment of resistant cases of tuberculosis.

Compound 33,355 Mestranol (see EE3ME).

Compound 38,174 Pronethanol hydrochloride (= Pronetalol HCl; Nethalide). A beta-adrenergic blocking agent, with actions similar to those of propranolol hydrochloride by which it has been superseded. Pronethalol has been found to be carcinogenic in the mouse, and because of the possibility of similar implied effects in man it is no longer used.

Compound 38,389 Levopropicillin potassium (= Potassium levopropylcillin). The levorotatory isomer of propicillin potassium with similar antimicrobial properties (see BRL 284).

Compound 40,602 Cephaloridine (see Ceph 87/4). A broad-spectrum bactericidal antibiotic, used in the treatment of serious infections due to streptococci or staphylococci, including penicillin-producing strains in patients, who are sensitized to penicillin, and in the treatment of urinary tract infections due to sensitive strains of coliform organisms.

Compound E Cortisone (= Kendall's Cortisone).

Compound E Acetate Cortisone acetate (= Cortisoni Acetas; Kendall's cortisone acetate; 11-Dehydro-17-hydrocorticosterone acetate).

Compound F Hydrocortisone (= Hydrocort; Cortisol; Kendall's hydrocortisone; 17-Hydroxycorticosterone; Hydrocortisonum).

Compound G-11 Hexachlorophene.

Compound P Nitrobenzoyl chloride pyridine.

Compound S (1) 11-deoxycortisol (a 17-OH-CS) (= Compd S); (2) Azidothymidine (also called Compound S) (see AZT).

Compr Compress(ion) (see Comp).

COMS Cerebro-oculomuscular syndrome.

COMT Catechol-O-methyltransferase.

COMTRAC Computer-based (case) tracing.

COMUL Complement-fixation murine leukosis (test).

CON Certificate of need.

Con Concanavalin.

CoN Committee on Nutrition (AAP).
con against (L. contra).
con- prefix meaning with or together (L.) (= com-; cor-).
CO_2 N Carbon dioxide narcosis.
CONA Canadian Opium and Narcotic Act.
Con A Concanavalin A. (antigens or allogeneic lymphocytes).
Con A-HRP Concanavalin A-horseradish peroxidase.
Conc Concentrate (= Concentr); Concentrated (= Concd; Concentr); Concentration (= Concentr; Concn); Conclude (= Concl); Conclusion (= Concl; Concn).
C-onc Cellular oncogene.
Concd Concentrated (see Conc).
Concentr Concentrate/ Concentrated/ Concentration (see Conc).
Conch Conchology.
concis cut (L. concisus).
Concl (see Conc) Conclude; Conclusion.
Concn (see Conc) Concentration; Conclusion.
Cond; cond Condensation/se(d); Condition(ed)/(s); Conduction/tivity/tor (see Conduc).
Cond ref Conditioned reflex.
Cond resp Conditioned response.
Conduc Conduction/tivity/tor (= Cond; cond).
Conf; conf Confection (L. confectio); Conference; Confine(d)/(ment); Confuse/sion.
Conflict 1. Mental conflict resulting from conflicting thoughts, ideas, goals, or desires; 2. A painful state of consciousness caused by such conflicting forces. Kinds of conflict include:
Approach-approach conflict (AAC) - a conflict caused by the need to choose between two or more things that are wanted.
Approach-avoidance conflict (AAC) - a conflict caused by something that is both wanted and not wanted.
Avoidance-avoidance conflict (AAC) - a conflict resulting from the confrontation of two or more events that are equally undesirable. Also called DAC or Double-avoidant conflict.
Double-avoidant conflict (DAC) - as above.
Extrapsychic conflict (EPC) - Emotional conflict unconnected with or outside oneself.
Intrapsychic conflict (IPC) - Emotional conflict within oneself.
Confuc Confucian.
Cong; cong Congested/tion; Congregationalist; Gallon (L. congius).
congen congenital.
$CO(NH_2)_2$ Urea.
coniz conization.
Conj, conj Conjugated/tion (see Conjug); Conjunction; Conjunctiva(l).
Conjug Conjugated/tion (= Conj; conj).
CONPADRI Cytoxan (cyclophosphamide), Oncovin (vincristine), Phenylalanine, Adriamycin (doxorubicin), and mustard.
CONPADRI I Vincristine, doxorubicin, and melphalan.
CONPADRI II Cytoxan (cyclophosphamide), Oncovin (vincristine), Phenylalanine, Adriamycin (doxorubicin), Melphalan (nitrogen mustard) (= CONPADRI I), plus high-dose Methotrexate.
CONPADRI III Conpadri I plus intensified doxorubicin.
CONS; Cons Consult(ant)/ation/ing (see Consult).
cons conservation/ive; consult(ation)/ing (see consult); keep, save (L. conserva); tinkling (L. consonans).
CONSENSUS Cooperative North Scandinavian Enalapril Survival Study.
CONSORT Consolidated Standards of Reporting Trials.
consperg dust, sprinkle (L. consperge).
const constant (see C).
Constit; constit Constituent; Constitution(al).
Consult; consult Consultant (journal); Consultant/ation/sulting (= CONS; Cons; cons).
Cont; cont Against (L. contra); Bruise(d) (see Contus); Contagion/ious (see Contag); Contain(s); Containing (see Contg); Contents; Continuation/ue/uously (see Contin); Contused/sion (see Contus); Let it be continued/ to be continued (see Contin).
Contac Contacto (NERF journal).
Contag Contagion/ious (= Cont; cont).
conter rub together (L. contere).
Contg Containing (= Cont; cont).
Contin; contin Continuation/ue/uously; Let

it/the medicine be continued; to be continued (L. continuetur) (= Cont; cont).

Contr; contr Contracted/tion.

contra contraindicated.

contra- contra-indicated; prefix meaning opposed to or against (L).

Contracep Contraception (journal).

Contraceptives in common use, their modes of action, and female/ male involvement (see Table).

contralat contralateral.

cont rem continue the medicine/ let the medicine be continued (L. continuantur/ continuetur remedia/ium).

contrib contributory.

contrit broken, broken down, ground (L. contritus).

CONTU Contusion (see Contus).

Contus; contus Bruise(d), Contused/sion (L. contusus) (= Cont; cont).

conv convalescence/scent/scing; convenience/nt; convention(al); convergence/nt (see converg); convulsion(s)/ive.

converg convergence/nt (= conv).

conv strab convergent strabismus.

COO Chief operating officer.

COOD Chronic obstructive outflow disease.

COOH Carboxyl group (characteristic of organic acids).

COOHC(OH)(CH_2.COOH)$_2$ Citric acid (=$C_6H_8O_7$).

COOP Cooperative.

coord coordinated/tion.

CO-ORD Albutoin.

COP American slang for Policeman (from the copper helmet worn by the law in Great Britain); Capillary osmotic pressure; Carbon monoxide poisoning (= CMP); Change of plaster; Chronic obstructive pulmonary (disease) (see COLD; COPD); Cicatricial ocular pemphigoid; Coefficient of performance; Colloid oncotic/ osmotic pressure; Cytotoxan (cyclophosphamide), Oncovin (vincristine), and prednisone (= CVP).

CO P Carbon monoxide poisoning.

CoP Code of Practice (Factory Inspectorate and NRPB).

Cop Commissura posterior (thalamus).

COP 1 Copolymer I (a synthetic peptide).

COPA Center for Occupational and Professional Assessment (ETS); Council on Postsecondary Accreditation.

COPAP Committee Opposing Psychiatric Abuse of Prisoners.

COPC Committee oriented primary care.

COPD Chronic obstructive pulmonary disease (see COLD); Cyclophosphamide, Oncovin, Prednisone and Doxorubicin (Chemotherapy).

COPE Chronic obstructive pulmonary emphysema; Committee on Political Education (AFL/CIO).

COPH Congress of Organizations of the Physically Handicapped.

COP_i Colloid osmotic pressure in interstitial fluid.

Copilot Dexedrine tablet (see Amphet).

COPP Cytoxan (cyclophosphamide), Oncovin (vincristine), Procarbazine, and Prednisone.

COP_p Colloid osmotic pressure in plasma.

copr- prefix meaning dung (Gr. kopros) (see copro-).

CoPreX Coprecipitation for X-ray.

COPRO; Copro Coproporphyrin.

copro- Prefix meaning dung (Gr. kopro-) (= copr-).

COPT Circumoval precipitin test (a serological test for diagnosing *Schistosoma* japonicum infection).

CoQ Coenzyme Q (Ubiquinone) (see CoQ-10).

coq boil (L. coque).

CoQ-10 Coenzyme Q-10 or Ubiquinone. A weak antioxidant manufactured by the body, and essential in converting food into energy (= CoQ).

coq in s a boil in sufficient water (L. coque in sufficiente aqua).

coq s a boil properly (L. coque secundum artem).

coq simul boil together (L. coque simul).

COR Body (L. corpus) (see Cor); Cardiac output recorder; Comprehensive outpatient rehabilitation; Conditioned orientation reflex (audiometry); Consensual ophthalmotonic reaction; Coronary observation radio; Corrosion/ive (see Cor); Cortical (see Cort); Corticosterone/ Cortisone (see Cort); Custodian of records.

Contraceptive	Woman	Man	Mode of action	Involvement time	
				Periodic	Daily
Natural family planning Rhythm/calendar	X		Couple cooperation: abstinence during fertile periods	Mathematic formula calculated once every month	
BBT (Basal body temperature)	X		Couple cooperation: abstinence during fertile periods	Ovulation determined from daily record of BBT	X
Cervical mucus	X		Couple cooperation: abstinence during fertile periods	Ovulation determined from daily record of cervical mucus characteristics	X
Symptothermal	X	Assists	Couple cooperation: abstinence during fertile periods	Combination of BBT, cervical mucus observation, and record of secondary symptoms by couple	X
OC (Oral conceptives)	X		Suppress ovulation by inhibiting hypothalamus & pituitaryat	Ingestion of OC same time each day; gynecol. exam. every six months	X
Norplant	X		Suppresses ovulation and alters cervical mucus and endometrium maturation	Capsules inserted subcut. into arm by local anesthetic. Effective for 5 years	
IUDs (Intrauterine devices) (unmedicated)	X		Prevention of ovum implantation within the uterus	Inserted into uterus by gynecologist. IUD changed every 2-3 years	
Mechanical barriers (Diaphragms)	X		Prevention of sperm migration into the uterus	Inserted into vagina over cervix before intercourse	
Cervical cap	X		Prevention of sperm migration into the uterus	Inserted into vagina over cervix before intercourse	
Condoms		X	Prevention of sperm migration into the uterus	Applied to penis before intercourse	

Contraceptive	Woman	Man	Mode of action	Involvement time	
				Periodic	Daily
Chemical barriers: foams, gels, suppositories	X	X	Destroy sperms or make them immobile within vaginal vault	Inserted into vagina before each intercourse; applied with diaphragm or condom	
Fertility awareness	X	X	Family planning plus barrier method of contraception		
Vaginal sponge	X		Releases spermicide, blocks cervial opening, absorbs semen	Inserted into upper vagina before intercourse; can be retained for 24 hours	

CoR Congo red.
Cor; cor Body (L. corpus) (= COR); Coronary; Corrected/tion; Corrosion/ive (= COR); Cortical (see Cort); Corticosterone/ Cortisone (see Cort); Heart (L. cordis).
cor- combining form meaning doll, small image, or pupil (Gr. kore); with or together (L. con) (see con-).
CORA Conditioned orientation reflex audiometry.
Co-Ral Coumaphos (see Bayer 21/199).
CORD Chronic obstructive respiratory disease (see COLD); Commissioned Officer Residency Deferrment (Program).
COREC Central Office for Research Ethics Committee (DoH, UK).
CORH Council on Rural Health (AMA).
cor L corrosive liquid.
Corp Corporation.
corpor- combining form meaning body (L. corpus).
CORR Clinical Orthopaedics and Related Research (journal).
corr correspondence/ding.
CORS Canadian Operational Research Society; Cronholm Ottosson rating scale.
CORT Certified Operating Room Technician; Cortical (see Cort); Corticosterone/ Cortisone (see Cort).
Cort cort. Bark (L. cortex); Cortex; Cortical (= COR; Cor; cor; CORT); Corticosterone/ Cortisone (= COR; Cor; cor; CORT).
cortic- prefix meaning bark or rind (L. cortex, corticis).
COS Canadian Ophthalmological/ Otolaryngological Society; Cheiro-oral syndrome; Chief of staff; Clinical Orthopaedic Society; Clinically observed seizure(s); Committee on Shock (NAS-NRC); Controlled ovarian stimulation (Gyn/Obs); Cross-over study.
CoS Canal of Schlemm (or Schlemm's canal, a tiny vein at the corner of the eye that drains the aqueous humor and funnels it into the bloodstream. Its blockage can result in glaucoma).
cos cosine.
COSA Clinical Oncological Society of Australia.
COSATI Committee on Scientific and Technical Information (US Govt).
COSMIS Computer System for Medical Information Systems.
COSPAR Committee on Space Research.
cost- combining form meaning rib (L. costa).
COSTAR Computer-Stored Ambulatory Record.
COSTART Coding Symbols for Thesaurus of Adverse Reaction Terms (system); Computer-Stored Ambulatory Record Tabulation/

Technology/ Terminology.

COSTEP Commissioned Officer Student Training and Extern Program.

COSV Cardiac output stroke volume.

COT Cadaveric organ transplant; Colony overlay test; Committee on Toxicology (AMA); Committee on Trauma (NAS-NRC); Content of thought; Contralateral optic tectum; Critical off-time; Crossover trial; Cyclic oral therapy/ treatment.

CO T Carbon monoxide toxicity (= CMT).

CO_2 T Carbon dioxide therapy (as in stimulating the CNS, controlling hiccups, etc).

COTA Certified Occupational Therapy Assistant.

COTD Cardiac output by thermodilution.

COTe Cathodal opening tetanus (see CaOTe).

COTH Council of Teaching Hospitals.

COTRANS Coordinated Transfer Application System.

CotSD Captain-of-the-ship doctrine (the idea that the doctor is personally responsible and accountable for her/ his patients' care).

COTX Cast off to x-ray.

COU Cardiac observation unit; Cerebral oxygen uptake (CMRO); Coronary observation unit.

coul coulomb.

Courage Barbiturate pill (see Barb).

COV Concentrated Oil of Vitriol (of commerce = H_2SO_4; Sulfuric acid); Cross-over value (genetics).

COVA Chronic obstructive ventilatory alteration (see COPD).

COVESDEM Costovertebral segmentation defect with mesomelia (syndrome).

CoVF Cobra venom factor.

CoW Circle of Willis.

COWS Cold to opposite and warm to same side.

COX Coxsackie (virus); Cyclooxygenase (a prostaglandin synthetase); Cytochrome c oxidase.

COX-1 Cyclooxygenase-1 (see COX).

COX-2 Cyclooxygenase-2 (see COX).

COX-2 I Cyclooxygenase-2 inhibitors (such as Celebra [Searle] and Vioxx [Merck] - antiprostaglandin enzymes, now used in the treatment of arthritic diseases).

COXD Cyclooxygenase-dependent.

CP Canadian Podiatrist (journal); Candle power (unit) (see cp); Canine Practice (journal); Capillary pressure; Cardiac pacing/ performance/ pool; Cardiopulmonary; Caudate putamen; Cell passage; Central pit; Centric position; Cerebellopontine (angle); Cerebral palsy; Certified Paramedic/ Prosthetist; Ceruloplasmin (see CPL); Charge-parity (violation/ symmetry); Chas Pfizer & Co code for experimental substances; Chemically pure (see cp); Chest pain; Child Psychiatry/ Psychology; Chloropurine; Chloroquine-Primaquine (see C-P); Chlorpropamide; Chondrodysplasia punctata; Chondromalacia patella; Chronic pain/ pancreatitis/ polyarthritis/ pyelonephritis; Cicatricial pemphigoid; Cisternal puncture; Cleft palate; Clinical Pathology/ Pediatrics/ Proceedings (journals); Clinical pathology; Clock pulse; Closing pressure (spinal tap); Cochlear potential; Code of practice; Cold pressor; Color perception; Combination product; Combining power; Commando procedure (see RNP); Communication patient; Compensated pace; Compound (see Cpd); Comprehensive Psychiatry (Am Psychopath Assn journal); Compressed (tablet); Congenital porphyria; Constant pressure; Contemporary Psychoanalysis (journal); Convenience package; Coproporphyrin; Cor pulmonale (see cp); Coracoid process; Coronary perfusion; C peptide; Creatine phosphate (= Phosphocreatine)/ phosphokinase; Cross-linked/ Crude/ Cytosol protein; "Crutch palsy" (due to radial nerve compression by long crutches, when weight is borne in the axilla); Current Podiatry (journal); Current practice; Cyclophosphamide (= CPA; CPM; CTX; CY; Cy; CYC; CYCLO; Cyclo; Cyto; Cytoxan); Cyclophosphamide and Platinum compound (cisplatin)/ and prednisone; Right ventricular failure (L. cor pulmonale) (see cp).

C-P Chloroquine with primaquine (= CP); Chronic-progressive.

Cp Ceruloplasmin (see CPL); Chickenpox; Corynebacterium parvum; Peak concentration; Phosphate/ Plasma clearance (see C_p).

cP Centipoise (= cp; CPS; 10^{-2} poise). A poise is the unit of viscosity of a liquid, in grams per centimeter per second.

cp candle power (= CP); centipoise (see cP); chemically pure (= CP); compare; cor pulmonale (radiograph symbol) (= CP).

C_p Constant pressure (= CP; c_p); Phosphate/ Plasma clearance (= Cp).

c_p Constant pressure (see C_p).

C/P Cholesterol/phospholipid (ratio); Cost plus.

C&P Compensation and pension; Complete and pain free (joint movement); Complete and pushing; Cystoscopy and panendoscopy/ pyelography.

CPA Canadian Paraplegic/ Pharmaceutical/ Physiotherapy/ Psychiatric Association; Cardiopulmonary arrest; Carotid phono/ photo angiography; Center for Professional Advancement (non-degree continuing technical education); Cerebellar pontine/ Cerebellopontine angle; Certified public accountant; Chemo preventive/ prophylactic agent (= CPD); Child Protection Act; Chlorophenylalanine; Chromophobic adenoma; Chronic progressive arthritis; Circulating platelet aggregate; Committee on Chemistry and Public Affairs (ACS); Complement proactivator (see C'3PA; C3PA); Conditioned play audiometry; Consumer Protection Administration/ Agency; Costophrenic angle; Cyclophosphamide (see CP); Cyproterone acetate.

CpA Cytidylyl phosphate adenosine.

C'3PA; C3PA Complement (C'; C3) proactivator (= CPA).

CPAF Chlorpropamide-alcohol flushing.

C_{PAH}; C_{pah} Para-aminohippurate clearance (procedure/ renal function test) (see KFT).

CPAIR Committee on Protection Against Ionizing Radiation (MRC).

CPAJ Canadian Psychiatric Association Journal.

CPAP Continuous positive airway pressure.

c parv a teaspoonful (L. cochleare parvum) (see coch/cochl parv).

CPAT Cerebellopontine angle tumor; College of Podiatry Admission Test (ETS).

CPB Carboxypeptidase B (anaphylatoxin inactivator); Cardiopulmonary bypass; Cetylpyridinium bromide; Charged particle beam (see CPBs); Competitive protein binding (assay/ method).

CPBA Competitive protein-binding analysis/ assay.

CPBs Charged particle beams (such as electron and protein particles in the latest laser weapons).

CPBV Cardiopulmonary blood volume.

CPC Cancer patient care; Carboprostacyclin; Central posterior curve; Cerebellar Purkinje cell; Cerebral Palsy Clinic; Cetylpyridinium chloride; Child-Pugh Class(ification) (A, B, or C - for mild, moderate, or severe grades of hepatic cirrhosis/ dysfunction/ insufficiency); Choroid plexus cyst (Obs & Gyn); Chromaffin precursor cell; Chronic passive congestion; Chronic productive cough; Circumferential pneumatic compression; Clinical Pathological Conference; Clinical-pathological correlation; Clinicopathologic(al) conference; College Placement Council; Competent patient's consent (to treatment) (see CRT); Cortisol-producing cortex (of the adrenal/suprarenal gland); Council on Pharmacy and Chemistry (AMA); Pulmonary venous confluence (see PVC).

CpC Cytidylyl phosphate cytidine.

CPCA Canadian Palliative Care Association; Carboprostacyclin analogue (used in the treatment of PAOD).

CP/CD Cardiac pool/(transverse) cardiac diameter (ratio).

CPCL Congenital pulmonary cystic lymphangiectasia.

CPCP Chronic progressive coccidioidal pneumonitis.

CPCR Cardiopulmonary cerebral resuscitation.

CPCS Circumferential pneumatic compression suit; Clinical pharmacokinetics consulting service.

CPD Calcium pyrophosphate deposition/ disease; Calvé-Perthes disease; Cancer predisposition; Cardiopulmonary disease; Cephalopelvic disproportion; Chemopreventive/ prophylactic drug (see

CPA); Childhood/ Congenital polycystic disease; Chorionic prostaglandin dehydrogenase; Chorioretinopathy and pituitary dysfunction; Chronic peritoneal dialysis; Chronic protein deprivation; Citrate-phosphate-dextrose (an anticoagulant and preservative for donor blood); Commonly prescribed drug; Compound (see Cpd); Contact potential difference; Contagious pustular dermatitis; Continuing/uous professional development; Critical point drying; Cumulative probability of death; Cyclopentadiene; Cyst protein disease; Cytapheresis device.

Cpd Compound (= CP; CPD; cpd).

cpd compound (see Cpd); cycles per degree.

CPDA Citrate-phosphate-dextrose-adenine.

CPDD Calcium pyrophosphate deposition disease; Cis-platinum-diamine-dichloride.

Cpd E; cpd E Compound E (cortisone).

Cpd F; cpd F Compoune F (hydrocortisone; cortisol).

CPDL Cumulative population doubling level.

CPDS Clinical pharmacodynamic service/ study (= CPS).

Cpd S; cpd S Compound S (11-deoxycortisol, a 17-OH-CS).

CPDX Cefpodoxime.

CPDX-PR Cefpodoxime proxetil.

CPE Cardiac/ Cardiogenic pulmonary edema; Cardio-protective effect; Chronic pulmonary emphysema; Clinicopathologic entity/ entry; Clot-producing enzyme (e.g. thrombin); Clubbing, pitting, or edema; Compensation, pension, and education; Complete physical examination (see CPX); Complex partial epilepsy (= complex partial seizure; Psychomotor epilepsy/leptic seizure; Temporal lobe seizure); Compliance, effective; Conventional polyethylene (low density); Corona-penetrating enzyme; Cytopathic/ Cytopathogenic effect(s).

CPEHS Consumer Protection and Environmental Health Service (PHS).

CPEO Chronic progressive external ophthalmoplegia.

CPES Comprehensive Program for Elective Surgery (= CHS).

CPF Casein-predominant formula (for infants); Central perivenous fibrosis (see PVF); Clot-promoting factor; Contraction peak force.

CPFS Council on Physical Fitness and Sports.

CPG Capillary blood gases; Cardinal position of gaze; Cardiopneumographic recording; Carotid phonoangiogram; Clinical-practice guideline; Controlled pore glass; Copper binding globulin (= Ceruloplasmin) (see LFT iv); Craniopharyngioma; Cyanide-producing glycoside (present in food such as cassava; one of the causes of chemically/ drug-induced NIDDM).

CpG Cytidylyl phosphate guanosine.

CPGN Chronic proliferative glomerulonephritis.

CPH Careful personal hygiene; Certificate in Public Health; Chief physician (see CPh); Chronic paroxysmal hemicrania; Chronic persistent hepatitis; Chronic primary headache; Chronic pulmonary histoplasmosis; Committee on Perinatal Health (AAFP; AAP; ACOG; AMA); Corticotropin-releasing hormone; Cox proportional-hazards (model) (Orthopedics); Cutter protein hydrolysate (see CPH 5).

CPh Chief physician (= CPH).

CPH 5 Cutter protein hydrolysate, 5% in water (= CPH).

CPHA Canadian Public Health Association (ACHP); Commission/ Committee on Professional and Hospital Activities; Cox proportional-hazards analysis (Statistical analysis of respiratory failure).

CPHA-PAS Commission/ Committee on Professional and Hospital Activities-Professional Activity Study.

CPHD California Public Health Department; Child Psychiatry and Human Development (journal).

CPHJ Canadian Public Health Journal.

CPHL Central Public Health Laboratory (London).

CPHLD Conference of Public Health Laboratory Directors.

C_{phos} Phosphorus clearance (see KFT).

CPI California Personality/ Psychological Inventory; Cancer Potential Index; Chronic placental insufficiency (Obstetrics); Chronic pulmonary insufficiency; Congenital palatopharyngeal incompetence; Constitutional psychopathia inferior/pathic inferiority; Consumer price index; Control of Patient Information (Health Service Regulation, UK); Coronary prognosis/stic index; Cysteine proteinase inhibitor.

C pi Corpus pineale (thalamus).

CPIB Chlorophenoxyisobutyrate.

CPID Chronic pelvic inflammatory disease.

CPIP Chronic pulmonary insufficiency of prematurity.

CPIR Cephalic-phase insulin release.

CPJ Canadian Pharmaceutical Journal; Cleft Palate Journal.

CPK Creatine phosphokinase (isoenzyme serum - laboratory/ chemistry) (CK).

CPK-1; CPK_1 Brain CPK isoenzyme (= BB).

CPK-2; CPK_2 Hybrid muscle-brain CPK isoenzyme (= MB).

CPK-3; CPK_3 Muscle CPK isoenzyme (= MM).

CPKD Childhood polycystic kidney disease.

CPKS Clinical pharmacokinetic service/ study (= CPS).

CPL Caprine placental lactogen; 2-Ceruloplasmin (= CP; Cp); Chemical Pharmacology Laboratory (NIH); Chemistry and Physics of Lipids (journal); Conditioned/ning pitch level; Congenital pulmonary lymphangiectasia/sis; Criminal procedure law; Cystic periventricular leukomalacia (a major cause of CP - Cystic palsy in neonates).

cpl complete(d).

C/PL Cholesterol/phospholipid (ratio).

CPLM Cysteine-peptone-liver (infusion) medium.

CPM Calcipotriene monohydrate (= [5Z,7E,22E,24S]-24-cyclopropyl-9,10-secochola-5,7,10,[19],22-tetraene-1α,3β 24-triol mononhydrate; $C_{27}H_{40}O3H_2O$) - a synthetic analogue of Vitamin D3, used as a cream in the topical treatment of plaque psoriasis and other dermatoses; Cardiac pacemaker; Catecholamine producing medulla (of the suprarenal gland) (see SRG); Cationic polar molecule; Central pontine myelinolysis; Chlorpheniramine maleate; Chronic pulmonary mycosis; Circumscribed pretibial myxedema; Clinical Pharmacy Manager; Clinical Practice Model; Continue present management; Continuous passive motion; Counts/ Cycles per minute (sec cpm); Critical path method; Cyclophosphamide (see CP).

cpm counts/ cycles per minute (= C/Min; c/min; CPM).

CP_{max} Peak or maximum serum concentration.

CPMC Columbia Presbyterian Medical Center.

CPMD Continuous passive motion device (Orthopedics).

CPMDI Computerized pharmacokinetic model-driven drug infusion.

CP_{min} Minimum or trough serum concentration.

CPMM Constant passive motion machine.

CPMP Complete patient management problems.

CPMS Chronic progressive multiple sclerosis.

CPMV Cowpea mosaic virus.

CPN Cephapirin; Chronic polyneuropathy(ies)/ progressive neurosis/ pyelonephritis; Clinical Psychiatry News; Common peroneal nerve (see PNE; PNG; PNP; PNR).

CPNM Corrected perinatal mortality.

CPOHCS Circadian pattern of plasma corticosteroid (levels).

CPP Calcified pleural plaque (as in asbestosis); Cancer proneness phenotype; Canine pancreatic polypeptide; Cardiac/ Cerebral perfusion pressure (during basic CPR); Central precocious puberty; Choroid plexus papilloma; Chronic-pain patient (see CPS); Chronic pelvic pain/ peritonitis; Chronic pigmented purpura; Chronic plaque psoriasis; Circulatory pathophysiology (e.g. of trauma - Orthopedics); Clinicopathological presentation; Committee on Private Practice (AMA); Committee on Professional Performance (GMC); Common peroneal palsy; Computing in the Physician's Practice (survey, US); Current Problems in Pediatrics (journal); Cyclic polypeptide; Cyclopenteno-phenanthrene; Dl-2[3-(2'-chlorophenoxy)phenyl]-propionic (acid).

CPPB Continuous positive pressure breathing

(respiratory therapy).

CPPB=5 Continuous positive pressure breathing with 5-cm H_2O end-expired pressure.

CPPD Calcium pyrophosphate deposition disease (see CPPDDD); Calcium pyrophosphate dihydrate deposition (syndrome); Cisplatin.

CPPDDD Calcium pyrophosphate dihydrate deposition disease (= CPPD).

CPPF Chronic progressive pulmonary fibrosis.

CPPS Calcium Polyp Prevention Study (Dietary calcium in the prevention of cervical adenomata in women).

CPPT Cardiopulmonary physical therapy.

CPPV Continuous positive pressure ventilation (respiratory therapy).

CPR Calcium-phosphorus ratio (in the daily diet; for calcium balance); Cardiac and pulmonary rehabilitation (= ARC); Cardiac pulmonary/ Cardiopulmonary reserve; Cardiopulmonary reaction/ recorder/ resuscitation (= ARC); Centripetal rib; Cerebral-cortex perfusion rate; Chlorophenyl red; Chlorpromazine (see CPZ); Clinicopathologic(al) review; Committee on Patients' Rights; Complete pathological response; Cortisol production rate; Cumulative patency rate; Current Problems in Radiology (journal); Customary, prevailing, and reasonable (rate); Cytoplasmic ribosome (see PPF).

c-PR Cyclopropyl.

CPRAM Controlled partial rebreathing anesthesia method.

CPRCA Constitutional pure red cell aplasia.

CPRD Committee on Prosthetics Research and Development (NAS-NRC).

CPRG Coronary Project Research Group.

CPRP Cancer Pain Relief Program (WHO).

CPRS Children's Psychiatric Rating Scale; Comprehensive Psychopathological/gy Rating Scale.

CPS California Physicians' Service; Canadian Paediatric/ Physiological Society; Carbamyl phosphate synthetase; Cardioplegic perfusion solution; Cardiopulmonary support; Carpopedal spasm; Central Prescription Services (Appalachian Region); Centipoise (see cP); Cerebral Performance scale; Cervical/ Chest pain syndrome; Characters per second; Child Personality Scale; Child Protective Services; Child-Pugh score (for hepatic insufficiency); Chloroquine, pyrimethamine, and sulfisoxazole; Chronic pain sufferer/ syndrome; Chronic prostatitis syndrome; Clinical performance score; Clinical pharmaco dynamic (see CPDS)/ kinetic (see CPKS) service/ study; Clinical Pharmacy Services; Clinicopathologic(al) seminar/ study; Clinics in Plastic Surgery (journal); Coagulase positive Staphylococcus; Compendium of Pharmaceuticals and Specialities; Complex partial seizures; Constitutional psychopathic state; Contagious pustular stomatitis; Counts/ Cycles per second (see cps); C-polysaccharide; Cricopharyngeal sphincterotomy; Cumulative probability of success; Current population survey; Current Problems in Surgery (journal).

cps counts per second (per culture) (= CPS; C/S; C/Sec); cycles per second (double vebrations) (= CPS; C/S; C/Sec).

C5pS Chromosome 5p-syndrome (p = short arm of chromosome) (see CCS).

CPSC Congenital paucity of (secondary) synaptic clefts (syndrome); Consumer Products Safety Commission.

CPSD Center for Pediatric Sleep Disorders.

CPSM Council for Professions Supplementary to Medicine (GMC; UK).

CPSO College of Physicians and Surgeons of Ontario.

CPSP Central poststroke pain.

CPT Camptothecin (a naturally occurring plant alkaloid compound, and anticancer drug); Cardiac-pacemaker therapy; Carnitine palmityl transferase; Carotid pulse tracing; Cerebellopontine tumor; Chemoprevention therapy; Chest physiotherapy (respiratory therapy); Child protection team; Ciliary particle transport; Clinical Pharmacology and Therapeutics; Clinical pharmacology trial; Cold pressor test; Combining power test; Complex pharmacological treatment; Continuous performance test; Craniopagus twins (see pagus); Current Procedural Terminology (AMA (journal); Cytoplasmic transfer.

Cpt Let the patient take (L. capiat) (see Cap).

CPTC Chronic-Pain Treatment Center.

CPTH Chronic post-traumatic headache.

CPTN Culture-positive toxin-negative.

CPTP Culture-positive toxin-positive.

CPTX Chronic parathyroidectomy.

CPU Caudate putamen; Central processing unit (of computer); Cryophake unit (Keeler - Ophthalmology); Culture protective unit(s).

CPUE Chest pain of unknown etiology.

CPV Canine parvovirus; Carcinogenic papilloma virus (esp. HPV 16 or 18 - both associated with cancer of the cervix); Chicken pox vaccine/ virus (see HZV); Childhood-polio(myelitis) vaccination/ vaccine; Conjugate pneumococcal vaccine (hepatovalent) (see HCPV; PCV); Critical prognostic value; Cytoplasmic polyhedrosis virus.

CPVD Congenital polyvalvular disease.

CPX Complete physical examination (= CPE).

CPZ Cefoperazone; Chlorpromazine (hydrochloride) (test; tranquillizing drug) (= CHL; Chl; CPR); Compazine.

CQ Chloroquine (= CHL; Chl); Chloroquine-quinine; Circadian/ Conceptual quotient.

C'q A fragment of the first component of serum complement (see C'r; C's).

CQHCA Committee on Quality Health Care Assurance.

CQI Continuous quality improvement.

CQM Chloroquine mustard.

CQT Carroll Quantitative Test (of upper extremity function).

CQTS Congenital QT syndrome (see Q-T).

CQUCC Commission on Quantities and Units in Clinical Chemistry.

CR Calculation rate; Calculus removed; Calorie-restricted; Cancer/ Carbohydrate/ Cardiovascular/ Circulation Research (journals); Cardiac rate/ rehabilitation/ resuscitation/ rhythm; Cardiac Rehabilitation (AMA journal); Cardiorespiratory; Cardiorrhexis; Cardiovascular Review (journal); Caries-resistant; Case reports; Catalytic-regulatory (chains); Cathode ray; Cellular rejection; Centric relation; Cervical rib; Chemical Reviews (journal); Chest and right arm (ECG lead) (see CR 1); Chest radiogram/graph(y); Chest roentgenogram/aphy; Chief resident; Child-resistant (bottletop); Chiropody Review (journal); Choice reaction; Choroidoretinitis; Chromium (see Cr); Chronic rejection; Citrovorum rescue (Citrovorum or folinic acid [see CF] used to rescue patients from the effects of chemotherapy that cause anemia); Clinical Radiology (UK journal); Clinical record/ research; Closed reduction; Clot retraction; Coefficient of (fat) retention; Colon resection; Colonization resistance; Colony reared (animal); Colorectal; Complement receptor; Complete remission/ response; Conditioned reflex/ response; Congenital rubella; Congo red; Consciousness-raising (group) (see CR group); Consumer Reports (publication); Contact record; Continuous reinforcement; Controlled release/ respiration; Conversion/ Cooling rate; Cortico-resistant; Cosmic rays; Cough reflex; Creatinine (see Creat); Cremaster reflex; Cresyl red (an indicator); Critical ratio/ response; Cross-reaction/ reactivity; Crown-rump (length/ measurement of baby/ fetus) (see C-R); Cytosolic receptor (= CSR).

Cr Chromium (Z = 24) (= CR) (see Elements - Chromium); Cranial/ium (see cran); Creatine/ Creatinine (see Creat); Crown (on tooth).

cr cream(ed); creatinine (see Creat); credit; tomorrow (L. cras).

C_r Renal clearance (= C_k) (see KFT - C_r).

C-R Crown-rump (length/ measurement of baby/ fetus) (= CR; CRD; CRL; CRM).

C&R Convalescence and rehabilitation; Cystoscopy and retrograde.

C'r Fragment of first component of serum complement (see C'q; C's).

CR 1 Chest lead with indifferent electrode on right arm (= CR).

CR^1 First cranial nerve (= CN I).

^{51}Cr; Cr-51 Radioactive chromium (nuclear medicine).

CRA Cancer related anemia; Carbon rod atomizer (spectroscopy); Cardiorespiratory arrest; Central retinal artery; Central reviewer assessment; Chinese restaurant asthma; Chronic rheumatoid arthritis; Civil Rights

Act; Colorectal adenoma/ anastomosis; Computer risk assessment; Constant relative alkalinity; Cross-reactive antibody; Gamma 1 protein found in heavy chain disease; Sandoz Pharmaceuticals code for experimental substances.

CRAA Current Researches in Anesthesia and Analgesia (journal).

CRAB Central Registry at Bethesda (Maryland).

CRABP Cellular retinoic acid-binding protein.

Crack Cocaine (see Erythroxylum).

CRAG Cerebral radionuclide angiography.

CRAMS Circulation, Respiration, Abdomen, Motor, and Speech.

Cran Crandial.

cran cranial (nerve/ves) (= Cr); cranium (= Cr).

Cr&Br Crown and bridge.

crani- prefix meaning skull (Gr. kranion; L. cranium).

Craniol Craniology.

Crank Amphetamine (see Amphet).

CRAO Central retinal artery occlusion.

CRAP Chronic recurrent abdominal pain (occurs in PS or Periodic syndrome (see CV; FMF).

CRARM Commission on Risk Assessment and Risk Management.

CRAS Comptes Rendus de l'Académie des Sciences.

crast for tomorrow (L. crastinus).

CRB Chemical, radiological, and biological; Cholinergic receptor blocker; Critical Reviews in Bioengineering (CRC journal).

CRBBB Complete right bundle branch block (ECG).

CRBC Chicken red blood cell.

CRBP Cellular retinol-binding protein; Chicago Regional Blood Program.

CRC Canadian Red Cross; Cancer Research Campaign (UK); Cardiovascular reflex conditioning; Cardiovascular/ Clinical Research Center; Chemical Rubber Co.; Child-resistant container; Chronic relapsing course (of a disease); Chronic respiratory condition; Cigar Research Council; Civil Rights Commission; Clinically relevant change; Colorectal carcinoma; Concentrated red (blood) cells; Concentration-response curve (of a drug) (= RCC; RCR); Conservation and Research Center (Smithsonian Institute, Washington, DC); Cross-reacting cannabinoids; Cytokine receptor chain.

CR&C Closed reduction and cast.

CRCB Cardiovascular Research Center Bulletin (journal).

CRCCRB Cardiovascular Research Center (CRC) Critical Reviews in Bioengineering (journal).

CRCCRT CRC Critical Reviews in Toxicology.

CrCl Creatinine clearance.

CRCLS Critical Reviews in Clinical Laboratory Sciences (journal).

CRCRNM Critical Reviews in Clinical Radiology and Nuclear Medicine (journal).

CRCS Cardiovascular reflex conditioning system.

C-RCU Cardiac-respiratory care unit.

CRD Cancer-related death; Cardiorespiratory drug; Cardiovascular-related death (= CVRD); Central respiratory depression; Child restraint device; Childhood rheumatic disease; Chorio-retinal degeneration; Chronic renal damage; Chronic renal/ respiratory disease; Clinically relevant dose; Coronoradiographic documentation; Complete reaction of degeneration; Computer-related disorder; Congenital rubella deafness; Cone-rod dystrophy; Corticosteroid-responding/ responsive dermatitis/ dermatoses/ dermatosis/ disorder; Corticoid-responsible disease/ disorder (see SRC); Crown-rump distance (= C-R); Currently recommended dose.

CRD 401 Diltiazem (= MW 450). A benzothiazine derivative, calcium antagonist and coronary vasodilator, with actions similar to those of nifedipine and verapamil.

CRDB Chronic Respiratory Diseases Branch (PHS).

CRDC Clinically relevant drug concentration.

CR-DIP Chronic relapsing demyelinating inflammatory polyneuropathy.

CRDN Chronic relapsing demyelinating neuropathy.

CRDP Center for Research in Disease Prevention Chronic Renal Disease Program.
CRE Chronic refractory eczema; Clinically relevant effect; Cross-reactive epitope; Clinical research experience; Cumulative radiation effect.
Cre Creatine/tinine (see Creat).
Crea Creatine/ Creatinine (see Creat).
Crea P; Creat P Creatine/ Creatinine phosphate (Cr P).
Creat Creatine/ Creatinine (= CR; Cr; cr; Crea; CTN).
creat- prefix meaning flesh or meat (Gr. kreas, kreat) (= creo-; kreo-).
CREG Cancer Research Emphasis Grant (NCI).
crem cremaster (muscle/ reflex).
creo- prefix meaning flesh or meat (see creat-).
Crep; crep Crepitation/itus (L. crepitus).
-crescent suffix meaning grow (L. cresco, crescentis).
CREST Calcinosis cutis, Raynaud's phenomenon, esophageal involvement, sclerodactyly, and (eosinophilia) telangiectasia/sis (syndrome).
cret- combining form meaning distinguish/ separate/ grow (L. cretus) (= crin-).
CRF Cardiorespiratory fitness/ function; Case report form; Chief/ Coronary risk factor; Chronic renal/ respiratory failure; Coagulase-reacting/ releasing factor; Compromised renal function; Continuous reinforcement; Controlled release formulation; Corticotropin-releasing factor (see Hormones - CRF).
CRFK Crandell feline kidney cells.
CRG Cardiorespirogram; Council for Responsible Genetics.
CR group Consciousness-raising group (= CR).
CRH Cardio-renal health; Corticotropin-releasing hormone (see Hormones - CRH); Council on Rural Health (AMA).
CRHL Collaborative Radiological Health Laboratory.
CRHP Council for the Regulation of Healthcare Professionals (GMC; UK).
CRHR2 Corticotropin releasing hormone receptor 2.
CRHS Counter-regulatory hormone secretion (of insulin - the Somogyi effect).
CRHV Cotton-tail rabbit herpes virus.
CRI Cancer/ Clinical Research Institute; Cardiac Risk Index; Catheter-related infection; Chemical/ Concentrated rust-inhibiting (germicide); Chronic renal/ respiratory impairment/ insufficiency; Clinically relevant impairment (of kidney/ liver function, etc.); Cold running intelligibility (hearing test for continuous speech); Community Research Initiative; Composite Risk Index; Congenital rubella infection; Corticosteroid-responsive illness (see CSRI); Cross-reaction idiotype.
CRIE Crossed radioimmunoelectrophoresis.
crin- combining form meaning distinguish or separate (Gr. krino) (see cret-).
CRISP Computer Retrieval of Information on Scientific Projects (PHS).
Crit; crit Hematocrit (laboratory/ hematology) (= crt; H'crit; Hct; PCV).
Crit Doc Criteria document.
CRL Cell repository line; Certified Record Librarian; Cholera Research Laboratory (Dacca); Clinically relevant level(s); Complement receptor location/ lymphocyte; Crown-rump length (see C-R).
CRLM Circulating radiolabelled metabolite.
CRM Center for Reproductive Medicine; Certified Reference Materials; Chloroquine-resistant malaria; Counting rate meter; Cross-reacting material; Crown-rump measurement (see C-R).
CRM + Cross-reacting material positive.
CRMA Conseil de Recherches Medicales Actualites (Canada, also MRCN).
CRMC Cycle-related myometrial contraction(Obs/Gyn).
CRMCCA Collège Royal dès Médecins et Chirurgiens du Canada Annales (journal).
CRMM Chemoreceptor-mediated mechanism (see CMM).
CRMN Chemotherapy-related myeloid neoplasm.
CRMO Chronic recurrent multifocal osteomyelitis.
CRMP Connecticut Regional Medical Program.

CRMS Childhood rhabdomyosarcoma.
CRN Chronic reflux nephropathy; Clinical-research network (see CTN); Complement requiring neutralization.
CRNA Certified Registered Nurse Anesthetist; Complement-requiring neutralizing antibody.
cRNA Chromosomal ribonucleic acid.
CRNF Chronic rheumatoid nodular fibrositis.
CRNI Certified Registered Nurse Intravenous.
CRN/N Complement-requiring neutralizing (antibody)/ complement.
Cr Nn; Cr nn; cr nn Cranial nerves.
CRNP Certified Registered Nurse Practitioner.
CRO Cathode ray oscilloscope; Centric relation occlusion; Contract-research organization; Controlled-release opioid.
CROI Conference on Retroviruses and Opportunistic Infections (Washington, DC).
CROM Cervical range of motion; Control read-only memory.
CROS Committee for Radiation Oncology Studies; Contralateral routing of signal(s).
Crossroad Amphetamine tablet (see Amphet).
CRP Cancer/ Civilian Research Program; Cardiac Rehabilitation and Prevention (department/ facility/ unit); Cardiac/ Coronary rehabilitation program; Certified Radiological Physicist; Characteristic release profile (drug absorption); Choking rescue procedure (= HM; VM); Cholestasis-related pruritus; Chronic radiation proctitis; Chronic relapsing pancreatitis/ polyneuritis; Clinical research program/ protocol; Compressive rehabilitation program; Corneal-retinal potential; C-reactive protein; Cross-reacting protein; Cyclic AMP receptor protein (see AMP; cAMP); Cytostolic receptor protein.
Cr P Creatine/ Creatinine phosphate (see Creat P).
CRPA C-reactive protein agglutination/ antiserum.
CRPBI Children's Report of Parent Behavior Inventory.
CRPD Chronic restrictive pulmonary disease.
CRPF Chloroquine-resistant PLASMODIUM falciparum; Contralateral renal plasma flow.
CRPS Chronic regional pain syndrome (= RSD); Columbia Relapse Prevention Study (for anorexia nervosa).
CRR Cardiac-related rehospitalization; Compensatory renin release; Congo red retention.
CRS Cardiorespiratory support; Catheter-related sepsis; Catholic Relief Services; Caudal regression syndrome; Chemical Registry System (CAS); Chinese restaurant syndrome (headaches, heart palpitations and sweating, supposedly but without scientific corroboration associated with the ingestion of MSG - Monosodium glutamate, a flavor enhancer commonly used in Chinese restaurants); Cirrhosis-related syndrome; Clinical Radioassay Society; Colon and rectum/ Colon-rectal surgery; Compliance of the respiratory system; Congenital rubella syndrome; Congressional Research Service (LC); Contamination Reduction System; Council of the Royal Society; Cytokine release syndrome (associated with severe dyspnea, bronchospasm, angioedema, urticaria, etc.).
CRSM Cherry red spot myoclonus.
CRSP Comprehensive renal scintillation procedure.
CrSp Craniospinal.
CRSSB Comptes Rendus des Seances de la Societe de Biologie.
CRST Calcinosis cutis, Raynaud's phenomenon, sclerodactyly, and telangiectasia/sis syndrome.
CRT Cadaver renal transplant; Cardiac resuscitation team; Cathode-ray tube; Cellular-response test (for viral diseases such as AIDS); Central/ Choice reaction time; Certified/fy; Certified Record Techniques; Chemoresistant tumor (see CRC); Chromium release test; Colorectal tumorigenesis; Commission on Radiation Therapy (CMSI of ACR); Competent refusal of treatment (of the patient) (see CPC); Complex reaction time(r); Computer remote terminal; Computer/ized renal tomography; Controlled room temperature; Copper reduction test; Correct(ed); Corrected retention time; Cortisone resistant thymocyte; Cranial radiation therapy; Critical Reviews in Toxicology (CRC journal); Cytoreductive therapy (as in chemotherapy, surgery, or by x-ray).

crt hematocrit (laboratory/ hematology) (see Crit).
CRTP Conciousness Research and Training Project.
CrTr Crutch training.
CRTS Committee on Radiation Therapy Studies (NCI).
CRTT Certified Respiratory Therapy Technician.
CRTX Cast removed take x-ray.
CRU Cardiac rehabilitation unit; Clinical Rehabilitation Unit; Clinical research unit.
CRUI Catheter-related urinary infection.
crur- combining form meaning leg or shin (L. cruris).
CRUS Congenital radio-ulnar synostosis (Orthopedics).
CRV Central retinal vein.
CRVF Congestive right ventricular failure.
CRVO Central retinal vein occlusion.
CRVS California Relative Value Studies.
cry- prefix meaning cold (Gr. cryos).
cryo cryogenic; cryoglobulin; cryoprecipitate; cryosurgery; cryotherapy.
crypt;- crypto- prefix meaning hidden or secret (Gr. kryptos) (= krypto-).
Crys Crystal, Crystalline, Crystallize(d) (see crys; Cryst; cryst); Methamphetamine (see Amphet).
crys; Cryst; cryst Crystal, Crystalline, Crystallize(d) (= Crys).
Crystal Any soluble amphetamine/ desoxyn/ methedrine (see Amphet).
Crystall Crystallography.
CS Caesarean/ Caesarian/ Cesarean/ Cesarian section (see C/S); Calabar swelling (found in loiasis and caused by the filarial worm *Loa* loa. It probably represents a reaction to the discharge of uterine contents or pheromones from the adult worm; transmission is by the bite of the orange-yellow horse-fly, *Chrysops* silacea and C. dimidiata); Calf/ Cobra/ Control serum; Campomelic/ Caplan's/ Carcinoid/ Climacteric/ Cockayne/ Compression/ Crush/ Cushing's syndrome; Camptothecin sodium; Cannabis sativa (see CANNABIS); Cantu syndrome (Onychotrichodysplasia with neutropenia) - Mild mental retardation with chronic neutropenia - an autosomal recessive, ectodermal dysplasia); Cardiogenic shock; Caries-susceptible; Carotid sheath/ sinus; Casualty Simulation (journal); Casualty station; Cataract surgery; Cat scratch (disease/ fever) (see CSD); Celiac sprue; Central service/ supply; Centrosome (a structure found just outside the nuclear membrane of a cell); Cockayne's syndrome (facial 'butterfly' erythema by age two, photosensitivity, long limbs and large heads, mental retardation, death during second decade - an autosomal recessive, congenital hypotrichosis) (= PAS); Cerebrospinal; Cervical spine (= Csp; C-spine)/ stimulation; Cervical spondylosis; Chemical Society (London); Chest strap; Chief of staff; Cholesterol stone; Chondroitin sulfate; Chorionic somatomammotropin/ somatotropin; Christian Scientist; Chronic schizophrenia; Church of Scotland; Cigarette/ Current smoker; Citrate synthetase/ synthase; Civil service; Clinic staging; Clinical Science/ Symposia (journals); Clinical scientist/ specialist/ stage; Close supervision; Coblenz Society; Coffin-Siris (syndrome) (absence of distant phalanges, broad nose, delayed dentition with small teeth, etc. - an autosomal dominant, ectodermal dysplasia); Cold sore (see HL); Colla sinistra (L.) - with the left hand; Colorimetric solution; Complete stroke; Concentrated strength of drugs/ solutions; Conditioned stimulus; Congenital syphilis; Conjunctival secretion; Conjunctiva-sclera (see C&S); Conscious(ness); Constant spring; Consultation/ C. service; Contact sensitivity; Contemporary Surgery (journal); Continue same; Contrast sensitivity; Control subject; Convalescence/nt; Convalescent status; Coronary sclerosis/ sinus/ stent(ing); Corpus striatum; Corticoid-sensitive; Corticosteroid (= CTS); Cromolyn sodium/ disodium (cromoglycate) (see DSCG); Cullen's sign (periumbilical discoloration in an acute abdomen, seen in ruptured abdominal aortic aneurysm and acute pancreatititis); Current strength; Cycloserine (TB); Cyclosporine (= Cs; CSP); Cytostatic (see CSACA); Interceptive (stimulus); With the left hand (L. colla sinistra).

CS# Cervical spine fracture (see CSF).

Cs Case(s) (see cs); Caesium (= Cesium) (Z = 55) (see Elements - Caesium); Cell surface; Conscious(ness) (see cs); Cyclosporine (see CS); Standard clearance (see C_s); Static respiratory compliance (see C_s).

cS centistoke (viscosity) (= cs).

cs case(s) (= Cs); centistoke (see cS); chromosome; conscious(ness) (= Cs).

C_s Standard clearance (Urea clearance test) (see KFT - UCl) (= Cs); Static respiratory compliance (= Cs).

C/S Caesarean/ Caesarian/ Cesarean/ Cesarian section (operation/ obstetrics) (= Caesarean/ Cesarian s; CS; C-S; C-sect; C-section); Counts/ Cycles per second (see cps).

C-S Cesarean section (see C/S).

C&S Calvarium and scalp; Conjunctiva and sclera (eye examination); Culture and sensitivity (laboratory/ sensitivity).

C's Fragment of first component of serum complement (see C'q; C'r).

^{137}Cs Radioactive caesium/ cesium (see Cs).

CS_2 Carbon disulfide.

C_4S Chondroitin-4-sulfate.

CS IV Clinical stage 4.

C_6S Chondroitin-6-sulfate.

CSA Canadian Standards Association; Canavaninosuccinic acid; Cancer-specific antigen; Carbonyl salicylamide; Cardioselective agent; Cavosurface angle (dentistry); Cell surface antigen; Central sleep apnea (see OSA); Chi-square analysis; Chrondroitin sulfate-A; Chronic stable angina; Colony-stimulating activity; Community Services Administration (SRS); Compressed spectral assay; Compression screw arthrodesis (e.g. of the metatarsophalyngeal joint) (Orthopedics); Computer systems analyst; Computerized spectral analysis; Congenital spinal anomalies/ly; Controlled substance analogue; Controlled Substances Act; Coronary spastic angina; Cross-section(al) area; Cyclosporine A (see CsA); Cytostatic activity.

CsA Cyclosporine A (= CSA).

CSAA Child Study Association of America.

CSAC Cancer Survivorship Advisory Council.

CSACA Cytostatic anticancer agent (= ACA; ACD; ANA; AND).

CSAD Center for the Study of Aging and Development.

CSAF Calcium-sodium alginate fiber.

CSAG Confidentiality and Security Advisory Group (for England/ Scotland/ Northern Ireland); Philips Roxane Laboratories code for experimental substances.

CSAHD Center for the Study of Aging and Human Development.

CSAP Chronic stable angina pectoris.

CSAT Center for Substance Abuse Treatment (Alcohol, Drugs, etc. - USA).

CSAVP Cerebral subarachnoid venous pressure.

CSB Caffeine sodium benzoate; Cheyne-Stokes breathing; Clinically significant benefit; Cold/ Cooling sponge bath; Contaminated small bowel.

csb chromosome break.

CBS I & II Chemistry Screening Batteries I and II.

CSBF Coronary sinus blood flow.

CSBG Corticosteroid-binding globulin (see CBG).

CSBS Contaminated small bowel syndrome.

CSC Canada Safety Council; Cancer supportive care; Cervical spinal cord; "Chain of survival" concept (AHA); Civil Service Commission; Clinically significant change; Collagen sponge contraceptive; Complete subligamentous calcification; Concern with self-competence (index); Cord-serum concentration (of a drug); Cord stem cell; Cornea, sclera, and conjunctiva; Corticostriatocerebellar; Coup sur coup (Fr.) - "blow on blow" (administration of small amounts of drugs at short intervals; giving a drug in small doses at short intervals in order to secure rapid, complete, or continued action; small freqent doses of medicine); Cryogenic storage container; Cumulative survival curve.

CSCB Canadian Society for Cell Biology.

CSCC Canadian Society of Clinical Chemists.

CS & CC Culture, sensitivity and colony count.

CSCD Center for Sensory and Communication Disorders (North Western

University Medical School, US); Center for Sickle Cell Disease; Coil-spring contraceptive diaphragm (see ASCD; Contraceptives).
CSCI Continuous subcutaneous infusion.
CSCR Central Society for Clinical Research.
CSCS Compressive spinal cord syndrome.
CSCT Combined sequential chemotherapy.
CSD Cardiac-support device; Carotid sinus denervation; Cat scratch disease (= CS; CSF); Caudal sympathetic denervation; Chemical Sensitivity Disorders (see MCS); Chronic sinus disease; Chronic skin disease/ disorder; Chronic sleep deprivation; Clinically significant decrease (see CSR); Closed suction drain; Coil spring diaphragm (contraceptive device); Colloidal Silicone Dioxide; Combined system disease/ disorder (= SCID) (a severe combined immune deficiency, characterized by abnormalities affecting the pluripotential lymphoid stem-cell system. Some deficiencies are inherited as autosomal recessive, others as x-linked traits. Biochemically, one group has been characterized by the lack of a particular enzyme, adenosine deaminase); Conditionally streptomycin-dependent; Conduction system disease; Controlled symmetrical distraction (of the epiphyseal plate) (Orthopedics); Cortical spreading depression; Craniospinal defect; Cross-sectional data; Critical stimulus duration; Cystathionine synthase deficiency.
CS&D Cleaned, sutured, and dressed.
CSDB Cat scratch disease bacillus.
CSE Central sedative effect/ stimulatory effect; Chronic synovial effusion; Clinical side/ Clinically significant effect; Clinical-symptom/ self-evaluation (questionnaire); Cone-shaped epiphysis; Consistent systemic exposure (to drugs) (see FI - Fluctuation Index); Cross-sectional echocardiography.
C/Sec Counts/ Cycles per second (see cps).
C-sect; C-section Cesarean section (see C/S).
CSEM. Colorized scanning electron micrograph(y).
CSEP Cortical somatosensory evoked potential.
CSER Committee for the Scientific Examination of Religion; Cortical somatosensory evoked response.
CSF Canadian Schizophrenia Foundation; Cancer family syndrome; Capillary stress failure (as in alveolar overdistention in ventilator-induced lung injury); Cat scratch fever (see CSD); Cerebrospinal fluid (= C); Cervical spine fracture (= CS#); Chronic fatigue syndrome (= CFIDS); Cold stability factor; Colony-stimulating factor (= see HGF); Colored single female; Coronary sinus flow; Cortisol secretion flow (rate); Cyanide-sensitive factor.
CSF-GOT Cerebrospinal fluid - glutamic oxalacetic transaminase.
CSFH Cerebrospinal fluid hyper/hypotension.
CSFI Cholesterol saturated fat index.
CSFM Cause-specific fetal mortality.
CSFN Canadian Schizophrenia Foundation Newsletter.
CSFP Cerebrospinal fluid pressure.
CSFV Cerebrospinal fluid volume.
CSF-WR Cerebrospinal fluid - Wassermann reaction (see STS).
CSG Chronic secondary/ simple glaucoma; Clinically strategic goal(s); Council of State Governments.
csg chromosome gap.
CSGBI Cardiac Society of Great Britain and Ireland.
CSGBM Collagenase soluble glomerular basement membrane.
CSGUS Clinical Society of Genito-Urinary Surgeons.
CSH Carotid sinus hypersensitivity; Catheterization-site hematoma; Cholestatic hepatitis; Chronic subdural hematoma; Congenital subluxation of the hip (Orthopedics); Cortical stromal hyperplasia.
C-Sh Chair shower.
CSHEP Constriction, sclerosis, hemorrhage, exudate, and papilledema (eye examination).
CSHH Congenital self-healing histiocytosis.
CSHN Central sclerosing hyaline necrosis (in chronic liver disease).
CSHP Center for the Study of Human Polymorphisms (Paris, France).
CSHSQB Cold Spring Harbor Symposia on Quantitative Biology (books).
CSI Calculus surface index; Canadian Society for Immunology; Cancer serum index;

Cavernous sinus infiltration; Cervical-spine injury (= CST); Cholesterol saturation index; Cholesterol synthesis inhibitor; Clinically significant increase; Colloquium Spectroscopicum Internationale; Computerized severity of illness (index); Confirmed silent ischemia; Continuous sedative infusion; Coronary sinus intervention; Coronary stent insertion; Corticosteroid insufficiency; Cross species infection; Cutaneous staphylococcal infection.

CSICU Cardiac surgical intensive care unit.

CSIEM Committee for the Study of Inborn Errors of Metabolism (NRC).

CSII Continuous subcutaneous insulin infusion.

CSIIP Continuous subcutaneous insulin infusion pump.

CSIN Chemical Substances Information Network.

CSIRO Commonwealth Scientific and Industrial Research Organization (Australia).

CSIS Clinical supplies and inventory system.

CSIT Committee on Social Implications of Technology (IEEE).

CSJ Cholestatic jaundice.

CSL Cardiolipin synthetic lecithin (test) (see STS); Chromosome specific library; Conference of State Legislatures; Corticosteroid liposome.

CSLM Confocal scanning light microscopy.

CSLP Center for Short-lived Phenomena.

CSLT Canadian Society of Laboratory Technologists.

CSLU Chronic stasis leg ulcer.

CSM Carotid sinus massage (cardiology) (= CSNS; CSP; CSS); Cause-specific mortality; Cell-surface molecule (such as CD34; E-selectin, ICAM-1, P-selectin, VCAM-1, etc.); Cerebrospinal meningitis; Circulation, sensation, and motion; Colored single male; Committee on Safety of Medicines (UK); Corn-soy milk (food blend - corn meal; soya/soy bean).

CSMA Chemical Specialities Manufacturers Association; Chronic spinal muscular atrophy.

CSMB Center for the Study of Multiple Births.

CSMC Cedars-Sinai Medical Center (LA, Ca).

CSME Cotton spot macular edema.

CSMEH Center for the Safety of Medical Ethics and Humanities (US).

CSMM Clinical Science and Molecular Medicine (journal).

CSMMG Chartered Society of Massage and Medical Gymnastics (British).

CSMP Chloramphenicol-sensitive microsomal protein; Continuous system modeling program.

CSMS Connecticut State Medical Society.

CSMT Center for Sexual and Marital Therapy; Chorionic somatomammotropin.

CSN Cardiac sympathetic nerve; Carotid sinus nerve; Chronic sensory neuropathy.

CSNA Congenital sensory neuropathy with anhidrosis (syndrome).

CSNB Congenital stationary night blindness.

CS(NCA) Clinical Laboratory Scientist Certified by the National Certification Agency for Medical Laboratory Personnel.

CSNM Cause-specific neonatal mortality.

CSNRT; cSNRT Corrected sinus node recovery time.

CSNS Carotid sinus nerve stimulation/ator (see CSM).

CSO Claims services only; Common source outbreak; Copied standing orders.

CSOM Chronic serous/ suppurative otitis media.

CSOP Coronary sinus occlusion pressure.

CSOS Cross-species organ sharing.

CSP Cancer Surveillance Program (LA); Capsular shift procedure (orthopedic surgery); Carotid sinus pressure (see CSM); Catatonic schizophrenia; Cavum septi pellucidi; Cell surface/ Cerebrospinal protein; Cellulose sodium phosphate; Chartered Society of Physiotherapists/py (UK); Chemistry screening panel/ profile; Chondroitin sulfate protein; Christian Science Practitioner; Clinical symptomatological parameter(s); Cochlear's speech processor; Comparable safety profile; Computerized Speech Processor; Contact-sensitizing potential (see CAP); Contralateral spastic paralysis/ paraparesis/ paraplegia; Cooperative

Statistical Program (for IUD data); Criminal sexual psychopath; Cyclosporin (see CS).

Csp; C-spine Cervical spine (see CS).

CSPED Center for Surrogate Parenting and Egg Donation (Ca).

CSPI Center for Science in the Public Interest.

CSPP Cancer Screening & Prevention Program (see COP).

CSPS Continual skin peeling syndrome.

CSR Carotid sinus reflex/ rhythm; Cell surface receptor (on the surface of lymphocytes: including CD3, CD4, CD8, Complement, Fc, Hormone, Interleukin, Mitogen, Virus and other receptors); Center of Stereotactic Radiosurgery (New Jersey Med. School, US); Central supply room; Cheyne-Stokes respiration; Clinically significant reduction (= CSD); Clinical sucess rate; Continued stay review; Corrected sedimentation rate; Corrective septorhinoplasty; Corrective/ Curative surgical resection; Cortical/ Corticosterone/ Cortisol secretion rate (of the adrenal gland); Cross-sensitivity reaction; Cumulative survival rate; Cytosolic receptor (see CR).

CSRA Clinical Scholar Research Award.

CSRC Corticosteroid-responsible condition (= see SRC).

CSRD Corticosteroid-responsive dermatoses/sis.

CSRDF Civil Service Retirement and Disability Fund.

CSRI Corticosteroid-responsive illness (= CRI).

CSRP Commission on Standards in Radiologic Practice (ACR).

CSRS Cooperative State Research Service.

CSRT Canadian Society of Radiological Technicians; Canadian Society of Respiratory Technologists; Corrected sinus recovery time.

CSS Cancer Surveillance System; Cardiac standstill (= Asystole; Cardiac arrest; CPA); Carotid sinus stimulation (see CSM); Carotid/ Cavernous sinus syndrome; Cerebrospinal shunt; Cervical-spine screening; Central sterile supply; Chewing, sucking, and swallowing; Christian Science sanatorium; Chronic/ Constant/ Continuous sensory stress; Chronic subclinical scurvy; Churg-Strauss syndrome; Clinical scurvy syndrome; Committee on the Skeletal System (now absorbed into CPRD); Cross-sectional study (see CST); Cranial sector scan; Creatinine (concentration in) steady-state serum; Cross-sectional study/ survey (see CST).

CSs Appetitive conditioning.

CSSA Crop Science Society of America.

CSSD Central sterile supply department.

CSSDC Canadian Society for the Study of Diseases of Children.

CSSM Chicago Stritch School of Medicine; Complete skin-sparing mastectomy.

CST Cardiac/ Contraction stress test; Cavernous sinus thrombosis; Central standard time; Cerebral seizure threshold; Cervical-spine trauma (see CSI); Chemosensitive tumor; Chi-square(d) test (a parametric test for caterogical variables in statistical analysis) (see KWT; PMT); Cholestatic jaundice; Christ-Siemens Touraine (syndrome); Chromosomal trisomy (21 - Down's syndrome; 18 - Exomphalos; 13 - Open scalp defect); Clinical screening test; Clinical selection theory (see AbST - Antibody specific theory); Clonal selection theory (see AST - Antibody specific theory); Clonidine suppression test (for pheochromocytoma); Committee on Science and Technology (USHR); Compartment syndrome of the thigh (Orthopedics); Compliance, static (see Cst); Computer scatter tomography; Contraction stress testing (in oligohydramnios of pregnancy - see BPP; NST); Convulsive shock therapy; Corticospinal tract; Corticosteroid therapy/ treatment; Cortisol/ Cortrosyn stimulation test (for secondary hypoadrenalism); Cosyntropin stimulation test; Cross-sectional trial (see CSS); Cytostatic therapy (= CCT; CTC; CTCT).

Cst; C_{st}; C_{stat} Static compliance (measure of lung elasticity) (= CST) - reduced in pulmonary fibrosis, and increased in emphysema.

cSt centistoke.

cst chi-square test (of treatment group variables).

CSTI Clearinghouse for Scientific and Technical Information.

CSTT Cold-stimulation time test.
CSU California State University; Cardiac surgery/ surveillance unit; Cardiovascular surgery unit; Casualty staging unit; Catheter specimen of urine; Central statistical unit; Clinical speciality unit.
C subst Complex carbohydrate substrate (of streptococci).
CSUF Continuous slow ultrafiltration.
CSUK Chemical Society of the United Kingdom.
CSUN California State University Northridge (see NCOD).
CSV Chick syncytial virus; Coxsackievirus (B).
CSVS Clinical Society for Vascular Surgery.
CSW Certified Social Worker; Current sleep walker.
CSWE Council of Social Work Education.
CSWG Clinically significant weight gain.
CT Calcitonin (see Ct); Calf testis; Calliper tape; Cardiac tamponade; Cardiotachometer; Cardiothoracic (ratio) (see CTR); Carotid tracing; Carpal tunnel (syndrome); Casoni test (intradermal test for hydatid cyst); Cell(ular)/ Cognitive/ Continue/ Corrective/ Cytotoxic therapy/ treatment; Cephalic tetanus; Cerebral thrombosis/ tumor; Cervical traction; Cervicothoracic; Chain-terminating; Chemotherapy; Chest/ Continuous-flow tube; Chewable tablet; Chicken/ Combined tumor; Chlamydia trachomatis; Chlorothiazide (see CTZ); Cholera/ Cobra/ Coley's toxin; Cholesterol, total; Chordae tendineae; Chronic thyroiditis; Chymotrypsin; Circulation/ Clotting/ Coagulation/ Contraction/ Crest time; Classic/ Contraceptive technique; Clinic Toxicology (journal); Closed thoracotomy; Coated tablet (see GRCT); Coil/ Coombs' test; Collecting tubule; Colon, transverse; Committee on Trauma (Am Col Surg); Compressed tablet; Compression threshold (hearing); Computed/ Computer-assisted/ Computerized (transaxial) tomography (see CAT); Connective tissue; Controlled temperature; Copper toxicosis (see CBG; WD); Corneal/ Cortical thickness; Corneal transplant; Coronary thrombosis; Corrected transposition; Corrective therapist; Cough threshold; Cyclothymia (a milder form of manic-depressive illness); Cystine-tellurite (medium); Cystitome (used to open the lens capsule - Ophthalmology); Cystotome (used to incise the bladder - Urology); Cytarabine and thioguanine; Cytoplasmic transfer (of cytoplasm or cell material from one woman's ovum to another's, thus enhancing the chances of successful fertilization); Cytotechnologist (ASCP); Unit of attenuation (number).
CT# Comminuted torsional fracture (see CTF).
Ct Calcitonin (= CT; CTN); Carboxyl terminal; Ctenocephalides (a genus of fleas).
ct carat; chromatid; count.
C/T Compression/traction (ratio).
C&T Color and temperature.
CT 871 Bialamicol hydrochloride (= Biallylamicol HCl; Biethylamicol HCl; PAA 701; SN 6771). Used as an alternative to emetine and bismuth iodide, and to supplement emetine HCl in the treatment of acute and chronic amebiasis.
CT 879 Sulfamethoxypyridazine (= RP 7522; SMP). A long-acting sulfonamide, rapidly absorbed (with a maximum blood level in 5 hours), and slowly excreted; it is detectable in serum even after 4 days.
Ct 1824; $C_{T\text{-}1824}$ Clearance of Evans blue (T-1824) (see KFT).
CTA Canadian Tuberculosis Association; Cancer Therapy Abstracts (SIS); Catamenia (menses); Center for Traditional Acupuncture; Chemotactic/ Chronotropic activity; Chemotherapeutic/ Cytotoxic (= CTD) agent; Chromotropic acid; Clear to auscultation; Clinical Trends in Anesthesiology (journal); Committee on Thrombolytic Agents; Commission on Technologist Affairs (ACR); Congenital triangular alopecia (a minor hypotrichosis of sporadic inheritance, with triangular areas of hair loss from birth in frontotemporal regions, extending to frontal hair line); Congenital trigeminal anesthesia; Coumarin-type anticoagulant; Cuff-tear arthropathy (shoulder joint); Cyanotrimethylandrosterone; Cyproterone acetate; Cystine trypticase agar; Cytoplasmic tubular aggre-

gate/s; Cytotoxic agent/ antibiotic (e.g. Daunorubicine; Epirubicin, etc.); Cytotoxic assay.

CTa; Cta Menses/ Menstruation (L. catamenia).

C II TA Class II transactivator (gene, of MHC - Major-histocompatibility complex).

CTAB Cetrimide (= Cetrimonium bromide) (consists chiefly of tetradecyltrimethyl-ammonium bromide); Cetyltrimethyl-ammonium bromide (see CTBM).

C-TAB; C-tab Cyanide tablet.

CTAC Cancer Treatment Advisory Committee (HEW).

cTAL cortical thick ascending limb.

c tant with the same amount (L. cum tanto).

CTAP Computed tomography during arterial portography; Connective tissue activating peptide.

CTAT Computerized transaxial tomography (see CAT).

CTB Ceased to breathe; Current Topics in Bioenergetics (annual volumes).

ctb chromated break.

CTC Calcium-tris-citrate (buffer); Cardiac transplant center; Carpal tunnel compression (see CTS); Chemotherapy clinic; Chlortetracycline; Clinical Trial Certificate; Common Toxicity Criteria (NCI); Computer-aided tomographic cisternography; Constant temperature circulator; Cultured T cells; Cytotoxic chemotherapy (see CST).

CtC Cell-to-cell (spread of destruction/ infection/ inflammation etc.).

CTCD Combined treatment for chronic depression (i.e. medication with psychotherapy).

CTCL Cutaneous T-cell lymphoma.

ctCO$_2$ Carbon dioxide concentration.

CTCR Continued care; Current Topics in Cellular Regulation (annual volumes).

CTCT Cytotoxic chemotherapy (e.g. the new and highly active drugs such as Capecitabine, Docetaxel, Paclitaxel, Vinorelbine, etc., used in the treatment of metastatic breast cancer) (= CST); Cytotoxic dose/ drug (see CTA).

CTD Carpal tunnel decompression (operation/ orthopedics); Chemotherapeutic drug (see CTA); Chest tube drainage; Chronic tissue disease/ disorder; Claw toe deformity; Clinical trial data; Congenital thymic dysplasia; Connective tissue disease/ disorder; Corrective therapy department; Cumulative trauma(tic) disorder.

CtD Consent to Donate (Blood, Bone marrow, etc.); Cup-to-disk (ratio) (in eye examination).

CT&DB Cough, turn, and deep breathe.

CTDG Clinical Trials Discussion Group.

ctDNA Chloroplast deoxyribonucleic acid.

CTDW Continues to do well.

CTE Calf thymus extract; Cerebral thromboembolism; Chronic telogen effluvium (hair loss) (see ACT); Clinical trial experience; Congenital talipes equinovarus (Orthopedics); Cultured thymic epithelium.

CTEC Chemical Transportation Emergency Center (MCA).

CTEM Conventional-transmission electron microscope/py (see CEM).

CTEV Congenital talipes equino-varum (clubfoot).

CTF Cancer therapy facility; Certificate (see ctf); Chemotactic/ Cytotoxic factor; Chemotherapy Foundation; Colorado tick fever (a relatively mild virus infection carried to humans by the bite of a tick, not the *Rickettsia* infection of RMSF or Rocky Mountain spotted fever (= AMF or American mountain fever. Also called Mountain fever and Mountain tick fever, these names also given to RMSF); Comminuted torsional fracture (e.g. of the tibia) (Orthopedics) (see CT#).

ctf certificate (= CTF).

CTFA Cosmetic, Toiletry, and Fragrance Association.

CTFE Chlorotrifluoroethylene.

CTFS Complete testicular feminization syndrome.

CTG Cardiotomography; Cardiotonic glycoside; Cervicothoracic ganglion; Chemotherapy group (of patients); Chymotrypsinogen; Combined treatment group; Connective tissue growth.

ctg chromated gap.

C/TG Cholesterol/triglyceride (ratio).

CTGA Complete transposition of the great

arteries.

CTH Ceramide trihexoside; Chondrotropic hormone (see Hormones - GH; CTH i); Chromatophorotropic hormone (see Hormones - CTH ii); Chronic tension headache; Clot to hold; Council of Teaching Hospitals (AAMC).

CTh Carrier-specific T-helper (cell).

^{14}C-9-THC ^{14}C-delta-tetrahydro-cannabinol.

CTHD Chlorthalidone.

C thickness Cortical thickness.

CTI Cardiac treponin I (an inflammatory marker of coronary risk, where serum levels are often elevated in myocarditis, as is Cardiac treponin T) (see CTT); Certification of terminal illness; Chronotropic incompetence (inadequate heart rate response to exercise).

CTIA Calcified tissue and implant analysis (see CTR).

CTIC Chemotherapy-induced cancer.

CTIN Chemotherapy-induced nausea.

CTIS Chemotherapy-induced stomatitis - Disease Staging: Stage 0 - no ulcers; Stage 1 - oral pain with no ulcers; Stage 2 - oral pain with ulcers but the ability to eat is retained; Stage 3 - liquid diet only; Stage 4 - inability to eat or drink.

CTITA Current Tiles in Immunology, Transplantation, and Allergy (journal).

CTIV Chemotherapy-induced vomiting.

CTJ Clinical Trials Journal; Clinical-trials junkie (in AIDS and similar fatal diseases).

CTK Cell and Tissue Kinetics (journal).

CTL Cervico-thoraco-lumbar; Complementary transistor logic; Cytotoxic T-lymphocyte.

CTLA-4 Cytotoxic T-lymphocyte antigen 4 (a polymorphism, associated with Graves' disease).

CTLL Cytotoxic lymphoid line.

CTLS Cardiac and trauma life support.

CTM Cardiotachometer; *Chlamydia* transport media; Chlortrimeton; Conjugating toxic metabolite; Connective tissue massage; Cricothyroid muscle.

CTMI Current Topics in Microbiology and Immunology (books).

CTMM Computed tomographic metrizamide myelography.

CTMM-SF California Test of Mental Maturity - Short Form.

CTMP Carboxyl-terminal modulator protein (an important regulator of PKB or Protein kinase B) (see PKB).

CT/MPR Computed tomography with multiplanar reconstructions.

CTN Calcitonin (see Ct); Cephalothin; Clinical Trials Network (see CRN); Computer tomography number; Continuous noise (condition); Creatine/ Creatinine (see Creat).

C&TN BLE Color and temperature normal, both lower extremities.

cTNM Tumor node staging (q.v.), as determined by clinical non-invasive examination (see TNM).

CTO Cell turnover.

CTP California Test of Personality; Cardiac transplant patient; Cell transplantation procedure; Clinical teaching program; Clinical trial population/ program; Combination-therapy patient; Community transmission parameters; Comparator-treated patient; Comprehensive treatment plan; Concentration-time profile (drugs); Cytidine/ Cytosine triphosphate.

C-TPN Cyclic total parenteral nutrition.

CTPP Cerebral tissue perfusion pressure.

CTPVO Chronic thrombotic pulmonary vascular obstruction.

CTR Calcaneal tendon reflex (= Ankle reflex) (see ATR); Calcified tissue research (see CBC; CTIA); Cardiac-transplant recipient; Cardiothoracic ratio (= CT); Carpal tunnel release; Central tumor registry; Chemotherapeutic/py regimen; Clinical Trends in Rheumatology (journal); Cooper type regimen (Cyclophosphamide, Methotrexate and 5-Fluorouracil) - chemotherapy in disseminated breast carcinoma; Corneal transplant rejection; Current Therapeutic Research (journal); Cutaneous tumor response (to chemotherapy).

Ctr; ctr Center/tral/tric.

CTRB Chymotrypsinogen B.

CTRDAB Canadian Tuberculosis and Respiratory Disease Association Bulletin.

CTRT Chemotherapy plus radiotherapy (see

CCTRT).
CTRX Ceftriaxone.
CTS Carpal tunnel surgery/ syndrome; Cardiothoracic surgeon/ery; CardioThoracic Systems; Cellular transport system; Chronic toxicity studies/dy; Coal tar solution; Communications Technology Satellite (US/Canadian); Composite treatment score; Computed/terized tomographic scan(ner); Computerized tomography of the spine (Five standard views: 1. anteroposterior; 2. cross table lateral; 3. left oblique; 4. open-mouth; and 5. right oblique); Contralateral threshold shift; Cooperative Tests and Services (ETS); Corticosteroid (see CS); Cubital tunnel syndrome; Cystathionine synthase (see HCU).
Cts Catalase.
CTSNFR Corrected time of sinoatrial node function recovery.
CTSP Called to see patient.
CTT Cancer-treatment trial; Carbohydrate tolerance test; Cardiac troponin T (an inflammatory marker of coronary risk, besides others such as C-reactive protein, etc.) (see IMCR); Cardiothoracic technique/ technology / transplant; Cefotetan; Cell-transplantation therapy/ treatment; Central tegmental tract; Central transmission time; Chemotherapeutic treatment; Compressed tablet triturate; Computerized transaxial tomogram/aphy (see CAT); Conventional tumor therapy; Cricothyroidotomy; Critical tracking time; Cytotoxic therapy/ treatment.
CTTC; CTT-C Cytotoxic T (thymus) cell.
CTTH Chronic tension-type headache (= CCH).
CTTR California Tumor Tissue Registry.
CTTT Carotid-thyroid transit time.
CTU Cardiac-thoracic unit; Celsius/ Centigrade thermal unit; Constitutive transcription unit.
CTV Cardiotropic virus; Central thoracic vessel; Cervical and thoracic vertebrae; Conventional tidal volume (see TTV).
CTW Central terminal of Wilson; Children's Television Workshop; Combined testicular weight.
CTX Cefotaxime; Cerebrotendinous xanthomatosis; Chemotaxis; Cholera toxin (gene/ virus) - invades the bacterial DNA of Vibrio cholerae and causes cholera; Costotendinous xanthomatosis; Cyclophosphamide (Cytoxan) (see CP).
CTx Cardiac transplant(ation); Conotoxin.
CTXN Contraction.
C-type RNA Large-size RNA molecule.
CTZ Chemoreceptor trigger zone (see CT zone); Chlorothiazide (a diuretic) (= CHTZ; CT); Co-Trimoxazole (sulfamethoxazole-trimethoprim).
CT zone Chemoreceptor trigger zone (vomiting area in the medulla) (= CTZ).
CU Cardiac/ Casein/ Chymotrypsin/ Clinical/ Color/ Conduit (ileal - after cystectomy)/ Convalescent unit; Cause undetermined (see CUD); Cause unknown (see CUK); Chloasma uterinum (see CG - Chloasma gravidarum); Citrullinuria (an autosomal recessive, hypotrichosis with bamboo hair, mental retardation, neonatal lethargy, irritability and convulsions); Contact urticaria.
Cu Copper (Z = 29) (L. cuprum) (see Elements - Copper); Curie (unit of radioactivity (see C).
C_u Urea clearance (see KFT).
cu cubic; cup.
^{61}Cu Radioactive copper.
^{64}Cu Radioactive copper.
CUA Congenital uterine anomaly.
CuB Copper band (dentistry).
Cube LSD-25 on sugar (see LSD).
CUC Chronic ulcerative colitis.
cu cm cubic centimeter (see cc).
CUCPS Columbia University College of Physicians and Surgeons (NY).
CUD Cause undetermined (= CU); Compulsive use of drugs (see CDUD; EUD; RUD); Congenital urinary (tract) deformity.
CuD Copper deficiency.
CUE Cumulative urinary excretion.
cu ft cubic foot (= ft^3).
CUG Catch-up growth; Cystidine, uridine, and guanidine; Cystourethrogram/aphy (see KFT).
CUI Cox-Uphoff International (tissue expander).
cu in cubic inch (in3).
cuj of any/ of which (L. cujus).

cuj lib of any/ of whatever you please (L. cujus libet).
CUK Cause unknown (= CU).
Culd Culdoscopy.
Cult; cult Culture (bacteriology).
cult- prefix meaning tend (L. cultus).
cum cumulative.
cu m cubic meter (= m^3; M^3).
CUMC Cornell University Medical College.
CUMITECH Cumulative Techniques and Procedures in Clinical Microbiology.
cu mm cubic millimeter (= c mm; microliter; m^{-6} l; μl; mm^3).
cune- combining form meaning wedge (L. cuneus).
CUNY City University of New York.
CuO Cupric oxide.
CuO_2 Cuprous oxide.
CUP Carcinoma unknown primary.
Cupid's bow Bow of the upper lip.
CUPS Carcinoma of unknown primary site (= CUP).
CUR Curettage; Cystourethrorectal.
cur curative; cure; current.
Cura Heroin (Sp. cure) (see Diamorph HCl).
Curat A dressing (L. curatio).
CURB Campaign for the Use and Restriction of Barbiturates.
CURE Clinical Unit of Recent Expirations.
C_{urea} Urea clearance (see KFT).
CURN Conduct and Utilization of Research in Nursing.
CUS Cardiac ultrasound; Carotid ultrasound examination; Catheterized urine specimen; Chronic undifferentiated schizophrenia; Contact urticaria syndrome.
CuS Copper supplement.
CUSA Cavitron ultrasonic surgical aspirator (Waller).
CuSCN Cuprous thiocyanate.
Cush Cushing's (syndrome).
CUSS University Center for the Health Services.
CUT Chronic undifferentiated type (schizophrenia).
cut- combining form skin (L. cutis).
Cutis (journal).
CuTS Cubital tunnel syndrome.
CUV Catch-up vaccination (between age 4 and 12 months) such as Polio, MMR, Varicella, etc.).
cu yd cubic yard (= yd^3).
CV Calici/ Corona (see ECV) virus; Cardiac/ Cell/ Closing/ Concentrated/ Corpuscular volume; Cardiovascular; Carotenoid vesicle; Central venous (pressure); Central vein; Cerebral vasculitis; Cerebrovascular; Cervical vertebra; Chikungunya virus; Cisplatin and Vepeside (etoposide - VP); Coefficient of variation; Color vision; Conducting vein; Conduction velocity; Conjugata vera; Conjugate vaccine; Consonant-vowel (syllable); Contrast ventriculography; Conventional ventilation; Conversational voice; Cornell Veterinarian (journal); Costovertebral; Cresyl/ Crystal violet; Curriculum vitae; Cutaneous vasculitis; Cyclical vomiting (occurs in PF) (see CRAP; FMF); Tomorrow evening (L. cras vespere) (see cv); True conjugate diameter of the pelvic inlet (L. conjugata vera).
Cv; C_v Constant volume (specific heat at).
cv cavity (radiograph symbol); cras vespere (L.) - tomorrow evening (= CV); cultivar.
C/V Compression/Ventilation (ratio) (in CPR); Coulomb per volt; Current-to-voltage (conversion).
CVA Cardiovascular/ Cerebrovascular accident/ assessment; Chronic villous arthritis; Coronary vasospastic angina; Costovertebral angle; Cyclophosphamide, Vincristine, & Adriamycin.
CVAH Congenital virilizing adrenal hyperplasia.
CVAP Cerebrovascular amyloid peptide.
CVAs Cardiovascular anomalies (such as coarctation of the aorta, hypoplastic left ventricle, pulmonic valve atresia, single umbilical artery, single ventricle, and transposition of the great vessels) (see DRM).
CVAT Costovertebral angle tenderness.
CVB Chorionic villi biopsy.
CVC Cardiovascular collapse; Cardio/ Cerebrovascular complication; Central venous catheter/ circulation; Color vision change; Consonant-vowel-consonant; Covalent chromatography; Crying vital capacity.
CV cath Central venous catheter.

CVCC Consonant-vowel-consonant-consonant (utterance).
CVCT Cardiovascular computed tomography.
CVD Cardiac valve disease; Cardio/Cerebrovascular damage/ death/ disease/ disorder/ drug; Central visual defect; Cerebrovascular disease (= CBVD); Chronic venous disease; Collagen vascular disease; Color vision deficiency (see ACVD)/ deviant/ deviate (anomalies of color vision).
cvd curved.
CVE Cardio/Cerebrovascular emergency/ episode/ evaluation/ event (see CVA); Cardiovascular fiberscope; Central vision function; Consistent vigorous exercise.
CVEB Cisplatin, vinblastine, etoposide, and bleomycin.
CVF Cardiovascular failure/ function; Central vision field; Cervicovaginal fluid; Chronic ventricular failure (see COLD; COPD); Cobra venom factor.
CVG Contrast ventriculography; Coronary venous graft (operation/ cardiac); Cryolife valvular graft (Cryolife Inc. - preserves living homografts for cardiothoracic surgery); Cutis verticis gyrata (see HDA).
CVH Cardio/Cerebrovascular health/ history/ homeostasis; Cerebroventricular hemorrhage; Cervicovaginal hood; Combined ventricular hypertrophy; Common variable hypogammaglobulin(emia).
CVHD Chronic valvular heart disease.
CVI Carboplastin, Vepeside (etoposide-VP), and ifosfamide; Cardiovascular/ Cerebrovascular incident/ insufficiency; Chronic viral infection; Chronic venous insufficiency; Common variable immunodeficiency (see CVID); Continuous venous infusion.
CVID Common variable immunodeficiency (= CVI).
C Vinar A wineglass(ful) (L. cyanthus vinosus/ cyathus vinarius) (= Cyanth vin; Cyath vin).
C-virus Coxsackie virus.
CVJ Canadian Veterinary Journal (CVMA).
CVK Compocillin - VK (= phenethicillin potassium; phenoxymethylpenicillin potassium) (a proprietary drug).
CVL Central venous line; Clinical vascular laboratory (= CVLT); Complete vision loss (see CLV).
CVLT California Verbal Learning Test; Clinical vascular laboratory (see CVL).
CVM Cardiovascular medicine/ monitor; Cardio/ Cerebrovascular malformation(s)/ morbidity/ mortality; Center for Veterinary Medicine (FDA); Cerebral venous malformation; Cerebral ventriculomegaly (fetal Obstetrics); College of Veterinary Medicine; Cyclophosphamide, vincristine, and methotrexate.
CVMA Canadian Veterinary Medical Association.
CVMP Committee on Veterans Medical Problems.
CVN Central venous nutrient.
CVO *Candida* vertebral osteomyelitis (see FVO); Cardio/ Cerebrovascular outcome; Central vein occlusion; Central venous oxygen; Chief Veterinary Officer; Obstetric conjugate diameter of the pelvic inlet (L. conjugata vera obstetrica).
CVO_2 Mixed venous oxygen content.
CVOD Cerebrovascular obstructive disease.
CVOR Cardiovascular operating room.
CVP Bioflavinoids; Cardio/ Cerebrovascular pathology/ physiology/ problem; Cardiovascular pharmacology/ parkinsonism; Cardioventricular pacing; Cell volume profile; Central venous polyethylene (catheter)/ pressure; Cyclophosphamide, vincristine, and prednisone (see COP).
$cvPO_2$; cvP_{O2} Cerebral venous partial pressure of oxygen.
CVPP CCNU (CeeNu or lomustine), vinblastine, procarbazine, and prednisone.
CVR Canadian Veterinary Record; Cardio/ Cerebrovascular regulation; Cardiovascular-renal (disease) (see CVRD); Cardiovascular Research (journal); Cardiovascular-respiratory (disease/ system) (see CVRD); Cardiovascular resistance/ resuscitation/ risk/; Craniovascular receptor; Cephalic vasomotor response; Cerebrovascular resistance.
CVRD Cardiovascular-related death (see CRD); Cardiovascular-renal/-respiratory disease (= CVR).

CVRF Cardiovascular risk factor.
CVRI Coronary vascular resistance index.
CVRR Cardiovascular recovery room.
CVS Cardiac/ Coronary vasospasm; Cardiovascular status/ support/ surgery/ system; Cerebral vascular/ Cerebrovascular stenosis; Cerebral vasospasm; Cervicovaginal secretion; Challenge virus strain; Chorionic villus sample/ sampling (at 9-12 weeks' gestation, first trimester); Clean voided specimen (procedure/ urine culture) (see KFT); Current vital signs; Strain of rabies vaccine (attenuated).
CVs Cancer vaccines (including Dendritic cells, Gangliosides, Heat-shock proteins, Nucleic acids, Peptides, Viral and bacterial vectors, and Whole cancer cells).
$CVSO_2$ Central venous oxygen saturation (see PFT).
CVSU Cardiovascular specialty unit.
CVT Cardiovascular toxicity; Central venous temperature/ thrombosis; Congenital vertical talus.
CVTR Charcoal virus transport medium.
CVUG Cysto-void urethrogram.
CVVC Cerebrovascular vasoconstriction.
CW Cardiac work; Careful watch; Case work(er); Cell/ Chest wall; Chemical warfare/ weapon; Children's Ward; Clockwise (see cw); Cold water; Compare with (see C/W); Continuous wave (ultrasound); Crutch walking.
cw clockwise (= CW).
C/W Compare/ Consistent with.
C-W Worst case (damage).
CWA Clean Water Act (1972).
CWB Cell wall biosynthesis.
CWBG Capillary whole-blood glucose.
CWBTS Capillary whole blood true sugar.
CWC Cardiac work capacity.
CWD Cell wall defect; Continuous-wave Doppler.
CWDF Cell wall-deficient (bacterial) form(s).
CWE Cottonwool exudate(s).
CWF Cornell Word Form (test).
CWG Core wire guide (cardiac catheterization).
CWH Caffeine-withdrawal headache; Cardiomyopathy and wooly haircoat (syndrome).
CWHB Citrated whole human blood.
CWHM Current Work in the History of Medicine (journal).
CWI Cardiac work index.
CWL Continuous wave laser; Cutaneous water loss.
CWLA Child Welfare League of America.
CWMD Cerebral white matter disease.
CWMS Color, warmth, and movement sensation.
CWOP Childbirth without pain (see CWP).
CWP Cellular waste product(s) (normally removed by the kidneys); Childbirth without pain (= CWOP); Coal worker's pneumoconiosis.
CWPEA Childbirth Without Pain Education Association.
CWPEAN Childbirth Without Pain Education Association Newsletter.
CWR Cog-wheel rigidity (in Parkinsonism).
CWRU Case Western Reserve University.
CWS Cell wall skeleton; Chemical Warfare Service; Chest wall stimulation; Child welfare service; Cogwheel sign (see BoaS Obs/Gyn); Cold water-soluble; Comfortable walking speed; Cotton wool spots.
CWT Cold water treatment.
Cwt; cwt Hundredweight (centweight - 100 lb average).
CWXSP Coal Workers' X-ray Surveillance Program.
CX Cervix (see Cx); Chest X-ray (= CXR); Critical experiment.
Cx Cancel; Cervix (gynecology) (= CX; cx); Circumflex; Clearance; Complaint; Complex (= cx); Convex (= cx); Culture.
cx cervix (see Cx); complex (see Cx); convex (see Cx); cylinder axis.
CXL Carotene xylose level.
CxMT Cervical motion tenderness.
CXR Chest X-ray (see CX).
CXTX Cervical traction.
CY Casein-yeast (autolysate) (medium); Cyclophosphamide (see CP).
Cy Copy; Cyanogen; Cyclonium (chemical symbol - obsolete); Cyclophosphamide (see CP); Cyst; Cytarabine; Cytoplasm(ic) (see Cyt).

cy cyanosis (= cyan).
C&Y Children and youth (projects).
CY 116 Epsilon aminocaproic acid (see EACA).
CyA Cyclosporine A.
CYADIC Cyclophosphamide, Adriamycin (doxorubicin), and DTIC (dacarbazine).
cyan cyanosis (see cy).
cyan- combining form meaning blue (Gr. kyanos).
cyanth a glassful (L. cyanthus) (see cyath).
cyanth vin a wineglass(ful) (L. cyanthus vinosus) (see C Vinar).
cyath a glassful (L. cyathus) (see cyanth).
cyath vin a wineglass(ful) (L. cyathus vinarius) (see C Vinar).
CYC Cyclophosphamide (see CP).
Cyc; cyc Cyclazocine; Cycle; Cyclotron.
cycl- prefix meaning circle or cycle (Gr. kyklos).
CYCLA Cyclacyllin anhydrous.
cyclin AMP adenosine 3'5'-cyclic monophosphate (see cAMP).
CYCLO; Cyclo Cyclophosphamide (see CP); Cyclopropane (anesthetic).
Cyclo C Cyclocytidine hydrochloride.
Cyd Cytidine.
CYE Charcoal yeast extract (agar).
CYL Casein yeast lactate (medium).
Cyl; cyl Cylinder; Cylindrical lens.
CyMD Cytoplasmic malate dehydrogenase (= cyt MDH).
CYN Cyanide.
CYP Cyanopindolol (a â-adrenoceptor blocking agent); Cyproheptadine. Cytochrome P (CYP 3A4 is the major enzyme responsible for formation of the oxidative metabolites).
C&Y projects Children and youth projects.
CYS Cystoscopy (procedure/ urology) (= Cys; Cysto) (see KFT).
Cys Cyclosporine; Cysteine; Cystoscopy (see CYS).
Cys A Cysteic acid.
Cys-Cys; Cys-cys Cystine.
CysLT1 Cysteinyl leukotriene 1 (receptors - such as LTC4, LTD4 and LTE4) (see CLT).
CysLT2 Cysteinyl leukotriene 2 (receptor) (see CLT).
cyst- combining form meaning bladder or sac (Gr. kystis).
CYSTO Cystogram.
Cysto Cystoscopy (see CYS).
CYT Cytochrome; Cytoxan (= Cyclophosphamide) (see CP).
Cyt; cyt Cytological/gy (= Cytol; cytol); Cytoplasm(ic) (= Cy); Cytosine.
cyt cytological/gy; cytoplasm(ic) (see Cyt).
cyt- combining form meaning cell or hollow (Gr. kytos).
CytaBOM Cytarabine, bleomycin, Oncovin (vincristine), and methotrexate (chemotherapy).
cyt MDH Cytoplasmic malate dehydrogenase (see CyMD).
Cytobios (journal).
Cytogen Cytogenetics (journal).
Cytokines Include: Granulocyte colony-stimulating factor (G-CSF), Interleukin-1α, 1β, 6, 8, etc., Tumor necrosis factor α (TNF-β), etc.
Cytol; cytol Cytological/gy (see Cyt).
cyt syst cytochrome system.
CY-VA-DIC Cyclophosphamide, vincristine, Adriamycin, and dacarbazine.
CZ Cefazolin.
Cz Central midline placement of electrodes in electroencephalography.
CZI Crystalline zinc insulin (see Insulin - CZI).
CZN Chlorzotocin.
C_{Zn} Zinc clearance.
CZP Clonazepam.
Cz. P Czechoslovak Pharmacopoeia (Ceskoslovensky Lekopis).

D

D Absorbed dose - aspartic acid; Cholecalciferol; Coefficient of diffusion; Da (L.) give; Dacryon; Dagga (Marijuana - see Cannabis); Date; Daughter; Day (see d); Dead/ Deceased/ Died (see d); Dead air space; Debye; Deca (prefix for 10) or 10' (e.g. Dg or Decagram/ 10 grams); Deci - or 10^{-1} (see d); Deciduous; Decimal reduction time; Degree; Dehydroepiandrosteron; Democrat; Density: 1. Quality: compactness or denseness; 2. Quantity of: electricity in a given area, time, or volume/ insects per room, etc. (e.g. mosquito d.)/ matter in a given space/ parasites per age group, etc. (parasite d); Dental; Department (see Dept); Depression; Dermatologic/gist/gy; Details (Rorschach); Detur (L.) let it be given; Deuterium (= 2H) - The mass two isotope of hydrogen (Heavy Hydrogen), e.g. D. oxide or Heavy water; Deuteron; Develop(ed)/ment; Deviation; Dexter (L.) right; Dextro; Dextrose; Di (two); Diabetes; Diagnosis - The art of determining the nature of a disease (e.g. Pathological d - Diagnosis based on observing the structural lesions present); Diagonal; Dialysance (ml/min); Diameter (= D); Diarrhea; Diastole; Diathermy; Diathesis (Gr.) arrangement/ disposition (e.g. Gouty d - predisposition to gout); Didymium (see Di); Died (see d); Difference; Diffusing (capacity); Diffusion coefficient/ constant; Dihydrouridine; Dilution (rate); Diopter (= d) (the refractive power of a lens with a focal distance of one meter/ a unit of refraction); Dioptry (eye examination); Diplomate; Disease; Dispense (on prescription); Displacement (loop); Distal (remote) (= d); District (Administrator/ Attorney); Diuresis; Diurnal (= d); Divergence; Diverticulum; Divorced; Doctor; Dog (Veterinary medicine); Dominion Rubber Co. code for experimental substances; Donor; Doriden (Trade name for Glutethimide); Dorsal (L. dorsum) (= Back or posterior, e.g. in Vertebral numbers - D. spines, etc.) (= d); Dose (L. dosis) - A quantity to be given at one time (e.g. Divided d; Lethal d; etc.); Drachma; Dream; Drive/ D state; Drug; Dual; Duct; Duodenal/num; Duration (= d); Dwarf; Electric displacement; Give (L. da) (= d; DA; da); Let it be given (L. detur); Mean dose; Rh gene; Right (L. dexter) (= d); Spectral line of sodium (γ = 5893 A); Vitamin D potency (Unit of) (e.g. of cod liver oil) (see Vitamins - D).

d allelic form of Rh gene; atomic orbital with angular momentum quantum number 2; day (L. dies); dead/ deceased/ died (= D); deci- (prefix for 0.1) (e.g. dg = decigram, 1/10 gram, 10^{-1} gram); decomposes; decrease(d); degree; density (see D); deoxy(ribose); detur (L.) let it be given (= D); dexter (L.) right (= D); dextro (= D); dextrorotatory (see D-); dies (L.) day (= D); diameter (see D); differential; diopter (see D); distal (see D); diurnal (see D); dorsal (see D); dose (see D); dosis (L.) dose; doubtful; duration (see D); dyne; give (see D); right (L. dexter) (see D).

$\bar{D}$ Mean dose.

Δ Greek capital letter delta.

δ delta - the fourth letter of the Greek alphabet; Immunoglobulin D.

D- Dextrorotatory (= d). 1) A chemical prefix (small capital = d-), which designates that a substance has the configuration of a glyceraldehyde. 2) In carbohydrate nomenclature, the symbol designates the configuration of the highest numbered asymmetric carbon atom (e.g. D-glucose). 3) In aminoacid nomenclature, the symbol designates the configuration to which the lowest numbered asymmetric carbon atom belongs (e.g. D-threonine).

d- Chemical abbreviation for dextro, to the right or clockwise, especially with reference to the direction in which a plane of polarized light is rotated: i.e. dextrorotatory (see D-).

/d/ Mean absolute between co-twins (statistics).

1-D One-dimensional/ One dimension.

2-D Two-dimensional/ Two dimensions.

1/d Once a day/ Once daily.

2/d Twice a day/ Twice daily.

3-D Diarrhea-dementia-dermatitis (pellagra);

Three dimensional/ Three dimensions.

2,4-D 2,4-dichlorophenoxyacetic acid. A plant hormone which stimulates growth at a concentration of 10 ppm. Higher strengths stimulate abnormal growth and the plant becomes distorted and dies. Strengths of 100 to 1,000 ppm. are widely used as selective herbicides, being particularly effective for broad-leaved plants (see Hormones - 2,4-D).

17-D A modified yellow fever virus.

D_1 Daunomycin (see Dauno); Diagonal one; Dopamine receptor 1; First dorsal vertebra; Vitamin D_1 (see Vitamins - D_1).

D_2 Daunomycin metabolite; Diagonal two; Dopamine receptor 2; Second dorsal vertebra; Vitamin D_2 (see Vitamins - D_2).

D_3 Cholecalciferol (Vitamin D_3) (see Vitamins - D_3); Third dorsal vertebra.

D1, D2 receptors Two types of dopamine receptors, located on nerve terminals of the brain (such as the cortex in the stratum, accumbens, and amygdala).

D/3 Distal third.

D4 Fourth digit.

D6 Detroit 6 (cells).

$D_{1,2,3,4,...12}$ First to twelth dorsal vertebrae.

D_{10} Decimal reduction time.

D 40 Uroselectan B (lopax). A compound used in radiography.

D 50 50% dextrose injection.

D 201 Isothipendyl hydrochloride. An antihistamine drug more potent than promethazine HCl ("Phenergan"), but with a shorter duration of action, and causing less sedation.

D 206 Prothipendyl hydrochloride. A tranquillizing drug with sedative and anti-emetic actions.

D 365 Verapamil hydrochloride (= Iproveratril HCl; Isoptin HCl; MW 455). A calcium antagonist and coronary vasodilator, used in the treatment of cardiac arrhythmias, angina pectoris, and hypertension.

D 600 Metoxy-verapamil. A calcium antagonist and slow channel cardiac blocking agent.

D 860 Tolbutamide (= Butamide; Orinase; Tolbut; Tolbutamidum; Tolglybutamide; U 2043). An oral hypoglycemic and antidiabetic sulphonylurea compound, with a shorter duration of action than chlorpropamide. The blood-sugar level falls within 2 to 4 hours and the reduced level is maintained for 8 to 10 hours. Used in the treatment of diabetes mellitus.

DA Dark adaptation; Dark agouti (rat); Date of admission (see D/A); Daunomycin (see Dauno); Daunorubicin (see Dauno); Degenerative arthritis; Degree of analgesia; Delayed action; Delivery awareness; Delta agent/ antigen (= HBsAG-associated antigen) (see HBsAG); Dental assistant; Dental Assistant (ADAA journal); Deoxyadenosine; Developmental age; Diabetic acidosis/ amyotrophy; Diagnostic arthroscopy; Dietetic assistant; Differential analyzer; Differentiation antigen; Digital to analog (see D/A); Diphenylamine-arsine chloride (= Adamsite; DM; Diphenylchlorarsine) - a war gas; Diploma in Anesthetics; Direct admission/ agglutination; Disability assistance; Disaggregated; Dopa; Dopamine (= DM; DPM); Dopamine agonist (e.g. bromocriptine); Drug abuse/ addict (= AD)/ addiction/ aerosol; Ductus arteriosus; Duodenal atresia; Give (L. da) (see D).

da daughter; day; give (L.) (see D); ten/ deca- (Gr. deka), e.g. dag = decagram/ dekagram/ 10 grams.

Da Dalton (see Dal).

D/A Date of accident; Date of admission (= DA); Digital-to-analog (converter) (= DA; DAC); Discharge and advice.

D-A Donor-acceptor.

D&A Dilatation and aspiration.

DAA Decompensated autonomous adenoma; Dementia associated with alcoholism; Diabetes-associated anomalies/ly (see DRMs); Dialysis-associated amyloidosis; Diaminoanisole; Diuretic-associated azotemia (e.g. with Thiazide, etc.); Dopamine-agonist agent; Dopamine antagonist activity.

DA/A Drug/alcohol addiction.

DAAO d-Amino acid oxidase (= diaminoacid oxidase).

DAB Days after birth; 3,3'-diamino-benzidine; Diamino-butyric acid (see DABA); Dimethylamino-azobenzene (= 4-DAB) a carcinogen; Dysrhythmic aggressive behavior.

DAB-6 Benzinum petrolii (= Petroleum benzine).

DABA 2,4-diaminobutyric acid (= DAB).

DABD Diabetes-associated birth defect(s) (Obstetrics).

DAC Digital-to-analog converter (= see D/A); Disabled adult child; Disaster assistance center; Division of Ambulatory Care; Double-avoidant conflict (see Conflict); Drug Abuse Control/ Council/ Counseling; Drug-associated change(s) (see DRC).

dac dacryon.

DACA Dissecting aneurysm of the coronary artery; Drug Abuse Control amendment of 1965 (Harris-Dodd Act, USA).

DACB Drug Abuse Control Bureau (FDA).

DACH Diamino-cyclohexane.

DACL Depression Adjective Check List.

DACM N-(7-diamethylamino-4-methyl-3-coumarinyl) maleimide.

dacry- prefix meaning tear (Gr. dakry).

DACS Data acquisition and control system; Director of ambulatory care services.

DACT Dactinomycin.

dactyl- Combining form meaning finger or toe (Gr. daktylos).

DAD Daily average dose; Delayed after depolarization; Dial-a-Diagnosis; Diffuse alveolar damage; Diffuse axonal injury; Dispense as directed; Doctor-assisted death; Dopamine antagonist drug; Dose adjustment design.

DaD Drunk and disorderly.

DADA Dichloroacetic acid diisopropylammonium salt (= Diisopropylamine-dichloroacetate).

DADAVS Deputy Assistant Director Army Veterinary Services.

DADDS Diacetyl diamino-diphenylsulfone (= 4,4'-DADDS).

DADMS Deputy Assistant Director of Medical Services (Armed Forces).

dADP Deoxy-adenosine-diphosphate.

DADPS Dapsone (= DDS; Diamino-diphenyl sulfone; Diaphenylsulfone; Disulone; Sulfonyldianiline). An antileprotic drug.

DADS Director Army Dental Service(s).

DADSG Direct access digital scan generator (SEM).

DADT 'Don't ask, don't tell' (policy).

DAE Diabetes-associated embryopathy (see DEP); Diphenylanthracene endoperoxide; Diving air embolism.

DaE Diet and exercise.

DAEA Drug Abuse Education Act.

DAF Decay-accelerating factor; Delayed auditory feedback; Drug-adulterated food.

DAG Diacylglycerol; Dianhydrogalactitol; Disease-associated gene.

dag decagram (10 grams) (see da).

DAGT Direct antiglobulin test.

DAH Disordered action of the heart (= NCA - Neurocirculatory asthenia or Da Costa's syndrome).

DAHEA Department of Allied Health Education and Accreditation.

DAHM Division of Allied/ Associated Health Manpower (HRA).

DAHP Division of Associated Health Professions (HRA).

DAI Daily alcohol intake.

DaI Drunk and incapable (of driving).

DAIB Dry air-induced bronchospasm (see DAS).

DAL Drug analysis laboratory.

Dal Dalton (= Da) (see Amu - Atomic mass unit).

dal decaliter (10 liters) (see da).

DALA; δ-ALA Delta-aminolevulinic acid.

DALE Drug Abuse Law Enforcement.

DAM Data-associated message; Decision-analytic model; Degraded amyloid; Diabetes-associated malformation; Diacetyl monoxime ($C_4H_7NO_2$) (used as an adjunct to atropine in the treatment of poisoning by cholinesterase inhibitors; also in myasthenia gravis); Diacetylmorphine; Dictionary of Abbreviations in Medicine; Disseminated acute mycosis.

dam decameter (10 meters) (see da).

DAMA Discharged against medical advice.

DAMD Dry age-related macular degeneration (milder, atrophic type) (see WAMD).

DAMP Bisacodyl.

dAMP Deoxy/ Deoxyadenylate adenosine monophosphate.

DAMPS Department of Allied Medical Professions and Services (AMA).

DAN Diabetic autonomic neuropathy.

Dan. Disp Danish Dispensary 1963

(Dispensatorium Danicum).

DANA Drug-induced antinuclear antibodies.

D and C See D&C (before DAC).

dand to be given (L. dandus).

D and E See D&E. (before DEA).

DANS 1-Dimethylaminonaphthalene-5-sulfonyl chloride.

DAO Diamine oxidase; Duly authorized officer.

DAo Descending aorta.

DAP Data acquisition processor; Depolarizing afterpotential; Diabetes-associated peptide; Diaminopimelic acid; Diaminopyrimidine (derivatives, such as trimethoprim, pyrimethamine); Diastolic aortic pressure; Dihydroxyacetone phosphate; Diminished antibody production; Dipeptidylaminopeptidase; Direct agglutination pregnancy (test) (see DAPT); Draw-a-Person (test) (see DAP Test); Drug abuse program.

DAP&E Diploma of Applied Parasitology and Entomology.

DAPI Diamidino-phenyl-indole.

DAPRE Daily adjustable progressive resistive exercise.

DAPRU Drug Abuse Prevention Resource Unit (NIAAA).

DAPS Department of Applied Pharmaceutical Sciences (Rhode I. Univ, US).

DAPST Denver Auditory Phonemic Sequency Test.

DAPT Diaminophenylthiazole (= Amiphenazole; Amphenazole hydrochloride; 2,4-Diamino-5-phenylthiazole HCl) - an analeptic with action similar to that of leptazol; Diphtheria alum precipitated toxoid; Direct agglutination pregnancy test (= DAP) - a latex agglutination test (laboratory/ serology).

Dapt Daptazole.

DAP Test Draw-a-Person Test (= DAP) (psychology).

DAQ Diagnostic Assessment Questionnaire.

DAR Daily affective rhythm; Damage-and-repair (cycle); Death after resuscitation; Delayed adaptive response; Diacereine; Differential absorption ratio; Distal absolute reabsorption (e.g. DAR_{NA} of sodium); Drug adverse reaction.

DaR Dip-and-Read (reagent strip/ test).

DARE Drug Abuse Research and Education.

DARP Drug abuse rehabilitation/ reporting program.

DARPA Defence Advanced Research Projects Agency.

DART Data acquisition real time; Depression, awareness, recognition, and treatment (a psychotherapeutic project); Diet and reinfarction trial.

DARTS Drug and Alcohol Rehabilitation Testing System.

DAS Data acquisition system; Dead air space; Death Anxiety Scale; Decreased/ Diminished acid secretion; Definite anxiety state; Delayed anovulatory syndrome; Development apraxia of speech; Dextroamphetamine sulfate (see Amphet); Diagnostic anoscopy; Died at scene; Doctor-assisted suicide; Double-armed suture (see Sut); Drug addiction service; Dry air stimulus (Bronchosensitivity to) (see DAIB).

DASAJ Dental Association of South Africa Journal.

DASAR Data acquisition storage and retrieval.

DASC Diabetic Association of Southern California.

DASD Direct access storage device.

DASE Denver Articulation Screening Exam.

DASH Dietary Approaches to Stop Hypertension (sodium intake and blood pressure trial); Distress Alarm for the Severely Handicapped.

DASL Data access system language.

DASP Double antibody solid phase.

DAT Daunorubicin, ARA-C (cytarabine), and thioguanine; Delayed-action tablet; Delayed antibiotic therapy; Dementia Alzheimer's type; Dental Admission/ Aptitude Test; Desktop analysis tool (TSL); Diacetylthiamine; Diamniotic twin (Obstetrics); Diet as tolerated; Differential agglutination titer/ test (an immunological assay for Rheumatoid factor or the Rose Waaler test); Differential Aptitude Test; Diphtheria antitoxin; Direct agglutination/ antiglobulin test; Disaster Action Team; Dopamine-agonist therapy/ treatment;

Thiocarlide.

DATC Di-allate.

DATDA; DATD Diallyl-tartardiamide.

DATE Dental auxiliary teacher education.

DATP Drug abuse treatment programme (UK) (see DTP).

DATP; dATP Deoxy-adenosine-triphosphate.

DATRC Drug addict treatment and rehabilitation center.

DATS Data acquisition time-sharing.

DATTA Diagnostic and therapeutic technology assessment.

DAU 3-Deazauridine; Dental Auxiliary Utilization.

Dau; dau Daughter.

Daun Daunorubicin (see Dauno).

Dauno Daunomycin (= D_l; DA; DNR; DRB; Daunorubicin).

DAV Data valid; Diamond anvil cell (spectroscopy); Disabled American Veterans; Duck adenovirus.

DAVIT Danish Verapamil Infarction Trial.

DAvMED Diploma in Aviation Medicine.

DAVP Deamino-arginine vasopressin.

DAV&RS Director Army Veterinary and Remount Services.

DAW Dispense as written.

DAZ Deleted in azoospermia (a sperm-producer, sex gene found on the Y chromosome).

DAZL DAZ-like (gene) found on chromosome 3, in both males and females, and precursor of the DAZ gene (see DAZ).

DB Baudelocque's diameter (external conjugate diameter of the pelvis); Data bank/ base; Date of birth (see db); Deep breath; Dependents benefit; Dense body; Developmental Biology (journal); Dextran blue; Diabetes/tic (see Db); Diagonal band; Diet beverage; Direct bilirubin; Disability; Distobuccal; Division for the Blind (LC); Double-blind (study); Dropping bottle; Dry bulb (temperature); Dutch belted (rabbit); Duodenal bulb; Dye baseline.

Db Diabetes/tic (= DB; db); Dubhium (chemical symbol for) - now known as Ytterbium - Yb (Z = 70) (see Elements - Ytterbium).

dB decibel (= db) - a unit of hearing or audition.

db date of birth (= DB); decibel (see dB); diabetes/tic (see Db).

D_b Body density.

DBA Data base administration/ analysis; Detoxification-based approach; Diamond-Blackfan anemia; Dibenzanthracene; Dibromoanthracene; Digital biplane angioscope/py; Dolichos biflorus agglutinin; Dopamine blocking action/ activity/ agent; 'Double-barreled' aorta (= Aortic dissection).

dbA; dBA decibel-A (decibels in the A level; a unit on the noise scale weighted for high freqencies).

dba doing business as.

DBAE Dihydroxyborylaminoethyl.

DBC Detectable breast cancer/ carcinoma; Dibencozide; Double-blind comparison/ condition(s); Dye-binding capacity.

DB&C Deep breathing and coughing.

DBCL Dilute blood clot lysis (method).

DBCOS Double-blind cross-over study (see DBCS).

DBCOT Double-blind cross-over trial (see DBCT).

DBCP Dibromo-chloropropane.

DBCS Double-blind comparative/ controlled/ cross-over study (see DBCOS; DBS).

DBCT Double-blind controlled/ cross-over trial (see DBCOT; DBT).

DBD Azinphos-methyl (= Bayer 17,147; Gasathion; Guthion). A benzotriazin-phosphorothiolothionate derivative and an organophosphorus insecticide (see Bayer 17,147); Definite brain damage; Degenerative brain disease/ disorder (e.g. Huntington's disease); Delayed body development; Dibromodulcitol; Disruptive behavioral disorder (see ADHD); Dopamine-based drug (such as Carbidopa, Levodopa, Selegiline, etc.); Double-blind design.

DBDG Distobuccal developmental groove.

DBE Deep breathing exercise; Double-blind experiment; Dibromoethane; Division of Biological Effects; Duck-bill elevator (Otolaryngology); A synthetic estrogen.

DBED Dibenzyl-ethylenediamine; Penicillin G benzathine.

DBEMOS therapy Dietary, Behavioral, Educational, Medicinal, Occupational, and Speech therapy (in the treatment of Autistic diseases).

DBF Decreased/ Diminished blood flow; Doppler blood flow (Obstetrics) (see DBFV; UADV); Double-blind fashion.

DBFV Doppler blood flow velocimetry (used in the assessment of fetal growth, multiple pregnancy, placental insufficiency, etc.) (see UADV).

DBG Dextrose-barbital-gelatin (buffer).

DBH; DβH Benzene hexachloride; Dopamine beta-hydroxylase (= Dopamine β-hydroxylase) - the enzyme that converts dopamine to norepinephrine.

DBI Debilitating brain illness; Development-at-birth index; Dumb-bell incision (refers to shape of incision); Phenformin hydrochloride (= PBI; PEBG; PEDG; Phen; Phenethylbiguanide HCl; N'-Phenethyldiguanide HCl) - proprietary or trade name for a diguanide derivative drug, used as an oral hypoglycemic agent in the treatment of diabetes mellitus.

DBIL Direct bilirubin (= DB).

DBIOC Data base input/ output control.

DBI-PT Long acting (prolonged-time) capsule of DBI.

DBIR Directory of Biotechnology Information Resources.

DBI-TD Trade name for long-acting (timed disintegration) DBI.

dBk decibels above 1 kilowatt.

DBL Diastolic baseline.

dbl double.

DB Lozenges Domiphen Bromide Lozenges (a proprietary drug).

DBM Data base management; Decreased/ Diminished bone mass; Demineralized bone matrix; Diabetic management; Dibromomannitol; Disseminated blastomycosis; Dobutamine.

dBm decibels above 1 milliwatt.

DBMB Department of Biochemistry and Molecular Biophysics (CUSPS) (CUCPS = Columbia University College of Physicians and Surgeons, NY).

DBMC Di-tert-butyl-m-cresol; Donor bone marrow cell.

DBMCS Double-blind multicenter study.

DBMS Data base management system(s).

DBO Distobucco-occlusal.

db/ob diabetic obese (mouse).

DBP Damaged body part(s); Diastolic blood pressure; (Vitamin) D-binding protein; Dibutylphthalate (insect repellant); Distobuccopulpal; Dohle body panmyelopathy; Double-blind phase/ procedure (see DBS).

DBPC Di-tert-butyl-p-cresol (= BHT; Butylated hydroxytoluene).

DBPCCS Double-blind placebo-controlled clinical study.

DBPCMCT Double-blind placebo-controlled multicenter trial.

DBPCT Double-blind placebo-controlled trial.

DBPH Division for the Blind and Physically Handicapped (LC). Library of Congress (see LCDB).

DBQ Debrisoquin.

DBR Decreased/ Diminished bone resorption; Distorted breathing rate; Drug Equivalence Report (FDA).

DBRMS Double-blind randomized multicenter study.

DBRS Double-blind randomized study.

DBS Data base system; Decreased/ Diminished blood supply; Deep brain stimulation; Denis Browne splint; Despeciated bovine serum; Diamond-Blackfan syndrome; Double-blind studies/dy; Drimosalicil (= Dibromosalicylanolide); Diminished breath sounds; Direct bonding system; Division of Biological Standards (FDA).

DBSP Drug Bioequivalence Study Panel.

DBT Detoxification-based therapy/ treatment; Double-blind therapy/ treatment/ trial; Dry-bulb temperature.

DBTP Double-blind treatment phase.

DBTS Double-blind treatment study.

D_B urea Dialysance of urea (in ml/min) (see KFT - $D_{B\ urea}$).

DBV DNA-based vaccine (elicits a more vigorous, aggressive response from the immune system with increased mobilization of killer T cells); Buformin (= N'-Butyldiguanide; W 37) - an oral hypoglycemic agent.

DBW Dead/ Desirable/ Dry body weight.

dBW decibels above 1 watt.

DBZ Dibenzamine.

DC Daily census; Data communication/ conversion; Daunorubicin and cytarabine; Day center; Decoy cell (see VIB); Decrease (see dc); Deep compartment; Dendrochronology; Dental Concepts (journal); Dental Corps; Deoxycholate; Descending/ Distal colon; Developed/ping country; Dextran charcoal; Diabetic clinic; Diagnostic center/ code; Diagonal conjugate; Differentiated cell; Digit copying; Digital computer; Dilatation and curettage/ curettement (see D&C); Dilatation/ Dilating/ Dilation catheter (Coronary angioplasty); Diphenylarsine cyanide (= Diphenylcyanoarsine) - a war gas; Direct Coombs' (test); Direct current (= dc); Discharge(d) (see dc); Discontinue (see D/C); Discontinued (see D/c'd; dc'd); Distocervical; District of Colombia; Doctor of Chiropractic; Donor cells/ corpuscles; Dressing change; Druggists Circular (journal); Duodenal cap; Dupuytren contracture; Dyskeratosis congenita; Electric defibrillator using DC discharge.

Dc Critical dilution rate.

dC Deoxycytidine.

dc decrease (= DC); direct current (see DC); discharge(d) (= DC); Discontinue (see D/C).

D/C Discontinue (= DC; dc).

D&C (= D and C) Desiccation and curettage; Dilatation and curettage/ curettement (= DC) (= Dilatation of the cervix and curettement of the uterus); Direct and consensual; Distance and convergence (eye examination); Drugs and Cosmetics; Dyes and Colorants/ Cosmetics (coal-tar dyes used in the Cosmetic Drug and Food industries).

DC 65 Darvon compound 65.

DCA Deep cystic acne; Deoxycholate-citrate agar/ sugar; Deoxycholic acid; Deoxy/Desoxy corticosterone acetate (see DOCA); Dichloroacetate; Dosimeter Corporation of America; Double-contrast arthrogram/graph(y).

Dca Dialysate calcium (see KFT - D_{ca}).

DCAA Defence Contract Audit Agency.

DCABG Double coronary artery bypass graft (= DCAG).

DCAG Double coronary artery graft (see DCABG).

DCB Department of Cell Biology; Deutan color-blindness; Dichlorobenzidine (a carcinogen); Dichlorobenzonitrile; Dilutional cardio-pulmonary bypass.

DCBE Double contrast barium enema.

DCBF Dynamic cardiac blood flow.

DC(B)L 306 Phenbenicillin potassium (= Phenoxybenzylpenicillin) - an antimicrobial agent of the family of penicillins.

DCC Data-coordinating center; Day Care Center; Detected in colon cancer; Dextran-coated charcoal; N,N'-Dicyclohexylcarbodiimide; Disaster control center; Dorsal cell column; Double concave (see DCc).

DCc Double concave (= DCC).

DCCF Dural carotid-cavernous fistula.

DCCMP Daunomycin, cyclocytidine, 6-mercaptopurine, and prednisolone.

DC_{CO2} Diffusing capacity for carbon dioxide.

DCCP Division of Cancer Cause and Prevention (NCI).

DCCT Diabetes Control and Complications Test.

DCCV Direct current cardioversion (= DCEC).

DCD Day Care doctor/ dose; Digital computing densitometer; Diploma in Chest Diseases; Division of Chronic Diseases (USPHS).

D/C'd; dc'd Discontinued (= DC).

DC-DA Dichorionic-diamniotic (triplet pregnancy) (see DDTP).

dCDP Deoxycytidine diphosphate.

DCE Data communications equipment; Delayed contrast-enhancement; Designated compensable event; Digital cervical examination (Gynecology/ Obstetrics); Double contrast enema.

DCEC Direct current electroconversion (see DCCV).

DCET Dicarboxyethoxythiamine (= Dicethiamin).

DCF Decompensated cardiac failure (= DHF); 2-Deoxycoformycin (= Pentostatin) - a new anti-cancer drug, used in the treatment of hairy cell leukemia (see CdA); Direct centrifugal flotation (Lane's method for diagnosing hookworm infection in feces); Dopachrome conversion factor.

DCFS Department of Children and Family Services.

DCG Deoxy/Desoxy corticosterone glucoside;

Disodium cromoglycate (see DSCG); Displacement cardiograph; Dual cell gravity; Dynamic electrocardiogram/graphy (a Holter monitor magnetic-tape recording); Dysconjugate gaze (dysjugate movement of the two eyes - not focusing together, or moving in opposite directions).

DCGH District of Columbia General Hospital.

DCH Delayed cutaneous hypersensitivity; Department of Child Health (Kings College Hospital, London); Diploma in Child Health (English Conjoint Board).

DCh Doctor of Surgery (L. Doctor Chirurgiae).

DCHFB Dichlorohexafluorobutane.

DCHHE Department of Community Health and Health Education (DS-EA).

DCHN Dicyclohexylamine nitrite.

DChO Doctor of Ophthalmic Surgery.

DCI Damage-control ion (i.e. Magnesium); Decompensated cardiac insufficiency; Dichloroisoprenaline; Dichloroisoproterenol; Drug and Cosmetic Industry (journal).

DCIP Dichlorophenol-indophenol.

DCIS Ductal carcinoma in situ.

Dck Duck.

DCL Decompensated cirrhosis of the liver (see DHC); Dense cellular layer (e.g. of fibrous tissue); Dicloxacillin; Diffuse/ Disseminated cutaneous leishmaniasis.

DCLS Deoxycholate citrate lactose saccharose (agar culture medium).

DCM Dichloromethane; Dichloromethotrexate; Decreased/ Diminished child mortality (see DIM); Dilated cardiomyopathy; Disseminated chronic mycosis; Doctor of Comparative Medicine; Dyssynergia cerebellaris myoclonica.

DCML Dorsal column medial lemniscus.

DCMP Daunomycin, cytosine arabinoside, 6-mercaptopurine, and prednisolone.

dCMP Deoxycytidine monophosphate.

DCMT Doctor of Clinical Medicine of the Tropics.

DCMX 2,4-Dichloro-m-xylenol (= Dichloroxylenol).

DCMXT Dichloromethotrexate.

DCN Darvocet N; Data collection network; Deep cerebral nucleus; Delayed conditioned necrosis; Depressed, cognitively normal; Dorsal column nucleus; Dorsal cutaneous nerve.

DCNA Dental Clinics of North America; 2,6-Dichloro-4-nitro-aniline.

DCNB 2,4-Dinitrochloro benzene (used in test for immune competence).

DCNU Chlorozotocin.

DCO Decreased/ Diminished cardiac output; Dermoid cyst of the ovary; Diploma of the College of Optics.

D_{CO} Diffusing capacity for carbon monoxide (see PFT - D_{CO}).

DCOG Diploma of the College of Obstetricians and Gynaecologists (UK).

DCP Day-care program; Decompensatory cardiopathy; Department of Clinical Pathology/ Pharmacology/ Psychology; Dicalcium phosphate; Dichorionic placenta; Dicrotic pulse (an arterial pulse with two separate peaks, the second slightly weaker than the first) (see BFP); Diploma in Clinical Pathology/ Psychology; Direct cortical response; District Community Physician; Division of Cancer Prevention (NCI); Dual chamber pacemaker/ pacing (= atrial/ physiologic pacing) (see SCAP; SCVP); Dynamic compression plate; Dyschondroplasia (= Enchondromatosis; Ollier's disease) (Orth); Dyskinetic cerebral palsy.

DCPA Defense Civil Preparedness Agency (DOD); Department of Chemistry and Public Affairs (ACS); 2,4-Dichlorophenoxyacetic acid (see PAH); Dimethyl-1-2,3,5,6-tetrachloroterephthalate.

DCPC Di(p-chlorophenyl)methylcarbinol (= DMC).

DCPM Daunorubicin, cytarabine, prednisolone, and mercaptopurine.

DCPN Direction-changing positional nystagmus.

DCR Dacryocystorhinostomy; Data conversion receiver; Delayed cutaneous reaction; Direct coronary revascularization; Direct cortical reponse; Diseases of the Colon and Rectum (journal); Division of Clinical Research (FDA); Drug-company representative.

DCRI Duke Clinical Research Institute (Duke Univ., N. Carolina, USA).

DCRT Division of Computer Research and Technology (NIH).

DCS DaCosta's syndrome (see Asthenia; NCA); Data collection/ communication system; Decompression sickness; Dense canalicular system; Diffuse cortical sclerosis; Dorsal column/ cord stimulation/tor; Doubtful clinical significance; Dynamic condylar screw; Dyskinetic cilia syndrome.

DCSA Double contrast shoulder arthrography.

DCT Daunorubicin, cytarabine, and thioguanine; Deep chest therapy; Dendritic-cell therapy (for cancer); Desferrioxamine chelation test (for iron in urine); Diarrheagenic cell tumor; Dichorionic twin; Digito-cancellation task; Dipstick chemical test; Direct Coombs' test; Distal convoluted tubule (of kidney); Diurnal cortisol test; Dynamic computed tomography.

dct boiled down (L. decoctum).

DCTD Diffuse connective tissue disease (e.g. PAN - Polyarteritis nodosa).

DCTL Direct-coupled transistor logic.

DCTM Delayed computer tomographic myelography; Department of Clinical Tropical Medicine.

DCTMA Deoxy/Desoxy corticosterone trimethylacetate.

DCTP Dichorionic twin pregnancy.

dCTP Deoxycytidine triphosphate.

DCTPA Deoxy/Desoxy corticosterone triphenylacetate.

DCU Dental care unit; Dichloral urea.

DCVO Deputy Chief Veterinary Officer.

DCX Double charge exchange.

DCx Double convex (lens).

DCYH D-cystathionine.

DD Dangerous drug; Data definition; Day of delivery; Degenerated disc; Degenerative/ Di Guglielmo's/ Dupuytren's disease; Degree-day; Delusional depression (psychotic depression with depressive delusions); Delusional/ Depressive/ Digestive/ Dysthymic disorder; Dependent drainage; Detrusor dyssynergia; Developmental disability; Developmentally disabled; Dialysis dementia; Died of the disease; Differential/ Discharge diagnosis; Diploma (of the American Board) of Dermatology; Disc/ Disk diameter (= dd) - eye exam; Discharged dead; Doctor of Divinity; Dog dander; Dose-dependent; Double diffusion (test); Down the drain; Drug dependence; Dry dressing; Duchenne's dystrophy; Duncan disease (after the Duncan family, in which the condition was first described. An X-linked lymphoproliferative disease with a defective gene at Xq 25, evoked by infection with the Epstein-Barr virus or EBG, the causal agent in infectious mononucleosis); Give/ Let it be given to (L. detur ad) (= dd).

Dd Unusual detail response (Rorschach).

dd daily (L. de die); disc/ disk diameter (see DD); give/ let it be given to (see DD); very small detail response (Rorschach).

D-D Diagnosis-delivery (interval).

D → D Discharge to duty.

D&D Diarrhea and dehydration.

D6D Delta-6-desaturase.

DDA Dangerous Drugs Act; Dichlorodiphenyl acetate/ acetic acid (an acetic metabolite of DDT excreted in the urine); Dideoxyadenosine (see ddA); Disabled Drivers' Association (UK); Downward dose adjustment.

ddA 2',3'-dideoxyadenosine (= DDA).

DDAE Dose dependent adverse event.

DDAVP; dDAVP 1-Deamino-8-D-arginine-vasopressin (= Desamino-d-arginine vasopressin).

DDB Drug database.

DDBE Duchenne de Boulogne.

DDC Dangerous drug cabinet; Decreased/ Diminished drug clearance; Dewey Decimal Classification (system); Dideoxycytidine (see ddC); Diethyl-dithiocarbamate/mic acid/mine; Direct display console; Diverticular disease of the colon; Dopa decarboxylase.

DDc Double concave.

ddC Dideoxycytidine or Zalcitabine (treatment for AIDS) (= DDC).

DDCI Dopa decarboxylase inhibitor.

DDCRTU Drug Dependence Clinical Research and Treatment Unit (UK).

DDD AV universal (pacemaker); Daily dose difference (see TDDD); Defined daily dose; Degenerative disc/ Dense deposit/ Denver dialysis/ Dowling-Degos disease; De/Dihydroxydinaphthyl disulfide; Dementia, diarrhea, and dermatitis (the three D's of pellagra); Diagnostic Devices Division (BMD of HPB); Dichlorodiphenyl-dichloroethane (= TDE) - an insecticide; Fully automatic pacing.

o,p'DDD Ortho-para-prime DDD {= 1,1-Dichloro-2,2-di(p- chlorophenyl)ethane} - has been used as an antineoplastic agent in the treatment of adrenocortical tumors and metastases.

DDD CT Double-dose-delay computed tomography.

DDDIC Department of Defense Disease and Injury Code.

DDE Dichlorodiphenyldichloroethylene (= Dichlorophenyl-dichloro-ethylene; 1,1-dichloro-2,2-bis ethylene) - a derivative of DDT stored in fat.

DDF Dumdum fever (= Assam fever; Black fever; KA or Kala-azar; Ponos; Visceral leishmaniasis).

DDG Deoxy-D-glucose; Digital delay generator.

DDGB Double-dose gallbladder (test).

DDH Diploma in Dental Health; Dissociated double hypertropia; Division of Dental Health (USPHS).

DDHT Double dissociated hypertropia.

DDI Daily dietary intake; Dideoxyinosine (see ddI); Doctor's Data, Inc.; Dopa decarboxylase inhibitor (= benserazide, carbidopa, etc); Dose-dependent increase (of abnormalities/ variants due to drugs)/ inhibition (of bone resorption); Dressing dry and intact; Drug-disease/ drug interaction(s); Drug-dependency insomnia; Drug-drug interaction (see DDIA; DDIS).

ddI Didanosine (an antiviral drug used in the treatment of AIDS); Dideoxyinosine (= DDI) - an AIDS drug and chemical analogue of AZT (see AZT).

DDIA Drug-drug interaction (see DDIS).

DDIB Disease Detection Information Bureau.

dd in d from day to day (L. de die in diem) (= de d in d).

Δ^5-diol Δ^5-androstenediol.

DDIS Drug-drug interaction study.

DDL Digital data logger.

DDLW "Detected distance from the left ear, of a watch", i.e. distance at which the ticking of a watch is detected by the left ear (see HDLW).

DDM Diaminodiphenylmethane; Diploma in Dermatological Medicine; Doctor in Dental Medicine; Drug delivery method; Dyke-Davidoff-Masson (syndrome).

DDMS Deputy Director of Medical Services (Armed Forces).

dDNA Denatured deoxyribonucleic acid (see DNA).

DDNTP Dideoxynucleoside triphosphate.

DDO Development Disabilities Office (HEW); Diploma in Dental Orthopaedics (UK).

D-D op Dupuy-Dutemps operation.

DDP Cisplatin (= Cisplatinum) - a cytotoxic drug; Decreased/ Diminished detrusor pressure (of the urinary bladder); Degradative deribosylation pathway (of metabolism) (see RPP); Density-dependent phosphoprotein; Diabetic dietary prescription; Dialysis-dependent patient; Diaminodichloroplatinum (= Cisplatin-platinum complex/ compound); Dichorionic dizygotic pregnancy (Obstetrics); Difficult denture patient; Digital/ Distributed data processing.

DDp Drug dependence.

DDPA Delta Dental Plans Association.

DDPD Delusional Dominating Personality Disorder (= JWS; MPD).

DDPI Department of Defence Polygraph Institute (US).

DDQ Dichloro-dicyano-benzoquinone.

DDR Diastolic descent rate; Diploma in Diagnostic Radiology; Doctor of Dental Radiology; Donor Deferral Register; Dose-dependent reaction/ reduction.

DDRB Doctors' and Dentists' Review Body.

DDRDC Desperate diseases (may) require desperate cures (e.g., cancer).

DDRW "Detected distance from the right ear, of a watch" i.e. distance at which the ticking of a watch is detected by the right ear (see

HDRW).

DDS Damaged disc syndrome; Dataphone Digital Service; Dendro-dendritic synaptosome; Dental distress syndrome; Depressed DNA synthesis; Dialysis disequilibrium syndrome; Diaminodiphenylsulfone (see DADPS); 4,5-Dihydro-drospirenone-3-sulfate (the major metabolite of the progestogen preparation, Drospirenone); Directional Doppler sonography; Director of Dental Services; Disability determination service; Disease-Disability Scale; Doctor of Dental Surgery; Dodecyl sulfate; Dose-dependent selectivity; Double decidual sac; Double dummy study (= DDT); Drug delivery system; Drug dependence syndrome; Drug dependency service; Dystrophy-dystocia syndrome.

DDSA Developmentally Disabled Society of America.

DDSc Doctor of Dental Science.

DDSE Dose-dependent stimulatory effect (e.g. on the transformation of choline to PTC - Phosphatidycholine or to Lecithin).

DDSI Digital damage severity index.

DDSO Diaminodiphenylsulfoxide.

DDST Denver Developmental Screening Test (pediatrics).

DDT Definitive diagnostic test; Dichloro-diphenyl-trichloro ethane (= Chlorophenothane; Chlorphenan; Dicophane; Parachlorocide; Penticide) - an insecticide and larvacide; Double-dummy technique/ trial (see DDS); Drug-delivery technology; Ductus deferens tumor.

pp'-DDT The predominant isomer in DDT (see DDT).

DDTN Dideoxy-didehydrothymidine.

DDTP Dichorionic diamniotic triplet pregnancy (Obstetrics).

ddTTP Dideoxythymidine triphosphate.

DDU Dermo-distortive urticaria.

DDV Dog distemper virus.

DDVF See DDVP.

DDVP Dimethyl-dichloro-vinyl phosphate (= DDVF; 2,2-Dichlorovinyl dimethyl phosphate; Dichlorvos; Nuvan; Vapona) - an organophosphorus insecticide.

DDW Double-distilled water.

D/DW Dextrose in distilled water.

D 5% DW 5 5% Dextrose in distilled water.

DDx Differential diagnosis.

DE Dental Economics (journal); Dentino-enamel (junction); Department of the Environment (Canada); Deprived eye; Diabetic extremity; Diagnostic error/ evaluation; Dialysis encephalopathy; Diethylaminoethyl; Digestive energy; Disc electrophoresis; Dose equivalent (radiation); Dream element(s); Drug evaluation; Duck embryo; Duke Endowment (hospital assistance); Duration of ejection.

de deciduous (teeth); edge detail (Rorschach).

de- prefix meaning down or from (L.).

D/E Dermal/epidermal.

2DE Two-dimensional echocardiography.

D&E Dilatation/ Dilation and evacuation (= D and E) (operation/ gynecology).

D_5E_{48} 5% Dextrose and Electrolyte 48.

D_5E_{75} 5% Dextrose and Electrolyte 75.

DEA Dehydroepiandrosterone; Diethanolamine; Diethylamine; Dihydrogenated ergot alkaloid; Drug Enforcement Administration/ Agency (Dept of Justice) (see DEA #).

DEA # Drug Enforcement Administration/ Agency number (physician's narcotic number).

DEAE Diethyl-aminoethanol; Diethyl-aminoethyl (cellulose).

DEAE-D Diethylaminoethyl dextran.

Dearg pil Let the pills be silvered/ silverized (L. deargentur pilulae).

Deaur pil Let the pills be gilded (L. deaurentur pilulae).

DEB Diepoxybutane; Diethylbutanediol; Division of Environmental Biology; Dystrophic epidermolysis bullosa.

deb debridement.

DEBA Diethylbarbituric acid (see Barb).

debil debilitated/itation/ity.

DEBRA Dystrophic Epidermolysis Bullosa Research Association.

DEBS Dominant epidermolysis bullosa simplex.

deb spis of the proper consistency (L. debita spissutudine).

DEC Decant or Pour off (see dec); Deceased

(see dec'd); Deciduous; (see dec); Decompose(d) (see decomp); Decrease(d) (see decr); Degenerative eye change(s); Deoxycholate citrate; Department of Environmental Conservation; Diethylcarbamazine; Digital Equipment Corporation; Dynamic environmental conditioning; Dysplastic erythroid cell (in erythrodysplasia).

Dec Decalin; Decant or Pour off (see dec); December; Decoction (see decoct).

dec decant or pour off (L. decanta) (= DEC; Dec); dead/ deceased (see dec'd); deciduous (= DEC); decimal; decompose(d)/sition (= decomp); decrease(d) (see decr).

dec- prefix meaning ten (Gr. deka) or one-tenth (L. decem).

deca ten (Gr. deka).

DECAFS Department of Children and Family Services.

dec'd; decd dead/ deceased (= DEC; dec).

Decel Deceleration.

DECG Dynamic electrocardiogram/graph(y).

deci- 10^{-1}; d; one-tenth; 0.1 (Gr. deka) (see d → deci-).

decoct decoction (L. decoctum) (= Dec).

decomp decompensate(d)/tion (heart disease); decompose(d)/sition (= DEC; dec).

decr decrease(d) (= DEC; dec).

DECRS Diabetic embryopathy-caudal regression syndrome (= CDS or Caudal dysplasia sequence/ syndrome) (see CDS, CRS, DEP - Obstetrics).

decub lying down (L. decubitus).

DED Date of expected delivery; Defined exposure dose; Delayed erythema dose; Diabetic eye disease; Distal epiphyseal distraction (Orthopedics) (see CSD); Dopaminergic ergoline derivative.

de d in d from day to day (L. de die in diem) (see dd in d).

DEE Diabetic eye examination.

Deeda LSD-25 (see LSD).

DEEG Depth electroencephalogram/graphy.

DEER Diet and Exercise for Elevated Risk (Study, on heart disease).

DEET Diethyl toluamide.

DEF Decayed, extracted, and filled (deciduous or primary teeth). Dental formula expressing caries in deciduous/ primary teeth: d = number of (decayed) teeth indicated for filling; e = number of teeth indicated for extraction; f = number of filled (deciduous or primary) teeth.

Def; def Defecate/tion; Defer(red); Deficiency/nt (see defic); Define/nite/nition; Deformed/mity (see deform).

DEFD Dynamic equinus foot deformity (see DFD; EFD).

defib defibrillate/tion.

defic deficiency/nt (= Def; def).

deform deformed/mity (= Def; def).

DEFT Direct epifluorescent filter technique.

DEG Diethylene glycol.

Deg; deg Degeneration/ive (see degen); Degree.

degen degeneration/ive (= Deg; deg).

deglut let it be swallowed; swallow it (L. deglutiatur).

DEH Dental enamel hypoplasia; Diethylhexyl; Dysplasia epiphysealis hemimelica.

DEHP Di(2-ethylhexyl)phthalate.

DEHS Division of Emergency Health Services (USPHS).

DEHT Developmental hand function test.

dehyd dehydrated/tion.

DEJ Dentinoenamel junction (= ADJ) - the plane of meeting between the dentin and enamel on a crown of a tooth.

DEJ; dej Dento-enamel junction.

déjà vu French - already seen.

deka ten (metric prefix).

Del; del Delete/tion; Delivery (room); Delusion.

Delhi boil A skin disease caused by *Leishmania* tropica (see Aleppo boil).

deliq deliquescence/nt.

DeLPS Deesterified lipopolysaccharide(s).

Delt Deltoid.

delta See δ.

De lun inq (L. de lunatico inquirendo) - a commission or jury appointed by a court to investigate the mental condition of a person whose sanity is under dispute.

delusion A false belief which cannot be corrected, rectified, or withdrawn by reason: Depressive delusion, with feelings of futility, uneasiness, unworthiness, etc.; expansive delusion, a false belief in one's own greatness, goodness or power (present in the manic form of manic-depressive psychosis); delusion of Grandeur, of one's own importance, power, wealth, etc. (as in general paresis); delusion of Negation, of one's own body, body parts, etc., or the world in general); nihilistic delusion, with denial of the existence of something or everything; delusion of Persecution, mistreatment, slander, injury, etc. by known or unknown enemies, as in paranoia (see paranoia); delusion of Reference, and similar ideas; somatic delusion, of some alteration in the patient's bodily organ or its function); systematized delusion, formulated by the patient in a logical manner (characteristic of true paranoia); unsystematized delusion, made up of disconnected parts.

DEM Decreased(sing)/ Diminished(hing) eye movement; Demerol (see Dem); Department of Emergency Medicine; Diethylmaleate.

Dem Demerol (= DEM; Meperidine hydrochloride).

dementia Among the organic causes are: AD: Alzheimer's dementia; BI: Brain injury; CA: Cerebral atrophy; CJD: Creutzfeldt-Jakob disease (= MCD); GPI: General paralysis of the insane (Tertiary syphilis); HD: Huntington's disease (genetic defect on chromosome 4); LBD: Lewy body dementia; MBC: Metastatic brain cancer; MCD: Mad cow disease (see CJD); MID: Multi-infarct dementia (i.e. vascular causes); NPH: Normal pressure hydrocephalus; PD: Parkinson's/ Pick's disease; VD: Vascular dementia/ disease (other causes besides MID).

DEN Denervation; Dengue; Department of Energy (UK); Dermatitis exfoliativa neonatorum; Diethylnitrosamine.

denat denatured.

dendr- combining form meaning tree (Gr. dendron).

Denom Denominator.

de novo Latin - appearing anew or unrelated.

DENT Dental Exposure Normalization Technique.

Dent; dent Dental/tist(ry)/tition; Dentistry, A Digest of Practice (journal); Give/ Let it be given (L. dentur) (see det).

dent- combining form meaning tooth (L. dentis).

DENTCAP Dental Civic Action Program.

DENTS Dental Examiners National Testing Service.

dent tal dos give of such doses (L. dentur tales doses).

DENTALPROJ Dental Research Projects.

DEP Diabetes education program; Diabetic embryopathy (associated with factors such as Altered metabolid fuels, Free oxygen radicals, Genetic susceptibility, Material hyperglycemia, hyperketonemia, hypoglycemia or other maternal factors, Somatomedin inhibitors, etc.) (see DRMs) (see scheme); Diethylpropanediol; Diethylpyrocarbonate (see DEPC); Dilution end point; Drug elimination procedure; Dyserythropoiesis.

Dep; dep Dependent(s); Depilate/tor(y) (see depil); Deplete(d)/tion (see depl); Depolarization/ze(d) (see depol); Deposit; Depreciate(d)/tion (see deprc); Depressed/sion/sor (see depr); purified (L. depuratus).

DEPA Diethylene phosphoramide.

DEPC Diethyl pyrocarbonate (= DEP) - used as an antimicrobial agent in wine and soft drinks.

depil depilate/tor(y) (= Dep; dep).

depl deplete(d)/tion (= Dep; dep).

depol depolarization/ze(d) (= Dep; dep).

depr; deprs depressed/sion/sor (= Dep; dep).

deprc depreciate(d)/tion (= Dep; dep).

DEPS Diabetes in Early Pregnancy Study (see DIEP); Distal effective potassium secretion.

DEP ST SEG Depressed ST segment (on the electrocardiogram).

Dept; dept Department (= D).

DEQ Depression Experiences Questionnaire.

DER Dermatome evoked response; Disulfiram-ethanol reaction; Doll's eyes reflex (positive in total coma); Dual energy radiography.

DeR Reaction of degeneration (see RD).

der derivative (chromosome).

DeRisi Version II A microarrayer or new high-tech robot used to battle disease (COH, Ca, US).

deriv derivative; derived (from).

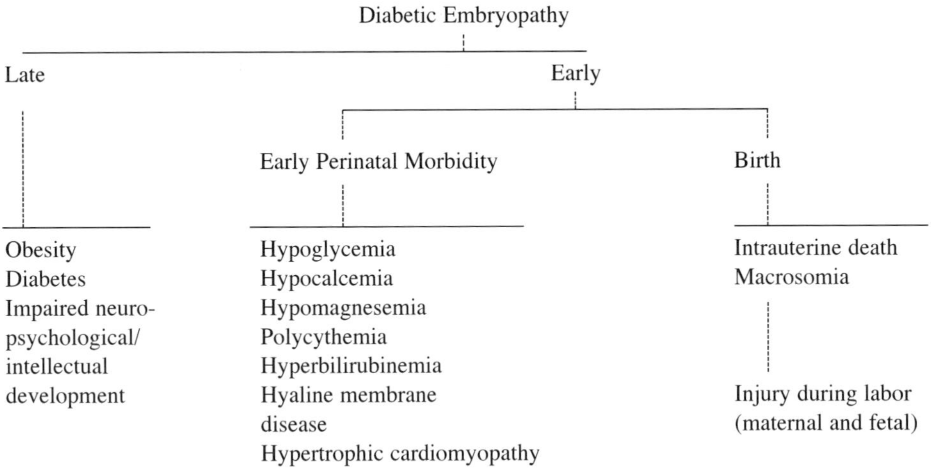

Perinatal morbidity in offspring of diabetic mothers

Derm; derm Dermatitis; Dermatological/gist/gy; Dermatome.

derm- combining form meaning skin (Gr. derma).

DES Dermal-epidermal separation; Dialysis encephalopathy syndrome; Diethylstilbestrol (= DIES; DS); Differential Emotional Scale (Izard); Diffuse esophageal spasm; Disequilibrium syndrome; Doctor's Emergency Service; Dry eye syndrome.

des; desat desaturate(d)/tion.

desc descendant/dent/ding.

Desc Ao Descending aorta.

DESI Drug efficacy study implementation; Drug Efficiency Study and Implementation (FDA).

desm- combining form meaning band or ligament (Gr. desmos).

desq desquamation.

DEST Denver Eye Screening Test; Dichotic Environmental Sounds Test.

dest; destil distil (L. destilla); distilled (L. destillatus).

DET Diethyltoluamide (an insect repellent); Diethyltryptamine (see DET,N); Diminished exercise tolerance; Dipyridamole echocardiography test.

det determination/ne(d) (see determ); Give/ Let it be given (L. detur) (see Dent; dent).

Det-6 Detroid-6 (human sternal marrow cells).

determ; determin determination/ne(d) (= det).

det in dup; det in 2 plo give twice as much/ let twice as much be given (L. detur in duplo).

detn detention.

DET,N N=diethyltrytamine (=DET).

detox detoxification (of drugs).

det s; d et s give and label/ let it be given and labelled (L. detur et signetur).

DEUV Direct electronic urethrocystometry.

DEV Deviant (see dev); Deviate/tion (see dev); Duck egg/ embryo vaccine/ virus (e.g. rabies).

dev deviant (= DEV); deviate/tion (= DEV); develop(ed)/(ment) (see devel).

devel develop(ed)/ment (= dev).

DevPd Developmental pediatrics.

DEX Dexamethasone (see Dex).

Dex Dexamethasone (= DEX); Dexedrine (see Amphet - Dex).

dex dexterity; dextrorotatory; right (L. dexter).

DEXA Dual-energy x-ray absorptiometry.

dexie Dexamyl (= Drinamyl) - proprietary tablet containing 5 mg dexamphetamine sulfate and 32 mg amylobarbitone (see Amphet - dexie; Barb - dexie); Dexedrin tablet (see Amphet - dexie).

dextr- combining form meaning right hand (L.

dexter).

DF Decapacitation (sperm)/ Decontamination/ Deficiency/ Distribution factor; Decayed and filled; Deferoxamine/ Desferrioxamine (see DFM); Defined flora (animal); Degree of freedom (of movement) (see DoF); Dengue fever; Dermatology Foundation; Diabetic father; Diastolic filling; Dietary fibers; Digital fluoroscopy; Discriminant/ating/ation function; Disseminated foci; Dorsiflexion; Drug/ Dye free.

Df Dermatophagoides farinae.

df degrees of freedom (see DoF).

DFA Deep femoral artery (= Arteria profunda femoris - L.); Desferrioxamine; Deuterofluoroalanine (= 2-deutero-3-fluoro-D-alanine) - an antibiotic; Diet for age; Difficulty falling asleep; Direct fluorescent antibody; Direct fluorescence assay (in skin biopsy for detection of RMSF and other rickettsial diseases); Director of fiscal affairs; Dorsiflexion assistance; Dried Fruit Association.

DFACT Desferrioxamine chelation test (for urinary iron in hemochromatosis).

DFB Dinitrofluorobenzene; Dysfunctional bleeding.

DFC Desferrioxamine chelation (test - see DFACT); Developmental field complex; Diabetic Foot Clinic (UK); Dry-filled capsule.

5'-DFCR 5'-deoxy-5-fluorocytidine (a metabolite of Capecitabine, an anti-neoplastic drug, which is converted by the enzyme Cytidine deaminase [Cyd deaminase] into 5'-deoxy-5-fluorouridine) (see 5'DFUR).

DFD Defined formula diet(s); Delayed functional development (of the fetus, offspring, etc.); Disopropyl phosphorofluoridate; Distal femoral diaphysis; Dynamic foot deformity (see DEFD; EFD).

DFDD Difluoro-diphenyl-dichloro-ethane.

DFDT Difluoro-diphenyl-trichloro-ethane (a powerful insecticide) (see GIX).

dF/dt First derivative of Force development (= Rate of Force development).

DFE Diabetic foot examination; Diffuse fasciitis with eosinophilia; Distal femoral epiphysis.

DFECT Dense fibroelastic connective tissue.

DFF Distal femoral fracture.

DFG Direct forward gaze; Discordant fetal growth; Down's flow generator (Device for maintaining continuous positive airway pressure {PAP}).

DFHom Diploma of the Faculty of Homeopathy.

DFI Disease-free interval;. Drug-food interaction; Drug-free interval (see DFP).

DFM Decreased fetal movement; Department of Family Medicine; Desferrioxamine (hydrochloride or mesylate) (= Ba-29837; Ba-33112; Deferoxamine; DF; DFO; DFOH; DFOM) - an iron chelating agent (see Ba-33112); Disease-fighting mechanism

DFMC Daily fetal movement count.

DFMO Difluoromethylornithine.

DFMR Daily fetal movement record.

DFO Definitely favorable opinion; Desferrioxamine (see DFM); Director of Field Operations; District Finance Officer.

DFOH Desferrioxamine hydrochloride (see DFM).

DFOM Desferrioxamine mesylate (see DFM).

DFP Diastolic filling period; Dichorionic fused placenta (Obstetrics); Di-isopropyl fluorophosphate (= Disopropyl fluorophosphate; Dyflos; Fluostigmine; Isofluorophate) - a powerful cholinergic drug with prolonged anti-cholinesterase action, used in treating glaucoma and myasthenia gravis; Di-isopropyl-fluorophosphonate; Drug-free period (= DFI).

DFP^{32}; $DF^{32}P$ ^{32}P-(radio)labeled diisopropyl fluorophosphate (= Isofluorophate P32) - a radioactive form used in measuring the life span of erythrocytes and blood platelets.

DFPP Double filtration plasmopheresis.

DFPV Disseminated focal perivasculitis.

DFR Diabetic floor routine; Distal femoral resection (Orthopedics); Distal functional reabsorption; Disturbed family relationship.

DFRC Deglycerolized frozen red cells.

DFRI Dihydrofolate reductase inhibitor (see DRI).

DFS Differential fluorescent staining; Disease-free survival; Dry Floatation System (cushion for decubitus ulcer in wheelchair patients).

DFSP Dermatofibrosarcoma protuberans.

DFT Defibrillation threshold; Dense fibrous tissue; Diagnostic function test; Dialyzable fraction of/ free thyroxine/ triiodothyronine (see DFT_3; DFT_4); Discrete Fourier transform.

DFT_3 Dialyzable fraction of/ free triiodothyronine (= DFT_3) (laboratory/ endocrinology).

DFT_4 Dialyzable fraction of/ free thyroxine (= DFT_4) (laboratory/ endocrinology).

DFU Dead fetus in uterus; Diabetic foot ulceration; Dideoxyfluorouridine.

5'-DFUR 5'-deoxy-5-fluorouridine (an antineoplastic drug) (see DFU; FUDR).

DFV Diarrhea with fever and vomiting.

DFW Dexide face wash; Disease-fighting weapon.

DG Darkground; Dentate gyrus (in the hippocampus) (= GD); Deoxyglucose (see 2DG); Diagnose/sed/sis (see dg); Diastolic gallop; Diglyceride; Distogingival.

dg decigram (= dgm; 10^{-1} gram; 0.1 gram; a tenth part of a gram); diagnose(d)/sis (= DG).

2DG 2-deoxy-D-glucose (= Deoxyglucose; DG).

DGAVP Desglycinamide-9-(Arg-8)-vasopressin.

DGBG Dimethylglyoxal bisguanyl-hydrazone.

DGCCPB Dental Guidance Council for Cerebral Palsy Bulletin (UCPA journal).

dGDP Deoxyguanosine diphosphate.

DGE Delayed gastric emptying; Dermamesh graft expander (Plastic and Reconstructive Surgery); aa-Di-(p-ethoxyphenyl)-beta-phenyl bromoethylene.

dge drainage.

DGF Delayed graft function; Duct growth factor.

DGG Department of Gerontology and Geriatrics; Dysgammaglobulinemia.

DGI Dentinogenesis imperfecta (a hereditary disorder of the teeth in which dentin overgrows and fills in the center of the tooth. Often associated with OGI or Osteogenesis imperfecta) (see AGS); Disseminated gonococcal infection.

DGLA Dihomogamma-linolenic acid.

DGM Department of Geriatric Medicine; Ductal glandular mastectomy.

dgm decigram (see dg).

DGMMD Department of Geriatric Medicine and Metabolic Diseases (Univ of Naples, Italy).

dGMP Deoxyguanosine monophosphate.

DGMS Director General of Medical Services (Armed Forces); Division of General Medical Sciences (NIH).

DGN Diffuse glomerulonephritis (proliferative) (= DGPG; DPG; DPGN).

DGO Diploma in Gynaecology and Obstetrics.

dGOPOPCP β,γ-methylene-deoxyguanosine triphosphate.

DGP Degradation product(s); Deputising general practitioner (UK); 2,3-diglycerophosphate.

DGPG Diffuse proliferative glomerulonephritis (see DGN).

DGR Duodenogastric reflux.

DGRC Deglycerolized red cell(s); Diabetes and Genetic Research Center (COH).

DGS Developmental Gerstmann's syndrome; Diabetic glomerulosclerosis; Di George's syndrome (Congenital aplasia of the thymus).

DGT Decreased/ Diminished glucose tolerance; Diabetes gene theory.

dGTP Deoxyguanosine triphosphate.

DGV Dextrose-gelatin-Veronal (buffer).

DH Daily habits; Day Hospital; Dehydrocholate/lic acid; Dehydrogenase; Delayed hypersensitivity; Dental Hygiene (ADHA journal); Dental Hygienist (journal); Department of Health; Dermatitis herpetiformis; Developmental history; Diabetogenic hormone (see Hormones - DH i); Diaphragmatic hernia; Diastolic hypertension; Disseminated histoplasmosis; Diuretic hormone (see Hormones - DH ii); Dominant hand; Dorsal horn; Ductal hyperplasia; Dunkin-Hartley (guinea-pig).

D/H Deuterium/hydrogen (ratio).

DHA Dehydroacetic acid; Dehydroascorbic acid; Dehydroepiandrosterone; Digital hearing aid; Dihydroacetic acid; Dihydroxyacetone (= Ketotriose) - used as an artificial suntan lotion; District Health Authority; Docohexanoic acid;

Docosahexaenoic acid (a polyunsaturated fatty acid).

DHA 180 Dihydroergocornine (see DHO 180).

DHAD Dihydroxy-bis-amino-anthraquinone dihydrochloride; Mitoxantrone hydrochloride.

DHAE Dihydrogenated alkaloids of ergotamine.

DHAP Dihydroxyacetone phosphate.

DHAP-AT Dihydroxyacetone phosphate acyltransferase.

DHAS Dehydroandrostenedione (= Dehydroepiandro-sterone sulfate; Androst-5-en-17-on-3b-yl sulfate) (= DHEA; DHEAS).

DHASCO Docosahexaenoic acid - (rich) single-cell oil (dietary fat in infant formula).

DHB Duck hepatitis B (vaccine/ virus) (= DHBV).

2-4 DHBA 2-4-dihydroxybenzoic acid.

3-4 DHBA 3-4-dihydroxybenzoic acid.

DHBE Dihydroxybutyl ether.

DHBG Dihydroxybutyl guanine.

DHBS Dihydrobiopterin synthetase.

DHBV Duck hepatitis B vaccine/ virus (see DHB).

DHC Decompensated hepatic cirrhosis (= DCL; DLC); Dehydrochalcone; Dehydrocholate; Dehydrocholesterol; Digital-healthcare; Dihydrocodeine; Dorsal horn cell.

DHCA Deep hypothermia and circulatory arrest.

1,25 DHCC 1,25 dihydroxychole-calciferol.

DHCS Department of Health Care Services.

DHD District Health Department; Down's hand dermatome (Plastic and Reconstructive Surgery).

DHE Dedehydro-ergotamine; Defence for Health Environment; Dehydroemetine (hydrochloride) (= 2,3-Dehydroemetine HCl; Ro 1- 9934) - a potent amebicide; Dihematoporphyrin ether; Dihydroergotamine (mesylate) (see DHE 45); Direct harmful effect.

DHE 45 Dihydroergotamine (mesylate; methanesulfonate) - used in the treatment of migraine.

DHEA Dehydroepiandrosterone (see DHAS); Dehydroxycorticosterone E acetate.

DHEAS Dehydroepiandrosterone sulfate (see DHAS).

DHEC Dihydroergocryptine.

DHEP Diclofenac Hydroxyethylpyrrolidine.

DHES Division of Health Examination Statistics.

DHESN Dihydroergosine.

DHEW Department of Health, Education, and Welfare (US).

DHF Decompensated heart failure (see DCF); Dengue hemorrhagic fever (caused by the dengue virus serotypes 1, 2, 3, or 4, of the viral family *Flaviviridae*, and transmitted from man to man by the mosquito, AEDES aegypti); Dorsi-hyperflexion.

DHF/DSS Dengue hemorrhagic fever/ dengue shock syndrome.

DHFR Dihydrofolate reductase (an enzyme essential for the synthesis of DNA).

DHG Department of Human Genetics (UCLA).

DHg Doctor of Hygiene (see DHyg).

DHGG Deaggregated human gamma-globulin.

DHHS Department of Health and Human Services (US).

DHI Dental Health International; Dihydroxyindole.

DHIA Dairy Herd Improvement Association; Dehydroisoandrosterol/erone.

DHIC Dihydroisocodeine.

DHIPU Department of Health Information Policy Unit (UK).

DHL Diffuse histiocytic lymphoma.

D-HL Durham-Humphrey Law (amends FFDCA).

DHLY; dHLY d-hydroxylysine.

DHM Dihydromorphine; Dichloroacet-p-hydroxy-N-methylanilide (= Diloxan; Diloxanide; RD 3803) - used as an intestinal amebicide; Dix-Hallpike maneuver (positional test for nystagmus) (= HDM; NBM); Doll's head manoeuvre (used for assessing eye movements in the unconscious patient. Rolling of the head to one side causes counter-rolling of the eyes to the other side, if the brain stem is intact).

DHMA Dehydroxymandelic acid (= 3,4-dihydroxymandelic acid).

DHM Fur Diloxanide Furoate (more potent

and less toxic than diloxanide in the treatment of amoebiasis).

DHMO Division of Hematology and Medical Oncology.

DHN Department of Hospital Nursing.

DHO Deuterium hydrogen oxide (protium oxide); Dihydroergocornine (see DHO 180).

DHO 180 Dihydroergocornine (= DHA 180; DHO).

DHP Dehydrogenated polymer; Diffuse hypersensitivity pneumonia (also called Allergic alveolitis, Bagassosis, EAP or Extrinsic allergic pneumonia) (see AIP); Dihydroprogesterone; Dihydropyridine(s); Dried human plasma.

DHPA Dihydroxypropyl adenine.

DHPC Dallas histopathological criteria.

DHPG Dihydroxyphenylglycol; Dihydroxyproproxymethylguanine; Ganciclovir.

DHPh Diploma in Homeopathic Pharmacy.

DHPR Dihydropteridine reductase.

DHR Delayed hypersensitivity reaction; Detrusor hyperreflexia (i.e. of the bladder muscle) (see OAB).

DHRA Director of Human Research Affairs.

DHS Delayed hypersensitivity; Department of Health/ Human Services; Dextrose in Hartman's solution (see D-5-HS); Diabetic hyperosmolar state; Dihydrostreptomycin (see DHSM); Division of Health and Safety (US Bureau of Mines); Dried human serum; Duration of hospital stay; Dynamic hip screw.

D-5-HS; D/5 HS Dextrose (5%) in Hartman's solution (= DHS; D-5-HS) - intravenous solution (for drip/ infusion).

DHSC Director(ate) of Health and Social Care (UK).

DHSM Dihydrostreptomycin (= DHS; DHSS).

DHSS Department of Health and Social Security/ Services (UK); Dihydrostreptomycin sulfate (see DHSM).

DHST Delayed hypersensitivity test.

DHT Damaged heart tissue; Dehydrotestosterone; Dihydroergotoxine; Dihydrotachysterol (an analogue of vitamin D) (see AT-10; Vitamins - D); Dihydrotestosterone (see DHTP); Dihydrothymine; Dihydroxytryptamine (see 5,7-DHT); Dissociated hypertropia.

5,7-DHT 5,7-dihydroxytryptamine (= DHT).

DHTN; Dias Htn Diastolic hypertension.

DHTP Dihydrotestosterone propionate (= DHT).

DHTR Dihydrotestosterone receptor.

DHV Disk heart valve (Hufnagel prosthesis).

DHW Department of Health and Welfare (Canada).

DHWU Drug and Hospital Workers Union.

Dhyg; Dhy Doctor of Hygiene (= DHg; DHy; DrHyg).

DHZ Dihydralazine.

DI Dalanated insulin (see Insulin - DI; SN 44); Date of injury; Debrix/ Decontamination/ Deoxyribonucleic acid/ Deterioration/ Dye/ Dyskaryosis index; Defective interfering (particle); Dental implant; Dentinogesis imperfecta; Department of the Interior; Detrusor instability; Diabetes insipidus; Diagnostic imaging; Dialized iron; Disability insurance; Disto-incisal; Dorso-iliac; Double indemnity; Drug-induced; Drug information/ interaction(s); Dry ice (solid CO_2).

Di Didymium (= D) (Gr. didymos - twin). A rare metal, formerly considered an element but later found to be a mixture of two rare-earth elements, Neodymium (Nd) and Praesodymium (Pr). Usually found associated with the elements, Cerium (Ce) and Lanthanum (La) (see Elements - Ce, La, Nd, and Pr); Diego blood group (see DiA; Di a).

di inside detail (Rorschach test); marked distortion of intrathoracic organs (radiographic symbol).

di- prefix meaning two (L. di), through or apart (L. dia), and apart or away from (L. dis).

D&I Dry and intact.

DIA Depolarization-induced automaticity; Diabetes/tic (see Diab); Diagnostic imaging agent; Diazepam; Drug-induced abnormality; Drug-induced acne (caused by anabolic steroids, corticosteroids, androgenic hormones and various other drugs such as phenytoin, rifam-picin, lithium and vitamin B12); Drug Information Association; Drug interaction.

Dia; dia Diabetes/tic (see Diab); Diakinesis; Diathermy (see Diath).
DiA; Di a Diego antigen (blood group) (= Di).
dia- prefix meaning through, between, across, apart, complete (Gr.).
Diab Diabetes/tic (= DIA; Dia; dia; diab); Diabetes (journal); Diabetologia (journal).
diab diabetes/tic (seee Diab).
DIAC Diiodothyroacetic acid.
Diag; diag Diagnosis/ostic; Diagonal; Diagram.
DIAGNO Differential diagnosis (by computer) (see diff diagn).
Dial Allobarbital (see Barb).
Dialog Dialogue (United Nurses journal, Canada).
DIAM Drug-induced allergic myocarditis.
Diam; diam Diameter.
Diamorph Diamorphine hydrochloride or Heroin. A potent analgesic and narcotic, with properties resembling those of morphine, and producing intense euphoria, but with fewer side-effects such as constipation, nausea, and vomiting; hence the greater danger of addiction. Used in the relief of severe pain in the terminal stages of cancer. Other names include: A-Bomb (a cigarette prepared from a mixture of marijuana and heroin - see Cannabis); Bang; Blanco; Bonita (with milk sugar to dilute heroin); Boy; Brother; Brown; Caballo; Ca-ca (counterfeit heroin); Cat; C&H (cocaine and heroin; Chick; Chinese white (concentrated heroin); Cura (Sp.) cure i.e. heroin; Diacetylmorphine HCl; Diamorph HCl; Diamorphine HCl: dogie; doojie; duji; Duster (heroin cigarette); Dynamite (cocaine and heroin mixture); Dyno (high-potency heroin); Frisco speedball (= FS; mixture of heroin, cocaine, and LSD-25); FS (= Frisco speedball); Girl; H; Harry; H-cap (heroin in a gelatine capsule); Henry; Heroin (symbol H); Heroin hydrochloride (Heroin HCl); Him; HMC (Heroin, morphine, and cocaine); Horse; Junk; Mojo (Heroin, morphine, or cocaine); Skag (chief, low-grade heroin); Smack; Speedball (a mixture of cocaine and heroin); Tecata; White lady (name also used for cocaine); WL (white lady).
diaph Diaphragm.
DIAR Dextran-induced anaphylactic reaction.
DIAS Drug-interaction study.
dias diastole/lic.
DIAS BH Diastolic blood pressure.
Diath; diath Diathermy (= Dia; dia).
Diath SW Diathermy short wave.
DIAZ Diazepam.
DIB Butyl-diiodo-hydroxy-benzoate (= Butyl 3:5-di-iodo-4-hydroxybenzoate); Diagnostic interview for borderlines; Disability insurance benefit(s); Dot immunobinding; Duodeno-ileal bypass.
DIBA Domestic and International Business Administration (Department of Commerce).
Dib alt On alternate days (L. diebus alternis) (see Dieb alt).
diBr-HQ 5,7-dibromo-8-hydroxy-quinidine.
Dib secund Every second day (see Dieb secund).
Dib tert Every third day (see Dieb tert).
DIC Adriamycin, cyclophosphamide, imidazole carboxamide; Diagnostic Imaging Center; Dicarbazine; Dependency and indemnity compensation (VA); Differential interference contrast (microscope/py); Diffuse/ Disseminated intravascular coagulation/ coagulopathy/ fibrin deposits; Dimethyl triazeno imidazole carboxamide; Drug information center.
dic dicentric.
DICD Dispersion-induced circular dichroism; Distal ileal Crohn's disease.
Dick Ethyldichloroarsine (a war gas); Test for susceptibility to scarlet fever.
DICP Drug Intelligence and Clinical Pharmacy (journal).
Dict Dictionary.
DID Deadly infectious disease; Dead of intercurrent disease; Deeply-invasive disease; Delayed-interval delivery; Delayed ischemia deficit; Dietary/ Drug -induced diuresis; Double immunodiffusion (technique); Drug-induced disease/ disorder / dyspepsia (= DII).
DIDD Dense intramembranous deposit disease.
DIDMOA Diabetes insipidus-diabetes mellitus-optic atrophy (syndrome).
DIDMOAD Diabetes insipidus, diabetes mellitus, optic atrophy, deafness (syndrome).

didym- combining form meaning twin (Gr. didymos).

DIE Died in emergency (department/ room); Drug-induced edema/ epilepsy (diurctics - acetazolamide, etc.).

Dieb alt On alternate days (L. diebus alternis) (= Dib alt).

Dieb secund Every second day (L. diebus secundus) (= Dib secund).

Dieb tert Every third day (L. diebus tertis) (= Dib tert).

DIEDI Diisopropylamine-dichloroacetate.

DIEP Diabetes in Early Pregnancy (Study) - Israel (= DEPS, DIEPS).

DIEPS Diabetes in Early Pregnancy Study (see DIEP).

DIES Diethylstilbestrol (see DES).

DIF Diffuse interstitial fibrosis; Direct immunofluorescence; Dose increase factor.

DIFF, diff difference/ent(ial); differential (blood count); diffuse/sion.

diff diagn; diff diag; dif diag Differential diagnosis (= DIAGNO).

DIFO Dimefox (= BFPO; tetramethyl-phosphorodiamidic fluoride) - an organophosphorus insecticide (see BFPO).

DIFP Diffuse interstitial fibrosing pneumonitis; Disopropyl fluorophosphate/phosphonate.

DIG Digital image processing/cessor (Echocardiographic, etc.); Digitalis/ Digoxin (see Dig); Digoxigenin (-labelled oligonucleotide/ riboprobe); Digoxin Investigation Group (trial); Disablement Income Group; Drug-induced galactorrhea/ glaucoma (from diuretics such as acetazolamide, etc.).

Dig Digitalis/ Digoxin (= DIG; dig).

dig digitalis/ digoxin (see Dig); let it be digested (L. digeretur).

digit- combining form meaning finger or toe (L. digitus).

DIH Died in hospital; Diploma in Industrial Health; Diuretic-induced hypokalemia/ hypomagnesemia/ hyponatremia; Drug-induced hepatitis/ hypotension.

DIHE Drug-induced hepatic encephalopathy.

diHETE Dihydroxyeicosatetraenoic acid.

DIHom Diploma of the Institute of Homeopathy.

DIHPPA Diiodohydroxyphenylpyruvic acid.

DIHT Drug-induced hepatotoxicity.

16α,18-dihydroxy-DOC 16α,18-dihydroxy-deoxycorticosterone.

DII Dense inflammatory infiltrate; Drug-induced illness (see DID).

DIIT Diabetes Institute for Immunology and Transplantation (Univ. of Minnesota, USA).

DIJ Drug-induced jaundice; Drug Information Journal (DIA).

DIJOA Dominantly inherited juvenile optic atrophy.

DIL Dilantin (see Dil); Drug-induced lupus (see DILE).

Dil Dilantin (= diphenylhydantoin) - used in the treatment of epilepsy (= DIL).

dil dilatation/late(d) (= dilat); dilute(d)/tion (L. dilue, dilutus) (= dild; diln; dilut); dilution (ratio; unit of).

dilat dilatation/late(d) (see dil).

DILC Dialysis-induced leg cramps (= DLC).

DILD Diffuse infiltrative lung disease.

dild diluted (see dil).

DILE Drug-induced lupus erythematosus.

Dillie Dilaudid (= dihydro-morphine hydrochloride) (see Papaver).

diln dilution (see dil).

Diluc; diluc At daybreak (L. diluculo).

dilut dilute(d)/tion (see dil).

DIM Decreased/ Diminished infant mortality (see DCM); Department of Internal Medicine; Divalent ion metabolism; Medium infective dose (L. dosis infectionis media) (see MID).

Dim Dimension (= dim).

dim dimension (see Dim); diminished/ diminutive (L. diminutus); one-half (L. dimidius).

D-IM Diplomate - American Board of Internal Medicine (= Dip).

DIMA Device for Multi-Analysis.

DIME Division of International Medical Education.

DIMIT 3,5-dimethyl-3'-isopropyl-L-thyronine.

DIMOAD Diabetes insipidus, diabetes mellitus, optic atrophy, deafness.

DIMS Disorders of initiating and maintaining sleep.

DIN Dental Industry News (journal); Drug-induced neurogenesis.

din damage inducible (gene).
DINF Do-It-Now Foundation (drugs).
D-in-L Daughter-in-law.
d in p aeq; d in p ae; d in par aeq divide/ let it be divided into equal parts (L. divatur/ divide/ dividetur in partes aequales) (= d in p ae; d in par aeq; div in p ae; div in p aeq; div in par aeq).
DIO Diet-induced obesity.
1,25-diOHCC 1,25-dihydroxy-cholecalciferol.
DIOP Isopropylidene-dihydroxy-bis-diphenylphosphino butane.
Diop Diopter.
DIP Decrement-increment pattern (see CMAP); Desquamative interstitial pneumonia; Dichlorophenol-indophenol; Diffuse interstitial pneumonia; Diisopropyl phosphate; Diisopropylamine (see DIPA); Diisopropylfluoro phosphate; Diphtheria (see Diph); Dipyridamole (see DIPY); Distal interphalangeal (joint) (= IPD); Dose-induction period; Drip infusion pyelogram/raphy; Drug-induced parkinsonism; Dual-in-line package.
Dip Diplomate (see D-IM).
dip diploid; diplotene.
DIPA Diisopropylamine (= DIP).
Dip Amer Bd P&N Diplomate, American Board of Psychiatry and Neurology.
DipBact Diploma in Bacteriology.
DIPC Diffuse interstitial pulmonary calcification.
DipChem Diploma in Chemistry.
DipClinPath Diploma in Clinical Pathology.
DIPD Drug-induced peptic disease (= DIPU).
Diph; diph Diphtheria (= DIP).
Diph-Tet Diphtheria-tetanus (toxoid).
Diph-Tox Diphtheria-toxoid (plain).
Diph-Tox AP Aluminium precipitated diphtheria toxoid.
DIPJ Distal interphalangeal joint.
diplo- prefix meaning two (Gr. diploos).
DipMicrobiol Diploma in Microbiology.
DipSocMed Diploma in Social Medicine.
DIPU Drug-induced peptic ulcer(ation) (e.g. NSAIDs - see DIPD).
DIPY Dipyridamole (DIP; DP; DPM; DPY; Persantin).
DIR Depressed/ Distorted/ Disturbed immune response; Double isomorphous replacement; Durable immune reconstitution (in HIV infection).
Dir Director.
dir direct(ion)/ions (L. directione).
DIRAC Direct action (interactive data management language).
DIRC Drug Information Research Center.
DIRD Drug-induced renal disease.
DIRECT Diabetic Retinopathy Candesartan Trial.
DIRLINE Directory of Information Resources On-Line.
dir prop with proper direction (L. directione propria) (= direct prop).
direct prop See dir prop.
DIRTY *D.* Distance (of fast runs); *I.* Interval (of rest or recovery between fast runs); *R.* Repetitions (of fast runs); *T.* Time (of fast runs); *Y.* Your activity (walking or jogging between fast runs).
DIS Diagnostic Interview Schedule; Direct image storage (SEM); Drug-induced state; Drug-interaction study.
DI-S Debris index, simplified.
Dis; dis disability/bled; discharge(d) (see disch); disease; dislocate(d)/tion (see disl; disloc); dissolve (see diss); dissolved (see dissd); distal/tance/tant (see dist).
dis- prefix meaning apart or away from (L.).
DISC Diagnostic Interview Schedule for Children; Dietary Intervention Study in Children.
disc discontinue(d).
disc- prefix meaning disk (Gr. diskos).
disch discharge(d) (= Dis; dis).
DisChest Diseases of the Chest (journal).
DisChr Disciples of Christ (member).
DISH Diffuse idiopathic skeletal hyperostosis.
DISI Dorsal intercalated segmental instability.
DISIDA Disopropyl-iminodiacetic acid.
disinfect disinfected/tion.
disl; disloc dislocate(d)/tion (= Dis; dis).
dism dismiss(ed).
disod disodium.
D_5 ISOM 5% Dextrose and Isolyte M.
D_5 ISOP 5% Dextrose and Isolyte P.
disord disorder.
Disp Dispensary.

disp dispensary/nsatory/nse(d) (L. dispensa).
dispar (L.) unequal.
Dispens The Dispensatory of the United States of America (book).
DISS Diameter Index Safety System (instrumentation).
diss dissolve (= Dis; dis); dissolved (see dissd).
dissd dissolved (= Dis; dis; diss).
dissem disseminate(d)/tion.
dist distal/tance/tant (= Dis; dis); distill(ed) (L. distilla); distillation (see distn); distribute(d)/ution; disturbance/bed.
dist f distinguished from.
distn distillation (= dist).
DIT Deferoxamine infusion test; Diet-induced thermogenesis; Digital imaging technique; Diiodotyrosine; Drug-induced thrombocytopenia/ toxicity.
DITC p-phenylene-diisothio-cyanate.
dITP Doxyinosine triphosphate.
Ditto Name given to one of two cloned rhesus monkeys (see Neti).
DIV Double inlet ventricle.
Div; div Diverge(nce)/nt; Divide(d)/vision (L. divide) (= divid); Divorce(d).
DIVA Digital intravenous angiography.
DIVBC Disseminated intravascular blood coagulation.
DIVC Disseminated intravascular coagulation.
DIVD Diabetes-induced vascular disease.
DIVH Disseminated intravascular hemolysis.
divid divide(d) (see Div; div).
div in p ae; div in p aeq; div in par aeq divide/ let it be divided into equal parts (see d in p aeq).
DIVOTS Data Input Voice Output Telephone Service/ System.
DJD Degenerative joint disease; Dental Journal Dentaire (Canadian Dental Association).
DJOA Dominant juvenile optic atrophy.
DJS Degenerative joint symptom(s); Dubin-Johnson syndrome.
DJs Dormescent jerks (appearing with sleep apnea).
DK Dark (see dk); Decay; Diabetic ketoacidosis (see DKA); Diet kitchen; Diseased kidney; Dog kidney (cells).
dk dark (= DK); deka.
DKA Diabetic ketoacidosis (= DK); Didn't keep appointment.
DKB Deep knee bends.
DKFZ German Cancer Research Center (Ger. Deutsche Krebsforschungszentrum), Heidelberg, Germany.
dkg decagram/ dekagram (= 10 grams).
DKINM Deutsches Krebsforschungszentrum Institut für Nuklearmedizin (Germany). German Cancer Research Center, Institute for Nuclear Medicine.
dkl decaliter/ dekaliter (= 10 liters).
dkm decameter/ dekameter (= 10 meters).
DKP Dikalium phosphate (= Dibasic kalium/ potassium phosphate).
DKS Deoxyketosteroid; Disseminated Kaposi's sarcoma.
DKT Distal kidney tubule (see DRT).
DKTC Dog kidney tissue culture.
DKV Deer kidney virus.
DL Danger/ Disabled list; De Lee (catheter); Deep lobe; Detection limit; Developmental/ Drug level; Diagnostic laparoscopy; Diastolic length; Difference limen (test/ threshold); Diffusion lung (= Diffusing capacity of the lung) (see D_L); Direct laryngoscopy; Disabled list; Distolingual; Donath-Landsteiner (see D-L; DL antibody); Equimolecular mixture of the dextrorotatory and levorotatory enantimorphs; Lethal dose (L. dosis lethalis) (see LD).
dl; dL deciliter (= decilitre; 10^{-1} liter; 100 ml; one tenth of a liter).
D_L Diffusing capacity of the lung(s) (= DL) (see PFT - D_L).
D-L Donath-Landsteiner (antibody) (= DL) (see DL antibody); Dorsolateral.
DLA Decreased/ Diminished locomotor activity (= LLA); Distolabial (see DLa); Dominant lethal assay.
DLa Distolabial (= DLA).
DLAI; DLaI Distolabioincisal.
DL antibody Donath-Landsteiner antibody (hemolysin/ test) (blood bank/ laboratory) (= DL; D-L).
DLAP; DLaP Distolabiopulpal.
DLB Dementia with Lewy bodies.
DL&B Direct laryngoscopy and bron-

choscopy.

DLBD Diffuse Lewy body disease.

DLC Decompensated liver cirrhosis (see DHC); Dental Laboratory Conference; Dialysis leg cramps (see DILC); Differential leukocyte count; Double/ Dual lumen catheter.

DLCO; D_LCO; DL_{CO} Diffusing capacity of the lungs for carbon monoxide (= Carbon monoxide diffusion in the lung; Single-breath diffusing capacity [see DLCO-SB]; Total lung capacity ratio) (see PFT - DLCO).

DLCO-SB; $DL_{CO\text{-}SB}$; DL_{CO}SB Single-breath diffusing capacity of the lungs for carbon monoxide (= DLCO) (see PFT - DLCO-SB).

DLCO-SS; $DL_{CO\text{-}SS}$; DL_{CO}SS Steady-state diffusing capacity of the lungs for carbon monoxide (see PFT - DLCO-SS).

DLD Decompensated liver disease (see IHF); Division of Lung Disease (NHLI).

DLE Delayed light emission; Dialyzable leukocyte extract; Discoid/ Disseminated lupus erythematosus; Disulfiram-like effects (of alcohol oxidation, such as abdominal cramps, nausea, vomiting, headache, or flushing of the face from acetaldehyde accumulation).

D_1 LE Diagonal 1 lower extremity.

D_2 LE Diagonal 2 lower extrmity.

DLF Difference limens for frequency; Digitalis-like factor; Disabled Living Foundation; Dorsolateral funiculus.

DLG Distolingual groove.

DLHP Dual-lock hip prosthesis (DuPuy).

DLI Distolinguoincisal; Double label index.

DLIF Digoxin-like immunoreactive factors.

DLIS Digoxin-like immunoreactive substance.

DLK Dorsolumbar kyphosis.

DLL Dihomo-gammalinoleic acid.

DLLI Dulcitol lysine lactose iron (agar).

DLM Disturbed lipid metabolism; Drug-level monitor(ing).

DLMP Date of last menstrual period.

DLN Double-lumen needle (e.g. to accomodate a fetoscope and a laser fiber) (Obstetrics).

DLNMP Date of last normal menstrual period.

DLO Diploma in Laryngology and Otology; Distolinguo-occlusal.

D_{LO2} Diffusing capacity of the lungs for oxygen.

DLP Delipidized serum protein (see DSP); Development learning problem(s); Diagnostic lumbar puncture; Direct linear plotting; Dislocation of patella; Distolinguopulpal; Dorsal lithotomy position (Obs/Gyn); Dysharmonic luteal phase; Dyslipoproteinemi; Isotactic polypropylene.

DLR Disulfiram-like reaction ("Antabuse").

D_5LR Dextrose in 5% lactated Ringer's solution.

DLS Daily living skills; Dorso-lumbar support.

DLT Dental Laboratory Technician; Dihydroepiandrosterone loading test; Dominant lethal test (in laboratory animals); Dose-limiting toxicity.

DLT_{36} Distal latency time at 36°.

DLV Defective leukemia virus.

DLW Dry lung weight.

Dly Daily.

DM Deficience Mentale (CAMR journal); Dental Management (journal); Dermatomyositis; Descemet's membrane; Dextromaltose; Dextromethorphan; Diabetes mellitus; Diabetic mother; Diastolic murmur; Difference of the means; Diffusing capacity of a membrane; Digital mammography; Diphenylamine-arsine chloride (Adamsite - a war gas) (see DA); Disease-A-Month (journal); Distal metastases; Doctor of Medicine (L. Doctor Medicinae) (see MD); Dopamine (see DA); Dorsomedial (see D-M); Dose modification; Double membrane/ minute (chromosome); Duodenal mucosa; Dry matter; Dystrophia myotonica (an autosomal dominant, hereditary hypotrichosis with myotonia and muscle wasting {onset in the third decade}, dry skin and loss of subcutaneous fat) (= SD - Steinert's disease).

dm decimeter (= 10 cm; one tenth of a meter); dorsomedial (see D-M).

D_m Membrane component of diffusion.

D-M Dorso-medial (= DM; dm).

DM2 Type 2 diabetes mellitus.

dm^2 square decimeter.

dm^3 cubic decimeter.

DMA Decreased/ Diminished mental acuity; Dimethylacetal; Dimethyladenosine; Dimethyladipimidate; Dimethylamine; Dimethylaniline; Dimethylarginine; Dimethylnaphthylamine (see DMANA); Direct memory access (computer).

DMAB; DMABA Dimethylaminobenzaldehyde.

DMAC N,N-dimethylacetamide.

DMAD Disease-modifying antirheumatic drug (see DMARD).

DMAE Dimethylaminoethanol.

DMAM Dimethylaminomethylene.

DM-ANA N,N-dimethyl-1-naphthylamin (= DMA).

4DMAP 4-dimethylaminophenol.

DMAPN Dimethylaminoproprionitrile.

DMARD Disease-modifying anti-rheumatic drug(s) - such as gold salts, antimalarial agents (e.g. hydroxychloroquine), methotrexate, cyclosporin, interferon, interleukin, etc.

DMB Department of Medical Bacteriology; Department of Molecular Biology.

dMb Disseminated (non-tuberculous) mycobacteriosis).

DMBC Department of Molecular Biology and Chemistry (TSRI).

DMBA Dimethylbenzathracene [= 7,12-dimethylbenz(a)anthracene]; Dimethylbenzylamine.

DMC Dactinomycin, methotrexate, and cyclophosphamide; Demeclocycline; Di(p-chlorophenyl)methylcarbinol (see DCPC); Depressive mood change(s); Dimethylcarbinol (an insecticide); Dimite (an acaricide) - [1,1-bis(p-chlorophenyl)ethanol]; Dimethylcysteine (= Penicillamine) - used in the treatment of copper and lead poisoning, and in Wilson's disease; Direct microscopic count; Division of Medicinal Chemistry (ACS); Double minute chromosome (= Minichromosome); Down-state Medical College (New York); Duration of muscle contraction; Dysplastic myeloid cell (in myelodysplasia).

DMCC Direct microscopic clump count.

DMCDX Desmethylchlordiazepoxide - the major metabolite of chlorodiazepoxide (CDX), and a benzodiazepine tranquillizer.

DMCL N-dimethylclindamycin; Dimethylclomipramine.

DMCS Dimethylchlorosilane; Dimethyl-dichlorosilane (see DMDCS).

DMCT; DMCTC Dimethylchlortetracycline (= Demeclocycline HCl) - an antibiotic produced from the growth of Streptomyces aureofaciens.

DMD Degenerative muscle/ muscular disease; Department of Membership Development; Depressive mood disturbance; Disease-modifying drug; Doctor of Dental Medicine; Duchenne's muscular dystrophy (= Pseudohypertrophic muscular dystrophy) (= PMD); Dystonia musculorum deformans.

DMDC Dimethyldithiocarbamate.

DMDCS Dimethyl-dichlorosilane (= DMCS).

DMDS Dimethyl-disulfide.

DMDT Dimethoxydiphenyl trichloroethane (= Dimethoxy-DT; Marlate; Methoxychlor; Methoxy-DDT) - a chlorinated insecticide.

DMDZ Desmethyldiazepam.

DME Degenerative myoclonus epilepsy; Diabetic macular edema; Dimethoxyethane; Dimethyl diester/ diether; Diphasic meningoencephalitis; Director/ Doctor of Medical Education; Dolichomegaesophagus; Dropping mercury electrode; Drug-metabolizing enzyme; Dulbecco's modified Eagle's (medium) (see DMEM); Durable medical equipment.

DMEM Department of Molecular and Experimental Medicine (TSRI); Dulbecco's modified Eagle's medium (= DME).

DMEZ Drug metabolizing enzyme system (e.g. Cytochrome P450-linked).

DMF Decayed, missing, and filled (teeth) (in dentistry, a formula representing the number of decayed, missing, and filled permanent teeth); Depressed myocardial function; N,N-dimethylformamide; Diphasic milk fever.

DMF rate Decayed-Missing-Filled teeth rate (see DMF).

DMFS Decayed, missing, filled surfaces (see DMF).

DMFT Decayed, missing, filled teeth (see DMF).

DMG 6-demethyl griseofulvin; Department of Medical Genetics; Dimethylglycin;

Dimethylglyoxime (spot test for nickel); Dominant mutant gene; Dosage/ Dose Modification Guideline(s).

DMGBL Dimethyl-gammabutyrolactone.

DMGG Metformin (= N,N-dimethyldiguanide hydrochloride; LA 6023) - an oral anti-diabetic agent (see LA 6023).

DMH Department of Mental Health; Department of mental hygiene; Diffuse mesangial hypercellularity (see DMP); Dorsal/ Dorso medial hypothalamus.

DMHA Directional microphone hearing aid.

DMHO Disease Management & Health Outcomes (journal).

DMHP Dimethylheptyl pyran.

DMHS Director Medical and Health Services.

DMI Defence Mechanism Inventory; Desmethylimipramine (= Desipramine HCl; GMI; JB 8181) - an antidepressant drug similar to imipramine; Diagnostic Medical Instruments; Diaphragmatic myocardial infarction; Direct migration inhibition; Disseminated mycotic infection; Duodenal mucosal injury.

DMID Diagnostic Microbiology and Infectious Diseases (journal).

dmil decimil (= decimilliliter; 10^{-1} ml; 1/10 cc; 0.1 cc; 10^{-4} liter).

dmin double minute.

DMJ Diploma in Medical Jurisprudence.

DMKA Diabetes mellitus ketoacidosis.

DML Distal motor latency.

DMM Decreased/ Diminished muscle mass; Desmethyl metabolite (of Esomeprazole) (see HMM); Dimethylmyleran; Disproportionate micromelia; Disseminated malignant melanoma; Dry mucous membrane.

DM2-MV Type 2 diabetes mellitus - macrovascular (disease).

DMN Diabetic mononeuropathy; Dimethylnitrosamine (see DMNA); Dorsal motor nucleus; Dysplastic melanocytic nevus.

DMNA Dimethylnitrosamine (= N-nitroso-dimethylamine) - a carcinogen (= DMN).

DMNL Dorsomedial hypothalamic nucleus lesion.

DMO Dimethyl-oxazolidine-dione (= 5,5-dimethyl-2,4-oxazolidine-dione; Dimethadione); District Medical Officer.

D_{mO2} Membrane diffusing capacity for oxygen.

DMOA Diabetes mellitus - optic atrophy (syndrome).

DMOOC Diabetes mellitus out of control.

DMOS Double-diffused metal-oxide semiconductor.

DMP Decision-making process; Dental Market Place (journal); Diffuse mesangial proliferation (see DMH); Dimercaprol; Dimethylphosphate; Dimethylphthalate (an insect repellent).

DMPA Depo-medroxy-progesterone/ Depot medroxyprogesterone acetate.

DMPE; DMPEA Dimethoxyphenyl-ethyl-amine (see 3,4-DMPEA).

3,4-DMPEA 3,4-dimethoxy-phenyl-ethyl-amine (= DMPE; DMPEA).

DMPOPOP Dimethyl-paraphenylene-phenyloxazole (= Paraphenylene-methyl-phenyl-oxazole) (scintillator).

DMPP Dimethylphenylpiperazinium.

DMPS 2,3-Dimercapto-1-propane sulfonate (water soluble analogue of dimercaptol [BAL]) - used in the treatment of inorganic mercury poisoning (see DMSA - Dimercaptosuccinic acid); Dysmyelopoietic syndrome (= DMS).

DMR Deuteron magnetic resonance; Diploma in Medical Radiology; Drug Metabolism Reviews (journal).

DMRD Diploma in Medical Radio-Diagnosis (UK).

DMRE Diploma in Medical Radiology and Electrology.

DMRF Dorsal medullary reticular formation.

DMRHD Daily maximum recommended human dose.

DMRI Diffusion magnetic resonance imaging.

DMRT Diploma in Medical Radio-Therapy; Doppelt mathematical reasoning test.

DMS Dartmouth Medical School; Delayed match-to-sample; Delayed micro-embolism syndrome; Demarcation membrane system; Department of Medicine and Surgery (see DM&S); Dermatomyositis; Diffuse mesangial sclerosis; Dimethyl-suberimidate; Dimethylsulfate; Dimethylsulfide; Dimethylsulfoxide (see DMSO); Direct medical supervision; Director/ Doctor of Medical Services (Armed Forces); District Management Service; Division of Medical Sciences (NAS-NRC); Doctor of Medical Science (see DMSc); Dysmorphic syndrome (= MFS - Malformation syndrome); Dysmyelopoietic syndrome (see DMPS).

DMs Doctor of Metaphysics (= MsD).

DM&S Department of Medicine and Surgery (= DMS).

DMSA Dimercaptosuccinic acid; Disodium monomethanearsonate.

DMSc Doctor of Medical Science (= DMS; MEDScD; MScD; MSD).

DMSO Dimethylsulfoxide (= DMS; Methyl sulfoxide; SQ 9453). Used as an industrial solvent for organic and inorganic chemicals. Also used in medicine as a solvent for Idoxuridine (IDU) in topical preparations; also as a linament in arthritis.

DMSS Director of Medical and Sanitary Services.

DMSSP Dithio-bis-dimethyl-propioimidate.

DMSSS Department of Medicine and Surgery Supply Service (VA).

DMT Dermatophytosis; Dimethyl-terephthalate; N,N-dimethyl-tryptamine (= BMLH); Diploma in Medical Technology (= MTD); Disease-modifying therapy; Disruptive muscular trauma; District Management Team; Doctor of Medical Technology; *Drosophila* melanogaster (the Vinegar-fly) test (a sex-linked recessive lethal mutation test on Fruit-flies); Drug monitoring technique.

DMTU Dimethylthiourea.

DMU Data management unit; Dimethanolurea.

DMV Damaged mitral valve; Doctor of Veterinary Medicine.

DMWP Distal mean wave pressure.

DMX Diathermy, massage, and exercise.

DN Deiter's nucleus; Dextrose/nitrogen (ratio) (see D/N); Diabetes in the News (journal); Diabetic nephropathy (see CFD, DNP); Diabetic neuropathy; Diagnosis News (see IMNDN); Dibucaine number; Dicrotic notch; Dinitrocresol (see DNOC); Diploma in Nursing/ Nutrition; Director/ Doctor of Nursing; District Nurse; Doctor of Naturopathy (= ND); Down; Dysplastic nevus.

Dn Dekanem (= 10 nems) (see nem).

dn decinem (= 10^{-1} nem; one tenth of a nem), i.e. the nutritive value of 1 decigram of milk.

D/N Dextrose/nitrogen (ratio), i.e. the ratio of urinary dextrose to nitrogen (= DN; D/N R; D:N Ratio) (see G/N).

D&N Distance and near (vision).

DNA Defense Nuclear Agency; Deoxyribonucleic acid (= Animal nucleic acid; Desoxypentose nucleic acid; Desoxyribonucleic acid; Desoxyribose nucleic acid; dorna; DRNA; DS; DSRNA; Thymus nucleic acid). In France, known as ADN. DNA is a nucleotide polymer found in the cell nuclei of living tissue, consisting of a number of chemical building blocks - a sugar, a phosphate and four bases, adenine (A), cytosine (C), guanine (G), and thymine (T): A-T:G-C. In DNA's precise architecture, the famed double helix unraveled by Watson and Crick in 1953, lies the secret of how the molecule conveys the message of heredity from one generation to the next. The twisted double-stranded DNA resembles a spiral staircase, with each step formed by a pair of bases - A always binding with T, G always with C, acting very much like a computer tape. Every three steps serve as a code word for one of the 20 essential aminoacids found in all life on earth. Strings of code words in turn, provide the sequence for linking these aminoacids into proteins, the basic building blocks of living things. DNA thus carries the entire genetic blueprint for assembling any organism, from bacterium to man (see RNA; rDNA or Recombinant DNA); Did not answer/ attend; Does not apply.

DNA/G Deoxyribonucleic acid content per genome.

DNAP Deoxyribonucleic acid phophorus; Dinosam {= DNOSAP; DNSAP; 2-(1-methylbutyl)-4,6-dinitrophenol} - an insecticide derivative of dinitrophenol.

DNAPI Deoxyribonucleic acid polymerase inhibitor (e.g. Acyclovir, Valaciclovir, etc.).

DNAR Decision not to attempt resuscitation (order - UK).

DNA-RA Deoxyribonucleic acid-repair assay.
DNA-RG Deoxyribonucleic acid-repair gene.
DNAse; DNase Deoxyribonuclease.
DNAse B; DNase B Deoxyribonuclease B.
DNAV DNA vaccine (see DNA).
DNB Digital nerve block; Dinitrobenzene; Diplomate of the National Board (of Medical Examiners); Doctor's Nurse Bulletin (AADN journal); Dorsal non-adrenergic bundle.
DNBC Dinitrobenzoyl chloride.
DNBP Dinitrobutyl phenol (= Dinitro-o-s-butyl-phenol; Dinoseb; DNOSBP; DNSBP; 2-s-butyl-4,6-dinitrophenol) - an insecticide derivative of dinitrophenol.
DNC Damaged nerve cell; Damaged/ Decreased/ Defective/ Diminished/ Disturbed nerve conduction; Did not come; Dinitrocarbanilide (see DNOC); Dinitrocresol (see DNOC); Disaster Nursing Chairman.
DNCB Dinitrochlorobenzene (= Dinitrochlorbenzene) - used externally in the treament of warts.
DND Degenerative neurological disease; Diabetic nerve damage (see DN - Diabetic neuropathy); Died a natural death; Do not disturb.
dNDP Deoxyribonucleoside diphosphate.
DNE Director/ Doctor of Nursing Education; Dorsal norepinephrine.
DNFA Dinitrofluoroaniline.
DNFB Dinitrofluorobenzene.
DNH Daily nasal hygiene.
DNHW Department of National Health and Welfare (Canada).
DNI Do not intubate.
DNIP Dinitroiodophenyl.
DNK Did not keep (appointment).
DNKA Did not keep appointment.
DNLL Dorsal nucleus of lateral lemniscus.
dNMP Deoxyribonucleoside monophosphate.
DNMS Director of Naval Medical Services.
DNO District Nursing Officer.
DNOC Dinitro-ortho-cresol/ Dinitrocresol (= Dekrysil; Dinitrocarbanilide; Ditrosol; DN; DNC; Effusan; K III; K IV; 2-methyl-4,6-dinitrophenol; Prokarbol) - an insecticide derivative of dinitrophenol.
DNOCHP Dinitro-o-cyclohexyl-phenol (= 2-cyclohexyl-4,6-dinitrophenol; Dinex; SN 46) - an insecticide derivative of dinitrophenol.
DNOIPP Dinitro-o-isopropyl-phenol (= Dinoprop; 2-isopropyl-3-methyl-4,6-dinitrophenol) - an insecticide derivative of dinitrophenol.
DNOSAP Dinosam (see DNAP).
DNOSBP Dinoseb (see DNBP).
DNP Deoxyribonucleoprotein (Deoxyribonucleic acid protein); Diabetic nephropathy (see CFD, DN)/ neuropathy (= DN); Diiodonitrophenol; Dinitrophenol (see 2,4-DNP); 2-4-dinitrophenyl (group); Dinitrophenylhydrazine (see DNPH); Do not publish.
2,4-DNP 2,4-Dinitrophenol (= DNP).
DNPA Dineopentyl acetal.
DNP-CAP-PE Dinitrophenylamino-caproyl-phosphatidyl-ethanolamine.
DNPH Dinitrophenylhydrazine.
DNPM Dinitrophenol-morphine (= Dinitrophenylmorphine).
DNR Daunorubicin (= Daunomycin) (see Dauno); Did not respond; Do not report/ resuscitate; Dorsal nerve root.
D/N R Dextrose-to-nitrogen ratio (see D/N).
D:N Ratio Ratio of glucose (dextrose) to nitrogen in (diabetic) urine (see D/N).
DNS Delayed neurological sequelae; Deviated nasal septum; Diaphragmatic nerve stimulation; Do/Did not show (for appointment); Dinitrosalicylate; Dinoyl sebacate; Diseases of the Nervous System (EPA journal); Doctor of Nursing Services; Doyle nasal splint (nasal reconstruction); Dysplastic nevus syndrome.
D-NS Diplomate - Neurosurgery (American Board of).
D_5 1/2NS Dextrose 5% in 0.45% sodium chloride (injection).
DNSAP Dinosam (see DNAP).
DNSG Diabetes and Nutrition Study Group (Israel).
DNSP Doctor did not see patient.
D_5NSS; D_5/NSS Dextrose (5%) in normal saline solution (for IV use).
DNT Damaged/ Decreased/ Defective/ Diminished/ Disturbed neuromuscular transmission (see ANT); Did not test; Doctor/nurse team; Dopaminergic neurotransmission.

DNTC Dimethyl-amino-naphthyl isothiocyanate.

DNTM Disseminated non-tuberculous mycobacterial (infection).

DNTP Diethyl-nitrophenyl thiophosphate (= Diethyl p-nitrophenyl phosphorothionate; E 605; Etilon; Niran; Paraphos; Parathion; SNP). Parathion is a well-known, widely used, organophosphorus insecticide.

dNTP Deoxyribonucleoside triphosphate.

DNU Diabetic neuropathic ulcer.

DNV Dorsal nucleus of vagus nerve.

DO Diabetes Outlook (journal); Diamine oxidase; Diet order; Digoxin; Diploma in Ophthalmology/ Osteopathy; Dispensing Optician (UK, ADO journal); Dissolved oxygen; Disto-occlusal; Doctor of Ophthalmology/ Optometry/ Osteopathy; Doctor's orders; Documenta Ophthalmologica; Drugs only (visits).

do as before/ ditto/ the same (L. dictum) (see Symbols - 5-do).

D_o Diffusing capacity of oxygen/ Oxygen diffusion (see PFT - D_o).

D-O Diplomate - Ophthalmology (of the American Board of); Directive-organic (psychiatrist).

D/O Disorder.

D_2O Deuterium oxide (Heavy water).

D_{O2} Oxygen delivery.

DOA Date of admission (see DoA); Dead on arrival (= BID) (see DoA); Department of Agriculture; Differential optical absorption; Dominant optic atrophy; Duration of action (see DoA).

DoA Date of admission (= DOA); Dead on arrival (= BID; DOA); Dissection of the aorta; Duration of action (= DOA).

DOAC Dubois oleic albumin complex (bacteriology).

DOA-DRA Dead on arrival despite resuscitative attempts.

DOB Dangle out of bed; Date of birth; (R- and S-) Desethyloxybutinin (a pharmacologically active metabolic product of the antispasmodic, anticholinergic agent, Oxybutinin) (see PCHGA); Distal occlusal buccal (tooth); Dobutamine; Doctor's order book.

DObstRCOG Diploma of the Royal College of Obstetricians and Gynaecologists (= DRCOG).

DOC Date of conception; Deoxycholate; Deoxycorticosterone (see DOCA); Department of Commerce (see DoC); Diabetes out of control; Died of other causes; Disorders of cornification; Dissolved organic carbon; Drug of choice.

DoC Department of Commerce (= DOC).

Doc; doc Doctor; Document(ation).

DOCA Desoxycorticosterone acetate (= 21-acetoxypregn-4-ene-3,20-dione; $C_{23}H_{32}O_4$; Decortone/ Deoxycorticosterone/ Deoxycortone/ Desoxycortone acetate; Deoxycort acet; Desoxycortoni acetas; DOC) (see Hormones - CS).

DOCG Deoxycorticosterone glucoside.

DOCLINE Documents On-Line.

DOCS Deoxycorticoids; Deoxycorticosteroids.

DOcSc Doctor of Ocular Science.

DOD Daily oral dose; Date of death (see DoD); Dead/ Diead of disease (see DoD); Dementia (syndrome) of depression; Dissolved oxygen deficit; Drug over-dose.

DoD Date of death (= DOD); Dead/ Died of disease (= DOD); Department of Defence/ Dietetics; Director of development; Division of Dentistry (HRD).

Δ OD 450 Deviation of optical density at 450.

DOE Date of examination; Department of Energy; Desoxyephedrine; Direct observation evaluation (test); Dyspnea on exercise/ exertion; Taking illicit drugs (origin of abbreviation unknown).

DOES Disorder(s) of excessive sleepiness/ somnolescence.

DOET Dimethoxyethyl amphetamine (= 2,5-dimethoxy-4-ethyl amphetamine) (see Amphet - DOET).

DoF Degree(s) of freedom (i.e. of movement) (= DF; df).

DOFOS Disturbance of function occlusion syndrome.

DOG Department of Obstetrics and Gynecology.

D-OG Diplomate - American Board of Obstetrics and Gynecology.

dogie heroin (see Diamorph).

DOH; DoH Department of Health.
1,25 D, OHCC 1,25 dihydroxy-cholecalciferol (a form of cholecalciferol: vitamin D3) (see Vitamins - D3).
DOI Date of injury; Demineralized osseous implant (Orthopedics); Died of injuries.
DoI Department of the Interior.
DOJ Department of Justice.
DOL Distal occlusal lingual (tooth).
DoL Department of Labor.
Dol; dol Pain (L. dolor) - a unit of pain intensity.
D-OL Diplomate - American Board of Otolaryngology.
DOL #2 Second day of life.
DOLD Diffuse obstructive lung disease.
doll Amphetamine or barbiturate pill (see Amphet; Barb).
dollie Dolophine pill (= Methadone hydrochloride).
DOLLS Double-loop locking suture (Lee's).
Dolly Name given to the world's first cloned sheep (= Lamb 6 LL3).
DOLV Double outlet left ventricle.
DOM Deaminated-O-methyl metabolite; Department of Medicine; Dimethoxymethyl amphetamine (= BZ; 2-5-dimethoxy-4-methyl-amphetamine; Methyldimethoxy-methylphenethylamine; STP) (see Amphet - DOM); Dissolved organic matter; Division of Medicine (HRD); Dominance/ant (see dom); Dysostosis multiplex (a syndrome of radiological abnormalities in MPS or Mucopolysaccharidoses disorders).
dom domestic; dominance/ant (= DOM).
DOMA Dihydro(xy) mandelic acid.
DOMF 2'7'-dibromo-4'-(hydroxymercuri)fluorescein (= Merbromin).
DOMS Diploma in Ophthalmic Medicine and Surgery.
DON Diazo-oxonorleucine (= Diazooxo-L-norleucine); Director/ Division of Nursing (HRD).
don until (L. donec).
don alv sol ft; donec alv sol fuerit until the bowels are open(ed), i.e. until a bowel movement takes place (L. donec alvus soluta fuerit).
doojie heroin (see Diamorph).
DOOR Deafness, onycho-osteodystrophy, (mental) retardation (syndrome).
DOP Dopamine (see DA; DOPA).
Dop Doppler.
DOPA; dopa Dihydroxyphenylalanine (= 3:4-dihydroxy-phenylalanine; Laevo-DOPA; L-dihydroxyphenylalanine; L-DOPA) - a transmitter amine, being an intermediate product in the synthesis of ephedrine and melanin, with unequivocal antidepressant activity in man (= dopa). The major metabolic pathways of the transmitter amines, NA (Noradrenaline), DA (Dopamine), and 5-HT (5-Hydroxytryptamine) (see Scheme).
DOPAC Dihydroxy-phenyl acetic acid (= Dihydrophenylacetic acid; 3,4-hydroxyphenyl acetic acid).
DOPAD L-dopa decarboxylase.
DOPAMINE Dihydroxy-phenyl-ethylamine (see DA; DM; DOPA) (see Scheme).
dopase; DOPAse dopa oxidase (= Dihydroxyphenylalanine oxidase).
DOPC Determined osteogenic precursor cell.
DOph Doctor of Ophthalmology.
DOPP Dihydroxyphenylpyruvate (= Dihydroxy-phenyl-pyruvic acid).
DOPS Diffuse obstructive pulmonary syndrome; Dihydroxyphenylserine.
DOPS$_i$ Irreversible diffuse obstructive pulmonary syndrome.
DOR Drop-out rate.
DoR Detachment of the retina.
dor dorsal (see Dors).
DORIS Doctor Registration Inquiry Service (UK).
DORNA; dorna Desoxyribonucleic acid (= Desoxyribose nucleic acid) (see DNA).
Dors Dorsal (= dor).
dors- combining form meaning back (L. dorsum).
dorsum rotundum Latin - rotational deformity of the spine.
DOrth Diploma in Orthodontics/ Orthoptics.
DORV Double outlet right ventricle.
DORx Date of treatment.
DOS Day of surgery; Deoxystreptamine; Department of Orthopedic Surgery; Disk operating system (computer); Division of Operational Safety; Doctor of Ocular/ Optical

DOPAMINE (and the major metabolic pathways of the transmitter amines)

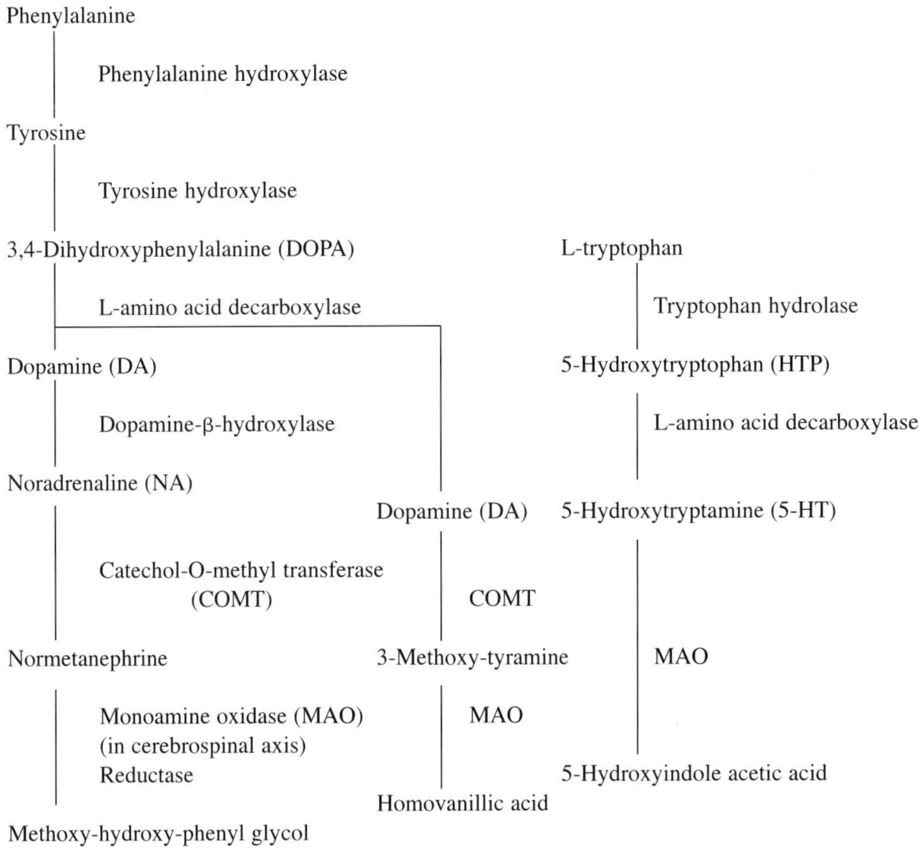

Science; Dosage (see dos).
dos dosage; dose (L. dosis).
D-OS Diplomate - American Board of Orthopedic Surgery.
DOSC Dubois oleic serum complex (bacteriology).
DOSS Distal over-shoulder strap; Dioctyl sodium sulfosuccinate; Docusate sodium.
DOT Date of transcription/ transfer; Dictionary of Occupational Titles (US Dept of Labor Employment Service); Died on table; Domain-tip technology (computer); Domiciliary occupational therapist/py; Doppler ophthalmic test.
DoT Department of Transportation.
DOTC Dameshek's oval target cell; Diethyloxatricarbo-cyanine.
DOTS Directly Observed Treatment, Short-course (of Tuberculosis).
dowager hump spinal deformity due to osteoporosis in post-menopausal women (= dromedary hump).
downer barbiturate (see Barb).
Dox Doxorubicin.
Doxy Doxycycline.
doz dozen (= 12; twelve).
DP Data processing; 'Dawn phenomenon' (increase of blood sugar or hyperglycemia in the early morning hours: a problem in the treatment of diabetes); Deep pulse; Definitive procedure; Degredation product; Degree of polymerization; Dementia praecox/ pugillisti-

ca; Dental Practice (UK journal); Dental Practitioner (journal, now J of Dentistry); Dental prosthodontics/ prosthesis; Dermatology in Practice (journal); Developmental Psychology (journal); Dexamethasone pretreatment; Dew point; Diastolic/ Diffusion pressure; Diffuse precipitation; Digestible protein; Diphosgene (a war gas); Diphosphate; Dipropionate; Dipyridamole (see DIPY); Directional preponderance; Disability pension; Discharge papers (see DS); Discharge planning. Discrimination power; Disopyramide phosphate; Displaced person; Disrhythmic phonation; Distal pancreatectomy/ phalanx/ pit; Distopulpal; Doctor of Pharmacy/ Podiatry; Donor's/ Dried plasma; Dorsal premammilary (nucleus); Dorsalis pedis (artery/ pulse); With proper direction (L. directione propria).

Dp Dyspnea.

D_p pattern difference.

DPA Data Protection Act 1998 (GMC, Britain); Department of Public Assistance; Dichloropropionanilide; Dihydroxy-progesterone acetate; Diphenadione (an anticoagulant); Diphenolic acid; Diphenylalanine; Diphenylamine; Dipicolinic/ Docosapentaenoic acid; Dipropylacetate/acetic acid; Dorsalis pedis artery; D-penicillamine (see D-PA); Dual photo(n) absorptiometry; Dynamic physical activity.

D-PA D-penicillamine (= DPA); Diplomate - American Board of Pathology.

DPB Days post-burn; Diffuse panbronchiolitis; Diphenylbenzene (acid); Dynamic patellar brace (Palumbo).

DPBC Depolarizing bipolar cell.

DPBP Diphenylbutylpiperidine.

DPBS Department of Psychiatry and Behavioral Sciences.

DPC Day-patient care/ clinic; Debilitating prolonged convalescence; Delayed primary closure; Desaturated phosphatidylcholine; Desert Protective Council; Diethylpyrocarbonate; Direct patient care; Discharge planning coordinator; Distal palmar crease; Division of Poison Control (OPS/FDA).

DPC4 Depleted in pancreatic cancer (= Smad4) - signalling molecule or tumor-suppressor gene.

DPCL 1'-dimethyl-dipropyl clindamycin.

DPCM Digital pulse-code modulation.

DPCMS Dynamic Processes in Condensed Molecular Systems.

DPCRT Double-blind placebo-controlled randomized clinical trial.

DPD Department of Public Dispensary (UK); Depression pure disease; Depressive pseudodementia (= Affective psychosis); Desoxypyridoxine; Diethylphenylenediamine; Diffuse pulmonary disease; Dihydropyrimidine dehydrogenase; Diphenamid; Diploma in Public Dentistry; Distal phalangeal depth; Dual-photon densitometer/metry (of bones, etc.); Dysfunctional prolonged delivery (Obstetrics).

DPDA Phosphoro-diamidic anhydride.

DPD/IPD Distal phalangeal/interphalangeal depth (width) ratio.

DPDL Diffuse poorly differentiated (lymphocytic) lymphoma.

DPDT Dichotic pitch discrimination test (= DPT).

dpdt double-pole, double-throw (switch).

dp/dt diastolic pressure/ diastolic time (= a measure of left ventricular cardiac contractility/ stroke work, a first derivative of left ventricular pressure development, or a ratio of change of left ventricular pressure to change in time).

dp/dt/p/max peak first derivative of pressure.

DPE Dipiperidinoethane; Dipivalyl epinephrine; Doctor/patient encounter (= PPE) (see DPR); Drip-proof equipment (MET-501).

DPer/Vac Diphtheria and Pertussis Vaccine (= Diphtheria-Whooping cough Prophylactic) - a mixture of Diphtheria Vaccine Formol Toxoid and Pertussis Vaccine, used for active immunization against diphtheria and whooping cough, and may be substituted for the constituent prophylactics.

DPF Defective platelet formation/function; Dental Practitioners' Formulary; Dilsopropyl fluorophosphate.

DPFC Distal palmar flexion crease.

DPFR Diastolic pressure-flow relationship.

DPG Diffuse proliferative glomerulonephritis (see DGN); Diphosphoglycerate (= 2,3-diphospho-glycerate) (see 2,3-DPG); Displacement placentogram.

2,3-DPG; 2-3 DPG 2,3-Diphosphoglycerate (= DPG; DPGA).

DPGA Diphosphoglycerate (see 2,3-DPG).

DPGM Diphospho-glycero-mutase (see 2,3-DPGM).

2,3-DPGM 2,3-diphosphoglycerate mutase (= Diphospho-glyceromutase; DPGM).

DPGN Diffuse proliferative glomerulonephritis (see DGN).

DPGP Diphosphogylcerate phosphatase.

DPH Department/ Director of Public Health; Diphenhydramine; Diphenylhexatriene; Diphenylhydantoin (Dilantin); Diploma in Public Health; Doctor of Public Health/ Hygiene; Dopamine betahydrolase.

DPh Doctor of Philosophy.

DPHB Department of Psychiatry and Human Behavior.

DPhC Doctor of Pharmaceutical Chemistry.

DPhc Doctor of Pharmacology.

DPHD Duchenne's pseudohypertrophic dystrophy (= PHD).

DPHN Department/ Doctor of Public Health Nursing.

DPHS Department of Public Health Sciences.

DPhys Diploma in Physiotherapy.

DPhysMed Diploma in Physical Medicine.

DPI Daily permissible intake; Days post incubation; Dietary protein intake; Diphtheria-pertussis immunization; Disposable personal income; Dose-proportional increase; Drug prescribing/iption index; Dynamic Personality Inventory.

Dpi Dermatophagoides pteronyssinus (see HDM).

DPJ Dementia paralytica juvenilis.

DPK Dysplastic kidney.

DPKA Defective phosphokinase activity.

DPL Dacron prosthetic ligament (made for shoulder repair); Diagnostic peritoneal lavage; Dipalmitoyl lecithin; Distopulpolingual.

DPLa Distopulpolabial.

DPLGN Diffuse proliferative lupus glomerulonephritis (= DPLN).

DPLN Diffuse proliferative lupus nephritis.

DPM Department of Preventive Medicine; Digital panel meter; Diploma in Psychological Medicine; Discontinue previous medication; Doctor of Physical/ Podiatric/ Preventive/ Psychiatric Medicine; Dipyridamole (see DIPY); Dopamine (see DA); Dose-proportional manner.

dpm disintegrations (radioactivity)/ drops per minute.

D-PM Diplomate - American Board of Physical Medicine.

D-PMR Diplomate - American Board of Physical Medicine and Rehabilitation.

DPN Dermatosis papulosa nigra; Diabetic peripheral neuropathy; Diabetic polyneuropathy; Diphosphopyridine nucleotide (now NAD) (see Co-1); Disabling pansclerotic morphea.

DPNA Diphosphopyridine nucleotide anhydrate.

DPNase Diphosphopyridine nucleonase.

DPNB Dorsal penile nerve block.

DPNH Diphosphopyridine nucleotide-reduced form (= Dihydronicotinamide adenosine dinucleotide; NADH; Nicotinamide adenine dinucleotide reduced; Reduced DPN; Reduced nadide).

DPO Dimethoxyphenyl penicillin.

dP_{O2} Rate of pressure change (see PFT - dP_{O2}).

DPOAE Distortion products otoacoustic emission (see TEOAE).

DPP Defensive Publication Program (US Patent Office); Diabetes Prevention Program; Diabetic pregnant patient (see PDP); Diastolic perfusion pressure; Differential pulse polarography; Dimethylphenyl penicillin; Dysphonia puberum (voice change taking place in teen-age boys).

DPPA Diphenylphosphoryl azide.

DPPC Dipalmitoylphosphatidyl choline; Double-blind placebo-controlled trial.

DPPD Diphenylphenylenediamine (= Diphenyl-p-phenylenediamine).

DPPH Diphenylpicryl hydrate.

DPQ Diphenylbenzoquinone.

DPR Decreased/ Diminished pulmonary reserve; Decreased pupillary reflex; Dental

Products Report (journal); Doctor-patient relation(ship).

D-PR Diplomate - American Board of Proctology.

DPS Data processing system; Descending perineum syndrome; Dimethylpolysiloxane; Division of Pharmaceutical Sciences (FDA); Drug Program Support (CIC - Clinical Interventions Catalogue); Dysesthetic pain syndrome.

dps disintegrations per second (radioactivity).

D-PS Diplomate - American Board of Plastic Surgery.

DPSC Defence Personnel Support Center.

DPSG Diabetes Pregnancy Study Group (EASD).

dpst double-pole, single-throw (switch).

DPT Demerol, Phenergan, and Thorazine; Depth perception test (Ophthalmology = sTt; TST - Titmus stereo test); Diabetic pseudotabes (diabetic neuropathy with associated sensory ataxia); Dichotic pitch (discrimination) test (see DPDT); Differential pressure transducer (used to measure ventilatory flow rate) (see VFR).Diphenylthiourea (= SU 1906; Thiambutos; Thiambutosine; Thiambutoxine; Thiocarbanilide - used in the treatment of leprosy; Diphosphothiamine; Diphtheria-pertussis-tetanus (vaccine); Diphtheritic pseudotabes; Dipropyltryptamine; Dissatisfied Parents Together (against the risks of Pertussis vaccination); Driver Performance Test; Dumping provocation test.

Dpt House dust mite (= Dermatophagoides pteronyssinus) (see HDM).

DPTA Diethylenetriamine penta-acetate/-acetic acid (see DTPA).

DPTI Diastolic pressure time index.

DPTPM Diphtheria, pertussis, tetanus, poliomyelitis, and measles (vaccine).

Dptr Diopter.

DPTZ Dysplasia-prone transition zone (anal/ cervical canal).

DPU Delayed pressure urticaria; Duodenal peptic ulcer.

DPUD Duodenal peptic ulcer disease.

DPV Disabling positional vertigo; Drug plasma value(s) (such as AUC, Cmax, etc.).

DPVS Denver peritoneovenous shunt.

DPW Distal phalangeal width.

DPX Dibutylphthalate (a mounting medium used in bacteriology, replacing Canada balsam).

DPY Dipyridamole (see DIPY).

DQ Deterioration quotient; Developmental quotient (pediatrics).

Dq D quotient - the ratio of glucose to nitrogen in the urine (see KFT - Dq).

D/Q; D-Q Oxygen-diffusing capacity/perfusion (ratio) (see PFT - D/Q, D-Q).

DQD Digital quadrature detection.

DQE Detective quantum efficiency.

DQF Double quartan fever (a form of malaria).

DQV-K Penicillin V-potassium salt.

DR Degeneration reaction (with reference to muscle fibers) (see RD); Delayed release (tablet); Delivery room; Dental Record (journal, now J. of Dentistry); Deoxyribose (see dRib); Depart dose; Detector response; Diabetic retinopathy; Diagnostic radiology; Dining room; Diploma in Radiology; Direct recording/ repeat; Distribution/ Dose ratio; Diurnal rhythm; Doctor (see Dr); Dorsal raphe; Dorsal root (see dr); Dose-/Drug-related; Drug receptor.

Dr Doctor (= DR).

dr dorsal root (of spinal nerve) (= DR); drachm/ dram (symbol: z) - a unit of weight i) in the apothecaries' system: = 60 grains or 1/8 ounce ii) in the avoirdupois system: = 27.34 grains or 1/16 ounce; drain; dressing.

D_R Difference between rates of inflow and outflow.

D-R Diplomate - American Board of Radiology.

DRA Dextran-reactive antibody; Disability Rights Advocates; Dopamine receptor agonist(s) - e.g. Apomorphine, Bromocriptine and Dopamine; Dopamine receptor antagonist(s) - e.g. the Neuroleptic drugs such as: Phenothiazines (e.g. chlor promazine), Thioxanthines (e.g. flupenthixol), Butyrophenones (e.g. haloperidol) and Metoclopramide; Dopamine releasing agent; Dose-response assessment/ association; Drug-related admission(s)/ alopecia.

DRACOG Diploma of the Royal Australian College of Obstetricians and Gynaecologists.
DRACR Diploma of Royal Australian College of Radiologists.
DRAE Dose/ Drug-related adverse event(s)/ experience(s).
Drags Dragees.
DRAM Dynamic random access memory.
dr ap drachm/ dram apothecary/apothecaries' weight (see dr).
DRAR Dose/ Drug-related adverse reaction(s) (see DRAE).
DRAT Differential rheumatoid agglutination test.
dr av drachm/ dram avoirdupois weight (see dr).
DRB Daunorubicin (see Dauno); Dichloro-ribofuranosylbenz-imidazole; Dopamine-receptor blocker; Drug Research Board; Drug-resistant bacteria/ium.
DRBA Dopamine receptor blocking activity.
DRBC Denaturated/ Dog/ Donkey red blood cell.
DRBS Dopamine receptor binding site (in the brain).
DRC Damage-risk criteria/rion; Dendritic reticulum cell; Digito-reno-cerebral (syndrome); Disease-related complication; Dorsal root, cervical; Dose-response characteristic(s)/ curve; Drug-related cataract/ change(s) (see DAC).
DRCOG Diploma of the Royal College of Obstetricians and Gynaecologists (see DObstRCOG).
DRCPath Diploma of the Royal College of Pathologists.
DRD Dairy-rich diet; Diabetic renal disease; Dorsal root dilator; Dose response data; Drug-related death/ disease/ disorder (= DRI).
DRDCIS Drug Research and Development Chemical Information System (NCI - CAS).
DRDT Diabetes Research Detection Therapy (journal).
DRE Digital rectal examination; Dilated retinal examination; Disease-related edema; Dose-related efficacy/ elevation (e.g. of body temperature); Dose-response effects; Drug-related effect(s)/ event.
DREF Dose rate effectiveness factor.
DREZ Dorsal root entry zone.
DRF Daily Rating Form; Daily replacement factor (of lymphocytes); Deafness Research Foundation; Decreased/ Diminished renal function; Diastolic reverse flow (heart); Dose-range finding (see PCDRFS); Dose reduction factor; Dose-related fashion (see DRM).
DRG Diagnosis-related group; Division of Research Grants (NIH); Dorsal respiratory group; Dorsal root ganglion; Drug-resistant gene/ gonorrhea; Duodenal-gastric reflex gastropathy.
drg; drge drainage.
DRH Detroit Receiving Hospital; Division of Radiological Health (USPHS); Division of Reproductive Health (CDC); Dose-related hyptension (see DRHtn).
DrHC; Drhc Doctor honoris causa (L.).
DRHtn Dose-related hyptension (= DRH).
DrHyg Doctor of Hygiene (see DHyg).
DRI Diabetes Research Institite (Univ of Miami, Florida); Diabetic renal insufficiency; Differential refractive index; Dihydrofolate reductase inhibitor (e.g. Trimitrexate); Discharge Readiness Index/ Inventory; Dopamine reuptake inhibitor; Dose-related incidence/ increase; Drug-related illness (see DRD); Drug-resistant infection.
dRib Deoxyribose (= DR).
DRID Double radial immunodiffusion; Double radioisotope derivative.
DRIS Diagnostic Radiology Information System (ACR).
DRL Different randomization list; Dorsal root, lumbar; Drug-related lupus.
D_5RL 5% dextrose in Ringer's lactate (solution).
DRM Disease-related mutation(s) (in genes); Dose-related manner (see DRF); Drug-resistant microbe/ mutant (gene/ viral protein/ virus).
DRME Division of Research in Medical Education.
Dr Med Doctor of Medicine (see MD).
DRMF Disease related marrow fibrosis.
DRMFCR Damon Runyon Memorial Fund for Cancer Research, Inc.
DRMGE Department of Reproductive

Medicine & Gynecologic Endocrinology (Maribor Teaching Hospital, Slovenia).

DRMS Drug reaction monitoring system.

DRMs Diabetes-related malformations (congenital malformations found in IDMs or Infants of Diabetic mothers, involving the cardiovascular, central nervous, gastrointestinal, genitourinary, and skeletal symptoms: *Skeletal and central nervous system anomalies*: Anencephaly with/without herniation of neural elements, Caudal regression syndrome, Microcephaly, Neural tube defects excluding ancephaly, etc. *Cardiac anomalies*: Atrial septal defect, Cardiomegaly, Transportation of the great vessels with/without Ventricular septal defect or Patent ductus Arteriosus, etc. *Renal anomalies*: Hydronephrosis, Renal agenesis, Ureteral duplication. *Gastrointestinal anomalies*: Anorectal/Duodenal atresia, Meckel's diverticulum, Small left colon syndrome, etc. *Other anomalies*: Potter facies, Single umbilical artery, etc. (see CVAs, DAA, DEP, GuAs, HIMs, NAMs, SAs).

DRMT Dosage/ Dose-related maternal toxicity.

DrMT Doctor of Mechanotherapy.

DRN Diabetic retinopathy and nephropathy; Dorsal raphe nucleus.

DRNA Deoxyribose nucleic acid (see DNA).

DRNDP Diribonucleoside-3',3'-diphosphate.

DRnt Diagnostic roentgenology.

DRO Department of Radiation Oncology; Differential reinforcement of other (behavior); Disablement Resettlement Officer.

drom- combining form meaning course (Gr. dromos).

dromedary hump See dowager hump.

DRP Decreased/ Diminished renal perfusion; Dental Radiography and Photography (journal); Deutsches Reichs Patent (German patent); Diabetic retinopathy (see DR); Digoxin reduction product; Disease-related protein; Dose-response pharmacology; Dose-retention period; Dorsal root potential.

dRp Deoxyribose-phosphate.

DrPH Doctor of Public Health/ Hygiene.

DRQ Discomfort relief quotient.

DRR Division of Research Resources (NIH); Dorsal root reflex; Dose-related reduction/ risk; Dose-response relationship.

DRS Descending rectal septum; Disease/ Dose/ Drug-related symptom(s); Division of Research Services (NIH); Dose-ranging/ response study; Drowsiness; Drug resistant strain (of bacteria, parasites, etc.); Dry rough skin; Duane retraction syndrome; Dynamic renal scintigraphy; Dyskinesia Rating Scale.

DRSCS Depth resolved surface coil spectroscopy.

DRSE Drug-related side effect(s).

drsg dressing (= dsg).

Dr SUMEX See SUMEX-AIM.

DRT Disaster response team; Distal renal tubule (= DKT); Dorsal root, thoracic; Dose-related toxicity; Dynamic-response test (to therapy).

DRUB Drug screen-blood.

DRUJ Distal radioulnar joint.

DRV Drug-resistant virus.

DRVO Deputy Regional Veterinary Officer.

DRW Antigen matching system.

DS Data system; Dead air space (see PFT - DS); Dead space; Deep sedative/ sleep; Defined substrate; Degree of substitution; Dehydroepiandrosterone/ Dermatan/ Dextran sulfate; Delayed sensitivity; Dendritic spine; Density standard (optical density s - now, absorbance s); Dental Student/ Survey (journals); Dental surgery; Deprivation/ Devic's/ Down's (Mongolism)/ Dumping syndrome; Dermatology and syphilology (see D&S); Desynchronized sleep; Dextrose/ D. and saline (see D/S); Dextrose stick; Diaphragm stimulation; Diastolic (murmur); Diethylstilbestrol (see DES); Differential stimulus; Diffuse scleroderma; Digit span (psychology); Dihydrostreptomycin (see DST); Dilute strength (of a solution); Dioptric strength (refractive power of a lens); Disaster services; Discharge summary (= DP); Discrimination score (hearing test); Disoriented; Disseminated sclerosis (see MS); Dissolved solids; Doctor of Science (see DSc); Doctor of Surgery (see ChD); Donor's serum; Doppler sonography; Double standard (sexual mores); Double-stranded (see DNA); Double strength (of a drug/ solution); Down's syndrome (21-chromosome trisomy; "Mongolism"); Drawer sign (A test for ligamentous instability or ruptured cruciate ligaments of the knee joint) (also called ADS - Anterior drawer sign; RS - Rocher's sign); Dressler's syndrome (see BIP; PIS); Drug store; Dry swallow (medication order); Duncan syndrome (see DD; DSHP; SH2D1A); Duplex scan (Ultrasound of the carotid arteries); Duration of systole.

D/S Dextrose/saline, i.e. dextrose in saline solution (for intravenous use) (= DS); Dominance and submission.

D-S Dejerine-Sottas (disease); Diplomate - American Board of Surgery; Doerfler-Stewart (test for hearing).

D&S Dermatology and syphilology (see DS); Diagnostic and surgical; Dilation and suction.

D_5/S; D-5-S Dextrose (5%) in saline solution (for IV use).

ds double-stranded (see ds; DNA).

DS# Displaced sacral fracture (see DSF).

DSA Deep-seated abscess; Detailed sectional anatomy; Digital signal/ spectrum analyzer; Digital subtraction angiography; Digital subtraction angiogram/graph(y)/ arteriogram/raph(y); Discrete sample analyzer.

DSAA Dental Surgery Assistants Association (UK).

DSACT; D-SACT Direct sinoatrial conduction time.

DSAP Disseminated superficial actinic porokeratosis.

DSAS Discrete (form of) subaortic stenosis.

DSB Distal small bowel (ileum); Drug safety board; Drug-seeking behavior.

Dsb Single-breath diffusion (capacity).

DSBFI Doppler sonographic blood flow imaging.

DSBL Disabled.

DSBT Donor-specific blood transfusion.

DSC Damaged spinal cord (in SCI); Data Sheet Compendium (UK); Decussation superior cerebellar; Definitive surgical care; de Sanctis-Cacchione (syndrome); Desquamating/ Dry skin change/ condition; Differential scanning calorimeter; Disodium cromoglycate (see DSCG); Doctor of Surgical Chiropody; Donor stem cell; Down's syndrome child.

DSc Doctor of Science (= DS; ScD).

DSCF Doppler-shifted constant frequency.

DSCG Disodium cromoglycate (= Cromolyn sodium/ disodium; CS; DCG; DSC; DSCS; DSTG).

DSCS Disodium cromoglycate (see DSCG).

DSCT Dorsal spinocerebellar tract.

DSD Departmental Science Development (program) (NSF); Depression sine depression (L. sine = without); Depression spectrum disease; Designer sex drug (e.g. Sildenafil {Viagra}); Diabetic sclerodactyly; Dietary salt depletion; Digestive system disease/ disorder; Diminished sexual desire; Discharge summary dictated; Drug Safety and Disposition; Drug Standards Division (USP); Dry sterile dressing.

DSDB Direct self-destructive behavior.

DSDDT Double sampling dye dilution technique.

dsDNA double-stranded deoxyribonucleic acid.

DSE Dangerous side effect(s); Direct sexing of embryo(s). Division of Solar Energy (ERDA); Doctor of Sanitary Engineering.

DS-EA Division of Socio-Economic Activities (AMA).

DSF Differential spectrofluorometer; Displaced sacral fracture (= DS#) (see SIJD); Morpholine salicylate.

DSG Dry sterile guaze.

dsg dressing (see drsg).

DSH Deliberate self harm; Dexamethasone suppressible hyperaldosteronism.

DSHE Dietary Supplement Health and Education (Act of 1994, US).

DSHEA Dietary Supplement Health and Education Act (1994 - US).

DSHP Duncan syndrome human protein (see DD; SH2D1A).

DSHR Delayed skin hypersensitivity reaction.

DSI Deep shock insulin; Depression Status Inventory; Disaccharidase inhibitor (for treatment of type II Diabetes); Down Syndrome International; Drug-seeking index; Dry skin irritation/ itching.

DSIM Doctor of Science in Industrial Medicine.

DSIP Delta sleep-inducing peptide.
DSL Deep scattering layer (ocean); Desired sensation level (hearing aid); Distal sensory latency.
D Sleep Deep (rapid eye movement)/ REM sleep (see REM).
DSL M-U Distal sensory latency - median-ulnar.
dslv dissolve.
DSM Dextrose solution mixture; Diagnostic and Statistical Manual (of Mental Disorders) (CNS - Am Psychiat Assn); Diploma in Social Medicine; Disease-specific mortality; Drink skim milk.
DSM III Diagnostic & Statistical Manual, 3rd Edition (see DSM).
DSMC Data and Safety Monitoring Committee.
DSMMD Diagnostic and Statistical Manual of Mental Disorders (see DSM).
DSMP Drug shortage monitoring program (ASHP + FDA).
DSMPD Diagnostic and Statistical Manual of Psychiatric Disorders.
DSN Dental Student News (AADS journal)/ Newsletter; Direct solids nebulizer.
DSNCL Dopamine-secreting neural cell line.
DSO Diffuse spinal osteopenia; Distal subungual onychomycosis.
DSP Decreased sensory perception; Delayed sleep phase; Delipidized serum protein (= DLP); Dibasic sodium phosphate; Dietary-supplement product(s) (see DSS); Digital signal processor; Digital subtraction phlebography; Disruption of symphysis pubis.
dsp died without issue (L. decessit sine prole).
DSPC Disaturated phosphatidylcholine.
DSPN Distal sensory/ symmetrical polyneuropathy; Distal symmetrical peripheral neuropathy.
DSPS Delayed sleep phase syndrome.
DSR Delayed stress reaction; Diaper skin rash; Dietary salt restriction; Distal splenorenal; Double simultaneous recording.
DSRF Drainage subretinal fluid.
DSRNA; dsRNA Double-stranded ribonucleic acid (see DNA).
DSRS Distal spleno-renal shunt.
DSRU Drug Safety Research Unit (GMC, UK).
DSS Decompression sickness syndrome (= the Bends; Caisson disease) (see ANB; CAD); Delayed stress syndrome (a mental illness arising years after its cause has ceased, e.g. the Vietnam war, among US army veterans of this conflict); Dengue shock syndrome; Department of Social Services; Dermal sensitisation study; Developmental Sentence Score; Dietary-supplement substance(s) (= DSP); Dioctyl sodium sulphosuccinate (= Aerosol OT, a wetting agent lowering surface tension; used as a fecal softening agent and mild laxative); Disability Status Scale; Division of Safety Services (OPS/FDA); Division of Special Services (PHS); Docusate sodium; Doppler shift signal; Double simultaneous stimulation.
DSSc Diploma in Sanitary Science.
DSSEP Dermatomal somatosensory evoked potential.
DSSNY Dental Society of the State of New York.
DSST Digit Symbol Substitution Task/ Test.
DST Daylight-saving time; Decreased/ Diminished skin turgor; Desensitization test; Developmental sentence types; Dexamethasone suppression test; Dihydrostreptomycin (= DS); Disk susceptibility test (of bacteria to antibiotics); Display storage tube; Disproportionate septal thickening; Donor-specific transfusion.
DSTG Disodium cromoglycate (see DSCG).
DSU Day surgery unit.
DSUH Direct(ed) suggestion under hypnosis.
DSur Doctor of Surgery (see ChD).
DSV Digital subtraction ventriculography.
DSVP Downstream venous pressure.
DSWI Deep surgical wound infection.
DSy Digit symbol (psychology).
DT Dead/ Diastolic time; Decision tree; Defibrillation threshold; Delirium tremens (see DT's); Dental Technician (UK journal); Dental/ Dietetic technician; Depression of transmission; Dialysis and Transplantation (journal); Digitoxin; Diphtheria-tetanus (see dT); Diphtheria toxin/ toxoid; Discharge tomorrow; Dispensing tablet; Distance test (hearing); Dorsalis tibialis; Double tachycar-

dia; Doubling time (tumor); Dream time (see D time); Duration tetany (see Dt); Dye test.

Dt Duration (of) tetany (= DT).

dT Deoxythymidine (see dTDP; dTMP; dTPM; dTTP); Diphtheria-tetanus (booster toxoid) (= DT; double Toxoid); Due to.

dt dystonic.

D/T Date of treatment; Deaths:total (ratio) (total ratio of deaths).

D&T Diagnosis and treatment.

DT3 Detrothyronine (= D-Triiodothyronine; SKF-D 2623) - has been used in the treatment of hypercholesterolemia, but its toxic effects outweigh any therapeutic advantage (see Hormones - TH iiB).

d4T Stavudine (anti-HIV drug).

DT4 Dextrothyroxine sodium (= d-thyroxine; T4; Tetraiodothyronine) (see Hormones - TH iiB).

DT 21 Downs Trisomy 21 (syndrome) (with mental retardation, congenital heart malformations, unique facial appearance, fixed erythema of cheeks, hypotrichosis with alopecia areata at times, livedo reticularis with short limbs and fingers and keratosis pilaris).

DT 104 A virulent antibiotic-resistant strain of *Salmonella* typhimurium, affecting both farm and other animals and man.

DT 327 Clopamide - a diuretic with actions and uses similar to those of chlorthiazide.

DTA Differential thermal analysis.

DTAP Diphtheria, tetanus, and pertussis (see DTP).

DTaP Diphtheria, Tetanus toxoids, and acellular Pertussis (vaccine) (see DTAP; DTP; DT Per/Vac).

DTB Dedicated time block.

DTBC d-tubocurarine (see dTc).

DTBN di-tert-butyl/ di-t-butyl nitroxide.

DTBP Di-tert-butyl/ di-t-butyl peroxide.

DTC Day treatment center; Diagnostic thoracentesis; Dibenzoxepin tricyclic compound (e.g. Doxepin); Differential thyroid carcinoma; d-tubocurarine (see dTc).

DtC Difficult-to-control.

dTc d-tubocurarine (test) (= DTBC; DTC).

DTCD Diploma in Tuberculosis and Chest Diseases.

DTCH Diploma in Tropical Child Health.

DTD Diet-treated diabetes/tic.

DtD Day-to-day (change/ variation).

dtd; DTD give such a dose/ give of such doses (= DTD) (L. datur talis dosis/ dentur tales doses).

DTD #4 Dispense 4 such doses (see dtd No: iv).

dtd No: iv let four such doses be given (L. dentur tales doses No: iv) (= DTD #4).

dTDP Deoxythymidine diphosphate.

DTE Data terminal experiment; Desiccated thyroid extract; Dithio-erythritol.

DTES Distal tubular exchange site (of the kidney nephron).

DTF Daytime frequency (of micturition); Detector transfer function; Drug Tariff Formulary.

DTG Derivative thermogravimetry; Discordant twin gestation (Obstetrics); Dopamine-transporter gene.

DTH Delayed-type hypersensitivity; Diploma in Tropical Hygiene.

DTI Dipyridamole-thallium imaging; Direct thrombin inhibitor (see SRDTI).

DTIC Dacarbazine; Dimethyltriazenylimidazole carboxamide (= Dimethyl-triazeno-imidazole carboxamide).

DTICH Delayed traumatic intracerebral hemorrhage.

D time Dream time (= DT).

DTL Deep tissue loss (as in 4th degree burns); Diode-transistor logic.

DTLA Detroit Test of Learning Aptitudes.

DTM Department of/ Diploma in Tropical Medicine; Dermatophyte test medium.

DTMA Desoxycorticosterone trimethylacetate.

DTM&H Diploma in/ Diplomate of/ Doctor of Tropical Medicine and Hygiene (UK).

dTMP; DTMP Deoxythymidine monophosphate (= dTPM; Thymidylate).

DTN Diphtheria toxin, normal; Dystonia.

DTNB Dithiobis-nitrobenzoic acid {= 5,5'-dithiobis-(2-nitrobenzoic) acid}; Dithionitrobenzene.

DTO Deodorized tincture of opium (medication order).

d tox toxic dose (L. dosis toxica).

DTP Diphtheria-tetanus-pertussis (vaccine) (=

Diphtheria and tetanus toxoids and pertussis vaccine mixture; DT Per/Vac); Distal tingling on percussion (= Formication or Tinel's sign); Drug treatment program.

DTPA Diethylenetriamine penta-acetate/ pentacetic/ penta-acetic acid (= DPTA) - a medicinal chelating agent.

DT Per/Vac Diphtheria-tetanus-pertussis vaccine (see DTP).

DTPH Department of Tropical Public Health; Diploma in Tropical Public Health.

dTPM Deoxythymidine monophosphate (see dTMP).

DT Pol/Vac Diphtheria-tetanus-poliomyelitis vaccine.

DTR Decreased/ Diminished treatment response; Deep tendon reflex (DTRs include ATR or Achilles tendon reflex, Biceps reflex, BRR or Brachioradialis reflex, Patellar reflex, Triceps reflex, etc); Desired therapeutic response.

DTRTT Digital temperature recovery time test.

DTS Dense tubular system; Developmental toxicity study (for teratogenicity); Diphtheria toxin sensitivity; Direct tissue sampling; Donor transfusion, specific; Dose-titration study.

DTs; DT's Delirium tremens.

D-TS Diplomate - American Board of Thoracic Surgery.

DTT Diagnostic and therapeutic team; Difficult to treat (patient); Diphtheria-tetanus toxoid; Direct transverse traction; Dithio-threitol.

dTTP Deoxythymidine triphosphate.

DTUS Diathermy, traction, and ultrasound.

DTV Due to void.

DT-VAC Diphtheria-tetanus vaccine.

DT/Vac/APT Diphtheria-tetanus vaccine with alum precipitated toxoid.

DT/Vac/FT Diphtheria-tetanus vaccine with formol toxoid.

DT/Vac/PTAH Diphtheria-tetanus vaccine with purified toxoid aluminium hydroxide.

DT/Vac/PTAP Diphtheria-tetanus vaccine with purified toxoid aluminium phosphate.

DTVM Diploma in Tropical Veterinary Medicine.

DTVMI Developmental test of visual motor integration.

DTVP Developmental test of visual perception.

DTW Dog tapeworm (= *Echinococcus* granulosus); Dwarf tapeworm (= *Hymenolepis* nana).

DTX Detoxification.

DTZ Diatrizoate.

DU Decubitus/ Dermal/ Duodenal/ ulcer; Density unknown (i.e. optical density, now absorbance); Dental Update (UK journal); Deoxyuridine (see dU); Diabetic urine; Diabetic ulcer (see DNU; IDU); Diagnosis undetermined/ unknown; Diazouracil; Dog unit (with reference to adrenal cortical hormones); Duroxide uptake; Dutch (see Du).

Du Dutch (rabbit) (= DU; Dut).

dU deoxyuridine (= DU).

du dial unit.

D-U Diplomate - American Board of Urology.

DUA Doppler ultrasonic angiography; Dorsal uterine artery.

DUAV Doppler umbilical artery velocimetry (in APS - Antepartum fetal surveillance).

DUB Dubowitz (score); Dysfunctional uterine bleeding.

duby marijuana (see Cannabis).

-ducent; -duct suffix meaning lead or conduct (L. ductus).

DUD Duodenal ulcer disease (see PUD).

dUDP Deoxyuridine diphosphate.

DUE Drug Use Evaluation(s) (see DUR).

D_1 UE Diagonal 1 upper extremity.

D_2 UE Diagonal 2 upper extremity.

DUF Doppler ultrasonic flowmeter; Drug use forecast.

DUI Driving under the influence (of alcohol).

DUID Driving under the influence of drugs.

DUII Driving under the influence of intoxicants (= DUID).

DUIL Driving under the influence of liquor (= DUI).

duji heroin (see Diamorph).

DUL Diffuse undifferentiated lymphoma.

dulc sweet (L. dulcis).

DUMC Duke University Medical Center.

dUMP Deoxyuridine monophosphate (= Diocyuridylate).

DUNHL Diffuse undifferentiated non-Hodgkins lymphoma.
DUO Daily urinary output (= DUV).
Duod; duod Duodenal/num.
dup duplicate/tion.
DUR Drug use review; Drug Utilization Review (CIC - Clinincal Interventions Catalogue).
dur duration; during/ hard (L. duris).
dur- combining form meaning during or hard (L. durus).
dur dolor while the pain lasts (L. durante dolore).
DUS Directly under supervision; Doppler ultrasound.
3DUS Three-dimensional ultrasound.
DUSA Dispensatory of the United States of America (Am Pharmac Assn).
DUSG Doppler ultrasonography.
DUSN Diffuse unilateral subacute neuroretinitis.
Duster Heroin in cigarette (see Diamorph).
Dut Dutch (see Du).
Dut Ref Dutch Reformed (Church member).
DUV Daily urinary volume (see DUO); Damaging ultraviolet (radiation).
DUVD Doppler ultrasonic velocity detector.
DV Dependent variable; Difference in volume; Digital vibration; Dilute volume (of solution); Distemper virus; Domiciliary visit; Dorsoventral; Double vibration(s) (see dv); Distance/ Double vision; Ductus venosus (see DVBF); Maximum segmental volume change per heart beat.
dv double vibration(s) (= DV; sound wave unit; unit for measurement of sound waves).
D_v Pulse volume.
D&V Diarrhea and vomiting.
DVA Decreased(sing)/ Diminished(hing) visual acuity; Department of Veterans Affairs; Developmental venous anomaly; Distal visual acuity (eye examination); Duration of voluntary apnea (test); Vindesine.
D-VAC Pollens Depot Pollen Vaccine - 12 varieties of common grass pollens of the Bencard Allergy Division (UK) - a proprietary product.
DVAMC Department of Veterans Affairs Medical Center (US).
DVB Divinylbenzene.
DVBF Ductus venosus blood flow (Obstetrics).
DVBS Domestic violence battering syndrome (see BWS, DVPTG).
DVC Deep vein/ venous clotting (see DVT); Diabetic vascular complication(s); Direct visualization of (vocal) cords (see DVVC); Divanillylcyclohexane (= Divanillylidene-cyclohexanone).
DVCC Disease Vector Control Center.
DVD Dissociated vertical deviation.
DV&D Diploma in Venereology and Dermatology.
dVDAVP 1-deamine-4-valine-D-arginine vasopressin.
DVE Duck virus enteritis.
DVetHom Diploma in Veterinary Homeopathy.
DVH Diploma in Veterinary Hygiene; Division for the Visually Handicapped.
DVI Deep venous incompetence; Digital vascular imaging; Doppler velocity index; AV sequential (pacemaker).
DVIS Digital vascular imaging system.
DVIU Direct-vision internal urethrotomy.
DVL Deep vastus lateralis.
DVLA Driver and Vehicle Licensing Agency (UK).
DVM Department/ Doctor of Vascular/ Veterinary Medicine; Digital voltmeter; Doctor of Veterinary Medicine; DVM (journal).
DVMS Doctor of Veterinary Medicine and Surgery.
DVN Dorsal vagal nucleus.
DVO Deep venous obstruction.
DVP Daunorubicin, vincristine, and prednisone; Déjà vu phenomenon (already seen); Diabetic vasculopathy.
DVPA; DVP-Asp Daunorubicin, vincristine, prednisone, and asparaginase.
DVPTC Domestic Violence Prevention and Treatment Center (Beer Sheva, Israel) (see BWS, DVBS).
DVR Decreased/ Diminished ventilatory response (to hypercapnia, hypoxia, etc.); Deep venous reflux; Department/ Division of Vocational Rehabilitation; Digital vascular

reactivity; Doctor of Veterinary Radiology; Double valve replacement; Double ventricular response.

DVS Daily vitamin supplement; Decreased/ Diminished vibration sense; Division of Vital Statistics; Doctor of Veterinary Science (see DVSc)/ Surgery.

DVSA Digital venous subtraction angiography.

DVSc Doctor of Veterinary Science (= DVS).

DVSM Diploma in Veterinary State Medicine.

DVT Deep vein/ venous thrombosis; Diastolic ventricular volume.

DVV Descending vertical vein (Obstetrics).

DVVC Direct visualization of the vocal cords (= DVC).

DW Daily/ Dead/ Dry weight; Defenders of Wildlife (Association); Deionized/ Distilled water; Dental World (journal); Dextrose in water (see D/W); Doctors of the World (emergency relief project); Doing well; a Rorschach score.

dw dwarf (mouse).

D/W Dextrose in water (= DW) (intravenous solution).

D_5/W; D5/W; D-5-W 5% Dextrose in water (intravenous solution).

D10W 10% Aqeous dextrose solution.

DW 62 Dimefline hydrochloride (= Rec 7-0267). An analeptic agent which has been used in the treatment of acute respiratory failure and in chronic respiratory diseases such as bronchitis, emphysema, and silicosis.

DWA Died (from) wounds (in) action (i.e. died from wounds by the action of the enemy); Doppler waveform analysis (Obstetrics).

Dwarf An abnormally undersized or short human being:

Achondroplastic dwarf - with early bone fusion or Achondroplasia - a hereditary, congenital or familial disturbance of epiphyseal chondroblastic growth and maturation.

Amsterdam dwarf = de Lange's syndrome, with severe mental retardation and other defects (see Infantile dwarf).

Aortic dwarf - underdevelopment as a result of severe aortic stenosis.

Asexual dwarf - an adult dwarf with deficient sexual development.

Ateliotic dwarf - with an infantile skeleton due to non-union of epiphyses and diaphyses.

Bird-headed dwarf = Nanocephalic dwarf.

Brissaud's dwarf - a dwarf with infantile myxedema or cretinism (see Cretin dwarf).

Cretin dwarf - a thyroid-deficient dwarf (= Brissaud's dwarf; Hypothyroid dwarf).

Deformed dwarf - who is both abnormally undersized as well as deformed.

Diastrophic dwarf - Dwarf with shortness of height caused by various deformities of the bones and joints.

Hypophysial dwarf = Pituitary dwarf.

Hypothyroid dwarf = Cretin dwarf.

Infantile dwarf - with severe retardation of mental and physical development (as in Amsterdam dwarf).

Levi-Lorain dwarf = Pituitary dwarf.

Micromelic dwarf - a dwarf with very small limbs (see Thanotophoric dwarf).

Nanocephalic dwarf - Nanocephaly, a growth defect characterized by a very small head (= Bird-headed dwarf).

Normal dwarf - a person who is abnormally undersized, but perfectly formed (= Physiologic dwarf; Primordial dwarf; Pure dwarf; True dwarf).

Paltauf's dwarf = Pituitary dwarf.

Phocomelic dwarf - a dwarf with abnormally short diaphyses of the long bones.

Physiologic dwarf = Normal dwarf.

Pituitary dwarf - with retarded development due to hypofunction of the anterior pituitary gland (Hypophysis cerebri) (= Hypophyseal dwarf; Levi-Lorain dwarf; Paltauf's dwarf).

Primordial dwarf = Normal dwarf.

Pure dwarf = Normal dwarf.

Rachitic dwarf - a dwarf having rickets, with bent long bones, high forehead, prominent bosses, etc.

Renal dwarf - a dwarf whose condition is associated with renal osteodystrophy.

Russell dwarf - a person with Russell's syndrome, an inherited disorder in which short stature is accompanied by defects of the head, face, and skeleton, with various degrees of mental retardation.

Sexual dwarf - an adult dwarf with normal

sexual development.
Silver dwarf - a dwarf with Silver's syndrome, a disorder present at birth in whom each side of the body has a different size, and there are numerous deformities of the head, face, and skeleton.
Thanatophoric dwarf - an infant with Micromelia (severe shortness or smallness of the limbs, flattened chest and vertebrae, and breathing problems, the latter usually causing death shortly after birth) (= Micromelic dwarf).
True dwarf = Normal dwarf.

DWB Doctors Without Borders (an international relief organization).

DWD Dashe water deprivation (test for diabetes insipidus) (= WDT); Died with disease.

DWDL Diffuse well-differentiated lymphocytic lymphoma.

DWG Decreased/ Delayed/ Diminished weight gain.

DWI Diffusion-weighted imaging (= see MR-DWI); Driving while impaired/ intoxicated.

DWL Delayed weight loss.

DWM Dandy-Walker malformation (see DWS).

DWMRI Diffusion-weighted magnetic resonance imaging.

DWRC Denver Wildlife Research Center (FWS).

DWRT Delayed work recall test.

DWS Dandy-Walker syndrome; Disaster/ Drug warning system; Drug withdrawel syndrome (see AWS).

DWT Dichotic word test.

dwt pennyweight (apothecary, 24 grains).

DX Dexamethasone (see DXM); Dextran; Diagnosis (see Dx); Dicloxacillin.

Dx; dx Diagnosis (= DX).

DXA Dual-energy x-ray absorptiometric (measurement of BMD - Bone mineral density).

2-DXA 2-Deoxyadenosine.

DXD; dxd Discontinued.

DXM Dexamethasone (= DX) (suppression test for adrenocortical function).

DXR Deep X-ray.

DXRT Deep X-ray therapy (= DXT).

DXT Deep X-ray therapy (see DXRT); Dextrose.

dXTP deoxyxanthine triphosphate.

DY Dense parenchyma; Double Y (hepateiportico-jejunostomy).

Dy Delivery; Dysprosium (Z = 66) (Elements - Dysprosium).

dy dystrophia muscularis (mouse).

DYF Drag your feet.

dyn dynamic; dynamometer; dyne.

Dynam Dynamics.

dynam- combining form meaning power (Gr. dynamis).

Dynamite cocaine and heroin mixture (see Erythroxylum; Diamorph); concentrated marijuana (see Cannabis).

Dynein The protein responsible for ciliary motion. Its suppression causes ciliary dyskinesia or ciliary immotility, and is said to be the basis of the bronchiectasis in Kartagener's syndrome (see BHS; BPD; KS; MLA; MLS; RMLS).

dynia- suffix meaning pain.

Dyno High-potency heroin (see Diamorph).

dys- prefix meaning bad, difficult, disordered, improper, painful (Gr).

Dyscal Dyscalculia.

Dyslex Dyslexia.

Dysp Dyspnea.

Dyspep Dyspepsia.

Dysphagia Difficulty in swallowing (Gr. dys - combining form signifying difficult, disordered, painful, etc. + Gr. phagein - to eat) - D. inflammatoria - dysphagia due to inflammation of the esophagus; D. lusoria - dysphagia caused by compression of the esophagus, as in developmental anomaly (lusus naturae); D. nervosa or Esophagism - dysphagia due to hypochondria, nervous tension, etc.; D. paralytica - dysphagia due to paralysis of the esophageal muscles, as occurs frequently in CVA; Sideropenic D. or the Plummer-Vinson syndrome - with glossitis, hypochromic anemia, spenomegaly, and atrophy of the mouth, pharynx, and upper end of the esophagus; D. spastica or Esophagism - due to any cause; Tropical D. or the Brazilian Entalacao or Mal d'engasgo, also known as tropical vasospasm; Vallecula D. - dysphagia caused by lodgement of food above or at the sides of the epiglottis; D. valsalviana - dysphagia due to subluxation of the major cornu of the hyoid bone.

DZ Diazepam (= DZP); Dizygotic/ous; Dizziness.

dz disease; dozen.

DZA Dizygotic twins reared apart.

DZM Dorsal zone of membranelle.

DZP Diazepam (see DZ); Dizygotic pregnancy.

DZT Dyzotic twins reared together (also called Binovular twins, Biovular twins, Dissimilar twins, False twins, Fratermal twins, Heterologous twins).

DZ twins Dizygotic/ Dizygous twins (i.e. fraternal twins).

E

E Air dose; Cortisone (Compound E); Each; East; Ectopia (Dislocation, displacement or malposition), e.g. E. lentis - displacement of the crystalline lens; Edema; Einstein (a unit of energy); Elastance; Electric charge; Electric field vector; Electrode potential (A medium used between an electric conductor and the object to which the current is to be applied), e.g. Therapeutic E. - a carbon electrode filled with materials for medication; Electromagnetic force; Electromotive force (A force which gives rise to an electric current as a result of a flow of electricity from one point to another, due to difference in potential. It is measured in volts [= EMF]); Electron (the unit of negative electricity), e.g. Free E. - a "moving" electron which is not bound to the nucleus of an atom; Element (A primary substance which cannot be decomposed by chemical means), e.g. Radioactive E. - an element which emits corpuscular or electromagnetic radiations, transforming itself spontaneously into another element as a result of this radiation (see Elements); Embryo; Emmetropia (A state of correct refraction of the eye, with exact focusing of light on the retina - symbol E; = EM; Em); Emphysema; Emplastrum - A plaster (L. Gr. emplastron), e.g. E. belladonnae (belladonna plaster); Encephalitis; Endangered (animal/ species); Endogenous; Endoplasm; Enema; Energy; Engorged; Entamoeba; Enterococcus; Enzyme; Eosinophil; Epicondyle; Epinephrine (see Epi); Equivalent (see Eq), e.g. RE (= REq) - Retinal equivalent; Error; Erythrocyte - RBC (Red Blood Cell/ Corpuscle) (= Er; Erc; Ery); Erythroid; Erythromycin (see ERY); Erythroxylum (see Erythroxylum); Escherichia (see Esch); Esophagus; Esophoria (eye exam.); Ester; Estradiol; Ethanol; Ethyl; Examination; Expectancy (wave); Expected frequency in a cell of a contingency table; Experiment, e.g. Control E. - mode under standard conditions to test the correctness of other observations; Experimenter; Expiration; Expired air/ gas (A pulmonary function test) (see PFT - E); Extract(ed)/tion; Extraction fraction; Extralymphatic; Eye (The organ of vision), e.g. Black E (subcutaneous periorbital hemorrhage or contusion), Pink E (acute conjunctivitis); Glutamicacid (symbol: E); Internal/ Kinetic energy; Mathematical expectation; Redox potential; Rh gene (symbol E) (see e); Stereodescriptor to indicate the configuration at a double bond (Ger. entgegen = opposite); Unit (Ger. Einheit); Vitamins E (Tocopherol) (see Vitamins - E).

ϵ epsilon (5th letter of the Greek alphabet); heavy chain of IgE; permittivity; specific absorptivity.

e allelic form of Rh gene; base of natural logarithms, approximately 2.7182818285; egg transfer; electric charge (amount of charge on an electron); electron; elementary charge; erg; ex (L.) - from; exchange.

E* Lesion on the erythrocyte cell membrane at the site of complement fixation.

$\bar{\mathbf{E}}$ Average beta energy.

e- negative electron; prefix meaning out from (L. e; ex).

e+ positron.

η Greek letter "eta"; Absolute viscosity.

$\mathbf{E_0}$ Electric affinity.

$\mathbf{E_1}$ Estrone (laboratory/ endocrinology).

$\mathbf{E_2}$ Estradiol (= 17-estradiol; 17β-estradiol) (laboratory/ endocrinology) (see E_{11}).

$\mathbf{E_3}$ Estriol (laboratory/ endocrinology).

E3 Lachesine Chloride (= Laches Chlor). A dimethylammonium compound with mydriatic and cycloplegic properties. Used as eyedrops (1% sol.) as a substitute for atropine or hyoscine in patients with an idiosyncrasy to these drugs.

4E Four-plus edema.

$\mathbf{E_{11}}$ Estradiol (i.e. 11-estradiol) (laboratory/ endocrinology).

E 107 Avertin.

E 605 Parathion (see DNTP).

E 1059 Demeton (see Bayer 8169).

E 2020 Donepezil hydrochloride (a reversible inhibitor of the enzyme acetylcholinesterase, with an empirical formula of $C_{24}H_{29}NO_3HCl$) - used in the treatment of Alzheimer's

Disease; see ACE) (= AchE-I).

EA Early antigen (induced by the Epstein-Barr virus); Eaton agent (= *Mycoplasma* pneumoniae); Educational age; Egg albumin; Elbow-aspiration; Electric affinity; Electroacupuncture (see EAC); Electroanesthesia; Electrophysiological abnormality; Embryonic antibody; Emphysema Anonymous; Endocardiographic amplifier; Endometriosis Association; Energy Abstracts (journal); Enteral alimentation; Enteroanastomosis; Enthalpimetric analysis; Enteropathic arthritis (see BSS; ERA); Enzymatically active; Epiandrosterone; Epilepsy Abstracts (journal); Epileptics Anonymous; Erythrocyte antibody (= Antibody-coated sheep erythrocyte - an immune complex) (see EAC); Erythrocyte antiserum; Esophageal atresia; Estivo-autumnal (e.g. EA malaria); Ethacrynic acid; Ethyl acetimidate; Parke, Davis & Co code for experimental substances.

ea each.

Eα Kinetic energy of alpha particles.

E → A Say E.E.E... (on chest auscultation) → comes out as A.A.A... (in lung consolidation).

E&A Evaluate and advise.

EAA Electroacupuncture analgesia; Electrothermal atomic absorption; Emergency assistance to adults; Epilepsy Association of America; Erosive azotemic arthropathy (see EAOA); Essential Amino Acid(s): Histidine; Isoleucine; Leucine; Lysine; Methionine; Phenylalanine; Threonine; Tryptophan; and Valine (see NEAA); Established asthma(tic) attack; Estrogenic-alkylating agent (= Estramustine); Extrinsic allergic alveolitis.

eAAA Endochondral AAA (bone regeneration) (see AAA).

EAACI European Academy of Allergology and Clinical Immunology.

EAAMP European Agency for the Evaluation of Medicinal Products.

EAB Elective abortion; Ethics Advisory Board.

EABV Effective arterial blood volume.

EAC Editorial Advisory Committee; Erlich ascites carcinoma; Electroacupuncture (= EA); Electroanalytical chemistry; Energy-absorbing capacity; Epithelioma adenoides cysticum (= AAC; Trichoepithelioma); Erythema annulare centrifugum; Erythrocyte, antibody, complement (= Erythrocyte antibody-coated complement or antibody-coated sheep erythrocyte bound to C [complement] receptor); Exterior/ External auditory canal.

EACA Epsilon-aminocaproic acid (= Aminocaproic acid; 6-aminohexanoic acid; ε-aminocaproic acid (CY 116; JD 177) - an antifibrinolytic agent.

EAC binding lymphocytes β cells.

EACD Eczematous allergic contact dermatitis.

EAC_{hu} Erythrocyte antibody complement (human).

EACL L'Énergie Atomique du Canada Limitée (AECL).

EAC rosette(s) Erythrocyte antibody complement rosette(s) - Rosette(s) with a complement component (C3) bound to antibody-coated sheep erythrocytes (EA), on the surface of bone-marrow derived (B) cells or lymphocytes.

EAD Early afterdepolarization; Extra-articular disease/ disorder; Extracranial arterial disease.

ead the same (L. eadem).

EA-D Early antigen diffuse (component).

E-ADD Epileptic attentional deficit disorder.

EADS Early amnion deficit spectrum/ syndrome.

EAE Esophageal adverse experience(s); Experimental allergic/ autoallergic encephalomyelitis; Experimental autoimmune encephalitis; Experimental (model of) allergic encephalitis.

EAEC Enteroadherent Escherichia coli; European Atomic Energy Community (Euratom).

EAF Emergency assistance to families.

EAG Electroantennogram; Electroarteriography; Epidemic acute gastritis.

EAHF Eczema, allergy/ asthma, and hay fever.

EAHFc The symptom complex of eczema, asthma, and hay fever (= EAHF complex).

EAHLG Equine antihuman lymphoblast globulin.

EAHLS Equine antihuman lymphoblast serum.

EAI Emphysema Anonymous, Inc.; Endocrine autoimmune/nity; Energy-adjusted intake; Erythrocyte antibody inhibition; Excessive alcohol intake; Extended action insulin (see Insulin).

EAIT Enzyme-associated immunoassay technique (for measuring drug levels in body liquids).

EAK Electronic acupuncture kit; Ethyl amyl ketone.

EAM Electrical accounting machine; External acoustic/ auditory meatus.

EAMG Experimental autoimmune myasthenia gravis.

EAN Energy-adjusted nutrient; Epiphyseal avascular necrosis (Orthopedics); Experimental allergic neuritis.

EAO Endarteritis obliterans; Experimental allergic orchitis.

EAOA Erosive azotemic osteoarthropathy (seen in long-term chronic renal failure) (= EAA).

EAP Early/ Expanded Access Program; Electric acupuncture; Employee/yment Assistance Program; Epiallo-pregnanolone (an androgen in pregnancy urine); Erythrocyte acid phosphatase; Evoked action potential; Extrinsic allergic pneumonia (see DHP).

EAQ Eudismic affinity quotient.

EAR European Association of Radiology; Expired air resuscitation (mouth to mouth).

EaR; Ea R Reaction of degeneration (Ger. Entartungsreaktion) (see RD).

EARC Early advanced resuscitative care.

EAROM Electrically alterable read-only memory (computer).

EARR Extended aortic root replacement.

EARS Environmental Action Reprint Service.

EAS Eastern Analytical Symposium; Edinburgh Artery Study (see MLR); Elemental analysis system; Endarterectomy spatula (Wylie - vascular surgery); Excessive acid secretion (see APG; GAS); External anal sphincter; Extra-articular symptom(s).

EASD European Association for the Study of Diabetes (1988).

EAST Elevated-arm stress test; Emory angioplasty vs. surgical trial; External rotation, abduction stress test.

EAT Eating Attitudes Test; Ectopic atrial tachycardia; Ehrlich ascites tumor; Electroaerosol therapy; Empirical antibiotic therapy/ treatment; Epidermolysis acuta toxica; 2-ethyl-amine-1,3,4-thiadiazole; Experimental autoimmune thymitis/ thyroiditis; Experiments in Art and Technology.

EATC Ehrlich ascites tumor cell.

EAU Experimental autoimmune uveitis.

EAV Enteric adenovirus; Equine abortion virus.

EAVC Enhanced atrioventricular conduction.

EAVM Extramedullary arteriovenous malformation.

EAVN Enhanced atrioventricular nodal (conduction).

EB Elective abortion; Elementary body; Endometrial biopsy; Epidermolysis bullosa; Epstein-Barr (virus) (see E-B); Esmarch bandage (used as an exsanguinating tourniquet); Esophageal body; Essays in Biochemistry (annual volumes); Estradiol benzoate; Evans blue.

Eb Enterobacteria.

E_B Binding energy in ev (electron-volt).

E-B Epstein-Barr (virus). The causal agent in infectious mononucleosis (= EB; EBV; E-BV). EBA.

Eβ Epoetin beta (see r-HuEPO).

EBA Empirically-based assessment (= EBM); Epidermolysis bullosa acquisita/ atrophicans; Epstein-Barr antibodies/dy (in association with Infectious mononucleosis and Burkitt's lymphoma); (ortho)-Ethoxybenzoic acid.

EBAA Eye-Bank Association of America.

EBAB Equal breath sounds bilaterally.

EBAM Electron-beam-accessed memory.

EBC Early brain/ breast cancer; Esophageal balloon catheter.

EBCDIC Extended Binary Coded Decimal Interchange Code.

EBCT Electron-beam computed tomogram/aph(y).

EBD Epidermolysis bullosa dystrophica.

EBDC Ethylene-bis-dithio-carbamate (pesticide).

EBDD Epidermolysis bullosa dystrophica dominant.

EBDR Epidermolysis bullosa dystrophica recessiva.

EBEA Epstein-Barr early antigen.

EBF Ectopic bone formation (see MCAs); Endometrial blood flow (Obs/Gyn); Erythroblastosis fetalis; External biliary fistula.

EBG Electroblepharogram/graphy; Endochondral block graft (Orthopedics)/ bone growth (in children); Evidence-based guideline(s).

EBI Electron beam irradiation; Emetine bismuth iodide (= Emetine and Bismuth Iodide; Emet Bism Iod) - used in the treatment of amebiasis; Enzyme-based interaction (e.g. with cytochrome P450 enzymes, etc.); Erythroblastic island; Estradiol binding index.

EBK Embryonic bovine kidney; Evidence-based knowledge (see EBM).

EBL Erthroblastic leukemia; Estimated blood loss.

eBL Endemic Burkitt's lymphoma.

EBL/S Estimated blood loss during surgery.

EBM Editorial board member; Electrophysiologic behavior modification; Empirically-based measure (see EBA); Endo/Epithelial basement membrane (Pulmonary alveolus); Environmental Biology and Medicine (journal); Evidence-based/ Evidence-biased medicine; Expressed breast milk.

EBNA Epstein-Barr virus-associated nuclear antigen.

E/BOD Electrolyte biochemical oxygen demand.

EBP Elevated blood pressure (see HTN); Engineering biophysics; Epidural blood patch; Erythroblastopenia (= PRCA or Pure red cell aplasia); Estradiol binding protein; Evidence-based practice (see EBM).

EBPC Effective blood pressure control.

EBR Endosteal bone repair (see EPBR); Evidence-based review; External-beam radiation (therapy for prostate cancer) (see EBT).

EBRT Electric beam radiotherapy.

EBS Education-based study; Elastic back strap; Electric brain stimulation/tor; Emergency Bed Service; Emergency broadcast system; Epidermolysis bullosa simplex; Evidence-based symposium; Experimental brain surgery.

EBSR Eye-bank for Sight Restoration (Association).

EBSS Earle's balanced salt solution.

EBT Electron beam tomogram/raph(y) (see EBTS); Erythromycin breath test (IV test); Evidence-based therapy/ treatment; Exchange blood transfusion; External beam therapy.

EBTS Electron beam tomography scan (see EBT).

EBV Effective blood volume; Epstein-Barr virus (see E-B).

E-BV Epstein-Barr virus (see E-B).

EBVCA Epstein-Barr virus, capsular antigen.

EBVEA Epstein-Barr virus, early antigen.

EBVNA Epstein-Barr virus, nuclear antigen.

EBW Electric blood warmer (an electric device for heating blood before transfusion) (see BWC).

EBZ Epidermal basement zone.

EC Effective concentration; Eisenmenger complex (congenital heart anomaly); Ejection capacity (see EF)/ click; Electrocautery; Electrochemical; Electron capture (a mode of radioactive decay involving the capture of an orbital electron by its nucleus); Embryonal carcinoma; Endemic cretinism; Endocrine cells; Endocrinological Communications (journal); Endothelial cell; Energy charge; Enteric coated/ting (tabl.); Entering complaint; Enterochromaffin; Entorhinal cortex; Environment Canada (journal); Enzyme Commission; Epidermal/ Epithelial cell; Equalization-cancellation; Error correction; Escherichia coli (see E coli); Esophageal carcinoma; Ether-chloroform (mixture) (see E-C); Ethylene chlorohydrin; European Communities; Excitation-contraction (see E-C); Exclusion chromatography; Experimental control; Expiratory center; External carotid (artery)/ conjugate; Extracellular; Extracellular concentration; Extracranial; Eye care; Eyes closed; Worthington Biochemical Corp code for experimental substances.

Ec Ectoconchion.

E-C Ether-chloroform (mixture) (= EC);

Excitation-concentration (coupling) (= EC).
E/C Endocystoscopy; Estrogen/creatinine (ratio).
EC 1.1.4.3.1 Phenylalanine 4 hydroxylase.
EC 2.7.1.1 Hexokinase.
EC 2.7.1.11 Phosphofructokinase.
EC 3.1.2 Phosphate-dependent glutaminase.
EC_{50} Median effective concentration.
ECA Effective/ Efficatious chemotherapeutic agent; Electrical control activity; Electrocardioanalyzer; Endothelial cell adhesion; Endothelial cytotoxic activity; Enteric coated aspirin; Enterobacterial common antigen; Environmental Control Administration; Epidemiological catchment area; Epithelial cell apoptosis; Erythrocyte cholinesterase activity; Ethacrynic acid (a diuretic); Ethylcarboxylate adenosine; External carotid artery.
E-CABG Endarterectomy and coronary artery bypass graft.
ECAO Enteric cytopathogenic avian orphan (virus).
ECB Enteric-coated beadlet.
ECBB Extracortical bone bridging.
ECBD Exploration of common bile duct.
ECBM Extracellular choriodecidual basement membrane.
ECBO Enteric cytopathogenic bovine orphan (virus).
Ecbo V Ecbo virus (see ECBO).
ECBR Ethics Committee on Biological Research.
ECBV Effective circulating blood volume.
ECC Electrocorticogram/graphy; Embryonal cell carcinoma; Emergency/ Enhanced cardiac care; Endocervical canal (Obs/Gyn)/ cone/ curettage; Enterochromaffin cell (a cell found in the brain and intestines, that releases the strong vasoconstricting agent Serotonin [= HT, SHT or 5-Hydroxytryptamine]; also named Argentaffin cell [AAC] or Kulchitsky's cell); Estimated creatinine clearance; External cardiac compression; Extracorporeal circulation (cardiopulmonary bypass).
ECCC Emergency Cardiac Care Committee (AHA).
ECCE Extracapsular cataract extraction (operation/ ophthalmology).
ECCL Encephalocraniocutaneous lipomatosis (a sporadic, inherited hypotrichosis with lipomas of scalp, alopecia, ocular lesions and unilateral cerebral malformations); Endocervical canal length (Obstetrics).
ECCLS European Committee for Clinical Laboratory Standards.
ECCO Enteric cytopathogenic cat orphan (virus).
$ECCO_2R$ Extracorporeal carbon dioxide removal.
ECD Early coronary detection; Elective cesarian delivery (see PCD) (Obstetrics); Electrochemical detector; Electron capture detector; Endocardial cushion defect; Endothelial cell dysfunction; Enzymatic cell dispersion; Ergot(amine)-containing drug (= ECP); Estimated conception/ confinement date (see EDC); Extracardiac disorder (e.g. flushing, vascular disorder, etc.); Extracompartmental disease.
ECDL Early Childhood Development and Learning (White House Conference).
ECDO Enteric cytopathogenic dog orphan (virus).
Ecdo V Ecdovirus (see ECDO).
ECE Equine conjugated estrogen.
ECEMG Evoked compound electromyography.
ECEO Enteric cytopathogenic equine orphan (virus).
ECF Early cardiac failure; Effective capillary flow; Endothelial cell function; Entero/Esophagocutaneous fistula; Eosinophil(ic) chemotactic factor; Erythroid colony formation; Extended care facility; Extracellular fluid.
ECFA; ECF-A Eosinophil(ic) chemotactic factor of anaphylaxis.
ECFC; ECF-C Eosinophil(ic) chemotactic factor complement (system).
ECFMG Educational Commission on/ Council for Foreign Medical Graduates.
ECFMS Educational Council for Foreign Medical Students.
ECFV Extracellular fluid volume.
ECG Echocardiogram/graph(y); Electrocardiogram/graph(y) (= EKG).

ECGAS Electrocardiographic-auscultatory syndrome (= Barlow's syndrome - an abnormal heart condition characterized by a murmur and a click due to prolapse of the mitral valve).
ECGF Endothelial cell growth factor.
ECG-LVH Electrocardiographic left ventricular hypertrophy.
ECGS Endothelial cell growth supplement.
ECH Environmental Child Health (journal).
-ech- combining form meaning have, hold, or be (Gr. echo).
ECHINO Echinocyte.
ECHO Echogram/graph(y) (see Echo); Electronic computing hospital-oriented (program); Enteric/tero cytopathic/thogenic human orphan (virus) (see ERC); Etoposide, cyclophosphamide, Adriamycin, and vincristine; Evidence for Community Health Organization.
Echo Echogram/graph(y) (= ECHO; Sonogram; Ultrasound; Ultrasonogram), e.g. Echocardiogram/graph(y) or EchoCG (procedure/ cardiology); Echoencephalogram or Echo-Eg (procedure/ neurology); Echoplacentogram (procedure/ obstetrics); etc. (= Sonocardiogram; Sonoencephalogram; Sonoplacentogram; etc).
EchoCG Echocardiography (see ECHO).
Echo-Eg Echoencephalography (see ECHO).
Echo-RNV Echoradionuclide ventriculography.
Echo-VM Echoventriculometry.
ECHR European Convention on Human Rights (Article 2 requires that a person's right to life be protected by law, Article 3 prohibits inhuman and degrading treatment, and Article 8 requires respect for private and family life).
ECHSCP Exeter Community Health Services Computer Project.
ECI Electrocerebral inactivity; Eosinophilic cytoplasmic inclusions; Extracorporeal irradiation.
ECIB Extracorporeal irradiation of blood.
EC-IC Extracranial-intracranial.
ECIL Extracorporeal irradiation of lymph.
ECIS Equipment control information system.
ECK Eckankar (soul travel); Extracellular potassium (kalium).
ECL Emitter-coupled logic; Endoscopic cord ligation (in selective feticide) (Obstetrics); Enterochromaffin-like (type); Epithelial cell; Extent(ion) of cerebral lesion; Extracapillary lesion(s); Euglobulin clot lysis (see ECLT).
Eclec Eclectic.
ECLT Euglobulin clot lysis time (laboratory/ hematology) (= ECL).
ECM Effective contraceptive measure; Egg crate mattress (for decubital ulcers); Embryonic chick muscle; Erythema chronicum migrans (associated with Lyme disease) (see LD); Experimental cerebral malaria; External cardiac massage; Extracellular contrast media/ium (MRI); Extracellular material/ matrix; Extracranial malformation(s).
ECMO Enteric cytopathic/thogenic monkey orphan (virus); Extracorporeal Mechanical/ Membrane Oxygenation/tor (artificial lung) (= ECOS).
Ecmo V Ecmovirus (see ECMO).
ECMP Extracellular-matrix protein (see CAP - Cell-adhesion protein; TGF-β).
ECN Extended care nursery.
Eco Ecology (see Ecol); Economic(al)/(s) (see Econ).
E co Escherichia coli (see E coli).
ECochG Electrocochleography.
ECOG Eastern Cooperative Onconology Group.
ECoG Electrocorticogram/aphy.
Ecol Ecology (= Eco).
E. coli *Escherichia* coli (= EC; E co) (see EAEC; EHEC; EIEC; EPEC; ETEC).
E. coli O157:H7 *Escherichia* coli O157:H7 verotoxin (a toxin produced by E. coli and found in the stool, causing severe diarrhea, and often resulting in HUS or Hemolytic uremic syndrome).
Econ Economic(al)/(s) (= Eco).
ECOP Extension Committee on Organization and Policy.
ECOS Extracorporeal oxygenator support (see ECMO).
ECP Ectrodactyly-cleft palate (syndrome); Effector cell precursor; Effusive-constrictive pericarditis; Elective cardiac procedure (coronary angioplasty, stenting, or coronary bypass surgery); Electron channeling pattern (SEM);

Emergency contraceptive pill; Encephalopathy; Endocardial potential; Endogenous cortisol production; Eosinophil cationic protein; Epidural catheter placement; Epiphysial cartilage plate (Orthopedics); Ergotamine-containing preparation (see ECD); Erythrocyte coproporphyrin; Erythrocyte cytoporphyrin (= Free cytoporphyrin in erythrocytes); Erythroid committed precursor; Escherichia coli polypeptide; Estradiol cyclopentane propionate; European Cancer Prevention (Organization study group); External cardiac pressure; External counterpulsation.

ECPD Endocrinopathic disease/ disorder; External counterpressure device.

ECPO Enteric cytopathic/thogenic porcine orphan (virus).

ECPOG Electrochemical potential gradient.

ECPR External cardiopulmonary resuscitation.

ECR Effectiveness-cost ratio; Electrocardiographic response; Emergency cardiopulmonary resuscitation; Emergency chemical restraint; Experimental Cell Research (journal); Extensor carpi radialis.

ECRB Extensor carpi radialis brevis.

ECRI Emergency Care Research Institute.

ECRL Extensor carpi radialis longus.

ECRO Enteric cytopathogenic rodent orphan (virus).

Ecro V Ecrovirus (see ECRO).

ECS Elective cosmetic surgery; Electrical conducting system (of the heart); Electrocerebral shock/ silence; Electroconvulsive shock; Electroshock; Emergency cesarian section; Enchondrosarcoma (see CCS); Epidemic-causing strain (of a parasite); Essential community services; Extracardiac shunt; Extracellular space.

ECSO Enteric cytopathic/thogenic swine orphan (virus).

Ecso V Ecsovirus (see ECSO).

ECSP Epidermal cell surface protein.

Ecstasy Methylenedioxy methamphetamine (see Amphet; MDMA).

ECT Ecological competition theory; Electroconvulsive therapy/ treatment (= Electroplexy; EST); Embryonic carcinoma of the testis; Emission/ Enhanced computed/er tomogram/aphy; Endrophonium chloride test (IV test used in myasthenia gravis); Enteric coated tablet; Epithelial cell turnover; Euglobulin clot test; European compression technique; Extracorporeal thrombosis/ thrombus.

ect ectopic/py.

ect- prefix meaning outside (Gr. ektos) (see ecto-).

ECTA Embryo cell Transformation Assay (Syrian Hamster) (see SHECTA); Everyman's Contingency Table Analysis.

-ectasis suffix meaning stretch or dilate (Gr. ektasis).

ECTEOLA Epichlorohydrin-triethanolamine (treated cellulose for TLC/ thin-layer chromatography).

ecto- prefix meaning outside (Gr. ektos) (= ect-).

-ectomy suffix meaning surgical removal (Gr. ektome).

ECU Environmental control unit; Extended care unit; Extensor carpi ulnaris.

ECV Elective/ Electrical cardioversion; Enteric coronavirus; Epithelial cell vacuolization; Extracellular/ Extracorporeal volume.

ECVD Emergency/ Enhanced cardiovascular care (= ECC); Extracellular volume of distribution.

ECW Extracellular water; Exuding cavity wound.

ED Early differentiation; Economically deprived; Ectodermal dysplasia; Ectopic depolarization; Effective/ Erythema dose; Ehlers-Danlos (syndrome) (see EDS); Ejaculation/ Emotional disorder; Elbow disarticulation; Electrodialysis; Electron diffraction; Ellis-Dawber (syndrome) (see EDS); Embryonic death; Emergency department; Emery-Dreifuss (syndrome) (see (EDS); Emotionally disturbed; End diastole; Endogenous depression (see ID); Energy dissipation; Entering diagnosis; Entner-Doudoroff (metabolic pathway) (see EDP); Enzyme deficiency; Epidural; Epigastric discomfort; Epileptiform discharge; Equine dermis (cells); Erectile dysfunction (i.e. impotence) (= EDF); Esophageal dilator; Ethyl dichlorarsine (a war gas); Ethynodiol; Evidence of disease; Exertional dyspnea; Exogenous depression (see RD); Extensive disease; Extensor digitorum; External diameter; Extra-low dispersion.

Ed Edit(ed)/ion (see Edn); Editor.

ed edema; edit (see Edn).

E_d Depth dose.

E-D Ego-defense.

ED 50 Expected death (rate of) 50%.

ED_{50} Mean/ Median effective dose.

E/D 50 50% egg infective dose.

EDA Early-detection activity; Economic Development Administration; Electrodermal activity/ audiometry; Electrolyte-deficient agar; Electron donor acceptor; End diastolic area; Enteral drug administration; Epidural anesthesia; Extradural abscess.

EDAC Ethyl-dimethyl-aminopropyl carbodiimide.

EDAM Electron-dense amorphous material.

EDAP Emergency Department Approved for Pediatrics.

EDAX Energy dispersive x-ray analysis.

EDB Early dry breakfast; Electron-dense body; Epidural block (see EDA); Ethylene dibromide; Extensor digitorum brevis.

EDBP Erect diastolic blood pressure.

EDC Effective dynamic compliance; Emergency decontamination center; Emotionally Disturbed Children (OAEDC journal); End-diastolic count; Estimated date of conception (= ECD); Erythropoietin-dependent cell; Estrogen-dependent carcinoma; Expected date of confinement (= ECD); Expected delivery, cesarean; Extensor digitorum communis; Extensive daily contact.

ED&C Electrodesiccation and curettage.

EDCC Early Detection Coronary Care (area).

EDCF Endothelium-derived contracting factor.

EDCI Energetic dynamic cardiac insufficiency.

EDCS End-diastolic chamber stiffness; End-diastolic circumferential stress.

EDD Effective drug duration; Electron dense deposit; End-diastolic dimension; Endothelium-dependent (vaso)dilation (see EDV); Enzyme-digested delta (endotoxin); Estimated/ Expected date of delivery; Estimated due date (see EDL).

EDDA Expanded-duty dental assistant/ auxiliary.

EDE Extensive diagnostic evaluation.

ede- prefix meaning swell (Gr. oideo).

edent edentia/tulous.

EDF Ejaculatory dysfunction; Elongation, derotation, and flexion; End-diastole flow (see EDV); Environmental Defense Fund; Erectile dysfunction (see ED); Extradural fluid.

EDG Electrodermogram/aphy.

EDH Extradural hematoma.

EDI Epidural injection.

EDIM Epizootic diarrhea of infant mice.

E-diol Estradiol.

EDL Electrode-less discharge lamp; Emerging Diseases Laboratory (UCI); End-diastolic length/ load; Estimated date of labor (= EDD; EDOC); Extensor digitorum longus.

ED/LD Emotionally disturbed and learning disabled.

EDM Early diastolic murmur; Extramucosal duodenal myotomy.

EDMA Ethylene glycol dimethacrylate.

EDMD Emery-Dreifuss muscular dystrophy.

EDN Electrodesiccation; Eosinophil-derived neurotoxin; Estrogen dependent neoplasia/lasm.

Edn Edition.

EDNA Emergency Department Nurses Association.

EDNF Endogenous digitalis-like natriuretic factor; Extradural neurofibroma (= ENF).

EDNO Endothelium-derived nitric oxide.

EDOA Extradural opioid analgesia.

EDOC Estimated date of confinement (see EDL).

EDP Early detection program (cancer); Egg-donation/ donor program; Electron dense particle; Electronic data processing; Elevated diastolic/ End-diastolic pressure; Emergency department physician; Entner-Doudoroff pathway (metabolic) (= ED); Erb-Duchenne paralysis (= Erb's palsy) (see BPP).

EDPRESS Educational Press Association of America.

EDQ Extensor digiti quinti.
EDR Early diastolic relaxation; Edophronium; Effective direct radiation; Egg-donor recepient; Electrodermal response.
EDRA Environmental Design Research Association.
EDRF Endothelial/thelium-dependent/ -derived relaxant/ xing factor (now identified as Noxide, cGMP, and phosphodiesterases like PDE and PDIE, released from the endothelium of arteries).
EDS Eastern Dental Society (Bulletin); Edema disease of swine; Egg drop syndrome; Ehlers-Danlos syndrome (= ED); Electrodiagnostic study (Orthopedics); Ellis-Dawber syndrome (sparse hair, peg-shaped deciduous teeth and hypoplastic nails); Emergency department study; Emery-Dreifuss syndrome (= ED); Energy-dispersive spectrometry (see EDXS); Environmental dependency syndrome; Epigastric distress syndrome; Erectile dysfunction syndrome; Estrogen deficiency state; Excessive daytime sleepiness; Extradimensional shift.
EDs Ectodermal dysplasias.
EDSS Expanded disability status scale.
EDT Early distal tubule (or proximal portion of the second convuluted tubule in the renal cortex); End-diastolic thickness; Entire duration of treatment; Epipodophyllotoxin; Erythrocyte density test.
EDTA Ethylenediamine tetraacetic acid (= Acid Tetracemique; Disodium edetic acid; Disodium ethylenediamine tetraacetate; Edathamil; Edathauril; Edetic acid; EDTAA; Ethylenediamine tetraacetic acid; Ethylenediamine tetraacetate; Ethylene dinitrilo tetraacetic acid. A preservative; the calcium salt is used as a chelating agent in the treatment of lead poisoning); European Dialysis and Transplant Association.
EDTAA See EDTA.
EDTAP Dipotassium ethylenediamine tetraacetate.
EDTIAR Extended Duration Topical Insect/ Arthopod Repellent.
Educ Education.
EDV End-diastole velocity (e.g. in the umbilical artery - Obstetrics); End-diastolic volume; Endothelium-dependent vasodilation (of the coronary arteries).
EDVI End-diastolic volume index.
EDWTH End-diastolic wall thickness.
EDX; EDx; Edx Electrodiagnosis.
EDXA Energy-dispersive x-ray analysis.
EDXS Energy-dispersive x-ray spectrometer/metry (SEM - Scanning electron microscope) (= EDS).
EE Electrical engineer; Electron excitation; Embryo extract; End-to-end (anastomosis) (see EEA); End expiration; Energy expenditure; Enterobacteriaceae enrichment (broth); Equine encephalitis; Ethinyl estradiol; Expressed emotion; External ear; Eye and ear (see E&E).
E-E Erythema(tous)-edema(tous) (reaction).
E&E Eye and ear (= EE).
EE2 Ethinyl estradiol (= EE).
EEA Echo-enhancing agent; Electroencephalic audiometry; Elemental external alimentation; End-to-end anastomosis (= EE); European Economic Area.
EEC Ectrodactyly-ectodermal (dysplasia)-clefting (syndrome); End-expiratory closure (of atelectatic alveoli, in lung injury); Entero-enteric circulation; Enteropathogenic Escherichia coli; European Economic Community/ Council.
EECD Endothelial-epithelial corneal dystrophy.
EECG Electroencephalogram/graph(y) (see EEG); Exercise electrocardiogram/graph(y).
EECV Elective electric cardioversion (= EEC).
EED Endogenous estrogen depletion; Endoscopy esophageal dilator.
EEDQ Ethoxycarbonyl-ethoxy-dihydroquinoline.
EEE Eastern equine encephalitis/lomyelitis; Edema, erythema, and exudate; Experimental enterococcal endocarditis; External eye examination.
EEEP End-expiratory esophageal pressure.
EEEV Eastern equine encephalomyelitis virus.
EEG Electroencephalogram/graph(y) (= EEECG).
EEGA Electroencephalographic audiometry.

EEGCN Electroencephalography and Clinical Neurophysiology (journal).

EEG-CSA Electroencephalography with computerized spectral analysis.

EEGT Electroencephalograph technician.

EEI Edison Electric Institute.

EELS Electron energy loss spectroscopy.

EEM Ectodermal dysplasia, ectrodactyly, macular dystrophy (syndrome); Emission electron microscope; Erythema exudativum multiforme; Excessive eye movement; Extrinsic eye muscle.

EEME Ethinylestradiol methyl ether (see EE3ME).

EE3ME Mestranol (= Compound 33355; EEME; Ethinylestradiol methyl ether; Ethinylo-estradiol-3-methyl ether). Used (i) in disorders of menstruation, fertility and pregnancy, and (ii) in conjunction with a progestational agent, as a contraceptive.

EEMF Endocardial elastomyofibrosis.

EEMG Evoked electromyogram.

EENT Eye(s), ear(s), nose, and throat.

EENTM Eye, Ear, Nose, and Throat Monthly (journal).

EEO Electroendosmosis; Equal employment opportunity.

EEOA Equal Employment Opportunity Act.

EEOC Equal Employment Opportunity Commission.

EEOCC Equal Employment Opportunity Coordinating Council.

EEP End-expiratory pressure; Equivalent effective photon; Erythrodermic exfoliative psoriasis; Ethanolic extract of propolis; Expanded end point (e.g. CABG, PEP, PTCA, etc.).

EEPI Extraretinal eye position information.

EER Electroencephalic/lographic response; Energy efficiency rating; Experimental Eye Research (journal).

EES Endogenous estrogen secretion (= EOS); Erythromycin ethylsuccinate; Ethyl ethane sulfate.

EESG Evoked electrospinogram.

EESRT Entrance Examination for Schools of Radiologic Technology.

EEU Environmental Epidemiology Unit (MRC, UK).

EF Ectopic/ Epithelial/ Equivalent focus; Edema/ Ejection/ Emotional/ Encephalitogenic/ Endurance/ Exophthalmos-producing/ Exposure/ Extrinsic factor; Ejection fraction (or EC - Ejection capacity of the calf muscle pump): EF = EV/VV x 100 (EV = Ejection volume; VV = Functional venous volume). It is more than 60% in normal limbs; Elastic fibril; Electric field; Elongation factor (protein synthesis) (= EF2; EF-G; EF-T); Embryo-fetal; Embryo fibroblasts; Emergency facility; Endothoracic fascia; Engineering Foundation; Enteric fever; Environmental Fund; Eosinophilic fasciitis; Erythroblastosis fetalis; Erythrocyte/cytic fragmentation; Esophagoscope, fiberoptic; Etiologic fraction; Explosion fracture (see PF - Type III); Extended field (radiotherapy); Extra fine.

ef effusion (pleural).

ef- prefix meaning from or out of (Gr., L. ex).

EF2 Elongation factor 2 (host cell) (see EF).

EFA Epilepsy Foundation of America; Essential (polyunsaturated) fatty acid; Esterified fatty acid; Extrafamily adoptee.

EFAD Essential fatty acid deficiency.

EFAS Embryofetal alcohol syndrome.

EFC Elastin fragment concentration; Endogenous fecal calcium; Ephemeral fever of cattle.

EFD Embryo-fetal development; Equinus foot deformity (see DEFD; DFD); Exfoliative dermatitis.

EFDA Expanded function dental assistant.

EFE Embryofetotoxic effect(s); Endocardial fibroelastosis.

EFEx Ejection fraction (during) exercise (see ExEF).

eff effect(s); effective (see effect); efferent (see effer); efficiency/nt; effusion.

Eff Effervescent (tablet) (= Effervesc).

effect effective (= eff).

effer efferent (= eff).

Effervesc Effervescent.

EFFU Epithelial focus-forming unit.

EFG Excessive fetal growth (= Macrosomia).

EF-G Elongation factor G (see EF).

EFH Explosive follicular hyperplasia.

EFHBM Eosinophilic fibrohistiocytic (lesion

of) bone marrow.
EFI Electrolyte fluid imbalance.
EFL Effective focal length; External fluid loss.
EFM Elderly fibromyalgia; Electronic/ Extensive fetal monitoring; External fetal monitor.
EFMU Elliot Fraley Minnesota Urology (virus).
EFP Early follicular phase; Effective filtration pressure (see KFT - EFP); Endoneural fluid pressure.
EFR Effective filtration rate (see KFT - EFR).
EFR_{max} Maximum expiratory flow rate (see PFT - EFR_{max}).
EFS Effective field stimulation; Event-free survival.
EFSR Event-free survival rate.
EFT Electronic funds transfer (banking); Embedded Figures Test.
EF-T Elongation factor T (see EF).
EFTS Electronic funds transfer system (banking).
EFU Extended follow-up.
EFV Expiratory flow volume (see PFT); Extracellular fluid volume.
efv en face visualization (Endoscopy).
EFVC Expiratory flow-volume curve (see PFT - EFVC).
EFW Electrolyte-free water; Estimated fetal weight.
EF/WM Ejection fraction/ wall motion.
EG Ecthyma gangrenosum; Embryonic germ (cell); Enteroglucagon; Esophagogastrectomy; External genitalia.
eg for example (L. exempli gratia).
E-G Elated-grandiose (manic symptom).
EGA Enzymatic glucose assay; Estimated gestational age.
EGBUS External genitalia, Bartholin, urethral, Skene's glands.
EGC Early gastric cancer; Elution gas chromatography; Embryonic germ cell; Endometrial glandular cell; Epithelioid-globoid cell(s).
EGCG Epigallocatechin gallate (an antioxidant found in green tea).
EGD Early growth delay (Obstetrics); Esophago-gastro-duodenoscopy.
EGDF Embryonic growth and development factor.
EGF Epidermal growth factor; Epithelial growth factor (including HGF and KGF).
EGFR Epithelial growth factor receptor.
EGF-R Epidermal growth factor, receptor.
EGF-URO Epidermal growth factor, urogastrone.
EGG Electrogastrogram; Equine gamma globulin.
EGH Endogenous/ Epidermal/ Equine growth hormone.
EGJ Esophagogastric junction.
EGL Eosinophilic granuloma of the lung.
EGLT Euglobin lysis time.
EGM Electrogram; Extracellular granular material.
EGME Ethylene glycol monomethyl ether.
EGN Endogen(ous) glucagon secretion; Experimental glomerulonephritis.
EGOR Enzymatic glucose oxidase reaction (tape test for glucose).
EGOT Erythrocyte glutamic oxaloacetic transaminase.
EGP Endogenous glycoprotein (e.g. IFN - Interferon).
EGR Erythema gyratum repens; Erythrocyte glutathione reductase (see E-GR).
E-GR Erythrocyte glutathione reductase (= EGR).
EGRA Equilibrium-gated radionuclide angiography.
EGRAC Erythrocyte glutathione reductase activity coefficient.
EGS Electrogalvanic stimulation; Endogenic secretion; External guide sequence.
EGT Ethanol gelation test; Experimental gene therapy (see HGT).
EGTA Esophageal gastric tube airway; Ethylene glycol tetraacetic acid (= Ethylene-bis-oxyethylene-nitrilo-tetraacetic acid; Ethyleneglycol-bis-[β-aminoethylether]-N,N,N',N'-tetraacetic acid; Ethyleneglycol tetraacetate).
EGW External genital wart(s) (= Condyloma acuminata; PAW).
EH Eczema herpeticum (Kaposi's varicelliform eruption); Educationally handicapped; Elimination half-life; Enlarged heart (see eh);

Epidermolytic hyperkeratosis; Epoxide hydratase; Essential hypertension (= EHT); Estrogenic hormones (see Hormones - EH); Extramedullary hematopoiesis.

eh enlarged heart (= EH).

eH; E_h Oxidation-reduction or redox potential.

E/H; E&H Environment and heredity (psychology).

E-H Eder-Hufford (esophagoscope).

E&H Ear and Hearing (journal, US).

EHA Education of the Handicapped Act; Emotional Health Anonymous; Environmental Health Agency.

EHAA Epidemic hepatitis-associated antigen.

EHB Elevate head of bed; Erythrohydrobupropion (metabolite of bupropion, an anti-smoking drug).

EHBA Extrahepatic biliary atresia.

EHBD Extrahepatic bile duct.

EHBF Estimated hepatic/ Exercise hyperemic/ Extrahepatic blood flow.

EHC Embryonic human cell; Enamel hypocalcification (the enamel, although of normal amount, is soft and lacks calcium) (Dentistry); End-hole catheter; Enterohepatic circulation/ clearance/ cycling; Environmental Health Center; Essential hypercholesterolemia; Ethyl hydrocaffeate (an antoxidant); Ethylhydrocupreine hydrochloride; Extended health care; Extrahepatic cholestasis.

EHD Electrohemodynamics; Environmental Health Directorate (HPB); Epizootic hemorrhagic disease (of poultry); Exercise hemodynamics.

EHDP Ethane hydroxy-diphosphate (= Disodium ethane-1-hydroxy-1,1-diphosphate/diphosphonate; Sodium etidronate). A drug used recently in Paget's disease to inhibit bone mineralization.

EHDV Epizootic hemorrhagic disease virus.

EHE Epithelioid hemangioendothelioma; Estimated human exposure.

EHEC Enterohemorrhagic Escherichia coli (see E. coli).

EHEs Embryonated hens' eggs (yolk sac - culture medium for microorganisms such as *Rickettsiae*).

EHF Ebola hemorrhagic fever (caused by the filovirus, a filamentous mammalian virus found in African green monkeys); Epidemic hemolytic/ hemorrhagic fever; Exophthalmos-hyperthyroid factor; Extreme(ly) high frequency.

EHG Executive Health Group.

EHH Esophageal hiatal/tus hernia.

EHHAIT *Entameba* histolytica hemagglutination inhibition titer.

EHJ European Heart Journal.

EHL Effective half-life (of radioactive substances) (= RHL) (see Half-life); Electrohydraulic lithotripsy; Elimination half life (of a drug - pharmacokinetic parameter); Endogenous/ Essential hyperlipidemia; Environmental Health Laboratory (USAF); Extensor hallucis longus.

EHM Encephalohepatomyocarditis.

EHME Employee health maintenance examination.

EHMS Electrohemodynamic ionization mass spectrometry (see EIMS).

EHN Environmental Health Network; European Heart Network (Internet).

EHNA 9-erythro-2-(hydroxy-3-nonyl) adenine.

EHO Extrahepatic obstruction.

EHP Di-(2-ethylhexyl) hydrogen phosphate; Enamel hypoplasia (a defect of the teeth, in which the enamel is thin and lacking (see AGS); Environmental Health Perspectives; Excessive heat production; Extra-high potency.

EHPA Emergency Health Personnel Act.

EHPAC Emergency Health Preparedness Advisory Committee.

EHPH Extrahepatic portal hypertension.

EHPT Eddy hot plate test.

HER Enterohepatic recirculation.

EHS Emergency health service; Environmental Health Services (HEW); Environmental health specialist; Exploding head syndrome (a common and totally benign condition in which patients are alarmed by a sudden loud noise in the twilight stage of sleep).

EHSC Environmental Health Sciences Center (USC).

EHSD Emergency Health Services Digest (journal).

EHSDS Experimental Health Service Delivery System/ Services Development Systems.

EHT Electrohydrothermoelectrode; Essential hypertension (see EH).

EHTN Essential hypertension (= EH; EHT; PHTN).

EHV Electric heart vector; Equine herpes virus; Extra/ Extreme high voltage (up to 765 kv).

EI Electrolyte imbalance (Warning signs: drowsiness; dryness of mouth, gastrointestinal disturbances such as nausea or vomiting, hypotension, lethargy, muscle pain or cramps, muscular fatigue, oliguria, restlessness, tachycardia, thirst, weakness, etc.); Electron impact/ ionization; Emotionally impaired; Endocrinology Index (journal); Engineering Index (NYC); Environmental illness (see MCS); Enzyme inducer(uctor)/ inhibition(tor); Eosinophilic/ Excretory Index; Erectile impotence; Erythema infectiosum (caused by parvovirus B19 infection) (= Fifth disease); Ethylene-imine (a carcinogen).

E/I Expiration/inspiration (ratio) (see PFT - E/I).

E&I Endocrinology and infertility.

EIA Electroimmunoassay; Electronic Industries Association (formerly RMA); Energy Independence Authority; Enzyme immunoassay; Enzyme-inducing agent (e.g. Antibiotics such as rifampicin; Anti-convulsants such as carbamazepine, phenobarbitone and phenytoin) (= EID); Enzyme-inhibiting agent; Enzyme-linked immunosorbent assay; Equine infectious anemia; Erythroimmunoassay; Exercise-induced asthma; Extra-intestinal amebiasis (invasion of the liver, lungs and brain; also the skin, vulva, vagina, uterine cervix and penis); Interface between a computer and a system for transmitting digital information.

EIAB Extracranial-intracranial arterial bypass.

EIAP End-inspiratory alveolar pressure.

EIAV Equine infectious anemia virus (= EIVA).

EIB Electrophoretic immunoblotting; Exercise-induced broncho-constriction/ bronchospasm.

EIBC Exercise-induced bronchoconstriction (see EIA; EIB; EIBS).

EIBS Exercise-induced bronchospasm (see EIA; EIB).

EIC Elastase inhibition capacity; Enzyme inhibition complex; Epilepsy Information Center.

EID Egg infectious/tive dose; Electroimmunodiffusion; Electronic/ Emergency infusion device; Emerging Infectious Diseases (journal); Endothelium-independent (vaso)dilation (see EIV); Enzyme-inducing/ inhibiting drug (see EIA).

EIEC Enteroinvasive Escherichia coli; Estrogen-induced endometrial cancer.

EIEE Early infantile epileptic encephalopathy.

EIF Erythema-inducing factor; Erythrocyte initiation factor (see eIF); Eukaryotic initiation factor.

eIF Erythrocyte initiation factor (= EIF).

EIL Elevated insulin level (causes macrosomia in fetuses - see MSB).

EIM Excitability-inducing material.

EIMC Exercise-induced muscle cramp(s) (see EIMP).

EIMP Exercise-induced muscle pain (see EIMC).

EIMS Electron ionization mass spectrometry (see EHMS).

EIOP Elevated intraocular pressure.

EIP Electrical impulse propagation; Emergency Infections Program (CDC); End-inspiratory pause/ pressure; Endogenous insulin production (see EIS; Insulin); Extensor indicis proprius.

EIPS Endogenous inhibitor of prostaglandin synthase/thetase.

EIPVD Exercise-induced premature ventricular depolarization.

EIR Effective immune response; Environmental impact review.

EIRNV; EIRnv; EIR_{nv} Extra incidence rate in/of non-vaccinated groups.

EIRP Effective isotropic radiated power.

EIRV; EIRv; EIR_v Extra incidence rate in/of vaccinated groups.

EIS Early intervention service(service for autistic children, etc.); Electrolyte imbalance state (such as HCA, KDS & NaDS); Endogenous insulin secretion (see Insulin); Endoscopic injection scleropathy; Environmental Impact Statement; Enzyme-impregnated strip; Epidemic/ Epidemiology Intelligence Service (NCID); Epidemiological Investigational Service; Equivalent Institutional Service; European Immunology Society; Excessive inspiratory stretch (causing lung injury); Exercise-induced sweating.

EIT Erythroid iron turnover; Essential initial therapy (such as cardiac defibrillation); Excessive iron therapy; Exogenous insulin therapy.

EIV Endothelium-independent vasodilation (= EID); External iliac vein.

EIVA Equine infectious virus anemia (see EIAV).

EJ Elbow jerk (= Ej); Electroencephalography Journal (IFSECN); External jugular.

Ej Elbow jerk (see EJ).

EJB Ectopic junctional beat; European Journal of Biochemistry (formerly BZ).

EJC Engineers Joint Council; European Journal of Cancer (UK).

EJCMID European Journal of Clinical Microbiology and Infectious Diseases.

EJD Erosive joint disease.

EJI European Journal of Immunology.

EJLM European Journal of Laboratory Medicine.

EJP European Journal of Pharmacology; Excitation/atory junction potential.

ejus; ejusd of the same (L. ejusdem).

EK Enterokinase; Erythrokinase.

EKC Eastman Kodak Co; Epidemic kerato-conjunctivitis.

EKG Electrocardiogram/graph(y) (see ECG).

EKHSC East Kentucky Health Services Center.

EKO Electroencephalogram.

EKP Epikeratophakia (superficial corneal lens).

EKS Epidemic Kaposi sarcoma.

EKV Erythrokeratodermia variabilis.

EKY Electrokymogram/graph(y).

EL Early latent; Elbow (see Elb; elb); Electroluminescence; Encephalitis lethargica; Erythroleukemia; Exercise limit; External lamina.

El; el Elastase; Elixir.

E-L Eaton-Lambert (see ELS; MS); External lid(s).

EL-4 Chemically-induced lymphoma.

ELA Elastomer-lubricating agent; Endotoxin-like activity; Excimer laser ablation/ angio-plasty.

ELAS Extended lymphadenopathy syndrome.

ELB Early light breakfast; Elbow (see Elb; elb).

Elb; elb Elbow (= EL; ELB).

ELBW Extremely low birth weight.

ELC Eccentric laser catheter (see ELA; ELS); Endoscopic laser coagulation.

-elc- combining form meaning sore or ulcer (Gr. elkos).

ELD Egg lethal dose; Estrogen-like drug (such as SERM - e.g. Raloxifene) (see SERM).

Elec; elec Electric(al)/ity; Elective/tuary (see Elect; elect).

Elect; elect Elective (= Elec; elec); Electuary (L. electuarium) (= Elec; elec).

electr- prefix meaning amber (Gr. elektron).

Electromed Electromedica (journal).

ELEM Equine leukoencephalomalacia.

elem elementary.

Elements see Table.

Elephant Phencyclidine (see CI 395).

Elev; elev Elevate(d)/tion/tor.

ELF Elective low forceps; Elevated liver function; External labor force; Extremely low frequency (≤) 100 hz).

ELH Egg-laying hormone; Endolymphatic hydrops.

ELI Endomyocardial lymphatic infiltrates; Environmental Language Inventory; Exercise lability index; Extensive lymphocytic infiltration.

ELIA Enzyme-linked immunoassay.

ELICT Enzyme-linked immunocytochemical technique.

ELIEDA Enzyme-linked immunoelectron diffusion assay.

ELIS Environmental Language Intervention Strategy.

ELISA Enzyme-linked immunosorbent assay.

ELITE Evaluation of Losartan in the Elderly

Elements

Name	Symbol	Atomic no.	Atomic weight	Other Details and Remarks
Actinium	**Ac**	89	227.	(Gr. aktinos = ray) Decomposes into francium and helium. Discovered in 1899.
Aluminium	**Al**	13	26.9815	(L. Aluminum) Discovered in 1827.
Americum	**Am**	95	243.	Named after the Americas. Obtained by cyclotron bombardment of uranium and plutonium. Discovered in 1944.
Antimony	**Sb**	51	121.75	(L. Antimonium; Stibium) Discovered about 1450.
Argon	**Ar**	18	39.948	(Gr. argos = inert) Discovered in 1894.
Arsenic	**As**	33	74.9216	(Gr. arsen = strong; arsenikos = male) (L. Arsenicum; Arsenium; Arsenum) Discovered about 1250.
Astatine	**At**	85	210	(Gr. astatos = unstable) Obtained by cyclotron bombardment of bismuth atoms with helium nuclei. Discovered in 1940.
Barium	**Ba**	56	137.34	(Gr. barys = heavy/dense) Discovered in 1808.
Berkelium	**Bk**	97	247.	Named after Berkeley, the home of the University of California, where it was produced by bombardment of the isotope americium-241 - by helium ions. Discovered in 1949.
Beryllium	**Be**	4	9.0122	From the mineral, beryl (Gr. beryllos). Formerly known by the name Glucinium (Gl). Discovered in 1798
Bismuth	**Bi**	83	208.980	(Ger. Wisemuth = white mass; L. Bismuthum) Discovered in 1450.
Boron	**B**	5	10.811	(L. Borium) Discovered in 1808.
Bromine	**Br**	35	79.909	(Gr. bromos = stench; L. Brominium; Bromium; Bromum) Discovered in 1826.
Cadmium	**Cd**	48	112.40	(Gr. kadmia = earth) Discovered in 1817.
Caesium	**Cs**	55	132.905	Also called Cesium (L. caesius = sky-blue). Discovered in 1860.
Calcium	**Ca**	20	40.08	(L. calx = lime) Discovered 1808.
Californium	**Cf**	98	249.	After the state and University of California, where it was produced by irradiation of the isotope of curium (Cm) -242 with helium ions. Discovered in 1950.
Carbon	**C**	6	12.01115	(L. Carbo = charcoal) Prehistoric.
Cerium	**Ce**	58	140.12	Named after the asteroid, Ceres. Discovered in 1803.
Chlorine	**Cl**	17	35.453	(Gr. chloros = green or greenish-yellow; L. Chlorinum; Chlorum) Discovered in 1774.

Elements (continued)

Name	Symbol	Atomic no.	Atomic weight	Other Details and Remarks
Chromium	**Cr**	24	51.996	(Gr. chroma = color) Discovered in 1797.
Cobalt	**Co**	27	58.9332	(Gr. kobold = evil spirit {its poisonous ores were once treachorous to miners}; L. Cobaltum) Discovered in 1735.
Copper	**Cu**	29	63.54	(Gr. Kypros - ancient name for Cyprus, famed for its copper mines; L. Cuprum) Known by early man.
Curium	**Cm**	96	247.	In honor of Pierre and Marie Curie - pioneers in the field of radioactivity. Obtained by cyclotron bombardment of uranium (U) and Plutonium (Pu). Discovered in 1944.
Dysprosium	**Dy**	66	162.50	(Gr. dysprositos = hard to get) Discovered in 1886.
Einsteinium	**Es**	99	254.	After Albert Einstein; first discovered in debris from the 1952 H-bomb explosion at Eniwetok Atoll in the Pacific.
Erbium	**Er**	68	167.26	From Ytterby in Sweden. Discovered in 1843.
Europium	**Eu**	63	151.96	From Europe. Discovered in 1896.
Fermium	**Fm**	100	253.	After Emrico Fermi, Italian physicist; first discovered from the debris of the 1952 H-bomb test, from the fission of uranium.
Fluorine	**F**	9	18.9984	From fluor spar (L. fluore = to flow), from which it is derived. Discovered in 1771.
Francium	**Fr**	87	223.	From France; discovered by Marguerite Percy, a one-time assistant to Marie Curie, in 1939. A short-lived product of actinium (Ac), francium has never actually been seen. Formerly called Virginium (Vi), after the state of Virginia.
Gadolinium	**Gd**	64	157.25	From the mineral gadolinite, named after a Finnish chemist. Discovered in 1880.
Gallium	**Ga**	31	69.72	(L. Gallia = Gaul - the old name for France) Discovered in 1875.
Germanium	**Ge**	32	72.59	After Germany. Discovered in 1886.
Gold	**Au**	79	196.967	From the old English word geolo or yellow (L. Aurum). Prehistoric.
Hafnium	**Hf**	72	178.49	From (Latin) Hafnia or Copenhagen, where it was discovered in 1923 in a mineral, zircon by Coster and Hevesy of that city.
Hahnium	**Ha**	105	?	?

Elements (continued)

Name	Symbol	Atomic no.	Atomic weight	Other Details and Remarks
Helium	**He**	2	4.0026	(Gr. helios = sun) First detected in the sun in 1868, and is now obtained from natural gas.
Holmium	**Ho**	67	164.930	From (Latin) Holmia or Stockholm. Discovered in 1879.
Hydrogen	**H**	1	1.00797	(Gr. hydor = water, and gennan = to produce, i.e. water-forming) Discovered in 1766.
Indium	**In**	49	114.82	(L. indicum = indigo blue) Discovered in 1863.
Iodine	**I**	53	126.9044	(Gr. iodes = violet) A blue-black solid which turns into a violet vapor when heated. Discovered 1811.
Iridium	**Ir**	77	192.2	(L. iris = rainbow) From the tints of its salts. Discovered 1804.
Iron	**Fe**	26	55.847	From (Anglo-Saxon) iren - its old English name; (L.) Ferrum. First utilized by prehistoric man.
Krypton	**Kr**	36	83.80	(Gr. kryptos = hidden) Discovered in 1898.
Kurchatovium	**Ku**	104	?	?
Lanthanum	**La**	57	138.91	(Gr. lanthanein = to be hidden or concealed) Discovered in 1839.
Lawrencium	**Lw**	103	257.	After the American physicist, Ernest Orlando Lawrence, and produced in 1961 by bombardment of Californium (Cf) isotopes of mass 250, 251, and 252. Now used with the symbol Lr.
Lead	**Pb**	82	207.19	From (Anglo-Saxon) lead - its old English name (L. Plumbum). Also the origin of the word, plumber. Prehistoric.
Lithium	**Li**	3	6.939	(Gr. lithos = stone) Discovered in 1817.
Lutetium	**Lu**	71	174.97	(L. Lutetia = the ancient name for Paris) Discovered in 1907.
Magnesium	**Mg**	12	24.312	From (L.) Magnesia, the name of a city in ancient Lydia, Asia Minor (= Mag). Discovered in 1775.
Manganese	**Mn**	25	54.9380	From magnes or magnet. Its ore was first confused with magnetic iron ore (L. Manganesium; Manganum). Discovered in 1774.
Mendelevium	**Md**	101	256.	After Dimitri Ivanovich Mendeleyev who devised the periodic table. First discovered in 1952 in debris from a thermonuclear explosion.
Mercury	**Hg**	80	200.59	From the planet Mercury (L. mercurius) and (L. Hydrargyrum = liquid silver) - "quicksilver"; Prehistoric.

Elements (continued)

Name	Symbol	Atomic no.	Atomic weight	Other Details and Remarks
Mesothorium 1	**Ms-Th or MSTh**	88-90		A radioactive isotope of radium (Z = 88), formed from thorium (Z = 90) (= Mesothorium 1).
Mesothorium 2	**Ms-Th or MSTh**	89-90		A radioactive isotope of actinium (Z = 89), formed from thorium (Z = 90) (= Mesothorium 2).
Molybdenum	**Mo**	42	95.94	(Gr. molybdos = lead) First found in what was thought to be lead ore. Discovered in 1778.
Neodymium	**Nd**	60	144.24	(Gr. neos didymos = new twin) Discovered in 1885, together with Praseodymium (Pr).
Neon	**Ne**	10	20.183	(Gr. neos = new) First discovered in the air in 1898.
Neptunium	**Np**	93	237.	After the planet Neptune. Obtained by splitting the uranium atom with neutrons. Discovered in 1940.
Nickel	**Ni**	28	58.71	(Ger. Kupfernickel = false copper) A reddish ore containing nickel but no copper (L. Niccolum). Discovered in 1751.
Niobium	**Nb**	41	92.906	From Niobe, daughter of the mythical Greek king Tantalus (niobium is found with tantalum), who was turned into stone. Discovered in 1801. Until 1950 it was known as Columbium (Cb), from Columbia - a poetic name for America, where its ore was first discovered.
Nitrogen	**N**	7	14.0067	(Gr. nitron = niter + gennen = to produce, i.e. nitre-forming) Discovered in 1772.
Nobelium	**No**	102	254.	After Alfred Bernard Nobel. A 1957 claim of discovery is disputed, but nobelium was positively identified in 1958 by a team of California scientists, by bombardment of Curium (Cu)-246 with Carbon (C)-12 ions in a heavy ion linear accelerator.
Osmium	**Os**	76	190.2	(Gr. osmē = odor) A metal with a pungent smell. Discovered in 1804.
Oxygen	**O**	8	15.9994	(Gr. oxys = sour + gennan = to produce, i.e. acid-forming) It exists free in the air, and in combination in most non-elementary solids, liquids, and gases. It forms the characteristic constituent of most acids. Discovered in 1774.

Elements (continued)

Name	Symbol	Atomic no.	Atomic weight	Other Details and Remarks
Palladium	**Pd**	46	106.4	Named after the asteroid Pallas. Discovered in 1803.
Phosphorus	**P**	15	30.9738	(Gr. phos = light + phoros = carry or light bearer) It occurs in 3 forms: amorphous, metallic, and vitreous. Discovered in 1669.
Platinum	**Pt**	78	195.09	(L. platina = little silver) Discovered in the 16th century.
Plutonium	**Pu**	94	242.	After Pluto, the planet beyond Neptune. Obtained by splitting the uranium atom, which changes into neptunium and then into plutonium. Discovered in 1940.
Polonium	**Po**	84	210.	(L. Polonia = Poland) Discovered in 1898 by Pierre and Marie Curie in pitchblende.
Potassium	**K**	19	39.102	From potash, an impure form of potassium carbonate known to the ancients (L. Kalium). Discovered in 1807.
Praseodymium	**Pr**	59	140.907	(Gr. prasios didymos = green twin) From its green salts. Discovered in 1885, when it was separated from its rare earth-twin neodymium (Nd).
Promethium	**Pm**	61	147.	After Prometheus. Produced in nuclear reactors. Discovered in 1947. Formerly known as Florentium (Fl or Ft) or Illinium (Il.).
Protactinium	**Pa**	91	231.	(Gr. protos = first) It is the parent of actinium (Ac), which is formed by its radioactive decay. Also known by the symbol: UX2. Discovered in 1917.
Radium	**Ra**	88	226.	(L. radius = ray) So-called from its radiant quality. Discovered in pitchblende, by Pierre and Marie Curie, in 1898.
Radon	**Rn**	86	222.	Also called radium emanation. Obtained by the breaking up of radium. Heaviest gaseous element, it is emitted by radium, and is itself radioactive, decaying into radioactive polonium and alpha rays. Discovered in 1900. Formerly known as Niton (Nt).
Rhenium	**Re**	75	186.2	From the Rhine provinces of Germany. Discovered in 1925. Formerly known as Bohemium (Bo).
Rhodium	**Rh**	45	102.905	(Gr. rhodon = rose [its salts give a rosy solution]) Discovered in 1803.
Rubidium	**Rb**	37	85.47	(L. rubidus = red [the color its salts impart to flames]) Discovered in 1861.
Ruthenium	**Ru**	44	101.07	(L. Ruthenia = Russia) Discovered in 1844.

Elements (continued)

Name	Symbol	Atomic no.	Atomic weight	Other Details and Remarks
Samarium	**Sm**	62	150.35	From the mineral samarskite, named after a Russian mine official, Colonel V. E. Samarsky. Former symbol: Sa. Discovered in 1879.
Scandium	**Sc**	21	44.956	From Scandinavia. Discovered 1879.
Seaborgium	?	106	?	Discovered by the American chemist Glenn Seaborg, between 1940 and 1955. Produced a second time in 1974 by Albert Ghiorso, at the Lawrence Berkeley Laboratory. Finally confirmed in 1993 at the University of California at Berkeley. An unstable element produced in the accelerator, and surviving for not more than 30 seconds, before it decays into the lighter elements Curium (Z = 96) and Neon (Z = 10).
Selenium	**Se**	34	78.96	(Gr. selene = moon) Discovered in 1817.
Silicone	**Si**	14	28.086	(L. silex = flint) Discovered in 1823.
Silver	**Ag**	47	107.870	From (Anglo-Saxon) seolfor - its old English name (L. Argentum). Prehistoric.
Sodium	**Na**	11	22.9898	From soda (L. Natrium). Discovered in 1807.
Strontium	**Sr**	38	87.62	From Strontian, in Scotland. Discovered in 1790.
Sulphur or Sulfur	**S**	16	32.064	From sulphur or brimstone, its Biblical name. Recognized since ancient times.
Tantalum	**Ta**	73	180.948	From King Tantalus of Greek mythology. Discovered in 1802.
Technetium	**Tc**	43	99.	(Gr. technetos = artificial) The first man-made element, it was originally produced in 1937 by the atomic bombardment of molybdenum (Mo). Later it was found among the fission products of uranium (U). Formerly known as Masurium (Ma).
Tellurium	**Te**	52	127.60	(L. tellus = earth) It is "out of step" in the periodic table, having a lower atomic number (I = 53), but a higher atomic weight (I = 126.9044) than Iodine. Discovered in 1782.
Terbium	**Tb**	65	158.924	From Ytterby, Sweden - named after the town that also gave its name to three other elements: the rare earths ytterbium (Yb) and erbium (Er), and the transition metal yttrium (Y). Discovered in 1843.
Thallium	**Tl**	81	204.37	(Gr. thallos = a green shoot) Its spectrum is a bright-green line. Discovered in 1861.

Elements (continued)

Name	Symbol	Atomic no.	Atomic weight	Other Details and Remarks
Thorium	**Th**	90	232.038	From Thor, a Scandinavian war-god. A radioactive metal, it is the parent element of a radioactive disintegration series. Thorium emanation is called Thoron (symbol Tn). Discovered in 1828.
Thulium	**Tm**	69	168.934	From Thule, ancient name of Shetland. When irradiated in a nuclear reactor, it produces an isotope that gives off X-rays. Discovered in 1879. Formerly also abbreviated: Tu.
Tin	**Sn**	50	118.69	From the old English word, tin (L. Stannum). Prehistoric.
Titanium	**Ti**	22	47.90	From (Gr.) Titans - the supermen of Greek mythology (also L. titan = the sun). Discovered in 1791.
Tungsten	**W**	74	183.85	From (Swedish) tungsten = heavy stone. Symbol W from its German name, Wolfram. Also known as Wolframium. Discovered in 1783.
Uranium	**U**	92	238.03	After the planet Uranus. The heaviest atom among the natural elements; its common form has a half-life of 4,500 million years. Discovered in 1789.
Vanadium	**V**	23	50.942	From Vanadis, a Scandinavian goddess. Discovered in 1830.
Xenon	**Xe**	54	131.30	(Gr. xenos = stranger) An inert gas; the rarest gas in the atmosphere. Discovered in 1898.
Ytterbium	**Yb**	70	173.04	From Ytterby, in Sweden. Along with the other rare earths, it recently turned up in Russia, in a mineral called gagarinite, after the first astronaut, Yuri Gargarin. Formerly known as Dubhium (Db). Discovered in 1907.
Yttrium	**Y**	39	88.905	From Ytterby, in Sweden, where it was discovered in 1794. Former symbol: Yt.
Zinc	**Zn**	30	65.37	Probably from zin, German for tin (L. Zincum). Discovered by the alchemist Paracelsus in the 16th century, though brass (zinc-copper alloy) was already known to the ancients.
Zirconium	**Zr**	40	91.22	From zircon, the name of the semi-precious gem stone in which it was discovered in 1789.

(Hyertension Study - of Losartan, a specific angiotensin II receptor antagonist).
Elix; elix Elixir (L. elixir) (see elx).
ELL Epiphyseal leg lengthening (Orthopedics).
ELLIP Elliptocytosis.
ELM Epitheloid leiomyoma (= Bizarre leiomyoma - of the stomach); External labor market; External limiting membrane (eye cone); Extravascular lung mass.
ELN Electronic noise.
ELOP Estimated length of program.
ELOS Estimated length of stay.
ELP Elastase-like protein; Electrophoresis; Endogenous limbic potential.
E/LPO The LDL (Low density lipoprotein) vitamin E/Lipid peroxidase enzyme ratio.
ELPS Eaton-Lambert perineoplastic syndrome (= Carcinomatous myopathy); Excessive lateral pressure syndrome.
ELR External loop recorder (for monitoring heart rhythm).
ELS Eaton-Lambert syndrome; Electron loss spectroscopy; Endolymphatic syndrome (= Labyrinthine hydrops or Ménière's syndrome); Excimer Laser System (see ELA); Extracorporeal life support; Extralobar sequestration.
ELSO Extracorporeal Life Support Organization.
Elspar L-asparaginase.
ELSS Emergency life support system; Environmental Life Support Systems.
ELT Electrolytic therapy; Endless loop tachycardia; Euglobulin lysis time; Excimer laser treatment (cornea in RES - Refractive eye surgery).
ELV Erythroid leukemia virus.
elx elixir (L.).
EM Early memory; Ejection murmur; Elastic membrane/ modulus; Electromagnetic; Electron micrograph; Electron microscope/py (see E/M); Electronics/ Engineering in Medicine (journals); Electronique Médicale (journal); Electrophoretic mobility; Embden-Meyerhof (pathway) (see E-M); Emergency Medicine (also, journal); EM Laboratories (E Merck); Emmetropia (eye examination) (see E - Emmetropia; Em); Emotional(ly) (disorder)/ disturbed (see ED); Ergonovine maleate; Erythema migrans/ multiforme; Erythrocyte mass; Erythromycin (see ERY); Esophageal manometry/ motility; Evans Medical Ltd code for experimental substances; Excerpta Medica; Extensive metabolizers; Extracellular matrix; Membrane potential difference.
Em Emmetropia (eye examination) (= EM) (see E - Emmetropia).
em marked emphysema (radiograph symbol).
E_m Mid-point redox potential.
E/M Electron microscope/py (= EM; EMC).
e/m ratio of charge to mass (of an electron).
E-M Embden-Meyerhof (glycolytic pathway) (= EM).
em- prefix meaning in or on (Gr. en) (see en-).
-em- combining form meaning blood (Gr. aima).
E&M Endocrine and metabolic/ism.
EMA Electronic microanalyzer; Emergency assistance/nt; Endomysial antibody; Epithelial membrane antigen; Ethylene maleic acid/ anhydride; European Marketing Approval/ Authorisation.
EMA-CF Etoposide, methotrexate, Actinomycin D (dactinomycin), and Citrovorum Factor (Folinic acid or leucovorin).
EMA-CO; EMA CO Etoposide, Methotrexate, Actinomycin-D, Cyclophosphamide and Oncovin (Chemotherapy - for trophoblastic disease).
Eman Emanation (e.g. of a gaseous disintegration product given off by a radioactive substance).
EMAP Evoked muscle action potential.
E max The greatest energy of electrons emitted from radioactive nuclei spread over a spectrum.
EMB Electromagnetic beam (X-ray); Embryology; Endometrial/ Endomyocardial biopsy; Engineering in Medicine and Biology (Group - IEEE); Eosin-methylene blue (agar/ culture medium); Ethambutol (used in the treatment of resistant tuberculosis); Ethambutol-myambutol (tuberculous therapy); Explosive mental behavior.
Emb; emb Embolism (see Embol); Embryo;

Embryology (see Embryol).
EMBASE Excerpta Medica Database.
EMBGN Engineering in Medicine and Biology Group Newsletter (IEEE).
EMBL European Molecular Biology Laboratory.
EMBO European Molecular Biology Organization.
Embol; embol Embolism (= EMB; emb).
embolism (see AMPE); Muco-purulent excretion (sputum).
Embryol; embryol; Embry; embry Embryology (= Emb; emb).
EMBS Endomyocardial biopsy specimen (see EMB).
EMC Electron microscope/py (see E/M); Emergency medical care/ center/ coordinator; Emerging and other Communicable Disease Surveillance and Control (WHO); Encephalomyocarditis; Eosinophil-mediated cytotoxicity; Essential mixed cryoglobulinemia.
EMC&R Emergency medical care and rescue.
EMCRO Experimental Medical Care Review Organization.
EMCV Encephalomyocarditis virus.
EMD Electromechanical dissociation; Emergency Medical Division (DoT); Emery-Dreifuss muscular dystrophy; Endometrial/ Extramedullary (see EMM) disease; Esophageal mobility disorder; European Medical Directive; Extensive metastatic disease.
EME Emergency/ Enhanced medical equipment (= EMK); Encapsulated mediastinal effusion; Epidemic myalgic encephalomyelitis; Esomeprazole metabolising enzyme (= CYP2C19, a PPI or Protein Pump Inhibitor m.e.).
EMEM Eagle's minimal essential medium.
Emend Emended (L. emendatis).
EMER Electromagnetic molecular electronic resistance.
emer emergency.
-emesis suffix meaning vomit (Gr. emein).
Emet Bism Iod Emetine and Bismuth Iodide (see EBI).
EMF Electromagnetic field/ flowmeter; Electromotive force (see emf); Electron-microscopical finding; Emergency Medicine Foundation; Endomyocardial fibrosis; Erythema multiforme; Erythrocyte maturation factor (= Antianemic maturation factor) (see ESF); Evaporated milk formula.
emf electromotive force (= EMF).
EMFA Excerpta Medica Foundation of Amsterdam (Netherlands).
Emfac Emery Industries Inc code for experimental substances.
EMG Electrometrogram (the recording of changes in electric potential of the uterine muscle); Electromyogram/graph (the recording of changes in electric potential of muscle); Electromyography (journal); Electron micrograph; Essential monoclonal gammopathy; Exophthalmos-macroglossia-gigantism (syndrome); Eye movement guage.
Emg Emergency.
EMGN Extramembranous glomerulonephritis.
EMGS Exophthalmos-macroglossia gigantism syndrome (= BWG or Beckwith-Wiedemann syndrome; EMG syndrome).
EMH Endometrial hyperplasia; Exact medical history.
EMI Electromagnetic interference; Electronic and Musical Industries Ltd. (Brain Scanner); Electronics and Medical Instrumentation (Program - CDL) (also TERC); Emergency medical information; Extensive muscular injury; External muon identifier; Unit of X-ray attenuation coefficient.
-emia suffix meaning blood (Gr. haima).
EMIC Emergency maternal and infant care.
EMIC BACK Environmental Mutagen Information Center Backfile.
E-MICR Electron microscopy.
EMIS Emergency medical identification symbol (AMA).
EMIT Enzyme multiplication/plied immunoassay technique.
EMJH Ellinghausen-McCullough-Johnson-Harris (medium).
EMK Emergency/ Enhanced medical kit (see EME).
EML Erythema nodosum leprosum.
EMLB Erythromycin lactobionate.
EMM Erythema multiforme major; Extramedullary mass (such as chloroma,

myeloblastoma, and granulocytic sarcoma - in the mediastinum) (= EMD).

EMMA Eye movement measuring apparatus.

EMMV Extended mandatory minute ventilation.

EMNA Esterase-metabolised narcotic analgesic (e.g. Remifentanil).

EMO Epstein and Macintosh, Oxford (ether inhaler and bellow); Exophthalmos, myxedema circumscriptum praetibiale, and osteoarthropathia hypertrophicans (syndrome).

Emot; emot Emotion(al).

EMP Electric membrane property; Electromagnetic pulse (radiation from a nuclear explosion); Embden-Meyerhof pathway; Emergency medical personnel (see EMSS; ERP); Environmental management program; Esophageal motility probe (see EMS); Estramustine phosphate; Experimental and Molecular Pathology (journal); External membrane potential/ protein; Extramedullary plasmacytoma.

Emp; emp A plaster (L. emplastrum); As directed or after/ in the manner prescribed (L. ex modo prescripto).

EMPAC Empire Medical Political Action Committee.

EM pathway Embden-Meyerhof pathway.

EMPEP Erythrocyte membrane protein electrophoretic pattern.

EMPI Enzyme modification of porcine insulin.

emp vesic a blistering plaster (L. emplastrum vesicatorium).

EMPS Exertional muscle pain syndrome.

EMR Educable mentally retarded; Electromagnetic radiation; Emergency mechanical restraint; Emergency medical response; Empty, measure, and record; EMR Schlumberger Co; Essential metabolism ratio; Ethics of Medical Research; Eye movement record.

EMRA Effective mucoregulatory action (in lung diseases such as COPD); Emergency Medicine Residents Association.

EMRC Emergency-medical-response capability; European Medical Research Council.

EMS Early morning sickness (= EMV)/ specimen/ stiffness; Electrical muscle stimulation; Electromagnetic sensor; Electron microscope; Electronic Medical Service; Electron-microscopical study; Emergency Medical Service (UK); Emergency medical services/ system; Endometriosis; Eosinophilia myalgia syndrome (caused by an excess of L-trytophan in the diet); Ethyl methane-sulfonate; Environmental Mutagen Society; Enzymic marker study; Erythropoietic marrow scanning; Esophageal Motility Studies; Expected median survival; Experimental Medicine and Surgery (journal); Express Mail Service.

EMSA Emergency Medical Service Agency (LA).

EMSCS Emergency Medical Services Communications Systems.

EMSS Emergency-medical-services system(s) (see EMP; ERP).

EMSSA Emergency Medical Service Systems Act.

EMSSDA Emergency Medical Service Systems Development Act.

EMSU Early morning specimen of urine.

EMT Electron Microscopy Technician; Electron microscopy terminology; Emergency medical tag/ team/ technician/ training (as in cardiac defibrillation)/ treatment; Emergency Medicine Today (journal); Erythrocyte Mobility Test (the erythrocyte unsaturated fatty acid test for multiple sclerosis, which guages the reduction of erythrocyte electrophoretic mobility in the presence of linoleic acid).

EMTA Endomethylene tetrahydrophthalic acid.

EMT-A Emergency medical technician - ambulance.

EMT-I Emergency medical technician - intermediate.

EMT-MAST; EMT-M Emergency medical technician - military antishock trousers.

EMT-P Emergency medical technician - paramedic.

EMU Early morning urine; Emergency Medical Unit.

emu electromagnetic unit.

emul; emuls emulsion (L. emulsio).

EMV Early morning vomiting (see EMS);

Emergency motor vehicle; Eye, motor, voice (Glasgow coma scale).

EMVC Early mitral valve closure.

EMW Electromagnetic wave(s).

EN Electronarcosis; Emergency/ Enrolled nurse; Endo Laboratories Inc. code for experimental substance; Endoscopy; Endothelial (cell) nucleus; Enema (see en); Enteral nutrition; Enteric (coated tablet) (see EC); Epidemic nephritis; Erythema nodosum; Ethylene diamine (see en); Experimental Neurology (journal).

En Enema (see en).

en enema (= EN; En; Enem; enem); Ethylene diamine (= EN).

en- prefix meaning in or on (Gr. en) (= em-).

ENA Extractable nuclear antigen.

ENaC Epithelial sodium channel (transport mechanism in the pulmonary alveolus).

en bissac (Fr.) - Reducing a strangulated hernia by forcing it into a sac or diverticulum.

en bloc (Fr.) - As a whole.

ENC Environmental control; European Nutrition Conference.

Enc Encourage.

enceph- prefix meaning brain (Gr. encephalo).

END Early neonatal death; Endocrine/nology (see Endocrin); Endorphin; Enhancement Newcastle disease; Extranodal disease (e.g. lung cancer, etc.).

End Endocrine/nology (see Endocrin).

end endoreduplication.

end-; endo- prefix meaning inside (Gr. endon).

Endo Endocardial/ium; Endocrine/nology (see Endocrin); Endodontics; Endoscope/py; Endotracheal.

Endocrin Endocrine/nology (= END; End; Endo); Endocrinology (journal).

ENDOR Electron nuclear double resonance.

ENE Ethyl norepinephrine.

ENEA European Nuclear Energy Agency (Euratom).

ENeG Electroneurography.

Enem; enem Enema (see en).

ENF Enfamil; Extradural neurofibroma (see EDNF).

en face French - do opposite/ on the face of.

ENG Electronystagmogram/graph(y) (record of speed of eye movement/ procedure/ ophthalmology).

Eng England/lish; Engorged.

Engin Engineering.

ENH Endoneurial hypoxia.

ENI Elective neck irradiation; Equivalent noise input.

ENIAC Electronic Numerical Integrator And Computer.

ENK Enkephalin.

ENL Erythema nodosum leprosum/oticum.

ENM Extraneurological manifestation(s) (of disease).

En Met Environmental metrology.

ENMS European Nuclear Medicine Society.

Eno Enolase.

ENOG Electroneurography.

ENOSI Endogenous nitric oxide synthase inhibitor.

ENP Ethyl-p-nitrophenylthiobenzene phosphate; Extractable nucleoprotein.

en plaque French - plate-like.

ENR Eosinophilic non-allergic rhinitis; Epineural neurorrhaphy (Orthopedics); Extrathyroid(al) neck radioactivity.

ENS Enteral nutritional support; Ethyl-nor-suprarenin; European Nuclear Society.

ENT Ear, nose, and throat; Enzootic nasal tumor; Equilibrative nucleoside transporter; Extranodular tissue.

Ent Entomology (see Entom).

ent enterotoxin.

ent A enterotoxin A.

enter- prefix meaning intestine (Gr. enteron).

Entom Entomology (= Ent).

ENU N-ethyl-N-nitrosourea.

Enuc Enucleation.

Env; Environ Environment(al).

ENV gene Envelope gene, found in the AIDS virus (HIV-1) genome, coding for structural proteins and expressed as a glycoprotein (gp 160), which is cleaved to form two envelope proteins (gp 41, which extends across the viral membrane and gp 120, which forms the outer spike).

Enz Enzyme (journal); Enzymologia (journal).

enz enzymatic; enzyme.

EO Early onset; Elbow orthosis; Eosinophil(s) (see Eo); Eosinophilia; Ethylene oxide; Eyes open.

Eo Eosinophil(s) (= EO; EOS; Eos; Eosin; Eosins) (white blood count report).

E_0 Skin dose.

EOA Effective orifice area; Erosive osteoarthritis; Esophageal obturator airway; Examination, opinion, and advice.

EOAD Early-onset Alzheimer's disease.

EOB Emergency observation bed.

EOC Economic Opportunity Commission; Enema of choice; Epithelial ovarian carcinoma; Excessive oxygen consumption.

EOCA Early onset cerebellar ataxia.

EOD Emergency open drainage; End organ damage; Entry on duty; Every other day (see eod).

eod every other day (= EOD).

EODD Early-onset dysthymic disorder (see MDD; PDD).

EOE End-organ effect(s); Equal opportunity employer.

EOF End of file; Endogenous osteochondral fracture (see OCL).

E of M Error of measurement/ metabolism.

EOG Electronogram/graph(y); Electro-oculogram/graph(y); Electro-olfactogram/graph(y); Ethrane, oxygen, and gas (nitrous oxide).

EOGBS Early onset group B streptococcal (infection).

EOH End organ hypertrophy.

EOJ Extrahepatic obstructive jaundice.

EOL End of life.

EOLC End-of-life care.

EOM End of message; Energize output medium; Equal ocular movement; External otitis media; Extra-ocular movement/ muscle.

EOMA Emergency oxygen mask assembly.

EOMB Explanation of medical benefits.

EOMC Extraocular muscle cell.

EO-3-ME Erythropoietic stimulating factor (= ESF).

EOMI Extraocular muscles intact.

EOM NL Extraocular eye movements normal.

EOP Elevated ocular pressure; Excessively obese patient.

EOPD Early-onset Parkinson's disease (see parkin gene).

EOR Exclusive operating room.

EORA Elderly onset rheumatoid arthritis.

EORTC European Organization on Research and Treatment of Cancer.

E Ortho Eastern Orthodox (Church member).

EOS Elective orthopedic surgery; End of study; Endogenous oestrogen secretion (see EES); Eosinophil(s) (see Eo); European Optometric/ Orthodontic Society.

Eos; eos; Eosin; eosin Eosinophil(s) (see Eo).

Eosins Eosinophils (see Eo).

Eosm Effective osmolarity.

EOT Effective oxygen transport.

EoT End of therapy/ treatment.

EOU Epidemic observation unit.

EOVA Evident obstructive ventilatory alteration.

EOW Elderly obese woman/ women.

EOXCTE Evaluation of Oral Xemilofiban in Controlling Thrombotic Events (see EXCITE).

EP Eagan Program (Cyclophosphamide, Vincristine and Methotrexate - Chemotherapy); Ectopic pregnancy; Edible portion; Edinburgh Pharmacopeia (= PE); Electrophoresis; Electrophysiologic; Electroprecipitin; Elopement precaution; Emergency physician/ procedure; Endogenous pyrogen; Endoperoxide; Endorphin; Endoscopic papillotomy (endoscopic removal of bile duct stones, using a papillotome); Endpoint; Enteropeptidase; Environmental protection; Enzyme product; Eosinophilic pneumonia; Epicardial (electrogram); Epithelial/lium; Epoxide; Erythrocyte protoporphyrin (test); Erythrophagocytosis; Erythropoietic porphyria; Erythropoietin (= Ep); Esophageal/ Extreme pressure; Evoked potentials: i. Visual (see VEP); ii. Brain stem (see BSAEP); iii. Somatosensory (see SSEP); Existential Psychiatry (Am Ontoanal Assn journal); Experimental Parasitology (journal); Protoporphyrin (free in erythrocytes).

Ep Erythropoietin (see EP).

ep- prefix meaning upon, after, in addition (Gr. epi).

E&P Estrogen and progesterone.

E4P Erythrose 4-phosphate.

EPA Eastern Psychiatric Association; Ectopic pacemaker activity; Effective preventive/ prophylactic agent; Eicosapent aenoic/oneic acid (found in fish oil); Empiric phrase association; Endocrine pancreas adenoma; Endogenous peroxidase activity; Environmental Protection Agency (a federal agency in the US); Epidemic polyarthritis (see RRF - Ross River fever); Erect posterior-anterior; Erythroid potentiating activity; Extrinsic plasminogen activator.

EPAH Renal extraction of p-aminohippurate.

EPAP Expiratory positive airway pressure.

EPAQ Extended Personal Attitudes Questionnaire.

EPA/RCRA Environmental Protection Agency Resource Conservation and Recovery Act.

EPB Extensor pollicis brevis.

EPBI Exercise penile-brachial index.

EPBR Endosteal and periosteal bone repair (Mast cells in Orthopedics).

EPC Echophonocardiogram/graph(y); Effective pain control; Elevated plasma cortisol/sone; Elevated platelet count; Endogenous pyrogenic cytokine(s) (e.g. IL-1; IL-6; Interferon; TNF); End-plate current; End-points committee; Epilepsia partialis continua; Erosive prephloric changes; Erythroid pro-genitor cell (see CFU-E; HGF); Estrogen-progestogen combination/ contraceptive; External pneumatic compression; Extrapsychic conflict (see Conflict).

EPCA Energy Policy and Conservation Act; External pressure circulatory assistance.

Ep cell Epithelial cell(s) (see Epith).

EPCG Endoscopic pancreatocholangiography.

EPCT Extramedullary plasma cell tumor.

EPD Elastoplast pressure dressing; Electrocardiographic potential distribution(s); Epidemic pleurodynia (= Bornholm disease, Devil's grip, Epidemic myalgia, Epidemic myositis); Exocrine/nic pancreatic disease; Extrapyramidal disorder (see EPR).

EPDML Epidemiologic/gy.

EPE Erythropoietin-producing enzyme; Extrapancreatic/ Extrapyramidal effect.

EPEC Enteropathogenic Escherichia coli.

EPEG Etoposide.

EPF Early pregnancy factor; Endocarditis parietalis fibroplastica; Endothelial proliferating factor; Enfamil Premature Formula; Estrogenic positive feedback; Exophthalmos-producing factor.

EPG Eggs per gram (count/ parasitology); Electronic pupillography; Electropneumogram/graph(y); Ethanolamine phosphoglyceride.

EPH Edema-proteinuria-hypertension; Extensor proprius hallucis.

EPHRP Estrogen-progestogen hormone replacement therapy.

EPI Ectoparasitic infection/ infestation; Electron probe interface; Emotion Profile Index; Epicardial (see epicard); Epicillin; Epidemic (see epid); Epidemiology (see Epidem); Epilepsy/ptic (see epil); Epinephrine (see epineph); Episiotomy (see Epis); Epithelial/lium (see Epith); Epitheloid (cell); Evoked potential index; Exocrine pancreatic insufficiency; Expanded Programme of Immunization (WHO); Extra-pyramidal involvement; Eysenck Personality Inventory.

Epi; epi See EPI.

epi- prefix meaning after, at, in addition to, upon (Gr.).

epi-aid epidemic aid.

EPIC Evaluation for the Prevention of Ischemic Complications (trial).

epid epidemic (see EPI); Epidemiology (see Epidem).

Epidem Epidemiology (= EPI; epid).

EPIG Etoposide (= Etopoxide; Epipodopophyllotoxin; VP-16).

epil epilepsy/ptic (= EPI).

Epilep Epilepsia (ILAE journal).

EPILOG Evaluation in PTCR to Improve Long-term Outcome with Abciximab GP (Glycoprotein) IIb/IIIa Blockade (study).

epin epinephrine (see epineph).

epineph epinephrine (= EPI; epin).

Epis Episcopalian (Church member); Episiotomy (= EPI).

EPISTENT Evaluation of Platelet IIb/IIIa Inhibition in Stenting (study).

epistom a stopper (L. epistomium).

Epith Epithelial (cell) (= Ep cell; EPI; ep's); Epithelium, e.g. Germinal epith (= EPI).

EPL Effective patient's life; Environmental Planning Lobby (New York); Essential phospholipid; Extensor pollicis longus;

Extracorporeal piezoelectric lithotriptor.

EPLN Extrapleural lymph node.

EPM Encephalitic poliomyelitis (involving the motor cortex); Educational and Psychological Measurement (journal); Elderfield pyrimidine mustard; Electron probe microanalysis; Electronic pacemaker; Electrophoretic mobility; Energy-protein malnutrition.

EPN Emergency Product News (journal); O-ethyl O-p-nitrophenylphosphonothionate (= Ethyl-para-nitrophenyl-phenyl-phosphonothio) (a pesticide); Etiopathogenetic nuance(s) (= APN); Extrapontine neuron.

EPNM Early perinatal morbidity/ mortalilty.

EPO Earliest possible occasion; Erythropoiesis; Erythropoietin (see Hormones - EPO); Evening primrose-oil; Expiratory port occlusion.

EPOC Epidemiology of constipation (study, US).

EPP End-plate potential; Enzyme-precursor protein (= Complement); Equal-pressure point; Erythropoietic protoporphyria; External pressure palsy/ paralysis.

EPPB End positive-pressure breathing.

EPPS Edwards Personal Preference Schedule.

EPPs End-plate potentials.

EPQ Eysenck Personality Questionnaire.

EPR Early progressive resistance; Electron paramagnetic resonance; Electrophrenic respiration; Emergency physical restraint; Estradiol production rate; Extensor plantar response; Extraparenchymal resistance; Extrapyramidal reaction(s) (dyskinesia, dystonia, tremor, etc.).

EPR; E/PR Estradiol/Progesterone ratio.

EPRA Elevated plasma renin activity (as in Congenital adrenal hypoplasia) (see CAH).

EPRI Electric Power Research Institute.

EPROM Electrically-/ Erasable programmable read-only memory (computer).

EPRT Estrogen-progestin replacement therapy (see HRT).

EPS Elastosis performans serpiginosa; Electrophysiologic studies/dy (e.g. of the cerebral cortex, etc.); Endogenous prostaglandin synthesis; Endogenous pulmonary surfactant; Enzyme pancreatic secretion; European Physical Society; Excellent performance status; Exophthalmos-producing substance (of anterior pituitary); Expressed prostatic secretion(s); Extracellular polysaccharide; Extrapyramidal signs (akathisia, akinesia, cogwheel rigidity, hypertonia, hypokinesia, neck rigidity, and tremor)/ symptom(s)/ syndrome.

ep's epithelial cells (see Epith).

EPSDT Early and Periodic Screening, Diagnosis, and Treatment (Program - MSA).

EPSE Extrapyramidal side effects.

EPSEM Equal probability of selection method.

EPSP Excitatory post-synaptic potential.

EPSS E-point septal separation.

EPST Ergonovine provocation/ stimulation test (cardiac catherization - to induce coronary artery spasm).

EPT Early pregnancy test; Edrophonium test (Dimethyl [3-hydroxyphenyl] ammonium, a chemical used in motor nerve evaluation in myasthenia gravis; Edrophonium Chloride = Tensilon); Eidetic Parents Test; Empirical psychotherapy; Endoscopic papillotomy; Exercise pneumotachometer (used to measure ventilatory flow rate) (see VFR).

EPTB; EPTBC; EPTbc Extrapulmonary tuberculosis.

EPTE Existed prior to enlistment.

EPTFE Expanded polytetrafluoroethylene.

EPTM Extraperitoneal tumor mass.

EPTS Existed prior to service (military).

E/PUFA Vitamin E/polyunsaturated fatty acid (ratio).

EPV Entomopoxvirus.

EPXMA Electron probe x-ray microanalyzer.

EQ Educational/ Energy quotient; Encephalization Quotient - the ratio of actual brain size to the expected brain size of that particular species, based on the size of its body; Equal to; Eugenics Quarterly (journal).

Eq; eq Equation; Equivalent (= E; Equiv; equiv) - formula weight/valence, e.g. NEq (= NE; N Equiv; Niacin equivalent), REq (= RE; R Equiv; Retinol equivalent).

equilib equilibrium.

EQuiP; EquiP European Working Party on Quality in Family Practice.

equip equipment.
Equiv; equiv Equivalency/lent (see Eq; eq).
EQWA Eccentric quadrant walking aid.
ER Efficiency/ Enhancement ratio; Einhorn regimen (Vinblastine, Bleomycin, & Cisplatin (Chemotherapy); Ejection rate; Electroresection; Emergency room; Endoplasmic reticulum (see er); Energy Reporter (FEA journal); Enhanced reactivation; Environmental Research (journal); Environmental/ Extended resistance; Epigastric region; Equine rhinopneumonia; Equivalent roentgen (unit); Erythrocyte/ Estradiol/ Estrogen receptor; Etretinate; Evoked response; Expiratory reserve; Extended release (tablet); External resistance/ rotation.
er early; endoplasmic reticulum (= ER).
Er Erbium (Z = 68) (see Elements - Erbium); Erythrocyte (see E).
ER+ Increased estrogen receptor (substantial relative estradiol binding capacity).
ER- Decreased estrogen receptor (little or no relative estradiol binding capacity).
ER+/- Borderline relative estradiol binding capacity.
E&R Equal and reactive; Examination and report.
ERA Elective/ Electric/ Electroencephalic/ Evoked response audiometry; Electrical response activity; Electroshock Research Association; Emergency-response amulet; Enteropathic reactive arthritis; Equal Rights Agency; Estradiol/ Estrogen receptor assay.
ERB Endotheline receptor blocker.
ERBF Effective renal blood flow.
ERC ECHO (Enteric cytopathic human orphan)-rhino-coryza virus(es) (see ECHO); Empire Rheumatism Council; Employment Rehabilitation Center; Endoscopic retrograde cholangiography; Energy Resources Council; Erythropoietin-responsive cell; Estradiol-receptor complex; European Rheumatology Congress.
Erc Erythrocyte (see E).
ERCHD Enhancing Recovery from Coronary Heart Disease (NHLBI).
ERCP Endoscopic retrograde cholangio-pancreatography.
ERD Early retirement with disability; Energy reduced diet; Evoked response detector.
ERDA Energy Research and Development Administration.
ERDS Extended-release delivery system.
ERE Erosive reflux esophagitis (see GERD); External rotation in extension.
EREP Estrogen-related endometrial proliferation.
ERF Education and Research Foundation (AMA); Effective refractory period (Class III antiarrhythmias); Energy-rich food; Environmental risk factor; External rotation in flexion; Eye Research Foundation.
erf error function.
ERFC Erythrocyte rosette-forming cell(s); Évaluation rapide des fonctions cognitives (Fr.) (Rapid evaluation of cognitive functions) - in psychiatric illnesses.
E-RFC E-rosette forming cell.
ERFS Electrophysiological ring finger splinting.
ERG Electron radiography; Electroretinogram/graph(y).
erg- combining form meaning energy or work (Gr. ergon).
ERHD Exposure-related hypothermic death.
ERI Early renal impairment/ insufficiency; Ear Research Institute (Los Angeles); E-rosette inhibitor.
ERIA Electroradioimmunoassay.
ERIC Educational Resource(s) Information Center/ Clearinghouse (USOE).
ERISA Employee Retirement Income Security Act (1974).
ERK cell line.
ERL Effective refractory length; Emergency reference level (radiation); Enteric Reference Laboratory (London).
ERM Electrochemical relaxation method; Embryonal rhabdomyosarcoma; Extended radical mastectomy.
ERMD Energy reduced mixed diet.
ERMS Embryonal rhabdomyosarcoma.
ERN Estrogen-receptor-negative.
EROS Earth Resources Observation System.
ERP Early receptor potential(s); Effective refractory period; Elodoisin-related peptide; Emergency-response personnel (e.g. in car-

diac arrest) (see EMP; EMSS); Emergency room physician/ practitioner; Endoscopic retrograde pancreatography; Enzyme-releasing peptide; Equine rhinopneumonitis; Estrogen-receptor-positive; Estrogen receptor protein; Estrogen replacement therapy; Event-related (brain) potential.

ERPF Effective renal plasma flow (see KFT - ERPF).

ERPLV Effective refractory period of left ventricle.

ERR Energy reducing regimen (for weight loss).

ERS Economic Research Service; Emergency room service; Endoscopic retrograde sphincterotomy (in bile duct obstruction); Error-reduction system; Estrogen receptor study (see PBD); Evacuation of retained secretions; Extensive reconstructive surgery (Neuro, Orthopedic, Pediatric, Plastic, etc.).

ERSD Exertion-related sudden death.

ERSP Event-related slow potential.

ERT Electrical resistance thermometer; Electrolyte replacement therapy (see SML); Elevated renal threshold (e.g. for glycosuria); Elimination rate of transfusion; Emergency reperfusion therapy (in MI); Emergency room therapy/ treatment; Endemic/ Epidemic Rhodesian trypanosomiasis (caused by the protozoan parasite, *Trypanosoma* brucei rhodesiense and transmitted by the savannah/ riveine species respectively, of the tsetse fly *Glossina*); Enzyme-replacement therapy; Esophageal radionuclide transit; Estrogen replacement therapy; External radiation therapy.

ERU Endorectal ultrasound.

ERV Ebola-Reston virus (named after the Ebola virus outbreak in Reston, Virginia, US); Equine rhinopneumonitis virus; Expiratory reserve volume (see PFT - ERV).

ERY Erysipelas; Erythromycin (= E; EM; ETM).

Ery Erysipelothrix.

erythr- prefix meaning inflamed or red (Gr. erythros).

Erythroxylum A genus of South American plants, also cultivated in Indonesia, of the family Erythroxylaceae. Sometimes called by the generic name Erythroxylum. For example, E. coca, a shrub native to the Andes mountains of Peru and Bolivia. The dried leaves of this and other similar species of this genus, are known as Coca, which contains the alkaloid ecgonine, from which is prepared synthetically the crystalline alkaloid, methyl benzoyl ecgonine or Cocaine - the oldest local anesthetic known to man, causing systemic toxic effects (cocainism) and addiction. Its medical use today is almost enterely restricted to local application (local anesthesia) in ophthalmic surgery and surgery of the ear, nose and throat. Cocaine is also known by other names, abbreviations, and popular or slang expressions, such as: Bernie; Bolivian marching powder; Bouncing powder; Burese; C; Cocaine; C&H (cocaine and heroin); Charles; C&M (cocaine and morphine mixture); CO; Coke; Crack; Dynamite; Flake; Frisco speedball (mixture of heroin, cocaine and LSD-25); FS (= Frisco speedball); Gold dust; Heaven dust; Her; HMC (Heroin, morphine and cocaine); Incentive; Jam; Lady Snow; M&C (Morphine and Cocaine); Mojo (cocaine, morphine or heroin); Rock; Sniff; Snort; Speedball (a mixture of cocaine and heroin); Star dust; White lady (name also used for heroin).

ES Abbot Laboratories Ltd code for experimental substances; Ejection sound; Elastic suspensor; Electrical stimulation/lus; Electron spectrometer; Electroshock; Electrostimulation; Electrosurgery; Embolic stroke; Embryonic stem (cell) (see ESC); Emergency service; Emission spectrometry; Endocrine Society; Endometritis-salpingitis; Endoscopic sphincterotomy; Endostatin (= AAGA; AGI) (see AAGT); End-stage; End-to-side (shunt); Enema saponis (L) (see es); Enzyme substrate; Epileptic/ Exfoliation syndrome; Esophageal/gus; Esophageal scintigraphy; Esterase; Eugenics Society; Exanthema subitum (see RI - Roseola infantum); Expectation Score; Experimental study; Ex-smoker; Exterior surface; Extrasystole.

Es Einsteinium (Z = 99) (see Elements - Einsteinium); Estrid; Estriol.

es egg shell calcification of hilar or mediastinal lymph nodes (radiograph symbol); soap enema (L. enema saponis) (= ES).

ES 132 Bibenzonium bromide (= Diphenetholine b) - a cough suppressant.

ESA Ecological/ Electrolysis/ Entomological Society of America; End-to-side anastomosis; Esterase; European Space Agency; Excessive systemic absorption.

ESAN End-stage allograft nephropathy (see HPV; VIB).

ESAP Evoked sensory action potential (nerve).

ESAR Envelope-specific antibody response.

ESB Electrical stimulation of the brain; Eugenics Society Bulletin.

ESC Electromechanical slope computer; Electroskin conductance; Embryonic stem cell; Endosystolic count; Endothelial spindle cell (see ETC); Erythropoietin-sensitive stem cell; European Society of Cardiology.

ESCA Electron spectroscopy for chemical analysis.

ESCAD End-stage coronary artery disease (see ESHD).

ESCC Epidural spinal cord compression.

ESCD End-stage cardiac disease (see ESHD).

Esch Escherichia (= E.).

ESCN Electrolyte and steroid(-produced) cardiopathy (characterized by)/ (with) necrosis.

E Score Extraversion score (Eysenck Personlity Inventory).

ESCR Embryonic stem cell research.

ESCS Electrical spinal cord stimulation.

ESD Early-stage disease (as in cancer, etc.); Electronic summation device; Electrostatic discharge; Emergency Services Department; Emission spectrometric device; End-stage disease (as in cancer, AIDS, etc.); End-systolic dimension; Esophagus, stomach, and duodenum; Esterase-D; Exoskeletal device.

ESDR European Society for Dermatological Research.

ESE Electrostatic unit (Ger. elektrostatische Einheit); Emotionally stressful event; Epidemiological Studies of the Elderly (Arch. Intern. Med.).

ESEA Elementary Secondary Education Act.

ESECA Energy Supply and Environmental Coordination Act.

ESETCID European Study of Epidemiology and Treatment of Cardiac Inflammatory Disease.

ESF Electrosurgical filter; Erythropoietic stimulating factor (see EMF; EO-3-ME); External skeletal fixation.

ESFD External skeletal fixation device.

ESFL End-systolic force-length (relationship).

ESG Estrogen (see Esg); Exfoliation syndrome glaucoma; Eye surgery/ surgical gonioscopy.

Esg Estrogen (= ESG).

ESGIE European Society of Gastrointestinal Endoscopy.

ESHD End-stage heart (see ESCAD; ESCD)/ hepatic (see ESLD) disease.

ESHF End-stage hepatic failure (see ESLF).

ESHG European Society for Human Genetics.

ESI Electrospray ionization; Employee state insurance; Enzyme-substrate-inhibitor (complex); Epidural steroid injection.

ESIMV Expiratory synchronized intermittent mandatory ventilation.

ESKD End-stage kidney disease (see ESRD).

ESL End-systolic length; Engineering Societies Library (NYC); Extracorporeal shockwave lithotripsy.

ESLD End-stage liver disease.

ESLF End-stage liver failure.

ESLO European Society for Lingual Orthodontics.

ESM Ejection systolic murmur; Endoscopic specular microscope; Epley or Semont Maneuver (or ORP - Otolith Repositioning Procedure, employed in the treatment of BPPV - Benign paroxysmal positional vertigo, using gravity or a vibrator placed on the mastoid to move the calcium carbonate crystals [otoconia or otoliths], away from the nerve endings in the semi-circular canals and deposit them back into areas of the inner ear vestibule, where they can do no further harm); Ethibond/ Ethicon/ Ethiflex/ Ethilon suture material; Ethosuximide; Extraskeletal myelomatosis (Orthopedics).

ESMIS Emergency Medical Services Management Information System.

ESMO European Society of Medical Oncology.

ESN Educationally subnormal; Estrogen-stimulated neurophysin.
ESN(M) Educationally subnormal - moderate.
ESN(S) Educationally subnormal - severe.
ESO Electrospinal orthosis; Eosophagoscopy (see eso); Esophagus (see Esoph).
eso eosophagoscopy (= ESO); esophagus (see Esoph).
eso- prefix meaning inside (Gr.).
ESOC Early-stage ovarian cancer.
ESONE European Standards on Nuclear Electronics.
Esoph; esoph Esophagus (= ESO; eso).
ESP Early systolic paradox; Economic Stabilization Program; Effective sensory projection; Effective systolic pressure; Electrically susceptible patient (system); Electrosensor panel; Elizabeth S. Priori (virus); Endometritis-salpingitis-peritonitis; End-systolic pressure; Eosinophil stimulation promoter; Epidermal soluble protein; Especially (see esp); European Society for Pathology; Evoked synaptic potential; Excellent safety profile; Extrasensory perception.
esp especially (= ESP; espec).
ESPA Electrical stimulation-produced analgesia.
espec especially (see esp).
ESPEN European Society for Parenteral and Enteral Nutrition.
ESPID European Society for Paediatric Infectious Diseases.
ESPS European Stroke Prevention Study.
ESR Early-stage risk; Early surgical repair; Einstein stoke radius; Electric skin resistance; Electron spin resonance; Erythrocyte sedimentation rate (= BSR; SRT).
ESRD End-stage renal disease; End-Stage Renal Disease (Program).
ESRF End-stage renal failure.
ESRI End-stage renal insufficiency (see ESRD).
ESRS Extrapyramidal Symptom Rating Scale.
ESS Elementary Science Study (NSF funded); Empty sella syndrome (sella turcica) - associated with hyperprolactinemia; Endostreptosin; Erythrocyte-sensitizing substance; Euthyroid sick syndrome; Excited skin syndrome.
ess essential(ly).
ESSEC École Supérieure des Sciences Économiques et Commerciales.
ess neg essentially negative.
EST Eastern standard time; Electric shock threshold; Electron(ic) stethoscope; Electroshock therapy/ treatment (see ECT); Endometrial sinus tumor; Endoscopic sphincterectomy; Environmental Science and Technology (ACS journal); Epicardial ST (segment) (site/ electrocardiogram); Erhard Seminars Training (Inc); Ester(ase) (see Est); Exercise stress test; Expressed sequence tag (a method of decoding the entire sequence of a gene from a pool of complementary DNA); External standard technique.
Est; est Ester(ase) (= EST); Estimate(d)/mation.
ES&T Environmental Science and Technology (journal).
esth esthetic(s).
esthe- combining form meaning feel or perceive (Gr. aisthe).
ESTP Ether-soluble tar paste (proprietary drug used in the treatment of eczema and psoriasis).
ESTS Empty sella turcica syndrome (see ESS); Expressed sequence tags (genetic sequence decoding).
Est wt Estimated weight.
ESU Electrosurgical unit; Electrostatic unit (see esu).
esu electrostatic unit (= ESU).
E-sub; E subst Excitor substance.
ESV End-systolic volume; Esophageal valve.
ESVI End-systolic volume index.
ESVS Epiurethral suprapubic vaginal suspension.
ESWL Extracorporeal shock-wave lithotripsy (shock waves from outside the body used to shatter kidney stones).
ESWS End-systolic wall stress.
ET Educational therapy; Effective temperature; Ejection/ Endurance/ Expiration time; Electron transport; Electrotherapy; Emergency tracheostomy; Endotoxin; Endotracheal/ E. tube; End-tidal; Enterostomal therapist/py; Enterotoxin;

Epidermolytic/ Exfoliative toxin; Epithelial tumor; Esotropia (eye examination); Essential thrombocythemia/ tremor; Ethanol; Etiocholanolone test; Etiology (see Et); Eustachian tube; Exchange transfusion; Exercise test; Exercise treadmill (test).

Et Ethyl (chemical symbol for) (= et); Etiology (= ET).

Et Estradiol-17 B.

et and (Fr., L.); ethyl (see Et).

E(T) Intermittent esotropia.

ET3; ET-3 Erythrocyte triiodothyronine (= T-e) (see Hormones - TH ii).

ET4 Effective thyroxine (test).

ET 14 Etrolene (= Dow-Et-57; Fenchlorphos; Korlan; Nankor; Ronnel; Trolene; Viozene; Dimethyl 2,4,5-trichlorophenyl phosphorothionate) - an organophosphorus insecticide.

ET 495 Piribedil (an apomorphine-type agent, having a direct postsynaptic action).

ETA Electron transfer agent; Electrothermal analyzer; Embryotoxic agent; Employment and Training Administration (Dept of Labor); Endotracheal airway(s); Enthalpic thermal analyzer; Ethionamide; European Thyroid Association.

ETAB Extrathoracic assisted breathing.

Et Ac Ethyl acetate.

et al. and elsewhere (L. et alibi); and others (= L. et alia; et alii), e.g. for three or more co-authors or co-workers.

et alia; et alii See et al.

ETC Electrical Testing Company; Electron transport chain; Embryo tissue culture (see CETC); Embryo transfer cycle (see ETF); Endothelial tumor cell (as in Kaposi's sarcoma) (= ESC); Enterotest Capsule (developed by the HDC for retrieving parasites such as *Giardia* lamblia from jejunal aspirates - a diagnostic jejunal sampling procedure) (see HDC); Essential thrombocythemia; Estimated time of conception; Eustacian tube congestion.

etc and others of like/ similar kind, and so forth (L. et cetera).

ET_c Corrected ejection time.

ET_{CO2} End tidal carbon dioxide (see PFT - ET_{CO2}).

ETD Effective therapeutic dosage/ dose; Eustacian tube dysfunction; Extensive tissue destruction.

ETDR Effective therapeutic dosage regimen.

ETE End-to-end.

EtE End-to-end (e.g. anastomosis) (= ETE).

ETEA End-to-end anastomosis.

ETEC Enterotoxic/ Enterotoxigenic (strains of) Escherichia coli (= Enterotoxigenic E. coli, e.g. Salmonellae, Shigellae, Campylobacters, etc.).

$ETEO_2$ End-tidal expired oxygen (see ETO_2).

ETEP Existing thromboembolic process.

ETF Electron-transferring flavoprotein; Embryo transfer factor (IVF Obstetrics); Eustacian tube function.

ETFE Ethylene-tetrafluor-ethylene (= Tefzel).

ETH Eidgenössische Technische Hochschule (Zurich); Elixir terpin hydrate (medication order); Ethanol (see Eth); Ethionamide (see Etha); Ethmoid (see Eth); Ethnology (see Ethnol); Ethrane.

Eth Ether (see eth); Ethyl ether (see ET2O); Ethyl group; Ethanol (= ETH); Ethionamide (see Etha); Ethmoid (= ETH); Ethnology (see Ethnol).

eth ether (= Eth).

Etha Ethionamide (= ETH; Eth).

ETHC; ETH/C Elixir terpin hydrate with codeine (medication order).

ETHzC Elixir terpin hydrate with codeine (see ETHC).

Eth Cult Ethical Culture (Society member).

Ethilism Alcoholism (for ethyl alcohol).

Ethnol Ethnology (= ETH; Eth).

ETI Ejection time index; Endotracheal intubation; Extraterrestrial intelligence.

ETIBACK Environmental Teratology Information Center Backfile.

ETIO Etiocholanolone (= Etio).

Etio Etiocholanolone (see ETIO); Etiology (see etiol).

etiol etiology (= Etio).

ETIP Ethyl dithiolisophthalate (= Ditophal; Diethyl dithiolisophthalate) - used as an inunction in leprosy; Experimental Technology Incentive Program (NBS).

ETK Erythrocyte transketolase.

ETKA Erythrocyte transketolase activity.

ETKM Every test known (to) man.

ETKTM Every test known to man.

ETL Expiratory threshold load.

ETM Ergot-type medication; Erythromycin (see ERY) (on culture and sensitivity reports); Extrathorcic manifestation.

EtNU Ethyl nitrosourea.

ETO Estimated time of ovulation; Eustacian tube obstruction.

Eto Ethylene oxide.

ETO_2 End-tidal oxygen (= $ETEO_2$) (see PFT).

ET2O; ET_2O Ethyl ether (= Eth).

ETOH; EtOH Ethyl alcohol (= Aethanolum; ALC; Alc - 95 per cent; Alcohol 95%; Alcool Officinal; Ethanol; Ethanolum; Spiritus; Spiritus Aethylicus; Spiritus Alcoholisatus; Spiritus Concentratus; Weingeist; C_2H_5OH).

ETOP Elective termination of pregnancy (= ETP).

ETOX Ethylene oxide.

ETP Elective termination of pregnancy (see ETOP); Electron transfer/ transport particle; Embryo transfer program; Entire treatment period; Environmental Toxicology Program (NIEHS); Ephedrine, theophylline, phenobarbital (used in the treatment of asthma); Eustachian tube pressure.

ETR Effective therapeutic regimen; Effective thyroxine ratio (nuclear medicine); Existing treatment regimen.

ETRF Easy-to-read-format.

ETS Educational Testing Service (Princeton, NJ); Electrical transcranial stimulation; End-to-side; Environmental tobacco smoke; European Teratology Society; Extrathyroidal site (bone marrow, lymph node, etc.).

et seq and the following (L. et sequens); and those that follow (L. et sequentes).

ETT Endotracheal tube; Epinephrine/ Exercise tolerance test; Extrathyroidal thyroxine.

ETTN Ettriol trinitrate (= Propatyl nitrate; Trinettriol; Win 9317) - used in acute attacks of angina pectoris.

ETU Emergency and trauma unit; Emergency treatment unit.

EtU Easy-to-understand.

ETV Educational television; Extravascular thermal volume.

Etym Etymology.

EU Ehrlich unit (urobilinogen); Emergency/ Endotoxin/ Entropy/ Enzyme/ Esophageal ulcer; Esterase unit; Etiology unknown; European Union; Excretory urogram/aphy.

Eu Europium (Z = 63) (see Elements - Europium); Euryon.

eu- prefix meaning good or normal (Gr.).

EUA Examination under anesthesia/thetic (procedure/ gynecology).

EUCD Emotionally unstable character disorder.

EUD Experimental use of drugs (see EDUD; CUD; RUD).

EUG Excretion urogram/graph(y); Extrauterine gestation.

EUH Effective ulcer healing.

EUL Expected upper limit.

EUM External urethral meatus.

EUO External use only.

EUP Epidemiologically unrelated patient; Extrauterine pregnancy.

Eur Europe(an).

EURATOM European Atomic Energy Community - a consortium of Belgium, Denmark, France, Germany, Ireland, Italy, Luxembourg, the Netherlands, and the United Kingdom, for nuclear research.

EURONET European On-Line Network (European scientific data bank).

EUROTOX European Committee on Chronic Toxicity Hazards.

EUS Elevated urinary steroid(s); Endoscopic ultrasound; External urethral sphincter.

EUs Exposed uninfecteds (AIDS).

Eusol Edinburgh University solution (= Calcium hypochlorite solution; Chlorinated lime and boric acid solution; Liquor Acidi Hypochlorosi Compositus) - Chlorated lime 1.25 g, boric acid 1.25 g, water to 100 ml; contains not less than 0.25% weight/volume of available chlorine. Used as a general antiseptic.

Eust Eustacian.

EUT Efferent urinary tract.

EUV Extreme ultraviolet (laser/ spectroscopy).

EV Echovirus (Enteric cytopathogenic human orphan virus) - 33 distinct serotypes (= ECHO; ERC); Ejaculate/ Ejected/tion volume (see EF); Electron volt (see eV); Emergency vehicle; Enterovirus; Epidermodysplasia verruciformis (a rare wart disease); Esophageal varices; Estradiol valerate; Eversion (see Ev); Evoked (potential/ response); Excessive ventilation; Expected value; Extravascular; Extroversion (namely warmth, gregariousness, assertiveness, activity, excitement seeking and positive emotions) (see NEOAC); Ex vivo (studies, etc.).

Ev Event; Eversion (= EV; ev).

eV Electron volt (= EV; ev) - the kinetic energy acquired by an electron when accelerated through a potential difference of 1 volt.

ev electron volt (see eV); eversion (see Ev).

EVA Ethyl violet azide (broth); Ethylene vinyl acetate; French - Etude du Vieillissement Artériel (Arterial aging study); Extravehicular activity (in space).

EVAC Etoposide (VP-16), Vincristine, Adriamycin and Cytoxan (Cyclo phosphamide) (Chemotherapy).

evac evacuate(d)/tion.

eval evaluate(d)/tion.

evap evaporate(d)/tion.

EVAS Extravascular albumin space.

EVB Esophageal variceal bleeding.

EVC Ellis-van Creveld (syndrome); Extravascular compartment.

EVCI Expected value of clinical information.

EVD Endothelial vaso dilator/ motor dysfunction; Equinovarus deformity (Orthopedics); Excessive volume depletion; External ventricular drainage; Extravascular density (of lung).

EVE Evening.

EVER Everninomycin.

ever eversion/rt(ed).

EVF Endothelial vaso dilator/ motor function; Ethanol volume fraction; Extravascular fluid.

EVFMG Exchange visitor foreign medical graduate.

EVG Electroventriculography; Enterovirus genome.

EVI Endocardial, vascular and interstitial; Enteroviral infection.

EVIMEC Eastern Virginia Inter-hospital Medical Education Committee.

E-viton Effective ultra-violet radiation (unit) - the unit of quantity of biologically effective ultraviolet radiation.

EVJ Equine Veterinary Journal (BEVA).

EVLP Ex vivo liver perfusion.

EVLT Endovenous laser therapy/ treatment.

EVLW Extravascular lung water.

EVM Electronic voltmeter; Extravascular mass.

EVP Endovascular procedure; Enhanced visual perception; Episcleral venous pressure; Evoked visual potential; Executive vice-president.

EVR Evoked vertex/ visual response; Extensive vagal reaction.

EVRS Early ventricular repolarization syndrome.

EVS Endoscopic variceal sclerosis; Endovaginal sonogram/graph(y).

EVT Endovaginal transducer (used in TVS or Transvaginal sonography).

EVTV Extravascular thermal volume.

EW Elsewhere; Emergency Ward.

E-W Edinger-Westphal (nucleus).

EWB Emotional well-being; Estrogen withdrawel bleeding.

EWF External wound fistula.

EWG Environmental Working Group (FDA; EPA).

EWHO Elbow-wrist-hand orthosis.

EWI Experimental World Inventory.

EWL Egg-white lysozyme; Evaporation/ive water loss.

EWLMD European Workshop on Lipodystrophy and Metabolic Disorders.

EWS Early warning signs (of a heart attack)/ symptom(s).

EWSCLs Extended-wear soft contact lenses.

EWT Erupted wisdom teeth/ tooth.

EX Exfoliation; Exsmoker; Lakeside Laboratories Inc code for experimental substances.

E(X) Expected value of the random variable "X".

Ex; ex Exacerbation (see exac); Exaggerate(d)/tion (see exag); Examination (see exam); Examine(d)/r (see exam); Example; Except(ed)/ion (see exc); Exchange (see exch); Excipient (see Excip); Excise(d)/sion (see excis);

Exclude(d)/ding/usive (see excl); Excretion (see excr); Exercise (see exer); Exogenous (see exog); Exophthalmos (see Exoph); Expose(d)/sure (see Exp); Extract(ed)/ion (see Ext; ext).

ex- prefix meaning from or out of (L.; Gr.).

EX-10-029 Dihydromorphine (derivative) (see Papaver).

exa- metric prefix for 10^{18} (see Ten).

exac exacerbation (= Ex; ex).

ex aff of affinity (L. ex affinis).

EXAFS Extended x-ray absorption fine structure.

exag exaggerate(d)/tion (= Ex; ex).

exam examination (= Ex; ex); examine(d)/r (= Ex; ex).

EXBF Exercise hyperemia blood flow.

exc except(ed)/ion (= Ex; ex); excise/sion (see excis).

EXCEL Expended clinical evaluation of Lovastatin.

exch exchange (= Ex; ex).

Excip Excipient (= Ex; ex).

excis excise/sion (= Ex; ex; exc).

excl exclude(d)/ding/usive (= Ex; ex).

excr excretion.

Exec Executive.

EXEF; ExEF Exercise ejection fraction (i.e. e. fr. during exercise).

EXELFS Extended electron-loss line fine structure.

exer exercise (= Ex; ex).

ex gr of the group of (L. ex grupa).

exhib let it be given (L. exhibeatur).

exis exist(s)/ing.

EXCITE Evaluation of Oral Xemilofiban Controlling in Thrombotic Events (Trial - testing the use of GRA - Glycoprotein IIb/IIIa receptor anta- gonists such as xemilofiban, in protecting from death patients with MI - myocardial infarction, and from need of urgent revascularization).

EXO Exonuclease; Exophoria.

exo- prefix meaning outside (Gr.).

exog exogenous.

Exon An amino acid coding region of the human DNA (for the formation of peptide chains in the genetic code) (see Intron).

Exoph Exophthalmos (= Ex; ex).

exoph exophthalmia.

exos exostosis.

EXP Expiratory date.

Exp; exp Expand/ansion; Expect(ed)/ing (see expt); Expectorant/ate (see Expect); Experienced; Experiment (see expt); Experimental (see exptl); Expiration/atory/ire(d) (see expir); Exploration/atory/plore (see expl); Exponent; Exponential (function); Expose(d)/sure (= Ex; ex); Expression (see expn).

EXP-105-1 Amantadine hydrochloride (= 1-Adamantanamine hydrochloride) - an antiviral agent used in influenza and also, in the treatment of Parkinsonism.

Expect Expecting (journal); Expectorant/ate (= Exp; exp; expt).

exper experiment (see expt); experimental (see exptl).

Experi Experimentia (journal).

ExPGN Extracapillary proliferative glomerulonephritis.

expir expiration/atory/ire(d) (= Exp; exp).

expl Exploration/atory/plore (= Exp; exp).

exp lap exploratory laparatomy (operation/abdominal).

expn expression (see Exp; exp).

expt expect(ed)/ing (= Exp; exp); expectorant (see Expect); experiment (= Exp; exp; exper).

exptl experimental (= Exp; exp; exper).

EXREM External radiation-emission man (dose).

EXS External stent (graft) (see FPBG); External support.

EXT Exercise testing.

Ext; ext Extend (L. extendere); Extension/ive (L. extensum); Extensor (L. extensus); Exterior (L. exterior); External (L. externus); Extract (L. extractum); Extracted (see extd); Extraction (dentistry); Extreme/mity (L. extremum); Spread (L. extende).

extd extracted (= Ext; ext).

Ext D and C External drug and cosmetic (preparations) (dyes permitted for use in the United States).

Ext fl Fluid extract.

Ext mon External monitor.

extra- prefix meaning beyond or outside of (L.).

extrap extrapolate.
extrav extravasation.
ext rot external rotation.
extub extubation.
EXU Excretory urogram.
exud exudate/tion.
EY Egg yolk; Epidemiological/ology year.
EYA Egg yolk agar.
Eyeli Eyelights (IEF journal).
EYEF Educated Youth for Epilepsy Foundation.
EZ; Ez Eczema; Enzymology.

F

F Bioavailability: A cell that donates F factor in bacterial conjugation/ A conjugative plasmid in F+ bacterial cells; Cortisol (= Hydrocortisone; Compound F); Degree of fineness of abrasive particles; Dominion Rubber Co (Canada) and Eaton Laboratories code for experimental substances; Fac (L.) Make; Facial/ies; Factor; Fahrenheit (temperature/ thermometer scale) (see °F); Failure; Fair; False; Family; Farad (unit of electrical capacity); Faraday constant; Fascia; Fasting (test); Fat; Father; Feces; Fellow; Female (symbol ♀) (see Symbols - 1, 5); Fermentation; Fertility/ F. factor; Fiat (L.) Let it be made (see ft); Fibroblast; Fibrous (with reference to proteins); Field of vision (seen by the fixed eye); Filament; Filaria; Fine; Finger; Firm; Fixed (pupil); Flexion; Flow; Fluid; Fluorine (Z = 9) (see Elements - Fluorine); Flux; Focal length; Focus; Foil; Fontanel; Foot; Foramen; Force; Form; Forma; Former name (vitamin F) for fatty acids (see Vitamins - F); Formula (a specific statement of the composition of a substance, e.g. Chemical F); Formulary; Fornix; Fossa; Fourneau (see Fourneau); Fraction; Fractional (gas concentration); Fracture; Fragment; Free; French (catheter scale/ size), used for denoting the size of bougies, catheters and other tubular instruments (1 F has a diameter of 1/3 mm) (see Fr); Frequency; Frontal; Frontal electrode placement in electroencephalography; Full (diet); Function; Fundus; Furstenau; Fusiformis; Fusobacterium; Gilbert (unit of magnetomotive force); Helmholz free energy; Hydrocortisone (= Compound F; Cortisol); Immediate and good continuing function (see F^{AR}); Inbreeding coefficient; Left foot electrode in vector-cardiography; Make (L. fac; fiat); Phenylalanine; Variance ratio.

f atomic orbital with angular momentum quantum number 3; fac (L.) - make; farad (unit of electrical capacity) (= F); father; female (see F.); femto- (= 10^{-15}); fiat (L.) - let it be made; fiber; fibrous; fingerbreadth; fission; fissure; flexion; fluid; focal; foot; form (L. forma); formula; fostered (experimental animal); fraction; fracture; fragment; frequency (e.g. f. of breathing, i.e. respiratory ratio); from; frontal; function; fundus; make (L. fiat); numerical expression of the relative aperture of a camera lens.

φ Phi (pronounced "fye") - 21st letter of the Greek alphabet.

F+ a bacterial cell having an F plasmid; form response scores (Rorschach).

F- a bacterial cell lacking an F plasmid; form response scores (Rorschach).

F' a hybrid F plasmid.

°F degree Fahrenheit (temperature/ thermometer scale) (= F; Fahr).

F↑ Full upper denture.

↓F Full lower denture.

(F) Final.

F_0 Oligomycin-sensitivity-conferring factor (see OSCF).

F_1 First filial generation (produced by crossing two individuals); Fluorescent substance found in small amounts in normal urine, and in larger quantities in the urine of pellagrins.

F_1, F_2, F_3, etc First, second, third, etc. filial generation.

F_2 Fluorescent substance developing in urine after the addition of alkali, and also normally, after the ingestion of nicotinic acid); Second filial generation (produced by mating two members of the F_1 generation; Zinc oxide - eugenol cement (dentistry).

F I, F II, F III, etc Factors I, II, III, etc.

f-12 Freon (a refrigerant).

^{18}F Radioactive fluorine.

F 99 Vitamin F - a mixture containing the ethyl esters of linoleic and linolenic (unsaturated fatty) acids (see Fourneau; Vitamins - F).

F 190 Stovarsol (see Fourneau).

F 270 Tryparsamide (see Fourneau).

F 309 Supramine sodium (see Fourneau).

F 344 Fischer 344 (rat).

F 664 A synthetic organic compound closely resembling plasmochin and used in the treatment of malaria. It is 8-(3- diethylamino-2,2-dimethyl-propylamino)-6-methoxyquinoline, $CH_3OC_8H_5NNHCH_2C(CH_3)_2CH_2N(C_2H_5)_2$

(see Fourneau).

F 693 Pamaquine (see Fourneau).

F 710 1) Neostibosan (= Ethylstibamine) - a pentavalent antimony compound used in the treatment of filariasis (see Fourneau); 2) Plasmocide (= Fourneau 710; SN 3115) - 8-(3-Diethylamino-propylamino)-6-methoxyquinoline methylene-bis-salicylate. A synthetic antimalarial drug, with similar actions and uses to pamaquin, used in Russia. Has been reported to be extremely toxic to the central nervous system (see Fourneau).

F 883 2-diethylamino-ethyl-1,4-benzodioxan - an adrenolytic drug (see Fourneau).

F 933 Piperoxan hydrochloride (= 2-piperidinomethyl-1,4-benzodioxan) (see Compound 933 F; Fourneau).

F 1262 2-diethylamino-ethoxydiphenyl. A drug that slows heart action and lowers blood pressure (see Fourneau).

F 30066 Furapromidium. A parasiticide used in the treatment of schistosomiasis and clonorchiasis (see Fourneau).

F 30069 An analogue of furapromidium; has been tried in patients with schistosomiasis (see Fourneau).

FA False aneurysm; Families Anonymous; Fanconi's anemia (= Congenital hypoplastica; Fanconi's syndrome); Far advanced; Fatty acid; Febrile antigen; Femoral artery; Ferretin-agglutinin; Fibrinolytic activity; Fibroadenoma; Fibrosing alveolitis; Field ambulance; Filterable agent; Filtered air; First aid; Flameless atomizer; Fluorescent antibody/ assay; Fluoroacetate; Fluoroalanine; Folic acid; Follicular area; Food allegy; Forearm; Fortified aqueous (solution); Free acid; Freund's adjuvant; Friedreich's ataxia; Friere-Maia (syndrome) (hyperkeratosis of palms, soles, elbows and knees, dystrophic nails and deafness - an autosomal recessive, ectodermal dysplasia); Functional activity; Furnace atomizer; Serum folate.

fa fatty (rat).

F/A Fetus active.

FAA Fatal aplastic anemia; Federal Aviation Administration; Flameless atomic absorption; Fluorescent antinuclear antibody (test) (see FAT); Folic acid antagonist; Food Additives Amendment (FFDCA); Formalin, acetic acid, alcohol (see FAA sol); Free amino acid; Freund's adjuvant arthritis.

FAAH Fatty acid amide hydrolase (an enzyme that metabolizes endocannabinoids, including anandamide, and is a potential target for pain therapy).

FAAN Fellow of the American Academy of Nursing.

FAAO Fellow of the American Association of Optometrists.

FAAOCAS Federal Aviation Agency's Office of the Civil Air Surgeon.

FAAP Family assessment adjustment pass/ plan; Fellow of the American Academy of Pediatrics.

FAA sol Formaldehyde (Formalin), acetic acid, and alcohol solution (a fixative) (= FAA).

FAAT Fluorescent antinuclear antibody test (see FAT).

FAB Fast atom bombardment; Formalin ammonium bromide; Fragment antigen-binding (i.e. Antigen-binding fragments of immunoglobulins) = Fab; F(ab')2; French-American-British (carcinoma staging); Functional arm brace.

Fab fragment, antigen-binding (see FAB).

F(ab')$_2$ Fragment, antigen-binding (see FAB).

FABB Feline Advisory Bureau Bulletin (UK).

Fabc Fragment, antigen and complement binding (of immunoglobulins) (see Facb).

FABER Flexion in/ Full abduction and external rotation.

FABF Femoral artery blood flow.

FABP Fatty/ Folate/ Folic acid-binding protein.

FABS Fresh AB serum.

Fabs Antibody-binding fragments (see FAB; Fab).

FAC Familial adenomatosis coli; Familial astrocytoma; Femoral arterial cannulation; Ferric ammonium citrate; Flexion-adduction contracture (of the thumb, as in CP or Cerebral palsy, causing SND - Swan-neck deformity) (Orthopedics); Fluorescent affinity chromatography; 5-Fluorouracil, Adriamycin, and cyclophosphamide; Foamy alveolar cast; Fractional area changes/ concentration; Free

available chlorine; Fulminating amebic colitis.
Fac Factor.
fac facility; to make (L. facere).
FACA Federal Advisory Committee Act; Fellow of the American College of Anesthesiologists/ Anesthetists/ Angiology/ Apothecaries.
FACAG Fellow of the American College of Angiology (= FACA).
FACAI Fellow of the College of Allergy and Immunology.
FACAL Fellow of the American College of Allergists (= FACAl).
FACAl Fellow of the College of Allergists/gy.
FACAN Fellow of the American College of Anesthiologists (= FACA).
FACAS Fellow of the American College of Abdominal Surgeons.
Facb Fragment, antigen, and complement binding (of immunoglobulins) (= Fabc).
FACC Fellow of the American College of Cardiologists/ Cardology.
FACCP Fellow of the American College of Chest Physicians (= FCCP).
FACCPC Fellow of the American College of Clinical Pharmacology & Chemotherapy.
FACD Fellow of the American College of Dentists.
FACEM Fellow of the American College of Emergency Medicine.
FACEP Fellow of the American College of Emergency Physicians.
FACES Unique facies, anorexia, cachexia, and eye and skin lesions (syndrome).
FACET Fosinopril Versus Amlodipine Cardiovascular Events Randomized Trial.
FACFP Fellow of the American College of Family Physicians.
FACFS Fellow of the American College of Foot Surgeons.
FACG Fellow of the American College of Gastroenterology.
FACGE Fellow of the American College of Gastroenterology (= FACG).
FACH Forceps to after-coming head.
FACHA Fellow of the American College of Health/ Hospital Administrators.
faci- prefix meaning face (L. facies).
F acid 7-amino-2-naphthalene-sulfonic acid.
-facient suffix meaning make (L. facio).
FACLM Fellow of the American College of Legal Medicine.
FACMH Fellow of the American College of Medical Hypnotists.
FACMTA Federal Advisory Council on Medical Training Aids.
FACN Fellow of the American College of Nutrition.
FACNHA Foundation of American College of Nursing Home Administrators.
FACNP Fellow of the American College of Neuropsychopharmacology.
FACO Fellow of the American College of Otolaryngology.
FACOG Fellow of the American College of Obstetricians and Gynecologists/ Obstetrics and Gynecology.
FACOS Fellow of the American College of Orthopedic Surgeons.
FACOSH Federal Advisory Committee on Occupational Safety and Health.
FACP Fellow of the American College of Physicians.
FACPM Fellow of the American College of Preventive Medicine.
FACPRM Fellow of the American College of Preventive Medicine (= FACPM).
FACR Fellow of the American College of Radiologists/gy.
FACS Fellow of the American College of Surgeons; Fluorescence-activated cell sorter.
FACSM Fellow of the American College of Sports Medicine.
FACSS Federation of Analytical Chemistry and Spectroscopy Societies.
FACT Flanagan Aptitude Classification Test; Focus on Alternative and Complementary Therapies (Homeopathy); Functional Assessment of Cancer Therapy (ECOG study).
-fact- combining form meaning make (L. facio).
Factor Blood coagulation factors:
I. Fibrinogen (= Plasma thromboplastin factor I; PTAH).
II. Prothrombin.
III. Tissue factor (= Thromboplastin);

Selenium.
IV. Calcium ions.
V. Proacclerin (= Accelerator factor/ globulin; AcG; Ac-G; Ac-g; Ac-globulin; Labile factor; LF; PCF; Plasma converting factor; Prothrombin conversion factor; Thrombogen.
VI. Not assigned at this time.
VII. Proconvertin (= Autoprothrombin I; Cothromboplastin; Plasma prothrombin conversion accelerator/ factor; PPCA; PPCF; Prothrombinogen; Prothrombinokinase; Serum prothrombin conversion accelerator; SPCA; Stable factor.
VIII. Antihemophilic factor (= AHF; Antihemophiliac factor; Antihemophilic factor A; Antihemophilic globulin; AHG; Antihemolytic globulin; Antihuman globulin; Cryoprecipitate; Hemophilic factor A; Platelet cofactor 1; PF-1; Platelet cofactor A; PF-A; Thrombocytolysin; Thromboplastinogen).
IX. Plasma thromboplastin component (= PTC); Antihemophilic factor B; Autoprothrombin II; Christmas factor; Hemophilic factor B; Platelet cofactor 2; PF-2; Platelet cofactor B; PF-B; PTL).
X. Stuart-Prower factor (= SP-F); Autoprothrombin III; PTF; Stuart factor; Thrombokinase.
XI. Plasma thromboplastin antecedent (= PTA; Antihemophilic factor C; Hemophilic factor C).
XII. Hageman factor (= HF; Activation/ Contact/ Glass factor).
XIII. Fibrin stabilizing factor (= FSF; Fibrinase; Laki-Lorand factor; LLF; Plasma trans-glutaminase). Fibrin stabilizing factor - activated form (= FSF*).

FACTS Fosinopril Versus Amlodipine Comparative Treatments Study (AHA).

FACWA Familial amyotrophic chorea with acanthocytosis.

FAD Familial Alzheimer's Dementia/ Disease (Three genes have been identified so far, one each on chromosomes 1, 14, and 21) (see PS1; PS2); Familial autonomic dysautonomia/ dysfunction; Family Accessment Device; Fetal activity-acceleration determination; Fibric acid derivative; Flavin(e) adenine dinucleotide (= FADN) (see AAD); Folic acid deficiency; Forced acid/ alkaline diuresis; Fully automated/matic device.

FaD Food and drug.

FADA Frequency-amplitude domain analysis.

FADF Fluorescent antibody dark-field (test).

FADH; FADH$_2$ Flavin(e) adenine dinucleotide, reduced form.

FADIR Flexion in adduction and internal rotation.

FADN Flavin(e) adenine dinucleotide (see AAD; FAD).

FADS Fetal akinesia deformation sequence.

FAE Fetal alcohol effect (see FAS); Fetoscopic air embolization (in selective feticide of the affected twin) (Obstetrics); Functional autoimmune epitope.

FAF Fatty acid free; Fibroblast-activating factor.

FA/FE Fatty acid/fatty ester (ratio).

FAFQ Food Amount Frequency Questionnaire (see FFQ).

FAG Fluorescein angiogram/graph(y).

Fag; Faggot Homosexual (see Homo).

FAGA Female androgenetic alopecia (see FPAGA); Full-term appropriate for gestational age.

FAH Factor(s) affecting healing; Federation of American Hospitals.

FAHIA Fast-acting human insulin analogue (= Insulin aspartate; RAIA).

Fahr Fahrenheit (temperature) (see °F).

FAI First aid instruction; Folic acid inhibitor; Free androgen index; Functional aerobic impairment; Functional assessment inventory.

FAIH Fellow of the American Institute of Hypnosis.

fait accompli French - an accomplished fact/ cannot be changed.

FAJ Fused apophyseal joint.

FAL Fanconi anemia lymphocyte.

FALG Fowl antimouse lymphocyte globulin.

FALL Fallopian.

FALP Fluoro-assisted lumbar puncture.

FAM Fatty-acid metabolism; 5-Fluorouracil, Adriamycin, and mitomycin C.

Fam; fam Familial/mily.

FAMA Fellow of the American Medical Association; Fluorescent antibody to mem-

brane antigen (test).
FAMC Fatty acid-mediated effect(s); Fitzsimmons Army Medical Center.
Fam Doc Family doctor (= Fam Phys; FD).
FAME Fatty acid methyl ester; Fluorouracil, Adriamycin (doxorubicin), and methyl CCNU (somustine).
fam hist family history.
FAMMM Familial atypical multiple mole - melanoma (syndrome).
FAMOS Floating-gate avalanche-injection metal-oxide semiconductor.
Fam per par(al) Familial periodic paralysis.
Fam Phys Family physician (see Fam Doc).
FAMSO Methyl methylthiomethyl sulfoxide (see MMTS).
FAMU Florida A&M University.
FAN Fuchsin, amidoblack, and naphthol yellow.
FANA Fluorescent antinuclear antibody (see FAT).
F and R Force and rhythm (of pulse) (see F&R).
FANPT Freeman Anxiety Neurosis and Psychosomatic Test.
FANS Fellow of the American Neurological Society.
FANY First Aid Nursing Yeoman(ry).
FAO Fatal airway obstruction; Fatty acid oxidation (in the liver); Food and Agricultural Organization (UN).
FAO/WHO Food and Agricultural Organization - World Health Organization (UN).
FAP Familial achondroplasia (see APD); Familial adenomatous polyposis; Familial amyloid polyneuropathy; Family assistance plan; Fatty acid, polyunsaturated; Fatty acid poor; Femoral artery pressure (see FBP); Fibrillating/ Fixed action potential; Fibrin-associated plasminogen; Flaccid atrophic paralysis/ paraplegia/ paresis; Frozen animal procedure; Functional artificial pacemaker.
FAPA Fellow of the American Psychiatric/ Psychoanalytical Association.
FAPHA Fellow of the American Public Health Association.
FAPVS Familial absent pulmonary valve syndrome (Obstetrics).
FAR Fast-acting relaxant; Fatal allergic/ anaphylactic reaction (= FHR); Flight aptitude rating; Food-allergy reaction (see AFR); Fractional albumin rate.
Far; far Farad (unit of faradic current); Faradic.
F^{AR} Immediate good function with accelerated rejection.
FARE Federation of Alcoholic Rehabilitation Establishments.
FARI Fetal aorta resistance index (Acupuncture therapy Obstetrics).
FART Fellow of the Association of Radiological Technologists.
FAS Fatty acid synthetase; Federation of American Scientists; Fluorescent antibody stain; Foetal alcohol syndrome (a condition associated with mental retardation and growth deficiencies, caused by heavy drinking of alcohol by the mother during pregnancy) (= FAE); Foreign Agricultural Service.
FASC Free-standing ambulatory surgical center.
Fasc; fasc Bundle, Fascicular/lus (L. fasciculus), e.g. Fasc of Gowers (= Anterior spinocerebellar tract; Gowers' tract; Tractus spinocerebellaris anterior).
fasci- prefix meaning band or bundle (L. fascia).
FASEB Federation of American Societies for Experimental Biology.
FASEBFP Federation of American Societies for Experimental Biology, Federation Proceedings.
FASHP Federation of Associations of Schools of the Health Professions; Fellow of the American Society of Hospital Pharmacists.
FAST Flow-assisted, short-term (balloon catheter); Fluorescent antibody serum titer; Fluorescent antibody staining technique; Fluoro-allergosorbent test; Frenchay Aphasia Screening Test; Functional Assessment Staging Test.
FAT Family attitudes test; Fetal activity test; Fluorescent antibody technique/ test (for Entamoeba histolytica, sometimes called the Indirect fluorescent antibody test (= FAA; FAAT; FANA; IFA; IFAT); Fujirebio agglutination test (for HIV infection).

F_1 ATPase Soluble coupling factor of Racker.

FAV Feline ataxia virus; Floppy aortic valve; Fowl adenovirus.

FAVP Functional artificial ventricular pacemaker (= FVP).

FAW Foreskin-associated wart(s) (see EGW).

FAX; fax Facsimile.

FAZ Fanconi-Albertini-Zeelweger (syndrome); Foveal avascular zone; Fragmented (atrial) activity zone.

FB Family bureau; Farm Bureau; Fasting blood (sugar); Feedback; Fiberoptic bronchoscopy; Fingerbreadth; Fluidized bath/ bed; Foreign body (= for body); Fusobacterium.

F/B Forward bending.

FBA FBA Pharmaceutical Ltd code for experimental substances (Farbenfabriken Bayer AG - English subsidiary); Fecal bile acid; Fellow of the British Academy; Full-blown arthritis.

FBA 1420 Propanidid (= Propyl-4-diethyl-carbamoylmethoxy-3-methoxyphenylacetate). A short-acting anesthetic used intravenously, as an induction anesthetic in major surgery, and as the sole anesthetic agent in minor surgical procedures.

FBAL α-Fluoro-β-alanine; 2-Fluoro-B-alanine.

FBBC Full-blown brain control.

FBC Feedback control; Fetal blood concentration; Fiber-binding cell; Fibroblast cell; Foreign body cyst (Orthopedics); Full blood count; Functional bactericidal concentration.

FBCOD Foreign body of the cornea, oculus dexter (right eye) (L. ocula dextra).

FBCOS Foreign body of the cornea, oculus sinister (left eye) (L. ocula sinistra).

FBCP Familial benign chronic pemphigus.

FBD Fetal biparietal diameter (Obstetrics); Fibrocystic breast disease (see FCDB); Full-blown diabetes; Functional bowel disease/ disorder (see IBS).

FBDG Food-based dietary guidelines.

FBDH Familial bilateral diaphragmatic hernia (Obs/Pediat).

FbDP Fibrin degradation products.

FBE Fiberoptic bronchoscopic examination; Full blood examination.

FBEC Fetal bovine endothelial cell.

FBF Fetal blood flow; Forearm blood flow.

FBG Fasting blood glucose (= BFS; FBS) (see LFT iv); Fibrinogen (see fbg); Foreign body(-type) granulomata; Free bone graft (Orthopedics).

fbg fibrinogen (= FBG).

FBGCR Foreign-body giant-cell reaction (Orthopedics).

FBH Hydroxybutyric dehydrogenase.

FBHA Food-borne hepatitis A.

FBHH Familial benign hypocalciuric hypercalcemia.

FBI Fecal-borne infection; Federal Bureau of Investigation (Department of Justice); Flossing, brushing, and irrigation (dentistry).

FBL Fecal blood loss; Follicular basal lamina.

FBL-3 Friend helper virus-induced lymphoblastic leukemia.

FBM Fatty bone marrow; Fetal breathing movements.

FBMI Full-blown mental illness.

FBN Federal Bureau of Narcotics.

FBOA Fellow of the British Optical Association.

FBP Female breast pain; Femoral blood pressure (= FAP); Fetal biophysical profile; Fetal blood pressure/ protein; Fibrin-bound plasmin; Fibrin(ogen) breakdown product(s) (laboratory/ coagulation); Folate/ Fucose-binding protein; Foreign-born patient; Free base peptide (see AFBP).

FBPS Fetal biophysical profile score (see BPS).

FBPsS Fellow of the British Psychological Society.

FBRCM Finger(breadth) below right costal margin.

FBS Family-based study; Fasting blood sugar (= BFS) (see FBG; LFT iv); Feedback signal/ system; Fetal blood sampling; Fetal bovine serum; Full-body scan.

FBSS Failed back surgery syndrome.

FBT Fetal brain tumor; Foodborne transmission (of disease/ infection).

FBU Fingers below umbilicus.

FBW Fasting blood work; Fetal body weight.

ϕ BZ Phenylbutazone.

FC Family conference; Fasciculus cuneatus; Fast component (of a neurone); Febrile convulsion(s); Feline conjunctivitis; Ferric citrate; Fever, chills; Fibrocyte; Film coated; Financial class; Finger clubbing; Finger counting (eye examination); Flucytosine; Fludrocortisone (see F-cortef); Fluorocarbon; Fluorocytosine (see 5-FC); Foley catheter (see F cath); Foster care; Fowl cholera; Fragment portion of immunoglobulin G (IgG) (see Fc); Free cholesterol; French Codex (pharmacopeia); Frontal cortex (see FCx); Functional capacity/ castration/ class.

Fc Centroid frequency; Crystallizable fragment (of IgG) (= FC) - Portion of antibody molecule bound by membrane receptors.

fc foot candle(s) (see ft-c).

F'C; F'c Fragment portion of immunoglobulin M (or an immunoglobulin molecule = IgM) produced by papain digestion.

F&C Foam and condom.

5-FC Fluorocytosine (= FC).

F+C Flare plus cells.

FCA False-color angiogram; Fatal cardiac arrest; Federal Council on the Aging (OHD); Ferritin-conjugated antibodies/body; Fetal cardiac activity; Flow-cytometric analysis (of tumors, etc.) (see FCM); Follicular cell adenoma (of the thyroid gland, etc.); Freund's complete adjuvant.

FCAP Fellow of the College of American Pathologists.

FCaR Fluoride-calcium regimen (in the treatment of osteoporosis).

F cath Foley catheter (= FC).

FCB Fetal cord blood.

FCBD Fibrocystic breast disease (see FBD; FCDB).

FCC Familial colonic cancer; Federal Communications Commission; Femoral cerebral catheter; Fibrin-cefotaxim compound (used locally as an implant in the treatment of chronic osteomyelitis) (Orthopedics); Fluorochlorocarbon; Follicular center cells; Food Chemicals Codex (FDA); Fracture, comminuted compound; Frank circulatory compromise

fcc face-centered-cubic.

f/cc fibers per cubic centimeter (of air).

FCCL Follicular center cell lymphoma.

FCCP Carbonyl-cyanide-trifluoro-methoxyphenyl-hydrazone; Fellow of the (American) College of Chest Physicians (see FACCP).

FCCSET Federal Coordinating Council for Science, Engineering, and Technology.

FCD Feces collection device; Fetal cardiac disease (Obstetrics); Fibrocystic disease/ dysplasia; Fistulating/ Fistulizing Crohn's disease; Focal cytoplasmic degradation.

FCDA Federal Civil Defence Administration.

FCDB Fibrocystic disease of the breast (= FBD).

FCE Fatal coronary event; Fibrocartilaginous embolism; Flow-cytometric examination; Fluorouracil, cisplatin, and etoposide.

F cell Scavenger cell.

FCF Fetal cardiac frequency; Fetal cardiac function (Obstetrics); Fiber-containing food; Fibroblast chemotactic factor.

FCFC Fibroblast colony-forming cell.

FCG French catheter guage.

FCGP Fellow of the College of General Practitioners.

FCH Familial combined hyperlipidemia (see FCHL).

FCHA Florence Crittenton Homes Association.

FCHL Familial combined hyperlipidemia.

FChS Fellow of the Society of Chiropodists.

FCI Federation for Clinical Investigation; Fixed-cell immunofluorescence; Food chemical intolerance.

FCIM Federated Council for Internal Medicine.

FCIS Flat carcinoma in situ (urinary bladder see PTC).

FCJ Fibrocartilaginous joint (such as the symphasis pubica/ pubis).

FCL Fetoscopic cord ligation (Obstetrics); Fibroblast cell line; Fibular collateral ligament.

F-CL Fluorouracil and calcium leucovorin.

FCLM Fellow of the College of Legal Medicine.

fcly face lying.

FCM Federal Council of Medicine (Brazil); Flow cytometry; Focal chronic myocarditis.

FCMC Family centered maternity care.

FCMD Fukuyama-type congenital muscular dystrophy.

FCMHSA Federal Coal Mine Health and

Safety Act (of 1969).

FCMM Federal Commission on Medical Malpractice.

FCMN Family centered maternity nursing.

FCMNC Family-centered maternity/ newborn care.

FCMP Family and Community Medicine Program.

FCMS Fellow of the College of Medicine and Surgery; Foix-Chavany-Marie syndrome.

FCMW Foundation for Child Mental Welfare.

FCN Family-centered nursing.

FCNBC Family-centered newborn care.

FCO Fellow of the College of Osteopathy; Fick Cardiac Output.

F-cortef Fludrocortisone (Proprietary Drug name) (= FC).

FCP Final common pathway (neurology); "First-contact" patient; Functional Communication Profile.

FCPD Fibrocalculous pancreatic diabetes (one of the two subtypes of MRDM - see MRDM; PD; PDPD).

FCPS Fellow of the College of Physicians and Surgeons.

FCPSSA Fellow of the College of Physicians and Surgeons of South Africa.

FCR Fetal-cell research; Flexor carpi radialis (tendon); Fractional catabolic rate; Fusin coreceptor.

FcR Fc receptor (see Fc).

FCRA Fecal collection receptacle assembly; Fellow of the College of Radiologists of Australasia.

FCRB Flexor carpi radialis brevis.

FCRC Frederick Cancer Research Center.

FCS Familial cancer syndrome; Farmer Cooperative Service; Fecal containment system; Feedback control system; Fellow of the Chemical Society; Fetal calf serum; Fetal cord serum (umbilical); Flexible Careers Scheme (DoH, UK); Foot compartment syndrome.

FCs Fluorocarbons (see VSA).

FCSNVD Fever, chills, sweating, nausea, vomiting, and diarrhea.

FCSP Fellow of the Chartered Society of Physiotherapy.

FCST Federal Council for Science and Technology; Fellow of the College of Speech Therapists.

FCT Fetal cell transplant; Fibro-cartilagenous tissue; Fibrocystic tumor; Film-coated tablet (see FC); Fixed combination tablet; Food and Cosmetics Toxicology; Food composition table; Full conventional therapy.

FCTG Fetal cardiotocogram/graph(y).

FCU Flexor carpi ulnaris (tendon).

FCVD Functional cardiovascular disorder.

FCx Frontal cortex (= FC).

FD Fabry Disease (= AKCD or Angiokeratoma corporis diffusum) - a glycosphingolipid storage disorder caused by deficient activity of the lysosomal enzyme AGA or galactosidase A, resulting in accumulation of Gb3 or CTH (Globotriaosylceramide), the glycosphingolipid substrate for this enzyme (see AGA); Facial dystonia; Familial dysautonomia; Family doctor (see Fam Doc); Fan douche; Fatal dose (see LD); Fetal danger (see FDZ)/ death/ demise; Fibrin(ogen) derivative; Field desorption; Fluorescent densitometer; Focal distance (eye examination); Folin-Denis (assay); Follicular diameter; Foot drape/ drop; Forceps delivery; Freeze dried/ drying; Frequency deviation; Fucose dehydrogenase (a crystalline methyl pentose deoxygalactose); Full denture.

Fd The amino-terminal portion of the heavy chain of an immunoglobulin molecule; Ferredoxin.

fd fundus.

F-D Franklin-Dukes (method).

F&D Fixed and dilated (pupils).

FD_{50} Median fatal dose (that fatal to 50% of test subjects).

FDA Federal Department of Agriculture; Federal Drug Administration; Fetal development abnormality; Fluorescein diacetate; Food and Drug Administration; Right frontoanterior (L. Fronto-dextra anterior) (position of the fetus).

FDAA Federal Disaster Assistance Administration (HUD).

FDAC Federal Disaster Assistance Corporation; Food and Drug Administration Consumer (journal).

FDAD Foreign Demographic Analysis Division (Dept of Commerce).
FDB First (only erythema with no loss of epidermis)/ Fourth (with deep tissue loss - see DTL) -degree burn; Freeze-dried bone (Orthopedics).
FDBA Freeze-dried bone allograft (Orthopedics).
FDBL Fecal daily blood loss.
FDC Faculty Development Center (Stanford Univ., US); Familial dilated cardiomyopathy; First derivative computer; Fixed dose combination; Flexor digitorum communis; Follicular dendritic cell; Food coloring(s); Food, Drug and Cosmetic (Act) (see FD&C).
FD&C Food, Drug and Cosmetic (Act) (= FDC); Food, drug and cosmetic (preparations)/ drugs and cosmetics (colors or dyes), permitted for use in the United States.
FDCP Fixed-dose combination product.
FDCPA Food, Drug, and Consumer Product Agency.
FD&C red no. 2 Food additive dye (amaranth).
FD&C yellow no. 5 Yellow dye food coloring (tartrazine).
FDD Fetal drug dependence; Fiberoptic delivery device (in CAD); Food and Drugs Directorate (Canada).
FDDC Ferric dimethyldithiocarbonate (a fungicide).
FDDS Family Drawing Depression Scale.
FDE Female day-equivalent; Final drug evaluation; First-dose effect; Fixed drug eruption.
FDF Fast death factor.
FDFQ Food/Drink Frequency Questionnaire.
FDG Firm diffuse goiter; Fluorodeoxyglucose; Freeze-dried graft.
fdg feeding.
FDGF Fibroblast-derived growth factor.
FDGS Feedings.
FDH Familial dysalbuminemic hyperthyroxinemia; Fetal diaphragmatic hernia (Obstetrics); Focal dermal hypoplasia (skeletal defects, osteopathia striata on X-ray findings, raspberry papillomas, asymmetrical linear streaks of atrophy and telangiectasia - probably sex-linked, dominant, congenital hypotrichosis) (= GS - Goltz syndrome); Formaldehyde dehydrogenase.
FDI International Dental Federation (Fr. Fédération Dentaire Internationale).
FDIC Federal Deposit Insurance Corporation.
FDICS Familial diffuse infantile cerebral sclerosis (= KD - Krabbe's disease).
FDIN Fédération Dentaire Internationale News Letter (UK).
FDIU Fetal death in utero.
FDL Flexor digitorum longus.
FDLF Fleur-de-lis (skin) flap (iris-shaped).
FDLI Food and Drug Law Institute (UK).
FDLMP First day of last menstrual period.
FDLP Familial dyslipoproteinemia.
FDLV Fer de lance virus.
FDM Fetus of diabetic mother; Fibrous dysplasia of the mandible.
FDNB Fluorodinitrobenzene.
FDNY Fire Department New York.
FDO Fibrodysplasia ossificans (Orthopedics); Fleet Dental Officer.
FDP Fibrin(ogen) degradation product; Flexor digitorum profundus (tendon); Frontodextra posterior (L.) (right fronto-posterior - position of fetus); Fructose-1,6-diphosphate.
FDPase Fructose-1,6-diphosphatase.
FDPu Fibrin(ogen) degradation products in urine.
FDQB Flexor digiti quinti brevis.
FDR Fractional disappearance rate; Full dose range.
FDS Fellow in Dental Surgery; Fiber duodenoscope; Flexor digitorum superficialis (tendon); For duration of stay.
FDSRCSEng Fellow in Dental Surgery of the Royal College of Surgeons of England.
FDT Frontodextra transversa (L.) (right fronto-transverse - position of fetus).
FdUMP 5-Fluoro-2-deoxyuridine monophosphate (a metabolite of 5-FU).
FDUS Four-dimensional ultrasound (Obstetrics).
FDV Friend disease virus.
FDZ Fetal danger zone (= FD).
FE Fatty ester; Fecal emesis; Fetal erythroblastosis/ erythrocyte(s); Flame emission; Fluid extract; Fluorescent/cing erythrocyte(s) (red); Food engineering; Forced expiration; Formaldehyde-ethanol; Fractional excretion;

Friends of the Earth (association).
Fe Female (see fe); Ferret; Iron (L. ferrum) (Z = 26) (see Elements - Iron).
fe female (= Fe).
F-E Formal-ether.
^{59}Fe Radioactive iron.
FEA Federal Energy Administration.
FEB Federal employees' benefits.
Feb February.
feb febrile/ fever (L. febris).
feb agglut febrile agglutination (laboratory/ serology).
feb dur while the fever lasts (L. febre durante).
FEBP Fetal estrogen-binding protein.
febr- prefix meaning fever (L. febris).
FEBS Federation of European Biochemical Societies.
FEBSL Federation of European Biochemical Societies Letters (journal).
FEC Fluorouracil, etoposide, and cisplatin; Forced expiratory capacity; Free erythrocyte coproporphyrin (see FECP); Free-standing emergency clinic; Friend erythroleukemia cell.
FECFV Functional extracellular fluid volume.
FECG Fetal electrocardiogram/graph(y) (= FEKG).
FECL Functional endocervical length (Obstetrics).
$FeCl_2$ Ferrous Chloride.
$FeCl_3$ Ferric Chloride (= Ferr Perchlor; Ferri Perchloridi).
$FECO_2$ Fractional concentration of carbon dioxide in expired gas.
$FeCO_3$ Ferrous carbonate.
FECP Free erythrocyte coproporphyrin (= FEC).
FECT Fibroelastic connective tissue.
-fect- combining form meaning make (L. facio).
fe cult fecal culture.
FECV Feline enteric coronavirus.
FED Fetal electrolyte/ytic disturbance(s).
FeD Iron deficiency (anemia) (= Fe def).
Fed Federal (Reserve System)/ation.
FeDA Iron deficiency anemia (see Fe def A; HCA; IDA).
Fe def Iron deficiency (anemia) (see FeD).
Fe def A Iron deficiency anemia (see FeDA; HCA; IDA).
FEDRIP Federal Research in Progress (database).
Fed spec Federal specification(s).
FEE Forced equilibrating expiration.
FEEG Fetal electroencephalogram/graph(y).
FEF Forced expiratory flow (see PFT - FEF).
$FEF_{25\text{-}75\%}$ Forced midexpiratory flow (rate) - between 25% and 75% of forced vital capacity (FVC) (see PFT - FEF 25-75%).
FEF_{50} Forced expiratory flow at 50% of FVC (see PFT - FEF).
FEF_{50}/FIF_{50} Ratio of expiratory flow to inspiratory flow at 50% of FVC (see PFT - FEF, FIF).
FEFR Forced expiratory flow rate (l/sec) (see PFT - FEF).
FEFV Forced expiratory flow volume (see PFT - FEF).
$FEF_{x\text{-}y}$ Forced expiratory flow between two designated volume points in the forced vital capacity.
FEGO International Federation of Gynecology and Obstetricics.
FEHB Federal Employee(s) Health Benefits (program) (see FEHBP).
FEHBP FEHB Program.
FEI Federal Executive Institute.
FeI Ferrous Iodide.
FEKG Fetal electrocardiogram/graph(y) (see FECG).
FEL Familial erythrophagocytic lymphohistiocytosis.
Fel Fellow.
FELK Friend erythroleukemia.
FELS Complete sheet to measure development in children.
FeLV Feline leukemia virus (= FLV).
FEM Field emission microscope.
Fem; fem Female/minine; Femoral/mur (L. femoris) - thigh.
FEMA Federal Emergency Management Agency; Flavor and Extract Manufacturers Association.
Fem extern Outer side of the thigh (L. femoribus externus).
Fem intern Inner side of the thigh (L. femoribus internus).

Fem-pop Femoral popliteal (bypass).
femto- 10^{-15}. Symbol f (see F - femto-).
FEN Fluid, electrolytes, and nutrition.
FENa; FENa Fractional excretion of sodium.
Fen-phen A combination of fenfluramine ("Ponderax") and phentermine ("Novirasin") - treatment for obesity.
FEO Federal Energy Office.
FeO Ferrous oxide.
FE_{O2}, F_{EO2} Fractitional concentration of oxygen in expired gas.
Fe_2O_3 Ferric oxide.
$Fe(OH)_2$ Ferrous hydroxide.
$Fe(OH)_3$ Ferric hydroxide.
FEP Fair employment practice; Federal Employees' Program (Health); First-episode patient (see NTFEP); Fluorinated ethylene propylene (Teflon); Frail elderly patient/ people/ person; Free erythrocyte protoporphyrin (see FEPP).
FEPB Functional electronic peroneal brace.
FEPCA Federal Environmental Pest Control Act (of 1972) (EPA, also known as FIFRA).
$Fe_3(PO_4)_2$ Ferrous phosphate.
FEPP Free erythrocyte protoporphyrin (test in lead poisoning) (= FEP).
FER Flexion, extension, rotation; Forced expiratory ratio (= FEV/VC or Forced expiratory volume in 1 second/ Vital capacity) 1 (see PFT - FER).
FEREAC CODEN (six-letter code) for Federal Register (see CODEN).
-ferent suffix meaning carry (L. fero).
Ferm Female hermaphrodite (see Herm; Merm).
ferr- prefix meaning iron (L. ferrum).
fert fertilized (= fertd); fertility (= ferty).
fertd fertilized (see fert).
ferty fertility (see fert).
ferv boiling or hot (L. fervens).
FES Fat embolism syndrome; Femoral epiphysial slipping (see SFE); Fiberoptic endoscopic surgery; Flame emission spectroscopy; Forced expiratory spirogram (see PFT - FES); Fully electronic stethoscope (see CAS) (HP - Hewlett-Packard stethoscope); Functional electrical stimulation; Zearalenone.
FeS Iron status (see IS).
Fe/S Iron/sulfur (protein).
$FeSO_4$ Ferrous sulfate.
FeSV Feline sarcoma virus (= FSV).
FET Field-effect transistor; Field emission tube (X-rays); Fisher's exact test (in statistical analysis); Flasher Exact Test; Forced expiratory time (see PFT - FET).
FETE Far Eastern tick-borne encephalitis.
FETI Fluorescent energy transfer immunoassay.
Fe/TIBC Iron saturation/Total iron-binding capacity (serum transferrin) (ratio) (see TIBC).
FETS see FETs.
FETs Forced expiratory time in seconds (= FETS) (see PFT - FETs).
FEUO For external use only.
FEV Familial exudative vitreoretinopathy (see FEVR); Flexion-extension view (CT spine); Forced expiratory volume (the volume of maximally fast expiration starting at full inspiration, i.e. Peak flow {PF}. Subscript indicates time in seconds, during which the FEV is measured, e.g. FEV1/2, FEV 0.75, FEV1, or per cent vital capacity in a certain time period, e.g. FEV 1% or FEV 25-75%. The FEV is a test of the Forced vital capacity {FVC}) (see PFT).
FEV1/2; $FEV_{1/2}$ Forced expiratory volume in half a second (see PFT - $FEV_{1/2}$).
FEV0.75; $FEV_{0.75}$ Forced expiratory volume in 3/4 second (see PFT - $FEV_{0.75}$).
FEV1; FEV_1 Forced expiratory volume in 1 second (see PFT - FEV_1).
$FEV_{25\text{-}75\%}$ Maximal midexpiratory flow (see PFT).
$FEV_{1\%}$, $\%FEV_1$ Percent vital capacity in one second.
$\%{>}FEV_1$ Mean percentage decrease in one second forced expiratory volume (see PFT).
FEVB Frequent ectopic ventricular beat.
FEVR Familial exudative vitreoretinopathy (= FEV).
FEV1/VC Ratio of forced expiratory volume in one second to the vital capacity i.e. per cent vital capacity expired in one second (= FER or Forced expiratory ratio) (see PFT - FER).
FF Degree of fineness of abrasive particles (= FFF); Fat-free (diet); Father/ Fertility factor;

Fear of failure; Fecal frequency; Field of Forel; Fight or flight (psychological reaction); Filterable/ Filtration fraction; Fine fiber; Finger flexion; Finger-to-finger (test for coordination/ neurology); Fixation/ Fixing/ Follicular fluid; Flat fee/ feet; Flip-flop (see F/F); Fluorescent focus; Force(d) fluids (see ff); Forced feeding; Fore-arm flow; Forward flexion; Foster father; Free fluid/ fraction; French Foundation (see FFAR); French fried (potatoes) ("French fries"); Fresh frozen; Fundus firm.

ff following; force(d) fluids (diet order) (= FF).

F/F Flip-flop (circuit) (= FF).

ff+ fertility inhibition positive.

ff- fertility inhibition negative.

F&F Fixes and follows.

FFA Familial focal alopecia; Fellow of the Faculty of Anaesthetists; Flammable Fabrics Act (CPSC); Free fatty acid (non-esterified).

FFAC Friends For All Children.

FFAH Flower and Fifth Avenue Hospital (= F&FAve).

FFAP Free fatty acid phase.

FFAR French Foundation for Alzheimer Research.

FFARCS Fellow of the Faculty of Anaesthetists of the Royal College of Surgeons (UK).

FFAT Fecal fat absorption test.

F&FAve Flower and Fifth Avenue (Hospital) (see FFAH).

FFB Flexible fiberoptic bronchoscope/py; Foundation for Fighting Blindness.

FFBM Fat-free body mass.

FFC Fixed flexion contracture; Fluorescence flow cytometry; Free from chlorine; Formula-fed child.

FFCM Fellow of the Faculty of Community Medicine.

FFCRA Federal Fair Credit Reporting Act.

FFD Fatal fulminant disease; Fat-free diet; Fellow in the Faculty of Dentistry; Focus-film distance (X-rays); Forefoot deformity.

FFDCA Federal Food, Drug, and Cosmetic Act.

FFDSRCS Fellow of the Faculty of Dental Surgery of the Royal College of Surgeons (UK).

FFDW Fat-free dry weight.

FFE Fecal fat excretion.

FFEL Federal Family Education Loan (Program).

FFET Fecal fat elimination/ excretion test.

FFF Degree of fineness of abrasive particles (see FF); Femoral fracture fixation; Field-flow fractionation; "Fight, Flight, or Fright" (Panic disorder) (see APD; CFR; GAD; PD; PTSD); Flicker fusion frequency.

FFFF Fight Food Fads Foundation.

FFG Free fat graft; Fusiform gyrus (an area of the brain that specializes in the recognition of human faces).

FFH Fatal fulminant hepatitis.

FFHom Fellow of the Faculty of Homeopathy.

FFI Fast food intake; Fatal familial insomnia; Fatal fungal infection; Fat-free interval; Fluorescent focus inhibition; Formula-fed infant; Free from infection; Fundamental frequency indicator.

FFIT Fluorescent focus inhibition test.

FFL Firefly luciferase.

FFM Fat-free mass; Fellowship for Freedom in Medicine; Five finger movement.

FFN Fetal fibronectin; Fractured femoral neck (Orthopedics).

FFOM Fellow of the Faculty of Occupational Medicine.

FFP Federal financial participation; Fresh frozen plasma.

FFPS Fauna and Flora Preservation Society.

FFQ Food Frequency Questionnaire (see FAFQ).

FFR Fellow of the Faculty of Radiologists; Fibrinogen-fibrin-related (antigen) (= FR); Fight-or-flight response (see FFF).

FFRDC Federally-funded research and development centers (administered by universities).

FFROM Free and full range of motion.

FFS Fat-free solids/ supper; Fee-for-service(s); Flexible fiberoptic sigmoidoscope/py.

FFT Fast Fourier transform; Flicker fusion test/ threshold.

FFTP First full-term pregnancy.

FFTS Fetofetal transfusion syndrome (Obstetrics).
FFU Femur-fibula-ulna (syndrome); Focal forming unit; Future follow-up.
FFW Fat-free weight.
FFWC Fractional free water clearance.
FFWW Fat-free wet weight.
FG Fasciculus gracilis; Fast-glycolytic (fiber); Feeley-Gorman (agar); Festinant gait (hurrying gait, in Parkinsonism); Fiberguide; Fibrin glue; Fibrinogen (= FGN); Flammable gas (compressed); Flemish giant (rabbit); Function generator.
fg femtogram (= 10^{-15} gram).
FGC Fasting glucose concentration (see FBS); Fetal germ cell; Fibrinogen gel chromatography; Frontal gas chromatography.
FGD Fatal granulomatous disease (now CGD); Fetal growth delay/ disorder/ disturbance(s); First-generation drug; Flue gas desulfurization.
FgD Fibrin(ogen) degradation product(s), fragment D.
FgD_{neo} Fibrin(ogen) degradation products, fragment D degraded by plasma.
FgDP Fibrin(ogen) degradation product(s).
FGDS Fibergastroduodenoscope/py.
FgE Fibrin(ogen) degradation product(s), fragment E.
FGF Father's grandfather; Fibroblast growth factor; Fresh gas flow; Froimovich Geriatric Formula.
FGFR3 Fibroblast growth factor receptor-3 gene (Genetic amniocentesis - Obstetrics).
FGG Focal global glomerulosclerosis; Fowl gamma-globulin.
FGHL Fetal giant hemangiolymphangioma (Obstetrics).
FGIR Final global improvement rate.
FGL Fasting gastrin/ glucose level.
FGM Father's grandmother.
FGN Fibrinogen (see FG); Focal glomerulonephritis.
FGP Federation of General Practitioners; Fetal growth parameter(s) (Obstetrics); Foster Grandparent Program (ACTION); Fundic gland polyp.
FGR Fetal growth retardation.
FGRP Fertility and General Reproductive Performance (study).
FGS Fiber/ Fibro gastroscope/py; Focal glomerular sclerosis.
FGT Female genital tract; Fetal gene therapy (Obstetrics); Fluorescent gonorrhea test; Formolgel test (for Kala-azar); French gastrostomy tube (e.g. No: 16).
FGTS Female genital tract sepsis.
FGW Floppy guide wire (Coronary angioplasty).
FH Facial hemihyperplasia; Faith healing; Familial hypercholesterolemia; Family history (see FHx); Fasting hyperbilirubinemia; Federation of the Handicapped; Femoral hypoplasia; Fetal head/ heart; Fibromuscular/ Follicular hyperplasia; Follicular hormone (see Hormones - FH); Frankfort horizontal (plane of skull); Fundal height; Make a draft (L. fiat haustus) (see fh).
fH Vitamin H (Biotin) (see Vitamins - H).
fh fostered by hand (experimental animal); let a draft/ draught be made or make a draft/ draught (L. fiat haustus) (= FH).
FH+ Family history positive.
FH- Family history negative.
FH_2 Dihydrofolic acid.
FH_4 Tetrahydrofolic acid.
FHA Familial hypoplastic anemia; Federal Housing Administration/ Authority; Fellow of the Institute of Hospital Administrators; Fetal heart anomalies/ly; Filamentous hemagglutinin; Filterable hemolytic anemia.
FHB Fetal heartbeat.
FH/BC Frontal horn/bicaudate (ratio).
FHC Familial hypercholesterolemia; Familial hypertrophic cardiomyopathy; Family health center; Fibrous histiocytoma (a malignant bone tumor); Ficoll-Hypaque centrifugation; Fuchs' heterochromic cyclitis.
FHCF (Potassium) ferrihexacyanoferrate (= PB or Prussian Blue - used in the treatment of thallium poisoning).
FHCP Family Health Center Program (PHS).
FHD Familial histiocytic dermatoarthritis; Family history of diabetes; Fixed-head disk/ drum (computer memory); Fundamental host defect (in genetic disorders).
FHE Firsthand experience.
FHF Fetal heart frequency; Fulminant heart/

hepatic failure.

FHFA Family Health Foundation of America.

fHg Free hemoglobin.

FHH Familial hypocalciuric hypercalcemia; Family health history; Family history of hirsutism/ hypertension; Female hypothalamic hypogonadism; Fetal heart heard; Fetal hepatic hemangioma (Obstetrics).

FHI Fetal hyperinsulinemia (cause of fetal macrosomia) (see EFG); Fuchs' heterochromic iridocyclitis.

FHIP Family health insurance plan.

FHIT Fragile histidine triad (gene).

FHL Flexor hallucis longus; Focal hepatic lesion (= FLL); Frontal hair loss; Functional hearing loss.

FHM Familial hemiplegic migraine; Fathead minnow (cells); Fetal heart monitor.

FHN Family history negative; Fatal hepatic necrosis; Fulminant hepatic necrosis.

FHNH Fetal heart not heard.

FHoPP Familial hypokalemic periodic paralysis (= FHPP).

FHP Family history positive.

FHPP Familial hypokalemic periodic paralysis (see FhoPP).

FHR Familial hemophagocytic reticulosis; Familial hypophosphatemic rickets; Fatal hypersensitivity reaction (see FAR); Femoral hernia repair (Lotheissen); Fetal heart rate.

FHRNST Fetal heart rate non-stress test.

FHS Facial hemispasm; Female healthy subject; Fetal heart sound; Fetal hydantoin syndrome; First heart sound.

FHSA Federal Hazardous Substances Act (CPSC).

F-HSA Fluorescent human serum albumin.

FHSC Female homosexual couple.

FHT Fetal heart/ heart tissue/ heart tone/ hypothyrodism; Fourier-Hadamard transform; Freeman-Halton test (in statistical analysis).

FHTG Familial hypertriglyceridemia.

FH-UFS Femoral hypoplasia - unusual facies syndrome.

FHV Falcon herpes virus.

FHVDRR Familial hypophosphatemic vitamin-D resistant rickets.

FHVP Free hepatic vein pressure.

FHx Family history (= FH).

FI Face immersion; Factory Inspectorate (UK); Fasciculus inter/intra fascicularis; Fertilizer Institute; Fever (caused by) infection; Fibrin (see Fib; Fib); Fibrinogen (see Fibrin); Fibrinogen (antihuman reagent); Fibrous insulin (see Insulin - FI); Fixed internal (reinforcement) (psychology); Fixed interval; Flame ionization; Flow index (see VFI); Fluctuation Index (of drug concentration in plasma) %FI = (Cmax - Cmin / Cavg) X 100 = Peak-to-trough FI within a 24-hr period; Fluid imbalance (see EI - Electrolyte index); Follicular involution; Food intolerance; Forced inspiration; Frontoiliac.

FI# Fluoride-induced fracture (see FIF).

Fi Fibrin (see Fib; fib); Fibrin (degradation products test); Fibrinogen (see Fibrin).

FI 5853 Aminosidin sulfate (see Antibioto 1600).

FIA Federal Insurance Administration; Fluorescent/ Focal immunoassay; Freedom of Information Act (1967); Freund's incomplete adjuvant.

FIAC 2'-fluoro-5-iodo-aracytosine.

FIAH Fully implantable artificial heart (see AbioCor 2001).

FIAT Field Information Agency, Technical (US Reports).

FIAU Fialuridine.

FIAX Fluorescent Immunoassay.

FIB Fellow of the Institute of Biology; Fibrin (see Fib; fib); Fibrinogen (see Fibrin); Fibrinolyric-induced bleeding; Fibrositis; Fibula (see Fib; fib).

Fib; fib Fiber; Fibrillation (see Fibrill); Fibrin (= FI; Fi; FIB); Fibrinogen (see Fibrin); Fibula (= FIB).

fibr- combining form meaning fiber (L. fibra).

Fibrill Fibrillation (= Fib; fib).

Fibrin Fibrinogen (= FI; Fi; FIB; Fib; fib).

FIBRO-AHF Fibrinogen and antihemophilic globin.

FIC Federal International Center (GSA); Federal Insurance Contribution (SS) (Social Security); Fellow of the Institute of Chemistry; Fogarty International Center (NIH); Fractitional inhibitory concentration.

FICA Federal Insurance Contributions Act (Society Security).

FICB Fetal intracerebral bleeding (see FICH).
FICCPM Fogarty International Center Conference on Preventive Medicine.
FICD Fellow of the Institute of Canadian Dentists; Fellow of the International College of Dentists.
FI Ceram Fellow of the Institute of Ceramics.
FICH. Fetal intracerebral hemorrhage (= FICB); Fetal intracranial hemorrhage (see SFIH).
$FICO_2$; FI_{CO2} Fractional concentration of carbon dioxide in inspired gas (respiratory therapy).
FICS Fellow of the International College of Surgeons.
FICU Fetal intensive care unit.
FID Father in delivery; Flame ionization detector; Free induction decay; Functional iron deficiency; Fungal immunodiffusion; Furosemide-induced diuresis.
FIDE Foundation for International Dermatologic Education.
FIEPB Fédération Internationale d'Éducation Physique Bulletin.
FIF Feedback inhibition factor; Fibroblast interferon; Fluoride-induced fracture (Orthopedics) (= FI#); Forced inspiratory flow (formely MIF) (see PFT - FIF); Formaldehyde-induced fluorescence.
FiF Fetus-in-fetu (a rare malformation in twins).
FIFO First in, first out.
FIFR Fasting intestinal flow rate; Forced inspiratory flow rate (formerly MIFR) (see PFT - FIFR).
FIFRA Federal Insecticide, Fungicide and Rodenticide Act (of 1972) (= FEPCA).
Fig Figurative(ly); Figure.
FIGD Familial idiopathic gonadotropin deficiency.
FIGLU Formiminoglutamic acid.
FIGO International Federation of Gynecology and Obstetrics; Federation of International Gynecologists and Obstetricians.
FIH Familial isolated hypoparathyroidism; Fat-induced hyperglycemia.
FII Food Irradiation Information (journal).
FIL Fasting insulin level; Father-in-law.
Fil; fil Filament(ous); Filial.
fil- prefix meaning thread (L. filum).
Filt; filt Filter/trate/tration (L. filtra).
FIM Field ion microscopy; Functional independence measure.
FIMB French Institute of Molecular Biology (Paris).
FIMC Femoral intermedullary canal.
FIMLT Fellow of the Institute of Medical Laboratory Technology.
FIN Fibrosing interstitial nephritis; Fine intestinal needle.
FINCC Familial idiopathic non-arteriosclerotic cerebral calcification.
FIND Financial Information National Directory.
Finger Hashish/ Marijuana (see Cannabis).
F-in-L Father-in-law.
FInstSP Fellow of the Institute of Sewage Purification (= FISP).
F-insul; F-insulin Fibrous insulin (= Glucokinin; Plant insulin) (see Insulin - PI).
FIO Fibrogenesis imperfecta ossium.
FIO_2; FI_{O2} Fractitional concentration of oxygen in inspired air/gas (= F_1O_2).
FIP Feline infectious peritonitis.
FIPP Fair Information Practice Principles.
FIPV Feline infectious peritonitis virus.
FIQ Full-scale intelligence quotient.
FIR Far infrared (spectroscopy); Fetal immune response; Fold increase in resistance.
FIRDA Frontal, intermittent delta activity.
FIRL Franklin Institute Research Laboratories.
FIRMS Fourier ion resonance mass spectrometer.
FIRS First International Reference Standard (WHO).
FIS Familial idiopathic scoliosis; Family interaction scale; Fetal immune system; Fetal insulin secretagogue; Fictitious illness syndrome (= Munchausen's s.) (see MS); Forced inspiratory spirogram.
FISH Fluorescent in-situ hybridization (in genetic prenatal screening); Friends In Service Here (community volunteers).
FISL Federally-insured student loan(s).
FISP Fast imaging with steady (state) precision; Fellow of the Institute of Sewage Purification (see FInstSP).

fiss- combining form meaning split (L. fissus).
Fist; fist Fistula.
FIT Federal income tax; Fluorescein isothiocyanate (see FITC); Fourier integral transform; Fracture Intervention Trial (US and Multinational Studies); Fusion-inferred threshold (test for hearing); Latex agglutination.
FITC Fluorescein isothiocyanate (= FIT).
FIUG Fetal intrauterine growth (Obstetrics).
FIUO For internal use only.
FIV Feline immunodeficiency virus; Forced inspiratory volume.
FIV_1 Forced inspiratory volume in one second.
FIVC Forced inspiratory vital capacity (= FVIC).
F-J Fisher-John (melting point method).
FJN Familial juvenile nephrophthisis.
FJRM Full joint range of movement.
FJROM Full joint range of motion/ movement (= FJRM).
FJS Finger joint size.
FJW Flat juvenile wart.
FK Feline kidney.
FKA Formerly known as.
FKD Fatal/ Fibrotic kidney disease.
FL Fatty liver; Feline/ Friend leukemia; Fetal/ Focal length (= Fl); Fibers of Luschka; Fibrinogen level; Fibroblast-like; Filtered load; Filtration leukapheresis; Flammable liquid; Fluid (see FLD); Flutamide and leuprolide (acetate); Frontal lobe; Full liquid (diet); Functional length.
Fl Fetal/ Focal length (see FL); Flexible/xion/xor (see Flex); Florentium (also Ft) - chemical element now known as Promethium (Pm) (Z = 61) (see Elements - Promethium); Fluid (see fl); Fluorescence/ent (see fl).
fL foot Lambert (= fl).
fl femtoliter (= 10^{-15} liter; 10^{-15} l); filtered load; flexible/xion/xor (see Flex); flow; fluid (L. fluidium) (= Fl; FLD; fld), e.g. fl dram (see fl dr); fluoroscence/ent (= Fl); flutter; foot lambert (see fL).
FL-2 Feline lung (cells).
FLA Fatal lactic acidosis; First-line antibiotic; Fluorescent-labeled antibody; Fronto-laeva anterior (L.) - left frontoanterior (position of the fetus).
Fla; fla Do/ Let it be done, according to rule (L. fiat lege artis).
Fl-Abs Fluorescein-antibodies (labeled).
flac flaccid(ity).
FLAG Friends (Parents and) of Lesbians and Gays.
flagel- prefix meaning whip (L. flagellum).
Flake Cocaine (see Erythroxylum).
FLASH Fast low-angle shot.
flav yellow (L. flavus).
flav- combining form meaning yellow (L. flavus).
FLB Funny looking beat (electrocardiogram).
FLC Fatty/ Fetal liver cell; First-line chemotherapy; Friend leukemia cell; Funny looking child (pediatrics).
FLD Fatty liver disease; Fibrotic lung disease; Fluid (= FL); First-line data/ drug (see FLDT); Flutamide and leuprolide (acetate) depot; Frontal lobe defect/ disease/ disorder/ disturbance/ dysfunction.
FlD Full denture.
Fld; fld Fluid (see fl).
fld ext; fldxt fluid extract.
FLDP Fluorinated pyrimidine.
fl dr fluid drachm/ dram.
FLDT First-line drug therapy (in RA) - such as the NSAIDs.
-flect- combining form meaning bend or divert (L. flecto) (= -flex-).
fleur-de-lis flap Skin flap shaped like a fleur-de-lis (French) lily blossom, or "iris-shaped".
FLEX Federal Licensing Examination (Federation of State Medical Boards of the United States, for FMGs - foreign medical graduates).
Flex; flex Flexible/ Flexion/ Flexor (L. flexum = bend or turn aside) (= Fl; fl).
-flex- combining form meaning bend or divert (see -flect-).
FLF Fulminant liver failure.
FLGA Full-term, large for gestational age.
FLI Fibrotic lung injury; Flu-like illness.
FLK Funny looking kid (pediatrics).
FLKS Fatty liver and kidney syndrome.
FLL Focal liver lesion (see FHL).
FLM Fasciculus longitudinalis medialis; Fetal

lung maturity (see PTG).
FLO Fetoscopic laser occlusion (Obstetrics).
floc; flocc flocculation.
Flor Flowers (L. flores).
fl oz fluid ounce.
FLP Fetal lung prematurity (se PTG); First-line pharmacotherapy (= FLT); Fronto-laeva posterior (L.) - left frontoposterior position of the fetus.
FLR Funny looking rash.
FLS Fatty liver syndrome; Fellow of the Linnaean Society; Fetal lung surgery (Obstetrics); Fibrous long-spacing (collagen); First-line study; Flashing lights and/or scotoma; Flat lumbar spine; Flow-limiting segment; Flu-like syndrome; Foil-lined sachet; Frank lead system (electrocardiography); Free-Lock System (Zimmer) (for hip fixation).
FLSA Follicular lymphosarcoma.
FLSP Fluorescein-labeled serum protein.
FLT Alovudine (a new NARTI, anti-HIV drug, ten times more potent than AZT - Azidothymidine or Zidovudine); First-line therapy/ treatment (see FLP); Front-line therapy/ treatment; Fronto-laeva transversa (L.) - left frontotransverse position of the fetus.
FLU Flunitrazepam; Fluphenazine.
Flu; flu Influenza.
flu- combining form meaning flow (L. fluo).
FLU A Influenza A (virus).
fluor fluorescence/nt (see fluores); fluorometry; fluoroscope/py (see fluoro).
fluores fluoroscence/nt (= fluor).
fluoro fluoroscope/py (= fluor).
Fluoroquinolones A new group of quinolone antibiotics, which includes ciprofloxacin, enoxacin, norfloxacin, ofloxacin and perfloxacin (see Quinolones).
Fl up Flare-up; Follow up.
FLV Feline leukemia virus (see FeLV); Friend leukemia virus.
FLW Fasting laboratory work.
FLZ Flurazepam.
FM Face mask; Facial myokymia (see FMK); Facilities management; Family medicine; Feedback mechanism; Fetal/ Functional movement; Fibromuscular; Filtered mass; Flavin mononucleotide (see FMN); Flow meter; Foramen magnum; Forensic medicine; Formerly married; Foster mother; Frequency modulated/tion; Fusobacteria organism(s); Make a mixture (L. fiat mistura) (see ft mist); Nitrofurantoin (on culture and sensitivity reports); a Rorschach score.
Fm Fermium (Z = 100) (see Elements - Fermium); Maximal isometric force.
fm femtometer; femtomole; let a mixture be made/ make a mixture (L. fiat mistura) (see ft mist).
F-M Fetal minus material (pH differences).
f-M free metanephrine.
F&M Firm and midline (uterus).
FMA Florida Medical Association; Forward Mutation Assay (Mouse Lymphoma Cell) (see MLCFMA); Frankfort mandibular (plane) angle.
F-MA 11 Aluminium hydroxide - Magnesium carbonate co-dried gel. A co-precipitate of aluminium hydroxide (Al_2O_3) and magnesium carbonate (MgO), carefully dried to contain a critical proportion of water for high antacid activity.
FMAT Fetal movement acceleration test.
FMBS Fasting morning blood sugar.
FMC Family medicine center/ clerkship; Federal Maritime Commission; Federal Medical College (see USUHS); Fetal movement count; Flight medical clinic; Focal macular choroidopathy; Food Machinery Co.; Foundation for Medical Care (San Joaquin County Medical Society).
FMD Family medical doctor; Fibromuscular dysplasia; Flow-mediated (vaso)dilation (of the coronary arteries) (= FMV; FMVD); Flow-mediated dilatation (of bronchial artery) = (Vessel diameter after cuff deflation - resting vessel diameter) / (Resting vessel diameter) x 100%; Foot and mouth disease; Frontometaphyseal dysplasia.
FMDV Foot and mouth disease virus.
FME Full mouth extraction (operation/ oral surgery).
Fmed Median frequency.
FMEL Friend murine erythroleukemia.
FMEN Familial multiple endocrine neoplasia.
FMet; fMet; F-met Formyl-methionine.
FMF Familial Mediterranean Fever (=

Periodic disease {PD}; Periodic syndrome {PS}); Fetal Medicine Foundation (UK); Fetal movement felt; Flow microfluorometry; Forced midexpiratory flow.

FMG Fine mesh/ Five-mesh guaze; Foreign medical graduate.

FMGEMS Foreign Medical Graduate Examination in Medical Sciences.

FMH Family medical history; Fat-mobilizing hormone; Feto-maternal hemorrhage; Fibromuscular hyperplasia; Foederatio Medicorum Heleveticorum (Swiss Federation of Physicians).

FM/HA Frequency modulated/Hearing aid (microphone transmission system).

FmHA Farmers Home Administration.

FMI Ferromagnetic implant; Foods and Moods Inventory.

FMIS Financial Management Information System (NIAAA); Fungal metabolic immunosuppressant (e.g. Cyclosporin; Tacrolimus) (see ISA).

FMJ Freely movable joint (or synovial joint).

FMK Facial myokymia (= FM).

FML Flail mitral leaflet; Fluorometholone.

FMLP; f-MLP N-formyl-methionyl-leucyl-phenylalanine.

FMN First malignant neoplasm; Flavin mononucleotide (= FM); Frontomaxillonasal (suture).

FMND Familial motor neurone disease.

FMNH; $FMNH_2$ Reduced form of flavin mononucleotide.

FMO First/ Flight Medical Officer.

FMo Foramen interventriculare Monroi (thalamus).

fmol femtomole (= 10^{-15} mole).

FMP Fasting metabolic panel; Fetal malpresentation; First menstrual period; Fructose monophosphate.

FMPH French Ministry of Public Health.

2-FMPOCl Pralidoxime chloride (= 2-PAM chloride; 2-PAMCl; 2-Pyridine aldoxine chloride) (used as an adjunct to atropine in the treatment of poisoning of certain cholinesterase inhibitors, such as the quarternary ammonium or organophosphorus insecticides).

2-FMPOI Pralidoxime iodide (= PAM; P-2-AM; 2-PAMI; 2-PAM iodide; 2-Pyridine aldoxime iodide) (same uses as in pralidoxime chloride - see 2-FMPOCl).

2-FMPOMS Pralidoxime mesylate (= 2-PAMM; Pralidoxime methanesulfonate; Pralidoximi mesylas; P2S; 2-Pyridine aldoxime mesylate; RP 7676) (uses as in pralidoxime chloride, see 2-FMPOCl).

FMR Fetal movement record; Friend-Moloney-Rauscher (antigen/ virus).

fMRI Functional magnetic resonance imaging (technique).

FMRP Family medicine residency program (Israel).

FMS Fatal myelosuppression; Fat-mobilizing substance; Fellow of the Medical Society; Fibromyalgia syndrome; Fluorouracil, mitomycin, and streptozocin; Foramen magnum syndrome; Frankfurt-Marburg syndrome; Full-mouth series.

FMT Fetal maturity test; Floating mass transducer (part of the Vibrant Soundbridge, a new hearing device); Foundation for Medical Technology; Fuel-mediated teratogenesis (Obstetrics); Full maintenance therapy.

FMU Feto-maternal unit; First morning urine.

FMULC Free monoclonal urinary light chain(s).

F-MuLV Friend murine leukemia virus.

FMV Flow-mediated vasodilation (see FMD; FMVD); Fluorouracil, methyl-CCNU, and vincristine.

FMVD Flow-mediated vasodilation (see FMD).

FMX Full-mouth x-ray/ radiography (dentistry).

FN False negative (see Fneg); Fibronectin; Finger nail; Finger-to-nose (see F-N); Fluoride number.

F-N Finger-to-nose (test - neurological examination) (= FN).

FN# Femoral neck fracture (see FNF).

FNA Fine-needle aspiration.

FNAB Fine-needle aspiration biopsy.

FNAC Fine-needle aspiration cytology.

FNAH Familial non-autoimmune hyperthyroidism.

FNAL Fermi National Accelerator Laboratory.

FNB Food and Nutrition Board (NRC).

F.N. Belg Belgian National Formulary (Formulaire Nationale Belge).
FNC Family nurse clinician; Fatty nutritional cirrhosis.
FNCJ Fine-needle catheter jejunostomy.
FND Febrile neutrophilic dermatosis; Focal neurological deficit; Frontonasal dysplasia.
FNDS French National Dermatological Society.
f-NE free norepinephrine.
Fneg False negative (= FN).
FNF False-negative fraction; Femoral neck fracture; Finger-nose-finger.
FNH Familial nonhemolytic hyperbilirubinemia (Gilbert's syndrome - see UGT) (= GS); Focal nodular hyperplasia.
FNIF Florence Nightingale International Foundation.
f-NM free normetanephrine.
FNMA Federal National Mortgage Association.
FNNR Full power, Normal hi frequency, Normal low frequency, Reduce (Maximum-output hearing-aid setting).
FNP Facial nerve palsy (= Bell's palsy; Facial paralysis; VIIth. Cranial nerve palsy); Family Nurse Practitioner; Federal non-participating/ation.
FnP Fusion point.
FNPA Fluoro-nitrophenyl-azide.
FNR False negative rate/ result.
FNRC Federal Nuclear Regulatory Commission.
FNS Food and Nutrition Service (USDA); Frontier Nursing Service/ Station; Functional neurologic status; Functional neuromuscular stimulation.
FNSIM Federation of the National Societies of Internal Medicine (CIOMS).
FNT False neurochemical transmitter (adrenergic); Finger to nose test.
FNTT Fetal nuchal translucency thickness (Obstetrics).
f-number focal length (of a lens).
FO Fiberoptic(s); Fish oil; Foot orthosis; Foramen ovale (heart); Forced oscillation; Foreign object; Formula (see form); Fronto-occipital.
Fo; fo Foment(ation)/ing; Formula (see form).
F_0 Oligomycin-sensitivity-conferring factor (see OSCF).
$F_I O_2$ Inspired oxygen fraction (see FIO_2; FI_{O2}).
FOA Federation of Orthodontic Associations.
FOAD Fetal Origins of Adult Disease (Southampton Medical Centre, UK) (see FPT).
FOAM 5-Fluorouracil, Oncovin, Adriamycin, & Mitomycin-C (Chemotherapy).
FOAVF Failure of all vital forces.
FOB Father of baby; Fecal occult blood; Feet out/ Foot of bed; Fiber-optic bronchoscopy; Foldout bed; Free on board; Functional observational battery.
FOBL Fecal occult blood loss (= OFBL).
FOBT Fecal occult blood test.
FOC Father of child; Fiberoptic cable; Fluid of choice; Follicular/ Functional ovarian cyst; Fronto-occipital circumference.
FOCAL Formula calculation.
FOCMA Feline oncornavirus-associated cell membrane antigen.
FOCUS Family (Planning) Obstetrics Clinical Utilization System.
FOD Familial osteochondritis dissecans (Orthopedics); Fungal ocular disease.
FOD; FoD Free of disease.
FOE Federal Office of Education; Fiberoptic endoscope/py; Friends of the Earth.
FOEB Feet over edge of bed.
FoF Fight-or-flight (psychological reaction/ response); Fixation of femur.
FOG Fast oxidative glycolytic (fiber); Fluothane, oxygen, and gas (nitrous oxide); Full-on gain.
FOI Flight of ideas.
FOIA Freedom of Information Act (1966).
FOK First order kinetics.
FOL Fiber-optic light.
fol following; leaf (L. folium)/ leaves (L. folia).
FOLA Latin American Odontological Federation.
folie French - Psychosis: folie à deux, occurrence/ presence of psychosis simultaneously in two closely associated persons; folie circulaire, the circular form of manic-depressive psychosis; folie du doute, doubting mania,

pathological inability to make even the most trifling decisions; folie du pourquoi, constant psychopathological questioning; folie gemellaire, psychosis occurring simultaneously in twins; folie musculaire, with severe chorea; folie raisonnante, psychotic delusion.

FOM Faculty of Occupational Medicine (UK); Floor of mouth.

FOMi 5-fluorouracil, Oncovin (vincristine), and mitomycin C.

FOOB Fell out of bed.

FOOSH Fell onto (her/his) outstretched hand.

Football Diphetamine pill (see Amphet).

FOP Fetal organ perfusion (Obstetrics); Fibrodysplasia ossificans progressiva; Forensic pathology.

FOPR Full outpatient rate.

FOR Feco-oral route (of infection); Free oxygen radical.

FOR; For Forensic (pathology).

for foreign; formula (see form).

for- combining form meaning door or opening (L. foris).

for body foreign body (see FB).

Ford Ford Foundation.

Form Formulary.

form formation; formula (= FO; Fo; fo; for).

-form suffix meaning shape (L. forma).

Form FNP Formulaire de la Fédération Nationale Pharmaceutique (Paris 1965) (Fr.) (Formulary of the National Pharmaceutical Federation).

fort strong (L. fortis).

FORTRAN Formula translation (a computer programming language).

Forward Amphetamine pill (see Amphet).

FOS Fiberoptic scope/ sigmoidoscopy; Flip-off seal; Fractional osteoid surface; Fructooligosaccharide (a 'prebiotic' or non-digested sugar found in foods such as artichokes, asparagus, bananas, garlic, honey, onions and tomatoes).

fos-fa-tiddle phosphatidyl (glycerol) (test for fetal maturity, done on amniotic fluid).

FOT Fecal-oral transmission (of infection); Fiberoptic tube/ tubing (see FOS); Free on track.

Found Foundation.

Four Tylenol with codeine tablet (= acetaminophen with codeine). A proprietary drug, widely used in the US as an analgesic.

Fourneau Earnest François Auguste, French physician 1872-1949.

FOV Field of view.

FoV Field of vision.

FOVEA Field of view evaluation apparatus.

FOW Fenestration oval window (operation/ otology).

FP Factitious pyrexia; False positive; Family Physician/ Plans (journals); Family physician/ planning/ practice/ practitioner; Fanconi's pancytopenia; Federal Proceedings (FASEB journal); Feline Practice (journal); Femoropopliteal; Fibrinopeptide; Filling/ Filtration/ Fluid pressure; Filter paper; Flame photometer; Flash point; Flat plate (X-ray/ abdomen); Flavin phosphate (= riboflavin-5'-phosphate); Flavoprotein; Flexor pollicis/ profundus (= fp); Fluorescence polarization; Fluticasone propionate; Food for Peace (AID); Food poisoning; Foot-pound (see fp); Foot process (see Fp); Forearm pronated (see fp); Fowler procedure (for relief of boutonniere deformity, clawhand and mallet-finger); Freezing point (see Fp); Frontoparietal; Frozen plasma; Full period; Fusion point; Let a pill/ potion be made or Make a pill/ potion (see fp).

Fp Foot process (= FP); Freezing point (= FP; fp); Frontal (polar electrode) placement (in electroencephalography); Let a pill/ potion be made (see fp).

fp flexor pollicis/ profundus (see FP); foot-pound (= FP); forearm pronated (= FP); freezing point (see Fp); let a pill be made/ make a pill (L. fiat pilula) (= FP; Fp; F pil; f pil); let pills be made/ make pills (L. fiant pilulae) (= as in the singular); let a potion be made/ make a potion (L. fiat potio) (= FP; Fp).

F-P Femoral - popliteal (= FP).

F6P; F_6P; F-6-P Fructose 6-phosphate.

FPA Family Planning Association; Female-pattern alopecia (see FPAGA); Fibrinopeptide A; Filter paper activity; Fluorophenylalanine; Flying Physicians Association; Food protein allergy; Full psychiatric assessment.

FPAGA Female-pattern androgenetic alopecia

(= FAGA; FPA).

FPAL Full-term, premature, abortion, living.

FPAMN Family Planning Association Medical Newsletter (UK).

FPB Femoral popliteal bypass; Fibrinopeptide B; Flexor pollicis brevis.

FPBG Femoropopliteal bypass graft (= EXS graft).

FPC Familial polyposis coli; Family Planning Clinic; Family practice center/ consultant/ation; Family Practitioner Committee; Federal Power Commission; Fetal-pig cell (see FPCT); Fetal-placental circulation (Obstetrics); Fish protein concentrate.

FpCA 1-fluoromethyl-2-p-chlorophenyl-ethylamine.

FPCC Familial pheochromocytoma (see PCC).

FPCT Fetal pig cell therapy/ transplant (in Parkinson's disease).

FPD Familial Parkinson's disease (see parkin gene); Fetopelvic disproportion; Fetoplacental dysfunction; Fixed partial denture; Flame photometric detector.

FPE Fatal pulmonary embolism; First-pass effect; Full physical examination (= GPE).

FPEA Fast plasma estrogen assay.

FPF False-positive finding (see FPTR); Fibroblast pneumocyte factor; Flexion-plantarflexion (of the ankle).

FPG Fasting plasma glucose; Fluorescence plus Giemsa; Focal proliferative glomerulonephritis.

FPGC Fasting plasma glucose concentration (see BFS; FBG; FBS; FPG).

FPGS Folylpolyglutamate synthetase.

FPH Female pseudohermaphroditism; Flavin phosphate (reduced form) (see FPH2).

FPH2; FPH_2 Reduced form of flavin phosphate (= FPH).

FPHE Formaldehyde-treated pyruvaldehyde-stabilized human erythrocytes.

FPHx Family psychiatric history.

FPI Fasting plasma insulin; Femoral pulsatility index; Flossing performance index; Freiburger Personality Identification/ Inventory; Full Prescribing Information.

FPIA Fluoroscence-polarization immunoassay.

FPIAN Family Planning International Assistance Newsletter.

f pil Let a pill/pills be made (see fp).

f pil (xi) Make 11 pills (L. fac pilulas xi).

FPIQ Freiburger Personality Identification Questionnaire.

FPK Fructose phosphokinase.

FPL Fasting plasma lipids; Finned pacemaker lead; Flexor pollicis longus; Forced-choice preferential looking (acuity); Forest Products Laboratory (US Forest Service).

FPLA Fair Packaging and Labeling Act.

FPLP Fasting plasma lipoprotein.

FPM False positive mammogram; Feet per minute (see fpm); Fellowship of Postgraduate Medicine; Filter paper microscopic (test); First-pass metabolism; Full passive movements; Functional pacemaker.

fpm feet per minute (unit) (= FPM).

FPMA Family Practice of Medicine Act.

FPN Family Practice News (journal); Ferric chloride, perchloric acid, and nitric acid (reagent solution used to test for phenothiazines).

FPNA First-pass nuclear angiocardiography.

FPO Family planning organization; Federation of Prosthodontic Organizations; Freezing point osmometer.

FPP Familial periodic paralysis; Family Planning Perspectives (PPFA journal); Female perineal pain; Family-practice physician; Fitness to Practise Procedures (GMC); Free portal pressure.

FPPC Fitness to Practise Policy Committee (GMC, UK).

FPPH Familial primary pulmonary hypertension.

FPPR Family Planning/ Population Reporter (PPFA journal).

FPQ Family Planning Quarterly.

FPR False-positive rate; False-positive reaction/ reading/ result (see FPTR); Finger peripheral resistance; Flexor plantar response; Fluorescence photobleaching recovery; Fractional proximal resorption.

FPRA First pass radionuclide angiogram.

FPRG Fitness to Practise Review Group (GMC, UK).

FPRP Family practice residency program.
FPS Febrile pneumonitis syndrome; Fellow of the Pathological/ Pharmaceutical Society; Fetal PCB (polychlorinated biphenyl) syndrome; Final placement syndrome; Flexion, pronation and supination (at/ of the elbow); Footpad swelling; Frankly purulent sputum.
fps feet per second; foot-pound-second (system of units - English); frames per second (motion picture).
FPT fabere-Patrick (orthopedic) test (fabere = flexion/ abduction/ external rotation/ extension); Fetal-programming theory (associated with diseases later on in life) (see FOAD).
FPTR False-positive test result (= FP; FPF; FPR).
FPU Fetoplacental unit (Obstetrics).
FPV Fowl plague virus.
FPVB Femoral popliteal vein bypass.
FPZ Fluphenazine.
FPZ-D Fluphenazine decanoate.
FQHC Federally Qualified Health Center (US).
FR Faculty of Radiologists (UK); Failure rate (with reference to conception); Fasciculus retroflexus; Father; Father (priest); Febrile reaction; Federal Register; Feedback regulation; Fibrin(ogen)-related (antigen) (see FFR); Filtration/ Flow rate; Fischer-Race (notation); Fixed ratio; Flexor retinaculum; Flocculation reaction, e.g. Hanger's test: Cephalin-cholesterol flocculation test (CCFT); Fluid restriction/ retention; Fluoridation Reporter (ADA journal); Food Research (journal); Free radical; French (catheter guage) (see Fr); Frequency of respiration; Frequent relapses; Furious rabies (R with hydrophobia) (see PR - Paralytic rabies).
Fr Fraction; Fracture (see fract); Francium (Z = 87) (see Elements - Francium); Franklin (unit charge); Friends i.e. Society of Friends (Quakers); French (catheter guage/ size) (= F; FR).
fr from.
F&R Force and rhythm (of pulse) (= F and R).
Fr1 First fraction.
FRA Fibrinogen-related antigen; Fluorescent rabies antibody.
fra fragile (site) (see frag).
FRAC Food Research and Action Center.
frac fracture (see fract).
FRACON Framycetin sulfate, Colistine sulfate and Nystatin (a combination of oral non-absorbable antibiotics) (see GVN).
FRACP Fellow of the Royal Australian College of Physicians.
FRACS Fellow of the Royal Australasian College of Surgeons.
fract fraction; fracture (= Fr; frac; Fx) (see Symbols - 5).
fract- combining form meaning break (L. fractus).
Fract BB Fracture of both bones (= #BB; Fr BB; Fx BB) (see Symbols - 5).
fract dos in divided doses (L. fracta dosi).
FRACTS Fractitional urines.
frag fragile (as of RBC, site, etc.) (= fra).
FRAI Fellow of the Royal Anthropological Institute.
FRAME Fund for the Replacement of Animals in Medical Experiments.
FR antigen Fibrinogen-fibrin-related antigen (see FR; FFR).
FRAP Fluorescence recovery after photobleaching.
FRAT Free radical assay technique (test for heroin by-products such as morphine).
FRAX Fragile X (chromosome) (see fra{X}).
fra(X) fragile X chromosome (= FRAX); fragile X syndrome.
FRAX-MR Fragile X-mental retardation (syndrome).
Fr BB Fracture of both bones (see Fract BB).
FRC Federation Radiation Council; Forced reserve/ residual/ resting capacity i.e. the amount of gas remaining in the lungs at the resting experimental level, or the volume of gas in the lungs at the end of quiet respiration (see PFT - FRC); Forearm resistance circulation; Fracture-related complication; Frozen red cells; Functional reserve/ residual/ resting capacity (of the lungs) (= Forced R. capacity - above) (see PFT - FRC).
FRCA Fellow of the Royal College of Anaesthesiologists (UK).
FRCAP Fellow of the Royal College of Australian Physicians (see FRACP).

FRACS Fellow of the Royal College of Australian Surgeons (see FRACS).

FRCD Fellow of the Royal College of Dentists; Fixed ratio combination drug.

FRCGP Fellow of the Royal College of General Practitioners.

FRCOG Fellow of the Royal College of Obstetricians and Gynaecologists (UK).

FRCP Fellow of the Royal College of Physicians (UK).

FRCPA Fellow of the Royal College of Pathologists of Australia.

FRCPath Fellow of the Royal College of Pathologists (UK).

FRCP(C) Fellow of the Royal College of Physicians of Canada.

FRCPE Fellow of the Royal College of Physicians of Edinburgh.

FRCP(Glasg) Fellow of the Royal College of Physicians and Surgeons of Glasgow qua Physician (= Fellow of the Royal College of Physicians of Glasgow).

FRCPI Fellow of the Royal College of Physicians of/in Ireland.

FRCPsych Fellow of the Royal College of Psychiatrists (UK).

FRCS Fellow of the Royal College of Surgeons (UK) (= FRCSEng).

FRCS(C) Fellow of the Royal College of Surgeons of Canada.

FRCSE; FRCSEd Fellow of the Royal College of Surgeons of Edinburgh.

FRCSEng Fellow of the Royal College of Surgeons of England (see FRCS).

FRCS(Glasg) Fellow of the Royal College of Physicians and Surgeons of Glasgow qua Surgeon (= Fellow of the Royal College of Surgeons of Glasgow).

FRCSI Fellow of the Royal College of Surgeons of/in Ireland.

FRCT Factor-Referenced Cognitive Tests (ETS).

FRCVS Fellow of the Royal College of Veterinary Surgeons (UK).

FRD Fatal respiratory depression; Female reproductive disorder; Fever-reducing drug; Fiber-rich diet.

FRE Fast renal elimination (see RRE); Fatigue-related error; Fischer rat embryo; Flow-related enhancement.

FREIR Federal Research on (Biological and Health) Effects of Ionizing Radiation.

frem (vocal) fremitus (L. fremitus vocalis).

freq frequency/nt.

FRES Fellow of the Royal Entomological Society (UK).

F response Retrograde activation of motor neurones.

FRF Female reproductive function; Fertility Research Foundation; Fiber-rich food; Filtration replacement fluid; Follicle(-stimulating hormone-)releasing factor (see Hormones - FSH-RH).

FRFC Functional renal failure of cirrhosis.

FRFPSG Fellow of the Royal Faculty of Physicians and Surgeons of Glasgow.

Frg Frog.

FRH Follicle (-stimulating hormone-)releasing hormone (see Hormones - FSH-RH).

FRh Fetal rhesus (monkey kidney cell).

FRHS Fast-repeating high sequence.

FRI Framingham Risk Index (for CHD).

FRIC Fellow of the Royal Institute of Chemistry (UK).

frict friction (rub).

Fried Friedman (test for pregnancy).

Frig Frigidity; Refrigerator.

frig cold (L. frigidus).

FRIPHH Fellow of the Royal Institute of Public Health and Hygiene (UK).

FRISC Fragmin during Instability in Coronary Artery Disease (Sclerosis of the Coronary vessels - study group).

Frisco speedball Mixture of heroin, cocaine, and LSD-25 (see Diamorph HCl; Erythroxylum; LSD).

FRJM Full range joint movement.

FRLM Fixed reference lung model.

FRM Federal reference method (or principle/ chemical analysis); Fever-reducing medication.

FRMedSoc Fellow of the Royal Medical Society (UK).

FRMP Florida Regional Medical Program.

FRMS Fellow of the Royal Microscopical Society (UK).

FRO Free radical oxidant/ oxidizer.

FROM Full range of motion/ movement(s).

front- combining form meaning forehead or front (L. frontis).

FRP Faculty Research Participation (program - NSF); Fetal renal perfusion; Fiberglass-reinforced plastic(s); Functional refractory period.

Fr. P. French Pharmacopeia (Pharmacopée Française).

FRPP Flexi-rod penile prosthesis (semi-rigid).

FRPV Full-Range Picture Vocabulary (test).

FRS Fellow of the Royal Society; Female reproductive system; Ferredoxin-reducing substance; First-rank symptom(s); Furosemide.

FRSA Fellow of the Royal Society of Arts.

FRSC Fellow of the Royal Society of Canada.

FRSE; FRSEd Fellow of the Royal Society of Edinburgh.

FRSH Fellow of the Royal Society of Health (UK).

FRSPSG Fellow of the Royal Society of Physicians and Surgeons of Glasgow.

FRT Family Relations Test; Fantasy relaxation technique; Full recovery time.

Fru Fructose.

frust in little bits/ in small pieces (L. frustillatim).

FRW Fatigue-related weakness.

Frx Fracture (see Symbols - #).

FS Factor of safety; Family stability; Famous Sayings (psychology test); Fanconi/ Felty/ Fibromyalgia/ Fisher syndrome; Fast-scan; Fertility and Sterility (journal); Field stimulation; Fight for Sight, Inc; Fingerstick; Flammable solid; Flexible sigmoidoscope/py; Fluorescence; Flu syndrome (arthralgia, asthenia, chills, fever, headache, muscle ache and nausea); Focalizing sign(s) (neurology); Food service; Forearm supinated/tion; Forensic Science (Switzerland); Foreskin (human - cells); Forest Service (USDA); Fourier synthesizer; Fracture/ Fragile site; Friesinger score; Frisco speedball (mixture of heroin, cocaine and LSD-25) (see Diamorph; Erythroxylum; LSD); Frozen section; Fructosamine assay (measuring glycosylated serum proteins); Full scale (IQ); Full and soft (diet); Full strength; Function study; Simple fracture.

F/S Female, spayed (animal).

F&S Full and soft (diet) (= FS).

FSA Family Service Association; Federal Security Administration; Fellow of the Society of Actuaries; Fetal sulfoglycoprotein antigen; Food Safety Administration; Make skillfully (see fsa).

fsa let it be done/ made skillfully/ make skillfully (L. fiat secundum artem) (= FSA).

FSAA Family Service Association of America.

FSALO Fletcher suite after loading ovoids.

FSALT Fletcher suite after loading tandem.

fsar do it/ let it be made according to the rules of the art (L. fiat secundum artem regulas).

FSB Fetal scalp blood; Fetal skin biopsy.

FSBM Full strength breast milk.

FSBP Finger systolic blood pressure.

FSBT Fowler single breath test.

FSC Federal Safety Council; Fetal stem cell; Food Standards Committee (of the Ministry of Agriculture, Fisheries, and Food) (UK); Fracture, simple, and complete.

FSCD Flat-spring contraceptive diaphragm (see ASCD; Contraceptives).

FSD Fatal systemic disease/ disorder; Female sexual dysfunction (Four classes: a. Lack of desire; b. Insufficient arousal with vaginal dryness and lubrication/ sensation problems; c. Inability to reach orgasm; and d. Sexual pain, including involuntary contraction of the vaginal muscles & severe genital discomfort); Fetal sex differentiation; Fetal skeletal development; Fetal structural defect (Obstetrics); Flea- spread disease (such as plague); Focal/ Focus skin distance (x-rays); Fractional standard deviation; Fracture, simple, and depressed.

FSE Fast spin echo (see MRT); Fetal scalp electrode; Filtered smoke exposure; Flexible skin electrode (bipotential).

FSEB Federation of Societies for Experimental Biology.

FSF Fibrin stabilizing factor (see Factor XIII).

FSF* Fibrin-stabilizing factor (Factor XIII activated form) (see Factor XIII).

FSG Family/ Free support group; Fasting serum glucose; Focal segmental glomerulosclerosis (see FSGS); Forensic Science

Gazette (SWIFS).

FSGA Fetus/ Full-term - small for gestational age.

FSGHS Focal segmental glomerular hyalinosis and sclerosis.

FSGN Focal sclerosing glomerulonephritis.

FSGS Focal segmental glomerulosclerosis.

FSH Fascioscapulohumeral; Female sex hormone(s) (see Hormones - FSH i); Focal and segmental hyalinosis; Follicle-stimulating hormone (see Hormones - FSH ii).

FSHB Follicle-stimulating hormone, beta chain.

FSHD Fascioscapulohumeral dystrophy.

FSH/LR-RH Follicle-stimulating hormone and luteinizing hormone releasing hormone.

FSHMD Facioscapulohumeral muscular dystrophy (= FSHD).

FSHRF; FSH-RF Follicle-stimulating hormone-releasing factor (= FSH releasing factor) (see Hormones - FSHRF; FSH-RF).

FSH-RH Follicle-stimulating hormone-releasing hormone (= FSH releasing hormone) (see Hormones - FSH-RH).

FSHS Facioscapulohumeral syndrome.

FSI Female stress incontinence (urinary); Foam stability index; Food Sanitary Institute; Function status index; Fungal skin infection.

FSID Fellow of the Society for Investigative Dermatology; Foundation for the Study of Infant Death.

FSIQ Full-scale intelligence quotient.

FSIS Food Safety and Inspection Service (USDA).

FSL Fasting serum level; Flying spot laser (a narrow beam 2 mm wide contacting the eye at lightening speed; used in RES or Refractive eye surgery).

FSLA Federal Student Loan Authority.

FSM Female sexual medicine (see FSD); Flying spot microscope; Frameshift mutation (of genes) (i.e. Mutagenesis).

FSMB Federation of State Medical Boards (of the United States).

F-SM/C Fungus, smear, and culture.

FSO Fetal skeletal ossification.

FSP Familial spastic paraplegia; Fellowship and Stipends for the Professions (NEP); Female sex(ual) partner problem (see FSD); Femoral stem prosthesis (see OI/OP); Fibrin(ogen)/(olytic)-split products; Fine suspended particles; Flat smallpox (a form of Variola minor, where the skin remains smooth and does not pustulate); Full sexual potential.

F-SP Special form (L. forma specialis).

FSQ Functional Status Questionnaire.

FS&Q Functions, standards and qualifications.

FSR (Cortisol/ Compound F) secretion rate; Feedback shift register; Fellow of the Society of Radiographers; Female sexual response (see SAL); Fetal selective reduction (Obstetrics); Film screen radiography; Fragmented sarcoplasmic reticulum; Fusiform skin revision.

FSR-3 Isoniazid.

FSRP First-stage reconstructive procedure (bone surgery); French Society for Radiation Protection.

FSS Fear Survey Scale (test); Focal segmental sclerosis; Forensic Science Service (UK)/ Society (UK); Freeman-Sheldon syndrome; French steel sound; Frozen semen storage; Frozen shoulder syndrome; Full scale score; Functional somatic syndrome (see PSS).

FSSJ Forensic Science Society Journal (UK).

FST Foam stability test.

FSTPP Foreign Service Team Preceptorship Program.

FSU Family service unit; Florida State University; Functional spine unit.

FSV Fat-soluble vitamins (A,D,E,K); Feline sarcoma virus (see FeSV).

FSVC First-second vital capacity (see PFT - FSVC).

FSW Field service/ social worker.

FT Fallot's tetralogy; False transmitter; Family therapy; Family Therapy (FTIM journal); Farr test (DNA antibody test); Fast twitch; Fibrinolytic therapy - This includes Acylated plasminogen streptokinase activator complex (APSAC), Recombinant tissue plasminogen activator (rt-PA), Streptokinase, Urokinase and single chain urokinase-type plasminogen activator (scu-PA); Fibrous tissue; Filling time; Filum terminale (terminal tubular sheath of the spinal cord, formed from the arachnoid and dura mater) (see CE);

Finger temperature/ tip; Fog test (Used in cerebral palsy: greater associated movement of the affected upper limb, when walking on the lateral borders of both feet); Follow through (after Ba meal - X-ray/ intestines); Foot (see ft); Formol toxoid; Foundation of Thanatology; Fourier transform (spectroscopy); Free testosterone (see fT)/ thyroxine (see FT_4); Full term (obstetrics); Function test.

Ft Ferritin; Florentium (see Fl; Elements - Promethium); Make (see ft).

fT Free testosterone (= FT).

ft foot/ feet; let it/ them/ there be made/ make (L. fac; fiat; fiant) (= Ft).

ft^3 cubic foot (see cu ft).

FT_3 Free triiodothyronine.

F_3T Trifluorothymidine (= F3TDR).

FT_4, fT_4 Free thyroxine (= FT) (see Hormones - fT_4).

FT 81 Bendrofluazide (= Bendroflumethiazide; Benzydroflumethiazide). A thiazide diuretic similar to chlorothiazide, but with a more prolonged diuresis, which continues for about 18 hours.

FTA First-trimester abortion; Fluorescent titer antibody; Fluorescent treponemal antibody (Lues test) (see STS-FTA).

FTA-ABS; FTA-Abs Fluorescent treponemal antibody-absorbed/ absorption (test) - a reagin serological test for lues or syphilis (= TPFA) (see STS - FTA-ABS).

FTAG; F-TAG Fast-binding target-attaching globulin.

FTAT Fluorescent treponemal antibody test.

FTB Finger-tip blood.

FTBD Fit to be detained; Full-term born dead.

FTBE Focal tick-borne encephalitis.

FTBS Family Therapist Behavioral Scale.

FTC Federal Trade Commission; Focal triangular cataract; Frequency threshold curve.

ftc; ft-c foot candle (= fc).

ft cataplasm let a poultice be made/ make a poultice (L. fiat cataplasma).

ft cerat let a cerate be made/ make a cerate (L. cera = wax) (L. fiat ceratum).

ft chart let a powder be made/ make a powder (L. fiat charta).

ft chart ix let nine powders be made/ make nine powders (L. fiant chartulae ix).

ft collyr let an eyewash be made/ make an eyewash (L. fiat collyrium).

FTD Femoral total density; Fibrotic/ Fibrous tissue degeneration; Frontotemporal dementia; Full term delivery; Full-thickness defect(s) (e.g. as in articular cartilage) (Orthopedics).

F_3TDR Trifluorothymidine (see F_3T).

FTE Fetotoxic effect (Obstetrics); Full-time equivalent (scientist).

ft emuls let an emulsion be made/ make an emulsion (L. fiat emulsio).

ft enem let an enema be made/ make an enema (L. fiat enema).

FTF Finger to finger.

FTFTN Finger-to-finger-to-nose.

FTG Fetal-tissue graft; First trimester of gestation; Full-thickness graft (operation/ plastic surgery).

ft garg let a gargle be made/ make a gargle (L. fiat gargarisma).

FTH Familiar tension headache; Ferritin heavy chain.

ft haust let a draft/ draught be made/ make a draft/ draught (L. fiat haustus).

FTI Farnesyltransferase inhibitor (an anti-cancer drug); Finger-tip injury; Free thyroxine index (= FT_4x; fT_4x); Full-term infant.

FT_3I Free triiodothyronine index.

FTIM Family Therapy Institute of Marin.

ft infus let an infusion be made/ make an infusion (L. fiat infusum).

ft injec let an injection be made/ make an injection (L. fiat injectio).

FTIR Fourier transform infrared (spectroscopy) (see FTMS); Functional terminal innervation ratio.

FTJ Fibulotalar joint.

FTKA Failed to keep appointment.

FTL Ferritin light chain.

ftL; ft-L foot Lambert.

FTLB Full-term live birth.

ft lb; ft-lb foot pound.

FTLFC Full-term living female child.

ft linim let a liniment be made/ make a liniment (L. fiat linimentum).

FTLMC Full-term living male child.

FTLV Feline T-lymphotropic lentivirus.
FTM Fluid thioglycolate medium; Fractional test meal.
FtM Female-to-male (transmission of disease, esp. STD, as in AIDS).
ft mas let a mass be made/ make a mass (L. fiat massa).
ft mas div in pil let a mass be made and divided into pills/ make a mass and divide into pills (L. fiat massa dividenda in pilulae).
ft mas div in pil xv let 15 pills be made/ make a mass and divide into 15 pills (L. fiat massa et divide in pilulae xv) (see ft pil xv).
ft mist let a mixture be made/ make a mixture (L. fiat mistura) (= FM; fm).
FTMS Fourier transform mass spectroscopy (infrared) (= FTIR; FTS).
FTN Finger to nose; Full term nursery.
FTNB Full-term newborn.
FTND Full-term normal delivery.
FTNSD Full-term, normal, spontaneous delivery.
FTO Fructose-terminated oligosaccharide.
FTP Failure to progress; First trimester of pregnancy; Fitness to Practise (see FTPAP); Full-term placenta.
FTPAP Fitness to Practise Adjudication Panel (GMC, UK).
ft pil let a pill be made/ make a pill (L. fiat pilula).
ft pil xv let 15 pills be made/ make 15 pills (L. fiat pilulae xv).
ft pulv let a powder be made/ make a powder (L. fiat pulvis).
FTR Fetal tissue research/ response; For the record; Fractional tubular reabsorption; Fractional turn-over rate.
FTS Family tracking system; Feminizing testes/ testis syndrome; Fetal tissue sampling; Fetal tobacco syndrome; First-trimester screening (CVS; USE; Amnio, etc.); Fissured tongue syndrome; Flexor tendon sheath; Flexor-tenosynovitis; Forced titration study; Fourier transform spectroscopy (see FTMS); Full toxoid series (tetanus) (see TTS); Thymulin (Fr. facteur thymique sérique).
FTSG Full-thickness skin graft.
ft solut let a solution be made/ make a solution (L. fiat solutio).
ft suppos let a suppository be made/ make a suppository (L. fiat suppositorium).
FTT Failure to thrive; Fat tolerance test; Fetal thyroid status.
FTU Fluorescence thiourea; Formazin turbidity unit.
ft ung let an ointment be made/ make an ointment (L. fiat unguentum).
FTW Full-thickness wound.
FT_4x; fT_4x Free thyroxine index (see FTI).
FU Fecal urobilinogen (see LFT iv); Finsen unit (UV) unit of ultraviolet light (see Fu); Fluorouracil (an antimetabolite drug used in the treatment of carcinoma; also locally, in the treatment of warts) (= 5-FU; see also NSC 19893); Follow-up (see f/u); Fractional urinalysis (see KFT - FU); Fundus; Fundus at umbilicus (see F/U).
Fu Finsen unit (for ultraviolet rays) (= FU).
F/U Follow-up (see f/u); Fundus of umbilicus.
f/u follow-up (= FU; F/U).
F↑U Fingers above umbilicus.
F↓U Fingers below umbilicus.
F&U Flanks and upper quadrants.
5-FU 5-Fluorouracil (see FU; NSC 19893) (cancer chemotherapy).
FUB Functional uterine bleeding.
FUC Follow-up care.
Fuc Fucose.
FUCG Fetal ultrasonic cardiography.
FUCL Fetal umbilical cord ligation (Obstetrics).
FuD Full denture.
FUDR; FUdR Fluorodeoxyuridine (= 2-Deoxy-5-fluorouridine; Floxuridine; 5-Fluoro-2'-deoxyuridine; Fluorodesoxyuridine; 5-Fluorouracil deoxyriboside; 5-FUDR) (an antimetabolite drug used in the treatment of carcinoma).
5-FUDR see FUDR.
FUDR-MP Floxuridine monophosphate (see FUDR).
FUE Fever of uncertain/ undetermined/ unknown etiology (see PUO); Follow-up evaluation/ examination.
-fug suffix meaning avoid or flee (L. fugio).
FUH_2 5-Fluoro-5,6-dihydro-fluorouracil.
Funisitis. Infection of the umbilical cord (see Amnionitis; Chorioamnionitis; Villitis).

FUM 5-Fluorouracil and methotrexate; Fumarate (see Fum); Fumigate/tion.
Fum Fumarate (= FUM).
FUMP Fluorouridine monophosphate.
FUN Follow-up note.
funct function(al) (see FXN).
funct- combining form meaning function or serve (L. functus).
fund- combining form meaning pour (L. fundo) (see fus-).
FUNG-C Fungus culture.
FUNG-S Fungus smear.
FUO Fever of uncertain/ undetermined/ unknown origin (see PUO).
FUOV Follow-up office visit.
FUP Follow-up period.
FuP Fusion point.
FUPA 5-Fluoro-ureido-propionic acid.
FUR Fluorouracil riboside; Fluorouridine.
5-FURD 5-Floxuridine (see 5-FUDR).
FUS Feline urologic syndrome; First-use syndrome; Follow-up scan/ study/ survey; Fusion.
fus- combining form meaning pour (L. fusus) (see fund-).
FUT Fibrinogen uptake test (fibrinogen-labeled and radioactive iodine); Follow-up test(s).
FUTP 5-Fluorouridine triphosphate (a metabolite of 5-FU).
FUV Follow-up visit.
FV Fatiguing vigil; Femoral vein; Field of vision; Fluid volume; Friend virus.
FVA Friend virus anemia; Functional valve area (of heart valves on Doppler ultrasonography).
FV-1^b Gene that inhibits helper virus, indigenous to Friend leukemia virus.
FVC False vocal cord; Forced ventilatory/ vital capacity (= ventilatory/ vital capacity during forced expiration) (see PFT - FVC).
FVC_1 Mean forced vital capacity (expiratory volume) (see PFT - FVC_1).
FVE Forced volume expiration/ Forced volume, expiratory (see PFT - FVE; PFT - FEV).
FVFA Free volatile fatty acid.
FVFR Filled voiding flow rate.
FVH Focal vascular headache.
FVIC Forced inspiratory vital capacity (see FIVC).
FVL Femoral vein ligation; Flow volume loop; Force, velocity, length.
FVO Fungal vertebral osteomyelitis (see COM; CVO).
FVOP Finger venous opening pressure.
FVP Friend virus polycythemia; Functional ventricular pacemaker (see FAVP).
FVR Feline viral rhinotracheitis; Forearm vascular resistance.
FVS Fetal valproate syndrome.
fvs bleed the patient/ let the patient be bled (L. fiat venaesectio).
FVT Fibrovascular tissue.
FVV Functional venous volume (see VV).
FW Felix-Weil (reaction) (see FWR); Folin-Wu (method/ reaction) (see FWR); Formula weight; Forced whisper; Fragment wound; Fresh water (see fw).
Fw F wave.
fw fresh water (= FW).
FWA Family Welfare Association.
F waves Fibrillatory/ Flutter waves.
FWB Fetal well-being (dynamic assessment) (Obstetrics); Full weight bearing.
FWH Frank W. Horner Ltd (Canada) code for experimental substances.
FWH 114 Isobuzole (= Glybusol) (a sulfonylurea; an orally active hypoglycemic agent with similar actions and uses to chlorpropamide).
FWH 429 Troxonium tosylate (a hypotensive agent).
FWHM Full width at half maximum (resonance peak).
FWI Families and Work Institute.
FWPCA Federal Water Pollution Control Act (of 1972)/ Administration/ Agency.
FWR Felix-Weil reaction (laboratory/ serology) (= FW); Folin-Wu reaction (or method) (see FW).
FWS Fish and Wildlife Service (US Dept of Interior).
FWW Front wheel walker.
FX Factor X; Fluoroscopy; Fornix (see Fx); Fracture (see Fx); Frozen section (see Fx).
Fx; fx Fornix (= FX); Fractional urine; Fracture (= FX; see Fract; Symbols - 5 #);

Friction.

FxBB Fracture of both bones (see Fract BB; Symbols - 5 #BB).

Fx-dis Fracture-dislocation.

FXMR Fragile-X mental retardation.

FXN Function (= Funct).

FXR Fracture (see Fx).

FXS Fragile X syndrome.

FY Fiscal/ Full year.

F-Y Fibrinogen (qualitative test).

FyFy Duffy blood group negative human erythrocyte.

FYI For your information.

FZ Focal zone; Furazolidone.

Fz Frontal midline placement of electrodes in electroencephalography.

FZP Fresnel zone plate.

FZS Fellow of the Zoological Society.

G

G Acceleration (force); Conductance; Free energy; Gallop; Ganglion; Ganga - Marijuana (see Cannabis); Gap (in cell cycle); Gas; Gastrin; Gauge; Gauss (in magnetism); Gaussian function; Generation, e.g. Gcr. (of creatinine); Geometric efficiency; German (see Ger); Giga - 10^9, e.g. Gg = Gigagram, Megakilogram, Mkg, or 10^9 gram; Gingiva(l) - pertaining to the gums; Girl; Glabella; Globular (with reference to proteins); Globulin; Glucose; Glycine; Glycinine (an albuminoid globulin which constitutes 90-95% of the protein content of the soya bean); Glycogen; Goat (veterinary medicine); Gold inlay (dentistry); Gonidial - with reference to colonies of bacteria (Gr. gone = seed); Gonorrhea (a contagious inflammation of the genital membrane, transmitted during coitus, and due to Neisseria gonorrheae) (= GO; Gon); Good; Goose; Grade; Grafenberg (ring/ spot); Gram (Symbol: G; g; Gm; gm)/ Fr. gramme (see Gm) - the basic unit of a mass (weight) of the metric system; Grand ($1,000); Grass - Marijuana (see Cannabis); Gravida; Gravitation(al) constant (Newtonian constant); Gravity (Symbol: G; g; gr; grav) - Newtonian symbol of gravitation (see G - Symbol); Greek (see Gr); Green (an indicator color); Guanidine; Guanine; Guanosine; Guaza - Marijuana (see Cannabis); Gynecology; an Immunoglobulin (see Ig); a Rorschach score; Symbol 1) of the Newtonian constant of gravitation: G, and 2) for the Unit of Force exerted upon the human body during acceleration, i.e. in Aviation Medicine: G (= g; gr; grav); Unit of force of acceleration.

g acceleration (due to gravity)/ force (pull of gravity); gap; gauge (needle); gender; grain; gram (see Gm); gravity; group; ratio of the magnetic moment of a particle to the Bohr magneton; relative centrifugal force; standard acceleration due to gravity (9.80665 m/s^2).

γ i. gamma - the third letter in the Greek alphabet. ii. a carbon atom separated from the carboxyl group by two other carbon atoms. iii. a constituent of the gamma protein plasma fraction. iv. immunoglobulin/ immunogammaglobulin (heavy chain). v. a monomer in fetal hemoglobin. vi. microgram (= 10^{-6} Gm; 10^{-3} mg; mcg; μg) (see Symbols 5). vii. numerical expression of the degree of development of a photographic negative. viii. photon (a quantum of light energy, analogous to the electron). ix. unit of intensity of the magnetic field (γ = 0.00001 gauss).

G* Standard free energy.

G+ Gram-positive (see GM+).

G- Gram-negative (see GM-).

G 1-4 Grade 1-4.

G1 Primigravida (number of previous pregnancies).

G2 Secundigravida (number of previous pregnancies).

G3 Tertigravida (number of previous pregnancies).

G_0 Quiescent phase of cells leaving the mitotic cycle.

G_1 Presynthetic gap (phase of cells prior to DNA synthesis).

G_2 Postsynthetic gap (phase of cells following DNA synthesis).

G4 Dichlorophen (= Dihydroxy-dichlorodiphenyl urethane; Di-phenthane-70; Gelocast dichlorophene). A tenicide (taeniacide; taenicide; teniacide).

G 11 Hexachlorophene (= Hexachlorophane; K 34). A bactericide; used as an antiseptic in soaps and creams; also as a deodorant.

G 115 Ginseng standard extract.

G 5668 Prethecamide. A respiratory stimulant.

G 23350 Nicoumalone (= Acenocoumarin; Acenocoumarol). An anticoagulant.

G 24480 Diazinon (= Dimpylate). An organophosphorus insecticide.

G 25766 Clorindione (= Chlorophenindione). A synthetic anticoagulant.

G 27202 Oxyphenbutazone (= Hydroxyphenyl-butazone). An anti-inflammatory, anti-rheumatic, pyrazolone compound, derived from phenylbutazone.

G 28315 Sulfinpyrazone (= Sulphinpyrazone; Sulphoxyphenylpyrazolidine). An analogue of phenylbutazone, with a greater uricosuric action, but much weaker anti-rheumatic effect. Used in the long-term treatment of chronic gout.

G 30320 An isopropylimino-phenazine compound (see B 663).

G 32883 Carbamazepine (= Carbamoyl dibenzapine; CBZ; CBz; $C_{15}H_{12}N_2O$). Used as an anticonvulsant in the treatment of grand mal epilepsy.

G 33040 Opipramol Hydrochloride. A sedative and mild tranquillizer, used in the treatment of mild depression and emotional fatigue resulting from anxiety and nervous tension.

G 33182 Chlorthalidone (= Chlortalidone). A diuretic, which though chemically unrelated to the thiazides, has actions and uses similar to those of chlorothiazide.

G 35020 Desipramine Hydrochloride (see DMI).

GA Airway conductance; Gamblers Anonymous; Gastric analysis/ antrum; General anesthesia/ appearance; Gentisic/ Glucuronic acid; Gestational age; Gibberellic acid (= Gibberelin A3; $C_{19}H_{22}O_6$) - Plant growth stimulator obtained from culture filtrates of the fungus Gibberella fugikuroi. Has been used in horticulture to increase plant yields and active principles; Ginger ale (see G'ale); Gingivoaxial; Glucoamylase; Glucose/ acetone; Golgi apparatus; Gramicidin A; Granulocyte adherence; Granulomatous angiitis; Granuloma annulare; Guessed average; Gut-associated; Gyrate atrophy.

Ga Gallium (Z = 31) (see Elements - Gallium); Granulocyte agglutination.

ga ginger ale (diet order); guage (of needles).

G/A Globulin/Albumin (ratio).

^{67}Ga Radioactive gallium (nuclear medicine).

GAA Genotoxic alkylating agent; Gossypol acetic acid.

GAAS Goldberg Anorectic Attitude Scale.

GABA; gaba Gamma-aminobutyric acid (= γ-aminobutyric acid). An inhibitory aminoacid neurotransmitter.

GABAT; GABA-T Gamma-aminobutyric acid transaminase.

GABD Ganglionic adrenergic-blocking drug.

GABHS Group A beta-hemolytic streptococcus.

GABOA Gamma-amino-beta-hydroxybutyric acid.

GAC Genetic amniocentesis (Obstetrics); Glucoronic acid conjugation.

GAD Generalized anxiety disorder; Glutamic acid decarboxylase.

GADA Glutamic acid decarboxylase autoantibody (see AAB).

GADH Gastric alcohol dehydrogenase; Glutamic acid dehydrogenase (see GDH).

GADS Gonococcal arthritis/dermatitis syndrome.

GAE Tuberculin carbohydrate fraction.

GAF Gene-altered food; General adaptive functioning.

GAfREC Government Arrangements for Research Ethics Committees (DoH UK).

GAFS Global Assessment of Functional Scale/ Score (Psychiatry - see DSM).

GAG Galactosaminoglycan; Glycosaminoglycan (see GAGPS); Group-specific antigen gene.

GAG gene A gene coding for core or structural proteins in the AIDS virus (HIV-1) genome, expressed as a precursor protein (p 55), which is cleaved into three proteins (p 24, p 18 and p 15), that are found in the core and the shell of the HIV virus.

GAGPS Glycosaminoglycan polysulfate (= GAG). A mucopolysaccharide enzyme inhibitor of lysomal elastase, responsible for connective tissue breakdown in articular cartilage. Used locally by intra-articular injections in the treatment of degenerative arthritis.

GAHS Galactorrhea-amenorrhea hyperprolactinemia syndrome.

GAIPAS General Audit Inpatient Psychiatric Assessment Scale.

GAL Galactosemia; β-Galactosidase; Galactosyl; Glucuronic acid lactone.

Gal Galactose (= gal); Galen.

gal galactose (see Gal); gallon (L. congius). A measurement of volume - symbol: C (see C. Gallon).

galact- combining form meaning milk (Gr. galactos).

gal Br British imperial gallon.
GalC Galactocerebroside.
G'ale Ginger ale (= GA).
GALI-PUT Galactose-l-phosphate uridyl transferase (enzyme).
gal/min gallons per minute.
GalN Galactosamine.
Gal-nAc n-acetyl-galactosamine.
GALT Galactose-1-p-uridyltransferase; Gut-associated lymphoid tissue.
GALV Gibbon ape leukemia virus.
Galv; galv Galvanic.
GAM Genetically altered molecule.
gam gammon (a microgram = 10^{-6} gram) (see μg - under "M").
gam- combining form meaning marriage or union (Gr. gamos).
GAML Gesell adaptive maturity level.
Gamma M-FTH Gamma M-fluorescent treponemal antibody.
GAN Generalized anxiety neuroses/osis; Giant axon neuropathy.
Ganc Ganciclovir.
Ganciclovir An acyclic nucleoside and antiviral drug, used especially in CMV infections (= BIOLF-62; DHPG; Ganc; Z'NDG).
G and D Growth and development (see G&D).
gang; gangl ganglion(ic).
gangli- combining form meaning swelling (Gr. ganglion).
Gangster Marijuana (see Cannabis).
Ganja Marijuana (see Cannabis).
GANS Granulomatous angiitis of the nervous system.
GAO Gastric acid output (see APG; GAS); General Accounting Office (US).
GAP Gastric acid production/ pump (the proton-pump enzyme H+, K+ -ATPase); Glyceraldehyde phosphate (= D-glyceraldehyde-3-phosphate); Government-Assured Program; Group for the Advancement of Psychiatry; Guanosine triphosphatase activating protein.
GAPD Glyceraldehyde-3-phosphate dehydrogenase.
GAPDH Reduced glyceraldehyde-phosphate dehydrogenase.
GAPO Growth retardation, alopecia, pseudo-anodontia, and optic atrophy (syndrome).
GAPS Glycine amide phosphoribosyl synthetase (= GAPS).
Garg; garg A gargle (L. gargarisma).
GARGG Goat antibody to rabbit gamma globulin.
GARP Global Atmospheric Research Program (UN).
GARS Glycine amide phosphoribosyl synthetase (see GAPS).
GAS Galactorrhea-amenorrhea syndrome; Gastric acid secretion; Gastroenterology; General adaptation syndrome (stress); Generalized arteriosclerosis; Glasgow Assessment Schedule; Global Assessment Scale; Group A Streptococcus.
GASA Growth-adjusted sonographic age.
Gas Anal F&T Gastric analysis, free and total.
Ga scan Gallium scan.
GASI Gastic acid secretion inhibitor.
GASP Group Against Smoke/ Smokers'/ Smoking Pollution.
Gast Gastroenterology (journal).
gastr- prefix meaning stomach (Gr. gastros).
Gastroc Gastrocnemius (muscle).
GAT Gas antitoxin; Gelatin agglutination test; General abdominal tenderness; General American Transportation Co; Gentamycin acetyl transferase; Gerontological Apperception Test; Group adjustment therapy; Gynecocyte auto-test.
GATB General Aptitude Test Battery-1.
GAU Geriatric assessment unit; Glutaric aciduria (a genetic, metabolic deficiency disease).
GAW Airway conductance (see GAW-Vtg).
GAW/Vtg Specific airway conductance.
Gay Homosexual (see Homo).
GAZT Glucuronide derivative of azidothymidine.
GB Gallbladder; Glial bundle; Goofball/ Goof ball (barbiturate pill) (see Barb); Great Britain; Guillain-Barré (syndrome) (see GBS).
Gb Gilbert.
G&B Good and bad.
Gb3 Globotriaosylceramide (see FD).
GBA Ganglionic blocking agent;

Gingivobuccoaxial.

G-banding Giemsa banding (chromosome staining procedure in microscopy).

GBBS Group B beta hemolytic Streptococcus.

GBC Gruntzig balloon catheter (see ADC).

GBD Gallbladder/ Glass blower's disease; Gender behavior disorder; Genetic blood disease/ disorder; Granulomatous bowel disease.

GBDC Genetics and Birth Defects Center.

GBE Ginkgo biloba extract.

GBF Generalized bronchial fibrosis.

GBG Glycine-rich beta-glycoprotein; Gonadal steroid-binding globulin.

GBH Gamma-benzene hexachloride/ hydrochloride (see GBHC); Graphite benzalkonium heparin.

GBHA Glyoxal-bis-(2-hydroxyanil).

GBHC Gamma benzene hexachloride or hydrochloride (= Benhexachlor; Gamma-BCH; Gamma-HCH; GBH; HCH Officinal; Hexicide; Lindane; 666; $C_6H_6Cl_6$). An insecticide, larvicide and ascaricide used in pediculosis, scabies and other skin infestations as a cream, dusting-powder, lotion or shampoo.

GBI Globulin-binding insulin; Group for Biology Information.

GBIA Guthrie bacterial inhibition assay.

GBIT Gene-based immunotherapy (see HGT).

GBL Glomerular basal lamina; Goddard-Bennett-Lovelace (Unit/ infant hand resuscitator).

GBM Gene-based medicine (functional genomics); Glioblastoma multiforme (a malignant glioma); Glomerular basement membrane.

GBMC Greater Baltimore Medical Center.

GBMI Guilty but mentally ill.

GBP Galactose-binding protein; Gastric bypass; Gated blood pool.

GBPS Gated blood pool scan (a radioisotope scanning test for cardiac function).

GBS Gallbladder series (X-rays/ gallbladder)/ surgery; Gastric bypass surgery; Gay bowel syndrome (a venereally transmitted proctocolitis in homosexuals); Glycerine-buffered saline (solution); Grey baby syndrome (toxic hepatitis with cardiovascular collapse); Group B Streptococcus; Guide to Biomedical Standards; Guillain-Barré syndrome.

GB series Gallbladder series (see GBS).

GBSS Gey's balanced saline solution; Guillain-Barré-Strohl syndrome.

GBV Gene-bearing virus.

GB vis Gallbladder visualization.

GC Ganglion/ Goblet/ Golgi/ Granulosa cell; Gas chromatography; General circulation/ closure/ condition; Geriatric care/ chair (Gerichair); Genetic consequence(s)/ counselling; Germinal center; Glucocorticoid; Gonococcus/ Gonococcal/ Gonorrhea (= G; Gc; Gon); Gonorrhea culture; Granular casts; Granulomatous colitis; Group-specific component (see Gc); Guanine cytosine; Guanylcyclase; Guiding catheter (Coronary angioplasty); Guyon's canal (in the palm of the hand, through which the ulnar nerve and artery pass).

Gc Gigacycle; Gonococcus (see GC); Group specific component of blood (serum protein) (= GC).

G+ C Gram-positive cocci.

G- C Gram-negative cocci.

GCA Gastric cancer area; General care area (MET-501); Generalized cerebral atrophy; Geological Corporation of America; Giant cell arteritis; Giant condyloma acuminata (see B-L); Glucocorticoid/icosteroid activity; Goblet-cell atrophy.

g-cal gram calorie (= small/ standard calorie), i.e. the amount of heat required to raise the temperature of 1 gram of water 1 degree Celsius (centigrade).

GCB Gonococcal base.

GCBADL General, Cognitive, Behavioral and Activities of Daily Living (four areas of patient function).

GCBDS Gonococcal broth defined supplement.

GCBM Glomerular capillary basement membrane.

GCC General Chiropractic Council (UK); Germ cell component (of rhabdomyosarcoma) (see TCC; TMC); Giant cell carcinoma (= CGC); Glassy cell carcinoma (of the uterine cervix).

GCDFP Gross cystic disease fluid protein.

GCE General and Comparative

Endocrinology (journal).

GCES Glucose-containing electrolyte solution.

GCF Germinal-center formation (in lymph nodes); Growth-rate-controlling factor.

GCFT Gonococcal/ Gonorrhea complement fixation test.

GCI General Cognitive Index; Genetics citation index; Giant cell infiltration; Global cerebral ischemia; Global cognitive impairment (dementia); Glucocorticoid insufficiency (as in Addison's disease, etc.).

GCIIS Glucose controlled insulin infusion system.

GCIO Glucocorticoid-induced osteoporosis.

GCJ Gastric cancer secretions.

GCLO Gastric Campylobacter-like organism.

GCL Giant cell lesion.

GCM General cytochemical methods; Giant-cell myocarditis; Good central maintainance.

g-cm gram-centimeter.

GCMER General Council of Medical Education and Registration (of the United Kingdom; abbreviated to GMC after the year 1951).

GCMS; GC-MS Gas chromatography (coupled with) - mass spectrometry/scopy.

GCN Giant cerebral neuron.

g-coef generalizability coefficient.

GCP Genetic counceling program; Global Clinical Project; Good Clinical Practice(s) (EC/Europe Community guidelines).

GCPG Good clinical practice guideline(s).

GCR Galactic cosmic rays; Gastro-colic reflex (Samson Wright, UK) (Defecation reflex initiated in the stomach by food or drink) (see CCR); Global cell replacement (neural SCT); Glucocorticoid receptor; Group Conformity Rating.

GCRC General Clinical Research Centers (NIH).

GCRD Glucocorticoid receptor density.

GCRS Gynecological chylous reflux syndrome.

GCS General clinical service(s); Genetic counselling service(s); Gianotti-Crosti syndrome; Glasgow Coma Scale; Glucocorticosteroid; α-Glutamylcysteine synthetase; Granulocytic sarcoma.

GCs Glucocorticoids (cortisone, cortisol and corticosterone) (= CS).

GCSA Gross cell surface antigen.

G-CSF Granulocyte colony-stimulating factor (see HGF; Hormones - G-CSF).

GCT Gate-control theory (of pain); General care and treatment; Germ-cell tumor (see AMT); Giant cell thyroiditis; Giant cell tumor; Glomerular capillary thrombosis; Glucocorticoid therapy; Glucose challenge test (in pregnancy, with oral intake of 50 gms glucose within 2 minutes, and measurement of plasma glucose level after 1 hour); Granulocyte transfusion (for the treatment of granulocytopenia in leukemia patients receiving cancer chemotherapy) (= BCT or Buffy coat transfusion).

GC(T)A Giant cell (temporal) arteritis.

GCU Glucocorticoid use; Gonococcal urethritis.

GCV Ganciclovir; Gene-carrying virus; Great cardiac vein; Great cerebral vein (= Vein of Galen).

GCVD Genetic cardiovascular disorder.

GCVF Great cardiac vein flow.

GCW Glomerular capillary wall.

GCWM General Conference on Weights and Measures.

GCY Gastroscopy.

GD Dentate gyrus (see DG); Gastroduodenal; Gel destrainer (electrophoresis); General diagnostics/ dispensary; Gestational day; Gianotti's/ Graves' disease; Gonadal dysgenesis; Growth and development (see G&D).

Gd Gadolinium (Z = 64) (see Elements - Gadolinium).

gd good.

G'd God.

G&D Growth and development (= G and D; GD).

GDA Germine diacetate.

GDB Gas density balance; Guide dogs for the blind.

GDC General Dental Council; Geometric Data Corporation; Giant dopamine-containing cell; Guglielmi detachable coil (for operation on aneurysms).

GDD Gastroduodenal defence/ disease; Gross destructive disease.

Gd-DTPA Gadolinium-diethylene-triamine-pentaacetic acid.
GDE Gastroduodenal epithelium/ erosion.
GDF Gel diffusion (precipitin) (see GDP).
GDFB Guide Dog Foundation for the Blind.
GDH Glucose/ Glycerophosphate/ Glycol dehydrogenase; Glutamate/ Glutamic acid dehydrogenase (= GADH; GHD; GLD; GLDH; GLUD; GMD); Gonadotropic hormone (see Hormones - GDH i; GTH); Growth and differentiation hormone (in insects) (see Hormones - GDH ii).
GDID Genetically determined immunodeficiency disease.
g/dl grams per deciliter.
GDM Gestational diabetes mellitus; Glutathione-dependent mechanism.
2G/DM Glyceryl guaiacolate and dextromethorphan hydrobromide.
GDMO General Duties Medical Officer.
GDMP Gestational diabetes mellitus pregnancy.
GDP Gel diffusion precipitin (= GDF); General dissolution procedure; Gross domestic product; Guanosine diphosphate.
GDR General dosage recommendation(s); German Democratic Republic (the late); Global drug resistance.
GDS Geriatric Depression Scale; Global Deterioration Scale; Good delivery system; Gordon Diagnostic System (for attention disorders); Gradual dosage/ dose schedule.
GDT "Genetic dog tag" (for identification of American GIs killed in combat).
GDTS Gilles de la Tourettes syndrome (= TS).
GDW Glass-distilled water.
gdw gram dry weight.
GDXY (XY) Gonadal dysgenesis.
GE Gainfully employed; Gastric emptying; Gastroemotional; Gastroenteritis; Gastroenterology; Gastroenterostomy; Gastroesophageal (= GO); Gastrointestinal Endoscopy (journal); Gel electrophoresis; General Electric (Co.); Generalized epilepsy; Generator of excitation; Gentamycin (sulfate) (see GENT); Glandular epithelium; Glucose - electrolyte; Guanethidine.
Ge Gerbich red-cell antigen; Germanium (Z = 32) (see Elements - Germanium).
G/E Granulocyte/erythroid (ratio) (laboratory/ hematology).
g-e gravity eliminated.
GEA Gas-exchange abnormality (in lung injury).
GEB Garren-Edwards bubble (gastric bubble inflated in the stomach, for the treatment of morbid obesity).
GEC Galactose elimination capacity; Gastric/ Glomerular epithelial cell; Gastro-entero-colitis.
GECC Government Employees' Clinic Center.
GECH Gastric epithelial cell hyperplasia.
GEE Genetic, environmental, and endogenous (factors) (see GEEFs).
GEEFs Genetic, environmental, and endogenous factors (causing susceptibility to disease).
GEE-OPG Oculoplethysmography (test - Gee is the name of the physician who devised this test) (see OPG) (= OPG-GEE).
GEF Gastroesophageal fundoplication; Genetically engineered food(s); Glossoepiglottic fold; Gonadotropin enhancing factor (see Hormones - GEF; GTH).
gegenhalten German - "against holding", i.e. involuntary resistance to passive movements (Neurology).
GEH Glycerol ester hydrolase.
GEHI Genetically engineered human insulin.
GEJ Gastro-esophageal junction.
gel gelatin(ous).
gelat- combining form meaning freeze (L. gelatus).
gel quav in any kind of jelly (L. gelatina quavis).
GEM Gene editing machine (= Spliceosome) - the function of which is to select and splice together useful genetic information (see GEP; GES); Glucose electrolyte mixture (of Queen Elizabeth Hospital for Children, UK). A solution of dextrose and electrolytes such as calcium, magnesium, potassium and sodium chloride; potassium and sodium citrate, and sodium acid phosphate. Used orally in the treatment of acute dehydration in infants. Has an approximate reaction of pH 6.6.

Geological time table

ERA		Period (time) or System (rock)	Epoch (time) or Series (rock)	Approximate time in years from present
Cenozoic		Quaternary	Holocene (recent)	50,000
			Pleistocene (Glacial)	1,000,000
		Tertiary	Pliocene	12,000,000
			Miocene	30,000,000
			Oligocene	40,000,000
			Eocene	60,000,000
			Paleocene	70,000,000
Mesozoic (Secondary)		Cretaceous		120,000,000
		Jurassic		160,000,000
		Triassic		200,000,000
Paleozoic (Primary)		Permian		220,000,000
		Carboniferous (Am Pennsylvanian & Mississipian)		300,000,000
		Devonian		350,000,000
		Silurian		400,000,000
		Ordovician		500,000,000
		Cambrian		600,000,000
Pre-Cambrian	Proterozoic			1,300,000,000
	Archeozoic			2,300,000,000

GEMB Group on Engineering in Medicine and Biology (IEEE).
gemin- combining form meaning double or twin (L. geminus).
GEMS Global Environmental Monitoring System; Good emergency mother substitute.
GEMSAEC General Medical Sciences and Atomic Energy Commission (National Institute of joint activity).
GEN Gender; Generation.
Gen Genetic(s) (see genet); Genus (L. genus).
gen general (see gen'l); genital; genitive.
gen- combining form meaning become, originate, produce (Gr.).
GEN/ENDO General (anesthesia) with endotracheal (intubation).
genet genetic(s) (= Gen).
Genetics (journal).
GENETOX Genetic Toxicology (data base).
gen et sp nov new genus and species (L. genus et species nova).
-genic suffix meaning original, cause or create.
genit genital(ia).
gen'l general (= gen).
gen nov new genus (L. genus novum).
GENOVA Generalized analysis of variance.
gen proc general procedure.
GENPS Genital neoplasm - papilloma syndrome.
GENT Gentamycin (= GE; GM).
GENTA/P Gentamycin-peak.
GENTA/T Gentamycin-trough.
geog geography.
geol geology.
geom geometric/ry.
Geo time Geological time (see Table).
GEP Gastroenteropancreatic (system); Gene

editing process (see GEM; GES); Gene expression profile; Genetically engineered protein (see FGF); Gluten enteropathy (celiac sprue).

GEPG Gastroesophageal pressure gradient.

GEPH Genetically engineered plasmid hybrid.

GER Gastric emptying rate; Gastroesophageal reflex/ lux (= GOR); Geriatrics (see Ger); Granular endoplasmic reticulum.

Ger Geriatric(s) (= GER; Geriat); Geriatrics (journal) (= Geriat); German (= G).

GERD Gastroesophageal reflux disease (= GORD).

Geriat Geriatric(s) (see Ger); Geriatrics (journal) (see Ger).

GERL Golgi-associated endoplasmic reticulum lysosome.

GERM Groupe d'Étude pour une Réforme de la Médecine (Belgium).

Geront Gerontologic (= Gerontol); Gerontologist (= Gerontol - journal); Gerontology (= Gerontol).

Gerontol Gerontologic/gist/gy (see Geront).

Ger P German Pharmacopeia (= GP).

GERU Gastroenterology Research Unit (UK).

GES Gene editing studies/dy (see GEM; GEP); Glucose-electrolyte solution; Gradient echo sequences (see GRE).

GESP General extrasensory perception.

GEST Gastro-esophageal sphincter tone; Gestation.

gest- combining form meaning carry (L. gestus).

GET Gastric emptying time; General endotracheal (anesthesia); Glucose enzymatic test(s); Graded (treadmill) exercise test.

GET 1/2 Gastric emptying half-time.

GETA General endotracheal anesthesia.

GETS Glucose Enzymatic Test Strip.

GeV; GEV; Gev Billion electron volts (= 10^9 or giga electron volt) (Gr. = giant) (formerly BEV).

GEWO 339 Isoniazid aminosalicylate (used in the treatment of tuberculosis).

GEWS Gianturco expandable wire stent.

GEX Gas exchange.

GF Garden fracture (of femoral neck) - G I: incomplete or impacted racture, G II: complete fracture without displacement, G III: complete fracture with partial displacement, or G IV: complete fracture with total displacement; Gastric fistula/ fluid; General Foods (Corp); Genetic fingerprint; Germ/ Gluten - free; Glass factor (tissue culture); Globule-fibril; Glomerular filtrate/ ration; Gold foil (dentistry); Grandfather; Growth factor/ failure/ fraction/ function; Guaifenesin (= Guaiphenesin; GFS).

Gf General factor (in intelligence tests).

gf gram-force.

G-F Globular-fibrous (with reference to proteins).

GFA Glial fibrillary acidic (protein) (see GFAP).

G-Factor Gyro-magnetic value.

GFAES Graphite furnace atomic emission spectroscopy.

GFAP Glial fibrillary acidic protein (= GFA).

GFB Gastroscope for biopsy.

GFCP Gross fixed capital formation.

GFD Gluten-free diet; Goldmann-Favre disease (see VRD).

GFFS Glycogen and fat-free solid(s).

GFG Growth-factor gene.

GFH Glucose-free Hanks (solution).

GFI Glucagon-free insulin (see Insulin - GFI); Ground-fault interrupter; Growth-factor inhibitor.

GFL Giant follicular lymphoma; Glaucomatous field loss.

GFLA Giant follicular lymphadenopathy (= BSD or Brill-Symmer's disease, GFL or Giant follicular lymphoma, Symmer's disease).

GFM Gel filtration medium; Good fetal movement.

GFN Genitofemoral nerve.

G-forces Acceleration forces (Gravity forces).

GFP Gamma-fetoprotein; Gel-filtered platelet; Genetic fingerprinting; Glomerular filtered phosphate; Green fluorescent protein (a histone protein molecule that lights up when excited by a laser); Growth-factor protein.

GFR German Federal Republic; Glomerular filtration rate; Good functional result (Orthopedics); Growth factor receptor; Grunting, flaring, and retractions.

GFS Glandular fever syndrome; Global focal sclerosis; Guaifenesin (see GF).
GFT Fiberoptic gastroscope.
GG Gamma globulin; Genioglossus; Glyceryl guaiacolate; Glycylglycine.
γG Immunoglobulin G (see IgG).
γγ Micromicrogram (= picogram; 10^{-12} g; μμg).
GGA General gonadotropic activity.
GGAB; GGAb Goitrogenic antibody.
GGC Gastric glandular cyst.
GGCH Giant germinal center hyperplasia (ass. e benign lymphadenopathy).
GGCS Gamma-glutamyl cysteine synthetase.
GGCT Ground glass clotting time.
GGD Goitrogenic disease.
GGE Generalized glandular enlargement; Gradient gel electrophoresis.
GGFC Gamma-globulin-free calf (serum).
GGG; ggg Gamboge (= Cambogia; Gutti) (L. gummi guttae gambiae). A yellow gum-resin (cambogia), extracted from Garcinia hanburyi (family Guttiferae) and other guttiferous East Indian trees. A drastic hydragogue cathartic; Glycine-rich gamma-glycoprotein.
GGM Glucose-galactose malabsorption.
GGMS Grocott-Gromori methenamine silver (stain) (= GMS).
GG or S Glands, goiter, or stiffness (of neck).
GGPNA Gamma-glutamyl-p-nitroanilide.
GGRO Glossary of the General Register Office.
GGS Glands, goiter, and stiffness.
GGT Gamma-glutamyl transferase/ transpeptidase (see GGTP).
γ-GT Gamma-glutamyl transpeptidase (see GTP).
GGTP Gamma-glutamyl transpeptidase (= GGT).
GGVB Gelatin, glucose, and veronal buffer.
GH Gastric hyperacidity; General health; General Hospital; Genital herpes; Genetic hypertension; Genetically hypertensive (rat); Geniohyoid; Growth hormone (see Hormones - GH).
G/H Graft/host.
G+H Gibb & Helmholtz (equation).
GH_3 Gerovital H_3 ("youth" drug).
GHA Government health agency; Group Health Association.
GHAA Group Health Association of America.
GHB Gamma hydroxybutyrate; Glycohemoglobin (see GHb).
GHb Glycated hemoglobin; Glycosylated hemoglobin (= GLYCOS Hb).
GHBA Gamma-hydroxybutyric acid.
GHC Group Health Cooperative.
GHD General hospital doctor; Glutamic acid dehydrogenase (see GDH); Growth hormone deficiency.
GHDI Group Health Dental Insurance.
GHI Genital herpes infection; Group Health Insurance; Group Hospitalization Inc.; Growth hormone insufficiency (= GHD).
GH-IF Growth hormone-inhibiting factor (= GIF).
GH-IH Growth hormone inhibiting hormone (= Somatostatin) (see Hormones - GH-IH).
GHJ Glenohumeral joint.
GHMA General hepatic metabolic activity.
Ghost LSD-25 (see LSD).
GHPQ General Health Perception Questionnaire.
GHQ General Headquarters; General health questionnaire.
GHR Generalized hypersensitivity reaction(s); Granulomatous hypersensitivity reaction.
GHRF Growth hormone-releasing factor (see Hormones - GHRF).
GH-RH Growth hormone-releasing hormone (see Hormones - GH-RH).
GHRIF; GH-RIF Growth hormone-release inhibiting factor (= Somatostatin) (see CNP) (see Hormones - GH-IH).
GHRIH; GH-RIH Growth hormone-release inhibiting hormone (= Somatostatin) (see Hormones - GH-IH).
GHRSF; GH-RSF Growth hormone-release stimulating factor (see GH-RH).
GHT Growth hormone therapy; Graves' hyperthyroidism (see GD; GLD; GLM; GOP; SHT) - Manifestations of hyperthyroidism. *Symptoms*: Hyperactivity, irritability, altered mood, insomnia; Heat intolerance, increased sweating; Palpitations; Fatigue, weakness; Dyspnea; Weight loss with increased appetite (weight gain in 10% of patients); Pruritus; Increased stool frequency; Thirst and

polyuria; Oligomenorrhea or amenorrhea, loss of libido. *Signs*: Sinus tachycardia, atrial fibrillation; Fine tremor, hyperkinesis, hyperreflexia; Warm, moist skin; Palmar erythema, onycholisis; Hair loss; Muscle weakness and wasting; and rarely, Congestive (high output) heart failure, chorea, periodic paralysis (primarily in Asian males), psychosis. *Manifestations of Graves' disease*: Diffuse goiter; Ophthalmopathy; A feeling of grittiness and discomfort in the eye; Retrobulbar pressure or pain; Eyelid lag or retraction; Periorbital edema, chemosis, scleral injection; Exophthalmos (proptosis); Extraocular-muscle disfunction; Exposure keratitis; Optic neuropathy; Localized dermopathy; Lyphoid hyperplasia; Thyroid acropachy. *Conditions associated with Graves' disease*: Type I diabetes mellitus; Addison's disease; Vitiligo; Pernicious anemia; Alopecia areata; Myasthenia gravis; Celiac disease; Other autoimmune disorders associated with the HLA-DR3 haplotype.

GHV Goose hepatitis virus.

GHz Gigahertz (= Ghz) (10^9 cycles/sec).

Ghz See GHz.

GI Gastrointestinal; Gelatin infusion (medium); General illness; Genito-intestinal; Gingival/ Glomerular index; Globin insulin (has an intermediate action between that of unmodified or regular insulin and protamine zinc insulin) (see Insulin - GZI); Glucose intolerance; Glycemic index (ratio of the AUC of blood glucose o a food, compared to the response following a standard meal); Government issue (US armed forces); Granuloma inguinale; Growth inhibiting/tion; Guillotine incision.

gi gill.

G/I Glucose/insulin (ratio).

GIA Gastrointestinal anastomosis/ absorption; General inhalation anesthesia/thetic; Goodwill Industries of America, Inc.

GIAE Gastrointestinal adverse effect/ event/ experience.

GIB Gastric ileal bypass; Gastrointestinal bleeding.

GIBF Gastrointestinal bacterial flora.

GIBL Gastrointestinal blood loss (see GIB).

GIC Gastrointestinal candidiasis/ care/ complaint(s)/ complication(s); General immunocompetence; Glucose-insulin cycle.

GICA Gastrointestinal cancer.

GICR Gastro-ileo-caecal reflex.

GID Gastrointestinal damage/ disease/ discomfort/ disorder/ distress/ disturbance/ dysfunction; Gender identity disorder.

GIDA Gastrointestinal Diagnostic Area.

GIE Gastrointestinal effect/ endoscopy/ enzyme/ event; Gluten-induced enteropathy (= Celiac disease, Celiac sprue, Non-tropical sprue).

GIF Gastrointestinal flora (bacterial)/ fullness/ function; Growth hormone-inhibiting factor (see GH-IF).

GIFL Gastrointestinal fluid loss.

GIFT Gamete intrafallopian transfer; Granulocyte immunofluorescence test.

giga- metric prefix for 10^9. Symbol: G (see G. Giga-).

GIGO "Garbage in, garbage out" (principle - associated with computers).

GIH Gastric inhibitory hormone; Gastrointestinal hemorrhage; General ill health; Growth-inhibiting hormone (see Hormones - GIH).

GII Gastrointestinal illness/ impairment/ infection/ intolerance/ irritation.

GIK Glucose-insulin-potassium (therapeutic intravenous solution).

GIL Gastrointestinal loss (e.g. of bicarbonate).

GILRV GIL Rubella Virus.

GIM Gastrointestinal malabsorption/ malignancy/ moniliasis/ motility; General internal medicine; Gonadotropin-inhibiting/tory material; Growth-inducing molecule (see HSC).

GIMD Gastrointestinal malabsorption/ motility disorder.

GIN Gastrointestinal narrowing (iatrogenic/ pathologic).

Ging; ging Gum(s) (= Gingiva/val) (L. gingiva).

GIO Gastrointestinal obstruction/ oncology; Glucocorticoid-induced osteoporosis.

GIOD Gastrointestinal obstructive disease/ disorder.

g-ion gram-ion.

GIP Gastric inhibitory peptide/ polypeptide; Gastrointestinal pain/ perforation (duodenum, colon, etc.)/ problem(s); Giant cell interstitial pneumonia; Glucose-dependent insulinotropic peptide; Gonorrheal invasive peritonitis.
GIPKA Gastrointestinal prokinetic agent (such as Cisapride, Metoclopramide, etc.).
GIR Gastrointestinal reaction (nausea, mucosal erosion, etc.); Gastrointestinal reflux; General improvement rate; General(ized) immune reaction; Glasgow Institute of Radiotherapeutics; Global improvement rating; Growth inhibitory response.
Girl Heroin (see Diamorph HCl).
GIS Gas in stomach; Gastrointestinal secretion/ series (X-rays)/ spasm/ symptoms/ system (see GITS); Geographical information system.
GISC Gastrointestinal stromal cancer.
GISD Gastrointestinal system disorder (see GID).
GISE Gastrointestinal side-effects.
GISSI Gruppo Italiano per lo Studio della Sopravvivenza nell'Infarto (Miocardico Prevenzione) - The Italian group for the study of MI prevention and survival.
GIT Gastrointestinal stromal tumor (a deadly stomach cancer); Gastrointestinal tolerance/ toxicity/ tract; Gene immunotherapy (for cancer) (see HGT); Georgia Institute of Technology; Glucose-induced toxicity.
GITS Gastrointestinal therapeutic system (= GIS).
GITSG Gastrointestinal Tumor Study Group.
GITT Gastrointestinal transit time; Glucose insulin tolerance test.
GIU Gastrointestinal ulcer(ation)/ upset.
GIV Gastrointestinal volvulus.
giv given.
GIWU Gastrointestinal work-up.
GIX Difluoro-diphenyl-trichloroethane (= DFDT). A powerful insecticidal compound similar to DDT, but with fluorine replacing chlorine in the paraphenyl position.
GJ Gap junction; Gastric juice; Gastrojejunostomy.
GJA-S Gastric juice aspiration syndrome.
GK Galactokinase; Gamma Knife (radiosurgery); Glomerulocystic kidney; Glycerol kinase.
Gk Greek (see Gr).
gK Backward current.
GKAS Genucom Knee Analysis System (Montreal, Canada).
GKD Glycerol kinase deficiency.
GKM Glass knife maker (for a microtome).
GKMDT Graham Kendall Memory for Design Test.
GKN Grosse-Kempf nail (Orthopedics) (see IIN).
GKR Geometric knee replacement (see OI/OP).
GL Gastric lavage; Gene library; Gill (see gl); Gland (see Gl); Glomerular layer; Glycolipid (see GL-3); Glycosphingolipid; Glycyrrhizin; Greatest length (a measurement used for small flexed embryos); Gustatory lacrimation; Gut lavage (see WBI).
Gl Glabella; Gland(ular) (= GL; gl; Gln) (L. glandula); Glucinium (L. - obsolete chemical symbol) - now known as Beryllium (Be) (Z = 4) (see Elements - Beryllium).
gl gill (= GL); gland(ular) (see Gl).
g/l grams per liter (= gli; gm/l).
GL-3 Glycolipid (= GL).
GL 54 Athomin.
GLA Galactosidase A; Gamma-linolenic acid; Giant left atrium; Gingivolinguoaxial; Granulomatous lymphocytic adenohypophysitis (= GMH).
GL-1a Glucosylceramide.
GL-2a Lactosylceramide.
glac glacial.
GLAD Gold-labelled antigen detection.
Glam Glutamine (see Gln).
gland glandular (L. glandula = a gland).
gland- combining form meaning acorn (L. glandis).
GLAT Glutamic acid, lysine, alanine, and tyrosine.
GL-1b Galactosylceramide.
GLC Gas-liquid chromatography; Germ-line cell; Glaucoma (see glc).
Glc Glaucoma (see glc); Glucose (see Gluc).
glc glaucoma (= GLC; Glc).
GlcA Gluconic acid.
GLC-MS Gas-liquid chromatography - mass spectrometry.

GlcN Glucosamine.
Glc-nAc N-acetyl-glucosamine.
GlcUA D-glucuronic acid.
GLD Germ-layer differentiation; Glanders-like disease; Globoid leukodystrophy; Glucose-lowering drug; Glutamate dehydrogenase (see GDH); Granulomatous lung disease; Graves' localized dermopathy (see GD; GHT).
GLE Glucose-lowering effect.
GLGT Germ-line gene transfer.
GLDH Glutamic dehydrogenase (see GDH).
GLGT Germ-line gene therapy (= GLT) (see HGT).
GLH Germinal layer hemorrhage; Giant lymph node hyperplasia.
GLI Genetic linkage (analysis); Glicentin; Glucagon-like immunoreactivity.
gli grams per liter (see g/l).
-glia suffix meaning glue (Gr.).
GLM General linear model; Germline mutation (of genes); Graves' localized myxedema (see GD; GHT).
glm gallons per minute (see g/m).
Gln Gland(ular) (see Gl); Glucagon; Glutamine (= Glam; gLN; Glu) (see Glx).
gLN Glutamine (see Gln).
GLNH Giant lymph node hyperplasia.
GLO Glyoxylase.
GLO 1 Glyoxylase 1.
Glob; glob Globular; Globulin.
Glob G Globulin G (= Lysozyme). A mucopolysaccharidase, whose action against viruses resembles that of interferon. Used in the prevention and treatment of herpes zoster, mumps, and chicken-pox.
GLOH Greater Louisville Organization for Health (Kentucky).
gloss- combining form meaning tongue (Gr. glossa).
glott- combining form meaning language or tongue (Gr. glotta).
GLP Gambro Liendia Plate; Glucose-L-phosphate; Glycolipoprotein; Good laboratory practice; Group-living program.
GLPP Glucose, post prandial (laboratory/chemistry).
GLR Graphic level recorder; Gravity lumbar reduction.
GLS Generalized lymphadenopathy syndrome; General laser surgery; Gibbon lymphosarcoma (cell).
GLT Germ-line therapy (see HGT).
GLTN; GlTN Glomerulotubulonephritis.
GLTT Glucose-lactate tolerance test.
GlTT Glucose tolerance test (see GTT; LFT iv).
GLU; Glu; glu Glucose (see Gluc); Glucuronidase-β (see Glucur); Glucuronide (see Glucur); Glutamate/mic acid (see Glx); Glutamine (see Gln).
GLU-5 Five-hour glucose tolerance test.
GLUC Glucosidase.
Gluc; gluc Glucose (= Glc; Glu).
gluc- combining form meaning sweet (Gr. glukus).
Glucur β-Glucuronidase (= Glu); Glucuronide (= Glu).
GLUD Glutamate dehydrogenase (see GHD).
GluOx; GlucOx Glucose oxidase.
Glut Glutethimide.
glutin- combining form meaning glue (L. gluten).
GLV Gross leukemia virus.
Glx Glutamine and/or glutamic acid (see Gln).
GLY; Gly; gly; Glyc; glyc Glyceride/rine; Glycerite (L. glyceritum); Glycine.
glyc- combining form meaning sweet (Gr. glukus).
glyco- prefix meaning sugar.
GLYCOS Hb Glycosylated hemoglobin (see GHb).
GM Gastric mucosa; Geiger-Mueller/Müller (counter) (see G-M); General medicine; General Motors (Corp); Genetic manipulation; Gentamycin (see GENT); Geometric mean; Giant melanosome; Gowers' maneuvre ("walking up the legs", as in DMD); Gram (see Gm); Grand mal (epilepsy); Grandmother; Grand multiparity; Granulocyte-macrophage; Grating monochrometer; Growth medium; Monosialoganglioside.
Gm An allotype marker on the heavy chains of immunoglobins; Gram - the basic unit of mass of the metric system (= G; g; GM; gm; Grm; grm).
gm gamma; gram (see Gm).

G-M Geiger-Mueller/Müller (counter) (= GM).
g-m gram-meter.
GM+; Gm+ Gram positive (stain/ on bacteriology reports).
GM-; Gm- Gram negative (stain/ on bacteriology reports).
Gm% Grams per hundred milliliters (= Grams per cent).
Gm‰ Grams per liter (= Grams promil).
GM-1 Sygen or ganglioside (found naturally in cell membranes; an experimental drug used to grow neurons in spinal nerve injuries).
G_{M1} pseudo-Hurler's syndrome ganglioside.
G_{M2}; G_{M2} (G5) Tay-Sachs ganglioside (a ganglioside in the brain which causes Tay-Sachs disease).
G_{M3} Predominant ganglioside.
Gm 3 Hematoside.
GMA Gastric mucosal atrophy/ Gene mutation assay (CHO/HGPRT - Chinese hamster ovary/ Hypoxanthine-guanine phosphoribosyl transferase assay); Germine monoacetate; Glyceral/ryl methacrylate; Glycidyl methacrylate (see BIS-GMA).
GMB Betamycin sulfate; Gastric mucosal barrier; Granulomembranous body.
GMBF Gastric mucosa blood flow.
GMC Gene-modified cell; General medical care/ clinic; General Medical Council (UK); Glucosteroid-mineralocorticoid/ Grand-mal convulsion; Grant Medical College (Bombay); Green/ Grivet monkey cell (see GMK).
GMC_1 Gentamycin C_1 sulfate.
gm cal gram calorie (small c).
gm/cc grams per cubic centimeter (= g/ml).
GMCD Grand mal convulsive disorder.
GM-CFU Granulocyte - macrophage colony forming unit.
GMCHP Greater Marshfield Community Health Plan.
GMCR Genetic Mutant Cell Repository (NIGMS).
GM-CSF Granulocyte-macrophage colony-stimulating factor (see HGF) - a lymphokine.
GMD Geometric mean diameter; Glossary of Mental Disorders; Glucide metabolism disorder; Glutamate dehydrogenase; Glycopeptide moiety modified derivative.
GMDS Gel-matrix delivery system (with statin drugs such as Fluvastatin).
GME Graduate medical education.
GMENAC Graduate Medical Education National Advisory Committee.
GM-FTA Gamma-M fluorescent treponemal antibody.
GMG Generalized myasthenia gravis.
G_{M2} (G5) See G_{M2}.
GMH Germinal matrix hemorrhage; Granulomatous hypophysitis (see GLA).
GMHC Gay Men's Health Clinic/ Crisis.
GMI Desipramine hydrochloride (see DMI); Gastric mucosal injury/ ischemia.
GMK Green/ Grivet monkey kidney (cells) (= GMC).
GML Generalized malignant lymphoma; Gut mucosa lymphocyte.
g/ml grams per milliliter (see gm/cc).
gm/l grams per liter (see g/l).
GMM German Medical Monthly; Glucose-mediated macrosomia (in gestational diabetes); Gluteus maximus muscle.
gm-m gram-meter.
GMO General Medical Officer.
g-mole gram mole(cule).
GMP Gene-mapping procedure; Generate mountains of paperwork; Glucose monophosphate; Good manufacturing practices (FDA); Good Medical Practice (UK booklet); Guanosine monophosphate (= Guanosine 3'5'-monophosphate/-cyclic phosphate) (see cGMP); Guanylic monophophate.
3':5'-GMP Guanosine 3':5'-cyclic phosphate (see GMP).
GMR Gallops, murmurs, and rubs (heart); Glucose-monitoring regimen.
GMS General Medical Service(s); General medical support; General medicine and surgery (see GM&S); Gilbert-Meulengracht syndrome; Gomori methenamine silver (stain); Glyceryl monostearate (= Monostearin) - used as a stabilizer of water-in-oil and oil-in-water emulsions; Grand mal seizure.
GM&S General medicine and surgery (= GMS).
GMSAEC General Midical Sciences Atomic

Energy Commission.
GMSC General Medical Services Committee.
GM seizure Grand mal seizure.
GMT Geometric mean titer (precipitin titer); Gingival margin trimmer; Glutamate-transpeptidase; (p-)glycoprotein-mediated transport (of drugs); Greenwich Mean Time.
GMTs Geometric mean (antibody) titers.
GMV Glass mini-sample vial; Gram molecular volume.
GMW Gluteal muscle weakness; Gram molecular weight.
GN Gaze nystagmus; Geriatric Nursing (journal); Glomerular nephritis; Glomerulonephritis; Glucose nitrogen (ratio) (see G/N); Gnotobiote; Graduate Nurse; Gram-negative.
Gn Gnathion; Gonadotropin (= Gonadotr).
G/N Glucose/nitrogen (ratio - in urine examination) (= DN; D/N; D/N R; D:N Ratio; GN; G:N; G/N R; etc.).
G:N See G/N.
G-N Glenn-Nelson (procedure).
GNA General nursing assistance.
gnath- combining form meaning jaw (Gr. gnathos).
GNB Ganglioneuroblastoma; Gram-negative bacillus/ bacteria/ium.
GNBM Gram-negative bacillary meningitis.
GNBS Gram-negative bacterial sepsis.
GNC General nursing care/ Nursing Council/ Nutrition Center.
GND Glutamate neuronal degeneration (found in Alzheimer's disease); Gram-negative diplococci (see GNID).
Gnd Ground.
GNG Gluconeogenesis.
GNID Gram-negative intracellular diplococci (= GND).
GNMA Government National Mortgage Association.
gno- combining form meaning know (Gr.).
GNP Gerontologic nurse practitioner; Gram negative pathogen; Gross National Product.
GNR Gram-negative rods.
G/N R Glucose/nitrogen ratio (see G/N).
GnRF Gonadotropin-releasing factor (see Hormones - GnRF; GTH).
GnRH Gonadotropin-releasing hormone (see Hormones - GnRH; GTH).
GnRI Gonadotropin release inhibitor.
GNRP Guanine nucleotide regulatory protein.
GNS Gram-negative sepsis/ septicemia/ stain.
G/NS Glucose in normal saline (intravenous solution).
GNTD Gastro-enteropancreatic neuroendocrine tumor disease.
GO Gastro-oesophageal (see GE); Gonorrhea (see G); Glucose oxidase.
Go Gonion.
G&O Gas and oxygen.
GΩ gigohm (one billion ohms).
GOA Gonadorelin analogue (e.g. Leuprolide - a monopeptide used in the treatment of Endometriosis, Prostatic carcinoma, Uterine fibroids, etc.).
GOAT Galveston Orientation and Amnesia Test.
GOBAB Gamma-hydroxy-beta-aminobutyric acid.
GOC General Optical/ Osteopathic (see GOsC) Council (UK).
GOD Glucose oxidase.
God's medicine Morphine (see Papaver).
GOE Gas (nitrous oxide), oxygen, and ether (anesthesia/ mixture).
GOG Gynecologic Oncology Group.
GOH Geroderma osteodysplastica hereditaria.
GOI Gonadrotropin ovarian insufficiency (see HGOI; NGOI).
GOK Go'd only knows.
Gold Concentrated marijuana (see Cannabis).
Gold dust Cocaine (see Erythroxylum).
Gold sol Colloidal gold curve.
GOMER "Get Out of My Emergency Room" - a psychosomatic patient or Somatizer/ patients with Munchausen syndrome who feign illness in order to enter hospital.
GON Gonococcal ophthalmia neonatorum.
Gon Gonococcus; Gonorrhea (see G).
gon- combining form meaning become, produce, originate (Gr.).
Gonadotr Gonadotropin (see Gn).
Gonadotr Seric Serum gonadotropin (see Hormones PMSG).
GOND Glaucomatous optic nerve damage.
GOO Gastric outlet obstruction; Giant osteoid osteoma (Orthopedics).

Goofball Barbiturate pill (see Barb - GB).

GOP Grand Old Party (= Republican Party - USA); Graves' ophthalmopathy (see GD; GHT).

GOPOPCP β,γ-methylene-guanosine triphosphate.

GOQ Glucose oxidation quotient.

GOR Gastro-oesophageal reflex/ reflux (see GER); General operating room; Glucose oxidase reaction.

GORD Gastro-oesophageal reflux disease (see GERD).

Gorilla Barbiturate pill (see Barb).

GORT Gilmore Oral Reading Test.

G Ortho Greek Orthodox (Church member).

GOsC General Osteopathic Council (UK) (= GOC).

GOSS-SSIS Goal Oriented Social Services - Social Services Information System.

GOT Glucose oxidase test; Glutamic oxalacetic transaminase (enzyme) - now known as AST (Aspartate aminotransferase) (= Glutamate oxaloacetate transaminase) (see AST); Goal of treatment.

GOTM Glutamic oxalacetic transaminase, mitochondrial.

Gov Government(al).

Gow Opium (see Papaver).

GP Du Pont code for experimental substances; Gangliocytic paraganglioma; Gastroplasty; General paralysis/ paresis/ practice/ practitioner/ psychiatrist; General Practitioner (journal); Generator potential; Genetic prediabetes; Geometric progression; German Pharmacopeia (see Ger P); Globus pallidus; Glucose phosphate; Glutathione peroxidase; Glycerol phosphate; Glycerophosphate; Glycopeptide (see GP1); Glycoprotein (= gp); Goodpasture's (syndrome) (see GPS); Graduate in Pharmacy; Gram-positive; Group (see Gp); Group practice; Group Practice (journal); Guinea pig; Gutta percha.

Gp Group (= GP; gp; grp).

gp gene product; glycoprotein (see GP); group (see Gp).

G-P Greulich-Pyle.

G/P Gravida/para.

G_p Glomerular capillary pressure.

GP1 Glycopeptide (= GP).

G-1-P Glucose-1-phosphate.

G3P; G-3-P Glyceraldehyde-3-phosphate; Glycerol-3-phosphate.

G_4P_{3104} Four pregnancies (gravida), three went to term, one premature, no abortion/ miscarriage, and 4 living children.

G6P; G-6-P Glucose-6-phosphate.

GPA Geigy USA code for experimental substances; Goodpasture antigen; Grade point average; Group Practice Association; Guinea pig albumin.

GpA Guanylyl phosphate adenosine.

$G_1P_0AB_1$ One pregnancy, no birth (para 0), and one abortion.

GPAIS Guinea pig anti-insulin serum.

GPANA Glutaryl-l-phenylalanine-p-nitroanalide.

G6Pase; G-6-Pase Glucose-6-phosphatase (enzyme); Glucose-6-phosphate phosphohydrolase.

GPB Glossopharyngeal breathing; Gram-positive bacillus/ bacterium.

GPC Gastric parietal cell(s); Gel permeation chromatography; Giant papillary conjunctivitis; Gram-positive cocci; Granular progenitor cell(s); Guanylyl phosphate cytidine (see GpC); Guinea pig complement.

GpC Guanylyl phosphate cytidine (= GPC).

GPCR G (Globulin) protein-coupled receptor (e.g. thyrotropin receptor).

GPC-S Granular progenitor cells in DNA synthesis.

GPC/TP Glycerylphophorylcholine to total phosphate.

GPD Gallons per day; Glucose-phosphate dehydrogenase (see G6PD); Glyceraldehyde 3-phosphate dehydrogenase; Growth-promoting (anabolic) drug (such as Oxandrolone).

G5PD; G-5-PD Glucose-5-phosphate dehydrogenase.

G6PD; G-6-PD Glucose-6-phosphate dehydrogenase (= BBS: GPD; G-6-PD; G-sixPD; PD; PDG; PDH; PGD; 6-PGD; PGDH) - an enzyme of which, the deficiency or absence in the red cells, results in an acute hemolytic anemia; this is associated with the ingestion of the fava or broad bean, or exposure to small quantities of drugs such as barbiturates, sulfa drugs, and anti-malarial compounds.

The disease is known as favism, the broad-bean syndrome, or the G6PD syndrome.
G6PDA; G-6-PDA Glucose-6-phosphate dehydrogenase enzyme variant A.
GPDH Glycerol phosphate dehydrogenase.
G6PDH; G-6-PDH Glucose-6-phosphate dehydrogenase reduced.
GPDM Good practice in decision-making.
GPE General physical examination (see FPE); Growth promoting effect; Guinea pig embryo.
GPEP General Professional Education of the Physician.
GPF Glomerular plasma flow; Good practice framework; Granulocytosis-/ Growth-promoting factor; Gross pathological finding(s).
GPFD Genetic, phenotypic, and functional diversity (in SCID patients).
GPG Good practice guideline(s).
GPg Guinea pig.
GPGG Guinea pig gamma-globulin.
GPH Galactopoietic hormone (see Hormones - GPH; LH i).
GPh Graduate in Pharmacy.
GPHN Giant pigmented hairy nevus.
GPHV Guinea pig herpes virus.
GPI General paralysis/ paresis of the insane; Glucose phosphate isomerase; Glycoprotein I; Guinea pig ileum/ inoculation.
GpIb Glycoprotein Ib.
GPIMH Guinea pig intestinal mucosal homogenase.
GPIPID Guinea pig intraperitoneal infectious disease.
GPK Guinea pig kidney (antigen).
GPKA Guinea pig kidney absorption (test).
GPL Geriatric protein loss; Granulomatous pulmonary lesion; Growth-promoting ligament (see LKAL).
G-PLT Giant platelet(s).
GPLV Guinea pig leukemia virus.
Gply Gingivoplasty.
GPM General preventive medicine; Genetic polymorphism; Giant pigmented melanosome; Good patient management; Growth-promoting molecule (see SLAM).
GPMAL Gravida, para, multiple births, abortions, and live births.
GPMT Guinea pig maximisation test.
GPN Glossopharyngeal nerve/ neuralgia; Graduate Practical Nurse.
GPO General Post Office; Government Printing Office; Great Plains Organization.
GPOA Guild of Prescription Opticians of America, Inc.
GPOPH Great Plains Organization for Perinatal Health (Care).
GPP Global Pharmacy Practice; Glycated plasma protein; Gram positive pathogen.
GPPQ General Purpose Psychiatric Questionnaire.
GPPT Group Personality Projective Test.
GPRA General Practice Reform Association (GB).
GPRBC Guinea pig red blood cell.
GPRG General Practice Research Group (GB).
GPS Global positioning system (monitor/ satellite); Goodpasture's syndrome (= GP); Good performance status; Grass pollen sensitivity; Gray platelet syndrome; Growth-promoting substance; Guinea pig serum/ spleen.
GPT Glutamic-pyruvic transaminase (enzyme) (= Glutamate-pyruvate t.) - now known as ALT (see ALT); Gravindex pregnancy test; Group psychotherapy.
GpTh Group therapy.
GPU Guinea pig unit.
GpU Guanylyl phosphate uridine.
GPUT Galactose phosphate uridyl transferase.
GPx Glutathione peroxidase.
GQAP General question-asking program.
GR Gag reflex (occurs in SIV - Self-induced vomiting, as in bulimia); Gamma ray(s); Gastric resection; Gastrin receptor; General research; Generalized rash; Glucocorticoid receptor; Glutathione reductase; Gonda reflex (similar to Babinski); Reagent grade (see RG).
Gr Greek (= G; Gk).
gr gamma roentgen (unit); grade; graft; grain (L. granum) - the twentieth part of a scruple (ε or 0.065 g) (one gram = 15.432 grains); gram; graphite; gravity (see G. Gravity); gray/ grey; gross.
gr- gram-negative (see GrN).
gr+ gram-positive (see GrP).
G- R Gram-negative rods.

G+ R Gram-positive rods.
GRA Gated radionuclide angiography; Glucocorticoid-remedial aldosteronism; Glycoprotein-receptor antagonist (IIb/IIIa) (see PGRA); Gombart's reducing agent; Gonadotropin-releasing agent.
GRABS Group A beta-hemolytic streptococcal pharyngitis.
Grace Graphic Arts Composing Equipment.
Grad Graduate.
grad gradient; gradually (by degrees) (L. gradatim); graduate(d).
grad- combining form meaning walk (L. gradior).
GRAE Generally regarded as effective.
-gram suffix meaning record or write (Gr. graph).
GRAMEC Grand Rapids Area Medical Education Corporation.
GRAN Gombart's reducing agent negative.
gran granular/lated/le (L. granulatus).
gran- combining form meaning record or write (Gr. graph).
GRAS Generally recognized/ regarded as safe (with reference to food additives - FDA).
Graser Nuclear-pumped or gamma-ray laser.
GRASS Gradient recalled acquisition in the steady state.
Grass Marijuana (see Cannabis).
gravid gravid (pregnant); gravida (pregnancy); gravity (see G. Gravity).
grav I; grav i first pregnancy, pregnancy one, or primigravida.
grav II; grav ii etc. second pregnancy, etc.
grav I/Ab I one pregnancy, one abortion.
grav o no pregnancies.
GRAY Gombart's reducing agent positive (yes).
Gray A unit of ionizing radiation equal to 100 rads (see Gy).
Grb Gerbil. A small burrowing rodent, Gerbillus interonia, native on the veldt of South Africa, one of the chief agents transmitting plague.
GRBD General Reference and Bibliography Division (LC - Library of Congress).
GRC Gerontological Research Center (NIA); Glutathione redox cycle.
GRCT Gastro-resistant coated tablet.
GRD Gastroesophageal reflux disease; Gender-related difference; Gender role definition; Gene-related disease/ disorder; Gibson-Ross dermatome (for skin grafting).
grd ground.
GRE Gradient-recalled echo; Graduate Record Examination.
Green Marijuana (see Cannabis).
Grefa Marijuana (see Cannabis).
Greta Marijuana (see Cannabis).
GRF Gastrin-releasing factor; Gelatin resorcinol formaldehyde (adhesive); Genetically-related (macrophage) factor; Genetic risk factor; Glaucoma Research Foundation; Gonadotropin-releasing factor (see Hormones - GTH); Growth (hormone)-releasing factor (see Hormones - GH-RH).
GR-FA Grandfather.
GRG Gender-related gene; Glycine-rich glycoprotein.
GRH Gonadotropin-releasing hormone (see Hormones - GTH); Growth (hormone)-releasing hormone (see Hormones - GH-RH).
GRID Gay-related immune/ immuno deficiency (syndrome) (see AIDS).
GRIF Growth (hormone) release-inhibiting factor (see Hormones - GRIF; GH-IH).
Grifa Marijuana cigarette (see Cannabis).
GRISA Research Group on Automated Scientific Information (Fr. Groupe de recherches sur l'information scientifique automatique / part of Euratom).
GR-IH Growth (hormone) release-inhibiting hormone (see Hormones - GH-IH).
grippe Influenza (see la grippe).
GRK Gamma-radiation knife.
GRL Genetic Reference Laboratory.
Grm; grm Gram (see Gm).
GR-MO Grandmother.
GRN Granules.
GrN Gram-negative (= gr-).
Grn Green.
GRO General Register Office.
Gr Orth Greek Orthodox (Church member).
gros coarse (L. grossus).
Grow Growth (journal).
GRP Gastrin-releasing peptide; General reproductive performance; Glucose-regulated protein; Good research practice.

GrP Gram-positive (= gr+).
grp group (see Gp).
$Gr_1P_0AB_1$ One pregnany, no births, one abortion.
GRPS Gastrin-releasing peptide stimulation (see APG; GAS); Glucose-Ringer-phosphate solution.
GRR Good response rate.
GRS Glycopeptide resistant strain (of organisms, such as *Enterococcus*); Golabi-Rosen syndrome.
GRT Gastric residence time; Gastro-resistant tablet (film-coated); Graduate Respiratory Therapist.
Gr Tr Graphite treatment.
GRTT Graduate Respiratory Therapist Technician.
Grüner Türke Marijuana (see Cannabis).
GRW Giant ragweed (test).
gr wt gross weight.
GS Gallstone; Gamma scan (with use of gallium); Gardner/ Gilbert/ Goldenhar/ Goodpasture's syndrome; Gastric shield; "Geek" syndrome (also known as Asperger syndrome or the "little professor" syndrome, a form of genetic autism; see ORB; SMC); General semantics/ surgery; Generalized seizure; Gerontological Society, Inc.; Gingivostomatitis; Glomerular sclerosis; Glucose and saline (see G/S); Glucosamine sulfate; Glutamine synthetase; Goat serum; Goltz syndrome (see FDH); Gourmand syndrome (a neurological condition characterized by an unusual passion for eating); Gradenigo's syndrome (osteitis of the petrous apex); Graft survival; Gram stain; Granulocytic sarcoma; Grip strength; Group section; Group-specific (antigen - see G-S); Gynecology and Sociology (journal, now MGAS); Pfizer Ltd (England) code for experimental substances.
GS# Graft-site fracture (see GSF).
gs group-specific (see G-S).
G/S Glucose and saline (= GS).
G-S Gastrocnemius-semimembranosus (muscle); Group-specific (antigen) (= GS; gs).
g/s gallons per second.
G6S Glucosamine-6-sulfatase.
GS 95 Thiethylperazine maleate. Used as an anti-emetic in post-operative vomiting, and vomiting associated with pregnancy, malignant disease, radiotherapy, and treatment with cytotoxic drugs.
GS 2876 Methacycline hydrochloride. An antibiotic belonging to the tetracycline group.
GSA General Services Administration; General somatic afferent (nerve); Gerontological Society of America; Girl Scouts of America; Gross structural anomalies/ly (of the fetus - Obstetrics); Gross virus antigen; Group-specific antigen; Guanidinosuccinic acid.
GSA65 Gross virus antigen (= GSA).
GSB; γSB Gamma-secretase blocker (used in treating Alzheimer's disease).
GSBG Gonadal steroid-binding globulin.
GSC Gas-solid chromatography; General supportive care; Genome Sequence Center (Toronto, Washington, etc.); Gravity-settling culture (plate).
GSCN Giant serotonin-containing neuron (= GSN).
G score Gleason score (a calculation indicating prostate cancer's level of aggressiveness/ metastasis).
GSCP General standard of care provided.
GSD Genetically significant dose; Gerstmann-Sträussler disease; Glutathione synthetase deficiency; Glucogen/ Glycogen storage disease.
GSD-1 Glucocerebroside/ Glycogen storage disease, type 1.
GSD II Glycogenose type II.
GSD IV Glycogen storage disease-type IV (= Amylopectinosis; Andersen's disease).
GSE General somatic efferent (nerve); Genital self-examination; Gluten-sensitive enteropathy; Grip strong and equal.
GSF Galactosemic fibroblast; Genital skin fibroblast; Graft-site fracture (= GS#).
GSH Glomerular/ulus - stimulating hormone (see Hormones - GSH); Glutathione (reduced form) (= Reduced glatathione; Glutathione SH). A naturally occurring tripeptide in living tissue. Has been used in hepatic cirrhosis as a detoxicating agent; Golden Syrian hamster; Growth stimulating hormone.
GSH/GSSG Oxidized to reduced glutathione

ratio.

GSH Px Glutathione peroxidase (activity).

GSI Association for Heavy Ion Research (Ger. Gesellschaft für Schwerionenforschung); Genuine stress incontinence; Glucan synthesis inhibitor (an antifungal drug); Gunshot injury (see GSW).

g_{si} inward polarizing current in the "slow" channels.

GSIS Glucose-stimulated insulin secretion.

G-six PD Glucose-6-phosphate dehydrogenase (see G6PD).

GSK Glaxo Smith Kline (pharmaceutical firm).

GSM General supportive measure(s); Gene-sequencing machine; Genetically susceptible mice/ mouse; Glucose self-monitoring (see BGSM).

GSMP German Society of Medical Physics.

GSN Giant serotonin-containing neuron (see GSCN).

GSoA Gerontological Society of America.

GSOST Goldstein-Scheerer Object Sorting Test.

GSP Galvanic skin potential; General survey panel; Genome-sequencing project; Gonadal steroid production; Good safety profile; Good standards of practice.

GSpl Gibbon (normal) spleen.

GSPN Greater superficial petrosal nerve; Greater superficial petrosal neurectomy.

G Spot Gräfenberg Spot. A so-called, bean-shaped erogenous zone consisting of a patch of erectile tissue in the front wall of the vagina, directly behind the pubic bone, and said to act something like a second clitoris. This spot has been called the "female prostate gland", and when stimulated by deep pressure, has been known to produce vaginal orgasm, distinctly different from clitoral orgasm. The presence of this so-called "spot" is still controversial, and as yet, without any anatomical evidence of its existence in women.

GSR Galvanic skin reflex/ resistance/ response (compare with basal skin resistance BSR); Generalized Schwartzman reaction; 'Glue sniffer's rash' (erythematous spots around the mouth and nose) (see VSA); Glutathione reductase (= Gss Rase); Graft survival rate.

GSRI Gulf South Research Institute.

GSS Gamete-shedding substance; General Social Survey; Gerstmann-Sträussler-Scheinker (disease/ syndrome) - a spongiform encephalopathy, affecting humans; Gluten-sensitive steatorrhea.

GSSG Oxidized glutathione (see GSH).

GSSR Generalized Sandarelli-Schwartzman reaction.

Gss Rase Glutathione reductase (see GSR).

GST Gastric secretion test (see PST); General supportive therapy/ treatment; Glucagon stimulation test; Glutathione-S-transferase; Glycogen storage test (see LFT iv); Gold salt therapy; Gold sodium thiomalate; Gold standard test (for assessing renal and other organ function); Graphic stress telethermometry; Group striction.

GSTM Gold sodium thiomalate (= GST).

G-Strep Non-hemolytic streptococcus.

G suit Gravity suit.

GSV Greater saphenous vein.

GSW Gunshot wound.

GSWA Gunshot wound, abdominal.

GT Gait; Gait training; Gamma-glutamyl-transferase; Gastrostomy/rotomy (tube); Generation time; Gene therapy (see HGT)/ transfer; Genetic/ Group therapy; Gingiva treatment; Glanzmann's thrombasthenia (see GTA); Glucagon test (see LFT iv); Glucose therapy/ tolerance/ transport; Glucuronyl transferase; Glutamyl transpeptidase (see GTP); Glycityrosine; Gore-Tex (graft); Granulation time/ tissue (see g/t); Gravindex test (for pregnancy); Great toe; Greater trochanter; Group tensions; Shortened form for SGOT.

gt drop (L. gutta); granulation time/ tissue (see g/t).

g/t granulation time/ tissue (= GT; gt).

G&T Gowns and towels.

GT 41 Busulfan (= Busulphan; CB 2041; Myelosan; Tetramethylene dimethanesulfonate). A cytotoxic agent having a selective depressant action on bone marrow. Used in the treatment of chronic myeloid leukemia.

GTA Gene transfer agent; Genetic toxicology/

Genotoxic activity/ assay; Glanzmann's thrombasthenia (= GT); Glycerol teichoic acid.

GTB Gastrointestinal tract bleeding.

GTC Generalized tonic convulsion(s); Glycerol-tellurite culture (medium).

GTCC Generalized tonic-clonic convulsion(s).

GTCS Generalized tonic-clonic seizure.

GTD Genetically transmitted disease/ disorder (= GTI); Gestational trophoblastic disease.

GTE Gene therapy experiment.

GTF Gastrostomy tube feeding; Glucose tolerance factor; Glucosyltransferase.

GTFC Genetic testing of fertilized cell (see PGD).

GT1-GT10 Glycogen storage disease, types 1-10.

GTH Gonadotropic hormone (= Gonadotrophic h) (see Hormones - GTH).

GTHR Generalized thyroid hormone resistance.

GTI Genetically transmitted illness (see GTD); Genital tract infection.

GTM Generalized tendomyopathy.

GTN Gestational trophoblastic neoplasia; Glomerulotubulonephritis; Glyceryl trinitrate.

GTO Golgi tendon organ.

GTP Ganciclovir-triphosphate; Gene therapy patient/ procedure/ program/ protocol; General toxic phenomenona/menon; General toxicity profile; Genotoxic potential; Glucose transporter protein; Glucosyltransferase (enzyme); Glucuronyl transferase pathway; Glutamyl transpeptidase (= Gamma-glutamyl transpeptidase; GT; γ-GT) (activity); Guanosine triphophate.

GTPC Gene Therapy Policy Conference.

GTR Galvanic tetanus ratio; Gene therapy research; Granulocyte turnover rate.

GTS Generalized tonic seizure; Gene therapy study; Genital tract sample/ swab; Genotoxicity study; Getting to sleep; Gilles de la Tourette syndrome; Glucose transport system; Grey-Turner's sign (discoloration of the flanks and costovertebral angles, seen in ruptured abdominal aortic aneurysm and acute pancreatitis).

$GTS_{0\text{-}2\,hr}$ Glucose tolerance sum for two hours.

GTT Gastric (see GET)/ Gut transit time; Gelatin-tellurite-taurocholate (agar); Genotoxicity test; Glucose tolerance test (= GITT) (see LFT iv).

gtt drops (L. guttae).

GTT 3H Glucose tolerance test, 3 hours (oral).

gtts drops (see gtt).

GU Gastric/ Gravitational ulcer; Genitourinary; Glucose uptake; Glycogenic/ Gutman unit; Gonococcal urethritis; Guanethidine.

GUA Group of units of analysis.

Gua Guanine.

GUAs Genitourinary (Renal) anomalies (such as Double ureters, Hydronephrosis, Multicystic kidney, and Renal agenesis. These anomalies may exist alone or in combination with other abnormalities such as Duodenal atresia, Meckel's diverticulum, Potter facias, etc. (see DRMs).

Guaza Marijuana (see Cannabis).

GUC Genitourinary clinic; Glucose utilization curve.

GUD Gastric ulcer disease (see PUD); Genitourinary disorder.

GUI Genitourinary infection.

Guid Guidance.

GULHEMP General physique, upper extremity, lower extremity, hearing, eyesight, mentality, and personality.

GUM Genito-urinary medicine (Venereology) (UK).

Gum Raw opium (see Papaver).

GUMC Georgetown University Medical Center.

Gunga Marijuana (see Cannabis).

GUO Genito-urinary oncology.

Guo Guanosine.

GUP Genito-urinary procedure.

GUR Global utility rate.

GUS Genitourinary sphincter/ symptoms/ system.

GUSAP Group for Utilization and Study of Articular Prostheses.

GUSM Georgetown University School of Medicine.

GUSTO-1 Global Utilization of Streptokinase

and Tissue plasminogen activator for Occluded coronary arteries - 1 (trial).

GUT Genito-urinary tract.

Gut (journal).

gutt to the throat (L. gutturi).

guttat drop by drop (L. guttatim).

guttatai Little "bumps" on back of cornea (a degenerative condition).

gutt quibusd with a few drops (L. guttis quibusdam).

GUU Guanylyl uridylyl uridine.

GV Gastric volume; Gentian violet (dye); Genu valgum/ varum; Germinal vesicle; Granulosis/ Gross virus; Griseo-viridan/din.

GVA General visceral afferent (nerve).

GVB Gelatin-Veronal buffer.

GVBD Germinal vesicle breakdown.

GVE General visceral efferent (nerve).

GVF Goldmann/ Good visual field(s).

GVG Gamma-vinyl-gamma-aminobutyric acid; Greater vestibular gland (one of two small glands located on the lower vaginal wall, which help lubricate the vagina) (= Bartholin's gland).

GvG Graft-versus-graft (reaction).

GVGHA Genessee Valley Group Health Association.

GVH; GvH Graft-versus-host (see GvsH).

GVHD; GvHD Graft-versus-host disease.

GVHR; GvHR Graft-versus-host reaction.

GVL Graft-versus-leukemia.

GVN Gentamycin, Vancomycin, and Nystatin. A combination of oral non-absorbable antibiotics (see FRACON).

GvsH Graft-versus-host (homologous/ runt/ transplantation disease) (= GVH; GvH).

GVTY; Gvty Gingivectomy.

GVV *Gardnerella* vaginalis vaginitis (= bacterial vaginosis, *Haemophilus* vaginitis, or non-specific vaginitis/nosis) (see NSV).

GW General Ward; Germ warfare; Gigawatt (see Gw); Glucose/ Glycerin(e) in water (see G/W); Gradual withdrawel; Group work.

Gw Gigawatt (= 10^9 watt).

G/W Glucose in water (intravenous solution) (= GW); Glycerin(e) in water (enema) (= GW) (see GWE).

GWA Gunshot wound of the abdomen.

GWDC Guide wire and dilatation catheter (Coronary angioplasty).

GWE Glycerin(e)/rol and water enema (procedure/ enema) (= GW; G/W).

GWH Gunshot wound in the head.

GWI Gulf War Illness (a malady characterized by fatigue, headaches and arthritis, and supposedly caused by infection with *Mycoplasma* fermentans. Most of the symptoms are also present in, and the sickness confounded with, CFS (Chronic fatigue syndrome) and FMS (Fibromyalgia syndrome) (see GWS).

GWIA Goodwill Industries of America.

GWG Generalized Wegener's granulomatosus.

GWS Gulf war syndrome (Kuwait-Iraq border - 1991).

GWSF Georgia Warm Springs Foundation.

GWT Gunshot wound of the throat.

GWU George Washington University (Washington, DC).

GWUSM George Washington University School of Medicine.

GX Glycinexylidide.

GXP Graded exercise program.

GXT Graded exercise test (procedure/ cardiology).

Gy Gray/ Grey - a unit of ionizing radiation equal to 100 rads (= 1 J/kg).

GYN; Gyn; gyn Gynecologic/gist/gy.

gyn- combining form meaning female, wife, or woman (Gr. gyne).

gyr- prefix meaning circle or ring (Gr. gyros).

Gyro Gyroscope.

GZ Ground zero (the point on the earth's surface at the center of a nuclear explosion); Guilford-Zimmerman (personality test).

GZI Globin zinc insulin (see Insulin - GI; GZI).

GZMO Genzyme Molecular Oncology (US pharmaceutical firm).

GZTS Guilford-Zimmerman Temperament Survey.

H

H A draft (L. haustus); Bacterial antigen in serologic classification of bacteria (Ger. Hauch = film); Deflection in the His bundle in the electrocardiogram (spike); Electrically induced spinal reflex; Enthalpy; Flagella (with reference to antigens/ bacteriology); Fucosal transferase-producing gene; Halothane (an inhalation anesthetic/ chemical name: 2-bromo-2-chloro-1,1,1-trifluoroethane); Hanfkraut (Marijuana - see Cannabis); H antigen (Flagellar a. - see Hauch); Hashish (Marijuana - see Cannabis); Hauch (Ger.) = breath - denoting the flagellate or motile type of a microorganism, as contrasted with the O (ohne Hauch) or nonmotile type (e.g. H antigen or flagellar antigen); Haustus (L.) = a draft/ draught (= h; Haust) (e.g. H niger = black draft); Heart (see Ht); Heavy; Height (see ht); Hemagglutination; Hemisphere; Hemolysis; Hemophilus; Henry = unit of electric(al) induction/ inductance (= h); Heparin; Hernia (protrusion of an organ or tissue through an abnormal opening, popularly known as a "rupture", e.g. Inguinal H - a hernia into the inguinal canal); Heroin (see Diamorph); Herpes = an inflammatory skin lesion, characterized by the formation of small vesicles in clusters, e.g. H. zoster (= Acute posterior ganglionitis; shingles; zona; zoster) - an acute inflammation of the posterior nerve ganglion. It is caused by the virus of chicken-pox and produces clusters of inflamed vesicles in skin areas supplied by certain nerve trunks); High; His (potential) (see H potential); Histamine (see H-subst); Histidine; Histoplasma; Histoplasmosis; Hoffmann (reflex) (see H-reflex); Holzknecht (Unit) or H unit = a unit of X-ray dosage equal to one fifth (1/5) of the erythema dose; Homosexual (see Homo); Hora (L.) an hour (= h; Hr; hr); Horizontal (= h): i) Parallel to the plane of the horizon, ii) Upright position of the body (anatomical orientation); Hormone - any chemical substance produced in the body (but later the term has been applied to any substance having similar action, not necessarily secreted by an endocrine gland), which has a specific effect on the activity of a certain organ or organs (see Hormones); Horse (in veterinary medicine); Hospital; Hounsfield (unit); Hour (see h); H-response - exaggerated photic response (see H-response); Human (= h); Husband; Hyaluronidase; Hydrogen (Z = 1) (see Elements - Hydrogen); Hydrolysis; Hygiene; Hyoscine (scolopamine); Hypermetropia; Hyperopia; Hyperplasia; Hypo; Hypodermic (needle) (= h); Hypothalamus; Magnetic field strength; Magnetization; Mustard gas (a war gas); Oersted (a unit of magnetizing force); Planck's constant (see h); Quantum constant (= Planck's c) (see h); Sodium idohippurate; The region of a sarcomere containing only myosin (Ger. heller = lighter {band}).

h hand-rearing (of experimental animals); haustus (L.) a draft (see H. Haustus); heat transfer coefficient; hecto (prefix for 100) (see hecto-); height (see ht); henry (inductance unit) (see H. Henry); hora (L.) hour (see H); horizontal (see H. Horizontal); hormone (see H. Hormone; Hormones); hour (L. hora) (= H); human (see H); hundred; hypodermic (see H); negatively staining region of a chromosome; Planck's constant (represents the ratio of the energy of any quantum of radiation to its frequency) i.e. h = 6.55 x 10^{-27} erg seconds (= H; Quantum constant); Quantum constant (= H; Planck's constant).

H^+ Hydrogen ion.

$[H^+]$ Hydrogen ion concentration.

Ⓗ Hypodermic injection (medication order).

H_0 Null hypothesis.

H1; H^1; ^1H Protium (light hydrogen) (chemical symbol for).

H1 Alternative hypothesis.

H-1 Para-aminobenzoic acid.

2H Hiatal hernia.

H2; H^2; ^2H; H^b Deuterium (= Deutium) (chemical symbol for heavy hydrogen, or mass 2 isotope hydrogen).

H_2 (blockers) Histamine blockers.

H-2 Diethylaminoethanol; Mouse histocompatibility-2 complex.

h^2 heritability index.

3H High, hot, and a hellavu lot.

H3; H^3; ^{3}H Tritium.

H-3; H_3 Procaine hydrochloride. A 2% procaine solution buffered at pH 4.3, used in Prof. Anna Aslan claims for "treatment of old age and atherosclerosis" in Bucharest, Romania.

H-11; H_{11} Human urine extract containing growth-inhibiting substances or growth inhibitors. A non-toxic product, said to inhibit growth of cancerous tumors.

H 940 Ethosuximide (= PM 671; α-Ethyl-α-methylsuccimide; $C_7H_{11}NO_2$) - an anticonvulsant used in the treatment of petit mal epilepsy.

H 990 Oxymetazoline hydrochloride. Used in 0.05% solution as a local vasoconstrictor to relieve nasal congestion.

HA H antigen (flagellar a); Hakim-Adams (syndrome); Halothane anesthesia; Hartley (guinea pig); Headache; Health Affairs (journal); Health Authority; Hearing aid; Height age; Hemadsorption (virus) (see HA virus); Hemagglutinating antibody; Hemagglutination (see HAgg); Hemagglutinin (see HAgg); Hemagglutinin activity; Hemolytic anemia; Hemophiliac with adenopathy; Hepatic adenoma/ artery; Hepatitis A; Hepatitis-associated (virus); Heterophil antibody (e.g. in infectious mononucleosis); Heyden antibiotic; High anxiety; Hippuric/ Hyaluronic acid; Histamine; Histocompatibility antigen; Honeywill-Atlas Laboratories code for experimental substances; Horton's arteritis; Hospital administration/ admission/ apprentice; H substance (histamine-like action); Human albumin; Hydroxyapatite (see HAP); Hyperalimentation; Hyperandrogenism; Hypermetropic astigmatism; Hypersensitivity alveolitis; Hypothalamic amenorrhea.

Ha Absolute/tion hypermetropia; Hahnium (Z = 105) (see Elements - Hahnnium); Hamster; Hartmann number.

ha hectare.

H/A Head to abdomen.

H&A Health and accident (insurance) (= H&A Ins).

HA1 Hemadsorption (virus), type 1 (see HA virus).

HA2 Hemadsotption (virus), type 2 (see HA virus).

HA 560 (Honeywill-Atlas) A brand of macrogel 600 monostearate.

HA 621 (Honeywill-Atlas) A brand of propylene glycol monostearate.

HAA Hearing aid amplifier; Hemolytic anemia antigen; Hepatitis-associated antigen/ antibody - type B (= Australia antigen/ antibody); HbAb; HbAg); Heterocyclic acetic acid (NSAID); Hospital activity analysis; Human autoantibody; Hyperactive appetite (as in Prader-Willi syndrome).

HA Ag Hepatitis A antigen.

HAART Highly active anti-retroviral therapy (e.g. AZT, ddI and Indinavir combination).

HAAS Honolulu-Asia Aging Study (of risk factors in VaD - Vascular dementia) (= HHP).

HAB Antiheart antibody; Hemangioblastoma (see HLD; H-LD; HLS).

HABA Hydroxybenzeneazobenzoic acid.

HABF Hepatic artery blood flow.

habit habitat.

HABMT Human allogeneic bone marrow transplantation (= AMT).

HAC Hanging arm cast; High alcohol consumption; Human artificial chromosome; Hyperadrenocorticism/icoid.

HAc Acetic acid; Hemagglutin activitiy on chick.

HACA Human anti-chimeric antibody.

HACCP Hazard Analysis Critical Control Point (USDA).

HAChT High affinity choline transport.

HACI Hydroxyapatite-coated implant (see HACPD).

HACP Hydroxyapatite-coated prosthesis (see HACPD).

HACPD Hydroxyapatite-coated prosthetic device (= HACI; HACP).

HACR Hereditary adenomatosis of the cholon and rectum.

HACS Hazard Assessment Computer System (USCG); Hyperactive child syndrome.

hACSP Human adenylate cyclase-stimulating protein.

HAD Healthcare Advance Directive; Heart-assist device; Hereditary areflexic dysstasia

(Roussy-Lévy); Human adjuvant disease; Hypogonadic androgen deficiency.

HAD; HAd Hemadsorption (= Had); Hospital administration/ator.

Had Hemadsorption (see HAD; HAd).

Had 15 Hadamard Imaging Spectrometer.

HADD Hyperactive attention-deficit disorder (see ADD; ADDH; ADD/HA; ADHD).

HAd-I Hemadsorption-inhibition.

HADS Hospital Anxiety and Depression Scale.

HAE Health appraisal examination; Hearing aid evaluation; Hepatic artery embolism; Hereditary angioedema; Hereditary angioneurotic edema; Highly acidic environment.

haem haemolysis (with reference to blood fragility test).

haem- prefix meaning blood (Gr. aima).

haemat haematocrit; haematologist/gy (see haematol).

haematol haematologist/gy (= haematol).

haemorrh haemorrhage.

HAET Hippuric acid excretion test (see LFT iv).

HAF Healing Alternatives Foundation (San Francisco).

HaF Hageman factor.

Haff Myoglobinuria.

HAFMC Haight-Asbury Free Medical Clinic.

HAFMR Hellenic Armed Forces Medical Review.

HAFP Human alpha-fetoprotein.

HAG Heat-aggregated globulin; *Helicobacter*-associated gastritis (= Pangastritis) (see APG); Heterophil agglutination (test for mononucleosis); Human antihemophilic globulin.

HA_G Hemagglutinin activity on guinea pig.

HAGA Hereditary androgenetic alopecia.

HAGG Hyperimmune antivariola gamma globulin.

HAgg Hemagglutination/tinin (= HA) (e.g. Rubella HAgg).

HAGH Hydroxyacyl-glutathione hydrolase.

HAHTG Horse antihuman thymus globulin.

HAI Heavy/ High alcohol ingestion/ intake; Hemagglutination inhibition (laboratory procedure/ test - hematology); Hepatic arterial infusion; Histologic Activity Index; Hospital-acquired infection (see NCI); Humoral autoimmunity.

HAIC Hearing Aid Industrial Conference.

H&A Ins Health and Accident Insurance (see H&A).

HAIR-AN Hyperandrogenism, insulin resistance, and acanthosis nigricans (syndrome).

HAIT Hemagglutination inhibition test/ titer.

HaK Hamster kidney.

HAL Hepatic artery ligation; Hybridization assay limit (solution); Hyperalimentation; Hypoplastic acute leukemia.

Hal; hal Halogen; Halothane.

HALA Hemangiolymphangioma (see FGHL).

HALC High affinity-low capacity.

Half-life (= HL; T1/2; $T_{1/2}$; τ1/2; $\tau_{1/2}$; t1/2; $t_{1/2}$) 1. The time needed for a radioactive substance to lose half of its activity through decay; 2. The time needed for a drug's level in the blood stream to descend to one half of its former level. Examples are:

BHL - Biologic half-life (the time required for the body to eliminate one half of any drug or substance entering it) (= MHL).

EHL - Effective half-life (the time needed for a radioactive element in an animal body to be diminished 50% as a result of the combined action of radiooactive decay and biological elimination) (= RHL).

MHL - Metabolic half-life (= Biologic half-life - see).

RHL - Radioactive half-life (= Effective half-life - see).

Halluc; halluc Hallucination(s).

HALO Halothane.

HALP Hyperalphalipoproteinemia.

HaLV Hamster leukemia virus.

HAM Hearing aid microphone; Helical axis in motion; Hinge axis movement (one of two movements in opening of mouth); Human albumin microspheres; Human alveolar macrophage; Hyperabduction maneuver (i.e. sideward elevation of the arm beyond 90 degrees); Hypoparathyroidism, Addison's disease, and mucocutaneous candidiasis (syndrome).

HAm Human amnion.

Ham Hamster.

HAMA Hamilton Anxiety (scale) (see HAM-

A); Human anti-mouse/ anti-murine antibody.
HAM-A Hamilton Anxiety (scale) (= HAMA).
HAMD; HAM-D Hamilton Depression (scale).
HAMLET Human Alpha-lactalbumin Made Lethal to Tumor cells (see αLA).
Ha-MSV Harvey murine sarcoma virus.
HAN Heroin-associated nephropathy; Hyperplastic alveolar nodule(s).
HANA Hemagglutinin neuraminidase.
H and C Hot and cold (see H/C; H&C).
H and E Hematoxylin and eosin (stain).
Handicp Handicapped.
HANE Hereditary angioneurotic edema.
HANES Health and Nutrition Examination Survey (HRA).
hANF Human atrial natriuretic factor.
h-ANP Human atrial natriuretic polypeptide.
H antigen Flagellar antigen (the antigen localized in the flagella of motile bacteria - from the Ger. Hauch = breath) (see H. Hauch).
HANYS Hospital Association of New York State.
HAP Handicapped Aid Program; Heart-attack patient; Heredopathia atactica polyneuritiformis; High-amplitude peristalsis; Hip arthroplasty; Histamine acid phosphate; Hospital-acquired pneumonia; Humoral antibody production; Hydrolyzed animal protein; Hydroxyapatite (= HA).
HAPA Hemagglutinating anti-penicillin antibody.
HAPC High-amplitude peristaltic contraction; Hospital-acquired penetration contact.
HAPE High-altitude pulmonary edema.
HAPO Hyperglycemia and Adverse Pregnancy Outcome (study) (NIH).
HAPP Heart Attack Prevention Program; Hospital Admission Precertification Program.
HAPPAs High air-pollution-potential advisories.
HAPPHY Heart Attack Primary Prevention in Hypertension.
"Happy Pill" 5-adenosyl-L-methionine (see "Sammy").
HAPS Hepatic arterial perfusion scintigraphy.
hapt- prefix meaning to touch or seize (Gr. apto).
HAPTO Haptoglobin.
HAQ Headache/ Health Assessment Questionnaire.
HAR Heart-attack risk; Hematological adverse reaction(s); High-altitude retinopathy; Hyperacute rejection (of organ transplant).
H-Ara-C H-arabinosyl-cytosine.
HARC Human Affairs Research Center.
HAREM Heparin assay rapid easy method.
HARH High-altitude retinal hemorrhage.
HARM Heparin assay rapid method.
Harm Harmonic.
HARQ Hearing Attitudes in Rehabilitation Questionnaire (NHS).
Harry Heroin (see Diamorph HCl).
HARS Hamilton Anxiety Rating Scale (= HAS); Histidyl-RNA synthetase.
HART Heparin-Aspirin Reinfarction Trial.
Hart John A. Hartford Foundation.
HAS Hamilton Anxiety Scale (see HARS); Health advisory service; Health Application Systems; Highest asymptomatic (dose) (see HASD); Hospital adjustment scale; Hospital Administration Services; Hospital administrative/ advisory service(s); Hospital Albert Schweitzer (Deschapelles, Haiti); Hospital Ambulance Service; Human-adapted strain (of a parasite); Human adult serum; Human albumin solution; Human autopsy specimen; Hyperalimentation solution; Hypertension-associated stroke; Hypertensive arteriosclerotic.
HAs Highest asymptomatic (dose) (see HASD).
HASB Hospital and Ambulance Services Branch (USPHS).
HASCVD Hypertensive arteriosclerotic cardiovascular disease (= HASHD; H&ASHD; HCVD; HTCVD; HTHD; HTVD; HVD).
HASD Highest asymptomatic dose (= HAS; HAs).
Hash Hashish (see Cannabis).
HASHD Hypertensive arteriosclerotic heart disease (see HASCVD).
H&ASHD Hypertensive and arteriosclerotic heart disease (see HASCVD).
HASP Hospital Admissions and Surveillance Program.

HAT Halsted Aphasia Test; Head, arm and trunk; Hearing aid technology; Heart-allogenic transplant; Hemadsorption test (see Ha test); Heparin-associated thrombocytopenia; Hepatic n-acetyl-transferase; Heterophil agglutination test (for mononucleosis); Heterophil antibody titer; Hospital arrival time; Hypoxanthine, aminopterin/ azaserine, and thymidine.

Ha test Hemadsorption test (= HAT).

HATG Horse antihuman thymocyte globulin.

HATH Heterosexual Attitudes Toward Homosexuality (scale).

HATT Heparin-associated thrombocytopenia and thrombosis.

HATTS Hemagglutination treponemal test for syphilis (see STS).

HAU; HA unit Hemagglutinating/ation unit.

Haust; haust A draft/ draught (L. haustus).

HAV Hallux abductor valgus; Heart attack victim; Hemadsorption virus (see HA virus); Hepatitis A virus; Homovanillic (acid) (see HAVA).

HAVA Homovanillic acid. A major monoamine metabolite (= HAV).

HAVAB Hepatitis A virus antibody.

HA virus Hemadsorption virus (type 1; 2) (= HA; HA1; HA2; HAV).

HAWIC Hamburg-Wechsler Intelligence Test for Children.

Hay Marijuana (see Cannabis).

HAZ MAT Hazardous material.

HB Health board; Heart block (e.g. Adams-Stokes disease/ syndrome, Atrioventricular block, Bundle branch block, Cardiac conduction defect, Infranodal block, Intraatrial block, Intraventricular block, Sinoatrial block, etc.); Heel to buttock; Held back; Hemoglobin (see Hb); Hepatitis B; His bundle; Hold breakfast; Hormones and Behavior (journal); Hospital bed; Housebound; Human behavior; Hybridoma bank; Hyoid body.

Hb Ganglion habenulae (thalamus); Hemoglobin (= HB; Hbg; Hg; Hgb) - the oxygen-carrying pigment of the red blood cells. A molecule of hemoglobin contains four different polypeptide chains, α, β, γ, and δ, each containing several hundred aminoacids.

HbA: Adult hemoglobin (= Hemoglobin A; Hgb-A), normally predominant in the adult, designation: $Hb_{\alpha 2}A_{\beta 2}A2$.

HbA2: Found in adults in limited concentrations, designation: $Hb_{\alpha 2}A_{\delta 2}A2$.

HbA1, HbA1c: Glycohemoglobin/ Glycosylated hemoglobin.

HbAS, HbA/S: Group A sickle cell anemia (sicklemia) hemoglobin (= HgbAS/HgbA/S).

HbCO: Carboxyhemoglobin (= Hgb-CO)

HbCS: Hemoglobin Constant Spring (= Hgb-CS).

HBD: Hyperkinetic behavior disorder.

HbD punjab: Hemoglobin D punjab α2β2 (= Hgb-D punjab).

HbF: Fetal hemoglobin (predominant type in the newborn), designation $Hb_{\alpha 2}A_{\gamma 2}F$ (= HbP; Hemoglobin F; Hgb-F; Hgb-P; HgF).

Hb Kansas: Mutant hemoglobin with a low affinity for oxygen.

HbM: Hemoglobin Milwaukee.

HbMet: Methemoglobin (= HiHb).

HbO: Oxyhemoglobin (see HbO_2).

HbO_2: Oxyhemoglobin (= HbO; Hemoglobulin O_2; $HgbO_2$; Oxygenated Hb).

HbP: Primitive (fetal) hemoglobin (see HbF).

HbS: Sickle-cell hemoglobin (= Hemoglobin S; HbS-C; Hgb-S; HgbS-C).

HbS-C: Sickle-cell hemoglobin (see HbS).

HbSS: Hemoglobin SS.

Hb-A to S: Hemoglobin variants.

HbZ: Hemoglobin Z (= Hemoglobin Zürich).

Hgb-A: Adult hemoglobin (see HbA).

HgbAS: Group A sickle-cell hemoglobin (see HbAS).

Hgb-CO: Carboxyhemoglobin (see HbCO).

Hgb-CS: Hemoglobin Constant Spring (see HbCS).

Hgb-D punjab: Hemoglobin D punjab (see HbD punjab).

Hgb-F: Fetal hemoglobin (see HbF).

Hgb-O_2: Oxyhemoglobin (see HbO_2).

Hgb-P: Primitive (fetal) hemoglobin (see HbF).

Hgb-S, HgbS-C: Sickle-cell hemoglobin (see HbS).

HgF: Fetal hemoglobin (see HbF).

HHB: Reduced hemoglobin (see HHb).

HHb: Reduced hemoglobin (i.e. un-ionized

Hb) (= HHB; HHg; HHgb).
HHg, HHgb: Reduced hemoglobin (see HHb).
HiHb: Hemiglobin (= Methemoglobin) (see HbMet).

H^{b} Deuterium (Heavy hydrogen) (see H2).

1 HB First degree heart block.

HBA Histamine-blocking agent; Histaminergic blocking activity.

HbA Adult hemoglobin (= Hemoglobin A) (see Hb); X-hydroxybutyrate dehydrogenase.

HbA1 Glycohemoglobin/ Glycosylated hemoglobin (see Hb).

HbAb Hepatitis B antibody (see HAA) (= Hepatitis-associated antibody - type B; Australia antibody).

HBABA; Hbaba Hydroxybenzene-azobenzoic acid.

HBAC Hypodynamic beta-adrenergic circulatory.

HbA1c Glycohemoglobin/ Glycosylated hemoglobin (see Hb).

H-bag Hepatitis B antigen (see HBAg; HbAg).

HbAg Hepatitis B antigen (see HAA) (= Hepatitis-associated antigen - type B; Australia antigen).

HbAS; HbA/S Group A sickle cell anemia (sicklemia) hemoglobin (Sickle cell trait) (see Hb).

Hb-A to S Hemoglobin variants (see Hb).

HBB Hemoglobin beta-chain; Histomorphometric (HMM) bone biopsy (Orthopedics); Hospital blood bank; Hydroxybenzyl benzimidazole (see Hbb).

HbB Hemoglobin concentration in the blood.

Hbb Hydroxybenzyl benzimidazole (= HBB).

HbBC Hemoglobin binding capacity.

HBBW; HB/BW Hold breakfast for blood work.

HBC Health Board Committee; Hepatitis B core (antigen) (see HBc); Heterocyclic biphosphonate compound; Human body composition; Human brain/ breast cancer; Human brain cell; Hyperbaric chamber.

HBc; HB$_{c}$ Hepatitis B core (antigen) (= HBC).

HbC Hemoglobin C (see Hb).

HBcAg; HBCAG; HB$_{c}$Ag Hepatitis B core antigen.

HbCC Homozygous hemoglobin C disease; Human bone cell culture.

HBCG Heat-aggregated Calmette-Guérin bacillus.

HbCMet Cyanomethemoglobin (see CHbMet).

HbCO Carboxyhemoglobin (see Hb).

HbCS Hemoglobin Constant Spring (see Hb).

HBCT Human brain cell transplant (for Parkinson's disease).

HBCX Human breast cancer xenograft.

HBD Has been drinking; Hepatobiliary disease; High-bulk diet (see FRD; RRD); Hydroxybutyrate/ric degydrogenase (see HBDH); Hypophosphatemic bone disease; Hypoxic brain damage.

HbD Hemoglobin D (see Hb).

H2BD H2 - blocking drug.

HBDH Hydroxybutyrate/yric degydrogenase (an enzyme used in testing for myocardial infarction) (= HBD; α-HBDH; HDBH).

HBDT Human basophil degranulation test.

HBE His bundle electrogram.

HbE Hemoglobin E (see Hb); Hemoglobin entity (see MCHC).

HBeAg; HBEAG; HBeAg Hepatitis B early antigen.

HBF Hand/ Hemispheric/ Hepatic/ Hyperemic/ Hypothalamic blood flow; Hemoglobinuric bilious fever; Heterotopic bone formation.

HbF Fetal hemoglobin (= Hemoglobin F; HbP) (see Hb).

HBF 386 Actinomycin C (= Cactinomycin). Antimicrobial substances obtained from the culture of Streptococcus chrysomallus) (see Streptococcus).

HBFP Hematoxylin - basic fuchsin - picric acid (stain).

HBG Homogenous bone graft; Hormone-binding globulin (= CBG; SBG; TBG).

Hbg Hemoglobin (see Hb).

HBGC Hormone-binding globulin concentration.

HBGM Home blood glucose monitoring.

HBGR Hemoglobin-gamma regulator.

HBH Hypobaric hypoxia.

HbH Hemoglobin H (see Hb).

Hb-Hp Hemoglobin-haptoglobin (complex).
HBI Hemibody irradiation; Heterogenous bone implant; High (serum-)bound iron; Hydrophilic β-inhibitor (e.g. Timolol, etc.).
HBID Hereditary benign intraepithelial dyskeratosis.
HBIG; HBIg Hepatitis B immunoglobulin.
Hb_{Kansas} Mutant hemoglobin with a low affinity for oxygen (see Hb).
HBL Hepatoblastoma; High blood level.
HBLA Human B-cell lymphocyte antigen/ antibody.
HBLV Human B-cell lymphotropic virus.
HBM Haploidentical/ Human bone marrow; Health Belief Model; Heart bypass machine; High body mass; Human breast milk; Hyperbaric medicine; Hypertonic buffered medium.
HbM Hemoglobin Milwaukee (see Hb).
HBMC Hormone-based male contraception/ive (e.g. progestin, testosterone, etc.).
HbMet Methemoglobin (see Hb).
HBMetCy Cyanmethemoglobin (see Hb).
HBMCIT Haagen and Black Multiple Choice Intelligibility Test.
HBO Hyperbaric oxygen(ation).
HbO Oxyhemoglobin (see Hb; HbO_2).
HbO_2 Hyperbaric oxygen (= HbO); Oxyhemoglobin (see Hb).
H_3BO_3 Boric acid (L. acidum boricum).
HBOC Hemoglobin-based oxygen carrier; Hyperbaric oxygen chamber.
HbODC; HbO_2DC Oxyhemoglobin dissociation curve.
HBOT Hyperbaric oxygen therapy.
HBP Hepatic binding protein; High blood pressure.
HbP Primitive (fetal) hemoglobin (see Hb; HbF).
HBPM Home blood pressure monitoring.
HBR Hemocystine blood reducer.
HBr Hydrobromic acid.
HBRN Hepatobiliary radionuclide (scan - using Tc99m DISIDA).
HBS Health Behavior Scale; Heart-bypass surgery; Hepatitis B surface (antigen) (see HBsAG); Hepatobiliary system; High blood sugar; Hospital-based specialist/ specialty/ study; Human brain scan(ning); Hyperkinetic behavior syndrome.
HbS Hemoglobin S (Sickle-cell hemoglobin) (see Hb).
HBsAG; HBSAG; HBsAg Hepatitis B surface antigen (laboratory/ virology).
HBsAg/adr Hepatitis B surface antigen manifesting group-specific determinant "a" and subtype-specific determinants "d" and "r".
HBSC Hematopoietic blood stem cell.
HbSC; HbS/C A sickle-cell hemoglobin/ hemoglobin C disease.
HbSD A hemoglobin disease.
HBSS Hank's balanced salt solution.
HbSS Hemoglobin SS (see Hb).
2HBSS Two-hour blood sugar screen.
HbS/Thal Sickle cell/thalassemia.
HBT Hepatic biotransformation; Hepatobiliary toxicity; Homologous β-thalassemia (Obstetrics); Human brain thromboplastin/ tissue; Human breast tumor; Hydroxybenzotriazole.
HBV Hepatitis B vaccine/ virus; Honey-bee venom.
HBVD Hepatitis B virus antigen D.
HBVG Hepatitis B virus antigen G.
HBV-MN Membranous nephropathy associated with hepatitis B virus.
HBVY Hepatitis B virus antigen Y.
HBW High birth weight.
H/BW Heart-to-body weight (ratio).
HbZ Hemoglobin Z (= Hemoglobin Zürich) (see Hb).
HC Hair/ Hairy/ Horizontal cell; Handicapped (= HCAP; HCP); Head circumference/ compression/ constrictor; Healthy control; Heart Care (journal); Heat conservation; Heavy chain; Heel cords; Hemachromatosis (see ISD); Hemoglobin concentration; Hemorrhagic colitis; Hemostatic clamp (= HSC); Heparin cofactor; Hepatic catalase; Hepatocellular; Hereditary coproporphyria (= HCP); Hickman catheter; High calorie; Hippocampus; Histamine challenge; Histochemistry; Home care; Homocystinuria; Hospital Career (journal); Hospital Corps; House call; Huntington's chorea; Hyaline casts (urine); Hydraulic concussion; Hydrocarbon; Hydrocephalus/ly;

Hydrocortisone (= Hyd); Hydrophobic chromatography; Hydroxycorticoid; Hyoid cornu; Hypercholesterolemia; Hypertrophic cardiomyopathy; Hypoglycemic coma.

hc honoris causa (L.) - degrees.

Hc Hydrocolloid.

H/C; H&C Hot and cold (= H and C).

HC3 Hemicholinium No: 3.

HC 20-511 Ketotifen - An orally active, anti-anaphylactic, benzocycloheptathiophene compound, an H receptor (Histamine r) antagonist, asthma prophylactic and anti-allergic agent.

HCA Health-care access; Health/ Home care aide; Health Care Association (formerly ANHA - American Nursing Home Association); Heart cell aggregate; Hepatocellular adenoma; Heterocyclic amine; Histocompatibility antigen; Homocysteic/ Hydroxycitric acid; Hospital Corporation of America; Hydrocortisone acetate; Hyperosmolar contrast agent (see HyCoSy); Hyperchloremic acidosis (see EIS); Hypochloremic alkalosis; Hypochromic anemia (see FeDA).

HCAP Handicapped (see HC); Hospitalized Community Acquired Pneumonia.

H-CAP Hexamethylmelamine, cyclophosphamide, Adriamycin (doxorubicin), and Platinum compound (cisplatin).

H-cap Heroin in a gelatine capsule (see Diamorph).

HCB Hexachlorobenzene (an insecticide); Hollister colostomy bag; Hypercapnic breathing (see HCV).

HCBM Hypocellular bone marrow.

HCC Health and Community Care (UK); Health care campaign/ center/ chiropractor/ choice/ clinic(ian)/ cost/ coverage; Health Care Corporation; Hepatic copper concentration (in liver biopsy; a concentration greater than 250 μg/g of dry liver confirms the diagnosis of Wilson's disease) (see CT - Copper toxicosis); Hepatitis contagiosa canis (virus); Hepatocellular carcinoma; Histocompatibility complex; History of chief complaint; Human colon cancer; Husband-coached childbirth (= Bradley method - Obstetrics); Hydroxyxcholecalciferol (see Vitamins - D3).

25-HCC 25-hydroxycholecalciferol (peak IV metabolite of vitamin D3) (see Vitamins - D3).

21, 25 HCC 21, 25 hydroxycholecalciferol (peak V metabolite of vitamin D3 (see Vitamins - D3).

HCD Health care delivery/ doctor (see HCP); Heavy-chain disease; Hepatocellular damage; Hepatocerebral degeneration; High-calorie/ High-carbohydrate diet; Histologically confirmed diagnosis; Homologous canine distemper (antiserum); Human clinical dose (see RCD; RHCD); Hydrocolloid dressing; Hypercoagulable disease/ disorder.

^{3}HCd-R ^{3}H-deoxycytidine.

HCE Hard coal equivalent (unit of energy used in Euratom); Hormonal contraceptive exposure; Hypoglossal carotid entrapment.

HCF Health care facility; Hepatocellular failure; Hereditary capillary fragility; Highest common factor; Hyperkinetic cardiac failure; Hypocaloric carbohydrate feeding.

HCFA Health Care Financing Administration.

hCFSH Human chorionic follicle-stimulating hormone (see Hormones - hCFSH).

HCG Histocompatibility gene.

HCG; hCG Human chorionic gonadotropin (see Hormones - HCG; hCG).

HCH Hexachlorocyclohexane (see BHC); Hemochromatosis.

H chain Heavy chain (one pair of polypeptide chains making up an immuno-globulin molecule, which contains twice the number of amino acids and twice the molecular weight of the light chain) - subtyped alpha, gamma and Mu chains.

HCHO Formaldehyde.

HCH Officinal (Fr. P) Gamma benzene hexachloride (Lindane) - An insecticide (see GBHC).

HCHP Harvard Community Health Plan; Hydroxyapatite-coated hip prosthesis.

HCHWA Hereditary cerebral hemorrhage with amyloidosis.

HCI Health-care institution/ insurance; Hepatocellular injury; Human complement inhibitor.

HCIB Health Computer Information Bureau (Canada).

HcImp Hydrocolloid impression (dentistry).
HCID Humoral and cellular immunodeficiency (see AT).
HCIS Health Care Information System.
HCIST Health Care Information Systems and Technology (Division of) (HSR - Health Services Reseach).
HCL Hairy-cell leukemia; Hepatic cytolysis; Human cultured lymphoblasts.
HCl Hydrochloric acid; Hydrochloride.
HCLD Hepato-cellular liver disease.
HCLF High carbohydrate, low fiber (diet).
HCLHb Human cross-linked hemoglobin (see HXLHb).
HCLN High calorie liquid nutrition.
HCLs Hard contact lenses.
HCM Health care maintenance/ management; Host cell metabolism; Hypertrophic cardiomyopathy.
HCMA Hyperchloremic metabolic acidosis (see HMA).
HCMM Hereditary cutaneous malignant melanoma.
HCMT Homocysteine metyltransferase.
HCMTD Hypertrophic Charcot-Marie-Tooth disease (= HMSN Type I) (see HMSN).
HCMV Human cytomegalovirus (see CMV).
HCN Hederitary chronic nephritis; Hepatocellular necrosis/ neoplasm; Hydrocyanic acid; Hydrocyanide.
HCO Health-care organization (see HMO); Hematogenous CANDIDA osteomyelitis (= COM; OAC).
HCO_3 Bicarbonate ion/ radical.
H_2CO_3 Carbonic acid.
$(HCO_3)a$ Acid-base deficit.
HCOOH Formic acid (= CH_2O_2).
HCP Handicapped (see HC); Health care personnel/ physician/ policy/ practitioner/ profession(al)/ program/ promotion/ provider/ provision; Hepatocatalase peroxidase; Hereditary coproporphyria (see HC); Hexachlorophene; High cell passage; Homecare program; Hospital and Community Psychiatry (APA journal); Hospital Construction Program.
H&CP Hospital and community psychiatry.
HCPCS Health Care Financing Administrators Common Procedure Coding System.
HCPM Hypertrophic cranial pachymeningitis (in Sjogren's syndrome).
HCPV Heptavalent conjugate pneumococcal vaccine (see PCV).
HCQ Health care quality/ research/ resource.
HCR Heme-controlled repressor; Histochemical response (to injury); Host-cell reactivation/ receptor; Hysterical conversion reaction.
HCRE Homeopathic Council for Research and Education.
hCRH Human corticotropin-releasing hormone (see Hormones - hCRH).
Hcrit; H'crit Hematocrit (laboratory/ hematology) (see Crit; Hct).
HCS Hajdu-Cheney syndrome; Hamburger-coke syndrome (low Ca/P ratio); Hard-core science; Harvey Cushing Society; Hazard Communication Standard; Health care service(s)/ specialist/ support/ system; Healthy control subject; Hepatic cytochrome system (see P450); High calorie supplement; High clinical suspicion; Hospital Car Service; Hourglass contraction of the stomach; Human chorionic somatomammotropin (= hCS; HCSM; hCSM; HPL; hPL; HPL molecule) (see Hormones - HCS); Human cord serum (umbilical serum).
hCS Human chorionic somatomammotropin (see Hormones - HCS).
17-HCS 17-hydroxycorticosteroid.
HCSCST House of Commons Select Committee on Science and Technology.
HCSD Health Care Studies Division.
HCSM; hCSM Human chorionic somatomammotropin (see Hormones - HCSM).
HCSS Hypersensitive carotid sinus syndrome.
HCST Hematopoietic-cell-specific transmembrane (tyrosine phosphatase) - regulates src tyrosine kinases required for signal transduction of T- cell and B-cell receptors.
HCT Health care team/ technology; Health check test; Hematocrit (see Hct); Hematopoietic cell transplant(ation); Hepatic cell tumor; Histamine challenge test; Historic control trial; Homocytotropic (antibodies) - Immunoglobulin (long term HCT antibody or

IgE and short term HCT antibody or IgG); Human calcitonin (see hCT); Human cancer therapy; Human chorionic thyrotropin (= hCT; HPT; hPT) (see Hormones - HCT); Hydrochlorothiazide (= HCTZ); Hydroxycortisone.

Hct Hematocrit (= Crit; Hcrit; H'crit; HCT; Hemat; HMT; Hmt; PCV).

hCT Human calcitonin (= HCT); Human chorionic thyrotropin (see HCT).

HCTC Health Care Technology Center.

HCTD Hepatic computed tomography density.

HCTS High cholesterol and tocopherol supplement.

HCTU Home cervical traction unit.

HCTZ Hydrochlorothiazide (see HCT).

HCU Health Care Unit (UK); Health check-up; Homocystinuria (a recessively inherited disorder of methionine metabolism, caused by a deficiency of the enzyme cystathionine synthase); Hyperplasia cystica uteri.

HCV Hepatitis C virus; Hypercapnic ventilation (see HCB); Hypocontractile ventricle.

HCVA Hemorrhagic cerebrovascular accident; High-contrast visual acuity.

HCVD Hypertensive cardiovascular disease (see HASCVD).

HCW Healh care worker.

HCY Homocysteine (see tHCY).

Hcy; Hcys Homocysteine/ tine.

HcyT Homocysteine thiolactone.

HD Haab-Dimmer (syndrome); Hajna-Damon (broth); Haloperidol decanoate; Hansen's (leprosy)/ Hart's (= H dis)/ Heart/ Hemolytic/ Hirschsprung's/ Hodgkin's/ Huntington's/ Hydatid disease; Health Devices (journal); Hearing distance; Heaven dust (cocaine) (see Erythroxylum); Helix destabilizing (protein); Heloma durum; Hemidiaphragm; Hemodialysis; Hemodilution; Hemolyzing/ High dose; Hemorrhagic diathesis; Herniated disc; High density; Hip disarticulation; Hormone-dependent; Horror drug (any drug containing belladonna); Hospital day; House dust; Human diploid (cells); Huntington's disease (see HC); Hydatid disease; Hydroxydopamine (see HDA).

hd at bedtime (L. hora decubitus); head.

H&D Hunter and Driffield (curve).

HD_{50} Hemolyzing dose that lyses 50% of complement/red blood cells.

HDA Harris-Dodd Act (Drug Abuse Control Amendment of 1965); Hemodynamic action (venodilatation and arterial dilatation); Hepatitis delta antigen (see HDI); Hereditary diffuse alopecia - types include: AED - Anhidrotic ectodermal dysplasia, CHT - Congenital hypotrichosis, CVG - Cutis verticis gyrata, HHT - Hereditary hypotrichosis (Marie Unna type), HMI - Hypomelanosis of Ito, LGS - Langer-Giedion syndrome, TRPS - Trichorhinopharangeal syndrome; Huntington's Disease Association; Hydroxydopamine (= HD).

HDAC High-dose cytarabine (see HDARAC).

HDARAC High dose cytarabine (ara-C; cytosine arabinoside).

HDBH Hydroxybutyrate/tyric dehydrogenase (see HBDH).

HDC Health Development Corporation (California, USA) (see ETC); Hemodynamic compromise; High-dose chemotherapy (see HDTC); Highly desirable characteristic; Histidine decarboxylase; Human Development Center; Human diploid cell; Huntington's Disease Commission; Hygiéniste Dentaire du Canada (CDHA journal).

HDCS High dose calcium supplement; Human diploid cell strain (vaccine for the prophylactic treatment of rabies) (see HDCSV).

HDCSV Human diploid cell strain vaccine (= HDCS; HDCV; Merieux anti-rabies vaccine).

HDCV Human diploid cell (rabies) vaccine (see HDCSV).

HDD High-dosage depth; Higher Dental Diploma; Human daily dose.

HDE Hemodynamic effect; High-density electrode.

HDF Hemodynamic finding(s) (see HDS)/ function; Hepatic dysfunction; Hereditary Disease Foundation; High-dose fortification; High dry field (microscopy); Host defence factor; Human diploid fibroblast.

HDFP Hypertension Detection, (Treatment and) Follow-up Program.

HDG High-dose group.

HDH Hardening and darkening hormone; Heart disease history.

^{3}HDHA ^{3}H-dihydroalprenolol (a radiolabelled pindolol derivative).

HDI Hemodynamic imbalance (in shock syndrome); Hemorrhagic disease of infants; Hepatitis delta infection (caused by an incomplete virus particle associated with Hepatitis B and resulting in a severe form of hepatitis); Hexamethylene diisocyanate; Human Development Index; Hypothalamic diabetes insipidus.

HDIg Human diphtheria immunoglobulin.

H dis Hart's disease (see HD).

HDL High-density lipoprotein (a form of blood cholesterol) (= HDLP).

HDL-C HDL cholesterol (see HDL).

HDL-c High density lipoprotein - cell surface.

HDLL High density lipoprotein lipid(s).

HDL/(LDL + VLDL) The plasma lipid ratio (see HDL; LDL; VLDL).

HDLP High-density lipoprotein (see HDL).

HDLS Hereditary diffuse leukoencephalopathy with spheroids.

HDLs High density lipoproteins.

HDLW "Hearing distance from the left ear, of a watch" i.e. distance from which a watch ticking is heard by the left ear (= DDLW).

HDM Hallpike-Dix maneuver (see DHM); Hemodynamic monitor(ing); House dust mite (= Dermatophagoides pteronyssinus; Dpi; Dpt) - the major cause of house dust asthma; Hyperlabile diabetes mellitus (= 'Brittle' diabetes; HLD; IDDM; Juvenile diabetes; Type 1 DM).

HDMP High-dose methylprednisolone.

HDMR Holodiastolic mitral rumble.

HDMTX High-dose methotrexate.

HDMTX-CF High-dose methotrexate citrovorum factor.

HDMTX-LV High-dose methotrexate leucovorin.

HDN Hemolytic disease of the newborn; Hormone-dependent neoplasm.

hDNA Hybrid deoxyribonucleic acid.

HDP Habitual dislocation of the patella (Orthopedics); Hemo/ Home dialysis patient; Hemodynamic patient; Hexose diphosphate; Hexosediphosphoric acid { = $C_6H_{10}O_4(PO_4H_2)_2$ }(involved in the ossification of cartilage); High-density polyethylene; Hydrolytic depolymerization/zer; Hydroxydimethylpyrimidine; Hydroxymethyline diphosphonate; Hypertensive diabetic patient.

HDPAA Heparin-dependent platelet-associated antibody.

HDPC Health Data Policy Committee (HEW); Hormone-dependent prostatic cancer.

HDPE High density polyethylene (medicine bottle).

HDR Heart Disease Resources; Hemodynamically relevant (e.g. aortic/ mitral valve stenosis, etc.); Hemodynamic response; High-dose radiation/ rate/ recipient (chemotherapy, radiotherapy, etc.).

HDRF Heart Disease Research Foundation.

HDRS Hamilton Depression Rating Scale.

HDRT High-dose radiation therapy.

HDRV Human diploid rabies vaccine.

HDRW "Hearing distance from the right ear, of a watch" i.e. distance from which a watch ticking is heard by the right ear (= DDRW).

HDS Halobutyl disc seal (for injection cartridges); Hamilton Depression Scale; Hard disc storage (Computer memory); Healthcare Data Systems; Health Data Services; Health delivery system(s); Hemodialysis shunt; Hemodynamic status; Hemodynamically stable; Hemodynamic study (see HDF); Heparin/ Dextran solution; Herniated disc/ disk syndrome; Hospital-discharge summary; Hospital Discharge Survey; Host defence system.

HDST High-dose sequential therapy (as in neoplastic diseases).

HDSTT High dose, short term therapy (1-3 days).

HDT High-dose therapy; Hormonal-dependent tumor; Hypotensive drug therapy.

HDTC High-dose toxic chemotherapy.

^{3}H-dTHd Tritated thymidine.

HDU Hemodialysis unit.

HDV Hemodynamic variable(s); Hepatitis delta virus.

HDW Hearing distance with watch (see DDLW; DDRW; HDLW; HDRW).

HDZ Hydralazine.

HE Hard exudate; Hektoen enteric (agar);

Hemagglutinating encephalomyelitis; Hemagglutination enhancement; Hemoglobin electrophoresis; Hepatic encephalopathy; Hereditary eliptocytosis; Hernia equivalent; Herpes encephalitis; High exposure; Hollow enzyme; Human enteric (virus); Hydranencephaly; Hydroxyethyl (cellulose); Hyperextension; Hypogonadotropic eunuchoidism.

He Heart; Helium (Z = 2) (see Elements - Helium).

H&E Hematoxylin and eosin (stain); Hemorrhage and exudate; Heredity and environment.

HEA Hepatic encephalopathy due to alcohol (= AHE); Hexone-extracted acetone; Human erythrocyte antigen.

Headache (journal).

HEAL Health Education Assistance Loan.

Health (journal).

HEAR Hospital Emergency Ambulance Radio; Screening test: *H* Hearing concern? *E* Ear test results normal? *A* Awaken to sound? *R* Responses in the developmental and communication scales?

Heart Dexadrine heart-shaped tablet (see Amphet); Heart (journal).

HEAT Human erythrocyte agglutination test (laboratory/ hematology).

Heaven dust Cocaine (see Erythroxylum).

HEB Hepato-encephalic barrier.

Heb Hebrew (religion).

Hebdom A week (L. hebdomada).

hebet- prefix meaning puberty.

HEC Hamster embryo cell; Hand-eye coordination; Health Education Center/ Council; Hospital Ethics Committee; Human embryonic (see ESC)/ endothelial/ epithelial cell; Human ethics committee; Hydroxyergocalciferol (see Vitamins - D2); Hydroxyethylcelluloose.

HECP Hepatic encephalopathy (see HE).

hecto-; hect- metric prefix meaning 100 (Gr. ekt-) (= h; 10^2), e.g. hg = hectogram, 100 grams, or 10^2 grams.

HED Hereditary/ Hypohidrotic ectodermal dysplasia; Hospital emergency department; Hydrotropic electron-donor; Unit skin dose (of roentgen rays or X-rays) (Ger. Haut-Einheits-Dosis).

HEDH Hypohidrotic ectodermal dysplasia with hypothyroidism.

HEDIS Health Plan Employer Data and Information Set (CA).

HEDS HIV Early Detection Study.

HEENT Head, eyes, ears, nose, and throat.

HEEP Health effects of environmental pollutants.

HEF Hamster/ Human embryo fibroblast; Head extractor forceps (Murless - Obstetrics and Gynecology); Healthy elderly female.

HEG Hemorrhagic erosive gastritis; Human-engineered/ erythropoietin gene; Hyperemesis gravidarum.

HEGC Hyperechogenic change(s) - in the endometrium (Obs/Gyn).

HEH Hereditary enamel hypoplasia (see AGS).

HEHR Highest equivalent heart rate.

HEI Health Effects Institute; Hepatic eosinophilic infiltration; High-energy intermediate; Homogenous enzyme immunoassay; Human embryonic intestine (cells); Hyperextension injury (e.g. of the cervical spine, the knee joint, etc.).

HEIA Hepatic enzyme-inducing agent (e.g. Barbiturate, Phenytoin, etc.).

HEID Hepatic enzyme-induced drug (e.g. Carbamazepine).

HEIR Health effects of/ High-energy ionizing radiation.

HEIS High-energy ion scattering.

HEK Human embryo(nic) kidney (cell/ cell culture).

HEL Hen egg-white lysozyme; High energy laser; Human embryo(nic) lung (cell/ cell culture); Human erythroleukemia; Human Exercise Laboratory; Human exposure level.

HeLa cells Helen Lake/ Henrietta Lacks cells (human cervical carcinoma cells). A strain of human cancer or carcinogenic cells, after the name of the patient who died at the age of 31 years, from whose cancer (of the cervix uteri), the parent cells were isolated in 1951. They form a continuous cell line used for tissue cultures.

helc- prefix meaning sore or ulcer (Gr. elkos).

HELF Human embryo lung fibroblast.

helic- prefix meaning coil (Gr. helix).
helio- prefix meaning sun (Gr. helios).
HELLIS Health, Literature, Library and Information Services.
HELLP Hemolysis, elevated liver enzymes, and low platelet count (syndrome).
helo- prefix meaning callus, nail, or wart.
Heloma Growth (corn/ callosity) of the skin (H. durum = hard corn; H. molle = soft corn; H. milliare = seed corn; H. neuro = nerve corn; H. vasculare = blood corn).
HELP Health Education Library Program; Health Emergency Loan Program; Health Evaluation and Learning Program; Heat escape lessening posture; Heroin Emergency Life Project; Hospital Employees Labor Program; Hospital Equipment Loan Project.
HELs High energy lasers.
HELTA High-energy laser technology assessment.
HEM Healthy elderly male; Heterozygous extensive metaboliser (patient's reaction to drugs); Hysteria-enhanced migraine.
HEM; Hem Hematologist/ogy (= Hemat; Hematol); Hematuric (= Hemat); Hemorrhage (= Hemorrh); Hemorrhoids.
hem- prefix meaning blood (Gr. aima).
HEMA Health Education Media Association; Hydroxyethyl-methacrylate.
Hemat; hemat Hematocrit (see Hct); Hematologist/ogy (see HEM); Hematuric (see HEM).
Hematol; hematol Hematologist/ogy (see HEM).
HEMB Hemophilia B.
HEMC Hydroxyethyl-methylcellulose (an emulsifying and thickening agent).
Hemi; hemi Hemiparalysis; Hemiparesis; Hemiplegia.
hemi- prefix meaning half (Gr. emi).
Hemo Nur Hemodialysis Nurse.
Hemorrh Hemorrhage (see HEM).
HEMOSID Hemosiderin.
Hemp Marijuana (see Cannabis).
HEMPAS Hereditary erythroblastic/ erythrocytic multinuclearity with positive acidified serum (test).
HEMRI Hereditary multifocal relapsing inflammation.
HEMS Helicopter emergency medical services.
hen- prefix meaning one (Gr. enos).
HeNe; He-Ne Helium-neon (laser radiation).
Henry Heroin (see Diamorph).
HEOD Hexachloroepoxy-octahydro-dimethano-naphthalene. A chlorinated organic compound, being the main (85%) component of the insecticide dieldrin.
HEP Hemolysis end point; High egg passage (virus); High-energy phosphate; Histamine equivalent prick; Human epithelial cell (see Hep); Human epithelioid (see HEp).
HEp Human epithelial (cell) (= HEP); Human epithelioid (= HEP).
Hep Heparin; Hepatic/titis.
hEP Human endorphin.
HEp-1 Human cervical carcinoma cells.
HEp-2 Human laryngeal tumor cells; Human heteroploid cells.
HEPA Hamster egg penetration assay; High efficiency particulate air (filter) (see HEPAvac); Highly exaggerated pharmacological activity.
hepat- combining form meaning liver (Gr. epatos).
HEPAvac High Efficiency Particulate Air-Filtered Vacuum.
hep cap heparin cap.
HEPES N-2-hydroxyethylpiperazine-N-2-ethanesulfonic acid.
HEPM Human embryonic palatal mesenchymal (cell).
hept- prefix meaning seven (Gr. epta).
HER Hemorrhagic encephalopathy of rats; Hepatic endoplasmic reticulum; Hernia (see Hern).
HER-2 Human Epidermal Growth Receptor No: 2 (gene - involved in regulating cell growth. Its antagonist Herceptin is now used in the treatment of metastatic breast cancer) (= HER-2/neu / see CGs).
Her Cocaine (see Erythroxylum); Hernia (see Hern).
her hernia (see Hern).
HERA Hyperexcitable reflex arch(es).
Herb Marijuana (see Cannabis).
herb recent of fresh herbs (L. herbarium recentium).

HERC Health Economics Research Center.
Hered Hereditas (journal).
hered hereditary/ty.
hered- prefix meaning heir (L. heredis).
HERL Health Effects Research Laboratory (EPA).
Herm True hermaphrodite (see Ferm; Merm).
Hern; hern Hernia(ted) (= HER; Her; her).
HER2/neu gene (also known as HER2, neu, and c-erbB-2) (see HER2).
Heroin Symbol H (see Diamorph).
HERP Human exposure/rodent potency (index of cancer hazard).
HERS Health Evaluation and Referral Service; Heart and Estrogen-Progestin Replacement Study; Hemorrhagic (fever) with renal syndrome (see HFRS); Hysterectomy Educational Resources and Services (Foundation).
HES Health Education Service (AMA publication); Health Examination Survey (NCHS); Healthy elderly smoker/ subject; Hematoxylin-eosin stain; Hepatic enzyme system (e.g. microsomal cytochrome P-450 system); Human embryonic skin/ spleen; Human experimental study; Hydroxyethyl starch (used commercially in instant laundry starch preparations); Hypereosinophilic syndrome; Hyperprostaglandin E syndrome; Hypertonic electrolyte solution.
HESC Human embryonic stem cell.
HESCA; HeSCA Health Sciences Communications Associations.
HESCR Human embryonic stem cell research.
HESM Hospital electrical safety meter.
HET Health Education Telecommunications; Helium equilibration/rium time; High environmental temperature.
Het Heterophil.
het heterozygous.
HETE 5-Monohydroxy-eicosatetraenoic acid (an important product of the lipoxygenase pathway in bronchial asthma).
hetero- prefix meaning dissimilar (Gr.).
HETP Height equivalent to a theoretical plate; Hexaethyltetraphosphate.
HEV Health and environment; Hemagglutinating encephalomyelitis virus; Hepatitis E virus; Hepato-encephalomyelitis virus; High endothelial venule; Human enteric virus.
HEW Hardened ear wax; (Department of) Health, Education, and Welfare (US); Heavily exuding wound.
HEX Hexaminidase; Hexosaminidase.
Hex Hexamethylmelamine.
hex- combining form meaning have or hold (Gr. echo); prefix meaning six (Gr. ex).
HEX A; Hex A; hex A Hexosaminidase-A.
HEX B; Hex B; hex B Hexosaminidase-B.
HEX C; Hex C; hex C Hexosaminidase-C.
Hexa-CAF Hexamethylmelamine, cyclophosphamide, amethopterin (methotrexate), and fluroruracil.
HF Dorsey Laboratories code for experimental substances; Hageman factor (see Factor XII); Haplotype/ Hertz/ High (see hf) frequency; Hard feces; Hard-filled (capsule); Hay fever; Head of fetus; Head forward; Health facility; Heart failure; Helper factor; Hemofiltration; Hemophilia Foundation; Hemorrhage/gic factor/ fever; High fat (diet); High flow; House formula; Human Fertility (journal); Human fibroblast; Hydrogen fluoride; Hydrops fetalis (Obstetrics); Hyperflexion.
Hf Hafnium (Z = 72) (see Elements - Hafnium).
hf half; high frequency (= HF).
H-F Histamine-like factor (of Lewis).
HF 1927 Dibenzepin hydrochloride (a benzodiazepine compound used in the treatment of endogenous depression).
HFA Health facility administrator; Healthy Families America (National network program - US); Hearing field audiometry; Hepatic function abnormality; Hydrofluoroalcane.
HFAA Heptafluoro-butyric acid.
HFAC Human Factors Association of Canada.
HFAK Hollow-fiber artificial kidney.
HFB Heptafluoro-butyryl; High fat breakfast.
HFBI Heptafluoro-butyryl imidazole.
HFC Hard-filled capsule; High-frequency current; Hip flexion contracture (Orthopedics); Histamine-forming capacity.
HFCT Human fetal cell transplant.
HFD Hemorrhagic fever of diet; High-fiber

diet; High-flux dialysis; High forceps delivery; Hollow-fiber dialyzer (Hemodialysis); Hospital field director.

HFDK Human fetal diploid kidney.

HFDL Human fetal diploid lung.

HFE; HFe Hemochromatosis.

HFEA Human Fertilisation and Embryology Authority (UK).

HFEC Human foreskin epithelial cell.

HFF Human fetal foreskin; Human fibrin factor; Human foreskin fibroblast.

HFG Hand-foot-genital (syndrome).

HFGL High fasting glucose level.

HFH Hemifacial hyperplasia; Heterozygous familial hypercholesterolemia; High-frequency hearing; Homozygous familial hypercholesterolemia.

HFHD High flux hemodialysis.

HFHL High-frequency hearing loss.

HFHV High frequency/ volume.

HFI Hepatic functional impairment (see IHF); Hereditary fructose intolerance; High fiber/ fluid intake; Human fibroblast interferon (see HFIF).

HFIEPM Howard Florey Institute of Experimental Physiology and Medicine (Australia).

HFIF Human fibroblast interferon (= HFI).

HFIP Hexafluoro-isopropanol.

HFJV High-frequency jet ventilation.

HFL Human fetal lung; Hyperfibrinolysis; Hypotonic fluid loss.

H flu Hemophilus influenzae.

HFM Hemifacial microsomia.

HFMA Healthcare/ Hospital Financial Management Association.

HFMD Hand-foot-and-mouth disease (an enteroviral infection caused by coxsackievirus A16).

HFMI High-frequency microsatellite instability (see TMI).

HFO High-frequency oscillator; H/f oscillatory (ventilation).

HFO$_2$ High flow oxygen.

HFO-A High-frequency oscillatory (ventilation) - active (expiratory phase).

HFOV High-frequency oscillatory ventilation.

HFP Heart-failure patient; Hexafluoropropylene; High filling/ fluid pressure (vascular/ ventricular); High-frequency pulsation; Hypertonic feeding preparation; Hypofibrogenic plasma.

HFPM High-flux polyacrylonitrile membrane.

HFPPV High-frequency positive pressure ventilation.

HFR Healthy female relative; High-frequency recombination (see Hfr).

Hfr Heart/ High frequency; High-frequency (of recombination cells) (= HFR).

HFRNS High-frequency repetitive nerve stimulation.

HFRS Hemorrhagic fever with renal syndrome (caused by the hantavirus of the Bunyavirus group and transmitted by rodents) (= HERS; KHF) (see KHF).

HFS Hand-and-foot syndrome; Healthy female subject; Hemifacial spasm; High(er)-frequency sound; Hospital Financial Support.

hfs hyperfine structure.

HFSA Heart Failure Society of America.

HFSH; hFSH Human follicle-stimulating hormone (see Hormones - HFSH).

HFSS Heart Failure Survival Study.

HFST Hearing for speech test.

HFSWs High-frequency sound waves (= Echogram or Ultrasound).

HFT Hepatic Function Test(s) (see LFT); Hidden Figures Test (ETS); High-frequency transduction/ transfer (see Hft).

Hft High-frequency transfer (= HFT).

HFU Hand-foot-uterus (syndrome); Heat flow unit.

HFUPR Hourly fetal urine production rate.

HFV Healthy female volunteer; High-frequency ventilation; Human foamy virus; Hypofunctional ventricle.

HG Hand grip; Herpes gestationis; Heschl's gyrus; High gain (amplifier); High glucose; Human gonadotropin (see Hormones - HG)/ growth; Hypoglycemia.

Hg Hemoglobin (see Hb); Mercury (Z = 80) (L. hydrargyrum) (see Elements - Mercury).

hg hectogram (= 100 grams; 10 g); hemoglobin (see Hb).

H-G Hepa-Gent (test).

^{197}Hg; ^{203}Hg Radioisotopes of Mercury.

HGA Histalog gastric analysis (measurement of gastric acid); Homogentisate/sic acid;

Hyper/Hypoglycemic activity (of drugs).

Hgb Hemoglobin (see Hb).

Hgb-A Adult hemoglobin (see Hb).

HgbAS; HgbA/S Group A sickle-cell anemia (sicklemia)/ trait hemoglobin (see Hb).

Hgb-CO Carboxyhemoglobin (see Hb); Hemoglobin-carbon monoxide saturation.

HgbCS Hemoglobin constant spring (see Hb).

HgbD punjab Hemoglobin D punjab α β (see Hb).

Hgb-F Fetal hemoglobin (see Hb).

Hgb-O_2 Oxyhemoglobin (see Hb).

Hgb-P Primitive hemoglobin (see Hb).

Hgb-S; Hgb-SC Sickle-cell hemoglobin (see Hb).

HGC Hard gelatine capsule; Human genetic code; Human Genetics Commission (UK); Human Genome Center; Hypoglycemic coma/ convulsion(s); Hypogranular cytoplasm.

$HgCl_2$ Mercuric chloride (corrosive).

Hg_2Cl_2 Mercurous chloride (mild).

HGD Human genetic disorder; Hypoglycemic diabetic.

HGE Human granulocytic erlichiosis (a newly identified bacterial tick-borne disease); Hypoglycemic episode (see AHE).

HGF Hematologic/ Hematopoietic growth factor(s) (see Table). These include: BFU, Burst-forming unit. BFU-E, Erythroid cell BFU. BFU-ME, Myeloid/ Erythroid cell BFU. CFU, Colony-forming unit. CFU-C, CF-culture. CFU-E, Erythroid cell. CFU. CFU-Eo. Eosinophil CFU. CFU-GEMM, Granulocyte/ Erythrocyte/ Monocyte/ Megakaryocyte CFU. CFU-GM, Granulocyte/ Monocyte CFU. CFU-Meg, Megakaryocyte CFU. CFU-S, CFU-spleen. CSF, Colony-stimulating factor. EPO, Erythropoietin. G-CSF, Granulocyte colony-stimulating factor. GM-CSF, Granulocyte/ Macrophage CSF. IL 1,3,5,6, Interleukin 1, 3, 5, & 6. M-CSF, Macrophage colony-stimulating factor. TGF, Transforming growth factor (e.g. TGF-β) (see Hormones - HGF); Hepatocyte growth factor (see EGF); Human Growth Foundation; Hyperglycemic-gluco/-glyco genolytic factor (glucagon) - a polypeptide secreted by the alpha cells of the islets of Langerhans. Used chiefly in the treatment of insulin hypoglycemia as a hyperglycemic agent. Administered by injection (= HG factor).

Hg-F Fetal hemoglobin (see Hb).

HG factor Glucagon (see HGF).

HGG Herpetic geniculate ganglionitis; Human gamma globulin; Hypogammaglobulinemia.

HGGM Human gastric gel mucin.

HGH Harbor General Hospital (Torrence, California); Human growth hormone (see Hormones - HGH); Hypogonadotrophic hypogonadism.

hGH Human/ Hypophyseal growth hormone (see Hormones - hGh; HGH).

HGHRF Human growth hormone releasing factor (= see Hormones - HGHRF).

HGI Hyperglycemic index.

HgI_2 Mercuric iodide.

Hg_2I_2 Mercurous iodide.

HGL High glucose level.

HGM High-grade malignancy; Hog gastric mucosa; Home/ Human glucose monitoring; Human gene mapping.

HGMCR Human genetic mutant cell repository.

HGN Hypocomplementemic glomerulonephritis.

$Hg(NO_3)_2$ Mercuric nitrate.

HGO Hepatic/ Human glucose output; Hip guidance orthosis; Human Genome Organization.

HgO Mercuric oxide.

Hg_2O Mercurous oxide.

HGOI Hypogonadotrophic ovarian insufficiency.

HGP Hepatic glucose production; Human gene pool (eugenics); Human Genome Project; Hyperglobulinemia purpura.

HGPRT Hypoxanthine-guanine phosphoribosyl transferase (= HG-PRTase).

HG-PRTase See HGPRT.

HGPS Hereditary giant platelet syndrome; Hutchinson-Gilford progeria syndrome.

HGPT Hypoxanthine-guanine phosphoribosyltransferse (see HGPRT; LNS).

HGR High genetic risk; Human genome research.

H graft Refers to shape of graft (of spinous

HGF – Factors relevant to hematopoiesis identified to date:

Growth factor	Molecular wt. (Dalton)	Cell line stimulated	Localization of gene
GM-CSF	14,000-35,000	Granulopoiesis, monocyte line, eosinophils, basophils, erythropoiesis, megakaryocytes	Chromosome 5q23-q32
Interleukin-3	14,000-28,000	Granulopoiesis, monopoiesis, eosinophils, megakaryopoiesis and mast cells, basophils	Chromosome 5q23-q31
M-CSF	45,000-90,000	Monocyte line	Chromosome 5q23-q31
G-CSF	18,000-22,000	Granulopoiesis	Chromosome 17q11-q23
Interleukin-1	12,000-19,000	Pluripotent hematopoietic stem cells	Chromosome 2
Interleukin-5	130,000	Eosinophils.	Chromosome 5q31
Interleukin-6	26,000	Pluripotent hematopoietic stem cells; synergistic with interleukin-1	Chromosome 7p15
Erythropoietin	30,000	Erythropoiesis	Chromosome 7

processes of the vertebrae) (= Clothespin graft; Prop graft).

HGRC Human Genetics Research Center (Laval University, Montreal, Canada).

hGRH Human growth hormone-releasing hormone.

HGS High-grade sarcoma; Human Genome Sciences/ Human genome sequencing (HGP).

HgS Mercuric sulfide.

HGSG Helsinki Gastritis Study Group (Scandinavia) (for gastric cancer and premalignant lesions in atrophic gastritis).

$HgSO_4$ Mercuric sulfate.

Hg_2SO_4 Mercurous sulfate.

HGT Human gene therapy (see CGT; EGT; GBIT; GIT; GLGT; GLT; GT; SGT)/ transfer; Hypoglycemic therapy/ treatment.

HGV High genetic vulnerability.

HH Halothane hepatitis; Hard of hearing; Healthy hemophiliac/ human; Henderson and Haggard (inhaler); Hereditary hypotrichosis (scanty eyebrows and body hair, sparse and twisted later, scarring alopecia, folliculitis decalvans - an autosomal dominant, hereditary syndrome) (= MUSC; PAS); Hiatal hernia; Holistic/ Home health; Home Help; Homozygous; Human Heredity (journal, formerly AGSM); Hydroxyhexamide; Hypergastrinemic hyperchlorhydria; Hyperhidrosis; Hypogonadotropic hypogo-

All the lines in hematopoiesis are maintained by a pool of pluripotent stem cells that have the capacity to duplicate themselves. After the level of the pluripotent hematopoietic stem cells, hematopoiesis is rapidly differentiated to the stage of committed multipotent hematopoietic stem cells and committed multipotent lymphatic stem cells. The lymphatic stem cells are further differentiated into the T and B lines, whereas the multipotent hematopoietic stem cell differentiates into further committed precursor cells, which give rise to the erythropoietic, megakaryopoietic and granulopoietic lines, the monocyte line, eosinophils and basophils. The various committed precursor cells are named after the assays in which they can be detected. As may be seen from the following illustration, a number of different hematopoietic growth factors are involved in the expansion of the various hematopoietic lines and their maturation.

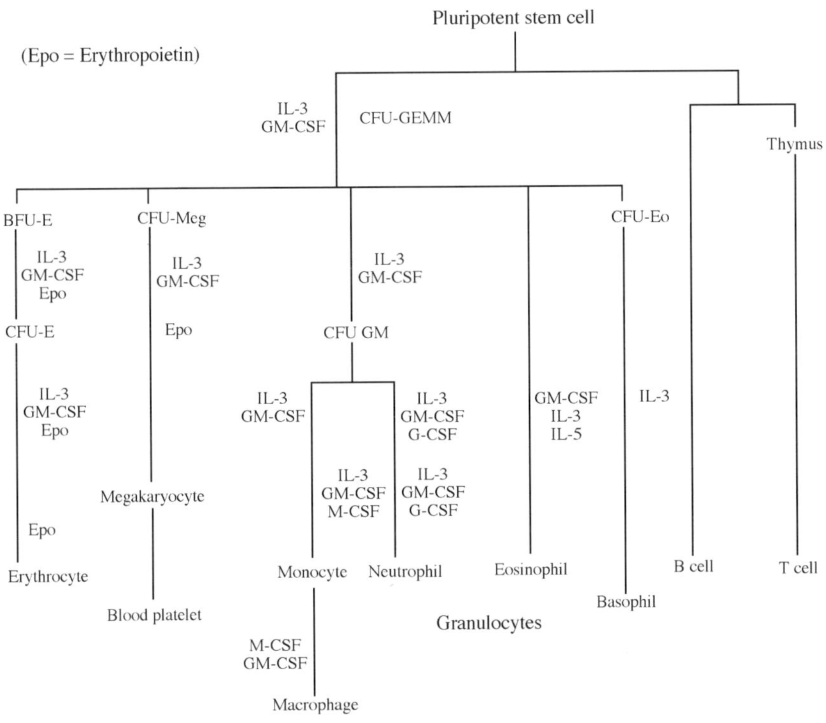

nadism; Hyporeninemic hypoaldosteronism.

Hh Heterozygous.

H&H Hematocrit and hemoglobin (laboratory/hematology).

HHA Health Hazard Appraisal; Hereditary hemolytic anemia; Home Health Agency/Aide; Hyperhydrosis axillae; Hypothalamo-hypophyseo-adrenal (system); Hypothalamus-hypophysial axis.

HHb Hypohemoglobinemia; Reduced hemoglobin (= Unionized Hb) (see Hb).

HHC Halogenated hydrocarbon; Harlem Hospital Center; Health and Hospitals Corporation (New York City); Home Health Care; Hygiene/nic home cleansing; Hyperglycemic hyperosmolar coma; Hyperhomocysteinemia.

HHCS High-altitude hypertrophic cardiomyopathy syndrome.

HHD High(est) human dose; High heparin

dose; Home hemodialysis; Hypertensive heart disease.

HHDE Hydro-hypodynamic environment.

HHDN Hexachloro-hexahydro-dimethano-naphthalene (a chlorinated insecticide).

HHE Health hazard evaluation; Hemiconvulsion(s)-hemiplegia-epilepsy (syndrome).

HHF Hypothalamus-hypophysis function.

HHFH Hypomelia, Hypotrichosis, Facial hemangioma (an autosomal recessive, congenital hypotrichosis with limb reduction defects such as pseudo-thalidomide syndrome, and facial capillary nevus).

HHFM High humidity face mask.

HHG Human haploid genome (consists of 3 billion = 3 x 10,000,000,000 base pairs of double-stranded DNA); Human hyperimmune globulin (see HHIG); Hypertrophic hypersecretory gastropathy.

HHH High, hot, and a helluva lot (enema); Hyperornithinemia, hyperammonemia, homocitrillinuria (syndrome).

HHHE 'Hit hard, hit early' (therapy).

HHHO Hypotonia, hypomentia, hypogonadism and obesity (Prader-Willi syndrome).

HHHS Halogenated hydrocarbon hepatitis syndrome.

HHI Hypercapnia-hypoxia interaction.

HHIE Hearing Handicap Inventory for the Elderly.

HHIE-S Hearing Handicap Inventory for the Elderly-Screening Version.

HHIG Human hyperimmune globulin (= HHG).

HHM Humoral hypercalcemia of malignancy.

H + Hm Compound hypermetropic astigmatism.

HHMC Howard Hughes Medical Center.

HHMI Howard Hughes Medical Institute.

HHN Hand held nebulizer.

HHNC; HHNK Hyperglycemic hyperosmolar non-ketotic coma/ koma (i.e. diabetic coma).

HHNS Hyperglycemic hyperosmolar non-ketotic syndrome (= HHS).

HHO Hypertonic hyperosmolality (in hypernatremia).

HHP Hidden health problem; Honolulu Heart Program (see HAAS).

HHR Hiatal hernia repair (= TP - Thal procedure); Hydralazine, hydrochlorothiazide, and reserpine.

HHRC Hypothalamic heat-regulating center.

HHRH Hereditary hypophosphatemic rickets with hypercalciuria; Hypothalamic hypophysiotropic releasing hormone (see Hormones - HHRH).

HHS Habitual heavy smoker (smoking)/ snorer (snoring); Hand-held syringe; Health and Human Services (Department of); Hearing Handicap Scale; Hereditary hemolytic syndrome; Hospital and Health Services; Human hypopituitary serum; Hyperglycemic hyperosmolar syndrome (see HHNS); Hyperkinetic heart syndrome.

HHSA Hospital Health Services Administration (ACHA journal).

HHSR Hospital and Health Services Review (journal).

HHSSA Home Health Services and Staffing Association.

HHT Head halter traction; Hereditary hemorrhagic telangiectasia; Hereditary hypotrichosis (Marie Unna type) (see HDA); Heterotopic heart transplantation; Homoharringtonine; Human heart transplant; Hydroxyheptadecatrienoic acid.

HHTC High-humidity tracheal collar.

HHTM High-humidity tracheal mask.

HHV Healthy human volunteer; Human herpes virus.

HHV4; HHV-4 Human herpesvirus 4 (= Epstein-Barr virus see E-B).

HHV6 Human herpesvirus 6 (a human B cell lymphotropic virus) (= HBLV) (see PVFS).

HHV8; HHV-8 Human herpes virus 8 (sexually transmitted among men who have sex with other men, and found predominantly in oropharyngeal secretions, but only infrequently in semen, the anal canal, and prostatic secretions. Also, an associated cause of Kaposi's sarcoma).

HI Head injury; Health insurance; Hearing impaired; Heart infusion; Hemagglutination/lutinin inhibition (see H-I); Hemophilus influenzae (see HIB); Hepatobiliary imaging; Hexamine insulin (see Insulin - HI i); High impulsiveness;

Histamine/ Histidine (see His); Hormone-independent; Hormone insensitivity; Hospital-induced; Hospital insurance; Human insulin (see Insulin - HI ii); Humoral immunity; Hydriodic acid; Hydroxyindole; Hyperglycemic index; Hypomelanosis of Ito; Hypothermic ischemia.

Hi Histamine (see His); Histidine (see His).

hi enlargement of hilar or mediastinal lymph nodes (radiograph symbol).

H-I Hemagglutination/lutinin inhibition (= HI).

HIA Hearing Industries Association; Heat infusion agar; Hemagglutination inhibition antibody/ assay; Hospital Insurance Act (Canada); Human insulin analogue; Hydroxyitraconazole (a bioactive metabolite of the azole-derivative, antifungal family of drugs).

HIAA Health Insurance Association of America; Hydroxyindoleacetic acid (= Hydroxylindoacetic acid) (see 5- HIAA).

5-HIAA 5-Hydroxyindoleacetic acid (= HIAA).

HIAC Hepatic intraarterial chemotherapy (for hepatic metastases in colorectal cancer) (= HAI).

HIB Heart infusion broth; Hemolytic immune body; Hemophilus influenzae B (type B - vaccine) (= HI; HITB; HiTB).

Hib *Hemophilus* influenzae type B (disease/ vaccine/ virus) (see HIB).

HIBAC Health Insurance Benefits Advisory Council.

HIC Handling-induced convulsions; Health Information Center (UK); Health insurance claim (number)/ company; Health Insurance Council; Hearing-impaired child(ren); Heart Information Center.

HICA Hydroxyisocaproic acid.

hi-cal high caloric.

HiCn Cyanomethemoglobin.

HI-CSFN Huxley Institute - Canadian Schizophrenia Foundation Newsletter.

HID Haploidentical donor; Headache, insomnia, depression (syndrome); Hereditary immunodeficiency; Herniated intervertebral disc; Human infectious dose; Hyperkinetic impulse disorder.

HID_{50} 50% Human infectious dose.

HIDA Health Industry Distributors Association; Hepato-iminodiacetic acid (= Lidofenin) (nuclear medicine scan).

hidr- combining form meaning sweat (Gr. idros).

HIE Health Insurance Experiment; Human intestinal epithelium; Hyper-IgE (syndrome) (see HIES); Hypoxic-ischemic encephalopathy.

HIES Hyper-IgE syndrome (= HIE).

HIF Haemophilus influenzae; Higher integrated/ integrative functions.

HIFBS Heat-inactivated fetal bovine serum.

HIFC Hog intrinsic factor concentrate.

HIG Human insulin gene ("Humulin").

HIG; HIg; hIG Human immunoglobulin.

HIg Human/ Hyper immunogobulin.

HIgMS Hyper-IgM syndrome (see HIM; X-l HIMS).

HIgS Human immunoglobin (IgG1) skeleton.

HIH Hypertensive intracerebral hemorrhage.

HIHA High impulsiveness, high anxiety.

HIHATIg Hyperimmune human anti-tetanus immunoglobulin (see HTIG).

HiHb Hemiglobin (methmoglobin) (see HbMet).

HII Health Industries/ Insurance Institute; Hemagglutination inhibitor immunoassay.

HIL Hypoxic-ischemic lesion.

HILA High impulsiveness, low anxiety.

HILS High-Intensity Learning Systems.

HIM Hemagglutination inhibition morphine (test) (see HIM test); Hepatitis-infectious mononucleosis; Hexosephosphate isomerase; Hyper-IgM (in immunodeficiency diseases); Viral-latex particle agglutination.

Him Heroin (see Diamorph HCl).

HIMA Health Industries Manufacturers Association.

Hi mag High magnification.

HIMC Hepatic intra-mitochondrial crystalloid(s).

HIMP High-dose intravenous methyl-prednisolone.

HIMs Hyperglycemia-induced malformations (see DRMs).

HIMT See HIM test.

HIM test Hemagglutination inhibition mor-

phine test (= HIM; HIMT).
HiN Hearing-in-Noise (multi-microphone hearing aid).
Hin Hindu (religion).
H inf Hypodermoclysis infusion.
Hint Hinton (flocculation test for syphilis) (see STS).
HIO Hepatic iron overload; Hypoiodide/iodism.
HIO_3 Iodic acid.
HIOMT Hydroxyindole-O-methyl transferase.
HIOS High index of suspicion.
HIP Health illness profile; Health Insurance Plan; Hepatically impaired patient; Homograft incus prosthesis; Hospital Insurance Program; Humoral immunocompetence profile; Hydrostatic indifference point.
HIPA Heparin-induced platelet activation.
HIPAA Health Insurance Portability and Accountability Act (1996, US).
HIPC Health Insurance Purchasing Cooperative.
HIPE Hospital Inpatient Enquiry.
HiPIP High potential iron protein.
HIPO Hemihypertrophy, intestinal web, preauricular skin tag, and congenital corneal opacity (syndrome); Hospital Indicator for Physicians Orders.
HIPPY Home Instruction Program for Preschool Youngsters (parenting and child development).
HIR Head injury routine; Host immune response; Humoral immune/ immunologic(al) response.
HIRMAN Human Instrumental Mannequin (Army project).
HIS Hanover Intensive Score; Health/ Hospital information system; Health Intention Scale; Health Interview Survey; Histamine/ Histidine (see His); Human/ Humoral immune system (= ABS + CMS); Hybrid immune-system (see ISH); Hyperimmune serum.
His Histamine/ Histidine (= HI; Hi; HIS; Hist; hist).
HISG Human immune serum globulin.
HISMS How I See Myself Scale.
HISN Heparin-induced skin necrosis.
HISSG Hospital Information Systems Sharing Group.
HIST Hospital in-service training.
Hist; hist Histamine/ histidine (see His); Histidinemia; Histology (see Histol); Histogram; Historical/ory.
hist- prefix meaning tissue (Gr. istos).
HISTLINE History of Medicine On-Line.
Histo Histoplasmin (skin test).
Histol; histol Histological/gist/gy (= Hist; hist).
HIT Heavy-ion therapy/ treatment (see RSP); Hemagglutination-inhibition test (for pregnancy); Heparin-induced thrombocytopenia; Histamine inhalation test; Hybridization identified transcript (virology); Hyperglycemia-induced teratogenesis (Obstetrics); Hypertrophic infiltrative tendonitis.
HITB; HiTB Hemophilus influenzae type B (see HIB).
HITF Hospital Insurance Trust Fund (SSA).
HITT Heparin-induced thrombocytopenia and thrombosis.
HITTS Heparin-induced thrombosis-thrombocytopenia syndrome.
HIU Head injury unit; Hyperplasia interstitialis uteri.
HIUPB Human intrauterine parabiotic syndrome (Obstetrics).
HIV Human immunodeficiency virus (see AIDS; HTLV-III).
HIVE Human immunodeficiency virus epidemic.
HIV I; HIV-I Human immunodeficiency virus type 1 (see HTLV III).
HIV Ag Human immunodeficiency virus antigen.
HIVAN Human immunodeficiency virus-associated nephropathy.
HIVD Herniated intervertebral disc.
HIV-G Human immunodefiency virus-associated gingivitis.
HIVRD HIV-related disease (see HIV).
HIVWS HIV wasting syndrome (see HIV).
HJ Hepatojugular (reflex/ reflux) (see HJR); Howell-Jolly (bodies).
HJB Howell-Jolly bodies.
HJD Hospital for Joint Disease (NY).
HJDMC Hospital for Joint Diseases and Medical Center.

HJR Hepatojugular (reflex/ reflux) (= HJ).

HJSR Hip joint surface replacement (St. Urban Berlin) (see OI/OP).

HK Hand-to-knee (see H-K); Heat-killed; Heel-to-knee (see H-K); Hexagonal keratotomy; Hexokinase; Human kidney (cells); Hypokinesia (slowness in the initiation and execution of voluntary movement, seen especially in Parkinson's disease, with impaired ocular convergence, mask-like facies, micrographia, monotonous speech - degenerating to virtual anarthria, reduced blinking, and reduced swinging of the arms while walking).

H-K Hand-to-knee (coordination); Heel-to-knee (distance).

HK^+ High potassium ion.

HKAFO Hip-knee-ankle-foot orthosis.

HKAO Hip-knee-ankle orthosis.

H+K+ATPase. Hydrogen potassium adenine triphosphatase (the protein pump enzyme).

HKC Herpetic keratoconjunctivitis; Human kidney cell.

HKD Hyperkeratotic dermatitis/atosis; Hyperkinetic disorder (see ADHD).

HKLM Heat-killed Listeria monocytogenes.

HKO Hip-knee orthosis.

HKS Heel, knee, and skin; Hyper/Hypo kalemic state; Hyperkeratotic skin; Hyperkinesis syndrome.

HL Hairline; Hairy leukoplakia; Half-life (of a radioactive element); Hallux limitus; Haloperidol; Harelip; Hayflick limit (to division of normal cells, which after about 50 divisions, enter the final state of senescence before natural death. Cells dividing beyond this limit are almost always cancerous. This limit was discovered by Leonard Hayflick, a cell biologist in the early 1960s, at the UCSF); Hearing level/ loss; Heparin lock; Herpes labialis (= CS - Cold sore); Hickman line; Histiocytic lymphoma; Histocompatibility locus; Hodgkin's lymphoma; Human leukocyte; Human, luteinizing (see Hormones - LH v); Hygienic Laboratory (USHL journal); Hyperlipidemia; Hypermetropia, latent (see Hl); Hyperopia, latent (see Hl); Hypertrichosis lanuginosa; Hypertriglyceridemia (hyperlipemia).

Hl Hypermetropia, latent (eye examination) (= HL); Hyperopia, latent (= HL).

hl hectoliter (100 liters; 10^2 liters).

H/L Hydrophil/lipophil (balance/number/ratio) (see HLB).

H&L Heart and Lung (AACCN journal); Heart and lung (machine); Heart and lungs.

HLA High local activity; Hilar lymphadenopathy (characteristic of sarcoidosis); Histocompatibility leukocyte/ locus antigen; Homologous leukocyte antibody; Human leukocyte/ lymphocyte antibody/ antigen (= Histocompatibility antegens; HL-A; Homologous leucocytic antibody; Human leucocyte antigen/ antibody; "Self-recognition" antigen). Important in the laboratory and in the field of serology, these antigens are associated with various immune-response diseases. They include: HLA - A 11: Systemic lupus erythematosus (SLE); B 1: Celiac disease; B 7 (+ DR 3): Very severe form of anti-glomerular basement membrane (GBM) nephritis; B 8: Addison's disease, Autoimmune chronic active hepatitis, Celiac disease, Dermatitis herpetiformis, Rheumatoid arthritis (RA), Sjögren's syndrome, Systemic lupus erythematosus (SLE); B 15: Hepatitis B virus, Polyarteritis nodosa; B 18 (+ DR 3): Very severe form of membranous glomerulonephritis; B 27: Ankylosing spondylitis, Reiter's disease, Other reactive arthrites; B 35: Hepatitis B virus, Polyarteritis nodosa, SLE; C: Spondylitis (some association reported); D 3: Sjögren's syndrome, Rheumatoid arthritis (RA), SLE; D 4: Sjögren's syndrome, Rheumatoid arthritis (RA), SLE; D 5: Scleroderma; DR: Rheumatoid arthritis (RA); DR 2: Anti-GBM (glomerular basement membrane) nephritis, RA; DR 2 (+ B 7): Very severe forms of Anti-GBM nephritis; DR 3: Autoimmune diseases such as Addison's disease, Chronic active hepatitis, Coeliac disease, Graves' disease, Insulin dependent diabetes mellitus (IDDM), Membranous glomerulonephritis, Myasthenia gravis, Rheumatoid arthritis (RA), Sjögren's syndrome, Systemic lupus erythematosus (SLE); DR 3 (+ B 18): Very severe form of Membranous glomerulonephritis; DR 4: Berger's disease,

Rheumatoid arthritis (RA) (very common); DRW 3: Celiac/ Coeliac disease, Dermatitis herpetiformis; DW 3: Celiac/ Coeliac disease; DW4: Rheumatoid arthritis (RA).

HL-A Human leucocyte antigen (see HLA).

HLAA; HLA-A Human leucocyte antigen A (see HLA).

HLAB; HLA-B Human leucocyte antigen B (see HLA).

HLAC; HLA-C Human leucocyte antigen C (see HLA).

HLAD; HLA-D Human leucocyte antigen D (see HLA).

HLA-LD Human lymphocyte antigen - lymphocyte defined (see HLA).

HLA-MAD Human leukocyte antigen-matched allogeneic donor.

HLA neg Heart, lungs, and abdomen negative.

HLA-SD Human lymphocyte antigen - serologically defined (see HLA).

HLB Hydrophil(ic)-lipophil(ic) balance (= H/L; H/L No; HL number or ratio) - with reference to surfactants; Hygienic Laboratory Bulletin (now BNIH); Hypotonic lysis buffer.

HLBI Human lymphoblastoid interferon.

HLC Heat loss center.

HLCA Human lymphocyte clastogenic assay.

HLCAA Human lymphocyte chromosomal aberration assay (for mutagenesis).

HLCL Human lymphoblastoid cell line(s).

HLCMA (TK6) Human lymphoblastoid cell mutagenesis assay.

HLD Haloperidol decanoate; Hepatolenticular degeneration (Wilson's disease) (also known as PLD or Progressive lenticular degeneration); Herniated lumbar disc/ disk; Hippel-Lindau disease (= HLS); Hyperkinesis learning disability (see H-LD); Hyperlabile diabetes (see HDM); Hyperlipidemia - Fredrickson's classification: Phenotype I - Elevated lipoproteins: Chylomicrons; Elevated lipids: Triglycerides. Phenotype IIa - Elevated lipoproteins: LDL; Elevated lipids: Cholesterol. Phenotype IIb - Elevated lipoproteins: LDL, VLDL, HDL; Elevated lipids: Cholesterol, Triglycerides. Phenotype III -Elevated lipoproteins: Chylomicron and VLDL remnants; Elevated lipids: Triglycerides, Cholesterol. Phenotype IV - Elevated lipoproteins: VLDL; Elevated lipids: Triglycerides. Phenotype V - Elevated lipoproteins: Chylomicrons, VLDL; Elevated lipids: Triglycerides, Cholesterol; Hypersensitivity lung disease; Hypoplastic lung development.

H-LD Hyperkinesis and learning difficulties/ disability (= HLD); (Von) Hippel-Lindau disease (commonly associated with multiple hemangioblastomas) (see HAB; HLD; HLS).

HLDE Harris Lateral Dominance Examination.

HLDH Heat-stable lactic dehydrogenase.

HLE Human lysosomal enzyme (= Beta-glucocerebrosidase, which catalyzes the hydrolysis of the glycolipid glucocerebroside to glucose and ceramide. Used in the treatment of Gaucher's disease) (see ARD; ART).

HLEG Hydrolysate lactalbumin Earle's glucose.

HLF Heat-labile factor; Human Life Foundation.

H-LG Hepta-decapeptide-like gastrin.

HLH; hLH Hemophagocytic lymphohistiocytosis; Human luteinizing hormone (see Hormones - LH v).

HLHS Hypoplastic left heart syndrome.

HLI Hand-lung incoordination (in the use of inhalers); Hemolysis inhibition; Human leukocyte interferon.

HLK; H-L-K Heart, liver, and kidneys.

HLL Hypoplastic left lung.

HLM Heart-lung machine; Hypolobulated megakaryocyte.

HLMO Heart-lung machine operator.

HLN Hilar lymph node; Hyperplastic liver nodule(s); Hypolobulated nucleus.

H/L No Hydrophile/lipophile number (see HLB).

HLOE Hallerian Lodge of the Order of Esculapius.

HLP Heart-lung pump (see HLM); Hepatic lipoperoxidation; Hind leg paralysis; Hyperkeratosis lenticularis perstans; Hyperlipoproteinemia; Hypolipoproteinemia.

HLPO Hydrolipoperoxide.

HLPS Hemolymphopoietic system.

HLR Heart-lung resuscitation; High-level resistance; High likelihood of recurrence.

HLS Health Laboratory Science (journal); Health Learning System; Heart Laser Surgeon/ System; Hemic and Lymphatic System; Herniated lumbar spine; Hippel-Lindau syndrome (see HLD); Hypertonic lactated saline (solution) (see HLSS).

HL service HeartLine service (system used to store a patient's most recent electrocardiogram in an Intromedix computer).

HLSS Hypertonic lactated saline solution (= HLS).

HLT Heart-lung transplantation; Human lipotropin; Human lymphocyte transformation.

Hlth Health.

HLTP Heart and Lung Transplant Programs (UCLA).

HLU Heaviside-Lorentz unit/ system of units.

HLV Half-value layer (see HVL); Heart, Lung, Vascular (Center); Herpes-like virus; High-level variability; Hypoplastic left ventricle.

HL-VAB Heparin-less venoarterial bypass.

HLVC Heart, Lung and Vascular Center (Scripps Clinic).

HLVS Hypoplastic left ventricle syndrome.

HL-X Human lymphocyte X.

HM Hand motion/ movements); Health maintenance; Heart murmur; Heavily muscled; Heimlich maneuver (for expelling food caught in the larynx) (see CRP); Hemifacial microsomia; Hemola molle; Hepatomegaly; History of Medicine (journal); Holter monitoring; Homosexual male; Homozygote(s); Hospital management; Hospital Medicine (journal); Human milk; Human monocomponent (insulin) (see Insulin - MCI); Hydatidiform mole; Hyperimmune mouse; Manifest hypermetropia/ hyperopia (see Hm).

Hm Manifest hypermetropia/ hyperopia (= HM).

hm hectometer (= 100 meters; 10^2 meters).

HMA Haemorrhages and microaneurysms; Hawaii Medical Association; Health Manpower Act; Homeostasis model assessment; Hydroxymethionine analog; Hyperchloremic metabolic acidosis (= HCMA); Hypochloremic metabolic acidosis; Hypochromic microcytic anemia.

HMAC Health Manpower Advisory Council.

HMAS History of Medicine and Allied Sciences, Inc.; Hyperimmune mouse ascites.

HMB Homatropine methobromide/ methylbromide.

HMBA Hexamethylene bisacetamide.

HMC Hair matrix carcinoma (see BCC); Hand-mirror cell; Health maintenance cooperative; Hepatic metabolic capacity (for a drug/ drugs); Heroin, morphine and cocaine (see Diamorph, Papaver, and Erythroxylum); Herzlia Medical Center (Haifa, Northern Israel); Histocompatibility complex, major; Home medical care; Hospital management committee; Human mast cell; Human metaphase chromosome; Hydroxymethyl cystosine; Hygiene Mentale au Canada (journal); Hypertelorism-microtia-clefting (syndrome).

HMCCMP Human mammary carcinoma cell membrane proteinase.

HMCH Hahnemann Medical College and Hospital.

HMCT Highly myelosuppressive chemotherapy.

HMD Heart-muscle disease; Home-monitoring device; Hyaline membrane disease (see RDS); α-Hydrazine-α-methyl-B-(3,4-dihydroxyphenyl) (= L-α-hydrazine-α-methyldopa; methyldopa hydrazine).

HMDP Health Manpower Development Program; Hydroxymethyline diphosphonate; Hypertensive microalbuminuric diabetic patient.

HMDS Hexamethyl-disilazane.

HME Health Media Education; Heat and moisture exchanger (see HMX); Heat, massage and exercise (see HMX); Hepatic microsomal enzyme; Histomorphometric evaluation (see BHM; QHM).

HMEA Hepatic microsomal enzyme activity.

HMEIP Health Manpower Education Initiative Project (HRA).

HMETSC Heavy metal screen.

HMF Health Maintenance Foundation; Human myocardial fibroblast; Hyaline membrane failure; Hydroxymethyl furaldehyde/ furfural.

HMFI Human milk-fed infant (see BFI).

HMG High mitral gradient (mean, 20 mm Hg)

(seen on DUSonography); High mobility group; Human menopausal gonadotropin (see Hormones - HMG) (= hMG); Human Molecular Genetics (US journal); Humegon; 3-hydroxy-3-methyl-glutaryl.

hMG Human menopausal gonadotropin (see HMG).

HMG CoA 3-Hydroxy-3-methylglutaryl coenzyme A (reductase) - enzyme, participating in the biosynthesis of cholesterol.

HMG-HCG Human menopausal gonadotropin - human chorionic gonadotropin (see Hormones - HMG-HCG).

HMI Healed myocardial infarct(ion); Human monocomponent insulin (see Insulin); Hypomelanosis of Ito (a hereditary hypotrichosis, with depigmentation, ocular and dental defects) (see HDA; IPA).

HMIS Hazardous materials identification system; Hospital medical information system.

HMK Homemaking; 'Housemaid's knee' (Patellar bursitis).

HML Human milk lysosome/ lysozyme.

HMLEs HIRUDO medicinalis - leech enzymes (such as: 1. the natural anticoagulant Hirudin; 2. Antibacterial peptides extracted from *Aeromonas* hydrophila, a bacterium living a synergistic existence in the leech's gut; 3. the 'spreading factor' Orgelase in the leech's saliva; 4. the enzyme Hementin, derived from the 18-inch (46-cm.) long Amazon leech, *Haementaria* ghilianii, and other anticoagulants and local anesthetics).

HMM Heavy meromyosin (of muscle); Hexamethyl(ol)-melamine; Hydroxymethyl metabolite (of Esomeprazole) (see DMM; 2-HMM).

2-HMM 2-Hydroxymethyl metabolite.

HMMA 4-Hydroxy-3-methoxymandelic acid.

HMMD Histomorphometric data.

HMN Hyperbaric Medicine Newsletter.

HMO Health Maintenance Organization; Heart minute output; House Medical Officer.

HMOA Health Maintenance Organization Act (of 1973); Hepatic mono-oxygenase activity.

HMOE Hepatic mono-oxygenase enzyme.

HMORDA Health Maintenance Organization and Resources Development Act (of 1973).

HMOSC Health Maintenance Organization of South Carolina.

HMP Heat-malleable plastic; Heavy metal poisoning (see ICF); Hexose monophosphate; Hexose monophosphate pathway; Home management plan; Hot moist pack(s).

HMPA Hexamethylphosphoramide.

HMPAO; HM-PAO Hexamethyl-propyleneamine-oxide/-oxime.

HMPG Hydroxymethoxy-phenylglycol.

HMPS Hexose monophosphate shunt.

HMPT Hexamethylphosphoro-triamide.

HMR Healthy male relative; High(er) mortality rate; Histiocytic medullary reticulosis.

HMRB Hazardous Materials Regulation Board.

H-mRNA H-chain messenger ribonucleic acid.

HMRTE Human milk reverse transcriptase enzyme.

HMS Harvard Medical School; Healthy male subject; Her Majesty's Service (UK); Hematomedullar status (in cytotoxic therapy); Hexose monophosphate shunt; Histamine-mediated symptom(s); Hypermobility syndrome; Medrysone.

HMs Humoral mediators or "Spasmogens" (= PMsI), chemicals released by mast cells and eosinophils in the allergic and/or asthmatic reaction, such as: Bradykinin, cAMP - Cyclic adenosine 3'-5'monophosphate, cGMP - Cyclic guanosine monophosphate, CLT; CysLT - Cysteinyl leukotrienes (LTC4, LTD4, LTE4), ECF-A - Eosinophil Chemotactic Factor of Anaphylaxis, Histamine, Kallikrein, LTR - Leukotriene receptor (see above, CLT; CysLT), NCF-A - Neutrophil Chemotactic Factor of Anaphylaxis, PAF - Platelet Activating Factor, PGs - Prostaglandins (F2α), Serotonin, SRS-A - Slow Reacting Substance of Anaphylaxis, Tryptase.

HMSA Health Manpower Shortage Area.

HMSAS Hypertrophic muscular subaortic stenosis.

hMSC Human mesenchymal stem cell.

HMSN Heriditary motor and sensory neuropathy.

HMSN Type I Hereditary motor and sensory neuropathy (hypertrophic type) (see HCMTD).

HMSN Type II Hereditary motor and sensory neuropathy (neuronal type) (see NCMTD).
HMSO Her Majesty's Stationary Office (UK).
HMSS Hospital Management Systems Society.
HMT Heart-monitoring test(s) (such as ECG, ELR, Holter monitor, Ult. S. (echocardiogram), TTT, etc.); Hematocrit (see Hct); Histamine-N-methyl-transferase; Hospital management team; Human molar thyrotropin.
Hmt Hematocrit (see Hct).
HMTA Health Manpower Training Act; Hexamethylenetetramine.
HMU Hydroxymethyl-uracil.
HMV Healthy male volunteer.
HMW High molecular weight.
HMWC High-molecular-weight component.
HMWFC High-molecular-weight fibrin(ogen) complex.
HMWGP High-molecular-weight glycoprotein.
HMW-γM High-molecular-weight immunoglobulin.
HMWK High-molecular-weight kininogen.
HMX Heat, massage and exercise/ Heat and moist exchanger (see HME).
HN Head and neck (see H&N); Head Nurse; Heberden's node (Osteoarthritic - with or without florid joint inflammation or tophi/tophaceous deposits within the joints); Hemagglutinin neuraminidase; Hematemesis neonatorum; Hemorrhage of newborn; Hereditary nephritis; High necrosis/ nitrogen; Hilar node; Histamine-containing neuron; Home nursing; Human nutrition; Hypertrophic neuropathy (see HN-CMT; HN-DS).
hn tonight (L. hoc nocte).
H&N Head and neck (= HN).
H1N1 A porcine/ swine influenza A virus (may be transmitted to humans).
HN2 Nitrogen mustard (= Chlorethazine hydrochloride; Chlormethine HCl; Mechlorethamine HCl; Mustine HCl; $C_5H_{11}Cl_2NHCl$). A war gas; used as a cytotoxic agent in neoplastic diseases, particularly those of lymphoid and hemopoietic tissues, such as in Hodgkin's disease.
HN3 Trichloro-triethylamine.
H3N2 Hong Kong virus.
H5N1 An influenza A subtype, chicken-borne virus (Hemagglutinin and Neuraminidase), causing disease in humans.
HNA Harrison Narcotics Act (1914); Heparin neutralizing activity (by plasma); Heparin neutralizing antibody.
HNaG Hypertonic sodium gain.
HNB Human neuroblastoma.
HNC Hypernephroma cell; Hyperosmolar non-ketotic coma; Hypothalamic/mo-neuro-hypophyseal complex.
HN-CMT Hypertrophic neuropathy of the Charcot-Marie-Tooth (type).
HNCO Cyanic acid (see CNOH).
HN-DS Hypertrophic neuropathy of the Dejerinesottas.
HNF1 Hepatic nuclear factor 1.
HNFH. Heterozygous non-familial hypercholesterolemia (= HNH).
HNG High nuclear grade (as in breast cancer).
HNH Heterozygous non-familial hypercholesterolemia (see HNFH).
HNI Human normal immunoglobulin.
HNKDC Hyperosmolar non-ketotic diabetic coma.
HNKDS Hyperosmolar non-ketotic diabetic state.
HNL Histiocytic necrotizing lymphadenitis.
HNLN Hospitalization no longer necessary.
HNM Hypernatremic myopathy.
HNMAb Human neutralizing monoclonal antibody (see IANA; NMAb).
HNO_2 Nitrous acid.
HNO_3 Nitric acid.
HNP Hereditary nephritic protein; Herniated nucleus pulposus; Human neurophysin.
HNPCC Hereditary non-polyposis colo-rectal cancer.
HNRCA Human Nutrition Research Center on Aging (USDA).
hnRNA Heterogenous nuclear ribonucleic acid (see RNA).
hnRNP Heterogenous nuclear ribonucleoprotein.
HNS Head and neck surgery; Head, neck, and shaft; Home nursing supervisor.
HNSCC Head and neck squamous cell carcinoma.

HNSHA Hereditary non-spherocytic hemolytic anemia.
HNT Habits of nervous tension.
HNTD Highest non-toxic dose.
HNV Has not voided.
HO Hand/ Hip orthosis; Hematology-Oncology; Heterotopic ossification (see HTO); High/ Hyperbaric oxygen; Holt-Oram (syndrome); House Officer (intern or resident physician/ surgeon).
Ho Holmium (Z = 67) (see Elements - Holmium); Horse.
ho honeycomb lung (radiograph symbol).
H/O History of.
(HO-) Hydroxy radical (= Hydroxyl group).
(HO_2) Hydroperoxy (free radical).
H_2O Water.
H_2O_2 Hydrogen peroxide (= H. dioxide).
HOA Healthy older adult; Hip osteoarthritis; Hypertrophic osteoarthropathy.
3-HOA 3-Hydroxy-anthranilic acid.
HoaRhLG Horse anti-rhesus lymphocyte globulin.
HoaTTG Horse anti-tetanus toxoid globulin.
HOB Head of bed (see HoB); Hyperbaric oxygen breathing (see HPO).
HoB Head of bed (= HOB).
HOBUPSOB Head of bed up for shortness of breath.
HOC Health Officer Certificate; Human ovarian cancer; Hydroxycorticoid; Hyperosmolar coma; Hypertrophic obstructive cardiomyopathy; Hypogonadal-obesity cycle.
HOCl Hypochlorous acid.
HOCM High-osmolar contrast media/ium (= HOM); Hypertrophic obstructive cardiomyopathy.
hocus-pocus Latin - hoc est enim corpus meum: "This is in fact/ truly My body" - A sacramental blessing of the Consecration of the Mass, i.e. any meaningless action or words meant to draw attention away from some trick or deception; Sleight of hand; Trickery.
hoc vesp this evening or tonight (L. hoc vespere).
HOD Hoffer-Osmond Diagnostic (score) (see HODS); Human oral dosing; Hyperbaric oxygen drenching.
hod- prefix meaning path (Gr. odos).
HODS Hoffer-Osmond Diagnostic Score (= HOD).
Hoechst 12,512 Prenylamine lactate (see B 436).
HOEI Hepatic oxidative enzyme inhibitor (e.g. the sulfonamides).
HOEW Heavy-oxygen-enriched water.
HOF Hepatic outflow; High osmolality fluid; Hyperosmotic feeding/ food.
H of F Height of fundus.
Hoff Hoffman (reflex).
HOG Halothane, oxygen, and gas (nitrous oxide); Hepatic output of glucose; Hyperosmolar glucose.
Hog Phencyclidine hydrochloride (= PCP).
HOGA Hyperornithinemia with gyrate atrophy.
HOH Hard of hearing.
^{3}HOH Tritiated body water.
HOI Hospital onset of infection.
HoIg Horse immunoglobulin.
hol- prefix meaning whole.
HOM High-osmolar (contrast) media/ium (see HOCM); Hospital outpatient management (= HOPM).
hom- prefix meaning same or similar (Gr. omos).
HOMA Homeostatic model assessment.
HOMI. Homeostatic model index.
HOME Home Observation for Measurement of the Environment.
Homeop Homeopathy.
HOMES Helping Our Mentally Ill Experience Success (a pioneering outpatient program).
HOMO Highest occupied molecular orbital; Homosexual (see Homo).
Homo Homosexual (= Exhaust; Fag; Faggot; Fairy; Gay; HOMO; Pansy; Queer, etc.).
homo- prefix meaning homogenous i.e. having a similar name, sound, or standing in the same relation (as in "homozygous").
Homolat Homolateral.
HON Hydroxy-oxo-norvaline.
HONDA Hypertensive, obese, Negro, diabetic, and arthritic.
HONKH Hyperosmolar non-ketotic hyperglycemia.
HOO House officer observer.

HOOCCOOH Oxalic acid ($C_2H_2O_4$).
HOOD Hereditary onycho-osteodysplasia.
HOODS HOOD syndrome.
HOP High oxygen pressure (respiratory therapy); Hydroxyproline.
Hop Opium (see Papaver).
HOPE Health Opportunity for People Everywhere; Health and Optimum Physical Education; Healthcare Options Plan Entitlement; Health-oriented physical education; Heart Outcomes Prevention Evaluation (Study/ Trial); Holostic orthogonal parameter estimation.
HOPI History of present illness.
HOPM Hospital outpatient management (see HOM).
HOPP Hepatic occluded portal pressure.
HOPT Hospital outpatient treatment (= HOT).
HOR Human organ replacement.
hor horizontal (= horiz).
hor decub at bedtime (L. hora decubitus) (see hor som).
hor interm at intermediate hours (L. horis intermediis).
horiz horizontal (see hor).
horm- prefix meaning impetus or impulse (Gr. orme).
Hormones Symbol H; Hs. These are chemical substances having specific effects on the activity of certain body organs. The term was originally applied to the secretions of the endocrine glands, but today many drugs are produced synthetically in the laboratory, having similar action on the target organs, and as such, are also called hormones.
ACH: Adrenocortical hormones = Adrenal cortical h (ACH); Cortical h. (CH) - secreted by the adrenal cortex. It includes androgens, corticosteroids, estrogens and progestogens.
ACTH: Adrenocorticotropic hormone (= ACTN). Secreted by the anterior lobe of the pituitary.
ACTH/MSH: Adrenocorticotropic hormone/ melanin stimulating hormone (see Hormones - ACTH; MSH b).
ACTN: Adrenocorticotropin (see Hormones - ACTH).
ACTP: Adrenocorticotropic polypeptide. A hydrolysate of ACTH.
ADH: i. Antidiabetic hormone. The Insulins (see Insulin). ii. Antidiuretic hormone. Antidiuretic substance (ADS); Vasopressin. Secreted by the posterior lobe of the pituitary (see Hormones - PPH).
ADP: Antidiabetic principle (see Insulin).
ADS: Antidiuretic substance (= ADH; Vasopressin) (see Hs - ADH ii).
AH: i. Adaptive hormones. Secreted during adaptation to unusual circumstances, such as stress: e.g. ACTH; CH (epinephrine), etc. ii. Anabolic hormones, e.g. Nandrolone; Stanozolol (= Win 14,833). iii. Androgenic hormones. The masculinization hormones, androsterone and testosterone.
AMH: Adrenomedullary hormones = Chromaffin hs. (= CH). Secreted by the adrenal medulla, and including epinephrine and nor-epinephrine.
AMSH: Alpha melanocyte-stimulating hormone - now used in the treatment of arthritis.
APH: Anterior pituitary hormones. Secreted by the anterior lobe of the pituitary; these include: i. Adrenocorticotropic h. (= ACTH). ii. Anterior pituitary extract (= APE). iii. Gonadotropic h. (= GTH). iv. Somatotropic h. (= STH). v. Thyrotropic h. (= TTH) (see Hormones - under the appropriate headings).
APL: Anterior pituitary-like (substance) (see Hormones - HCG i).
APLH: Anterior pituitary-like hormone (see Hormones - HCG ii).
APLS: Anterior pituitary-like substance (see Hormones - HCG iii).
AVP: Aqueous/ Argenine vasopressin (hormone).
A-ZH: Ascheim-Zondek hormone = Luteinizing h. (LH) (see Hormones - LH v).
BGH: Bovine growth hormone = Bovine somatotropin (see Hormones - GH i).
B Hormone: Melanin stimulating hormone (see Hormones - MSH. b ii).
BMSH: Beta melanocytic-stimulating hormone = B hormone - (see Hormones b i).
BTSH: Bovine thyroid stimulating hormone (see Hormones - TSH i).
CCK: Cholecystokinin. An intestinal hormone that mediates impulses from the digestive tract and helps produce satiety.

CG: Chorionic gonadotropins (= Chorion Gonadotr) (see Hormones - HCG v).
CGH: Chorionic gonadotropic hormone (see Hormones - HCG iv).
CGP: Chorionic growth hormone prolactin (see Hormones - GH iii).
CGT: Chorionic gonadotropins (see Hormones - HCG v).
CGTH: Chorionic gonadotropic hormone (see Hormones - HCG iv).
CH: i. Chromaffin hormones - secreted by the adrenalin medulla, viz. epinephrine and norepinephrine (see Hormones - AMH). ii. Cortical hormone = Adrenocortical hs (ACH) (see Hormones - ACH).
CLH: Corpus luteum hormone, e.g. Progesterone (see Hormones - LH iv; OH - iiia; PH iii).
CLSH: Corpus luteum - stimulating hormone.
CRF: Corticotropin-releasing factor - the hypothalamic hormone that activates the anterior pituitary gland in its production of ACTH.
CRH: Corticotropin-releasing hormone.
CS: Corticosteroids. a. Naturally occurring CS, secreted by the adrenal cortex. i. Glucocorticoids - influencing gluconeogenesis (carbohydrate-regulating action), glycogenesis (glycogen deposition), and protein and calcium metabolism, e.g. cortisone and hydrocortisone. ii. Mineralocorticoids - influencing electrolyte and water metabolism, e.g. aldosterone, deoxycortone acetate (DOCA), etc. iii. Sex corticosteroids - some estrogens and androgens. b. Synthetically produced CS. i. Mainly glucocorticoid action, e.g. betamethasone; methylprednisolone, prednisone, etc. ii. Both glucocorticoid and mineralocorticoid action, e.g. fludrocortisone, etc. iii. Both anabolic and androgenic action e.g. methandriol, nandrolone, etc.
CSH: Chromatophore-stimulating hormone.
CTH: i. Chondrotropic hormone = Growth h (GH) (see Hormones - GH ii). ii. Chromatophototropic hormone (= Intermedin) - A proteohormone secreted by the pars intermedia of the pituitary, producing color changes in the skin of fishes and reptiles placed in the dark.
2,4-D: Dichlorophenoxy-acetic acid - a plant hormone (see 2,4-D).
DH: i. Diabetogenic hormone - secreted by the anterior lobe of the pituitary; causes glycosuria. ii. Diuretic hormone.
EH: Estrogenic hormones - the naturally occurring estrogens (see Hormones - H ii).
EPO: Erythropoietin. A hormone that stimulates red blood cell production in a major capacity, and could replace transfusions for dialysis patients.
FH: Follicle hormone (= Follicular h) - an estrogenic hormone produced by the graafian follicle (see Hormones - OH ii).
FRF: Follicle releasing factor (= FSH-RF).
FRH: Follicle releasing hormone (= FSH-RH).
FSH: i. Female sex hormones (see Hormones - OH ii). ii. Follicle stimulating hormone - a gonadotropic hormone (GTH), secreted by the anterior lobe of the pituitary and acting on the graafian follicle.
FSH-RF: Follicle-stimulating hormone releasing factor (see Hormones - FRF).
FSH-RH: Follicle-stimulating h. releasing hormone (see Hormones - FRH).
FT4; fT4: Free thyroxine (see Hormones - TH. ii B).
G-CSF: Granulocyte colony-stimulating factor (see HGF ii).
GDH: i. Gonadotropic hormones (= GTH) (see Hormones - GTH). ii. Growth and differentiation hormone (in insects).
GEF: Gonadotropin enhancing factor (see Hormones - GTH ii).
GH: Growth hormone. Any substance stimulating growth (see Hormones - IGF), especially that secreted by the anterior pituitary. This includes: i. Bovine growth h. (= BGH). ii. Chondrotropic h. (= CTH). iii. Chorionic growth hormone prolactin (= CGP). iv. Human growth h. (= HGH; hGH). v. Hypophyseal growth h. (= HGH; hGH). vi. Immunoreactive growth h. (= IGH; IRGH). vii. Immunoreactive human growth h. (= IRHGH). viii. Pituitary growth h. (= PGH). ix. Porcine growth h. (= PGH). x. Somatotropic h. (= STH). xi. Somatotropin (= ST).

GH-IH: Growth hormone-inhibiting hormone. This includes: i. Growth hormone release-inhibiting factor (= GHRIF; GRIF). ii. Growth hormone-releasing inhibitory h. (= GHRIH). iii. Growth (hormone) release-inhibitory h. (= GR-H). iv. Somatostatin. v. Somatotropin release inhibitory factor (= SRIF).
GHRF: Growth hormone releasing factor (see Hormones - GH-RH i).
GH-RH: Growth hormone-releasing hormone - Secreted by the anterior lobe of the pituitary gland; also by the thalamus. Included are: i. Growth hormone releasing factor (= GHRF). ii. Growth hormone release stimulating factor (= GHRSF). iii. Growth (hormone) releasing factor (= GRF). iv. Growth (hormone) releasing hormone (= GRH). v. Somatotropin releasing factor (= SRF). vi. Somatotropin releasing h. (= SRH).
GHRIF: Growth hormone release inhibiting factor (see Hormones - GH-IH i).
GHRIH: Growth hormone-release inhibitory hormone (see Hormones - GH-IH ii).
GHRSF: Growth hormone-release stimulating factor (see Hormones - GH-RH ii).
GIH: Gastrointestinal hormone.
GM-CSF: Granulocyte-macrophage colony-stimulating factor (see Hormones - HGF iii).
GnRF: Gonadotropin-releasing factor (see Hormones - GTH iii).
GnRH: Gonadotropin-releasing hormone (see Hormones - GTH iv).
GPH: Galactopoietic hormone = Lactogenic h. (LH) (see Hormones - LH i).
GRF: i. Gonadotropin-releasing factor (see Hormones - GTH iii). ii. Growth (hormone) releasing factor (see Hormones - GH-RH iii).
GRH. i. Gonadotropin-releasing hormone (see Hormones - GTH iv). ii. Growth (hormone) releasing hormone (see Hormones - GH-RH iv).
GRIF: Growth (hormone) release-inhibiting factor (see Hormones - GH-IH i).
GR-IH: Growth (hormone) release-inhibitory h. (see Hormones - GH-IH iii).
GSH: Glomerular-stimulating hormone.
GTH: Gonadotropic hormones (= GDH; Gonadotrophic hs.). Secreted by the anterior lobe of the pituitary, and acting on the gonads. These include: i. Follicular-stimulating h. (FSH) (see Hormones - FSH ii). ii. Gonadotropin enhancing factor (= GEF). iii. Gonadotropin-releasing factor (= GnRF; GRF). iv. Gonadotropin-releasing h. (= GnRH; GRH). v. Human pituitary follicle-stimulating h. (= HPFSH; hPFSH). vi. Human pituitary gonadotropin (= HPG). vii. Lactogenic h. (LH) (see Hormones - LH i). viii. Luteinizing h. (LH) (see Hormones - LH v). N.B. Any hormone acting on the gonads is known as a gonadotropic h.
hCFSH: Human chorionic follicle-stimulating hormone.
HCG; hCG. Human chorionic gonadotropin. Produced in the placenta and extracted from the urine of pregnant women. In the Female, its action is predominantly that of the pituitary luteinizing h. LH). In the Male, it stimulates the interstitial cells of the testes and the secretion of androgens (ICSH). These hormones include: i. Anterior pituitary-like (substance) (= APL). ii. Anterior pituitary-like h. (= APLH). iii. Anterior pituitary-like substance (= APLS). iv. Chorionic gonadotropic h. (= CGH; CGTH; PH). v. Chorionic gonadotropin (= CG; CGT; PH). vi. Immunoreactive human chorionic gonadotropin (= IRHCG). vii. Pregnancy urine (hormone) (= PU). viii. Pregnancy urine h. (= PUH). ix. Urinary chorionic gonadotropin (= UCG). x. Chorion Gonadotr. (= CG) (see Hormones - CG).
hCRH: Human corticotropin-releasing hormone.
HCS: Human chorionic somatomammotropin (= HCSM; hCSM; HPL; hPL; HPL molecule) (see Hormones - HPL; IRHCS; IRHPL).
HCSM; hCSM: Human chorionic somatomammotropin (see Hormones - HCS).
HCT; hCT: Human chorionic thyrotropin (= HPT; hPT).
HFSH: Human follicle-stimulating hormone (see Hormones - HMG ii).
HG: Human gonadotropin (see Hormones - HMG iii).
HGF: Hematologic growth factors. These hormones include: i. Erythropoietin (= EPO)

- necessary for normal red cell production. ii. Granulocyte colony-stimulating factor (= G-CSF) - this increases neutrophil activity and may help treat infections and cancer, and aid in bone-marrow transplants. iii. Granulocyte-macrophage colony-stimulating factor (= GM-CSF) - this enhances production of macrophages, neutrophils, eosinophils, and possibly red blood cells. iv. Interleukin-3 (= IL-3) - this stimulates production of myeloid cells, and may be used to treat AIDS and promote recovery from burns, chemotherapy, and bone-marrow transplants. v. Macrophage colony-stimulating factor (= M-CSF) - this causes macrophages to proliferate and may cause them to produce GM-CSF. It may fight infections and cancer.

HGH; hGH: i. Human growth hormone (see Hormones - GH iv). ii. Hypophyseal growth hormone (see Hormones - GH v).

HGHRF; hGHRF: Human growth hormone-releasing factor.

HGRH; hGRH: Human growth (hormone) releasing hormone.

HHRH: Hypothalamic hypophysiotropic releasing hormone.

HL: Luteinizing hormone (see Hormones - LH v).

HLH; hLH: Human luteinizing hormone (see Hormones - LH v).

HMG: Human menopausal gonadotropin. A purified standardized extract of urine of post-menopausal women, containing primarily the follicle-stimulating hormone (FSH), with only a trace of the luteinizing hormone (LH). This includes: i. Follotropin. ii. Human follicle-stimulating hormone (= HFSH). iii. Human gonadotropin (= HG). iv. Hu Me Gon (see Hormones - HUMEGON). v. Menopausal gonadotropin (= MG). vi. Menopausal urine hormone (= MUH).

HMG-HCG: Human menopausal gonadotropin-human chorionic gonadotropin.

HPFSH; hPFSH: Human pituitary follicle-stimulating h. (see Hormones - GTH v).

HPG: Human pituitary gonadotropin (see Hormones - GTH vi).

HPL; hPL: Human placental lactogen - produced by the syncytiotrophoblast cells of the placenta (see Hormones - HCS; IRHPL).

HPr: Human prolactin (see Hormones - PRL; LH i).

hPRL: Human (pituitary) prolactin (see Hormones - PRL; LH i).

HPT; hPT: Human placental thyrotropin (see Hormones - HCT).

HPTH: Hyperparathyroid hormone (see Hormones - PTH i).

HTH: Homeostatic thymus hormone.

HTS: Human thyroid-stimulating (hormone).

HTSH: Human thyroid stimulating hormone.

HU-FSH: Human urinary follicle-stimulating hormone.

HUMEGON: Human menopausal gonadotropin (see Hormones - HMG iv).

IADH: Inappropriate antidiuretic hormone (= ISADH).

ICGH: Integrated concentration of growth hormone.

ICSH: Interstitial cell-stimulating hormone. It stimulates the interstitial or Leydig cells of the testes (see Hormones - LH v).

IGF: Insulin-like growth factor. Many actions previously attributed to growth hormone (GH), are known to be mediated by these secondary growth factors. Two such factors have been isolated in humans. They have aminoacid structures, and both react homologously to proinsulin. Both factors are bound in serum to proteins in a complex carrier system. Several abnormal patterns of these factors are found in various types of diabetes. They are: i. IGF I - identical to Somatomedin C. ii. IGF II.

IGH: Immunoreactive growth hormone (see Hormones - GH vi).

IH: Inhibitory hormone (= Inhibiting h.). Any substance that exerts a depressing influence on certain of its target organs.

ILH: Immunoreactive luteinizing hormone.

IL-3: Interleukin-3 (see Hormones - HGF iv).

IPTH: Immunoreactive parathyroid hormone (see Hormones - PTH i).

I R-ACTH: Immunoreactive adrenocorticotropic hormone.

I RGH: Immunoreactive growth hormone (see Hormones - GH vi).

I RHCG: Immunoreactive human chorionic

gonadotropin (see Hormones - HCG vi).
IRHCS: Immuno-radioassayable/ Immunoreactive human chorionic somatomammotropin (see Hormones - HCS).
IRHGH: Immunoreactive human growth hormone (see Hormones - GH iv).
IRHPL: Immunoreactive human placental lactogen (see Hormones - HCS; HPL).
ISADH: Inappropriate secretion of antidiuretic hormone (see Hormones - IADH).
JH: Juvenile hormone (of insects).
KH: Ketogenic hormone. Secreted by the anterior lobe of the pituitary, and producing ketones.
LGH: Lactogenic hormone (see Hormones - LH i).
LH. i. Lactogenic hormone (= LGH) - one of the gonadotropic hormones secreted by the anterior pituitary. These include: a) Galactin; b) Galactopoietic h. (= GPH); c) Human pituitary prolactin (= hPRL); d) Human prolactin (= HPr); e) Lactation h. (= LH); f) Lutein-stimulating h. (= LSH); g) Luteomammotropic h. (= LMTH); h) Luteotropic factor (= LTF); i) Luteotropic h. (= LTH); j) Mammogen m I. - stimulates growth of the mammary ducts; m II. - stimulates growth of the lobules of the mammary gland; k) Mammotropic h. (= MH; MTH); l) Mammotropin; m) Prolactin (= PRL). ii. Langerhansian hormones - secreted by the islets of Langerhans, i.e. insulin; glucagon (see Insulin). iii. Local hormone - a substance with hormone-like properties produced from blood or the body fluids, acting locally in the target tissues where needed. iv. Luteal hormone - secreted by the Corpeus Luteum and including a) Corpeus luteum h. (= CLH); b) Luteohormone; c) Progesterone (see Hormones - OH iiia). v. Luteinizing hormone - a gonadotropic h. of the anterior pituitary. Among these are: a) Ascheim-Zondek h. (= A-ZH); b) Hormone, luteinizing (= HL); c) Human luteinizing h. (= HLH; hLH); d) Interstitial cell-stimulating h. (= ICSH) - in the male.
LH/FSH/RH: Luteinizing hormone/ follicle-stimulating hormone/ releasing hormone.
LHRF: Luteinizing hormone-releasing factor (see Hormones - LH-RH).
LH-RH: Luteinizing hormone-releasing hormone (a peptide) - Now used in treatment of cancer of the prostate. i. Secrcted by the anterior lobe of the pituitary: a) Luteinizing hormone-releaing factor (= LHRF); b) Luteinizing releasing factor (= LRF); c) Luteinizing releasing hormone (= LRH). ii. Also produced synthetically: a) Synthetic gonadotropic-releasing hormone (= SGRH); b) Synthetic gonadotropin (= SG).
LMH: Lipid mobilizing hormone.
LMTH: Luteomammotropic hormone (see Hormones - LH i).
LPH: Lipotropic hormone (= Lipotropic pituitary h.; Lipotropin).
LRF: Luteinizing releasing factor (see LH-RH i).
LRH: Luteinizing releasing hormone (see LH-RH i).
LSF: Lymphocyte-stimulating factor (see Hormones - LSH ii).
LSH: i. Lutein-stimulating hormone (see Hormones - LH i); ii. Lymphocyte-stimulating hormone (= LSF).
LT: l-Thyroxine; l-Triiodothyronine (see Hormones - TH iiA).
LT3: Triiodothyronine (see Hormones - TH iiA).
LT4: Thyroxine (see Hormones - TH iiA).
LTF: Luteotropic factor (see Hormones - LH i).
LTH: Luteotropic hormone (see Hormones - LH i).
M-CSF: Macrophage colony-stimulating factor (see Hormones - HGF v).
MG: Menopausal gonadotropin (see Hormones - HMG v).
MH: i. Mammotropic hormone (see Hormones - MTH; LH i); ii. Melanophore hormone (see Hormones - MSH b viii).
MIF: i. Melanocyte-stimulating hormone inhibitory factor; ii. Melanotropin-release inhibiting factor.
MRF: Melanocyte (stimulating hormone) releasing factor (see Hormones - MSH b vi).
MRH: Melanocyte (stimulating hormone) releasing hormone (see Hormones - MSH b vii).

MSH: a. Male sex hormone (see Hormones - OH i); b. Melanin-stimulating hormone - a polypeptide derived from the pars intermedia of the pituitary. It stimulates the production of melanin and includes: i) Beta melanocyte-stimulating h. (= BMSH). ii) B hormone (= Melanin stimulating h.). iii) Chromatophore h. iv) Intermedin. v) Melanocyte/tic-stimulating h. (= MSH). vi) Melanocyte (stimulating hormone) releasing factor (= MRF; MSH-releasing factor). vii) Melanocyte (stimulating hormone) releasing hormone (= MRH; MSH-releasing hormone). viii) Melanophore h. (= MH). ix) Melanophore-stimulating h. (= MSH). x) MSH-releasing factor/ hormone (see Hs. - MSH b vi & b vii). xi) Pigment h.
MSHIF: Melanocyte-stimulating hormone inhibiting factor.
MSHRF: Melanocyte-stimulating hormone-releasing factor.
MSHRH: Melanocyte-stimulating hormone-releasing hormone.
MTH: Mammotropic hormone (see Hormones - LH i).
MUH: Menopausal urine hormone (see Hormones - HMG vi).
OCH: Oral contraceptive hormone.
OH: i. Orchidic hormones (The androgens or Male sex hs. - MSH; Testicular hs. - TH). a) Naturally occurring - secreted by the testes, e.g. Androsterone - found in the testes and male human urine; Dihydroandrosterone - found in male urine; Testosterone - isolated by the testes. b) Synthetic androgens, e.g. Fluoxymesterone; Stanolone. ii. Ovarian hormones (The estrogens or Estrogenic hs - EH; Female sex hs. - FSH; Follicular hs. - FH). a) Naturally occurring - secreted by the ovaries, e.g. Estradiol (= dihydroxy-esterone) - the hormone secreted in the follicular fluid of the ovary; also present in pregnancy urine. Estriol (= trihydroxy-estrone) - found in pregnant urine and in the placenta. Estrone (= ketohydroxy-estrone) - found in the urine of pregnancy. b) Synthetic estrogens. Not steroids, but have action similar to those of estradiol, e.g. Chlorotrianisene; Ethynylestradiol; Hexestrol; Mestranol; Quinestradol; Stilbestrol; etc. iii. The Progestogens. a) Naturally occurring, e.g. Corpus luteum h. (CLH); Luteo hormone; Progesterone (see LH iv). b) Synthetic progestogens - Chlormedinone; Dydrogesterone; Hydroxyprogesterone caproate; Medroxyprogesterone acetate; Megestrol acetate; Normethandrone; etc.
OIH: Ovulation-inducing hormone.
OLH: Ovine lactogenic hormone.
oLH: Ovine luteinizing hormone.
OP; oPRL: Ovine prolactin.
PGH: i. Pituitary growth hormone (see Hormones - GH viii). ii. Porcine growth hormone (see Hormones - GH ix).
PH: i. Phytohormone. A plant h. (see 2,4-D; 2,4,5-T). ii. Placental hormone - produced by the placenta during pregnancy. It includes Chorionic gonadotropin (CG; CGT); Relaxin; etc. (see HCG). iii. Progestational hormone - Progesterone. This prepares the endometrium for nidation of the fertilized ovum during conception, e.g. Corpus luteal h. (CLH); Luteal h. (LH).
PIF: Prolactin inhibiting factor (see Hormones - PIH).
PIH: Prolactin inhibiting hormone. Secreted by the anterior lobe of the pituitary; controls excessive milk secretion and engorgement of the breast (= PIF).
PMS: Pregnant mares' serum (see Hormones - PMSG).
PMSG: Pregnant mares' serum gonadotropin (= Gonadotr Seric; PMS; Serum Gonadotropin). Produced in the placenta and endometrium of the pregnant mare, and extracted from its serum.
PPH: Posterior pituitary hormones. Secreted by the posterior lobe of the pituitary. Includes Vasopressin (ADH, Anti-diuretic h, or Pitressin) and Oxytocin (= Pitocin).
PRF: Prolactin releasing factor (see Hormones - PRH).
PRH: Prolactin releasing hormone. Secreted by the anterior lobe of the pituitary; maintains milk secretion in the breast (= PRF).
PRL: Prolactin (= HPr; hPRL) (see Hormones - LH i).
PTH: i. Parathyroid hormone (= Parathormone) - secreted by the parathyroid

glands, and influences calcium and phosphorus metabolism and bone formation. ii. Parathyrotropic hormone (= Parathyreotrophic h) - secreted by the anterior lobe of the pituitary.
PU: Pregnancy urine (hormone) (see PUH).
PUH: Pregnany urine hormone (= PU) - contains Chorionic gonadotropin (CG) (see Hormones - HCG vii & viii).
SG: Synthetic gonadotropin (see Hormones - LH-RH ii).
SGRH: Synthetic gonadotropic/pin-releasing hormone (see Hormomes - LH-RH ii).
SH: Sex hormones. i. Androgenic activity hormones (= MSH or Male sex hs.) (see Hormones - MSH a; OH i). ii. Estrogenic activity hormones (= FSH or Female sex hs.) (see Hormones - FSH i; OH ii).
SMS: Somatostatin. A synthetic pituitary hormone which depresses thyroid function.
SRF: Somatotropin releasing factor (see Hormones - GH-RH v).
SRH: Somatotropin releasing hormone (see Hormones - GH-RH vi).
SRIF: Somatotropin release inhibitory factor (see Hormones - GH-IH v).
ST: Somatotropin (see Hormones - GH xi).
STH: i. Somatotropic hormone (see Hormones - GH x). ii. Supplemental throid hormone.
T_3: Triiodothyronine (see Hormones - TH iiA).
T_4: Tetraiodothyronine (see Hormones - TH iiB).
TH: i. Testicular hormones (= Testes hs.). Secreted by the testes (see Hormones - OH i). ii. Thyroid hormones. A. The laevo-isomers. They raise the metabolic rate, increase oxygen consumption, reduce cholesterol levels, and are used in the treatment of thyroid deficiency states, e.g. Thyroxine (= l-Thyroxine; LT; LT4). Triiodothyronine (= l-Triiodothyronine; LT3; T3). B. The dextro-isomers. They reduce serum cholesterol levels and increase oxygen consumption, but have a greatly reduced effect on the basal metabolic rate. They have been tried in the treatment of hypercholesterolemia, but may bave adverse effects on the heart, such as attacks of angina pectoris, e.g. Detrothyronine (= DT3; D-Triiodothyronine; SKF D-2623). Tetraiodothyronine (= DT4; Dextrothyroxine sodium; d-thyroxine; FT4; fT4; Free thyroxine). iii. Thyrotropic hormone (= TTH) (see Hormones - TSH ii).
THRF: Thyrotropic hormone-releasing factor (see Hormones - TRH ii).
TRF: Thyrotropin-releasing factor (see Hormones - TRH iii).
TRH: Thyrotropin-releasing hormone. Secreted by the anterior lobe of the pituitary, and includes: i. Thyroid stimulating hormone-releasing factor (= TSH-RF). ii. Thyrotropic hormone-releasing factor (= THRF). iii. Thyrotropin-releasing factor (= TRF).
TSH: Thyroid stimulating hormone. Secreted by the anterior lobe of the pituitary, and includes: i. Bovine thyroid stimulating hormone (= BTSH). ii. Thyrotropic hormone (= TH; TTH). iii. Thyrotropin (= TT).
TSH-RF: Thyroid stimulating hormone-releasing factor (see Hormones - TRH i).
TT: Thyrotropin (see Hormones - TSH iii).
TTH: Thyrotropic hormone (see Hormones - TSH ii).
UCG: Urinary chorionic gonadotropin (see Hormones - HCG ix).

Horse Heroin (see Diamorph).
hor som at bedtime (L. hori somni) (see hor decub).
Hort Horticulture.
hor un spatio at the end of one hour (L. horae unius spatio).
HOS Holt-Oram syndrome; Human osteosarcoma; Hyper/ Hypo-osmolar solution/ state.
HoS Horse serum.
H_2OsO_4 Osmic acid.
Hosp Hospital (= hosp); Hospitals (AHA journal).
hosp hospital (see Hosp).
Hosp Ins Hospital insurance.
HOST Hypo-osmotic shock treatment.
HOT Hands-on therapy (psychiatry); Hemoccult-test (selective for Hb - for detection of occult blood); Hospital outpatient treatment (see HOPT); Human old tuberculin (see Tuberculin - TO); Human organ transplant; Hyperbaric oxygen therapy;

Hypertension Optimal Trial (see HOTS; HOTT); Hypertensive Optimal Treatment (Study).

HOTS Hypercalcemia-osteolysis - T-cell syndrome; Hypertension Optional Treatment Study.

HOTT Hypertension Optimal Treatment Trial.

HP Halogen phosphorus; Handicapped person; Haptoglobin (see Hp); Hard palate; Hartmann procedure (sigmoid resection and colostomy); Harvard pump; Health Physics (journal); Health profession(al); Heat production; Heel to patella; Hemiparesis; Hemiparkinsonism; Hemipelvectomy; Hemiplegia (see Hp); Hemoperfusion; Hemophilus pleuropneumoniae; Heparin; Hewlitt-Packard (Co.); High potency/ power/ pressure/ protein; Highly possible/ probable/ purified; Hoffmann procedure (for reconstruction of forefoot); Horizontal plane; Horsepower (unit) (see hp); Hospital participation/ pharmacist/ physician/ practice; Hospital Physician/ Practice (journals); Hot pack/ pad; House physician; Human Pathology (journal); Human pituitary; Hydrogen peroxide; Hydrophilic petrolatum; Hydrostatic pressure; Hydroxypropyl; Hydroxypyruvate; Hyperparathyroidism; Hyperpathia (excessive pain experienced from a minor noxious stimulus); Hyperphoria; Hypersensitivity pneumonitis; Hypertension + proteinuria; Hypophoria; Smith & Nephew Pharmaceutical Ltd. code for experimental substances.

Hp Haptoglobin (= HP; α-2-haptoglobin); *Helicobacter* pylori (see HAG; NNC).Hematoporphyrin; Hemiplegia (= HP).

hp horsepower (unit of) (= HP).

H&P History and physical (examination) (= HPE).

HP 209 Ethoxybenzamide (= Ethenzamide; Ethylsalicylamide). Used as an analgesic.

HP 1275 Phenoxypropazine maleate - a monoamine oxidase inhibitor, used in the treatment of depression.

HPA 4-ethylsulphonyl-naphthalene-1-sulfonamide; Healthcare Power of Attorney; *Helix* pomatia agglutinin; Hemagglutinating penicillin antibody; Histoplasma capsulatum polysaccharide antigen; Hospital Physicists' Association (UK); Humeroscapular periarthritis; Hypoplastic anemia; Hypoproteinanemia; Hypothalamic-pituitary axis; Hypothalamic/mo-pituitary-adrenal/nocortical (axis, function, or system) (= HPAA; HPAC).

HPAA Hydroperoxyarachidonic acid; Hydroxyphenylacetic acid; Hypothalamo-pituitary-adrenal axis (see HPA).

HPAC Health Policy Advisory Center; Hypothalamo-pituitary-adreno-cortical (see HPA).

HPADU *Helicobacter* pylori-associated duodenal ulcer.

HPAGA uman protein galactosidase A (see AGA; FD).

HPAP Herpes zoster-associated pain; High peak airway pressure.

HPAPUD *Helicobacter* pylori-associated peptic ulcer disease.

HPB Health Programs/ Protection Branch (DNHW); High protein binding; Host:parasite balance.

HPBC Hyperpolarizing bipolar cell.

HPβCD Hydroxypropyl-β-cyclodextrin.

HPBDs Highly protein-bound drugs (such as Beta adrenergic blocking agents, Chloramphenicol, Coumarins, Monoxamine oxidase inhibitors, Probenecid, Salicylates, Sulfonamines, etc.).

HPBF Hepatotrophic portal blood factor.

HPBL Human peripheral blood leukocyte; Human Peripheral Blood Lymphocyte (chromosome aberration test, for mutagenicity).

HPC Hemangiopericytoma; High peak concentration; High-pitched cry; Hippocampal pyramidal cell; Histopathologic(al) change/ classification/ criteria; History of present complaint; Holoprosencephaly; Hydrophilic compound; Hydrophobic chromatography; Hydroxyphenyl-cinchoninic acid (= Oxycinchophen) - formerly used in the treatment of gout and rheumatism; Hydroxypropylcellulose.

HPC-1 Hereditary prostate cancer 1-gene.

HPCA Human progenitor cell antigen.

HPCC Human pancreatic/ pulmonary cancer cell.

HPCHA High (red-cell) phosphatidylcholine

hemolytic anemia.

HPCT Hematopoietic progenitor cell transplant.

HPCUS Homeopathic Pharmacopoeia Convention of the United States.

HPD Hearing protective device; Hemopoietic depression; Hepatic parenchymal disease; High-protein diet; Histopathological difference; Histrionic Personality Disorder; Home peritoneal dialysis; Hyperprolactinemic disorder(s) (with amenorrhea, galactorrhea, etc.); Hypothalamic-pituitary disease/ dysfunction.

H-PD Hough-Powell digitizer.

HPE Health ProfessionalEducation; Heavy physical exertion; Hepatic portoenterostomy; Hexosephosphoric ester (see HDP); High-permeability edema; Histopathological examination; History and physical examination (see H&P); Hydrostatic permeability edema.

HPEA Health Programs Extension Act (of 1973).

HPEAA Health Professions Educational Assistance Act.

HPEK Paul B Elder Co code for experimental substances.

HPER Health, physical education, and recreation.

HPETE Hydroxyperoxy-eicosotetranoic (acid).

HPF Heparin-precipitable fraction; Hepatic plasma flow; High-pass filter; High-power field (see hpf); High protection factor; Histopathological feature(s)/ finding(s); Hypocaloric protein feeding.

hpf high-power field (microscope/py) (= HPF).

HPFH Hereditary persistance of fetal hemoglobin.

HPFN High-pass filtered noise.

HPFS Health Professionals' Follow-up Study.

HPFSH; hPFSH Human pituitary follicle-stimulating hormone (see Hormones - GTH; HPFSH; hPFSH).

HPG Helicobacter pylori-associated gastritis.

HPG; hPG Human pituitary gonadotropin (see Hormones - HPG; GTH vi).

2hPG Two-hour plasma glucose.

3HPGA Tritium-labeled pteroylglutamic acid (drug therapy).

HPGF Hypothalamic-pituitary gonadotrophic function.

HPH Hemiplegic hypoglycemia.

HPHG Hyperprolactinemic hypogonadism.

HPI *Helicobacter* pylori infection (see NNC); Hepatic perfusion index; High protein intake; Highly purified insulin (see Insulin); History of present illness.

HPIP Health Practitioners Intervention Program (Williamsburg, Va).

HPL Habitual pitch level; Health-plan level; High plasma level (of a drug); Histopathologic lesion(s); Human parotid lysozyme; Human peripheral lymphocyte; Human placental lactogen - produced by the syncytiotrophoblast cells of the placenta (= hPL) (see Hormones - HCS; HPL); Human platelet lactogen (= hPL); Hyperplexia; Hyperprolactinemia.

hPL Human placental lactogen (see HPL); Human platelet lactogen (see HPL).

HPLA Hippurylphenyl-lactate; Hydroxyphenyl-lactic acid.

HPLAC High-pressure liquid-affinity chromatography.

HPLC High-performance/ -power/ -pressure liquid chromatography.

HPLD Hyperprolactinemic disease/ disorder/ dysfunction (see HPL).

HPLE Hereditary polymorphic light eruption.

HPL molecule Human placental lactogen molecule (see Hormones - HCS; HPL).

HPLO Health-promoting live organism (such as *Lactobacillus*, *Bifidobacterium*, etc., also known as the 'friendly bacteria/ium' or Probiotic) (see BFB; FOS; PB).

HPM Harding-Passey melanoma; Hemiplegic migraine; High-performance membrane; High-power microscope.

HPMC Human peripheral mononuclear cell; Hydroxypropyl-methylcellulose - used as an emulsifying, lubricating and thickening agent.

HPMG Human post-menopausal gonadotrophin (see HMG; PMG).

HPMT Histoplasma myecelial (serology) test.

HPN Home parenteral nutrition; Hypertension (= hpn).

hpn hypertension (see HPN); our own purgative draft (L. haustus purgans noster).

HPNS High pressure neurological syndrome.
HPO High pressure oxygen (respiratory therapy) (see HOB); Hydroperoxide; Hydrophilic ointment/ opioid (e.g. morphine); Hypertrophic pulmonary osteoarthropathy; Hypothalamic-pituitary-ovarian (axis) (see HPOA).
HPO_3 Metaphophoric acid.
H_3PO_2 Hypophosphorous acid.
H_3PO_4 Orthophosphoric acid (= Phosphoric acid).
$H_4P_2O_6$ Hypophosphoric acid.
$H_4P_2O_7$ Pyrophosphoric acid.
HPOA Hypothalamic-pituitary-ovarian axis (= HPO); Hypothalamus and preoptic area.
H potential His potential (symbol H).
HPP Hereditary pyropoikilocytosis; High pharmacological potency; History of presenting problems; Human pancreatic polypeptide; Human plasma protein; Hydroxyphenylpyruvate (= hPP) (see HPPA); Hydroxypyrazolo-pyrimidine (= Allopurinol; hPP; 4-HPP) - it reduces the production of uric acid by inhibiting xanthine oxidase, and is used in the treatment of gout (see BW 55-158); Hyper/ Hypo kalemic periodic paralysis.
hPP; 4-HPP Hydroxypyrazolopyrimidine (see HPP).
HPPA Hydroxyphenyl-pyruvic acid (see HPP).
HPPF Human plasma protein fraction.
HPPH Hydroxyphenyl-phenylhydantoin (= 5-{4-hydroxyphenyl}-5-phenylhydantoin; 5-phenyl-5-parahydroxyl-phenylhydantoin).
HPPO High partial pressure of oxygen; Hydroxyphenyl pyruvate oxidase.
HPR Haptoglobin-related gene; Health Policy Report; House Physician Reporter (journal).
HPr Heat-stable protein; Human prolactin (see Hormones - LH id; PRL).
HPRA High plasma renin activity (see PRA).
hPRL Human (pituitary) prolactin (see Hormones - LH ic; PRL).
Hpro Hydroxyproline.
HPRP Human platelet-rich plasma.
HPRT Hypoxanthine(-guanine) phospho-ribosyl-transferase. An enzyme found lacking in Lesch-Nyhan disease.
HPS Hantavirus pulmonary syndrome; Health Physics Society; Health promotion specialist; Hematopoietic system; Hematoxylin-phloxine-saffron; Hermansky-Pudlak syndrome; High-pressure sodium (lamp); High-protein supplement (diet order); His-Purkinje system; Histopathological study; Human Patient Simulator; Human platelet suspension; Hypertrophic pyloric stenosis; Hypothalamic-pituitary sarcoidosis; Hypothalamic pubertal syndrome.
HPSA Hyper/Hypo baric spinal anesthesia.
HPSAP Health Professions Student Assistance Program.
HPSL Health Professions Student Loan.
HPT Histamine provocation test; Home pregnancy test (based on detection of HCG in the urine); Human phage therapy (bacteriophage - "bacteria devouring"); Human placental thyrotropin (see Hormones-HPT); Hyperparathyroidism; Hypoparathyroidism; Hypothalamic-pituitary testicular (axis); Hypothalamo-pituitary-thyroid (system); Hysterical personality trait(s).
H2PteGlu Dihydrofolate.
H4PteGlu Tetrahydrofolate.
HPTH Hyperparathyroid hormone (see Hormones - HPTH).
hPTH Human parathyroid hormone (I_{34}-teriparatide).
HPTIN Human pancreatic trypsin inhibitor.
HPTM Home prothrombin time monitoring.
HPU Heater probe unit.
HPUS Homeopathic Pharmacopoeia of the United States.
HPV *Hemophilus* pertussis vaccine; Hepatic portal vein; Human papilloma virus; Human parvovirus; Human polyoma virus (types BKV and JCV, pathogens causing nephropathy in renal transplantation); Human pulmonary vasoconstriction.
HPVC High-production-volume chemical.
HPVD Hypertensive pulmonary vascular disease.
HPV-DE High-passage virus - duck embryo.
HPV-DK High-passage virus - dog kidney.
HPVG Hepatic portal venous gas.
HPW Hypergammaglobulinemia purpura of Waldenström.

HPX Hexachloroparaxylene (= Chloxyle; Hexachloroparaxylol). Used as an anthelmintic in the treatment of clonorchiasis, fascioliasis, and paragonimiasis; High peroxidase (content); Hypophysectomized.

HPY Histoplasma yeast (serology test).

HPZ High-pressure zone.

HQ Headquarters; Homeostasis Quaterly (AMRS journal); Hypnosis Quaterly (journal).

HQC High-quality care (see HQHC); Hydroquinone cream.

HQHC High-quality health care (= HQC).

(3H)QNB (3H)quinuclidinyl benzilate.

HR A buffer; Hallux rigidus; Harrington rod; Hazard ratio; Health Resources (see HRA; HRD; HRF; HRO; HRP; HRPP; HRS; HRSA); Heart rate (beats/minute) (= HRT; HRt); Hemorrhagic retinopathy; Hernia repair; Herxheimer reaction (of fat cells to Herxheimer stain); Heterosexual relations (scale); High resolution; Higher rate; Hormonal response; Hospital record/ report; House of Representatives (US Congress = HR + Senate); Hyperimmune reaction; Hypophosphatemic rickets; O-B-hydroxyethyl-rutosides (= HRs).

Hr Blood factor related to Rh; Hour (see hr).

hr hairless (mouse); host-range (mutant); hour (= Hr).

H&R Hysterectomy and radiation (operation/ gynecology).

HR1 House Resolution 1 (US House of Representatives).

H2R Histamine-2-receptor.

HRA Health Resources Administration (HEW) (formerly HSMHA); Health risk appraisal; Health Risk Assessment (test); Heart rate audiometry; Heart-related ailment (see HRC); High right atrium (see HRAE); High-risk activity; Histamine-receptor antagonist; Histamine release activity; Human Resources Administration.

H1RA H1 receptor antagonist(s) (Antihistamines).

H2RA H2 receptor antagonist(s) (gastric anticholinergic agents such as cimetidine, famotidine, ranitidine, etc.).

HRAE High right atrial/ atrium electrogram (= HRA).

HRANA Histone reactive ANA.

HRB High-risk behavior.

HRBC Horse red blood cell.

HRC Hattler respiratory catheter (used intravenously in acute lung injury, to oxygenate blood through one interior channel while drawing carbon dioxide out through another); Heart-related condition (= HRA); Heat-regulating center (hypothalamus) (see HHRC); High-resolution chromatography; Highest risk category; Horse red cell; Human rights committee.

HRCT; HR-CT High-resolution computed tomography.

HRD Health Resources Development (Bureau of) (HEW).

HRDD Human recommended daily dose (see RHDD).

HRDG Holographically recorded diffraction grating.

HRDI Hospital Reserve Disaster Inventory.

HRE Hepatic reticuloendothelial (cell); Herpes-related encephalitis; High-resolution electrocardiography; Hormone receptor enzyme.

H-reflx Hoffmann reflex (symbol: H).

HREH High-renin essential hypertension.

HREM High-resolution electron microscope/py.

H-response Exaggerated photic response to intermittent flashes of light (migraine) (symbol: H).

HRF Harris return flow; Health-related facility; Health Resources Fund; Histamine releasing factor; Humoral recognition factor(s); Hypercapnic/ Hypoxemic respiratory failure.

HRG Health Research Group (Consumer advocate group - Ralph Nader); High-risk group; HIV/ Human resistance/ restriction gene; Hypocretin-receptor gene (see ORG).

HR2G Hypocretin receptor 2 gene (= OR2G) (its mutation causes the sleep disorder, narcolepsy).

HRHP High-risk heart patient.

HRI High(er) resolution image (such as on BSE-imaging technique); Holt Radium Institute (UK).

HRIF Histamine releasing inhibitory factor.

HRIG; HRIg Human rabies immunoglobulin.
HRL Hair-removal laser; Head rotated/ation (to the) left.
HRLA Human reovirus-like agent.
HRLC High-resolution liquid chromatography.
HRLM High resolution light microscopy.
HRM Heart rate meter; Heart-related morbidity/ mortality (see HRMR); High-risk method.
HRMR Heart-related morbidity/ mortality rate.
HRN Health Rights News (journal).
hRNA Heterogeneous ribonucleic acid.
HRNB Halstead-Reitan Neuropsychological Battery; High-risk neuroblastoma.
HRO Health Resources Opportunity (HRA); Hip replacement operation.
HRP Health resources planning; High-risk patient/ population/ pregnancy; Histidine-rich protein; Hormone-replacement pill (see HRT); Horseradish peroxidase.
HRPC Hormone refractory prostatic cancer.
HRPD Hamburg Rating Scale for Psychiatric Disorders.
HRPP Health Resources Planning Program.
HRQL Health-related quality of life.
HRR Head rotated/ation (to the) right; Health-risk research; Heart rate range; High relative risk; Higher response rate.
HRRD Heart-rate and rhythm disorder.
HRRI Heart rate retardation index.
HRS Hamilton Rating Scale; Harm reduction strategy (in the management of problem drinkers) (= HRT); Health Resources and Services; Health resources statistics; Hepatic redox state; Hepato-renal syndrome; High rate of stimulation; High-resolution scan; High-risk source (of infection, etc.); Hip replacement surgery (Orthopedics); Histamine/ Hormone receptor site; Humeroradial synostosis.
HRs Hydroxyethylrutosides (see HR).
Hrs Hours.
HRSA Health Resources and Services Administration; High-risk sexual activity.
HRSD Hamilton Rating Scale for Depression (= HRS-D).
HRS-D Hamilton Rating Scale for Depression; Hirschsprung's disease.
HRSEM High-resolution scanning electron microscope.
HRT Harm reduction technique(s) (see HRS); Heart rate (see HR); High-risk therapy/ transplant; Hormone-refractive/-related tumor; Hormone replacement therapy.
HRt Heart rate (see HR).
HRTCP Heparin-related thrombocytopenia.
HRTE Human reverse transcriptase enzyme.
HRTEM High-resolution transmission electron microscope/py.
HRTI Hospital Research and Testing Institute.
HRU Hypertension Research Unit (Paris, France; Quebec, Canada; etc.).
HRUM Health Revolutionary Unity Movement.
HRV Heart rate variability; High resolution valve (gas flow); Human reovirus/ rotavirus.
HRVV Human rotavirus vaccine.
HRWCJ Highly respected and widely circulated journal.
HS At bedtime (see hs); Haber/ Hegglin's/ Horner's/ Hurler's/ Hypereosinophilic syndrome; Half-strength; Hamstring; Hand surgery; Hartmann's solution; Head sling; Healthy subject; Heart sound(s); Heat-stable; Heavy smoker; Heme synthetase; Henoch-Schönlein (purpura) (see HSP); Heparan sulfate; Hereditary spherocytosis; Herpes simplex; Hidradenitis suppurativa; High school/ sensitivity; Homeostasis; Home study; Homologous/ Horse/ Human serum; Horizontally selective; Hospital ship/ staff/ stay; Hours of sleep (see hs); House Supervisor/ Surgeon; Hyperkinetic syndrome (= ADD or Attention deficit disorder; MBD or Minimal brain damage; OBD or Organic behavior disorder); Hypersensitivity; Hypertonic saline; Sandoz (USA) code for experimental substances.
Hs Hormones (see Hormones).
hs at bedtime or just before sleeping (L. hora somni) (= HS; h som; hss); hours of sleep (= HS).
H/S Helper-suppressor (ratio).
H→S Heel to shin.
H&S Hemorrhage and shock; Hysterectomy and sterilization.
H_2S Hydrogen sulfide.

HSA Hair shaft abnormality (= HSD) - Four major categories: 1. Fracture; 2. Irregularity; 3. Coiling and twisting; 4. Extraneous matter, such as Tinea capitis, Trichomycosis axillaris or piedra, Pediculosis capitis and Peripilar cast; Hazardous Substances Act; Health Service Agency/ Area (see HSAs); Health Services Act/ Administration (HEW)/ Agencies (HEW); Health-system administrator; Health Systems Agency (HEW) (see HSAs); Hearing and Speech Action (journal); Hereditary sideroblastic anemia; Hereditary spastic ataxia (Marie); Highly strenuous activity; High sustained acceleration; High systemic activity; Horse/ Human serum albumin; Hospital Savings Association; Hospital Seminar on Audit (JCAH); Hypersomnia-sleep apnea.

HSAC Health Security Action Council; Health Services Advisory Committee (UK).

HSAG N-2-hydroxyethylpiperazine-N-2-ethanesulfonate-saline-albumin-gelatin.

HSA^{125} I Human serum albumin labeled with radioactive iodine.

HSAN Hereditary sensory and autonomic neuropathy.

HSAP Heat-stable alkaline phophatase.

HSArg High-speed autoradiography.

HSAS Hypertrophic subaortic stenosis.

HSAs Health service agencies/ areas (= HSA); Health systems agencies (= HSA).

HSB Human sexual/social behavior (normal/pathological).

HSBP Heyer-Schulte breast prosthesis.

HSBG Heel stick blood gas.

HSC Hand-Schüller-Christian (disease/ syndrome) (see HSCD); Hard shell capsule; Health and Safety Commission (UK); Health sciences/ screening center; Health Service Commissioner (NHS, Brit); Health Standards and Consultants (DNHW); Hematopoietic stem cell (= GF - Growth factor, GIM - Growth-inducing molecule, or IM - Inducing molecule); Hemostatic clamp (see HC); Hetero/ Homosexual couple; Hospital for Sick Children (London, UK) (Toronto, Canada); Human sex chromosome (X); Human skin collagenase; Human stem cell.

HSCA Health and Social Care Act (2001) (UK); Health Sciences Communications Association.

HSCD Hand-Schüller-Christian disease (= HSC).

HSCL Hopkins Symptom Check List.

HSCl High systemic clearance (in l/min).

HS-CoA Reduced coenzyme A.

HSCRC Health Services Cost Review Commission (Maryland).

hs-CRP High-sensitivity C-reactive protein (high blood level is associated with MI, CVA, and other vascular conditions).

HSCS Hysterosalpingo-contrast sonograph(y) (see HyCoSy).

HSCT Hematopoietic stem-cell transplant(ation).

HSD Habital shoulder dislocation (Orthopedics); Hair shaft defect (see HSA); Hallermann-Streiff syndrome (see MOFD); Hallervorden-Spatz disease; Hamilton Scale of Depression; Hemoglobin S disease (see SCD - Sickle cell disease); Hepatosplenic disease; Herniated spinal disk; Highly significant difference (see PSD); Honest significant difference; Human sleep disorder; Hydroxysteroid dehydrogenase; Hypersensitivity disorder; Hypoactive sexual desire.

H(SD) Holtzman Sprague-Dawley (rat).

HSDA Health Systems Development Act.

HSDB Hazardous Substances Data Bank.

HSE Harmful side effect(s); Herpes simplex encephalitis; Hemorrhagic shock and encephalopathy; High/ Human systemic exposure; Human serum esterase; Hypertonic saline enema.

HSEL High systemic exposure level.

HSES Hemorrhagic shock-encephalopathy syndrome.

HSF Hip screw fixation (Orthopedics).Histamine sensitizing factor; Hypothalamic secretory factor.

HSG Health and Safety Guidelines (DoH, UK); Herpes simplex genitalis; High sustained gravity; Histosalpingogram/graphy; Hysterosalpingogram/graphy.

hSGF Human skeletal growth factor.

HSGP Human sialoglycoprotein.

HSH Homologous serum hepatitis; Human

stress hormone (see ASH).
HSHC Hydrocortisone hemisuccinate.
HSI Heat stress index; Hetero/Homo sexual intercourse; Highly significant increase; Highway Safety Institute; Human seminal (plasma) inhibitor; Human specific immunoglobulin.
H_2SiO_3 Metasilicic acid.
H_2SiO_4 Orthosilicic acid.
HSJ Homologous serum jaundice.
HSK Herpes simplex keratitis.
HSL Herpes simplex labialis.
HSLC High-speed liquid chromatography.
HSM Hamstring muscle (= Biceps femoris); Hepatosplenomegaly; Holosystolic murmur.
HSMET Health Systems and Medical Engineering Technology (Committee).
HSMHA Health Services and Mental Health Administration (now HRA) (HEW).
HSN Hereditary sensory neuropathy.
HSO Health Service Ombudsman (GMC, UK); Health service organization(s).
H_2SO_3 Sulphurous acid (= Sulfurous a.).
H_2SO_4 Sulfuric acid.
hSOD Human superoxide dismutase.
h som at bedtime (L. hora somni) (see hs).
HSP Health-surveillance program; Health Systems Plan; Heat-shock protein (gene) (resistant to tumor cells = hsp); Heat-stable protein; Hemorrhagic smallpox (or Black pox, a form of Variola major, with black, unclotted blood oozing from the mouth and other body orifices; almost 100% fatal); Hemostatic screening profile; Henoch-Schönlein purpura (= HS; HSS); Hereditary spastic paraparesis; Hermetically sealed pacemaker (Starr-Edwards); Hospital Service Plan; Human serum prealbumin/ protein; Hypothalamus-specific peptide; Hysterosalpingography (see HSG).
hsp heat shock protein (gene).
HSPC Hormone-sensitive prostatic cancer.
HS-PG Heparan sulfate - proteoglycan.
HSPM Hippocampal synaptic plasma membrane.
HSPN Henoch-Schönlein purpura nephritis.
HSPP Health Services Planning Program; Heterosexual precocious puberty.
HSPR Health Sciences Public Relations (USC).
HSPS Health Sciences Placement Service.
HSQB Health Standards and Quality Bureau.
HSQR Health Services Quality Research (Division of) (HSR).
HSR Harleco synthetic resin; Health Service Regulation (Act, 2002, UK see CPI); Health Services Research (Bureau of HRA) journal; Heated serum reagin; High success rate; Homogeneously staining region; Hyperadrenergic stress reaction/ response; Hypersensitivity reaction(s).
HSRA Harvard-Smithsonian Reference Atmosphere; Health Services Research and Analysis (Division of) (HSR).
HSRC Health Services Research Center; Human Subjects Review Committee.
HSRD Health Systems Research and Development (Division of) (HSR); Hypertension secondary to renal disease.
HSRI Health Systems Research Institute.
HSRS Health-Sickness Rating Scale.
H-S rule Howland and Schweizer rule (44 milliequivalents of sodium given intravenously for every 5 pints of blood transfusion).
HSRV Human spuma retrovirus.
HSS Hallermann-Streiff syndrome (see MOFD; PAS); Hallervorden-Spatz syndrome; Heel spur syndrome (Calcaneal spur); Henoch-Schönlein syndrome (see HSP); Hepatosplenic schistosomiasis; Hetero/ Homosexual sex; Highly statistically significant; High-speed supernatant; Hospital for Special Surgery (New York); Human subject studies/dy; Hyperstimulation syndrome; Hypertrophic subaortic stenosis; Hysterosalpingoscintigram/graph(y).
hss to be taken at bedtime (L. hora somni sumendum) (see hs).
HSSCC Hereditary site-specific colon cancer.
HSSE High soap suds enema.
HSST Hypersensitivity skin test.
HST Hetero/ Homo sexual transmission; Hormone-sensitive tumor.
HSTC House Science and Technology Committee.
HSTF Human serum thymus factor.
HSTP Heyer-Schulte testicular prosthesis.
H-subst Histamine-like substance.

HSUS Humane Society of the United States.
HSV Herpes simplex virus; High selective vagotomy; Hop stunt viroid; Hypersensitivity vasculitis; Hyperviscosity syndrome.
HSV-1 Herpes simplex virus, type 1 (oral).
HSV-2 Herpes simplex virus, type 2 (genital).
HSVE Herpes simplex virus encephalitis.
HSVP Histamine-stimulated vascular permeability.
HSVtk Herpes simplex virus thymidine kinase.
HSyn Heme synthase.
HSZPC Hoppe-Seyler's Zeitschrift für Physiologische Chemie (journal).
HT A chromatogram packing; Half-thickness (see HVL); Hammer toe; Hand tremor; Hashimoto's thyroiditis; Hearing test/ threshold; Heart (see Ht); Heart transplant(ation); Hemagglutination titer; Hereditary tyrosinemia; High-frequency transduction; High temperature; High tension (see ht); Histologic technician; Histologic Technician (ASCR journal); Hollander test (see IHT - Insulin hypoglycemia test); Home/ Hospital treatment; Horizontal transmission (of disease, e.g. HIV, via breast milk and human bites) (see MFT); Hormone therapy; Hospitalization and treatment (see H&T); Hospital Topics/ Tribune (journals); Hubbard tank; Human thrombin; Hydrocortisone test; Hydrotherapy; Hydroxytryptamine (see 5-HT); Hydroxytryptophan (see HTP); Hypertension (see HTN); Hyperthyroidism; Hypertransfusion; Hypertropia; Hypodermic tablet; Hypothalamus (see HTH); Hypothermia; Hypothyroidism; Total hypermetropia/ hyperopia (see Ht).
Ht Heart (= H; HT; ht); Heart - height of (= ht); Heart tones (= ht); Height (see ht); Heterozygote(s); High tension (see ht); Hypothalamus (see HTH); Total hypermetropia (= HT; Hy); Total hyperopia (= HT; Hy).
ht a draft (L. haustus); heart (see Ht); heart - height of (see Ht); heart tones (see Ht); height (= H; h; Ht); high tension (voltage) (= Ht; HT).
H(T) Intermittent hypertropia.
H&T Hospitalization and treatment (= HT).
^{3}HT Tritiated thymidine (= ^{31}H-TDR).
5-HT 5-Hydroxytryptamine (= Enteramine; HT; HTA; Serotonin). A breakdown product of 5-Hydroxytryptophan (see HTP) (has been implicated in the etiology of migraine and allergic diseases); 5-Hydroxytryptophan (see HTP).
5-HT3 5-Hydroxytryptamine (antagonist, such as dolasetron and ondansetron) (see 5-HT).
HTA Halo traction apparatus (Orthopedics); Heterophil transplantation antigen (= HT-A); Human thymocyte antigen; Hydroxytryptamine (see 5-HT); Hypophysiotropic area; Hypothalamic amenorrhea.
HT-A Heterophil transplantation antigen (see HTA).
5-HTA 5-Hydroxytryptamine agonist (see 5-HT).
HTACS Human thyroid adenyl-cyclase stimulator.
ht aer heated aerosol.
HT(ASCP) Histologic Technician certified by the American Society of Clinical Pathologists.
HTAT Human tetanus antitoxin.
HTB Heat-treatment bacterium (e.g. *Thermus* aquaticus, a species isolated from the Yellowstone Hot Springs in the Yellowstone National Park, Wyoming, in the 1960s) (= HTM); Hospital trust board; Hot/ House tub bath; Hot/ House tube (feeding) (see HTF); Human trabecular bone; Human tumor bank.
HTBFL High tumor burden follicular lymphoma.
HTC Hepatoma cell(s); Hepatoma tissue culture; High-technology care; High total cholesterol; High(er) tissue concentration (of a drug); Homozygous typing cell; Hypertensive crisis.
HTCVD Hypertensive cardiovascular disease (see HASCVD).
HTD Hammertoe deformity (Orthopedics); Hepatotoxic drug; Highest tolerated dose; High tech dentistry; Human therapeutic dose; Hypertensive diabetic; Hypertonic dehydration.
HtD Hard-to-diagnose.
^{31}H-TDR Tritiated thymidine (see ^{3}HT).

HTDW Heterosexual development of women.
HTE Hepatotoxic effect(s) (including AHN, CSH, etc.).
5-HTergic Serotonergic (receptor).
H-Tetanase Hemolytic element in tetanus toxin.
HTF Heterothyrotropic factor; Hot/ House tube feeding (= HTB); Hpa II tiny fragments (specialized gene sequences; Hpa II is a restricting enzyme which digests the DNA into independent fragments); Hypotonic fluid (i.e. 0.2% or 0.45% NaCl) - used to correct hypernatremia).
HTG Hypertriglyceridemia.
HTGL Hepatic triglyceride lipase.
HTH Calcium hypochlorite; Homeostatic thymus hormone (see Hormones - HTH); Hypothalamic hormone; Hypothalamus (= HT; Ht; Hyp).
HTh High tension (voltage) hours (X-ray tube).
HtH Human-to-human (transfer-infection).
HTHD Hypertensive heart disease (see HASCVD).
HTHN Hypotonic hyponatremia (see AHH).
HTHP Human total hip prosthesis.
HTI Healthy term infant; Hemispheric thrombotic infarction.
HTIG Homologous/ Human tetanus immune globulin.
HTK Heel to knee.
HTL Hamster tumor line; Hearing threshold level; Histotechnologist; Human T-cell leukemia; Human thymic leukemia.
HTLA High-titer, low acidity; Human T-lymphocyte antigen.
HTL(ASCP) Histotechnologist certified by the American Society of Clinical Pathologists.
HTLS High thoracic left sympathectomy.
HTLV Human T-cell leukemia/ lymphoma/ lymphotropic virus; Human T-lymphotropic virus (see HTLV III).
HTLV-I Human T-cell leukemia virus - I. A retrovirus linked with chronic T cell leukemia of adults; Human T lymphocyte virus I.
HTLV-II similar to HTLV-I, and the second-known human retrovirus.
HTLV-III; HTLV-3 Human T-cell lymphotropic virus III (known as such in most of the US), or the AIDS virus - a retrovirus which kills the T cells of the immune system, causing AIDS or the Acquired immune deficiency syndrome (see AIDS). The virus is also known as: ARV - AIDS retrovirus; HIV - Human immunodeficiency virus; HIV-I - Human immunodeficiency virus - type 1; LAV - Lymphadenopathy-associated virus (known as such in France); LAV/HTLV III (a universal name); HTLV-3 (as above).
HTLV-MA Cell membrane antigen associated with the human T-cell leukemia virus.
HTLV-I-MA Human T-cell leukemia virus-I-associated membrane antigen.
HTM Haemophilus Test Medium; Heat-tolerant microbe (see HTB); Hepatotoxic medication (see HTD).
HTN Hantaan (-like virus); Hypertension (= HT; Hypn; hypn); Hypertensive nephropathy.
HTNP Hypothalamic neuropeptide.
HTO Hammertoe operation (Orthopedics); Heterotopic ossification (= HO); High turn over; High tibial osteotomy (for Genu varum or Varus deformity of knee); Hospital transfer order.
HTOH Hydroxytryptophol.
HTOR 5-hydroxytryptamine oxygenase regulator.
HTP Heart transplant patient; Heterotopic pregnancy; House-Tree-Person (drawing test) (see HVTA); Hydroxytryptophan (= HT; 5-HT; 5-HTP) - a transmitter amine and antidepressant drug, broken down by the enzyme l-aminoacid decarboxylase into 5-Hydroxytryptamine (see L-5HTP); Hypothromboplastinemia.
5-HTP 5-hydroxy-L-tryptophan (a precursor of serotonin) (see HTP).
HtPA Hexahydrophthalic anhydride.
HTPN Home total parenteral nutrition.
HTR Hammer toe repair; Heart-transplant recipient; Home treatment regimen; Hypotensive transfusion reaction.
HTRP Hypertensive retinopathy.
HTS Head traumatic syndrome; Heel-to-shin; Heterotaxy syndrome; High thoracic sympathicolysis; Human thyroid-stimulating (hormone) (see Hormones - HTS); Human thy-

roid stimulator; Hypertensive shock (see ACF; CGS); Hypertrophic scar (after deep tissue loss) (see DTL); Hypertrophic synovium (e.g. of the knee joint); Hysterical trance state (stupor or mute immobility).

HTSAB Human thyroid-stimulating antibody.

HTSH; hTSH Human thyroid-stimulating hormone (see Hormones - HTSH).

HTST High temperature (for a) short time (pasteurization).

HTT Hand thrust test; Hand tool test (see BHTT).

H-TTP H-thymidine-methyl-5'-triphosphate.

HTU Heart-transplant unit.

HTV Herpes-type virus.

HTVD Hypertensive vascular disease (see HASCVD).

HTX Histrionicotoxin.

HU Hampson/ Head/ Heat/ Hemagglutinating/ Hemolytic/ Holzknecht/ Hounsfield/ Hyperemia unit; Harvard University; Hebrew University (Jerusalem); Human urinary/ urine; Hydroxyurea (= HUR; HYD; Hyd).

Hu Human.

HUA Hyaluronic acid (see NaHA).

HUC Human umbilical cord; Hypertonic uterine contraction(s); Hypouricemia.

HUD Housing and Urban Development (Department of).

HUDAS Hereditary "urticaria/deafness/amyloid" syndrome.

HuEPO Human erythropoietin.

HU-FSH Human urinary follicle-stimulating hormone (see Hormones - HU-FSH).

HUGO Human Genome Organization (international = HGO).

HUI Headache unit index.

HUIFM Human (leukocyte) interferon meloy.

HuIFN Human interferon.

HUIS High-dose urea in invert sugar.

HUK Human urinary kallikrein.

Hum Humerus.

HumAB4D5-8 Humanized antibody used in cancer therapy, later named Trastuzumab or Traztuzumab (see CMA; MumAB).

HUMEGON Human menopausal gonadotropin (see Hormones - HMG iv; HUMEGON)

HUMP Howard University Mississippi Project.

Hung. P Hungarian Pharmacopoeia (Magyar Gyogyszerkonov).

HUP Hospital of the University of Pennsylvania; Hospital Utilization Project.

HUR Hemocystine urine reducer; Hydroxyurea (see HU).

HURA Health in underserved rural areas.

HURT Hospital utilization review team.

HUS Hemolytic uremic syndrome (caused by *Escherichia* coli - serotype 0157:H7); Husband (see husb); Hyaluronidase unit for semen.

HuSA Human serum albumin.

husb husband.

HUT *Helicobacter* urease test - a rapid urease test for H. pylori in gastric mucosa; Urease secreted by this curved, Gram-negative bacterium (with up to five unipolar flagella), splits the urea in the medium into ammonia and carbon dioxide, the former increasing its pH, which can be detected by a color change in a suitable pH indicator (see also UBT).

h ut histidine utilization (gene).

HUTHAS Human thymus antiserum.

HUV Human umbilical vein.

HUVEC Human umbilical vein endothelial cell.

HV Hallux valgus; Hantaan virus (causative agent of Korean hemorrhagic fever) (see KHF); Has voided; Health Visitor (HVA journal); Heart/ High volume; Hemovac; Hepatic vein; Herpes virus; High voltage; His ventricular (see H-V); Home/ Hospital visit; Hyperventilation (= OV); Hypovolemia.

H-V His-ventricular (interval/ time). Conduction time or interval through the His Purkinje system - from the Bundle of His to ventricular activation. The normal recording is less than 75 milliseconds.

H&V Hemigastectomy and vagotomy (operation/ stomach).

HVA Health Visitors Association (UK); Homovanillic acid (laboratory/ endocrinology).

HVAA Heated vaporization atomic absorption (spectroscopy).

HVAC Heating, ventilating, and air conditioning.

HVB Heavy vaginal bleeding.
HVBL High-volume bowel lavage.
HVC Health Visitor's Certificate; Hepatic vein catheterization.
HVD Heart valve disease; Homogeneous vaginal discharge; Hypertensive vascular disease (see HASCVD).
HVE Habitual vigorous exercise; Hepatic venous effluence; High-voltage electrophoresis.
HVG Host versus graft (disease) (see HVE).
HVGS High-voltage galvanic stimulation.
HVH Herpes virus hominis; Heterozygous variant hypercholesterolemia (= FCH or Familial hypercholesterolemia).
HVHMA Herpes virus hominis membrane antigen.
HVI Herpesvirus infection.
HVJ Hemagglutinating virus of Japan.
HVL Half-value layer (radiation shielding, i.e. of different types of material capable of acting as a barrier to absorb gamma radiation) (= hvl; HLV; HT; HVT).
hvl half-value layer (see HVL).
HVLP High volume, low pressure.
HVM High-velocity missile; Human viral myocarditis (see Table).
HVO Heart-valve operation (see HVR).
HVP Highly-vulnerable patient/person.
HVPC High-voltage pulsed current.
HVPE High-voltage paper electrophoresis.
HVPG Hepatic venous pressure gradient.
2HVPV Two-hour venous plasma value (see 2HBSS).
HVR Heart-valve replacement; Hypoxic ventilation response.
HVS Heart-valve surgery; Herpes virus of Saimiri; Herpes virus sensitivity; Hyperventilation/ Hyperviscosity syndrome (in the fetus or infant; may be accompanied by cyanotic spells, hypoglycemia, necrotizing enterocolitis, oliguria, polycythemia, respiratory distress, etc.); Hypovolemic shock (see HVSS).
HVSD Hydrogen-detected ventricular septal defect.
HVSS Hypovolemic shock syndrome.
HVSV Human vesicular stomatitis virus.
HVT Half-value thickness (see HVL); Hepatic vein thrombosis (= BCS - Budd-Chiari syndrome); Herpes virus of turkeys; Hormonal vaginal therapy.
HVTA House-Vehicle-Tree-Animal (drawing test) (see HTP).
HVTEM High-voltage transmission electron microscope/py.
HVUS Hypocomplementemic vasculitis urticaria syndrome.
HW Hay-Wells (syndrome) (see AEC - Ankyloblepharon EC); Healing/ Heparin well; Herpetic hitlow; Hot water; Housewife.
HWB; hwb Hot water bottle.
HWC Health and Welfare, Canada.
HWD Heartworm disease.
HWE Healthy worker effect; Hot water extract.
HWFE Housewife.
HWL Hen worker's lung (see PBD).
HWMC House Ways and Means Committee (US Congress).
HWP Hot wet pack.
HWS Hot water-soluble.
HWY Hundred woman years (unit of radiation exposure).
HX Histiocytosis X; Hydrogen exchange; Hypophysectomized.
Hx Hemopexin; History; Hospitalization; Hypoxanthine.
21-HXD 21-hydroxylase deficiency (the most common cause of Congenital adrenal hyperplasia) (see CAH).
HXIS Hard x-ray imaging spectrometry.
HXLHb Human cross-linked hemoglobin (= HCLHb).
HXM Hexamethylmelamine.
HXR Hypoxanthine riboside.
HY Hatha Yoga.
Hy Hyaluronic acid; Hypermetropia (see Ht); Hyperopia (see Ht); Hypophysis; Hypothenar; Hysteria/ical (see Hys).
hyal- prefix meaning glass (Gr. hyalos).
HyCoSy Hysterosalpingo-contrast sonography.
HYD; Hyd Hydralazine; Hydrated/tion; Hydrocortisone (see HC); Hydroxyurea (see HU).
hydat- prefix meaning water (Gr. ydatos) (= hydro-).

HVM – Human viral myocarditis

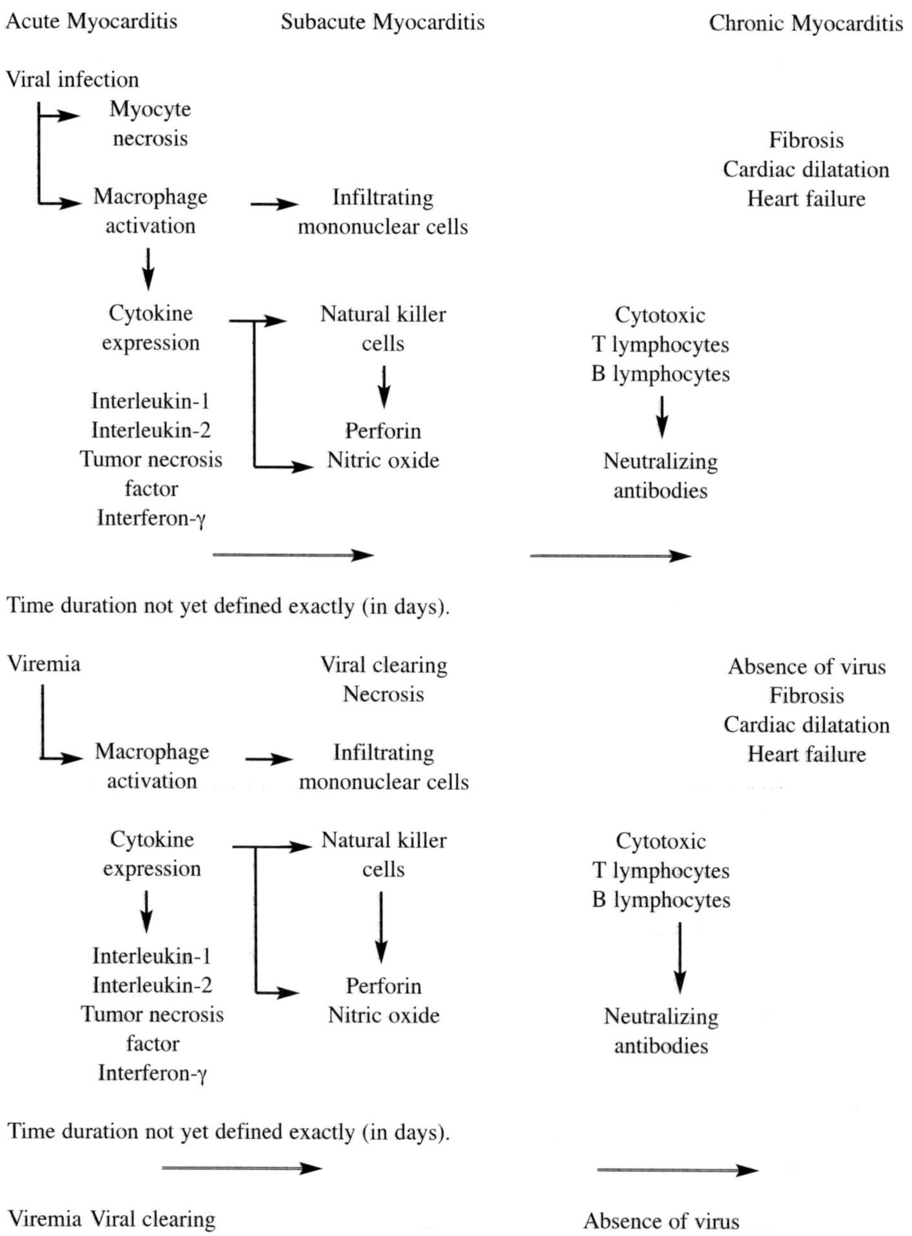

hydr hydraulic.
hydr- combining form meaning water (Gr. ydor).
hydrarg mercury (L. hydrargyrum) (see Elements - Mercury).
Hydro; hydro Hydrotherapy.
hydro- prefix meaning water (Gr.) (see hydat-).
Hydrox Hydroxyline.
HYF Healthy young female.
Hyg; hyg Hygiene/nic/nist.
HYL; Hyl Hydroxylysine.
hyl- prefix meaning material or substance (Gr. hyle).
HYM Healthy young male.
Hyo Hyoscine; Hyoscyamine (= Hyoscy); Hyoscyamus (a genus of plants, from which is extracted the alkaloids, hyoscyamine and scopolamine) (= Hyoscy).
Hyoscy Hyoscyamine/ Hyoscyamus (see Hyo).
HYP p-Hydroxybenzylpindolol (a beta-blocker) (= HYP); Hydroxyproline (see Hypro); Hypnosis/notism (= Hyp; Hypno; hypno; Hypnot).
Hyp p-Hydroxybenzylpindolol (see HYP); Hydroxyproline (see Hypro); Hyper-resonance; Hypertrophy; Hypnosis (see HYP); Hypothalamus (see HTH).
hyp hypophysectomy; hypophysis.
hyp- prefix meaning less or under (Gr. ypo) (see hypo-).
hyper- prefix meaning above or increased (Gr. yper).
HyperAl Hyperalimentation.
hyper-IgE Hyperimmunoglobulinemia E.
Hypn; hypn Hypertension (see HTN).
hypn- prefix meaning sleep (Gr. ypnos).
Hypno; hypno Hypnosis/notism (see HYP).
Hypnot Hypnotism (see HYP).
Hypo Hypochromasia (red blood cells); Hypodermic (injection) (medication order).
hypo- an injection (hypodermic); prefix meaning below, decreased, deficiency/ient, less, or under (Gr. ypo) (= hyp-).
hypopit hypopituitarism.
Hypox; hypox Hypophysectomized.
HypRF Hypothalamic releasing factor.
Hypro Hydroxyproline (= HYP; Hyp).
hypsi- prefix meaning high (Gr.).
hypso- prefix meaning height (Gr. hypsos).
HYR Hoehn-Yahr rating (in Parkinson's disease).
Hys; hys; Hyst; hyst Hysterectomy; Hysteria/ical (= Hy).
hyster- prefix meaning uterus (Gr. ystera).
HYV Healthy young volunteer; High-yielding variety (IRRI rice and wheat).
HZ Herpes zoster.
Hz; hz Hertz (one cycle/sec) - an electrical measurement/ unit of frequency.
HZI Histamine zinc insulin (see Insulin - HZI).
HZLTF Herpes zoster lymphocytic transfer factor (specific immune f).
HZM Hetero/ Homo zygous mutation (gene) (see CHM; SHM).
HZO Herpes zoster ophthalmicus; Hydrous zirconium oxide.
HZR Herpes zoster radiculitis.
HZV Herpes zoster vaccine/ virus(= CPV; Shingles v.).

I

I Electric current; Impression; Incisal; Incisor (permanent tooth); Independent; Indeterminate; Index; Indicated; Induction; Inertia; Infarct (an area of coagulation necrosis resulting from obstruction to the circulation, i.e. loss of arterial blood supply, e.g. Embolic I. - an infarct caused by an embolus; Mycocardial I. - as occurs in coronary thrombosis; Inhalation; Inhibition/or; Initial; Inosine; Insoluble; Inspiration; Inspired (gas); Insulin (see under Insulin); Intact (bag of waters); Intake; Intensity (of light/ magnetism); Intermediate; Intermittent; Internal medicine; Internist; Intestine; Iodine (Z = 53) (see Elements - Iodine); Ionic strength; Isoleucine; Isotope; Isotopenpraxis (journal); Permanent incisor (tooth); Region of a sarcomere that contains only actin filaments; Roman numeral one.

i impurity; incisor (deciduous tooth); insoluble; Iota - the ninth letter of the Greek alphabet (= IOTA) (see Symbols - 4, Greek Alphabet); isochromosome; optically inactive.

ι Greek letter "iota".

I_2 Iodine.

3-1 I 3-1 Insulin (see Insulin - 3-1 I).

^{123}I; ^{125}I; ^{128}I; ^{130}I Radioactive iodine.

^{131}I; I^{131}; I-131 Iodine-131 - a radioactive isotope of iodine with an atomic weight of 131, and a half-life of 8.04 days, used in radioactive uptakes.

^{132}I; I^{132}; I-132 Iodine-132 - a radioactive isotope of iodine with an atomic weight of 132, and a half-life of 2 to 4 hours.

IA Ibotenic/ Indolic/ Isonicotinic acid; Immune adherence (see IAT); Immunoadsorbent; Immunobiologic activity; Impedance/ Inferior angle; Impotence Anonymous; Incidental appendectomy (operation/ abdominal); Indolaminergic accumulation; Indulin agar; Infantile autism; Infected area; Inhibitory antigen; Interaural attenuation; Internal auditory (ear); International Audiology (journal, now Audiology/ Audiologie); Intestinal Absorption (journal); Intra-alveolar/ amniotic/ aortic/ arterial/ articular/ atrial/ auricular; Intrinsic activity; Investigator assessment (see PSA - Patient self assessment).

Ia Immune response gene-associated antigen.

-ia suffix meaning a condition or state.

I&A Irrigation and aspiration.

IAA Imidazoleacetic acid (= IAc); Indoacetic acid; Indoleacetic acid (= Indoacetic acid; Indole-3-acetic acid; Indolyle-3-acetic acid); Infectious agent, arthritis; Inferior alveolar artery (a branch of the maxillary artery, the (L.) Arteria alveolaris inferior or IAA, also called the Inferior dental artery [IDA] or the Mandibular artery); Insulin autoantibody (see AAB); International Allergy/ Antituberculosis Association; International Association of Allergology (CIOMS)/ Asthmology; Interruption of the aortic arch; Intraarticular adhesion; Iridocyclitis-associated arthritis.

I-3-AA Indole-3-acetic acid (see IAA).

^{131}IAA Radioiodinated aminoacid.

IAAA Intergroup Association of Alcoholics Anonymous; Intramembranous AAA (bone regeneration) (see AAA).

IAAAI International Archives of Allergy and Applied Immunology (CIA journal).

IAAAS International Agranulocytosis and Aplastic Anemia Study.

IAAF International Amateur Athletic Federation.

IAAM International Academy of Aerospace Medicine; International Association of Agricultural Medicine.

IAAP International Association of Applied Psychology.

IAAR Imidazoleacetic acid ribonucleotide.

IAATM International Association for Accident and Traffic Medicine.

IAB Industrial Accident Board; Internal antibody (= IB - Intrabody); Intra-abdominal; Intra-aortic balloon; Intra-atrial block.

IABA Intra-aortic balloon assistance.

IABC; IABCP Intra-aortic balloon counterpulsation (= IACP) (procedure/ cardiology).

IABM Idiopathic aplastic bone marrow.

IABMS Institute for the Advancement of Bloodless Medicine and Surgery (New Jersey,

US).

IABP Intra-aortic balloon pump(ing) (procedure/ cardiology) = IBP.

IABPA Intra-aortic balloon pumping assistance (= IBA).

IABS Institute for Applied Behavioral Science.

IAC Ineffective airway clearance; Internal auditory canal; International Anesthesiology Clinics (journal); International Association for Cybernetics; Interposed abdominal compression(s); Intra-arterial catheter/ chemotherapy.

IAc Imidazoleacetic acid (see IAA).

IAC-CPR Interposed abdominal compressions - cardiopulmonary resuscitation.

IACD Implantable automatic cardioverter-defibrillator; Interatrial conduction delay (finding in ECG); Intra-arterial conduction defect.

IACI Intra-arterial contrast injection.

IACL Interpersonal Adjective Checklist - Leary.

IACM Intra-arterial contrast medium.

IACP Intra-aortic counterpulsation (see IABC).

IACPAP International Association for Child Psychiatry and Allied Professions.

IACR Intra-articular cruciate reconstruction (Knee joint) (Orthopedics)

IACS International Academy of Cosmetic Surgery.

IACT Intra-articular corticosteroid therapy.

IACV International Association of Cancer Victims.

IACVF International Association of Cancer Victims and Friends, Inc.

IAD Immuno-allergic diathesis/ disease/ disorder; Inactivating dose; Internal absorbed dose.

IADCJ International Association of Dentistry for Children Journal (UK).

IADD Inherited adenosine deaminase deficiency.

IADFA International Association of Dento-Facial Abnormalities.

IADH Inappropriate antidiuretic hormone (= ISADH) (see Hormones - IADH).

IADHS Inappropriate antidiuretic hormone syndrome.

IADL Instrumental activities of daily living.

IADR International Association for Dental Research.

IAds Immunoadsorption.

IADSA Intra-arterial subtraction arteriography.

IAE Idiopathic angioneurotic edema; Important adverse event(s); Inflammation-associated enzyme (e.g. Cyclooxygenase - COX-1, -2; Prostaglandin, etc.).

IAEA International Atomic Energy Agency (UN).

IAET International Association of Enterostomal Therapy.

IAF Imidazole antifungal (e.g. Ketoconazole); Intermittent atrial fibrillation; Intra-abdominal fat; Intra-articular fracture.

IAFI Infantile amaurotic familial idiocy.

IAG Impedance audiogram (hearing test); International Association of Gerontology; International Academy of Gnathology.

IAGBIQJ Ileostomy Association of Great Britain and Ireland Quaterly Journal (see IAQJ).

IAGP International Association of Geographic Pathology.

IAGT Indirect antoglobulin test (= IAT).

IAGUS International Association of Genito-Urinary Surgeons.

IAH Idiopathic adrenal hyperplasia; Immune adherence hemagglutination (see IAHA); Implantable artificial heart; Intra-abdominal hemorrhage.

IAHA Idiopathic autoimmune hemolytic anemia; Immune adherence hemagglutination (= IAH).

IAHD Idiopathic acquired hemolytic disorder.

IAHS Infection-associated hemophagocytic syndrome; International Association of Hospital Security.

IAI Impact Assessment Institute; Intermediate acting insulin (see Insulin); Intra-abdominal/ amniotic infection; Intra-arachnoid/ arterial/ articular injection; Intra-articular injury; Irreversible aromatase inactivator/ inhibitor (see ISAI); Islet autoimmunity (pancreas); Israel Aircraft Industries.

IAIM International Association of Infant

Massage; International Association of Integrative Medicine.

IAIMS Integrated Academic Information Management System.

IAIS Insulin autoimmune syndrome.

IAL Insulin analog lispro; International Association of Laryngectomees; Intra-abdominal lesion; Intra-articular lesion (see IAT).

IALN International Association of Laryngectomees News.

IAM Immunization Action Month; Institute of Applied Microbiology (Japan); Institute of Aviation Medicine; Internal acoustic/ auditory meatus; Isolated articular melioidosis (caused by the Gram-negative bacillus, *Pseudomonas* pseudomallei).

i am intra-amniotic.

IAMAT International Association for Medical Assistance to Travelers.

IAMFES International Association of Milk, Food, and Environmental Sanitarians.

IAMLA International Association of Medical Licensing Authorities.

IAMLT International Association of Medical Laboratory Technologists.

IAMM International Association of Medical Musuems.

IAMRA International Association of Medical Regulatory Authorities (UK).

i-amniot intra-amniotical.

IAMS International Association of Microbiological Societies.

IAN Idiopathic aseptic necrosis; Indole acetonitrile; Intern admission note.

IANA International Academy on Nutrition and Aging (US).

IANA; IANAb Intravenously administered neutralizing antibody.

iANP Immunoreactive atrial natriuretic peptide.

IAO Immediately after onset; Intermittent aortic occlusion; International Academy of Orthodontics; International Association of Orthodontists.

IAOG Israel Association of Obstetrics and Gynecology.

IAOH International Archives of Occupational Health (journal).

IAOM International Association of Oral Myology.

IAOS International Association of Oral Surgeons (Denmark).

IAP Immunosuppressive acidic protein; Inosinic acid pyrophosphorylase; Institute of Animal Physiology (UK); Intermittent acute porphyria; Intermittent/ Intra-abdominal pain; International Academy of Pathology/ Proctology; Intra-abdominal pressure; Intra-articular preparation; Intracisternal A-type particle; Islet-activating protein.

IAPB International Association for Prevention of Blindness (CIOMS).

IAPG Interatrial pressure gradient.

IAPM International Academy of Preventive Medicine.

IAPMJ International Academy of Preventive Medicine Journal.

IAPP International Association for Preventive Pediatrics; Islet amyloid polypeptide.

IAPRD Israel Annals of Psychiatry and Related Disciplines (journal).

IAPS International Affiliation of Planning Societies.

IAQJ Ileostomy Association (of Great Britain and Ireland) Quaterly Journal (= IAGBIQJ).

IAR Immediate asthma reaction; Impaired adrenal reserve; Inhibitory anal reflex; Intractable allergic rhinitis; Iodine-azide reaction (see IAT); Ionizing atomic radiation (see Radionuclide[s]).

IARC International Agency for Research on Cancer (WHO); International Association for Research into Cancer.

IARF Ischemic acute renal failure.

IARS International Anesthesia Research Society.

IARSA Idiopathic acquired refractory sideroblastic anemia.

i-arter intra-arterial.

IAS Idiopathic ankylosing spondylitis; Image Analysis System (Cambridge Instruments, Cambridge, UK); Immunosuppressive acidic substance; Indirectly acting sympathomimetic (e.g. Ephedrine); Infant apnea syndrome; Institute of Accident Surgery; Institute for Advanced Study (Princeton, NJ); Insulin autoimmune syndrome; Interaction study; Interatrial septum/ shunting; Internal anal sphincter; International Abstract of Surgery (included in SGO journal); Intra-amniotic saline (infusion); Intra-articular surgery; Inversion ankle sprain.

IASA Interatrial septal aneurysm.

IASC Inter-American Safety Council.

IASD Interatrial/ Interauricular septal defect.

IASH Isolated asymmetric septal hypertrophy.

IASHS Institute for Advanced Study in Human Sexuality.

-iasis suffix meaning a morbid condition or process.

IASL International Association for the Study of the Liver.

IASP International Association for the Study of Pain; International Association of Social Psychiatry.

IASR International Academy of Sex Research.

IASS Intraarticular synovial sarcoma.

IAT Immune adherence test; Immunoaugmentive therapy; Implicit association test (developed by Professor (Ms.) Mahzarin Banaji, Dept. of Psychology at Harvard University, US); Indirect antiglobulin test (see IAGT); Innovation arrhythmia therapy/ treatment; Instillation abortion time; International Atomic Time (= TAI); Intra-articular tear (see IAL)/ therapy; Intra-operative autologous transfusion; Invasive activity test; Iodine-azide test (see IAR).

IATA International Air Transport Association.

IATJ Institute of Animal Technicians Journal (UK).

-iatr suffix meaning field of medicine (Gr. iatros).

-iatrist suffix meaning medical specialist (Gr. iatros).

IAV Intermittent assisted ventilation; Intra-arterial vasopressin.

IAVI International AIDS Vaccine Inititiative (US).

IAVM Intramedullary arteriovenous malformation.

IAW Intra-anal wart(s) (see IGW).

IB Ideal bypass; Idiopathic blepharospasm; Immune/ Inclusion body; Index of body build; Infectious bronchitis; Insect Biochemistry (journal); Institute of Biology; Intrabody (see IAB - Internal antibody); Isolation bed.

Ib A glycoprotein.

ib in the same place (L. ibidem) (see ibid).

IBA Individual benefit assessment; Inhaled beta agonist; Insulin-binding antibody; Intermittent bolus administration; Intra-aortic balloon pumping assistance (see IABPA).

IBAT Intravascular bronchoalveolar tumor.

IBB Intestinal brush border.

IBBB Intra-blood-brain barrier.

IBBBB Incomplete bilateral bundle branch block.

IBC Inflammatory/ Inoperable/ Invasive bladder/ breast cancer/ carcinoma; Institutional Biosafety Committee; Insulin-binding capacity (see MIBC); Involuntary bladder contraction(s); Iodine-/ Iron-binding capacity; Isobutyl cyanoacrylate (see IBCA).

IBCA Isobutyl-2-cyanoacrylate (= IBC).

IBCS International Breast Cancer Study.

IBD Infective/ Inflammatory/ Irritable/ Irritated/ Ischemic bowel disease (see IBS); Initial bolus dose (= IBI); Institute of Birth Defects (Albany, New York); Sandoz (USA) code for experimental substances; Irreversible brain damage.

IBE Immediate bowel evacuation/uator; Incomplete bladder emptying; Institute of Biomedical Engineering; International Bureau for Epilepsy.

IBED Inter-African Bureau for Epizootic Diseases.

IBEM Idiopathic benign essential myoclonus (see IBFM).

IB-EP Immunoreactive beta-endomorphin.

IBF Immature brown fat; Imminent bowel perforation; Immunoglobulin-binding factor; Inhibited bone formation; Insall-Burstein-Freeman (total knee instrumentation); Interbody fusion (of vertebrae).

IBFM Idiopathic benign familial myoclonus (= IBEM).

IBG Inlay bone graft (= RP - Russe procedure); Insoluble bone gelatin.

IBI Initial bolus injection (see IBD); Intermittent bladder irrigation (procedure/ urology); Intermittent bolus injection; Ischemic brain infarction.

ibid in the same place/ the same (L. ibidem)

(= ib) (author(s) of book or journal).
IBILI Indirect bilirubin.
IBK Infectious bovine keratoconjunctivitis.
IBL Impalpable breast lesion; Inoperable brain lesion.
IBM Inclusion body myositis; Institute of Behavioral/ Biological Medicine; International Business Machines Corp (Computers).
IBMC Incurable bone marrow cancer (e.g. Multiple myeloma).
IBMF Impaired bone marrow function.
IBMP International Board of Medicine and Psychology.
IBMX 3-Isobutyl-1-methylxanthine.
IBNR Incurred but not reported.
IBOW Intact bag of waters.
IBP Inflammatory back pain; International Biological Program; Intra-aortic balloon pump(ing) (see IABP); Iron-binding protein.
IB Paint Iodine-benzoic paint/ tincture. Weak iodine solution 3, compound benzoin tincture 3, camphor 1, chloral hydrate 1, and phenol 1 (Proprietary drug - Addenbrooke's Hospital, Cambridge, UK).
IBPMS Indirect blood pressure measuring system.
IBQ Illness Behavior Questionnaire.
IBR Increased/ Inhibited bone resorption; Infectious bovine rhinotracheitis; Insect bite reaction.
IBRD International Bank for Reconstruction and Development.
IBRDD Institute for Basic Research in Developmental Disabilities (NYS).
IBRMR Institute for Basic Research on Mental Retardation.
IBRO International Brain Research Organization.
IBRON International Brain Research Organization News (journal).
IBRS Impatient Behavior Rating Scale.
IBRV Infectious bovine rhinotracheitis virus.
IBS Imidazole buffered saline; Immunoblastic sarcoma; Impaired/ Insufficient blood supply; Incipient biliary stasis; Irritable bladder symptom(s); Irritable (Inflammatory or Irritated)/ Ischemic bowel syndrome (= CN; FBD; IBD; IC; ICS; SC); Isobaric solution; Isotope bone/ brain scan.
IBSA Iodinated (I^{131}) bovine serum albumin.
IBSN Infantile bilateral striated necrosis.
IBT Immune-based therapy; Ink blot test; Intensive behavior(al) therapy (in autistic and other nervous disorders); Isatin-beta-thiosemicarbasone.
IBU Ibuprofen; International benzoate unit.
i-Bu Isobutyl.
IBV Increased blood viscosity/ volume; Infectious bronchitis vaccine/ virus.
IBW Ideal/ Initial body weight; Infant birth weight.
IBWM International Bureau of Weights and Measures.
IC Icteric/rus; Immune complex; Immunoconglutinin (= IK); Immunocompetent; Immunocompromised; Immunoconjugate; Immunocytochemistry (see ICC); Immunocytotoxicity; Impedance cardiogram/raphy; Incomplete; Indirect calorimetry; Indirect Coombs' (method); Individual counseling; Inferior colliculus; Infirmière Canadienne (CNA journal); Inhibitory/ Integrated concentration; Inner canthal (distance); Inoculation chagoma (a furuncle-like lesion seen in Chagas' disease, when the portal of entry of the parasite, *Trypanosoma* cruzi is the skin) (see RS - Romana's sign); Inorganic carbon; Inspiratory capacity - the maximum amount of gas that can be inspired from the resting expiratory level (see PFT); Inspiratory center; Institute of Chiropodists (UK); Institutional/ Intensive/ Intermediate care; Integrated circuit; Intercibal (in between meals e.g. vomiting) (see ic); Intercostal; Intercourse; Intermittent catheterization/ claudication; Internal capsule; Internal carotid/ cerebral (artery) (see ICA); Internal conjugate; Internal conversion - the interaction of a gamma-ray photon emitted by a nucleus with an orbital electron of the same atom (see Ne/Nγ; ICC); International Classification (= Landsteiner's c.) - classification of blood types O, A, B, and AB, depending on the presence or absence of agglutinogens A and B in the erythrocytes; International Clinics (journal - now NIC); Interstitial cell (see ISC); Interstitial changes;

Intracapsular; Intracardiac; Intracarotid; Intracavitary; Intracellular; Intracerebral; Intracisternal; Intracranial; Intracutaneous; Ion chromatography; Iridocapsular; Irritable colon (see IBS); Islet cell(s); Isovolumic contraction (procedure/ heart) (see ICP).

IC# Intracapsular fracture (see ICF).

ic in between meals (L. inter cibos).

IC 50; IC_{50} Inhibitory concentration of 50% (blood concentration required to produce 50% inhibition), e.g. of gastric secretion, by the H2 receptor antagonist, cimetidine.

IC_{95} 95% inhibitory concentration.

IC 5902 Spiramycin (= NSC 64393). A mixture of basic antimicrobial substances produced by the growth of Streptomyces ambofaciens, and consisting of Spiramycin I, II, and III. Spiramycin is a narrow-spectrum antibiotic active against Gram-positive bacteria.

ICA Immersion-crystallization analysis (a qualitatitve data analysis); Immunocompetent/ promized adult; Important clinical application/ approach; Institute of Clinical Analysis; Intermediate care area; Internal carotid/ cerebral artery; International Chiropractors Association; Interstitial cell adenoma; Intracellular acidosis/ activity/ alkalosis/ antibody; Intracerebral anatomy; Intracranial aneurysm/ atherosclerosis; Ischemic cerebral attack (see TIA); Islet cell antibody (see ICAb); Islet cell autoantibody (see AAB); Isotonic contrast agent.

ICAA International Council on Alcohol and Addictions; Invalid Children's Aid Association; Islet cell auto-antibody (see ICAAb).

ICAAb Islet cell auto-antibody (= ICAA).

ICAb Islet cell antibody (= ICA).

ICAF Internal carotid/ cerebral artery flow (i.e. mean flow).

ICAM Intercellular adhesion molecule.

ICAM-1 Intercellular adhesion molecule - 1 (enables intercellular adhesion of the body cells; used in the treatment of rhinovirus infections like the common cold.

ICAMI International Committee Against Mental Illness.

ICAN International College of Applied Nutrition.

ICAO Internal carotid artery occlusion.

i-card intra-cardiac/ial.

ICAS Internal carotid artery stenosis; International Conference on Atomic Spectroscopy.

ICASHS International Center for Advanced Study in the Health Sciences (NIH).

I cav Intracavity.

ICAW International Commission on Atomic Weights.

ICB Iliac crest biopsy/ bone (Orthopedics); Internal carotid bypass; Intracerebral/ Intracranial bleeding.

ICBF Inner cortical blood flow.

ICBM International Consortium for Brain Mapping (UCLA).

ICBP Intracellular binding protein.

ICBR Increased chromosomal breakage rate.

ICBT Intercostobronchial trunk.

ICC Immunocompetent cells; Immunocompromised child; Immunocytochemistry (= IC); Inadequate cardiac contractility; Inadequate cerebral circulation; Indian childhood cirrhosis; Information Center Complex; Intensive coronary care; Intercanthal distance; Interchromosomal crossing (over); Interclass/ Intraclass correlation coefficient; Internal conversion coefficient (radiology) (see IC); International Certification Commission; International Congress of Chemotherapy; Interstate Commerce Commission; Intracervical (device) (see ICD); Islet-cell carcinoma.

ICCA Immunocytochemical analysis.

ICCB International Congress on Cell Biology.

ICCC International Conference of Culture Collections; International Congress on Clinical Chemistry.

ICCE Intracapsular cataract extraction (operation/ ophthalmology).

ICCE c̄ PI Intracapsular cataract extraction with peripheral iridectomy (operation/ ophthalmology).

iCCK Immunoreactive cholecystokinin.

ICCM Idiopathic congestive cardiomyopathy.

ICCND International Conference on Children and National Development.

ICCR International Committee for Contraceptive Research.

ICCU Intensive/ Intermediate coronary care unit.

ICD I-cell disease; Immune complex disease (as a result of: 1. Infections, such as meningococcal meningitis; 2. Exogenous antigens a) dietary, such as gluten sensitivity b) occupational, such as extrinsic allergic alveolitis; and c) drugs, as in serum sickness or penicillin allergy; 3. Neoplasms such as lymphoma or carcinoma; and 4. Autoimmunity a) IgG as in rheumatoid arthritis b) cytoplasmic antigen as in polyarteritis, c) nucleic acids as in systemic lupus erythematosus; etc.); Indigo carmine dye; Intercurrent disease (= ICI); Implantable cardioverter defibrillator; Induced circular dichroism; Instantaneous cardiac death; Institute for Chest Diseases; Institute for the Crippled and Disabled; International Center for the Disabled; International Classification/ Code of Diseases; International Classification of Diseases, Injuries, and Causes of Death; International College of Dentists; Intestinal carbohydrate dyspepsia; Intracervical device (= ICC); Intrauterine contraceptive device; Intrinsic claudication distance; Ischemic coronary disease; Isocitrate/ric dehydrogenase (see ICDH; LFT iv); Isolated conduction defect.

ICDA International Classification of Diseases, Adapted.

ICDC Implantable cardioverter - defibrillator catheter; Israel Center for Disease Control (Ministry of Health).

ICD-9-CM International Classification of Diseases - ninth revision - Clinical Modification.

ICDH Isocitrate/ric dehydrogenase (= ICD; IDH) (see LFT iv).

ICDN International College of Dentists Newsletter.

ICD-O International Classification of Diseases - Oncology.

ICDR Institute for Child Development Research.

ICDRC International Contact Dermatitis Research Center.

ICDS Immune complex deposition syndrome (SBE); Integrated Child Development Scheme.

ICDT Dimethyltriazeno.

ICE Iatrogenic cerebral edema; Ice, compression, elevation; Ichthyosis-cheek-eyebrow (syndrome); Individual career exploration; Institute of Cancer Epidemiology; Integrated color energy (Ultrasound see MCE); Internal carotid endarterectomy; Intracardiac electrogram; Intracellular enzyme/ event; Iridocorneal endothelial/theliopathy (syndrome) - a rare form of closed-angle, unilateral glaucoma; Islet cell engineering (see ICR).

i ce intracerebral.

ICEA International Childbirth Education Association.

ICEAN International Childbirth Education Association News (journal).

ICED International Conference on Eating Disorders (Denver, Co.).

ICEEGL Index to Current Electroencephalography Literature (in EEGCN).

ICES Information collection and evaluation system.

ICF Ileocutaneous fistula (between the ileum and the abdominal wall); Impending cardiac failure; Indirect centrifugal flotation; Inert complex formation (treatment of heavy metal poisoning with chelating agents); Intensive/ Intermediate care facility; Intercellular fluorescence; Interciliary fluid; International Cardiology Foundation; Intracapsular fracture (e.g. of the femoral neck) (= IC#); Intracellular fluid; Intravascular coagulation and fibrinolysis.

ICFA Incomplete Freund's adjuvant; Induced complement-fixation antigen; International Cystic Fibrosis Association [see ICF(M)A].

ICF(M)A International Cystic Fibrosis (Mucoviscidosis) Association.

ICF-MR Intensive-care facility for the mentally retarded.

ICG Impedance cardiograph; Indocyanine green (dye); Isotope cisternography.

ICGC Indocyanine-green clearance.

ICGH Integrated concentration of Growth

hormone (see Hormones - ICGH; GH).

ICGN Immune-complex glomerulonephritis.

ICH Iodochlorhydroxyquin (PBT-1 - Prana Biotechnology Ltd. of Australia) - used in the treatment of Alzheimer's disease (see Cdk 5); Idiopathic cortical hyperostosis; Immunocompromised host (as in AIDS, burns, hematological malignancies, malnutrition, organ transplant recipients on steroids, etc); Infectious canine hepatitis; Institute of Child Health; International Conference on Harmonisation (UK); Intracerebral hematoma/ hemorrhage; Intracranial hemorrhage/ hypertension; Iodochlorhydroxyquin (PBT-1 - Prana Biotechnology Ltd. of Australia - used in the treatment of Alzheimer's disease (see Cdk 5); Islet cell hyperplasia (see PICH).

ICHD Inter-Society Commission for Heart Disease (Resources) (see ICHDR).

ICH & DHC Information Center for Hearing and Disorders of Human Communication (Johns Hopkins University).

ICHDR Inter-Society Commission for Heart Disease Resources (= ICHD).

ICHE Infection Control and Hospital Epidemiology (journal).

ICHG International Congress of Human Genetics.

ICHHD Institute of Child Health and Human Development.

ICHTN Intracranial hypertension (Manifestations include bulging fontanelles, headaches, and bilateral papilledema) (see ICH).

ICHLS Inter-Society Committee on Health Laboratory Services.

ICHPPC International Classification of Health Problems in Primary Care.

ICHS International Haemoglobincyanide Reference Solution.

ICHS & DHC Information Center for Hearing, Speech, and Disorders of Human Communication (Johns Hopkins University).

Ichth Ichthyology.

ICI Immunocompetent individual; Imperial Chemical Industries Ltd. (England) code for experimental substances; Important clinical issue; Inflammatory cell (eosinophil) infiltrate/ation (as in bronchial asthma); Intercurrent illness (see ICD); Interstitial cellular infiltrate; Intracardiac infection/ injection; Intracavernosal/nous injection (into the Corpus cavernosum penis); Isovolumic contraction interval (see ICP).

ICi Intracisternal.

ICI 28,257 Clofibrate (= Ethyl Chlorophenoxy-isobutyrate) - a drug used in the treatment of atherosclerotic disease, in which elevated serum triglyceride and cholesterol levels are lowered by its action on low-density β-lipoproteins, particularly the triglyceride-rich pre-β subgroup.

ICI 31,397 Mebanazine (= α-Methylbenzylhydrazine) - a monoamine oxidase inhibitor used in the treatment of depressive disorders. It exerts a hypoglycemic action in diabetes mellitus.

ICI 32,865 Ethoglucid (= Etoglucid; Triethyleneglycol diglycidyl ether) - a cytotoxic agent used in the treatment of malignant diseases.

ICI 45,520 Propranolol hydrochloride (see AY 64,043).

ICI 46,683 Oxyclonazide - a hydroxybenzanilide derivative, and a veterinary anthelmintic used in the treatment of liver-fluke infestations in cattle and sheep.

ICI 50,123 A Butyloxycarbonyl-phenylalanine derivative; a synthetic pentapeptide. Like gastrin, it exerts a powerful stimulating effect on gastric secretion. It has been suggested for use as a test of gastric function. Given by intravenous infusion.

ICI 50,627 Tetramisole hydrochloride (= McN-JR 8299; R 8299) - a veterinary anthelmintic used in nematode infestation. In man it is reportedly active against Ascaris and Enterobius infections.

ICIA International Center of Information on Antibiotics.

ICIDH International Classification of Impairments, Disabilities, and Handicaps.

ICIG Institut de Cancérologie et d'Immunogénétique (Fr.) (Cancer and Immunogenetic Institute).

ICJ Intercarpal joint; Intrahepatic cholestatic jaundice.

ICK Intracondylar knee (see OI/OP).

ICL Idiopathic CD4 + T-cell lymphocytopenia (= CFS; CFIDS); Immunocompetent lymphocyte; Intracorneal/ Iris-clip lens; Intracranial lesion; Iris capsular lens; Isocitrate lyase.

ICLA International Committee on Laboratory Animals.

ICLC International Contact Lens Clinic (journal).

ICLH Imperial College, London Hospital.

ICLI Iris capsular lens implant.

ICM Idiopathic cardiomyopathy; Images in Clinical Medicine (journal); Inner cell mass; Institute of Clinical Medicine; Intensive care measure; Intensive Care, Medical; Intercostal margin; International Confederation of Midwives; Intracerebral mass; Intracranial mass; Intracytoplasmic membrane; Ion conductance modulator; Isolated cardiovascular malformation.

ICMBE International Conference on Medical and Biological Engineering (CIGMB).

ICMH Institute for Child Mental Health.

ICMI Inventory of Childhood Memories and Imaginings.

ICMJE International Committee of Medical Journal Editors.

ICMMP International Committee of Military Medicine and Pharmacy.

ICMP International Conference on Medical Physics.

ICMR Indian Council of Medical Research.

ICMSF International Commission on Microbiological Specifications for Foods.

ICMT Intracardiac mural thrombosis; Intracranial malignant tumor (= IMT).

ICN Immune complex nephritis; Infection control nurse; Intensive care, neonatal (see NIC); Intensive care nursery (= NIC); Intercondylar notch (lower femur); Intercostal nerve; International Congress of Nutrition; International Council of Nurses; Intracranial neoplasm; Intrinsic cortical neurotransmitter.

ICNa Intracellular concentration of sodium.

ICNBC International Committee on Nomenclature for Blood Coagulation.

ICNC International Chemical and Nuclear Corporation; Intracerebral nuclear cell.

ICNND Interdepartmental Committee on Nutrition in National Defence.

ICNS Interagency Conference on Nursing Statistics.

ICNV International Committee on Nomenclature of Viruses.

ICO Idiopathic cylic oedema; Impedence cardiac output; Improved clinical outcome; Increased cardiac output; International Commission for Optics; International Congress of Ophthalmology.

i-coch intra-cochlear.

ICP Immunocompetent/ Immunocompromised patient/ person; Incubation period; Inductively coupled plasma (spectroscopy); Indwelling catheter program; Infection-control practitioner; Infectious cell protein; Inflammatory cloacogenic polyp; Intensive-care physician/ procedure; Intermittent catheterization protocol; International Congress of Pediatrics; Intracranial pressure; Intractable chest/ chronic pain; Intracytoplasmic; Invasive cardiac procedure; Isovolumic contraction period (heart) (= IC; ICI; ICT).

ICPA International Commission for the Prevention of Alcoholism.

ICPB International Collection of Phytopathogenic Bacteria.

ICPE Idiopathic chronic pericardial effusion; Institute for Continuing Physical Education.

ICPEMC International Commission for Protection against Environmental Mutagens and Carcinogens.

ICPI Intersociety Committee on Pathology Information.

ICPM International College of Psychosomatic Medicine.

I,C,PM,M Incisors, canines, pre-molars, molars (teeth; when each is followed by a number, this expresses the formula of permanent dentition).

ICPP Intubated continuous positive pressure.

ICPQ Inductively-coupled plasma Quantometer (ARL).

ICPRT International Conference on Particles and Radiation Therapy.

ICPS International Center for Prison Studies (Kings College, London).

ICPSI Intra cell-penetrating/ cytoplasmic

sperm injection (IVF).

ICPSJ Irish College of Physicians and Surgeons Journal (formerly RCSIJ).

ICP test Imitation, Comprehension, Production test.

ICPT Intracranial pituitary/ primary tumor.

ICR Iliac crests (distance between); Illustrative case report; Immunochemical reaction/ reagent; Indirect cross-reference; Institute for/of Cancer Research (Mouse/UK); Intermittent catheter routine; International Congress of Radiology; Intracardiac catheter recording; Intracavitary radium; Intracorneal ring; Intracranial reinforcemet; Ion cyclotron resonance; Islet Cell Resource (Ten Centers for the study of Islet cell transplantation as a potential cure for Type I diabetes, located in Boston, Denver, Memphis, Miami, Minneapolils, New York, Philadelphia, Seattle, Southern California - COH, and St. Louis).

ICRC International Committee of the Red Cross.

ICRD Index of Codes for Research Drugs.

ICRDB International Cancer Research Data Bank (NCI).

ICRETT International Cancer Research Technology Transfer (Programme - ICRDB).

ICREW International Cancer Research Workshop (Programme - ICRDB).

ICRF Imperial Cancer Research Fund (London).

I-CRF Immunoreactive corticotropin-releasing factor.

ICRF-159 Razoxane.

ICRFL Imperial Cancer Research Fund Laboratories.

ICRISAT International Crops Research Institute for the Semi-Arid Tropics (India).

ICRO International Cell Research Organization.

ICRP International Commission on Radiation/ Radiological Protection.

ICRR International Congress of Radiation/ Radiological Research.

ICRS Index Chemicus Registry System; International Committee of the Red Cross.

ICRU International Commission on Radiation Units and Measurements (formerly, International Commission on Radiological Units and Measurements; International Committee for Radiological Units; International X-ray Unit Committee - IXUC).

ICS Ileocecal sphincter; Immotile cilia syndrome; Immunocompetent subject; Impaired cognition syndrome; Impulse-conducting system; Indian Civil Service (formerly, British Indian Empire); Individual clinical status; Infantile cerebral sclerosis (see FDICS); Intensive care sedation/ society/ support; Intensive Care, Surgical; Intercellular/ Intercostal space; Internal carotid shunt (Neurosurgery); International Cardiovascular Society (CIOMS); International Clinical Studies/dy; International College of Surgeons (CIOMS); Intracardiac shunt(ing); Intracoronary stent(ing); Intracranial sepsis/ stimulation/surgery; Irritable colon syndrome (see IBS); Islet cell transplantation (see ICR).

ICSA Islet cell surface antibody.

ICSB International Committee of Systematic Bacteriology.

ICSC Idiopathic central serous choroidopathy; Immunologically compatible stem cell.

ICSD Intrinsic conduction system disease (see LS).

ICSH International Committee for Standardization in Hematology; Interstitial cell-stimulating hormone (see Hormones - ICSH; LH v).

ICSI Intra-cytoplasmic sperm injection.

ICSM Instant corn-soya milk.

ICSO Intermittent coronary sinus occlusion.

ICSP International Congress on Social Psychiatry; International Council of Societies of Pathology.

ICSS Intracranial self-stimulation.

ICST Intracranial secondary tumor.

ICSTM Imperial College of Science, Technology and Medicine (London).

ICSU International Council of Scientific Unions.

ICT Icteric/rus (see Ict); Immunoreactive calcitonin (human) (see iCT); Indirect Coombs' test; Induction chemotherapy (for cancer); Inflammation of connective tissue; Insulating core transformer; Insulin coma therapy; Intensive care therapy/ treatment; Intensive conventional therapy; Intermittent calcitriol therapy (e.g. in hyperparathyroidism); Intermittent cervical traction; Interstitial/Islet cell tumor; Intracardiac thrombus; Intracranial tumor; Inulin clearance test (see KFT - ICT; INULA); Iron-chelation therapy; Islet cell transplantation (see ICR); Isovolumetric/mic contraction time (heart) (see ICP).

Ict Icteric/rus (jaundice) (= ICT).

iCT Immunoreactive calcitonin (human) (= ICT).

Ict Ind Icteric/rus index.

ICTMM International Congress on Tropical Medicine and Malaria.

ICTP Iodocytidine-triphosphate.

ICTS Idiopathic carpal tunnel syndrome.

ICTV International Committee for/on the Taxonomy of Viruses.

ICTX Intermittent cervical traction.

ICU Idiopathic chronic urticaria; Immunologic contact urticaria; Infant care unit; Intensive care/ coronary unit; Intermediate care unit (see IMCU).

ICUMSA International Commission for Uniform Methods of Sugar Analysis.

i-cut intra-cutaneous.

ICV Ileocecal valve; International Certificate of Vaccination; Intracellular volume; Intracerebro-ventricular.

icv intracervical.

ICVH Ischemic cerebrovascular headache.

ICVHI International Conference on Voluntary Health Insurance.

ICVI Intra-cardiovascular insufficiency.

ICVS International Cardiovascular Society.

ICW Intensive care ward; Intercellular/ Intracellular water.

ICWH International Conference on Women in Health.

ICx Immune complex.

^{125}ICYP ^{125}Iodocyanopindolol - a radiolabeled pindolol derivative.

ICZN International Commission on Zoological Nomenclature.

ID Identification/ I. donor; Identify/tity; Iditol dehydrogenase; Ifosamide, (mesnauroprotection), and doxorubicin; Immunodeficiency; Immunodiffusion (see ID test); Immunoglobulin deficiency; Inappropriate disability; Inclusion/ Infectious/ Interstitial disease; Index of Dermatology (journal); Index of discrimination; Individual/ Infective/ Inhibitory/ Initial/ Injected dose; Infant death; Initial diagnosis/ dyskinesia; Inside/ Internal diameter; Insufficient data; Interdigitating; Interhemispheric disconnection; Intradermal(ly) (injection site) (= i d; i-derm; idr); Intraduodenal; Involutional depression (= ED); Number of identities); Iridodialysis (the iris is torn free from its root).

Id Infradentale; Interdentale.

id ill-defined (image); the same (L. idem).

i d during the day (L. in diem); intradermal(ly) (see ID).

I-D Intensity - duration (curve) (= S-D).

id- suffix meaning resembling or the same (L. idem).

I&D Incision and drainage (operation/ skin).

ID_{50} Mean/ Median infective dose - the amount of pathogenic microorganisms producing infection in 50% of test subjects.

IDA Idiopathic diffuse alopecia; Image display and analysis; Iminodiacetic acid; Infectious Disease Association (Thailand); Inferior dental artery (see IAA); Injecting drug abuse(r); Institute for Defence Analysis; Insulin-degrading activity; Insulin dose adjustment; International Development Association; Irish/ Israel Dental Association; Iron deficiency anemia; Israel Defence Army (see IDF); Israel Diabetes Association.

IDAA International Doctors in Alcoholics Anonymous.

id ac the same as (L. idem ac).

IDAJ Irish Dental Association Journal.

IDAMS Integrated Drug Abuse Management System (NIAAA).

IDAP Illinois Drug Abuse Program.

IDAT Indirect antiglobulin test.

IDAV Immunodeficiency-associated virus.

IDBS Infantile diffuse brain sclerosis.

IDC Idiopathic dialted cardiomyopathy; Infectious Diseases Committee; Insulin-dosage computer; Interdigitating cell; Isocaloric diet change.

IDCE Institute for Dermatologic Communication and Education.

IDCI Intradiplochromatid interchange.
IDCM Idiopathic dilated cardiomyopathy.
IDCP Infectious Diseases in Clinical Practice (journal).
IdCTP Iododeoxycytidine-triphosphate.
IDD Immunodeficiency disease/ disorder (see IIDD); Infectious disease drug; Insulin-dependent diabetes (see IDDM); Intraluminal duodenal diverticulum; Intrathecal drug delivery (see ITDD); Inventory to Diagnose Depression.
IDDF Investigational drug data form.
IDDM Insulin-dependent diabetes mellitus (= IDD); Insulin-dependent diabetic mother.
IDDN Insulin dependent diabetic nephritis.
IDDP Insulin-dependent diabetic pregnancy.
IDDS Implantable drug delivery system.
IDDT Immune double diffusion test.
IDE Impaired drug excretion; In-depth evaluation; Investigational/ative device exemption.
-ide suffix meaning a binary chemical compound
idée (Fr.) idea (e.g. i. fixe = fixed idea).
IDEA Individuals with Disabilities Act.
IDEM Intradural extramedullary meningioma (= IEM).
idem (L.) the same (authors; titles).
i-derm intradermal(ly) (see ID).
IDES Image Dissector Echelle Spectrometer.
IDETM Intradural extramedullary thoracic meningioma (= IETM).
IDF International Dental Federation (CIOMS); International Diabetes Federation; Israel Defence Forces (= IDA).
IDFB International Diabetes Federation Bulletin (CIOMS).
IDFC Immature dead female child.
IDFNL International Dental Federation News Letter (UK).
IDFP Intradental fixation procedure.
IDG Interdisciplinary group; Intermediate dose group.
IDH Isocitric dehydrogenase (see ICDH; LFT iv).
Id Hypo P Idiopathic hypoparathyroidism.
IDI Idiopathic diabetes insipidus; Immunodeficiency of infancy; Immunologically-detectable insulin; Individualized dose initiation; Induction-delivery interval; Inter-dentale inferius; Interpersonal Dependency Inventory; Intradermal injection; Israel Drug Index.
idi- combining form meaning distinct, peculiar or separate (Gr. idios).
IDIC Internal Dose Information Center.
idic isodicentric.
Idiot Barbiturate pill (see Barb).
IDISA Intraoperative digital subtraction angiography.
IDJ International Dental Journal and Newsletter (IDF - CIOMS).
IDK Internal derangement of knee (joint).
IDL Index to Dental Literature; Interdigital lesion; Intermediate density lipoprotein.
IDLA Illinois Dental Laboratory Association.
IDLH Immediate danger to life and health.
IDM Idiopathic disease of the myocardium; Immune defence mechanism (= IDMC); Indirect method; Infant of diabetic mother; Intermediate-dose methotrexate.
IDMC Immature dead male child; Immune defence mechanism (see IDM); Institute on Disability and Managed Care (Washington, D.C.).
IDMD Idiopathic dystonia musculorum deformans (= ITD).
ID-MS Isotope dilution - mass spectrometry.
iDNA Intercalary deoxyribonucleic acid.
IDO-E d-alpha-tocopherol (see Vitamins - E).
idon vehic in a suitable vehicle (L. idoneo vehiculo).
IDP Immunodeficient patient; Immunodiffusion procedure (see ID test); Initial dose period; Inosine diphosphate; Insulin-dependent patient; Internal podalic version (see VAE).
IDPA Illinois Department of Public Aid.
IDPase Inosine diphosphatase.
IDPH Idiopathic pulmonary hemosiderosis; Illinois Department of Public Health.
IDPN Iminodipropionitrile (= β-imino-dipro-prio-nitrile); Inflammatory demyelinating polyneuropathy.
IDR Idiosyncratic drug reaction; Increased diabetic risk (= IRD); Initial dosing regimen; Institute of Dental Research; Intradermal reaction; Investigator-determined response.
idr intradermal(ly) (see ID).

IDRC International Development Research Center (Canada).

IDS Immune/nity deficiency state; Infant death syndrome; Infectious disease service; Infectious-diseases specialist; Inhibitor of DNA synthesis; Insulin delivery system(s), i.e. insulin therapy with long-term infusion; Intraduodenal stimulation; Investigational drug service; Investigative Dermatological Society.

IdS Interdentale superius.

IDSA Infections Disease Society of America.

IDSAN International Drug Safety Advisory Network.

IDT Immune diffusion test (see ID test); Immunodiagnostic test; Immunosuppressive; Initial drug therapy; Incomplete duplication twins (see pagus); Instillation delivery time; Intensive diuretic/ drug therapy; Intradermal typhoid (vaccine).

ID test Immune diffusion test (= ID; IDP; IDT).

IDTN International Drug Therapy Newsletter.

IDTP Interdigital tinea pedis (= ITP).

IDU Idoxuridine (= 2'-Deoxy-5-ioduridine; IDUR; 5 IDUR; IdUrd; Iodode-oxyuridine; 5-iodo-2'-deoxyuridine; IUDR; IUdR; SKF 14,287) - an antiviral agent inhibiting the formation of deoxyribonucleic acid (DNA) of the virus. Especially useful in the local treatment of herpes simplex (or dendritic) keratitis; Illicit/ Intravenous drug use(r); Injection drug user; Ischemic diabetic ulcer.

idu intraduodenal.

IdUA Iduronic acid.

IDUR Idoxuridine (see IDU).

5 IDUR Idoxuridine (see IDU).

IdUrd Idoxuridine (see IDU).

IDV Indinavir; Intermittent demand ventilation.

IDVC Indwelling venous catheter.

Idx Cross-reactive idiotype.

IE Idiopathic eosinophilia; Immediate-early (antigen/ protein) - a large protein molecule synthesized by the CMV (Cytomegalovirus), to protect it from the host's immune system and allow it to replicate; Immunizing unit (Ger. Immunitäts-Einheit); Immunoelectrophoresis; Induced emesis; Industrial/ Intern engineer; Infectious endocarditis; Inner ear; Intake energy; Internal elastica (see IEL); International unit (European); Intraepithelial; Involved epidermis; Isoenzyme.

i.e. that is or that is to say (L. id est).

I/E Inspiratory/expiratory (ratio) (see PFT - I/E); Internal/external.

I&E Internal and external.

IEA Immediate early antigen; Immunoelectroadsorption; Immunoelectrophoretic analysis; Infectious equine anemia; International Energy Agency; International Epidemiological Association (CIOMS); Intravascular erythrocyte aggregation.

IEB Infant evaluation at birth (see ASS).

IEC Indwelling epidural catheter (postoperative); Injection electrode catheter; International Electrotechnical Commission; Intestinal epithelial cell; Intraepithelial carcinoma (= Bowen's disease, BPD or Bowen's precancerous dermatosis, PCD or Precancerous dermatitis) (see IECa); Ion-exchange chromatography.

IECa Intraepithelial carcinoma (= IEC).

IECO Institute of Experimental and Chemical Oncology.

IED Idiopathic endomyocardial disease; Infectious/tive eczematous dermatitis; Inherited epidermal dysplasia; Inner ear disease/ disorder; Intestinal enzyme deficiency.

IEE Inner enamel epithelium; Institute of Electrical Engineers (England).

IEEE Institute of Electrical and Electronics Engineers.

IEEECS Institute of Electrical and Electronics Engineers Computer Society.

IEF International Eye Foundation; Isoelectric focusing.

IEH Immature egg harvest (immature eggs harvested from the ovaries, are cultured in the lab, fertilized and transferred back into the woman's womb).

IEI Inner ear infection (= OI - Otitis interna); Isoelectric interval.

IEL Internal elastic lamina (in the walls of arteries and veins) (= IE); Intraepithelial lymphocyte.

I-ELCAP International Early Lung Cancer Action Program (COH).
IELTS International English Language Testing System.
IEM Immuno-electron microscopy; Inborn error of metabolism; Institute of Environmental Medicine; Intradural extramedullary meningioma (see IDEM); Ion-exchange medium.
IEMG Integrated electromyogram (procedure/ physical medicine).
IEMS Institute of Experimental Medicine and Surgery (University of Montreal).
IEOP Immunoelectro-osmophoresis.
IEP Immunoelectrophoresis; Individualized education program; Insert earphone (hearing aid); Isoelectric point.
IEPP International Energy Policy Perspectives (journal).
IEPR International Economic Policy and Research.
IER Internal-external rotation (of the leg) (Orthopedics).
IER test Institute of Educational Research (intelligence) test.
IES Illuminating Engineering Society; Impulse, Ego, and Superego (see IES test); Inner Ear Specialist; Institute of Ecosystem Studies (NY); Institutes of Environmental Sciences.
IES test Impulse, Ego, and Superego test (= IES).
IET Immediate emergency therapy/ treatment; Isotretinoin Efficacy Trial (NCI).
IETM Intradural extramedullary thoracic meningioma (see IDETM).
IEU Individual education unit.
IF Idiopathic fibroplasia/ flushing; Ifosphamide (= IFOS); Immersion foot; Immunofixation; Immunofluorescence (= IFL); Indirect fluorescence; Infrared; Inhibiting/ Intrinsic factor; Initiation/ Initiating factor (= If) - factor or factors present in the alternative pathway of the activation of the complement reaction. They include: E. Erythrocyte(s), B and D. Enzymes of the alternative pathway, P. Properdin, A. IgG or IgM antibody, and Ina. Inactivator (see also Ind. - Inducers); Inspiratory force; Institute for the Future; Interfamilial (between families); Interferon (see IFN); Interior facet; Intermaxillary/ Internal fixation; Intermediate filament/ frequency; Interstitial fluid; Intrafamilial (within families); Involved field (radiotherapy).
If See IF.
IF1; IF2; IF3 Interferon 1, 2, 3.
IFA Idiopathic fibrosing alveolitis; Immunofluorescence assay; Immunofluorescent antibody; Impaired/ Inadequate/ Insufficient fat absorption; Incomplete Freund's adjuvant; Indirect fluorescent antibody/ assay (test for Entameba histolytica) (see FAT); Infant Formula Act (see IFF); International Federation of Anatomists; International Fertility/ Filariasis Association; Ischio-femoral arthrodesis (Orthopedics).
IFAC International Federation of Automatic Control.
IFAD International Fund for Agricultural Development.
IFAT Indirect fluorescent antibody test (see FAT).
IFC Individual food consumption; Infant Formula Council (baby foods); Intermittent flow centrifugation; Intrinsic factor concentrate.
4 IFC Four-interval forced-choice.
IFCA In-flight cardiac arrest.
IFCB International Federation for Cell Biology.
IFCC International Federation of Clinical Chemistry/ Chemists.
IFCM Iron-fortified cow milk.
IFCR International Foundation for Cancer Research.
IFCS Inactivated fetal calf serum.
IFD Intrauterine fetal death/ distress (see IUFD); Irrevocably fatal disease (such as AIDS, certain Cancers, etc.).
IFDC International Fertilizer Development Center.
IFDR Industry-funded drug research.
IFDS Isolated follicle-stimulating (hormone) deficiency syndrome.
IFDT Industry-funded drug trial (= MST).
IFE Immunofixation electrophoresis;

Interfollicular epidermis.

IFF Inner fracture face; Iron-fortified formula (for infants) (see IFIF).

IFFH International Foundation for Family Health.

IFG Immune-function gene; Impaired fasting glucose; Impaired fetal growth; Interfascicular graft(ing) (Orthopedics).

IFGO International Federation of Gynecology and Obstetrics.

IFGOJ International Federation of Gynecology and Obstetrics Journal.

IFGS Interstitial fluid and ground substance.

IFHP International Federation of Health Professionals.

IFHPMSM International Federation for Hygiene, Preventive Medicine, and Social Medicine.

IFIF International Foundation for Internal Freedom (founded by Timothy Leary and Richard Alpert in 1962; now defunct); Iron Fortification of Infant Formulas (AAP); Iron-fortified infant formula (= IFF).

IFIP International Federation for Information Processing.

IFIX Immunofixation.

IFL Immunofluorescence (see IF).

IFLrA Recombinant human leukocyte interferon A.

IFM Immediate family member (i.e. father/ mother, brother/ sister, or son/ daughter); Institute of Forensic Medicine; Instrumentation for Medicine (Inc); Interfetal membrane; Internal fetal monitor.

IFMBE International Federation for Medical and Biological Engineering (FIGMB; CIOMS) (formerly IFME; IFMEBE).

IFMC Illinois Foundation for Medical Care.

IFME In-flight medical emergency; International Federation for Medical Electronics (now IFMBE).

IFMEBE International Federation for Medical Electronics and Biological Engineering (now IFMBE).

IFMP International Federation for Medical Psychotherapy.

IFMSA International Federation of Medical Student Associations.

IFMSAN International Federation of Medical Student Associations News.

IFMSS International Federation of Multiple Sclerosis Societies.

IFN Interferon (= IF; INF; ITF) - Interferons are glycoproteins formed in response to foreign double-stranded RNA, and produced when T cells react with antigen, as part of the natural host defences to viral infections. Thus interferon produced by virus infection of one cell protects neighboring cells from infection; its protective ability is not specific for the virus inducing its production, but is limited to cells of the animal species in which it is induced. Interferon is a representative of a non-antibody class of mediators known as lymphokines (so also are the interleukins - see IL), and are released from activated lymphocytes and also other cells. Interferons have a molecular weight, ranging in the 30 to 40 thousands.

α-IFN Alpha-interferon, an α-chain glycoprotein with a molecular weight of 34,000, and a product of leukocytes.

β-IFN Beta-interferon, a β-chain glycoprotein with a molecular weight of 29,000, and produced by fibroblasts.

γ-IFN Gamma-interferon, a γ-chain (heavy) glycoprotein with a molecular weight of 44,000, and a product of activated T lymphocytes. It acts at the cell membrane of virus-infected cells to inhibit viral replication. Its main function is as a regulating factor in cell-mediated immune responses. Its main target is inducement of Ig secretion and stimulation of macrophages.

IFN α-2b Interferon alfa-2b (used with ribarin in the treatment of chronic hepatitis C infection).

if nec if necessary (see SOS).

IFNMT Interferon monotherapy (see IFN).

IFO Institute for Fermentation (Japan).

IFORL International Federation of Oto-Rhino-Laryngology (CIOMS).

IFOS Ifosphamide (see IF); International Federation of Ophthalmological Societies (CIOMS).

IFP Glycerol (= Glycer; Glycerin; Glycerinum; Glycerolum; Propane-1,2,3-triol; $C_3H_5[OH]_3$; $C_3H_8O_3$); Inflammatory fibroid polyp; Insulin, compound F (hydrocortisone), prolactin; Intermediate filament protein; Intrafunicular pressure (Obstetrics); Intrapatellar fat pad; Isolated fetal pyelectasis (Obstetrics).

IFPEB International Federation of Physical Education Bulletin.

IFPM International Federation of Physical Medicine (CIOMS).

IFPRA International Family Planning Research Association.

IFPRI International Food Policy Research Institute.

IFR Income fund reimbursable; Infrared; Inspiratory flow rate (see PFT - IFR).

IFRA Indirect fluorescent rabies antibody (test).

IFRP International Fertility Research Program (University of North Carolina and AID).

IFS Immunofluorescence study; Interstitial fluid space.

IFSC International Federation of Surgical Colleges (CIOMS).

IFSECN See IFSEEGCN.

IFSEEGCN International Federation of Societies for Electroencephalography and Clinical Neurophysiology (CIOMS) (= IFSECN).

IFSM International Federation of Sports Medicine.

IFSSH International Federation of Societies for Surgery of the Hand.

IFT Immunofluorescence/ent technique/ test; Institute of Food Technologists; Interferential therapy (= IT); International Frequency Tables; Ipsilateral Fallopian tube.

IFTC International Federation of Thermalism and Climatism.

IFU Interferon unit.

IFV Interstitial/ Intracellular fluid volume; Ischemic failing ventricle.

IFVHSF International Federation of Voluntary Health Service Fund(s).

IFWF Insulin-Free World Foundation (CA).

IG Immature granule; Immunoglobulin (see Ig); Intragastric (see Ig); Irritable gut; Isogram.

Ig Immunoglobulin (= Gamma globulin; γ-globulin; IG; Immune globulin) - a group of immunological protein antibodies, including:
IgA: (= gamma A; secretory immunoglobulin; thyroglobin antibody) found in mucous secretions.
IgA1, IgA2: subclasses of immunoglobulin A.
IgD: (= gamma D; immunoglobulin D).
IgD1, IgD2: subclasses of immunoglobulin D.
IgE: (= gamma E; reagin antibody; reaginic immunoglobulin) found on mast cells, and causing type I or immediate asthmatic reaction.
IgE1: subclass of immunoglobulin E.
IgE AR: immunoglobulin antiragweed.
IgE ND: immunoglobulin E ND (a myeloma protein).
IgE SH: immunoglobulin E Sha (myelome).
IgE YU: immunoglobulin E YU (a myeloma protein).
IgG: = gamma G; γG; immunoglobulin G.
IgG1, IgG2, IgG3, IgG4: subclasses of immunoglobulin G.
IgM: (= gamma M; maternal gamma globulin; rubella-specific antigen) found in blood vessel lymphocytes B, T, and K ("killer") cells, and macrophages. Causing type III, arthrus, or late asthmatic reaction.
(75)IgM: low molecular weight immunoglobulin M.
IgM1: subclass of immunoglobulin M.; Intragastric (= IG).

I-G Insulin-glucagon (molar ratio).

IGA Infantile genetic agranulocytosis; Inherited genetic abnormalities/ty; International Grenfell Association; Intragastric acidity.

IgA Immunoglobulin A (see Ig).

IgA1; IgA2 Subclasses of immunoglobulin A (see Ig).

IgAGN Immunoglobulin A glomerulonephritis.

IGAM Immunoglobulins G, A, and M (see Ig).

IgAN Immunoglobulin A nephropathy.

IGC Immature germ cell; Interdisciplinary Generalist Curriculum (Project); Intragastric cannula.

IGCM Idiopathic giant-cell myocarditis.

IGCN Irish Guild of Catholic Nurses.

IGD Iatrogenic disease/ disorder; Idiopathic growth (hormone) deficiency (see IGHD); Inherited genetic disease/ disorder; Interglobal distance; Isolated gonadotropin deficiency.

IgD Immunoglobulin D (see Ig); Immunoglobulin deficiency (see BCRD).

IgD1; IgD2 Subclasses of immunoglobulin D (see Ig).

IGDE Idiopathic gait disorder(s) of the elderly.

IGDM Infant of gestational diabetic mother/ infant (of mother) with gestational diabetic mellitus.

IGE Impaired gas exchange; Infective gastroenteritis.

IgE Immunoglobulin E (see Ig).

IgE1 Subclass of immunoglobulin E (see Ig).

IgE AR Immunoglobulin E antiragweed (see Ig).

IgEDAD Immunoglobin E-dependent allergic disease (such as allergic asthma, allergic rhinitis, etc.).

IgEDR Immunoglobin E-dependent reaction (see IgEDAD).

IgE ND Immunoglobulin E ND (a myeloma protein) (see Ig).

IGES International Genetic Epidemiological Society.

IgE SH Immunoglobulin E Sha (myeloma) (see Ig).

IgE YU Immunoglobulin E YU (a myeloma protein) (see Ig).

IGF Insulin-like growth factor - a secondary growth factor associated with the action of the growth hormone (see Hormones - IGF).

IGF 1 Insulin-like growth factor 1 (= Somatomedin C) (see Hormones - IGF 1).

IGF 2 Insulin-like growth factor 2 (see Hormones - IGF 2).

IGFBP Insulin-like growth factor binding protein.

IGFET Insulated gate field effect transistor.

IgG Immunoglobulin G (see Ig).

IGl Immunoglobulin (see Ig); Independent genetic influence(s).

IgG1; IgG2; IgG3; IgG4 Subclasses of immunoglobulin G (see Ig).

IGH Immunoreactive growth hormone (see Hormones - IGH).

IGHD Isolated growth hormone deficiency (see IGD).

IGIM Immune globulin, intramuscular.

IGIV Immune globulin, intravenous.

IGM Idiopathic granulomatous mastitis; Impaired gastric motility; Inherited genetic mutation; Institute for Genetic Medicine (USC); Internet Grateful Med.

IgM Immunoglobulin M (see Ig).

(75)IgM Low molecular weight immunoglobulin M (see Ig).

IgM1 Subclass of immunoglobulin M (see Ig); Immunoglobulin-mediated inhibition (e.g. of the binding of radio-labeled thyrotropin to thyrotropin receptors, in the assay for thyrotropin-receptor antibodies in the assessment and diagnosis of Graves' hyperthyroidism) (see GHT).

IgMN Immunoglobulin M nephropathy.

IGOSS Integrated Global Ocean Station System.

IGP Immunogenic glycoprotein (e.g. gp 35-37 of HHV8 - Human herpesvirus - 8); Intestinal glycoprotein.

IGR Immediate generalized reaction; Increased general resistance; Insect growth regulator; Integrated gastrin response; Intrauterine growth retardation.

IGRT Immune globulin-replacement therapy.

IGS Image-guided surgery; Immunogenetic susceptibility; Inappropriate gonadotropin secretion; Institute of General Semantics; Internal guide sequence; Isotonic glucose solution; Israel Gerontological Society.

Igs Immunoglobulins (see Ig).

IgSC Immunoglobulin-secreting cell.

IGT Impaired glucose tolerance; Infected/ Inflamed gum tissue; Inflammatory granulation tissue; Institute of Gas Technology; Integrative gene transfer.

IGTC International Glutamate Technical Committee.

IGTT Intravenous glucose tolerance test.

IGV Intrathoracic gas volume.

IGW Internal genital wart(s) - such as cervical, intra-anal, intravaginal, rectal, and urethral warts (see EGW).

IGY International Geophysical Year.

IH Idiopathic hemochromatosis (see IHC)/ hirsutism/ hyperaldosteronism (see IHA)/ hypercalciuria (see IHC); Immediate hypersensitivity; Incompletely healed; Indirect hemagglutination; Industrial hygiene/nist; Infantile hydrocephalus; Infectious hepatitis (virus A, short incubation); Infective hepatitis; Inguinal hernia; Inhibiting/tory hormone (see Hormones - IH); In/ Inpatient hospital; Inner half; Intermittent heparinization; Intracranial hematoma; Iron hematoxylin.

IHA Anti-microsomal antibody; Idiopathic hyperaldosteronism (= IH); Illinois Hospital Association; Immune hemolytic anemia; Immunohistologic assessment; Indirect hemagglutination (test)/ antibody; International Health Activities/ Agency.

IHAC Industrial Health and Advisory Committee.

IHB Industrial Home for the Blind; Irregular heartbeat (see AHR).

IHBT Incompatible hemolytic blood transfusion.

IHBTD Incompatible hemolytic blood transfusion disease.

IHC Idiopathic hemochromatosis/ hypercalciuria (= IH); Immobilization hypercalcemia; Immunohistochemical (examination/ staining/ study/ technique); In-hole catheter; In-hospital care; Inner hair cell; International Hematology Congress; Internet Healthcare Coalition; Intrahepatic cholestasis (= IHPC).

IHCA Isocapnic hyperventilation with cold air.

IHCE Immunohistochemical examination (of enzymes such as MGMT in tumor cells).

IHCI Irreversible hepatocellular injury.

IHCJ Intrahepatic cholestatic jaundice.

IHCL Immunohistochemical localization.

IHCP Information on Healthcare Performance (NHS, UK).

IHCP Istitute of Hospital and Community Psychiatry.

IHCS Immunohistochemical studies/dy.

IHD Inborn heart defect; In-center hemodialysis; In-hospital death; Intrahepatic duct(ule); Ischemic heart disease.

IHE Indirect harmful effect; Institute for the Health of the Elderly (Univ. of Newcastle upon Tyne, England); Insurance health expenditure.

IHEA International Health Evaluation Assocation.

^{125}I-HE Prot Radioactive-labeled encephalitogenic basic protein.

IHES Idiopathic hypereosinophilic syndrome (= IHS).

IHF Impaired hepatic function (= HFI) (see DLD); Industrial Health Foundation (Inc.); Integration host factor; Interhemispheric fissure (brain); International Hospital Federation/ Foundation.

IHG Immunoreactive human gastrin.

IHGD Isolated human growth deficiency.

IHGT Institute for Human Gene Therapy (Univ. of Pennsylvania).

IHH Idiopathic hypogonadotropic/ hypothalamic hypogonadism; Infectious human hepatitis.

IHHS Idiopathic hyperkinetic heart syndrome.

IHI Institute for Healthcare Improvement (Boston, MA); Interactive Haematology Imagebank; Internet Health Information.

IHL Initial half-life; International Homeopathic League.

Ihl Inhalation.

IHM In-hospital mortality.

IHMR In-hospital mortality rate.

IHN Institute of Human Nutrition.

IHO Idiopathic hypertrophic osteoarthropathy.

IHP Idiopathic hyperprolactinemia/ hypoparathyroidism/ hypopituitarism; Interhospitalization period; Inverted hand position.

IHPC Intrahepatic cholestasis (see IHC); Iron hydroxide polymaltose complex (= IPC).

IHPH Intrahepatic portal hypertension.

IHPL Idiopathic hyperprolactinemia (see HPL; HPLD).

IHPP Intergovernmental Health Project Policy.

IHR Immediate hypersensitivity reaction(s); Inguinal hernia repair; Inguinal herniorrhaphy; Institute of Hearing Research (MRC); Intrahepatic resistance; Intrinsic heart rate.

IHRA Isocapnic hyperventilation with room air.

IHRB Industrial Health Research Board.

IHS Idiopathic Headache Score; Idiopathic hypereosinophilic syndrome (see IHES); Inactivated horse serum; Indian Health Service; Information Handling Services (Englewood, Colorado); Institute of Health Services (UK); International Headache/ Health Society; Irritable heart syndrome (see Asthenia).

IHs Iris hamartomas.

IHSA Iodinated human serum albumin.

[^{131}I]HSA Human serum albumin tagged with radioiodine (nuclear medicine).

IHSC Immunoreactive human skin collagenase.

IHSM Institute of Health Services Management (UK).

IHSS Idiopathic hypertrophic subaortic stenosis; Insufficiency (tricuspid), hypertension (pulmonary), stenosis (tricuspid) and stenosis (orificial pulmonary).

IHT Iatrogenic hypothyroidism; Inpatient hospital treatment; Insulin hypoglycemia test (= HT - Hollander test); Intravenous histamine test; Ipsilateral head turning.

I5HT Intraplatelet serotonin.

IHV Intrahepatic vasculature.

IHW Inner heel wedge.

^{125}IHYP ^{125}Iodohydroxy-benzylpindolol (a radiolabeled pindolol derivative).

II Icterus index (see LFT iv); Image intensifier; Infection and Immunity (journal); Injection insulin/ Insulin injection (see Insulin - II i); Integrase inhibitor(s). A new class of drugs, reportedly cabable of disarming three of HIV's (the human immunosuppressive virus's) critical enzymes - reverse transcriptase, integrase, and protease - all at once, and still under research for the treatment of AIDS (see AIDS); Isophane insulin (see Insulin - II ii); Roman numeral two.

Ii Incision inferius.

I-i A blood group system.

I&I Illness and injuries.

I-1I Interleukin-1 inhibitor.

IIA Impotence Institute of America; Internal iliac artery; Invasive intestinal amebiasis.

IIAC Infrared Information Analysis Center (Ann Arbor, Michigan).

IIAP Innovation Information and Analysis Project.

IIASA International Institute for Applied Systems Analysis.

IIC Image-intensifier control (investigation of fractures - Orthopedics); Insulin-induced coma (see IST - Insulin shock therapy).

IICP Increased intracranial pressure.

IICU Infant intensive care unit.

IID Illicit injectable drug; Inflammatory intestinal disease; Informations sur l'Irradiation des Denrées (journal); Insulin infusion device (= IIP; IRCP); Insulin-independent diabetes (see IIDM).

IIDD Inherited immunodeficiency disease/ disorder (affecting B cells, complement proteins, natural killer cells, phagocytic cells, T cells, etc.) (see GDID; IDD; PIDD).

IIDJ International interdisciplinary journal.

IIDM Insulin-independent diabetes mellitus (= IID) (see NIDDM).

IIE Idiopathic ineffective erythropoiesis; Institute of International Education.

IIEF International Index of Erectile Function.

IIF Indirect immunofluorescence/ent (technique).

IIFT Itraoperative intra-arterial fibrinolytic therapy.

IIGR Ipsilateral instinctive grasp reaction.

IIH Infectious-immune hypothesis (in diseases such as myocarditis, etc.); Insulin-induced hypoglycemia.

IIHDS Israeli Ischemic Heart Disease Study.

III Inosinyl inosinyl inosine; Irreversible immunological injury; Isophane insulin injection (see Insulin - III); Roman numeral three.

IIIN International Institute for Infant Nutrition (Hadassah Medical Center, Jerusalem, Israel).

III-para Third pregnancy (L. tertipara).

IIIVC Infrahepatic interruption of the inferior vena cava.

IIL Integrated injection logic (= I^2L).

IIMA . Isoxazole immunomodulatory agent (e.g. Leflunomide).

IIME Institute of International Medical Education.

IIMT International Institute for the Management of Technology.

IIN Idiopathic inflammatory neuropathy (see

GBS or Guillain-Barré syndrome); Interlocking intramedullary nail(ing) (Orthopedics) (= IMNT).

IIP Idiopathic interstitial pneumonia; Idiopathic intestinal pseudo-obstruction; Implantable insulin pump (see IID); Incentive inspirometry program (blow-bottle, to keep lungs clear); Increased intracranial pressure; Insulin infusion pump (see IID).

II-para Second pregnancy (L. secundipara).

IIQM International Institute for Qualitative Methodology (Edmonton, Alberta, Canada).

IIR Immune insulin resistance (= MIR) due to a high titer of circulating IgG antibodies; Immunological inflammatory reaction; Impaired immune response; Increased insulin requirement(s)/ resistance.

IIS Iatrogenic/ Intensive immunosuppression; Impaired immune system; Increased insulin sensitivity; Infant Intelligence Scale (psychological test, assessing general motor and cognitive development); Institute for Interdisciplinary Studies; International Institute of Stress; Intra-ocular irrigation solution (see IOIS).

IIT Iloprost inhalation therapy (see AIP); India ink test (staining agent for *Cryptococcus*); Ineffective iron turnover; Intermittent infusion/ injection therapy; Intensive insulin therapy; Israel Institute of Technology (The Technion, Haifa, Israel).

IITA International Institute of Tropical Agriculture (Nigeria).

IITRI Illinois Institute of Technology Research Institute.

IIU International insulin unit.

IIV Inactivated influenza vaccine; Inter-individual variability/ variation (of drug absorption).

IIVT Initial intravenous therapy.

IJ Ileojejunal; Infectious/tive jaundice; Internal jugular; Intrajejunal; Intrajugular.

IJA International Journal of the Addictions.

IJAP International Journal of Air Pollution.

IJARI International Journal of Applied Radiation and Isotopes.

IJB International Journal of Biometeorology.

IJBC International Journal of Bio-Medical Computing.

IJBE International Journal of Biomedical Engineering.

IJC International Journal of Cancer (IUAC); International Journal of Cardiology; Israel Journal of Chemistry.

IJCEH International Journal of Clinical and Experimental Hypnosis (SCEH).

IJD Inflammatory joint disease; International Journal of Dermatology.

IJDM Israel Journal of Dental Medicine (IDA).

IJE International Journal of Epidemiology (IEA).

IJEP International Journal of Experimental Pathology.

IJFD International Journal of Forensic Dentistry (UK).

IJID International Journal of Infectious Diseases.

IJL International Journal of Leprosy.

IJLD International Journal for Language and Documentation.

IJLOMD International Journal of Leprosy and Other Mycobacterial Disease (ILA).

IJMH International Journal of Mental Health.

IJMS International Journal of Medicine and Surgery; Irish Journal of Medical Science (RAMI).

IJN International Journal of Neuroscience/ Nursing.

IJNMB International Journal of Nuclear Medicine and Biology.

IJO Idiopathic juvenile osteoporosis (mild form of OGI - Osteogenesis imperfecta); International Journal of Orthodontics (FOA).

IJOS International Journal of Oral Surgery (IAOS).

IJP Inhibitory junction potential; Internal jugular pressure; International Journal of Parasitology/ Psychoanalysis (IPAA).

IJPM International Journal of Psychiatry in Medicine.

IJPPR International Journal of Peptide and Protein Research.

IJPRD International Journal of Periodontics and Restorative Dentistry.

IJR Idiojunctional rhythm.

IJROBP International Journal of Radiation Oncology, Biology, and Physics.

IJRPC International Journal of Radiation Physics and Chemistry.

IJS Inflammatory joint symptom(s).

IJSP International Journal of Social Psychiatry.

IJT Idiojunctional tachycardia.

IJV Internal jugular vein.

IK Immobilized knee; Immune body (Ger. immune Körper); Immunokonglutinin (see IC); Infusoria killing (unit) (see IKU); Interstitial keratitis.

IKD Irreversible kidney damage (see IRD).

IKE Ion kinetic energy.

IKF Immature/ Impaired kidney function (see IRF).

I2KI Lugol's solution (= Iodine 5% with Potassium [Kalium] iodide 10% in water; Aqueous Solution of Iodine; Liquor Iodi Aquosus) - used in the treatment of thyrotoxicosis, simple goiter and after thyroidectomy.

IKIC Iodine potassium (kalium) iodide catgut.

IKU Infusoria killing unit (= IK).

IL Ileum; Iliolumbar; Immature lungs; Incisolingual; Independent laboratory; Insensible (weight) loss; Inspiratory load; Institute of Living (Hartford, Conn); Instrumentation Laboratory (Inc); Insulin lente (see Insulin - IL; IZS); Intensity load; Interleukin (see IL 1, 2, 3, etc.); Interlingua; Intralipid; Intralumbar; Israel; Ives Laboratories (USA) code for experimental substances.

Il Illinium (now Promethium - Pm; Z = 61) (see Elements - Promethium); Illustration.

il- prefix, i) meaning in or on (L.); ii) negating what follows.

IL 1, 2, 3, etc Interleukins 1, 2, 3, etc. are hormone-like substances or lymphokines, a non-antibody class of mediators released mainly by T and B lymphocytes, and also by macrophages and monocytes. The interleukins are so called because they act as signals between one leukocyte and another. They are released from activated lymphocytes and other cells. They act as growth and differentiation factors, as chemotactic and regulating factors, and can affect immune function.

IL 1 Interleukin-1. Main function: Growth factor; Main target: T cells, fibroblasts, killer cells. Also stimulates lymphokine release.

IL 2 Interleukin-2. Main function: Growth factor. Main target: T cells, thymocytes.

IL 3 Interleukin-3. Main function: Growth factor. Main target: Multipotential stem cells (man); Mast cells (mouse) (see Hormones - HGF; IL-3).

IL 4 Interleukin-4. Main function: Growth factor. Main target: Important role in IgE synthesis (mouse).

IL 5 Interleukin-5. Main function: Growth factor. Main target: B cells; Differentiation of eosinophils; Release of acute phase proteins.

IL 6 Interleukin-6. Main function: Regulating factor. Main target: Induces Ig secretion, but counteracts IL 4 effect on IgE.

IL 10 Interleukin-10. Main function: Inflammation suppressor affecting the cardiac muscle. Its release is stimulated by Cytokines and Progesterone, enabling quicker recovery from heart surgery, especially in women.

I^{2}L Integrated injection logic (see IIL).

IL 6001 Trimipramine (= RP 7162; Trimeprimine) - an antidepressant drug used in the treatment of endogenous depression.

ILA Impaired/ Increased locomotor activity; Indolyle-3-lactic acid; Insulin-like activity; International Leprosy Association (CIOMS); Intralesional administration.

ILa Incisolabial.

iLa intralaminar (nuclei of thalamus).

I-Lac Imidazole-lactic acid.

ILAE International League Against Epilepsy (see ILE).

ILAR Institute for Laboratory Animal Resources; International League Against Rheumatism (CIOMS).

ILB Infant, low birth (weight) (see ILBW); Infant lung burden; Intraluminal baloon (Angioplasty).

ILBBB Incomplete left bundle branch block.

Ilb-illa Glycoproteins found on platelet membranes.

ILBW Infant, low birth weight (= ILB).

ILC Icthyosis linearis circumflex; Incipient lethal concentration.

ILCA International Livestock Center for Africa (Ethiopia).

ILCT Intralesional corticosteroid therapy.
ILD Influenza-like disease; Interstitial/ Ischemic lung disease; Intestinal lipodystrophy (= WD - Whipple's disease); Irreversible liver damage; Ischemic leg disease; Isolated lactase deficiency.
ILE Increased life expectancy; Infantile lobar emphysema; International League (Against) Epilepsy (= ILAE); Isoleucine (see Ileu).
ILe/ Ile Isoleucine (see Ileu).
ile- prefix meaning ilium (L.) (see ili-).
i-lesion intra-lesional.
Ileu Isoleucine (= ILE; ILe; Ile; Ilu).
ILF Impaired liver function; Indicated low forceps (delivery); Internal labor force.
ILFC Immature living female child.
ILGF Insulin-like growth factor.
ILH Immunoreactive luteinizing hormone (see Hormones - ILH).
ILI Influenza-like illness; Intraocular lens implant (see IOLI).
ili- prefix meaning ilium (L.) (= ile-).
ILL Intermediate lymphocyte lymphoma.
Ill Illusion.
Illus Illustrated/ation.
ILM Impaired lipid metabolism; Institute of Laser Medicine (UCLA); Insulin-like material; Internal limiting membrane.
ILMC Immature living male child.
ILMI Inferolateral myocardial infarct.
ILN Inferior laryngeal nerve; Inguinal lymph node.
ILNR Intralobar nephrogenic rest.
ILO International Labor Organization (UN).
ILo Iodine lotion.
ILP Inadequate luteal phase; Insufficiency of luteal phase; Interstitial lymphocytic pneumonia.
ILQTS Idiopathic long QT syndrome.
ILR Industrial and Labor Relations; Intraligamentous repair (Orthopedics); Irreversible loss rate.
IL-1RA Interleukin 1-receptor antagonist.
ILRAD International Laboratory for Research on Animal Diseases (Kenya).
ILS Idiopathic leucine sensitivity; Idiopathic lymphadenopathy syndrome; Increase in life span; Influenza-like symptoms/ syndrome; Infrared liver scanner; Intermittent light stimulation; Intralobal/lobar sequestration.
ILSA Ion luminescence spectroscopy for analysis.
ILSI International Life Sciences Institute.
ILSMH International League of Societies for the Mentally Handicapped.
ILSS Integrated life support system; Intraluminal somatostatin.
ILT Iliotibial tract; Intraluminal thrombosis.
IL-TASS International long-term average speech spectrum (see SCNRL).
Ilu Isoleucine (see Ileu).
ILVEN Inflammatory linear verrucal epidermal nevus.
IM Idiopathic myelofibrosis; Immunosuppressive method; Index Medicus (NLM journal); Indomethacin (= IMT; IND; INDO); Inducing molecule (see HSC); Industrial medicine; Industrial Medicine (journal); Infection medium; Infectious mononucleosis (= MI; Mono); Inner membrane; Innocent murmur; Inspiratory muscles; Institute of Medicine (NAS); Interest maturity; Interface memory (computer); Intermediate; Intermediate megaloblast; Intermetatarsal; Intermodulation; Internal malleolus; Internal mammary (artery); Internal Medicine; Intramedullary; Intramuscular (= im; ims) (see IMI); Invasive mole; Involutional melancholia.
im intramuscular (see IM).
IMA Immunomodulating/ory action/ activity/ agent (Isoxazole IMA - Leflunomide); Indian/ Industrial/ Irish/ Israel Medical Association; Inferior mesenteric artery; Interchurch Medical Assistance; Intermetatarsal angle (see IMTA); Internal mammary artery; Intramedullary application (Orthopedics); Intramuscular administration.
IMAA Iodinated macroaggregated albumin (radioactive).
IMAB Internal mammary artery bypass (operation/ heart); International Medical Advisory Bureau.
IMAC Ifosfamide, mesnauroprotection, Adriamycin (doxorubicin), and cisplatin.
IMAG Internal mammary artery graft; Israel Medical Association Journal.
IMAI Internal mammary artery implant (oper-

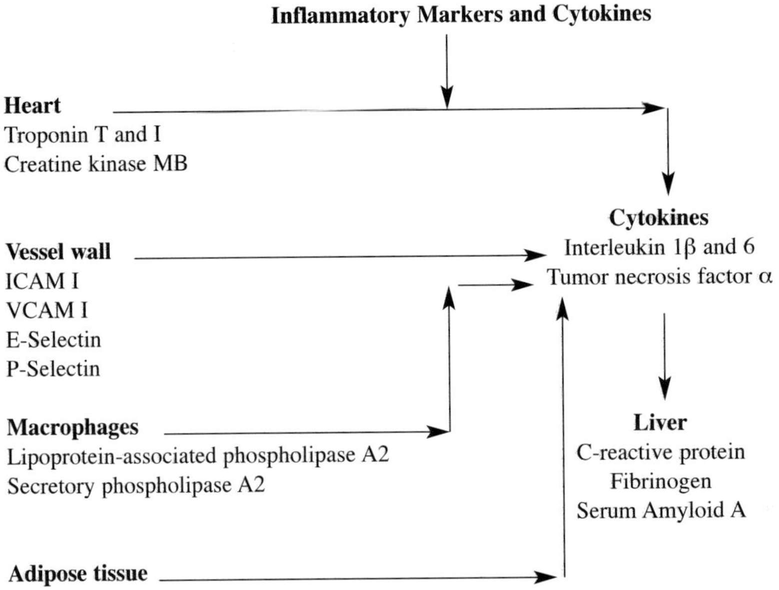

ation/ heart).

IMAJ Israel Medical Association Journal.

IMB Intermenstrual bleeding (i.e. metrorrhagia); Intermetatarsal bursa.

IMBC Indirect maximum breathing capacity (see PFT - IMBC).

IMBI Institute of Medical and Biological Illustrators.

IMBLMS Integrated Medical and Behavioral Laboratory Measurement System (NASA + HEW).

IMBR Internal Medicine Board Review.

IMC Immature (bone) marrow cell; Immunomodulating cytokine; Improved myocardial contractility; Inflammatory Markers and Cytokines (see Scheme); Interdigestive migrating contractions; International Medical Corps; Intestinal mast cell; Intramedullary canal (see IMS)/ catheter; Involuntary muscle/cular contraction(s) (as in Huntington's disease); Irregular menstrual cycle.

Imchem Immunochemistry (journal).

IMCI Integrated Management of Childhood Illnesses.

IMCR Inflammatory marker of coronary risk (including Cardiac troponin T, C-reactive protein, Serum fibrinogen, and Serum amyloid A).

IMCT Information-Memory-Concentration Test.

IMCU Intermediate/ (I. medical) care unit (= ICU).

IMD Immunologically mediated disease; Increased mineral demand; Inflammatory muscle disease; Inherited metabolic disorder; Inosine monophosphate dehydrogenase; International Medical Digest; Ipsilateral mediastinal disease (lung cancer, metastasis) (see MLN).

ImD_{50}; ImD_{50} Immunizing dose sufficient to protect 50% of the animals in a test group.

IMDC Intramedullary metatarsal decompression.

IMDD Idiopathic midline destructive disease.

IMDG International Maritime Dangerous Goods (code).

IMDP Imidocarb diproprionate.

IME Immunomodulatory effect; Independent medical examination/er; Institute of Medical Ethics; Isometric exercise.

IMEM Improved minimum essential medium.

IMER Institute for Medical Education and Research.

IMET Isometric endurance test.
IMF Idiopathic myelofibrosis; Ifosfamide, (mesnauroprotection), methotrexate, and fluorouracil; Immediate mechanical fixation (of fractures); Immunofixation; Immunofluorescence; Infant milk formula; International Medical Forum; Intermaxillary fixation; Intermediate filament; International Monetary Fund; Intramedullary fixation (e.g. of long bones) (Orthopedics).
IMFF Intramedullary fixation of femur (Schneider).
IMG Inferior mesenteric ganglion; Internal medicine group (practice); International medical graduate; Intramedullary glioma.
IMGG Intramuscular gammaglobulin.
IMH Idiopathic macular hole (retina); Idiopathic myocardial hypertrophy; Indirect microhemagglutination (test).
IMHD Immune-mediated heart disease.
IMHP 1-iodomercuri-2-hydroxypropane.
IMHRN International Mental Health Research Newsletter.
IMI Immediate medical intervention; Immunological(ly) measurable insulin (see Insulin - IMI); Impaired mucosal immunity; Impending/ Inferior myocardial infarction; Imperial Mycological Institute (Great Britain); Intermeal interval; Internal mammary implantation (Sewell procedure); Intramedullary injection (Orthopedics); Intramuscular injection (see IM); Ischemic myocardial injury.
Imi Imipramine.
^{123}I-MIBG ^{123}I-meta-iodobenzyl-guanidine (scintography for detecting chromaffin in pheochromocytoma and other tumors).
IMIC International Medical Information Center.
IMIG; IMIg Intramuscular immunoglobulin.
IMIP Industrial Modernization Incentive Program.
Imit Imitation/ative.
IMLA Intramural left anterior (artery).
IMLAD Intramural left anterior descending (artery).
IMLC Incomplete mitral leaflet closure.
IMLN Intramammary lymph node; Ipsilateral mediastinal lymph node (see MLN).
IMLNS Idiopathic minimal lesion nephrotic syndrome.
IMLT Institute of Medical Laboratory Technology (UK).
IMLTG Institute of Medical Laboratory Technology Gazette.
ImLy Immune lysis.
IMM Immune-mediated mechanism; Inhibitor-containing minimal medium; Institute for Molecular Medicine (CA); Intercellular-matrix macromolecular; Internal medial malleolus.
Imm Immune/nity/nization/nology (see Immun).
immat immature/rity.
IMMC Interdigestive migrating motor complex.
immed immediate(ly).
immob immobilize(d)/zation (see immobil).
immobil immobilization/ze(d) (= immob).
Immun Immune/ity/nization (= Imm; immun); Immunology (BSI journal); Immunology (= Imm; immun; Immunol).
immun immune/nity/nization (= Imm); immunology (see Immun).
Immunochem Immunochemistry (journal).
Immunol Immunology (see Immun).
IMN Internal mammary node; Intramedullary nail(ing) (stainless steel nail used in bone fracture repair, such as the treatment of transverse or short oblique fractures of the tibia).
IMNAS Institute of Medicine of the National Academy of Science.
IMNDN Internal Medicine News & Diagnosis News (journal).
IMNT Intramedullary nailing technique (Orthopedics) (see BWN; GKN;.IIN; IMN).
IMOS Inadvertent Modification of the Stratosphere (Federal Interagency Task Force on).
IMP Idiopathic myeloid proliferation; Immunomodulatory properties/ty; Impression; Incomplete male pseudohermaphroditism; Individual Medicade practitioner; Inosine 5'-monophosphate; Institute of Molecular Pathology (Vienna, Austria); Interface Message Processor; Intramembranous particle; Intramuscular compartment pressure; Invasive medical pro-

cedure.

Imp; imp Impacted/tion (see Impx); Impaired (see impair); Implant(ed); Important; Impressed (sion); Improve(ed).

IMPA Incisal mandibular plane angle.

IMPAC Information for Management, Planning, Analysis and Coordination.

IMPACT Integrelin to Minimize Platelet Aggregation and Prevent Coronary Thrombosis (trial).

impair impaired (= Imp; imp).

IMPC International Myopia Prevention Center.

IMPDH Inosine monophosphate dehydrogenase.

Imper Imperative; Imperial.

Impf Inoculated (Ger.), e.g. malaria, tetanus, etc.

Imprint (NSNA journal).

IMPS Inpatient Multidimensional Psychiatric Scale; Intact months of patient survival.

Impx Impacted/tion (= Imp; imp).

IMR Individual medical record; Infant mortality rate/ risk; Infectious mononucleosis receptor; Institute for Medical Research (NIA); Institution for the mentally retarded; Intramuscular route; Irrigating mushroom retractor (Ophthalmology).

IMRAD Introduction, methods, results, and discussion.

IMRS Inpatient Multidimensional Rating Scale.

IMRT Intensity-modulated radiation therapy (for prostate cancer).

IMS Immulogic marker study; Impaired mental status; Incurred in military service; Indian Medical Service; Industrial methylated spirit (= Alcohol Industriale; Industr Meth Spt). Alcohol (95%) 19 volumes with approved wood naphtha 1 volume; Information management system; Institute of Medical Sciences; Institutes for Medical Services; Integrated medical services; International Medical Systems (Ltd); International Meditation Society; International metric system; Intramedullary stem (bone); Ion mobility spectrometer.

ims intramuscular (see IM).

IMSP International Medical Society of Paraplegia.

IMSS In-flight medical support system; Instituto Mexicano del Seguro Social.

IMSSN Intramedullary stainless steel nail (Orthopedics).

IMT Immunomodulating/tory therapy/ treatment; Indomethacin (see IM); Induced muscular tension; Inspiratory muscle training; Intracranial malignant tumor (see ICMT).

IMTA Intermetatarsal angle (= IMA) (Orthopedics).

IMTGB International Medical Tribune of Great Britain (journal).

IMU Index of Medical Underservice; Irish Medical Union.

ImU International milliunit(s).

IMV Increased minute ventilation (see VFR); Inferior mesenteric vein; Intermittent mandatory/ mechanical ventilation (respiratory therapy); Isophosphamide, methotrexate, and vincristine.

IMViC; imvic; IMVPC Indole, methyl red, Voges-Proskauer, and citrate reactions/ tests used in bacteriology in classifying coliform bacteria.

IMVP Idiopathic mitral valve prolapse.

IMVP-16 Ifosfamide, (mesnauroprotection), methotrexate, and VP (etoposide).

IMVS Institute of Medical and Veterinary Science (Australia).

IMWIC International Maize and Wheat Improvement Center (Mexico, CIMMYT) (see CIMMYT).

IMWP Intramyocardial wall pressure (= IWP).

IN Icterus/ Impetigo neonatorum; Incidence; Industrial nurse; Infundibular nucleus; Insulin (see In); Interneuron; Interstitial nephritis; Intranasal; Irritation of nociceptors; Neisler Laboratories, Inc. code for experimental substances; Number of incompatibilities.

In Index; Indium (Z = 49) (see Elements - Indium); Inion; Insulin (= IN) (see Insulin); Into; Inulin.

in inch.

in- prefix meaning fiber (Gr. inos) or not, in, and on (L.).

in^2 square inch (see sq in).

in^3 cubic inch (see cu in).

^{111}**In** Radioactive indium.
IN 511 Phenyramidol hydrochloride - an analgesic agent.
INA Infectious nucleic acid; Inferior nasal artery; International Neurological Association; Jena Nomina Anatomica (see JNA).
IN a Indian a antigen (blood group of India).
Ina Inactivator (e.g. C1 Ina = Complement 1 inactivator).
INAA Instrumental neutron activation analysis.
inac inactive.
INAD Infantile neuroaxonal dystrophy.
INAH Interstitial nucleus of the anterior hypothalamus; Isonicotinic acid hydrazide (see INH).
INAM Istituto Nazionale per l'Assicurazione Control le Malattie (Italy).
INB Infranodal block (see HB); Internuclear bridging; Ischemic necrosis of bone.
inbr inbreeding.
INC Inside needle catheter; Internodular cortex; Intranasal corticosteroid.
inc incentive; incisal/se/sion (see incis); include(ed)/ding/usion/usive (see incl); incomparable (see incompar); incompatible/lity (see incompat); incomplete (see incompl); inconclusive (see inconclu); incontinent (see incont); incorporate(ed)/ting/tion/tive (see incorp); increase(d)/sing (see incr); increment (see incr); incur(red)/ incurable (see incur); *incision*:
ab externo incision (from externally inwards);
Auvray incision (for splenectomy);
Bar's incision (for cesarian section - midline abdominal incision);
Battle's incision (abdominal vertical incision - for the stomach, liver, gall-bladder, etc.);
Battle-Jalaguier-Kammerer incision (same as Battle's incision);
belt approach incision (a waistline incision);
Bergmann's incision (for exposure of the kidney);
Bevan's incision (for exposing the gall-bladder);
Bruner type incision (a zigzag incision - plastic and reconstructive surgery);
Bruser skin incision (knee surgery);
Buck-Gramcko incision (reconstructive hand surgery);
celiotomy incision (abdominal incision, for access to the peritoneal cavity);
Cheatle-Henry incision (in bilateral hernia repair);
Cherney incision (a low transverse abdominal incision);
Cherney-Winklesnit incision (abdominal incision);
chevron incision (exploratory laparotomy);
circular guillotine incision;
clitoris incision;
confirmatory incision (for confirming a diagnosis);
Conley incision (radical neck dissection);
crease incision (inguinal herniorrhaphy);
crucial incision (cross-shaped incision);
cruciate incision;
curvilinear incision;
Deaver's incision (for appendectomy);
Deaver skin incision (mastectomy);
deltopectoral incision;
dorsolateral incision;
double-Y incision;
Duhrssen's incision (obstetrics and gynecology);
dumb-bell incision;
Elsberg incision (general surgery);
endaural incision (otolaryngology);
Fergusson's incision (for excision of the upper jaw);
fishmouth incision;
Fowler's angular incision (for anterolateral abdominal section);
Fowler-Weir incision (general surgery);
Gibson (posterior muscle cutting) incision (in urology and total hip replacement);
Gibson-Foley type incision (groin incision in lower ureter surgery);
gingivolabial incision (used in the Caldwell-Luc operation);
grayline incision (eye surgery);
gridiron incision;
guillotine incision;
Gunter Von Noorden incision (ophthalmology);
Halstead/ Halstead-Meyer/ Halstead-Willie-

Meyer incision (radical breast surgery);
Heermann incision (otolaryngology);
Henry incision (general surgery);
hockey-stick incision (see Meyer's hockey stick incision);
house incision (eyelid, entropion repair);
infraumbilical incision;
Jackson incision (general surgery);
Kehr's incision (general surgery);
keratome incision (ophthalmology);
Kocher collar incision (thyroidectomy);
Kocher and Osborne incision (hip arthroplasty);
Kocher's incision (for the gall-bladder);
Kustner's incision (a semilunar abdominal incision);
Lahey incision (radical neck dissection);
Langenbeck's incision (for operations of the colon, kidney, spleen, tail of pancreas, etc);
Lateral rectus incision (abdomen);
lazy-S incision (orthopedics);
Lempert incision (radical tympanoplasty);
Leslie incision (shoulder);
Longuet's incision (for extraserous transplantation of the testicle for hydrocele and varicocele);
Mackenrodt's incision (a transverse semilunar abdominal incision);
McArthur's incision (a vertical upper transrectus incision);
McBurney's incision (appendectomy);
McIndoc incision (orthopedics);
median incision (in the midline of the body);
Meyer (Willie-Meyer) incision (general surgery);
Meyer's hockey stick incision (used in complicated appendicitis) (= hockey-stick incision);
Moynihan incision (intestinal surgery);
Ollier and Murphy incision (hip arthroplasty);
omega-shaped incision;
Orr incision (general surgery);
parainguinal incision;
paramedian incision (abdomen);
pararectus incision (general surgery);
parascapular incision;
Parker's incision (over the area of dullness in appendiceal abscess);
periareolar incision (general surgery);
periscapular incision (general surgery);
Perthes' incision (for the gall-bladder);
Pfannenstiel's incision (abdomen);
pubo-xyphoid incision;
Rambo endaural incision (otolaryngology);
relief incision (to relieve tension in a part);
rim incision (laparoscopy);
Risdon incision (submandibular);
Rockey-Davis incision (appendectomy);
Rodman incision (radical mastectomy);
S-shaped incision;
saber incision (general surgery);
saber-slash incision (general surgery);
scratch incision (general surgery);
serpentine incision;
Shea incision (otolaryngology);
Silovi incision (general surgery);
sinuous incision;
Skoog incision (palmar fasciectomy);
slot incision;
Smith-Petersen incision (total hip replacement);
Souttar incision (craniotomy);
stepladder incision;
T-incision (otolaryngology);
tepee incision;
transacromial incision;
Turner-Warwick incision (nephrectomy);
utility type incision (knee surgery);
Vischer's lumbo-iliac incision (above the center of the iliac crest);
Von Noorden incision (ophthalmology);
Warren's incision (across the thoracomammary fold);
Watson-Jones incision (orthopedics);
Wheeler incision (ophthalmology);
Wilde's incision (for exposure of the mastoid process; done for mastoid abscess);
Willie-Meyer incision (breast surgery).

INCAP Instituto de Nutrición de Centro America y Panama (Institute of Nutrition of Central America and Panama).

INCB International Narcotics Control Board (UN).

IncB Inclusion body.

INCD Infantile nuclear cerebral degeneration.

Incentive Cocaine (see Erthroxylum).

incis incisal/se/sion (= inc).

INCL Infantile/ Inherited neuronal ceroid

lipofuscinosis (a genetic illness caused by a mutation of a specific gene on Chromosome 1 and especially rampant in Finland, with early blindness in babies, progressive brain cell atrophy and leading to a slow, lingering death) (see NCL).
incl include(ed)/ding/usion/usive (= inc).
incompar incomparable (= inc).
incompat incompatible/lity (= inc).
incompl incomplete (= inc).
inconclu inconclusive (= inc).
incont incontinent (= inc).
incorp incorporate(ed)/ting/tion/tive (= inc).
incr increase(d)/sing (= inc); increment (= inc).
inc(R) increase (relative).
IncSpir Incentive spirometer.
incur incurable (= inc); incur(red) (= inc).
IND Daily (L. in dies) (see in d); In the name of God (L. in nomine Dei); Indomethacin (see IM); Inducer(s) - of the alternative pathway (to differentiate from the clinical pathway), in the activation of the complement reaction (They include: Endotoxins - liposaccharides from the cells of gram-negative bacteria, Polyanion - dextran sulfate, Zymosan - particulate constituents of yeast cell walls, Polyfructose - insulin, and Antigen-binding segments of antibody molecules); Industrial (medicine) (see Ind Med); Initial dose; Investigational new drug.
ind indefinite (see indef); independent (see indep); indeterminable/ate/ation/mined (see indeter); indicate(d)/ation (see indic); indigestion (see indig); indirect (see indir); individual (see indiv); induced; induction (see induct); industrial (see indust).
in d daily (L. in dies) (= IND).
InDDEx Investigation into Delay to Diagnosis of Alzheimer's disease with Exelon or ENA-713 (Rivastigmine) (study).
indef indefinite (= ind).
indep independent (= ind).
indeter indeterminable/ate/ation/mined (= ind).
Ind HA Indeterminate hyperaldosteronism.
Indian hay Marijuana (see Cannabis).
Indian hemp Marijuana (see Cannabis).
indic indicate(d)/ation (= ind).
indig indigestion (= ind).
indir indirect (= ind).
indiv individual (= ind).
INDM Infant of non-diabetic mother.
Ind Med Index Medicine; Industrial Medicine (= IND).
IND-NDA Investigation New Drug - New Drug Application.
Ind. N.F National Formulary of India (1960).
INDO Indomethacin (see IM).
INDOR Internuclear double resonance.
Ind P Indian Pharmacopoeia.
induct induction (= ind).
indust industrial (= ind).
INE Infantile necrotizing encephalomyelopathy.
INEX Inexperienced.
in ext at the point of death (L. in extremis).
INF Infant(ile) (see Inf); Infect(ed)/tion/tious/tive (see Infect); Infirmary (see Inf); Inflamed (see Inflam); Inflammation/tory (see Inflamm); Information (see Info); Infundibulum (see Inf); Infused/sion (see Inf); Interferon (see IFN); Isonicotinic acid methylfurfurylidene hydrazide; Intact neurological function.
Inf; inf Infant(ile) (= INF); Infarction (see Infarct); Infect(ed)/tion/tious/tive (see Infect); Inferior; Infinite/tive (see Infin); Infirmary (= INF); Inflamed (see Inflam); Inflammation/tory (see Inflamm); Influence(d) (see Infl); Information (see Info); Infundibulum (= INF); Infused/sion (L. infusum) (= INF); Pour in (L. infunde).
INF 1837 Flufenamic acid (see CI 440).
INF 3355 Mephenamic acid (see CI 473).
Infarct Infarction (= Inf).
INFC Infect(ed)/tion/tious/tive (see Infect).
Infect Infect(ed)/tion/tious/tive (= INF; Inf; inf).
Infect dis Infectious disease.
Infin Infinite/tive (= Inf; inf).
Infl Influence(d) (= Inf; inf).
Inflam Inflamed (= INF; Inf; inf).
Inflamm Inflammation/tory (= INF; Inf; inf).
Inf MI Inferior (wall) myocardial infarction.
Info Information (= INF; Inf; inf).
infra- prefix meaning less or under (L.).
Infus Infusion.

ING Isotope nephrogram.
ing inguinal.
√ **ing** checking.
InGP Indolglycerophosphate.
INH Inhalation/haler (see Inhal); Isonicotinic acid hydrazide (= INAH; Isoniaz; Isoniazid[um]; Isonicotinic hydrazide; Isonicotinoylhydrazine/tinylhydrazide[zine]; Pyridine-4-carboxy-hydrazide; Tubazid) - a bacteriostatic agent used in the treatment of tuberculosis.
Inh; inh Inhalation/haler (see Inhal); Inhibiting/tion/tory (see Inhib).
Inhal Inhalation/haler (= INH; Inh; inh).
INH-G Gatalone - the glucuronolactone of isonicotinic acid hydrazide (isoniazid). Has been used in the treatment of tuberculosis (see INH).
Inhib Inhibiting/tion/tory (= Inh; inh).
INI International News Items (WMA journal); International Nursing Index (journal); Intranuclear inclusion (agent).
INIS International Nuclear Information System (IAEA).
Initial Initially.
Inj; inj Inject(able)/ion (= Inject; inject); Injured/rious/ry; Injury (journal).
Inject; inject Injectable/tion (see Inj; inj).
inj enem give/ inject an enema or let an enema be given/ injected (L. injiciatur enema).
INK Injury not known.
INL Inner nuclear layer.
Inl Inlay.
in lit; in litt in correspondence (L. in litteris).
INLSD Ichthyosis and neutral lipid storage disease.
INM Infected/ Inflamed nasal mucosa; Institute of Naval Medicine (UK).
INN International Non-proprietary Names (WHO); Irish Nursing News (now IN Newsletter); Irish Nursing Newsletter (IGCN).
innerv innervated/tion.
innom innominate.
INO Internuclear ophthalmoplegia; Inosine (see Ino); Irish Nurses' Organization.
Ino Inosine (= INO).
INOC Isonicotinoyl-oxycarbonyl.
Inoc; inoc Inoculate(d)/tion.
inorg inorganic.
Inox Oxidized inosine.
INP Idiopathic neutropenia; Immunologically normal patient (= ICP - Immunocompetent patient).
INPAV Intermittent negative-pressure assisted ventilation (= INPV) (respiratory therapy).
INPC Isopropyl n-phenylcarbamate.
INPEA Isopropyl nitrophenyl-ethanolamine.
INPH Iproniazid phosphate.
INPRONS Information processing in the central nervous system.
INPS International Neuropsychological Society (see INS); National Institute of Social Providence (see NISP).
inpt inpatient.
in pulm in gruel (strained oatmeal) (L. in pulmento).
INPV Intermittent negative-pressure ventilation (see INPAV).
INQ Interior nasal quadrant.
INR International Narcotic Report (journal); International normalized ratio.
INREM Internal roentgen-equivalent, man (= Internal radiation dose in rem or Roentgen-equivalent-man units).
INS Idiopathic nephrotic syndrome; Immigration and Naturalization Service; Insurance (see Ins); International Neuropsychological Society (= INPS); International News Service.
Ins; ins Inches; Insert(ion); Insulin (see Insulin); Insurance/red (= INS).
insem insemination.
INSERM Institut National de la Santé et de la Recherche Médicine (National Institute for Health and Medical Research - France).
INSH Salinazid (= Salizid; o-Hydroxybenzal isonicotinyl hydrazone) - a bacteriostatic agent used in the treatment of tuberculosis.
in situ in natural or normal position (L.).
insol insoluble.
Insp; Inspir Inspiration/tory.
INSR Insulin receptor.
INST Instrumental (delivery).
Inst Institute.
instab instability.
INSTD Interlocking nail system with target

device (Russell-Taylor - Orthopedics).
instill instillation.
Instn Institution.
Instr Instruction/ctor/ctress; Instrument.
insuf; insuff insufficiency/ient; insufflation.
insul- prefix meaning island (L. insula).
Insulin (= I; In; INS; Ins; ins). A protein hormone produced by the islet cells of Langerhans in the pancreas and secreted into the blood, where it regulates carbohydrate metabolism. Also known as the antidiabetic hormone (ADH) (see Hormones - ADH i). The insulins include:
ARI: Acid regular insulin; Actrapid insulin (see Insulin - PI iii).
BI: Bovine insulin - prepared from cattle pancreas.
BII: Biphasic insulin injection. Insulin crystals suspended in a solution of insulin, buffered at pH 7 with sodium acetate. Incompatible with soluble insulin (SI). Maximum action at 6-8 hours; lasts 20-22 hours; especially of use in labile diabetes or brittle juvenile diabetes.
CZI: Crystalline Zinc Insulin (see Insulin - IZS cryst).
DI: Dalanated Insulin (= SN 44). An insulin derivative prepared by removal of C-terminal alanine from the B-chain of insulin. Human insulin has a C-terminal threonine instead of the alanine present in bovine and porcine insulins; removal of this terminal alanine does not affect insulin activity, but approximates it more to human insulin. This dalanated insulin has been suggested in the treatment of cases in which insulin resistance has developed.
FI: Fibrous Insulin (= F-insul; F-insulin) (see Insulin - PI ii).
GFI: Glucagon-free insulin.
GI: Globin insulin. Insulin combined with the globin of erythrocytes. Also known as Globin zinc insulin (see Insulin - GZI).
GZI: Globin zinc insulin (= Globin insulin). Insulin with added zinc chloride and globin. Intermediate period of action, midway between soluble insulin (SI) and Protamine zinc insulin (PZI). Acts within 1-2 hours; maximum action at 6-12 hours; lasts up to 20 hours.
HI: i. Hexamine insulin. Insulin combined with hexamine tetramine. Rapid action. Used in juvenile diabetes. ii. Human insulin - present naturally in man.
HZI: Histone zinc insulin. Insulin combined with histone and zinc.
II: i. Injection Insulin or Insulin Injection (= Insulin hydrochloride; Ordinary insulin; Regular insulin - RI; Rapid- acting insulin - RI; Soluble insulin - SI; Unmodified insulin - acts within 20-30 minutes; maximum action at 4-6 hours; lasts up to 8-10 hours. ii. Isophane insulin (= Isophane insulin injection - III; Neutral protamine Hagedorn insulin - NPH insulin). Insulin made from zinc-insulin crystals, modified by the addition of protamine (see Insulin - NPH insulin).
III: Isophane insulin injection (see Insulin - NPH insulin).
IL: Insulin lente (see Insulin - LI; IZS).
I MI: Immunological(ly) measurable insulin.
IPZ: Insulin protamine zinc (see Insulin - PZI).
I RI: Immunoreactive insulin (plasma In.).
IRP: Immunoreactive proinsulin (plasma In.).
IS: Insulin semilente (= Semilente insulin) (see Insulin - SI i; IZS amorph).
IT: Insulin tannate (see Insulin - TI).
IU: Insulin ultralente (see Insulin - UI; IZS cryst).
I Var: Insulin variable.
IZS: Insulin zinc suspension (= Lente insulin - LI; Insulin lente - IL) - a mixture of 3 volumes of IZS (amorph) and 7 volumes of IZS (cryst). Insulin suspensions are modified by the addition of zinc chloride. Acts within 1 to 2 hours; maximum action at 4-5 hours; lasts up to 24 hours.
IZS (amorph): Amorphous insulin zinc suspension (= Semilente insulin - SI; Insulin semilente - IS; Prompt IZS) - resembles Globin zinc insulin (GZI), but with quicker action. Acts within 30 minutes; maximum action at 2-3 hours; lasts 12-16 hours.
IZS (cryst): Crystalline insulin zinc suspension (= Ultralente insulin - UI; Insulin ultralente - IU; Extended IZS) - resembles Protamine zinc insulin (PZI), but with earlier

maximal effect. Acts within 4-6 hours; maximum action at 7-10 hours; lasts for 30-36 hours.
LI: Lente insulin/ Insulin lente (see Insulin - IZS).
MCI: Monocomponent insulin (= MC-insulin; SCI; SC insulin; Single component ins). Insulin in which the connecting peptide of the proinsulin molecule is split off by enzymatic action, leaving a pure insulin virtually free of impurities, such as altered insulin, insulin polymer, proinsulin, and peptides derived from proinsulin. This produces a non-antigenic or non-immunogenic insulin in its purest form with no antibody production as in the conventional or mono-species insulins (MSI).
MC-insulin: See Insulin - MCI.
MSI: Mono-species insulins or the conventional insulin preparations containing antigenic impurities, and resulting in the production of insulin antibodies. This causes allergy, local lipotrophy, high insulin requirement due to raised antibody-bound insulin (i.e. IBS or raised Insulin Binding Capacity), and insulin resistance. As a sequel to this, the new pure insulins, the Monocomponent insulin (MCI or MC-insulin) or Single Component insulin (SCI or SC-insulin) have been produced, particularly for patients sensitized to the conventional insulins (see Insulin - MCI).
MC-insulin: See Insulin - MSI.
NII: Neutral insulin injection. An isotonic solution of insulin buffered at pH 7, having a more rapid action than Soluble Insulin (SI) and with greater intensity of action during the first 4-6 hours. Particularly of value in the treatment of diabetic coma.
NPBI: Non-protein bound insulin.
NPH i: See NPH insulin.
NPH insulin: Neutral protamine Hagedorn insulin (= II or Isophane ins; III or Isophane ins inj); NPH i) - acts within 1 to 2 hours; maximum action at 10-20 hours; lasts up to 28-30 hours (see Insulin - II ii; III).
NRI: Neutral regular insulin.
OI: Oral insulin (= Peroral insulin - PI). Insulin used orally by the addition of a substance protecting it from the enzymes of the gastroin-testinal tract.
PI i: Peroral insulin (see Insulin - OI). ii. Plant insulin (= Fibrous insulin - FI; Glucokinin; Vegetable insulin - VI) - a hormone-like substance obtained from vegetable tissues and yeast, injections of which produce hypoglycemia in animals. iii. Porcine insulin - many of the newer insulins, prepared from the pancreas of pigs, such as Actrapid ins (ARI); Semilente ins (SI), etc. iv. Protamine insulin (= Insulin protaminate). Insulin precipitated from insulin hydrochloride (Soluble ins. - SI), plus a monoprotamine compound.
PZI: Protamine zinc insulin (= IPZ; ZPI). Insulin combined with protamine and zinc. Acts within 4-6 hours; maximum action at 15-20 hours; lasts from 24-36 hours.
RI: Regular insulin or Rapid-acting insulin (see Insulin - II i).
SCI: Single component insulin (see Insulin - MCI).
SC-insulin: See Insulin - SCI.
SI: i. Semilente insulin (= Insulin semilente - IS) (see Insulin - IZS amorph). ii. Soluble insulin (= Rapid-acting or Regular insulin - RI) (see Insulin - II i).
SPI: Single Peak Insulin.
Three-to-one I: See 3-1 Insulin.
3 to 1 Insulin, Three to One Insulin: See 3-1 I.
3-1 I: (= 3-1 Insulin; Three to One Insulin) - a combination of soluble insulin (3 parts) and protamine zinc insulin (1 part).
TI: Tannate insulin (= Insulin tannate - IT) - the insulin salt of tannic acid.
TIRI: Total immunoreactive insulin (= TIR insulin).
TIR insulin: See TIRI.
UI: Ultralente insulin (= Insulin ultralente - IU) (see Insulin - IZS cryst).
VI: Vegetable insulin (= Glucokinin) (see Insulin - PI ii).
ZPI: Zinc-protamine insulin (see Insulin - PZI).

INT; Int Integral; Integument (see INTEG); Intelligence (see Intell); Interject(ed)/ion (see Interj); Intermediate (see Intmd); Intermittent (see INTR); Intermittent needle therapy; Intern(ist)/ship; Internal (see intern);

International (see Internat); Interval; Intestinal/ne (see Intest); Intima; Intoxicated/tion (see INTOX); Intrathecal (see INTH); Intubation (see intub); Iodonitrotetrazolium (= p-iodophenyl-nitrophenylphenyl-tetrazolium chloride) (an analytical dye); Thoroughly (L. intime).

int al; int alia among others (L. inter alia).

int cib between meals (L. inter cibos).

INTEG Integument (= INT; Int).

Intell Intelligence (= INT; Int).

inter- prefix meaning among or between (L.).

Intercien Interciencia (journal).

Interface (journal).

Interj Interject(ed)/tion (= INT; Int).

InterMT Intermetatarsal (angle) (see IMA; IMTA) (Orthopedics).

Intern Internist (journal).

intern internal (= INT; Int).

Internat International (= INT; Int).

INTERP Interpretation.

Intervir Intervirology (journal).

intes intestinal/ne (see Intest).

Intest Intestinal/ne (= INT; Int; intes).

Int/Ext Internal/External.

INTH; Inth Intrathecal (= INT; Int).

Intmd Intermediate (= INT; Int).

Int Med Internal medicine.

Int mon Internal monitor.

int noct during the night (L. inter noctem).

intol intolerance.

INTOX; Intox; intox Intoxicated/tion (= INT; Int).

INTR Intermittent (= INT; Int).

intra- prefix meaning within (L.).

Intro Introduction.

intro- prefix meaning into or within (L.).

Intron An intervening sequence and non-coding region of the human DNA, interspersed with and larger than the exon, in the gene base of the genetic code (see Exon).

Int Rot Internal rotation.

Int trx Intermittent traction.

intub intubation (= INT; Int).

InU International Unit.

INULA The Elecampane plant (I. helenium) of the Daisy family, Compositae. Elecampane root is one source of the vegetable starch, known as Alant Starch, a polymerized form of fructofuranose (a polysaccharide), yielding levulose on hydrolysis, and is used in the preparation of special breads for diabetics; also as a diagnostic agent in the kidney function test ICT (Inulin clearance test) (see KFT - ICT).

in utero within the uterus (L.).

INV Inferior nasal vein.

InV Site on human immunoglobulins (abbreviation derived from a patient's name).

Inv; inv Inversion/erted; Involuntary.

inver inversion/erted (= Inv; inv).

invest investigate(d)/ating/ation.

Inv/Ev Inversion/Eversion.

inv ins inverted insertion.

in vitro within a glass vessel or test tube (L.).

in vivo within a living body (L.).

invol involuntary.

involv involve(d)/ment/olving.

inv(p+ q-); inv(p- q+) pericentric inversion.

IO Incisal/ Initial opening; Inferior oblique (muscle)/ olive; Internal os (cervix); Internist Observer (journal); Interorbital; Intestinal obstruction; Intraocular; Intra-operative; Investigative Ophthalmology (ARVO).

Io Ionium - a radioactive isotope of thorium (TH; Z = 90), of atomic weight 230.5. It emits both alpha & gamma rays (see Elements - Thorium).

I/O; I&O In and out; Input/Intake and output.

IOA Inner optic anlage; International Osteopathic Association.

IOAT International Organization Against Trachoma.

IOC In our culture; Intergovernmental Oceanographic Commission (UN); Interim Orders Committee (GMC, Britain); International Olympic Committee; International Ophthalmology Clinics (journal); International Organizing Committee (on Medical Librarianship); Intern on call; Intraoperative cholangiogram (see IOCG).

IOCG Intraoperative cholangiogram.

IOD Injured on duty; Inorganic dust (dry highly powdered particles of an inorganic substance, especially dust, and causing diseases such as Anthracosis, Asbestosis, Berylliosis, Pneumoconiosis, and Silicosis) (see MPC); Integrated optical density;

Interorbital distance.
IODM Infant of diabetic mother.
IOF Intraocular fluid.
IOFB Intraocular foreign body.
IOFNA Intraoperative fine needle aspirate/tion.
IOH Idiopathic orthostatic hypotension; Intraocular hemorrhage/ hypertension.
IOI Inadequate oral intake; Intraocular injection; Intraosseous infusion.
IOIS Intraocular irrigation solution (= IIS).
IOL Intraocular lens; Iron overload.
IOLF Intraocular lens forceps (Ophthalmology).
IOLI Intraocular lens implant (= ILI).
IOM Institute of Medicine (NAS); Internal oblique muscle (see OIA).
IOMD Intraoperative monitoring device (e.g. echocardiograph).
IOMP International Organization for Medical Physics.
ION Idiopathic osteonecrosis (see SON); Ischemic optic neuropathy.
ionto iontophoresis.
IOOL International Optometric and Optical League.
IOP Institute of Physics (UK); Intraocular pressure; Intraoperative patient; Intraosseous pressure (Orthopedics).
IOPE Intraocular pressure elevation.
IOPNSG Institute of Physics Neutron Scattering Group.
IOR Index of response.
IORT Intraoperative radiotherapy.
IOS Idiopathic oligospermia; International Organization for Standardization; Intraocular syringe; Intraoperative sampling (of bone) (Orthopedics); Intraoperative sonography; Iron overload syndrome.
IOSS Intraoperative skeletal scintogram/graph(y) (Orthopedics).
IOT Increased operating time; Internist-obstetrician team; Intraocular tension/ transfer; Intraoperative tachycardia/ therapy/ treatment; Ipsilateral optic tectum.
IOTA Information overload testing aid.
IOTT Institute of Operation Theatre Technicians (UK).
IOU I owe you; Illicit opioid use; Intensive (care/ therapy) observation unit; International opacity unit; Intraoperative use.
IOV Initial office visit.
IP Icterus praecox; Idiopathic parkinsonism (see PA; PD); Illif procedure (for correction of ptosis); Immune precipitate; Immunoblastic plasma; Immunoperoxidase (assay/ technique) (see IPA); Inactivated pepsin; Incisoproximal; Incisopulpal; Incontinentia pigmenti (a sex-linked dominant, congenital hypotrichosis with defects of teeth, bones, eyes and CNS, with skin hyperpigmentation); Incubation/ Induction period; Indices proprius (extensor muscle of index finger); Individualized plan; Induced/ Intracellular/ Ionic/nization potential; Infantile paralysis (poliomyelitis); Infection prevention (with reference to testing antiseptics); Infundibular process; Infusion pump; Inorganic phosphate; Inosine phosphorylase; Inpatient; Instantaneous pressure; Institute of Psychiatry (London); Interface principle; International Pathology (journal); International Pharmacopoeia (1967); Interpeduncular; Interphalangeal (joint) (see IPh); Interpupillary (see IPD); Interstitial pneumonitis; Intestinal pseudo-obstruction; Intraperitoneal(ly) (injection site) (= ip; i-periton); Intrapulmonary; Isoelectric point; Isoproterenol (see ISO); Isotopic purity; L'Institut Pasteur.
IP; IIP Incubation period; Intrinsic incubation period: The period of time between the moment of entrance of an infecting organism (bacterium, virus, etc.) into the body and the first appearance of the symptoms of the consequent disease.
Amebiasis (*Entameba* histolytica) - 3 days to several months;
Ascariasis (*Ascaris* lumbricoides hominis) - 2 months;
Brucellosis (Undulant fever)/ *Brucella* melitensis, abortus, or suis - one week to several months;
Cerebrospinal fever (Meningitis)/ *Meningococcus* (*Neisseria* meningitidis) - 2-10 days;
Chancroid (Soft chancre)/ *Hemophilus* ducreyi - 1-12 days;

Chickenpox (Varicella)/ virus - 14-21 days;
Cholera (*Vibrio* cholerae) - 1-5 days;
Diphtheria (*Corynebacterium* diphtheriae) - 1-5 days;
Dysentery (bacillary)/ *Shigella* sp. bacillus - 1-7 days;
Enterobiosis (Pinworm/ Threadworm infection)/ *Enterobius* vermicularis - 14-21 days;
Erysipelas (*Streptococcus* hemolyticus A) - 1-10 days;
German measles (Rubella)/ virus - 14-21 days;
Gonorrhea (*Neisseria* gonorrheae) - 2-10 days (Men), 7-21 days (Women);
Hepatitis (Acute viral) Virus A - 2-6 weeks;
(Serum) Virus B - 6-25 weeks;
Infectious Mononucleosis (Glandular fever)/ EBV (Epstein-Barr virus) - 4-14 days;
Influenza (A, B, subtypes)/ virus - 1-3 days;
Malaria (*Plasmodium* vivax - 14 days, ovale - 14 days, falciparum - 12 days, malariae - 30 days;
Measles (Rubeola)/ virus - 7-14 days;
Mumps (Epidemic/ Infectious Parotitis) virus - 14-24 days;
Plague (Bubonic, Pneumonic, Septicemic)/ *Pasteurella* pestis 1-6 days;
Pneumonia (Acute lobar pneumonia)/ *Pneumococcus* - 1-3 days;
(Mycoplasma)/ Eaton Agent - 7-21 days;
Poliomyelitis (Infantile paralysis)/ virus: Minor illness (First phase) - 3-5 days, Major illness (Second phase) - 7-14 days (major illness may be as long as 35 days);
Rabies (Hydrophobia)/ virus - 10 days to as much as 2 years;
Rocky Mountain Spotted Fever (*Rickettsia* rickettsii) - 3-10 days;
Scarlet Fever (Scarlatina)/ *Streptococcus* hemolyticus A) 3-5 days;
Smallpox (Variola)/ virus - 10-14 days;
Syphilis (*Treponema* pallidim/ *Spirochaeta* pallida) - 10-40 days;
Tetanus (*Clostridium* tetani) (usually 5-10 days) - 2-50 days;
Trichinosis (*Trichinella* spiralis) - 1-28 days;
Tularemia (*Pasteurella* tularensis) - 1-10 days;
Typhoid (Enteric) Fever (*Salmonella* typhi) - 5-25 days;
Typhus (Epidemic Louse-borne)/ *Rickettsia* prowazeki - 10-14 days;
(Endemic Murine Flea-borne)/ *Rickettsia* mooseri - 6-14 days;
Whooping Cough (Pertussis)/ *Bordetella* pertussis - 7-14 days;
Yellow Fever (virus) - 3-6 days.

ip Intraperitoneal(ly) (see IP).

IP3 Inositol triphosphate.

IPA Immunoperoxidase assay (= IP; IPT); Impaired platelet aggregation (see PAI); Incontinentia pigmenti achromians(see HMI); Increased physical activity; Independent/ Individual Practice Association; Infantile papular acrodermatitis; Inflammatory polyarthritis; Inhibition of platelet aggregation (= PAI); Interaction process analysis; International Pediatric/ Pharmaceutical/ Psychoanalytical Association; International Phonetic Alphabet; Intracellular parasitic agent; Intracellular phospholipid accumulation (or Phospholipidosis); Intraperitoneal administration; Intrapleural adhesion(s); Invasive pulmonary aspergillosis; Isopropyl alcohol.

IP-A Institute of Psycho-Analysis (UK).

IPAA International Psychoanalytical Association.

I-PAO Insulin (induced) peak acid output.

I-para Primipara (= first pregnancy).

IPAT Institute for Personality and Ability Testing (Cattel's Institute - France); Iowa Pressure Articulation Test.

IPB In-patient basis (of treatment).

IPBC Insulin-producing beta cell (in the pancreas).

IPBI Incompetent patient's best interest(s).

IPC Immature progenitor cell; Immunization Practices Committee (CDC - Centers for Disease Control); Inoperable prostatic cancer/ carcinoma; In-patient care; Insulin-producing cell (see IPBC); Intermittent pneumatic compression; Internal primary care; International Poliomyelitis/ Psychoanalytic Congress; Intrapartal/ partum care; Intrapsychic conflict (see Conflict); Ion pair chromatography; Iron (hydroxide) polymaltose complex (see IHPC); Isopropyl carbamate/ chlorophenyl/

N-phenylcarbamate (= IPPC; Propham) - a carbamate compound used as an agricultural insectiside or herbicide, and for the control of flies - A cholinesterase inhibitor.

ipc intraplacental.

4-IPC 4-isopropylcatechol.

IPCD Infantile polycystic disease.

IPCS Intrauterine progesterone contraceptive system (an IUD).

IPD Distal interphalangeal (joint) (see DIP); Idiopathic Parkinson's disease; Idiopathic protracted diarrhea; Immediate/ Intermittent pigment darkening; Impending preterm delivery; Increase in pupillary diameter; Incurable problem drinker; Inflammatory pelvic disease; Intermittent painless dysphagia; Intermittent peritoneal dialysis; Interpupillary distance (= PD); Interstitial pulmonary disease (= IPI); Invasive pneumococcal disease; Inventory of Psychosocial Development; Isolated Parkinson's disease (see parkin gene).

IPE Iatrogenic perforation of the esophagus; Idiopathic pericardial effusion (see ICPE); Infectious porcine encephalomyelitis; Institute for Physician Evaluation; Intermittent passive exercise (Orthopedics); Interstitial pulmonary emphysema.

IPEH Intravascular papillary endothelial hyperplasia.

i-periton intraperitoneal(ly) (see IP).

IPF Idiopathic/ Interstitial pulmonary fibrosis; Immunophenotypic feature(s); Important precipitating factor; Infection-potentiating factor.

IPFD Intrapartum fetal distress.

IPFM Integral pulse frequency modulation.

IPG Impedance phlebogram/ plethysmography/ pneumography; Individually polymerized grass; Inspiration-phase gas; Isopropyl (thio)galactoside.

iPGE Immunoreactive prostaglandin E.

IPH Idiopathic portal hypertension; Idiopathic primary haemochromatosis (= IHC); Idiopathic pulmonary hemosiderosis; Inflammatory papillary hyperplasia; Interphalangeal (joint) (see IPh); Intraparenchymal hemorrhage.

IPh Interphalangeal (joint) (= IP; IPH).

IPHR Inverted polypoid hamartoma of the rectum.

IPI Intermittent parenteral injection; Interphonemic/ Interpulse interval; Interstitial pulmonary involvement (see IPD).

IpI Inosinyl phosphate inosine.

IPIA Immunoperoxidase infectivity assay.

IPJ Interphalangeal joint.

IPK Intractable plantar keratosis.

IPKD Infantile polycystic kidney disease.

IPL "Ice-pick" lobotomy; Idiopathic preterm labor; Implantable pacing lead (Pacemaker); Inferior parietal lobe (brain); Inner plexiform layer; Intense pulsed light (Laser therapy for removal of acne scars, age spots, skin wrinkles, spider veins, etc.); Intrapleural (see ipl); Isopropyl alcohol (= Avantin, DMC or Dimethyl carbinol, Isopropanol) (an insecticide).

ipl intrapleural (= IPL).

IPLN Intrapleural lymph node.

IPM Impulses/ Inches per minute.

IPMA Infantile progressive muscular atrophy (see WHD - Werdnig-Hoffman disease); Impaired psychomotor activity.

IPMI Inferoposterior myocardial infarct.

IPMR Institute of Physical Medicine and Rehabilitation.

IPMS Induced post-menopausal status; Inhibited power motive syndrome.

IPN Infantile polyarteritis nodosa; Infectious pancreatic necrosis (of trout); Intern progress note; Interpeduncular nucleus; Interstitial pneumonitis.

IPNA Isopropyl noradrenalin.

IPO Improved pregnancy outcome.

IPOF Immediate postoperative fitting.

IPOP Immediate postoperative period/ prosthesis.

IPP Independent practice plan; Individual Physician Profile; Inflatable penile prosthesis; Influenza pandemic preparedness (see PIC); Inorganic pyrophosphate; Inosine, pyruvate, and (inorganic) phosphate; Intermittent positive pressure (respiratory therapy); Intrahepatic partial pressure; Isosexual precocious puberty.

IPPA Ispection, palpation, percussion, and auscultation.

IPPase Inosine pyrophosphate phosphoribosyltransferase.

IPPB Intermittent positive-pressure breathing (see IPPV).

IPPB-I; IPPB/I Intermittent positive-pressure breathing - inspiration/tory (see IPPV).

IPPC Isopropyl N-phenylcarbamate (see IPC).

IPPD Isopropyl phenylparaphrenylene diamine.

IPPF International Planned Parenthood Federation.

IPPH Intermittent positive pressure hyperventilation.

IPPI Interruption of pregnancy for psychiatric indication.

IPPNW International Physicians for the Prevention of Nuclear War.

IPPO Intermittent positive-pressure (inflation) with oxygen (respiratory therapy) (see IPPV).

IPPR Integrated pancreatic polypeptide response; Intermittent positive-pressure respiration (see IPPV).

IPPV Intermittent positive-pressure ventilation (respiratory therapy). Active inflation of the lungs during inspiration under positive pressure from a cycling valve (= IPPB; IPPB-I; IPPB/I; IPPO; IPPR).

IPQ Intimacy potential quotient.

IPR Increased platelet reactivity; Independent professional review; Institute of Pharmacologic Research (Milan); Insulin production rate; Intraparenchymal resistance.

ipr intraperitoneal.

i-Pr Isopropyl.

IPRF International Pediatric Research Foundation.

IPRL Isolated perfused rat liver/ lung.

IPRSO Illinois Professional Review Standards Organization.

IPRT Interpersonal reaction test.

IPS "Ice pick" scarring (seen in acne vulgaris); Idiopathic postprandial syndrome; Impaired performance status; Inches per second (see ips); Information-processing system (Brain); Infundibular pulmonary stenosis; Initial prognostic score; Institute for Professional Standards; Intermittent photic stimulation; Interpalpebral suture (see Sut); Intrapartum stillbirth; Intraperitoneal shock; Ischiopubic synchondrosis.

ips inches per second (= IPS).

IPSC Inhibitory postsynaptic current.

IPSC-E Inventory of Psychic and Somatic Complaints in the Elderly.

IPSF Immediate postsurgical fitting.

IPSID Immunoproliferative small intestine disease.

IPSP Inhibitory postsynaptic potential.

IPSS International Pilot Study of Schizophrenia (WHO).

IPT Image-processing technique; Immunoperoxidase technique (see IPA); Immunophenotype/ typing; Immunoprecipitation; Individual/ Interpersonal psychotherapy; Insulin pump therapy (see CLS); Interpersonal therapy (psycho); Interventional pain treatment; Isoproterenol (see ISO).

IPTG Isopropyl thiogalactose/side.

IPTH; iPTH Immunoreactive parathyroid hormone (see Hormones - IPTH).

IPTX Intermittent pelvic traction.

IPU Inpatient unit.

IPV Inactivated polio vaccine (Salk); Inactivated poliomyelitis vaccine (Salk) virus; Incompetent perforator vein; Infectious pustular vaginitis/ vulvovaginitis (of cattle); Inter-patient variability/ variation; Intrapulmonary vein.

IPVC Interpolated premature ventricular contraction.

IPW Interphalangeal width.

IPZ Insulin protamine zinc (see Insulin - PZI).

IQ Intelligence quotient.

IQB Individual quick blanch.

IQR Interquartile range.

IQ&S Iron, quinine, and strychnine.

IR Ileal resection; Immediate release (tablet); Immune response (see Ir); Immunization rate; Immunoreactive (= ir); Immunoreagent; Inactive renin; Index of response; Index of Rheumatology (journal); Individual/ Irritant reaction; Industrial Research (journal); Industrial revolution; Inferior rectus (muscle); Inflow/ Inspiratory/ Insulin/ Internal resistance; Information retrieval; Infrared (rays); Infrarenal; Inside radius; Insoluble residue; Inspiratory reserve; Institut du Radium (Canada); Internal rotation; International

Rectifier Co; Intrarectal (= ir); Intrarenal (= ir; irn); Inversion recovery; Inverted repeat; Investigative Radiology (journal); Ion retardation; Isovolumic relaxation; Voltage drop across a resistor produced by a current.

Ir Immune response (genes) (= IR); Iridium (Z = 77) (see Elements - Iridium); Irish.

ir immunoreactive/ intrarectal/ intrarenal (see IR).

ir- prefix meaning in, on, or not (L.).

I_R Digital inflow.

I-R Ito-Reenstierna (reaction).

I&R Insertion and removal.

IRA Ileorectal anastomosis; Immunoradioassay; Immunoregulatory alpha-globulin; Inactive renin activity; Individual retirement account (annuity/ arrangement); Individual risk assessment; Infantile renal acidosis; Insulin receptor antibody; Interns and Residents Association; Irish Republican Army.

IRAAD International Registry of Acute Aortic Dissection.

IR-ACTH Immunoreactive adrenocorticotropic hormone (see Hormones - IR-ACTH).

IRA-EEA Ileorectal anastomoses with end-to-end anastomosis.

IrANP Immunoreactive atrial natriuretic peptide.

IRAP International Review of Applied Psychology (IAAP journal).

IRAS Infrared astronomy (telescope); Insulin Resistance Atherosclerosis Study.

IR-AVP Immunoreactive arginine-vasopressin.

IRB Institutional Review Board; Insurance Rating Board; Investigational Review Board.

IRBBB Incomplete right bundle branch block (ECG).

IRBC Immature/ Infected red blood cell.

IRBP Interphotoreceptor retinoid-binding protein.

IRBS Interns and Residents Business Session.

IRC Impaired renal clearance; Indirect radionuclide cystography; Information Resources Center (for Mental Health and Family Life Education) (see IRCMHFLE); Inspiratory reserve capacity; Instantaneous resonance curve; Intensive respiratory care (see IRCU); International Red Cross; International Research Communications System; International Rescue Committee (Inc); International Resistance Co.

IRCA Intravascular red cell aggregation.

IRCC International Red Cross Committee.

IRCFPA International Reference Center for Fertility-Promoting Agents.

IRCM Institute of Research on Complementary Medicine (Jerusalem, Israel).

IRCMHFLE Information Resources Center for Mental Health and Family Life Education (MHMC) (= IRC).

IRCP Implantable remote-controlled pump (see IID).

IRCS-JMS International Research Communications System Journal of Medical Science (UK).

IRCS-MS International Research Communications System Medical Science (UK, series of journals) - Alimentary System; Anatomy and Human Biology; Anesthetics; Biochemistry; Biomedical Technology; Cancer; Cardiovascular System; Cell and Membrane Biology; Clinical Pharmacology and Therapeutics; Connective Tissue, Skin and Bone; Dentistry and Oral Biology; Endocrine System; Hematology; Immunology and Allergy; Kidneys and Urinary System; Library Compendium; Metabolism and Nutrition; Microbiology, Parasitology and Infectious Diseases; Neurobiology and Neurophysiology; Neurology and Neurosurgery; Pediatrics; Pharmacology; Physiology; Psychiatry and Clinical Psychology; Psychology; Radiology and Nuclear Medicine; Reproduction, Obstetrics and Gynecology; Respiratory System; Social and Occupational Medicine; Surgery and Transplantation; The Eye; Veterinary Science.

IRCU Intensive respiratory care unit.

IRD Increased risk of diabetes (see IDR); Infantile Refsum's syndrome; Inflammation-relieving drug; Intermittent rage disorder; Intrinsic renal disease; Irreversible renal damage (= IKD); Isorhythmic dissociation.

IRDB Institute for Reproductive Developmental Biology (London, UK).

IRDHC Institute for Research and

Development in Health Care.
IRDP Insulin-related DNA polymorphism.
IRDS Idiopathic/ Infant respiratory distress syndrome.
IRE Impaired renal excretion; Infusion-related effect(s) (see IRR); Internal rotation in extenxion; Intra-retinal exudate (Ophthalmoscopy).
IRF Identifiable/ Individual risk factor; Idiopathic retroperitoneal fibrosis; Immature/ Impaired renal function; Immediate release formulation (of a drug); Immunology Research Foundation; Independent risk factor (for CHD) (see MRF); Indirect risk factor (e.g. obesity, physical inactivity, etc. - for CVD); Internal rotation in flexion; Interstitial renal fibrosis (see CIRF).
IRG Immunoreactive gastrin; Immunoreactive glucagon (= IRGl).
IRGD Insulin-requiring gestational diabetic.
IRGH Immunoreactive growth hormone (see Hormones - IRGH).
IRGl Immunoreactive glucagon (see IRG).
IRH Institute for Research in Hypnosis; Institute of Religion and Health; Intrarenal/ Intraretinal hemorrhage.
IRHCG Immunoreactive human chorionic gonadotropin (see Hormones - IRHCG).
IRHCS Immuno-radioassayable/ radioreactive human chorionic somatomammatropin (see Hormones - IRHCS).
IRHGH; IRhGH Immunoreactive human growth hormone (see Hormones - IRHGH).
IRHPL; IRhPL Immunoreactive human placental lactogen (see Hormones - IRHPL).
IRI Immunoreactive insulin (plasma) (see Insulin - IRI); Insulin resistance index.
IRIA Indirect radioimmunoassay.
Irid Iridectomy (operation/ eye).
irid- combining form meaning colored circle or rainbow (Gr. iridos).
IRIG Inter-Range Instrumentation Group (electronic standards).
IRIg Insulin-reactive immunoglobulin.
IRIS Integrated Risk Information System; Interleukin regulation of immune system; International Research Information Service.
IRM Immunoregulatory molecule; Information and Records Management; Inherited/ Innate release/sing mechanism; Institute of Rehabilitation/tative Medicine (NY University).
IRMA Immission Rate Measuring Apparatus; Immunoradiometric assay; Intraretinal microaneurysm/ microvascular abnormalities.
IRMGPC International Record of Medicine and General Practice Clinics (journal).
IRMP Illinois/ Intermountain Regional Medical Program.
IRMR Institute of Research on Mental Retardation.
IRMS Immediate-release morphine sulfate.
irn intrarenal (see IR).
iRNA Immune/ Informational ribonucleic acid.
IRO Institute of Radiotherapy and Oncology (Australia); International Refugee Organization.
IROFMS International Reference Organization in Forensic Medicine and Sciences.
IROS Ipsilateral routing of signal.
IRP Immediate-release product; Immunoreactive plasma/ proinsulin (plasma insulin) (see Insulin - IRP); Incus replacement prosthesis; Infusion-related pain (including headaches, myalgia, & pain at the extremities); Institute of Radiation Physics (Stockholm); Insulin-releasing polypeptide; International Reference Preparation; International Review of Psychoanalysis (IP-A); Interstitial radiation pneumonitis; Intractable rest pain.
IRPA Immune-response-provoking antigen; International Radiation Protection Association.
IRPS Institute of Reconstructive Plastic Surgery.
IRR Immediate/ Initial rapid release (medication); Increased recurrence risk; Increased response rate (to medication); Infusion-related reaction (= IRE); Initial rapid release (medication); International Rehabilitation Review (ISRD journal); Intrarenal reflux.
Irr; irr Irradiation; Irritation.
IRRD Institute for Research in Rheumatic Diseases.
irreg irregular(ity).

IRRF Infection-related risk factor.
irrg irrigate(d)/tion (= irrig).
IRRI International Rice Research Institute (Philippines).
irrig irrigate(d)/tion (see irrg).
IRRPOS Interdisciplinary Research Relevant to Problems of Society (NSF).
IRS Immunoreactive secretion; Information Retrieval System (Software); Infrared spectrophotometry/ spectroscopy; Institutional review system; Insulin receptor site/ species; Insulin-resistant state; Insulin-resistance syndrome; Internal resolution site; Internal Revenue Service; International Referral System (UN environmental information); International Rhinologic Society.
IRSA Idiopathic refractory sideroblastic anemia; Iodinated rat serum albumin.
IRSCOT Infrared Structural Correlation Tables.
IRSS Immunoreactive somatostatin.
IRT Immunoreactive trypsin/ trypsinogen; Inter-response time; Irradiation-resistant tumor; Issues in Radial Therapy (journal).
IRTO Immunoreactive trypsin output.
IRTU Integrating regulatory transcription unit.
IRU Industrial Rehabilitation Unit; Interferon reference unit.
IRV Inactivated rabies vaccine; Inferior radicular vein; Inspiratory reserve volume (see PFT - IRV); Inverse ratio ventilation.
IS Ileal segment; Immediate sensitivity; Immune serum; Immunosuppression; Impingement syndrome; Incentive spirometer; Index of sexuality; Induced sputum; Infant size; Infantile spasms; Information system; Insertion sequence; In situ (see is); Insular sclerosis (see MS); Insulin secretion; Insulin semilente (see Insulin - IS; IZS amorph); Intercellular/ Intercostal space; Interictal spike; Internal standard; International Surgery (journal); Interspace; Interstitial space; Intracardial shunt; Intraspinal (see ITh); Intrasplenic; Intrastriatal; Intraventricular septum; Invalided from service; Inventory of systems; Ipecac(uanha) syrup; Iron status (= FeS; SF; TS); Isaac's syndrome (= Continuous motor activity s.) (see CMAS); Ischemic score/ stroke; Isoproterenol (see ISO); Israel (see Isr).
Is Incision superius; Island(s) (= is); Israel (see Isr).
is in situ (L.) - in the natural, normal, or original place (= IS); island(s) (see Is); islet; isolated.
I/S Instruct/supervise.
is- prefix meaning equal (Gr. isos).
I-10-S Invert sugar 10% in saline (solution).
IS 499 Poldine methylsulfate - an anticholinergic drug with actions similar to those of atropine. Used to inhibit gastric secretion in peptic ulcer and hyperacidity.
ISA Immune-system activator (such as γ/ gamma-interferon); Immunosuppressive activity/ agent (e.g. cyclosporin) (see ISC; ISD; PDA); Increased sexual activity; Injection site abscess; Instrument Society of America; International Society of Acupunture; International Society of Audiology (CIOMS) (SIA); Intracarotid sodium amytal; Intrinsic simulating/ sympathomimetic activity; Iodinated serum albumin; Ionic strength adjustor; Irregular spiking activity; Iron status assessment.
ISAB International Scientific Advisory Board.
ISADH Inappropriate secretion of antidiuretic hormone (see IADH; Hormones - ISADH).
ISAI Irreversible steroidal aromatase inactivator/ inhibitor (e.g. Exemestine, used in treatment of advanced breast cancer) (= IAI; SAI).
ISAP International Society of Art and Psychopathology (CIOMS).
ISAS Idiopathic subvalvular aortic stenosis.
ISB Immune-system booster; Incentive spirometry breathing; Infantile spastic bronchitis (see BAI); International Society on Biotelemetry.
ISBI International Society for Burn Injuries.
ISBN International Standard Book Number.
ISBP International Society for Biochemical Pharmacology.
ISBT International Society for/of Blood Transfusion (CIOMS).
ISC Immune system cell; Immunoglobulin-secreting cells; Immunosuppressant compound (e.g. azathioprine, cyclosporin,

rapamycin, etc); Infective/ Inflammatory skin condition; Insoluble collagen; Intensive supportive care; Intermediate stem cell; International Society of Cardiology/ Chemotherapy; International Statistical Classification; Intershift coordination; Interstate Sanitation Commission; Interstitial cell(s) (= IC); Intersystem crossing (spectroscopy); Iron sucrose complex; Irreversibly sickled cell(s); Isolette servo control; Itch scratch cycle.

ISCAT International Symposium on Computer-Assisted Tomography.

ISCB International Society of Cardiology Bulletin (CIOMS).

ISCC Inter-Society Color Council.

ISCD Indiana Scale of Clausal Development (speech/ audiology); Institute for the Study of Child Development.

ISCE International Society of Clinical Electroretinography.

ISCEH International Society for Clinical and Experimental Hypnosis.

ISCF Interstitial cell fluid.

ISCHDR Inter-Society Commission for Heart Disease Resources.

ischi- prefix meaning hip (Gr. ischion).

ISCLT International Society for Clinical Laboratory Technology.

ISCM International Society of Cybernetic Medicine.

ISCN International System for (Human) Cytogenetic Nomenclature.

ISCO Immunostimulating complex (vaccine).

ISCP Infection surveillance and control program; International Society of Comparative Pathology.

ISCT Immunosuppressive chemotherapy (see IST).

ISCTR International Scientific Committee for Trypanosomiasis Research.

ISD Ichthyosiform dermatitis/tosis; Immunosuppressant dose; Immune system disease/ disorder; Immunosuppressive drug; Information Services Division; Inhibited sexual desire; Initial sleep disturbance; Integrated safety database; International Symposium on Drugs (affecting lipid metabolism - US); Interventricular septal defect (see IVSD); Iron storage disease (= HC - Hemachromatosis); Isosorbide dinitrate (see ISDN).

ISDN Integrated service digital network; Isosorbide dinitrate (= ISD) - a long-acting nitrate used in the treatment of angina pectoris.

ISE Inhibited sexual excitement; International Society of Endocrinology/ Endoscopy; Ion-selective electrode.

ISEA Industrial Safety Equipment Association.

ISEE International Society for Electrosleep and Electroanaesthesia.

ISEF International Science and Engineering Fair.

ISEK International Society of Electromyographic Kinesiology.

ISELS Institute of Society, Ethics and the Life Sciences.

ISEM Immunosorbent electron microscope/py.

ISEP Instructional Scientific Equipment Program (NSF).

ISER International Society for Eye Research.

ISF Increased seizure frequency (epilepsy); Increased stool frequency; Interstitial fibrosis/ fluid.

ISFV Interstitial fluid volume.

ISG Immune serum globulin; Immune system gene (in the X chromosome); ternational Study Group.

ISGE International Society of Gastroenterology.

ISGP International Society of Geographical Pathology (CIOMS).

ISH Icteric serum hepatitis; Idiopathic skeletal hyperostosis (see DISH); Immune-system hybrid (donor-recipient immune system/ kidney transplant patients); Immunosuppressed host; Injection site hemorrhage (see ISR); In situ hybridization (see PCR-ISH); International Society of Hematology/ Homotoxicology; Intra-spinal hematoma; Isolated systolic hypertension.

ISHAM International Society for Human and Animal Mycology.

ISHD International Society of Hydatid Disease.

ISHM International Society of the History of Medicine (CIOMS).
ISI Independent scientific institution; Infarct size/ Initial slope/ Injury severity/ Insulin sensitivity index; Injection-site induration/ infection/ inflammation; Institute for Scientific Information; International Statistical Institute; Intersexual infant; Intersignal/ Interspike (ECG)/ Interstimulus interval.
ISIH Interspike interval histogram (ECG).
ISIM International Society of Internal Medicine.
ISIS International Study of Infarct/ Infant Survival.
ISJ Institute for Scientific Judgement.
ISKCON International Society for Krishna Consciousness.
ISKDC International Study of Kidney Diseases in Childhood.
ISL Inner scapular line; International Society of Lymphology (CIOMS); Interspinous ligament; Isoleucine.
Is Lang Islands/ Islets of Langerhans (see Is of Lang).
ISM Immunosuppressive medication; Industrial, scientific, and medical (equipment capable of causing interference - FCC); Institute of Sanitation Management; Intensive supporting measure(s); International Society of Microbiologists; Intersegmental muscle.
ISMA Infantile spinal muscular atrophy.
ISME Immunosuppressive measles encephalopathy.
ISMED International Society on Metabolic Eye Disorders.
ISMG Islet-specific monosialoganglioside (= anti-GM2 -1) (see AAB).
ISMH International Society of Medical Hydrology.
ISMHC International Society of Medical Hydrology and Climatology.
ISMID Immune system-mediated inflammatory disease (e.g. Asthma).
ISML Israel Society of Medicine and Law.
2-/5-ISMN 2-/5-isosorbide mononitrate.
ISMP Institute for Safe Medication Practices.
ISMRRD Institute for the Study of Mental Retardation and Related Disabilities (Univ. of Michigan).
ISMS Illinois State Medical Society.
ISN Injection site necrosis; International Society of Nephrology/ Neurochemistry; Interstitial nephritis.
ISNA Intersex Society of North America.
ISNC Intensive supportive (and)/ nursing care.
$[^{125}I]S^{NP}$ Radioactive iodine (tagged) soluble nuclear protein.
ISO Insurance Services Office; International Standards Organization (= International Organization for Standardization); Isoproterenol (= IP; IPT; IS; iso; ISP; isp).
iso isoproterenol (see ISO); isotropic.
Isoenz Isoenzyme.
Is of Lang Islands/ Islets of Langerhans (= Is Lang).
isol isolated; isolation (see isoln).
isoln isolation (= isol).
isom isometric.
ISOPP . International Society for Oncology Pharmacy Practitioners; International Symposium on Oncology Pharmacy Practice.
ISOR Immune-system overreaction (as in Sarcoidosis, the 'Chameleon' disease, and other autoimmune disorders).
ISP Distance between iliac spines (see ISp); Immunosuppressed patient; Immunosuppression potential; Immunosuppressive property/ protein; Improved safety profile; Independent study program; Injection site pain (see ISR); Intentional self-poisoning; Interesting sociological phenomenon; International Symposium on Pain; Interspace (see ISp); Intraspinal (see ISp); Invasive surgical procedure; Ipsilateral spastic paralysis/ paraparesis/ paraplegia; Isoproterenol (see ISO); Israel Society of Prosthodontics.
ISp Distance between iliac spines/ Interspace/ Intraspinal (= ISP; Isp; isp).
Isp Interspace/ Intraspinal (see ISp).
isp interspace/ intraspinal (see ISp); isoproterenol (see ISO).
ISPN International Society for Paediatric Neurosurgery.
ISPO International Society for Prosthetics and Orthotics.
ISPRAD International Symposium on the

Planning of Radiological Departments.

ISPT Interspecies (ovum) penetration test.

ISQ; isq As before/ Continue on/ Unchanged (L. in status quo).

ISR Idiosyncratic reaction/ response (see ADE; ADR); Immunosuppressive regimen; Improved/ Increased survival rate; Information storage and retrieval; Infusion site reaction; Injection site reaction: i. Local: Hemorrhage, infection, inflammation, nodules, oozing, pain, skin necrosis, etc.; ii. Systemic (allergic reaction.): Anaphylaxis, pruritus, urticaria, etc.; Institute for Sex Research; Institute of Surgical Research; Insulin secretion rate; Interdisciplinary Science Reviews (UK journal); International sanitary regulations; International Society of Radiology.

Isr Israel(i) (= IS; Is).

ISRAAM Israel Association of Alternative Medicine.

ISRCDVS International Society for Research on Civilization Diseases and Vital Substances.

ISRD International Society for the Rehabilitation of the Disabled (Rehabilitation International).

ISREC Swiss Institute of Experimental Research into Cancer.

ISRM International Society of Reproductive Medicine.

ISS Idiopathic structural sclerosis (Orthopedics); Iduronate sulphate sulphatase (enzyme) (deficient in Hunter's syndrome or MPS II - Mucopolysaccharidosis type II disease); Impact of Science on Society (journal); Index/ Injury Severity Score; International Society of Surgery; Intraspinal surgery; Ion-scattering spectroscopy; Ion surface scattering; Isotonic saline solution.

IS 10S 10% invert sugar in saline.

ISSA International Social Security Association; International Society of Stress Analysts.

ISSD Immunosuppressive steroid dose.

ISSN International Standard Serial Number (for journals).

IST Immune-system transplant; Immunostimulating/ suppressant/sive therapy/ treatment; Inappropriate sinus tachycardia; Incomplete Sentences Test (Rotter - psychological test); Insulin sensitivity test (procedure/ endocrinology); Insulin shock therapy (procedure/ psychiatry); Intensive speech therapy; International Society on Toxicology (UK); Interscapulothoracic (amputation/ resection) (see ISTR); Intraspinal tumor; Invasive surveillance technology; Isometric systolic tension.

ISTA International Society for Technology Assessment.

ISTD International Society of Tropical Dermatology.

IStd Insulin/ International standard.

ISTH International Society for Thrombosis and Hemostasis.

ISTR Interscapulothoracic resection (see TBR; TLP; TLR).

ISU International Society of Urologists/ Urology; International System of Units.

I-sub Inhibitor substance.

ISUIA International Study of Unruptured Intracranial Aneurysms.

ISUOG International Society of Ultrasound in Obstetrics & Gynecology.

ISV International Scientific Vocabulary; Inter/Intra-subject variability.

ISVAS Idiopathic subvalvular aortic stenosis.

ISW Interstitial water.

IS 10W 10% invert sugar in water.

ISWI Incisional surgical wound infection.

ISY Intrasynovial.

IT Imidazolyl-thioguanine (see ITC); Immunological/ Implantation/ Inhalation/ Intradermal test; Immunosuppressive/ Individual/ Inhalation/ Insulin/ Intensive therapy; Immunotherapy; Inferior-temporal; Insulin tannate (see Insulin - IT); Intention/ Intermittent tremor; Interferential therapy (see IFT); Intermittent traction; Interstitial tissue; Inter-tuberous (pelvic diameter); Intratesticular; Intra-thecal (= ITh; Ith: ith); Intrathoracic; Intratracheal (= ITR; ITr; Itr; itr); Intratracheal tube; Intratumoral (= i-tum); Intubercular; Ischial tuberosity; Isomeric transition; Isotope technician.

IT# Ipsilateral tibial fracture (see ITF).

I/T Intensity/Time (duration) ratio.

I&T Intolerance and toxicity.

IT-290 Indole analog of amphetamine (see Amphet - IT-290).

ITA Immunotherapeutic agent; Individual treatment assessment; Inferior temporal artery; Integrated therapeutic approach; Internal thoracic artery; International Tuberculosis Association; Intrathecal administration; Itaconic acid.

ITAG Internal thoracic artery graft.

ITAI Intrathyroidal autoimmunity.

ITAL Institute for the Use of Atomic Energy in Agriculture (Dutch: Instituut voor de Toepassing van Atoomenenergie in de Landbouw; part of Euratom).

Ital Italian; Italy.

ital italic(ize).

ITAP Intrathyroidal autoimmune process.

ITB Iliac trabecular bone; Iliotibial band.

ITBS Iowa Test of Basic Skills.

ITC Idiopathic thrombocytopenia; Imidazoylthioguanine chemotherapy; ImmunoTherapy Corporation; Incontinence Treatment Center; Interagency Testing Committee; Isothiocyanate (a chemical compound found in cruciferous vegetables such as broccoli, cabbage, etc., which inhibits enzymes producing carcinogens, and protects against colon cancer).

ITc International Table calorie (= IT cal) - a unit of heat, equivalent to 4.1868 joules.

IT cal See ITc.

ITCO Intertrochanteric compression osteotomy (Orthopedics).

ITCP Idiopathic thrombocytopenic purpura (see ITP).

ITCU Intensive thoracic cardiovascular unit.

ITCVD Ischemic thrombotic cerebrovascular disease.

ITD Idiopathic torsion dystonia; Induced thermogenesis/netic diet; Initial target dose; Insulin-treated diabetes/tic; Intensely transfused dialysis; Intrathoracic disease.

ITDD Intrathecal drug delivery (= IDD).

ITDM Insulin-treated diabetes mellitus (see IDDM).

ITDO Intertrochanteric displacement osteotomy (Orthopedics).

ITDR Initial target dose range.

ITE Improved therapeutic efficacy; Insufficient therapeutic effect; In the ear; In-training examination; Intrapulmonary interstitial emphysema.

ITED Iowa Tests of Educational Development.

ITEST Institute for Theological Encounter with Science and Technology.

ITET Isotonic endurance test.

ITF Interactive terminal facility (time-sharing computer); Interferon (see IFN); Ipsilateral tibial fracture (= IT#).

ITFS Iliotibial tract friction syndrome; Incomplete testicular feminization syndrome; Instructional television fixed service.

ITG Inferior temporal gyrus (in the lower cerebral cortex).

ITGC Intestinal-type gastric cancer.

ITGS Intrathoracic granulocytic sarcoma.

ITGV Intrathoracic gas volume.

ITh; Ith; ith Intrathecal (with reference to injections) (see IS; IT).

ItH Intermediate-to-high (level).

IThP Intrathyroidal parathyroid.

ITI Intertrial interval.

ITIC Intrathyroidal inflammatory cell.

ITIg Idiotypic immunoglobulin.

ITIR International Tumor Immunotherapy Registry (NCI).

-itis suffix meaning inflammation (Gr.).

ITJ Intertarsal joint.

ITL Intrathyroidal lymphocyte.

ITLC Instant thin-layer chromatography (glass fiber paper).

ITLC/SA Polysilicic-acid-impregnated glass filter paper (see ITLC).

ITLC/SAF ITLC/SA plus a fluorescent indicator.

ITLC/SG Silica gel impregnated glass fibers.

ITLN Intrathoracic lymph node.

ITM Improved Thayer-Martin (medium); Inappropriate therapeutic measure(s); Institute for Tropical Medicine (Antwerp); Instron testing machine (mechanical testing of prosthetic devices, for intact stiffness, fixed stiffness, and ultimate load to failure); Intrathecal methotrexate (= ITMTX); Intrathecal morphine (see ITOA); Israel turkey meningoencephalitis.

ITMTX Intrathecal methotrexate (see ITM).
ITN Ingrowing toe-nail.
ITO Intertrochanteric osteotomy (Hip joint) (see ITDO).
ITOA Intrathecal opioid analgesia (see ITM).
ITOU Intensive therapy observation unit.
ITP Idiopathic thrombocytopenic purpura (= ITCP); Immunogenic thrombocytopenic purpura; Inosine triphosphate; Interdigital tinea pedis (see IDTP); Interim treatment plan; Intrathecal pressure; Islet-cell tumor of the pancreas; Isolated testicular pain (a predominant symptom of AAAA - Acute abdominal aortic aneurysm); Isotachophoresis.
ITPA Illinois Test of Psycholinguistic Abilities/ty; Inosine triphosphatase.
ITPG Inflammation-type prostaglandin.
ITQ Inferior temporal quadrant.
ITR Immunotherapy research; Intraocular tension recorder; Intrathoracic rhabdomyosarcoma (see ITRMS); Intratracheal (see IT).
ITr; Itr; itr Intratracheal (see IT).
ITRMS Intrathoracic rhabdomyosarcoma (= ITR).
ITS Infective toxic shock; Intratracheal surfactant.
ITSHD Isolated thyroid-stimulating hormone deficiency.
ITSS Infective toxic shock syndrome.
ITT Identical twins (raised) together; Infratentorial tumor; Inhalation therapy technician; Insulin tolerance test (procedure/ endocrinology); Intention-to-treat (analysis/ basis); Internal tibial torsion; International Telephone and Telegraph Co.
ItT Intention-to-treat (analysis/ basis/ principle) (= ITT).
ITU Intensive therapy unit.
i-tum intratumoral (see IT).
ITV Inferior temporal vein.
ITVAD Indwelling transcutaneous vascular access device.
ITVOP Intrathoracic volume organ perfusion.
ITX Intertriginous xanthoma.
IU Immunizing/ International unit; In utero; Insulin ultralente (see Insulin - IU; IZS cryst); Intrauterine; Investigative Urology (journal); 5-iodouracil.
iu infectious unit.
IUA International Union of Angiology (CIOMS); Intraurethral/ Intrauterine adhesions/ administration/ assessment.
IUAC International Union against Cancer (CIOMS).
IUAT International Union against Tuberculosis (CIOMS).
IUAVDT International Union against Venereal Diseases and Treponematoses (CIOMS).
IUB International Union of Biochemistry.
IUBC Intrauterine balloon catheter.
IUBMB International Union of Biochemistry and Molecular Biology.
IUBS International Union of Biological Sciences.
IUC Idiopathic ulcerative colitis; Intrauterine cannula (Gynecology)/ catheter/ contraceptive (see IUCD; IUD).
IUCD Intrauterine contraceptive device (see IUD).
IUCNNR International Union for the Conservation of Nature and Natural Resources.
IUD Intrauterine death; Intrauterine device (= IUCD).
IUDR; IUdR Idoxuridine (see IDU).
IUF Isolated ultrafiltration.
IUFB Intrauterine foreign body.
IUFD Intrauterine fetal death/ distress.
IUFM Intrauterine fetal monitoring.
IUG Infusion urogram; Intrauterine growth.
IU/g International units per gram.
IUGR Intrauterine growth rate/ restriction/ retardation.
IUGS International Union of Geological Sciences.
IUHE International Union for Health Education (CIOMS).
IUHI Intrauterine hyperinsulinemia.
IUI Intrauterine infection/ injection/ insemination; Intraurethral injection; Involuntary urinary incontinence (or Enuresis).
IUIS International Union of Immunological Sciences.
IU/l International units per liter.
IUM Internal urethral meatus; Intrauterine (fetally/tus) malnourished/ (fetal) malnutrition; Intrauterine membrane.
IU/min International units per minute.

IUMP International Union of the Medical Press.
IUNS International Union of Nutritional Sciences.
IUP Intrauterine plasmapheresis/ pregnancy/ pressure.
IUPAC International Union of Pure and Applied Chemistry.
IUPAP International Union of Pure and Applied Physics.
IUPC Intrauterine pressure catheter.
IUPD Intrauterine pregnancy delivered.
IUPHAR International Union of Pharmacology.
IUPS International Union of Physiological Sciences/ Psychological Science.
IUPTB Intrauterine pregnancy, term birth.
IUP,TBCS Intrauterine pregnancy, term birth, cesarean section.
IUP,TBLC Intrauterine pregnancy, term birth, living child.
IUPU Indiana University - Purdue University (Medical Center).
IUR Intrauterine retardation (see IUGR).
IURES International Union of Reticuloendothelial Societies.
IURMS International Union of Railway Medical Services.
IUS In-use stability/ storage (of drugs); Irritant urinary symptom(s).
IUSSP International Union for Scientific Study of Population.
IUT International Union of Therapeutics (CIOMS); Intrauterine transfusion.
IUTM International Union against Tuberculosis Mycobacterium.
IUVDT International Union against Venereal Diseases and the Treponematoses.
IUVI Intrauterine viral infection.
IV Icthyosis vulgaris; Initial visit; Interventricular; Intervertebral; Intravaginal; Intravascular (= iv); Intravenous(ly) (= iv; ivn); Intraventricular (= IVT); Intravertebral; Invasive; In vitro; In vivo; Iodine value (= iv); Roman numeral four (= iv); Symbol for class 4 controlled substances.
iv (see IV - intravascular; intravenous(ly); iodine value; Roman numeral four.
I_V Volume inflow (see PFT - I_V).
IVA Intervir-A; Intra vaginal/ venous/ vesical administration/ application (see IVT); Intravenous angiogram/raph(y)/ anesthesia.
IVAC IV infusion control device.
IVAD Implanted vascular access device.
IVAP Implantable vascular access device; In-vivo adhesive platelet.
I Var Insulin variable (see Insulin - I Var).
IVB Intraventricular block (see IVHB); Intravitrial blood.
IVBA Intravenous bolus administration.
IVBAT Intravascular bronchioalveolar tumor.
IVBC Intravascular blood coagulation.
IVC Indwelling venous catheter; Inferior vena cava; Infused vein complication; Inspiratory/ Inspired vital capacity (see PFT - IVC); Integrated vector control; Intravascular coagulation/ compartment; Intravenous cholangiogram/graphy (= IVCH); Intraventricular catheter; Isolated venous congestion.
IVCC Intravascular consumption coagulopathy.
IVCD Intraventricular conduction defect/ delay/ disturbance (ECG).
IVCH Intravenous cholangiogram/graphy (see IVC).
IVCI Intravenous contrast injection.
IVCP Inferior vena cava pressure.
IVCR Inferior vena cava reconstruction.
IVCT Inferior vena cava thrombosis; Intravenously enhanced computed tomography; Isovolumic contraction time.
IVCUS Intravascular coronary ultrasound (= IVUS).
IVCV Inferior venocavography (X-ray/ vascular).
IVD Increased vitamin demand; Indwelling venipuncture device; Intervertebral disc/ disk; Intra vaginal/ venous/ vesical dose (see IVT); Intravenous drip.
IVDA Intravenous digital angiogram/raph(y).
IVDA/IVDU Intravenous drug abuse(r)/Intravenous drug use(r).
IVDS Intervertebral disc space.
IVF Idiopathic ventricular fibrillation (identified recently in people with a mutant gene, a sodium ion channel regulator, on chromosome 3); Impaired ventricular function; Interventricular/ Intervertebral foramen;

Intravascular/ Intravenous fluid(s); In vitro fertilization (see NORIF).

IVFC In Vitro Fertilization Clinic.

IVFE Intravenous fat emulsion.

IVF-ET In vitro fertilization - embryo transfer.

IVFT Intravenous fetal transfusion.

ivg intravaginal.

IVGG Intravenous gammaglobulin.

IVGT Intravenous glucose tolerance (see IVGTT).

IVGTT Intravenous glucose tolerance test.

IVH Intravascular hemolysis; Intravenous hyperalimentation; Intraventricular hemorrhage (brain); In vitro hyperploidy.

IVHB Intraventricular heart block (= IVB).

IVI Influenza virus isolate(s); Intravaginal/ vesical instillation (see IVT); Intravascular/venous infusion/ injection; In-vitro incompatibilities/ity; Irreversible visual impairment.

IVIC Venezuelan Institute for Scientific Investigation = (Span Amer. Instituto Venezolano de Investigaciones Científicas).

IVIG; IVIg Intravenous immunoglobulin.

IVIP Intravascular Imaging Program.

IVIT Intravesicular immunotherapy (for bladder carcinoma see IVT).

IVJC Intervertebral joint complex.

IVL Intravenous lock.

IVLBW Infant of very low birth weight.

IVM Intravascular mass; In Vivo Metric (Systems); In vitro maturation (of immature eggs - for use in IVF).

IVMP Intravenous methylprednisolone.

IVN Intravenous nutrition.

ivn intravenous(ly) (see IV).

IVNAA In vivo neutron activation analysis.

IVOM Isolated volitional oral movement(s).

IVOTTS Irvine viable organ - tissue transport system.

IVOX Intravascular oxygenator.

IVP Intermediate-vulnerable person; Intravascular/ Intraventricular pressure; Intravenous portal/ pressure/ push (dose); Intravenous pyelogram/aphy (X-ray/ kidneys) (see KFT - IVP).

IVPB Intravenous piggyback (IV infusion).

IVPF Isovolume pressure flow (curve).

IVPLS Isotope ventilation-perfusion lung scan (see VPLS).

IVPU Intravenous push (= IVP).

IVR Idioventricular rhythm; Intermittent vacuum regulator; Intravaginal ring; Isolated volume responder.

IVRS Intraventricular reservoir system (Neurosurgery).

IVRT Isovolumic relaxation time.

IVS Inadequate vascular supply (caused by atheromatosis); Inappropriate vasopressin secretion; Intervening sequence; Interventricular septum; Intervillous/ Intravascular space; Irritable voiding syndrome.

IVSA International Veterinary Students Association.

IVSD Interventricular septal defect (heart) (= IVD).

IVSE Interventricular septal excursion.

IVSS Intravenous Soluset.

IVSS Intravenous Soluset.

IVT Index of vertical transmission; Intravaginal/ venous/ vesical (in the urinary bladder) therapy (= IVA; IVD; IVI); Intravenous transfusion; Intraventricular (see IV); In vitro test/ tetraploidy; Isovolumetric time.

IVTA Idiopathic ventricular tachyarrhythmia.

IVTTT Intravenous tolbutamide tolerance test.

IVU Intravenous urogram/graphy (X-ray/ kidneys) (see KFT - IVU).

IVUS Intravascular ultrasound (coronary, etc.) (see IVCUS).

IVV Influenza virus vaccine; Intravascular volume; Intravenous vasopressin.

IVVD Intravascular volume depletion.

IVW Intra-vaginal wart(s) (see IGW).

IW Inner wall.

I-5-W Invert sugar (5%) in water.

IWC International Whaling Commission.

IWGMT International Working Group on Mycobacterial Taxonomy.

IWI Inferior wall infarct(ion) (see IWMI); Interwave interval.

IWL Insensible water loss.

IWMI Inferior wall mycardial infarct(ion) (= IWI).

IWML Idiopathic white matter lesion.
IWP Intramyocardial wall pressure (see IMWP).
IWS Improved/ Insufficient water supply; Index of Work Satisfaction.
IWT Impacted wisdom teeth/ tooth.
IX Ion exchange.
IXA International Xenotransplantation Association.
i(Xq) Long arm isochromosome.
IXUC International X-ray Unit Committee (now ICRU) (see ICRU).
IYS Inverted Y-suspensor.
IZ Infarction zone.
-ize suffix meaning action or treatment (Gr. -izo).
IZS Insulin zinc suspension (= Lente insulin) (see Insulin - IZS).
IZS (amorph) Amorphous insulin zinc suspension (= Semilente insulin) (see Insulin - IZS amorph).
IZS (cryst) Crystalline insulin zinc suspension (= Ultralente insulin) (see Insulin - IZS cryst).
IZSEPF Infarct zone subendocardial Purkinje fiber (heart).

J

J Dynamic movement of inertia; Electric current density; Flux density (see õ);Jerk (a sudden involuntary or reflex movement); Jew(ish); Joint; Joule (electrical measurement), i.e. the Meter-kilogram-second (MKS) unit of work or energy = Energy/ work/ quantity unit = kgm^2s^{-2}. Adopted in 1948 as the unit of heat (= j); Joule's equivalent (the mechanical equivalent of heat or the amount of work expanded on raising a pound of water through 1 °F = 772 foot-pounds); Journal; Juice; Juvenile (young, immature or "stab" forms of cells) - the term is commonly used to designate a juvenile neutrophil (immature polymorphonuclear leucocyte) in the differential white cell (WBC) count; Juxtapulmonary-capillary receptor; Magnetic polarization; Marijuana cigarette (see Cannabis); Polypeptide chain in polymeric immunoglobulins; Reference point following the QRS complex; Sound intensity; ST segment (at the beginning of the), in electrocardiography.

j in prescription writing, used as a Roman numeral - the equivalent of one (= i or j), or at the end of a number, e.g. ij (= ii), iij (= iii), xij (= xii), etc.; jaundice (rat); joule (see J); square root of minus one.

J Flux (density) (= J).

JA Jaccoud arthritis (see PRFS); Journal of Allergy/ Anatomy; Judgment analysis; Juvenile atrophy; Juxta-articular.

JAAA Journal of the American Academy of Audiology.

JAAC Journal of the Association of Analytical Chemists.

JAAD Journal of the American Academy of Dermatology.

JAAHA The Journal of the American Animal Hospital Association.

JAAMI Journal of the Association for the Advancement of Medical Instrumentation (now MIJ).

JAB Journal of Applied Bacteriology.

JAC Joint Accrediation Committee (Amer Hosp Assn); Joint arthrocentesis.

JACC Journal of the American College of Cardiology.

JACEPUAEMS Journal of the American College of Emergency Physicians and the University Association for Emergency Medical Services.

JACI Journal of Allergy and Clinical Immunology.

JACS Journal of the American Chemical Society; Journal of Autism and Childhood Schizophrenia.

jact- prefix meaning throw (L. iactus/ iectus).

JADA Journal of the American Dental/ Dietetic Association.

JADC Journal de l'Association Dentaire Canadienne (= JCDA).

JAE Journal of Anatomy and Embryology.

JAFC Journal of Agriculture and Food Chemistry.

JAGC Judge Advocate General's Corps.

JAGS Journal of the American Geriatrics Society.

JAHA Journal of the American Heart/ Hospital Association.

JAI Juvenile amaurotic idiocy.

JAIH Journal of the American Institute of Homeopathy.

JAISHR Journal of Acquired Immunodeficiency Syndromes and Human Retrovirology.

JAK 3; Jak 3 Janus kinase 3 (gene).

Jak3D Janus kinase 3 deficiency.

JAL Juxta-articular lesion (Orthopedics).

JAM Journal of Advancement in Medicine; Journal of American Medicine.

Jam Cocaine (see Erythroxylum).

JAMA Journal of the American Medical Association.

jamais vu French - never seen.

JAMC Journal de l'Association Médicale Canadienne (CMAJ).

JAMG Juvenile autoimmune myasthenia gravis.

JAMWA Journal of the American Medical Women's Association.

Jan January.

JAOA Journal of the American Optometric/ Osteopathic Association.

JAOAC Journal of the Association of Official Analytical Chemists (formerly JAO Agricultural Chemists).
JAOCS Journal of the American Oil Chemists' Society.
JAP Journal of Analytical Psychology (SAP); Journal of Applied Physics/ Physiology.
Jap Japan(ese).
JAPA Journal of the American Pharmaceutical/ Psychoanalytic Association.
JAPCA Journal of the Air Pollution Control Association.
Jap. N.F. National Formulary of Japan.
Jap. P Japanese Pharmacopoeia.
JAR Journal of Agricultural/ Auditory Research.
JARA Journal of the Academy of Rehabilitative Audiology (US).
JARF Journal of the Addiction Research Foundation.
JARP Japanese Association of Radiological Physicists.
Jarvik-7 Artificial heart (a mechanical device of molded polyurethane, the first artificial heart implanted in a human being in December 1982, at the University of Utah Medical Center in Salt Lake City, US. He was a retired dentist and was kept alive for 112 days).
JAS Jenkins Activity Survey; Journal of Abdominal Surgery (ASAS); Journal of Agricultural/ Animal Science.
JASA Journal of the Acoustical Society of America.
JASNDT Journal of the American Society for Non-Destructive Testing.
JASRP Journal of Applied Spectroscopy and Related Phenomena.
jaun; jaund jaundice.
JAVMA Journal of the American Veterinary Medical Association.
Jay Marijuana cigarette (joint) (see Cannabis).
JB Johanson-Blizzard (syndrome) (a probably autosomal recessive, hereditary hypotrichosis with hypopigmented, fine, sparse hair and aplasia cutis of scalp, multiple defects such as deafness, absence of teeth, short stature, mental retardation, pancreatic insufficiency and hypothyroidism); Journal of Bacteriology/ Biocommunications/ Biomechanics; Lakeside Laboratories, Inc code for experimental substances.
JB 251 Protokylol hydrochloride (= Protochylol HCl) - a sympathomimetic amine acting almost exclusively on beta receptors. It accelerates the heart rate, causes peripheral vasodilation and produces a fall in blood pressure; acts as a powerful antispasmodic in bronchial asthma.
JB 336 Methyl-piperidyl-benzitate hydrochloride (see LBJ).
JB 516 Pheniprazine hydrochloride (= Amphetamine hydrazide HCl) - a monoamine oxidase inhibitor formerly used in the treatment of depression. Toxic effects include severe jaundice and color blindness.
JB 8181 Desipramine hydrochloride (see DMI).
JBA Juvenile bronchial asthma.
JBC Joint Blood Council; Journal of Biological Chemistry.
JBE Japanese B encephalitis.
JBJS Journal of Bone and Joint Surgery.
JBMR Journal of Biomedical Materials Research.
JBP Jod-Basedow phenomenon (in hypothyroidism).
JBS Johanson-Bizzard syndrome; Journal of Biomedical Systems.
JBTEP Journal of Behavior Therapy and Experimental Psychiatry.
JC Jakob-Creutzfeldt (disease/ syndrome); Joint contracture; Journal of Chemotherapy/ Chromatography; Junior clinician (i.e. medical student).
jc juice (diet order).
J/C Joules per coulomb.
JC+ Jones criteria positive.
JC- Jones criteria negative.
JCA Juvenile chronic arthritis.
JCAE Joint Committee on Atomic Energy (US Congress).
JCAED Joint Committee on Audiology and Education of the Deaf.
JCAH Joint Commission on the Accreditation of Hospitals.
JCAHO Joint Commission on Accreditation of Healthcare Organizations.

JCAI Joint Council of Allergy and Immunology.
JCB Journal of Cell Biology; Journal of Cellular Biochemistry.
JCBB Journal of Cancer Biochemistry and Biophysics (UK).
JCC Joint Committee on Contraception; Journal of Clinical Chiropractice/ Clinical Computing; Juxtacortical chondroma (Orthopedics).
JCCP Journal of Cellular and Comparative Physiology (now JCP); Journal of Consulting and Clinical Psychology.
JCD Jakob-Creutzfeld dementia; Journal of Children's Dentistry/ Chronic Diseases/ Communication Disorders.
JCDA Journal of the Canadian Dental Association (see JADC); Journal of Clinical Data and Analysis.
JCDS Journal of Cutaneous Diseases including Syphilis.
JCE Journal of Chemical Education/ Clinical Endocrinology/ Clinical Engineering/ Clinical Ethics; Just-conceived embryo (see NCE).
JCEH Journal of Clinical and Experimental Hypnosis.
JCEM Journal of Clinical Endocrinology and Metabolism (Endocrine Society).
JCEMB Joint Committee on Engineering in Medicine and Biology.
JCEN Journal of Continuing Education in Nursing.
JCF Juvenile calcaneal fracture.
JCGC Journal Canadien de Génétique et de Cytologie.
JCH Journal of Community Health.
JCI Journal of Clinical Immunology/ Investigation.
JCIC Joint Committee on Intersociety Cooperation.
JCIS Journal of Colloid and Interface Science.
JCM Japanese Collection of Microorganisms; Journal of Clinical Microbiology.
JCML Juvenile chronic myelogenous leukemia.
JCN Journal of Child Neurology/ Clinical Nutrition/ Comparative Neurology (WIAB).
JCO Journal of Clinical Oncology/ Orthodontics.
JCP Journal of Cellular Physiology (formerly JCCP)/ Clinical Pathology (ACP)/ Clinical Pharmacology (formerly Journal of New Drugs, ACCP)/ Clinical Psychology/ Clinical Psychopharmacology/ Comparative Pathology (UK)/ Consulting Psychology/ Contemporary Psychotherapy/ Counseling Psychology; Juvenile chronic polyarthritis (= Felty's syndrome or Still's disease).
JCPDS Joint Committee on Powder Diffraction Standards (X-rays).
JCPHLD Journal of the Conference of Public Health Laboratory Directors.
JCPP Journal of Comparative and Physiological Psychology.
JCPT Journal of Cardiovascular and Pulmonary Technology; Journal of Comparative Pathology and Therapeutics.
JCPTGP Joint Committee on Postgraduate Training for General Practice.
JCQA Joint Committee on Quality Assurance.
JCR Journal of Chemical Research (CSUK).
JCS Joint Chiefs of Staff; Journal of Cell Science; Journal of Chromatographic Science (formerly JGC).
JCSC Joint Conference of Surgical Colleges.
JCSEA Joint Council of Socio-economics of Allergy.
JCSPPHLD Journal of the Conference of State and Provincial Public Health Laboratory Directors.
Jct; jct Junction.
JCU Journal of Clinical Ultrasound.
JCV Jamestown Canyon virus.
JD Jaundice; Jejunal diverticulitis; Journal of Dentistry (UK); Juvenile delinquent/ diabetes/tic.
JD 177 Epsilon aminocaproic acid (see EACA).
JDBP Journal of Developmental & Behavioral Pediatrics (US).
JDC Journal of Dentistry for Children (ASDC).
JDE Journal of Dental Education (AADS).
JDF Juvenile Diabetes Foundation.
JDFN Juvenile Diabetes Foundation, Inc. Newsletter.
JDL Jewish Defence League.

JDM Juvenile diabetes mellitus.
JDMS Juvenile dermatomyositis.
JDQ Journal Dentaire du Québec (ACDQ).
JDR Journal of Dairy Research/ Dental Research (IADR).
JDRF Juvenile Diabetes Research Foundation (NJH).
JDS Journal of Dairy Science.
JE Japanese encephalitis; Journal of Electrocardiology/ Endocrinology (SE)/ Endodontics (AAE); Junctional escape.
JEB Journal of Experimental Biology.
JEBL Junctional epidermolysis bullosa letalis.
JECH Journal of Epidemiology and Community Health.
ject- combining form meaning throw (L. -iectus).
JEDEC Joint Electron Device Engineering Council (EIA; NEMA).
JEE Japanese equine encephalitis; Journal of Economic Entomology (ESA).
JEEM Journal of Embryology and Experimental Morphology.
Jeh Wit Jehovah's Witness (church member).
Jej; jej Jejunum.
jejun- combining form meaning hungry (L. ieiunus).
JEM Journal of Electron Microscopy/ Experimental Medicine.
JEMBEC Agar plates for transporting cultures of gonococci.
jentac breakfast (L. jentaculum).
JEOL Japan Electron Optics Laboratory.
JEP Journal of Educational Psychology/ Existential Psychiatry (now Exist Psychiat).
JER Junctional escape rhythm.
JES Jacksonian epileptic seizure (= Focal s; Jacksonian epilepsy).
JET Journal of Enterostomal Therapy.
JEV Japanese encephalitis virus.
JEZ Journal of Experimental Zoology.
JF Joint fluid; Jugular foramen; Junctional fold.
JFD Junk-food diet.
JFET Junction field-effect transistor.
JFI Journal of the Franklin Institute.
JFP Journal of Family Practice.
JFS Jewish Family Service; Journal of Food Science/ Forensic Sciences; Jugular foramen syndrome.
JFSS Journal of the Forensic Science Society (UK).
JG Journal of Gerontology; Juxtaglomerular (see jg).
jg juxtaglomerular (= JG).
JGA Juxtaglomerular apparatus (kidney).
JGC Journal of Gas Chromatography (now JCS); Juxtaglomerular cell.
JGCT Juvenile granulosa cell tumor; Juxtaglomerular cell tumor.
JGD Juvenile Graves' disease.
JGI Jejunogastric intussuception; Juxtaglomerular granulation index.
JGM Journal of General Microbiology.
JGN Journal of Geriatric Neurology.
JGP Journal of General Physiology/ Genetic Psychology; Juvenile general paresis.
JGV Journal of General Virology.
JH Journal of Helminthology/ Hygiene; Juvenile hormone (of insects) (see Hormones - JH).
J_H Heat transfer factor.
J-H Jarisch-Herxheimer (reaction) (see JHR).
JHA Juvenile hormone analog.
JHC Journal of Histochemistry and Cytochemistry.
JHCC Joint Health Care Committee.
JHD Junior hospital doctor.
JHDA Junior Hospital Doctors Association.
JHDP Journal of Hospital Dental Practice (AAHD).
JHH Johns Hopkins Hospital.
JHI Journal of Hospital Infection.
JHM Journal of Hazardous Materials.
JHMAS Journal of the History of Medicine and Allied Sciences.
JHMI Johns Hopkins Medical Institutions.
JHMO Junior Hospital Medical Officer (also name of journal).
JHMR Journal of Hormone Metabolism Research.
JHOC Johns Hopkins Oncology Center.
JHPER Journal of Health, Physical Education and Recreation.
JHR Jarisch-Herxheimer reaction (= J-H).
JHS Journal of Human Stress.
JHSB Journal of Health and Social Behavior.
JHSM Johns Hopkins School of Medicine.

JHU Johns Hopkins University.
JI Jejunoileal/eitis/eostomy; Journal of Immunology.
JIAM Journal of the International Academy of Metabiology.
JIB Jejunoileal bypass.
JICR Journal of Interdisciplinary Cycle Research.
JICS Journal of the International College of Surgeons.
JID Journal of Infectious Diseases/ Investigative Dermatology (SID).
JIG Jejunoileal gastroplexy.
JIH Joint interval histogram.
JIHT Journal of Industrial Hygiene and Toxicology.
JIM Journal of Investigative Medicine.
JIMR Journal of International Medical Research.
"Jimson weed" The *Datura* stramonium plant, referred to as such in the US and containing the anticholinergic alkaloids atropine, hyoscine and hyoscyamine. Known as the 'mad apple' in the UK. The long flowers are sometimes called 'angels' trumpets'. Potent narcotics, associated with drug abuse.
JIS Jejunoileostomy; Joint Information Service (Am Psychiatric Assn); Juvenile idiopathic scoliosis.
Jitter Random variations in the latencies of consecutively firing single-fiber potentials or the variability in transmission time of a single motor end plate: increased in the muscles of patients with myasthenia gravis (see SFAP; SFEMG).
JJ Jaw jerk (neurological examination); Jejunojejunostomy; Joy juice (chloral hydrate) (see Chloral hydrate).
Jk a Kidd antigen (blood group).
J/kg Joules per kilogram.
JL Jet-lag (air-travel/ sleep/ time zone).
JL 1078 Dihexyverine hydrochloride - an antispasmodic, parasympatholytic drug acting on smooth muscle, and used for the relief of pain due to pylorospasm, peptic ulcer, dysmenorrhea, etc. Also for the relief of nausea and vomiting, prevention of motion sickness and the treatment of spasmodic cough.
JLCM Journal of Laboratory and Clinical Medicine (CSCR).
JLD Journal of Learning Disabilities.
JLHT Jacobs-Linde hemagglutination test.
JLM Journal of Legal Medicine (ACLM).
JLO Journal of Laryngology and Otology (UK).
JLP Juvenile laryngeal papilloma.
JLR Journal of Lipid Research.
JLS Journal of the Linnaean Society.
JM-9 Iproplatin.
JMA Japanese Medical Association; Juvenile muscular atrophy (see K-W - Kugelberg-Welander).
JMB Journal of Membrane/ Molecular Biology.
JMC Jefferson Medical College; Journal of Medicinal Chemistry (ACS).
JMCC Journal of Molecular and Cellular Cardiology.
JMD Juvenile macular degeneration.
JMDI Journal de Médecine Dentaire D'Israel (IDA).
JMDR Journal of Mental Deficiency Research (NSMHC, UK).
JME Journal of Medical Education (AAMC)/ Entomology/ Ethics.
JMH Journal of Mental Health.
JMM Journal of Medical Microbiology/ of Molecular Medicine.
JMPM Journal of Medical and Pharmaceutical Marketing.
JMR Joint medical research.
JMS Journal of Medical Science (IRCS)/ Mental Science; Journal of Molecular Structure; Junior medical student.
JMT Journal of Music Therapy.
JN Jamaican neuropathy; Journal of Neurochemistry/ Neurophysiology/ Neurosurgery (AANS); The Journal of Nutrition.
JNA Jena Nomina Anatomica (= INA) - with reference to anatomical terminology; Journal of Nursing Administration.
JNC Joint National Committee.
JNCI Journal of the National Cancer Institute.
JNCM Journal of New Chinese Medicine.
JND Just noticeable difference.
JNDS Journal of Near-Death Studies.
JNE Journal of Nursing Education.

JNEN Journal of Neuropathology and Experimental Neurology.
JNF Jewish National Fund.
JNIH Japanese National Institute of Health.
JNM Journal of Nature Medicine/ Nuclear Medicine (SNM)/ Nurse-Midwifery (ACNM).
JNMA Journal of the National Medical Association.
JNMD Journal of Nervous and Mental Disease.
JNMS Journal of the National Malaria Society.
JNMT Journal of Nuclear Medicine Technology (SNM).
JNN Journal of Neurosurgical Nursing (AANN).
JNNP Journal of Neurology, Neurosurgery and Psychiatry (UK).
JNS Journal of the Neurological Sciences (WFN)/ Neurosurgery.
Jnt; jnt Joint (= Jt; jt).
JO Journal of Opticianry (see RxO-JO); Journal of Orgonomy (AA Orgon).
JOC Journal of Organic Chemistry; Juvenile osteochondrosis.
JOD Juvenile-onset diabetes (Type I).
JODM Juvenile-onset diabetes mellitus.
JOGBC Journal of Obstetrics and Gynaecology of the British Commonwealth.
JOGNN Journal of Obstetric, Gynecologic and Neonatal Nursing (NAACOG).
Joint Marijuana cigarette (see Cannabis).
"joker" periosteal elevator.
JOM Journal of Occupational/ Oral Medicine (AAOM).
JOMAC Judgement, orientation, memory, affect, and cognition.
JOMACT Judgement, orientation, memory, abstraction, and calculation intact.
JOPD Juvenile-onset Parkinson's disease (see parkin gene).
JOPP Journal of Oncology Pharmacy Practice (UK).
JOR Journal of Oral Rehabilitation (UK).
JOS Journal of Oral Surgery (ADA journal, formerly JOSAHDS).
JOSA Journal of the Optical Society of America.
JOSAHDS Journal of Oral Surgery, Anesthesia and Hospital Dental Service (now JOS).
Jour; jour Journal.
Joy juice Chloral hydrate (see JJ; Chloral hydrate).
JP Jackson-Pratt (drain); Jarvis (artificial heart) pump; Jobst pump; Joining peptide; Joint protection; Journal of Parasitology/ Pathology (PSGBI)/ Pediatrics/ Periodontology (AAP, formerly JPP)/ Personality/ Physics/ Physiology (London)/ Psychology; Juvenile periodontitis.
JPB Journal of Pathology and Bacteriology; Junctional/ Juvenile premature beat.
JPC Joint Policy Committee (A Public HA); Journal of Pediatric Cardiology; Junctional premature contraction.
JPCRD Journal of Physical and Chemical Reference Data (ACS; AIP; NBS).
JPD Journal of Prosthetic Dentistry/ of Psychedelic Drugs; Juvenile Paget's disease; Juvenile plantar dermatosis.
JPET Journal of Pharmacology and Experimental Therapeutics.
JPG Journal of Psychoanalysis in Groups (AMGP).
JPGN Journal of Pediatric Gastroenterology and Nutrition.
JPHD Journal of Public Health Dentistry (AAPHD).
JPI Jackson Personality Inventory.
JPL Jet Propulsion Laboratory (CIT); Journal of Psychiatry and Law.
JPM Journal of Perinatal/ Pediatric/ Postgraduate/ Preventive/ Psychosomatic Medicine.
JPN Journal of Practical Nursing (NAPNES)/ of Psychiatric Nursing.
JPO Journal of Pediatric Ophthalmology.
JPOBD Joint Program Office for Biological Defence (DoD, US).
JPP Journal of Periodontology - Periodontics (now JP)/ of Pharmacy and Pharmacology.
JPR Journal of Psychiatric/ Psychosomatic Research.
JPS Joint position sense; Journal of Pediatric Surgery/ of Pharmaceutical Sciences (APA).
JPSA Joint Program for the Study of

Abortion.

JPSM Journal of Pain and Symptom Management.

JPSP Journal of Personality and Social Psychology.

JPT Journal of Parenteral Therapy.

JPTS Juvenile pancreatitis tropical syndrome.

JR Jolly reaction; Journal of Rehabilitation/ Rheumatology; Junctional rhythm.

Jr Junior.

JRA Juvenile rheumatoid arthritis.

JRAMC Journal of the Royal Army Medical Corps.

JRAN Junior resident admission note.

JrBF Junior baby food.

JRC Joint replacement center; Journal of Radioanalytical Chemistry.

JRCERT Joint Review Committee on Education in Radiologic Technology (ACR; ASRT).

JRCITT Joint Review Committee for Inhalation Therapy Training (AMA; AAIT).

JRCPL Journal of the Royal College of Physicians, London.

JRF Joint reaction force (orthopedics); Journal of Reproduction and Fertility (UK).

JRLD Job-related lung disease (see Pneumoconiosis).

JRM Journal of Reproductive Medicine.

JRNBS Journal of Research, National Bureau of Standards.

JROM Joint range of motion.

JRP Job-related pressure.

JRR Journal of Radiation Research.

JRRD Journal of Rehabilitation Research and Development (VA).

JRS Joint-replacement surgery; Journal of the Reticuloendothelial Society.

JRSM Journal of the Royal Society of Medicine (UK).

JRT Junctional recovery time.

JS Jejunal segment; Job syndrome; Junctional slowing.

J/s Joules per second.

JSAP Journal of Small Animal Practice (BSAVA).

JSB Journal of Steroid Biochemistry.

JSH Journal of School Health.

JSHD Journal of Speech and Hearing Disorders (ASHA).

JSHR Journal of Speech and Hearing Research (ASHA).

JSLHR Journal of Speech, Language and Hearing Research (US).

JSO Journal of Social Ophthalmology (IAPB)/ of Surgical Oncology.

JSP Journal of Social Psychology.

JSR Journal of Sex/ Surgical Research.

JSU Junkman-Schoeller unit (of thyrotropin).

JSV Jerry-Slough virus.

JSWC Journal of Soil Water Conservation.

JT Jejunostomy tube; Journal of Thanatology/ Trauma.

Jt; jt Joint (see Jnt; jnt).

J/T Joules per tesla.

JTB Journal of Theoretical Biology.

JTCS Journal of Thoracic and Cardiovascular Surgery (AATS).

JTD Juvenile-type diabetes/tic (type I DM).

JTEH Journal of Toxicology and Environmental Health.

JTF Jejunostomy tube feeding.

JTM Journal of Traffic/ Travel Medicine.

JTMH Journal of Tropical Medicine and Hygiene.

JTP Joint projection; Journal of Tropical Pediatrics (in ECH).

JTPS Juvenile tropical pancreatitis syndrome.

JTS Journal of Thoracic Surgery.

JTU Jackson turbidity unit.

J-Tube Jejunostomy tube.

JU Journal of Urology.

Ju Jugale.

JUA Joint Underwriting Association.

Juanita Marijuana (see Cannabis).

juc; jucund pleasantly (L. jucunde).

jug jugular.

jug- combining form meaning yoke (L. iugum).

Jug. P Jugoslav Pharmacopoeia 1951 (Farmacopeja FNRJ).

junct junction (see Jx).

junct- combining form meaning join or yoke (L. iunctus).

Jungle drug Ayahuaca/ Ayahuasca - a narcotic drink containing the alkaloids harmine and harmaline, expressed from the Latin American plant of the genus Tetrapteris, in

Bolivia, Ecuador, and Peru. Known as "Caapi" in Brazil and "Yage" in Columbia.

Junk Heroin (see Diamorph HCl).

JUR Journal of Ultrastructure Research.

Juscul Broth or soup (L. jusculum).

juv; juve juvenile.

juxt near (L. juxta).

JV Journal of Virology; Jugular vein/ venous; Junin virus.

JVAP Joint Vaccine Acquisition Program (DoD, US).

JVC Jugular venous catheter.

JVD Journal of Venereal Diseases (UK); Jugular venous distention.

JVDI Journal of Venereal Disease Information.

JVME Journal of Veterinary Medical Education (AAVMC).

JVP Jugular vein/ venous pressure/ pulse.

JVPT Jugular venous pulse tracing (procedure/ cardiology).

JVS Journal of Vascular Surgery.

JWC Journal Watch Cardiology (NEJM).

JWID Journal Watch Infectious Diseases (reviewer of medical journals).

JW Jehovah's witness.

JWB Jewish Welfare Board.

JWD Journal of Wildlife Disease (WDA).

J-wire Flexible angiographic wire catheter guide.

JWRR Journal of Water Resources Research.

JWS John Wayne syndrome (see DDPD).

Jx Junction (= junct).

JXG Juvenile xanthogranuloma.

JZAM Journal of Zoo Animal Medicine (AAZV).

K

K Absolute zero (see K. Kelvin); A thousand; Capsular antigen (Ger. Kapsel = capsule); Carrying capacity; Cathode; Chloromethyl chloroformate (war gas); Coefficient of heat transfer; Constant (see k); Electroencephalography (in, a burst of diphasic slow waves in response to stimuli during sleep); Electron capture; Electrostatic capacity; Equilibrium/ Ionization constant (see k); Kallikrein inhibiting unit; Kanamycin; Kathode; Kell (antigen, blood factor/ group/ system) (see K a); Kelvin - a thermodynamic temperature scale, an absolute scale (absolute zero), on which the unit of measurement equals that of the Celsius or Centigrade scale. Ice (freezing) point is at 273.15 degrees (i.e. 273.15 °K); Kerma; Kernenergie (German journal); Kidney; Killer (cell/ lymphocyte); Kilo- (see k); Kinetic energy; Klebsiella (= Kb; Klebs) - a genus of microorganisms of the family Enterobacteriaceae; Knee; Koch-Weeks bacillus (= Haemophilus aegyptius; H. conjunctivitidis); Lysine; Modulus of compression; Number (the) 1024 in computer core memory; Potassium (L. kalium) (Z = 19) (= Kal) (see Elements - Potassium); Vitamin K (see Vitamins - K).

k Boltzmann constant; constant (= K); Equilibrium/ Ionization constant (= K); kilo (a thousand); kilo- (prefix for one thousand = 10^3 = K); kilohm (see kΩ); septal Kerley lines (radiograph symbol).

Κ kappa (the tenth letter of the Greek alphabet); magnetic susceptibility.

°K Degree on the Kelvin scale (see K - Kelvin).

K° Kelvin degree (see K - Kelvin).

K_1 Phylloquinone; Phytonadione.

K_3 Menadione.

K_4 Menadiol sodium phosphate.

K-9 Canine.

K-10 Gastric tube.

K 17 Thalidomide (= α-phthalimidoglutarimide) - a non-barbituric hypnotic which was responsible for the teratogenic disaster with congenital deformities in children in the early 1960s (whose mothers had taken the drug in the early months of pregnancy). Has been shown to have immunosuppressive activity, and has been used in the treatment of cancer and lepra reactions.

17-K 17-ketosteroids (excretion/ test - laboratory/ endocrinology) (= keto; 17-KS).

K 34 Hexachlorophane (see G 11).

K 374 Cloponone - a chlorpropiophenone compound; has antibacterial, antiprotozoal and antifungal properties.

KA Alkaline phosphatase; Kainic/ Keto acid; Kala-azar (see); Keratoacanthoma; Ketoacidosis; Kinetic analyzer; King-Armstrong (unit) (see KAU); Koilocytotic atypia.

Ka Cathode (Ger. kathode) (= ka).

ka cathode (see Ka).

kA kiloampere.

K a Kell antigen (blood factor/ group/ system) (= K. Kell).

K_a Acid ionization constant/ Symbol for the dissociation constant of an acid.

K/A Ketogen(ic)/antiketogen(ic) ratio (diet) - ratio of ketogenic to antiketogenic substances in dieting or nutrition.

KAAD Kerosene, alcohol, acetic acid and dioxane (insecticide mixture).

KAB Knowledge, attitude, and behavior.

KABC Kaufman Assessment Battery for Children.

KABI 925 Emylcamate (= MK 250; 1-ethyl-1-methyl-propyl carbamate; 2-ethylbutyl carbamate) - a tranquillizing and muscle-relaxing agent.

KABINS Knowledge, attitude, behavior, and improvement in nutritional status.

KAC Keto-acidotic coma.

KAF Conglutinogen-activating factor; Killer-assisting factor; Kinase activating factor.

KAFO Knee-ankle-foot orthosis (= KFAO).

kaino- prefix meaning new (Gr. kainos).

kak- prefix meaning bad or ill (see cac-).

KAL Kallmann (syndrome).

Kal Potassium (L. kalium) (see K. Potassium).

kal- prefix meaning potassium (L. kalium).

Kala-azar or 'black disease' - Indian name given to visceral leishmaniasis, wherein pigmentation of the skin is one of the prominent features besides splenomegaly, fever, toxemia, anemia and severe emaciation, hepatomegaly, lymphadenopathy, etc. (= KA; Assam/ Black/ Dumdum fever; Ponos; Visceral leishmaniasis).

-kalemia suffix meaning blood potassium.

KAO Knee-ankle orthosis.

KAP Knowledge, aptitude/ attitude and practice(s) (with reference to fertility).

kappa A light chain of human immunoglobulins.

KAR Kidney allograft rejection.

kary- combining form meaning kernel, nucleus, or nut (Gr. karyon).

KAS Katz Adjustment Scales; Kennedy-Alter-Sung (syndrome).

KASH Knowledge, abilities, skills, and habits.

KASPA Kay's advanced spatial perception aid (a headband-like device invented by Leslie Kay of Sonic Vision, in Canterbury, New Zealand for 'sonocular vision perception' or seeing with sound).

KAT Kanamycin acetyltransferase.

kat katal (unit of enzyme activitiy); khat.

kat- prefix meaning against or down ((Gr. kata).

Katie drink A mixture of ice, yogurt and Jell-O (dietary supplement).

kat/l katals per liter.

KAU King-Armstrong unit (= KA).

KB Human oral epidermoid carcinoma cells; Kashin-Bek (disease); Ketone bodies/dy (laboratory/ urine); Kilobit/byte (see kb); Kleihauer-Betke (test); Komuro-Boyse (assay); Knee brace.

Kb Klebsiella (see K. Klebsiella).

kb kilobit/byte (1000 bits/ bytes, computer memory).

3kb kilobase (= 10 base pairs) (see bp).

K_b Base ionization constant/ symbol for the dissociation constant of a base.

KBG Syndrome of multiple abnormalities designated with the original patient's initials.

kbp kilobase pair.

kBq kilobecquerel.

KBr Potassium bromide.

KBS Klüver-Bucy syndrome.

KC Cathodal/ Kathodal closing (= CC); Keratoconus; Keratoconjunctivitis; Kinetochore (a specialized protein complex situated on chromosomes); King's Counsel; Knee-to-chest; Knuckle cracking; Krishna Consciousness (Society member); Kupffer's cell.

kC kilocoulomb.

kc kilocycle (= 10^3 cycles; 1000 cycles) - kilohertz or 1000 cycles per second (electrical measurement).

KCA Koilocytotic atypia (abnormal pattern of cell structure in cervix).

KCAC Krebs' citric acid cycle (A series of enzyme reactions in which the body uses carbohydrates, proteins, and fats to yield carbon dioxide, water, and energy for organ functions) (also called TAC or Tricarboxylic acid cycle).

K Cal; Kcal; kcal Carbohydrate calorie; kilocalorie (= kg/cal; kgcal; kilogram calorie; large calorie; 1000 calories) - the amount of heat required to raise the temperature of 1 kilogram of water 1 degree Celsius (centigrade).

K-capture The radioactive decay process in which an orbital electron from the K-shell of an atom is captured by the nucleus.

KCC Kathodal closing contraction (see CCC); Kulchitsky-cell carcinoma (= Argentaffinoma; Carcinoid).

KCCF Kolmer cardiolipin complement fixation (test) - reagin test for syphilis (see STS).

KCCT Kaolin-cephalin clotting time.

KCD Koilocytotic dysplasia (a finding on Pap smear).

KCE Killer-cell response (see KTC).

K cell Killer cell.

kCF kilo cubic feet (of gas) (see MCF).

KCG Kinetocardiogram (procedure/ cardiogram).

KCH Kings College Hospital (London).

KCHC Kings County Hospital Center (New York).

KCH-DMC Kings County Hospital - Downtown Medical Center (New York).

$KC_2H_3O_2$ Potassium acetate.

kCi kilocurie.

KCl Potassium chloride.

KClO Potassium hypochlorite.

$KClO_3$ Potassium chlorate.
KCN Potassium cyanide.
K_{CO} Pulmonary diffusion coefficient (see PFT).
K_2CO_3 Potassium carbonate.
KCPMD Kinetic continuous passive motion device.
kcps kilocycles per second (see kc/s).
KCR Killer-cell response (see KTC).
KCS Keratoconjunctivitis sicca; Kidney collecting system; Krishna Consciousness Society.
kc/s kilocycles per second (= kcps).
K+CSS Potassium-containing salt substitute (= PCSS).
KCT; KCTe Kathodal closing tetanus (see CCT).
KD Kathodal duration (see CD); Kawasaki's disease (see MCLNS; MCLS); Kidney disease; Keto Diastex; Kidney donor(s); Killed; Knee disarticulation; Krabbe's disease (see FDICS).
kd kilodalton (= kDa).
K_d Dissociation constant; Distribution/ Partition coefficient.
KDA Known drug allergies.
K+DA Potassium (L. Kalium) depleting agent (such as furosemide, diathiazides, amphotericin B, etc.).
kDa kilodalton (see kd).
KDC Kidney disease (treatment) center.
K+DE Potassium-depleting effect (see PDE).
KDM Kidney dialysis machine.
KDNA; K-DNA Kinetoblast deoxyribonucleic acid.
KDO Ketodeoxyoctonate.
KDP Potassium dihydrogen phosphate.
KDS Kaufman Developmental Scale; King-Denborough syndrome; Kocher-Debré-Semelaigne (syndrome); Potassium (L. Kalium) depletion state (see EIS).
KDT Kathodal (Cathodal) duration tetanus (see CDTe).
kdyn kilodyne.
KE Kendall compound E (cortisone); Kenetic energy.
K_e Exchangeable body potassium.
KEA Kinetic enzyme analyzer.
KED Kendrick extrication device.
Kegels Simple exercises for strengthening the muscles of the vaginal floor.
keno- prefix meaning empty (Gr. kenos).
kephal- prefix meaning head (see cephal-).
Kera Keratitis.
kerat- combining form meaning horn (Gr. keras; keratos).
KERV Kentucky equine respiratory virus.
KEs Kegel exercises (for stress incontinence).
keto 17-ketosteroids (see 17-K).
keV; kev kiloelectron volt (1000 eVs; 1.6 x 10^{-9} ergs; 3.82 x 10^{-17} gram calories (see eV).
Key A kilogram of illicit drug.
KF Cephalothin; Katayama fever (= Acute schistosomiasis); Kayser-Fleischer (see KFR); Kenner-fecal (medium); Kidney function; Klippel-Feil (syndrome).
kf flocculation rate/ speed in antigen-antibody reactions.
K-F Kayser-Fleischer (rings) (see KFR).
K_f Glomerular capillary filtration coefficient.
KFAB Kidney-fixing antibody.
K-factor The gamma-ray dose rate in roentgens per hour, at a distance of 1 centimeter from a point source of radiation, with an activity of 1 millicurie.
KFAO Knee-foot-ankle orthosis (see KAFO).
KFD Kayasanur Forest disease (a zoonotic hemorrhagic fever, of South India); Kinetic family drawings.
KFHP Kaiser Foundation Health Plan.
KFR Kayser-Fleischer ring(s) (of copper deposits in Descemet's membrane of the cornea, as is present in Wilson's disease) (= KF; K-F).
KFS Klippel-Feil syndrome; Kurtzke functional scale (for grading patients with multiple sclerosis).
KFT Kidney function test(s) (= RFT):
BUN: Blood urea nitrogen (= UN).
C_{alb}: Albumin clearance.
CC: Creatinine clearance (see C_{cr}).
C_c: Creatinine clearance (see C_{cr}).
CCMSU: Clean catch midstream urine.
C_{cr}: Creatinine clearance (= CC; C_c; CCT; Cl_{cr}).
CCT: Creatinine clearance test (see C_{cr}).
C_g; C_G: Glucose clearance test (= K_g; K_G).
C_k: Kidney/ Renal clearance (= C_r).

Cl_{cr}: Creatinine clearance (see C_{cr}).
C_m: Maximum clearance.
C_{PAH}; C_{pah}: Para-aminohippurate clearance.
C_{phos}: Phosphorus clearance.
C_r: Kidney/ Renal clearance (see C_k).
Cs; C_s: Standard clearance (see UCl).
$C_{t\text{-}1824}$: Clearance of Evans blue (T-1824).
C_u: Urea clearance (see KFT - UCl).
CUG: Cystourethrogram.
C_{urea}: Urea clearance (see KFT - UCl).
CVS: Clean voided specimen (for urine culture).
Cysto: Cystoscopy.
$D_{B\ urea}$: Dialyance of urea (in ml/min).
D_{ca}: Dialysate calcium.
D_q: D quotient - the ratio of glucose to nitrogen in the urine.
EFP: Effective filtration pressure.
EFR: Effective filtration rate.
ERFP: Effective renal plasma flow.
FU: Functional urinalysis.
ICT: Inulin clearance test.
IVP: Intravenous pyelogram/raphy.
IVU: Intravenous urogram/raphy.
K_g; K_G: Glucose clearance rate (see C_g).
KUB: Kidneys and urinary bladder (X-ray/ urology).
Lu_{creat}: Urine creatinine concentration, left kidney.
Lu_{Na}: Urine sodium concentration, left kidney.
micro: microscopic findings (in urinary sediment).
NAI: Net acid input (urinary).
NPN: Non-protein nitrogen (test).
PAH: Para-aminohippuric acid.
PSP: Phenolsulfonphthalein.
RPG: Retrograde pyelogram/raphy (X-ray/ kidneys).
RSIVP: Rapid sequence intravenous pyelogram/raphy.
Ru_{creat}: Urine creatinine concentration, right kidney.
Ru_{Na}: Urine sodium concentration, right kidney.
SG: Specific gravity (urine).
T_m: Maximum tubular clearance.
Tm_G: Maximum glucose reabsorptive capacity.
Tm_{PAH}: Maximum tubular excretory capacity for para-aminohippurate.
TRBF: Total renal blood flow.
TRP: Tubular reabsorption of phosphate.
TVC: Triple voiding cystogram.
TVU: Total volume of urine (in 24 hours).
UA: Urine acid; Urinanalysis (Urine analysis).
UAN: Uric acid nitrogen.
UC: Urea clearance (see UCl); Urine culture.
UCl: Urea clearance (test) (= Cs; C_s; UC; UCT; C_u; C_{urea}).
UCT: Urea clearance test (see UCl).
UFR: Urine flow rate (see V_o).
UN: Urea nitrogen (= BUN).
UUN: Urine urea nitrogen.
V: Urine volume/ unit time (see KFT - V_o).
VCU; VCUG: Voiding cystourethrogram (see KFT - VCU).
V_i: Average urine output.
V_o: Urine output (in milliliters per hour) (= UFR; V).
WBC/hdf: White blood cells per high power field (urinanalysis report).
XC: Excretory cystogram.
XU: Excretory urogram.

KG Ketogenesis; Ketoglutarate.
kg kilogram (= 10^3 grams; 1000 g; kgm).
kG kilogauss.
K_g; K_G Glucose clearing rate (see KFT - C_g; C_G).
KG-1 Koeffler Golde-1 (cell line).
KGC Keflin, gentamicin, and carbenicillin.
kg/cal; kg-cal kilogram-calorie (see K Cal; Kcal; kcal).
kg/cm^2 kilogram per square centimeter.
KGF Keratinocyte growth factor (see EGF).
kgf kilogram-force.
kg/l kilograms per liter.
kgm kilogram (see kg).
kg/m kilograms per meter.
kg-m kilogram-meter - the energy required to raise 1 kilogram of weight 1 meter vertically against gravitational force (= 7.2 foot pounds; 10^3 gram-meters).
kg-m/s^2 kilogram-meter per second squared.
Kgn Kininogen.
kgps kilograms per second.
KGS Ketogenic steroid.

17-KGS 17-ketogenic steroids/ 17-ketogenosteroids.

KH Ketogenic hormone (see Hormones - KH); Krebs-Henseleit (buffer/ solution) (see KHS); Kupat Holim (Sick Fund of the Histadrut or General Workers' Trade Union of Israel).

KH3 "Geriatricum" - a proprietary drug containing procaine hydrochloride and hematoporphyrin base. Used for countering nervous and tissue degeneration, and mental disturbances of advancing age (see "H3").

K24H Potassium, urinary 24-hour.

KHB Keyhole bypass (see MIDCAB); Krebs-Henseleit buffer.

KHb Potassium hemoglobinate.

KHC Kinetic hemolysis curve.

$KHCO_3$ Potassium bicarbonate.

KHD Kinky hair disease (= KHS).

KHF Korean hemorrhagic fever (= HERS; HFRS) caused by the Hantaan virus or hantavirus (named after the Hantaan river in Korea), of the Bunyavirus group and transmitted by rodents, principally *Apodemus*, *Rattus* and *Clethrionomys* sp).

KHIIS Knodell Histology Inflammation Index Score (for virologic and histologic response to treatment with interferon + other drugs).

KHM Keratoderma hereditaria mutilans.

KHN Knoop hardness number.

KHP Kaiser Health Plan; King's Honorary Physician (= HP to the King).

KH_2PO_4 Potassium dihydrophosphate.

K_2HPO_4 Potassium hydrophosphate (= Dipotassium phosphate; monoacid phophate).

KHS King's Honorary Surgeon (= HS to the King); Kinky hair syndrome (see KHD); Krebs-Henseleit solution.

$KHSO_4$ Potassium bisulfate (= Potassium acid sulfate).

kHz; khz kilohertz (= 1000 cycles/sec).

KI Karyopyknotic index; Kidney illness (i.e. chronic kidney disease); Knee immobilizer; Kroenig's/ Kronig's isthmus; Kupperman Index; Potassium iodide.

Ki a kilogram of illicit drug.

KIA Killed in action; Kligler iron agar (culture medium).

K-IAO Potassium gluconate.

KIC Ketoisocaproate; Keto isocaproic acid.

KICB Killed intracellular bacteria.

kick stick Marijuana cigarette (see Cannabis).

KID Keratitis, ichthyosis, and deafness (syndrome).

Kidney (journal).

Kief; Kif Cannabis (see Cannabis).

K III; K IV Dinitrocresol (see DNOC).

KIIM Keyword Index in Internal Medicine (journal).

kil- prefix meaning 1000 (Gr. chilioi).

Killer weed Potent marijuana (see Cannabis).

kilo a thousand; kilogram.

kilo- metric prefix meaning 1000 (see k).

Kilter Marijuana (see Cannabis).

KIMSA Kirsten murine sarcoma.

KIMSV; Ki-MSV Kirsten murine sarcoma virus.

K_{inc} Incorporation constant.

kine- prefix meaning move (see kino-).

King-Kong Barbiturate or other sedative pill (see Barb).

kino- prefix meaning move (Gr. kineo) (= kine-).

KIP Key intermediary protein.

KIS Knee Instrumentation System (see OI/OP).

KISS Key integrative social system(s); Potassium iodide saturated solution.

KIT Kahn Intelligence Test(s).

KIT: Exp Kahn Intelligence Tests: Experimental Form.

KIU Kallidogenase/ Kallikrein/ Krein inactivating/vation/vator unit; Kallikrein-inhibiting unit.

KIVA Keto isovaleric acid.

KJ Knee jerk (see kj).

kJ kilojoule (= kj).

kj kilojoule (see kJ); knee jerk (neurological examination) (= KJ; KK; kk).

KJI Knee joint instability (see PIK).

KJM Knee joint meniscus (Orthopedics).

KK; kk Knee kick (see kj).

kkat kilokatal.

KKS Kallikrein-kinin system.

KL Keratolens (freeze-dried lens implant); Kidney lobe; Klebs-Loeffler (bacillus); Kleine-Levin (syndrome); Krypton laser (ophthalmic).

kl kiloliter (1000 liters; 10^3 liters); Klang (Ger.) - a compound musical tone/ overtone.
KL bac Klebs-Loeffler bacillus (= diphtheria b).
KL-BET Kleihauer-Bctke.
Klebs Klebsiella (see Klebsiella).
Klebsiella A genus of microorganisms of the family Enterobacteriaceae. They consist of short gram-negative rods, and are part of the normal flora; may become pathogenic (= K; Kb; Klebs), e.g. K. pneumoniae (= Freidlander's bacillus; K. friedlanderi; Kb friedlanderi; Klebs f; Kb pneumoniae; Klebs p; KP; Pneumobacillus Friedlander) - part of the normal flora in the nose, mouth and intestines. May cause intestinal, respiratory, and other infections in debilitated or susceptible persons.
K-Lens A solution containing methylcellulose sodium bicarbonate and sodium polymetaphosphate for use as a contact lens wetting solution and as an eye lotion.
KLH Keyhole limpet hemocyanin.
KLS Kidney, liver, and spleen; Kreuzbein's lipomatous syndrome.
K l's Group of lines (others are L, M, N, O and P lines) in a roentgen-ray spectrum, determined by the stability level to which the replacement electron "drops". The K "lines" come from the level nearest the nucleus of the atom, and have the shortest wavelength.
KM Kanamycin.
km kilometer (= 1000 meters; 10^3 meters).
Km; K_m Michaelis-Menten constant.
K-M Kato-Muira (thick smear).
KM 65 Benzonatate - a butylaminobenzoate compound, used as an expectorant.
KMA Kaplan-Meier Analysis (statistical); Kentucky Medical Association.
kMc kilomegacycle (= kilomegahertz; kMcps; kMc/s) - a unit of 1 kilomegacycle (= 10^3 megacycles; 10^9 cycles) per second (as applied to the frequency of electromagnetic waves).
K-MCM Potassium-containing minimum capacitation medium.
kMcps; kMc/s kilomegacycles per second (see kMc).
KME Kaplan-Meier Estimates (of Overall Survival (see KMSC).
KMEF Keratin, myosin, eprdermin, and fibrin (class of proteins).
KMFTR Kotz modular femur-tibia reconstruction (prosthesis) - Orthopedics.
KMIS Keratomileusis in situ (a corneal eye operation for improving vision in severe myopia or hypermetropia).
$KMnO_4$ Potassium permanganate.
KMPAC Kansas Medical Political Action Committee.
kmps; km/s kilometers per second.
KMS Kwashiorkor-marasmus syndrome.
KMSA Kaplan-Meier survival analysis (product-limit method of) (see KMSC).
KMSC Kaplan-Meier survival curve (statistical analysis, as in cancer, chronic heart failure, etc.) (= KME; KMSA).
KMV Killed measles-virus vaccine.
KN Knee (see kn).
Kn Knee (see kn); Knudsen number.
kN kilonewton (= 1000 newtons).
kn knee (= KN; Kn).
K nail Küntscher nail.
KNB Kidney needle biopsy.
KND Known notifiable disease (see SND).
knem kilonem (= 1000 nems; 10^3 nems) - a unit of nutritive value, equivalent to 667 calories.
KNF Küntscher nailing of the femur (= K nail).
KNL Darrow's solution (anti-diarrhea potassium solution).
KNO Keep needle open.
KNO_3 Potassium nitrate.
Knork Combination knife and fork.
KNRK Kirsten sarcoma virus in normal rat kidney.
KO Keep on/ open (see K/O); Killed organism; Knee orthosis; Knock(ed) out.
K/O Keep on/ open (= KO).
KOC; KOCl Cathodal/ Kathodal open(ing) clonus/ contraction (see CaOC).
KOD Knockout drops (see Chloral hydrate).
KOH Potassium hydroxide.
kΩ kilohm (= k).
koilo- prefix meaning concave or hollow (Gr. koilos).
Kold Kap Scalp hypothermia to prevent hair

loss during chemotherapy.
kolp- prefix meaning pouch or vagina (Gr. kolpos) (see colp-).
κOP Kappa opiate receptor (see μOP).
KP Hot pack; Kaiser-Permanente (see K-P); Kaufmann-Peterson (base); Keratic/itic precipitate; Keratitis punctata; Kidney protein; Killed parenteral (bivalent vaccine); Kitchen police; Klebsiella pneumoniae (see Klebsiella); Korsakoff's psychosis.
Kp Body potassium.
K-P Kaiser-Permanente (Diet or Dietary plan (= KP) (see K-PMC).
kPa kilopascal (= 1000 pascals; 10^3 pascals) - a unit of pressure (see Pa).
kPa-s/l kilopascal seconds per liter.
KPB Ketophenylbutazone; Potassium phosphate buffer.
KPE Kelman phacoemulsification/ pharmacoemulsification.
KPF Keratinous plug formation.
KPI Kallikrein-protease inhibitor; Karyopyknotic index.
KPM Kilopondmeter.
K-PMC Kaiser-Permanente Medical Center.
KPMG Kaiser Permanente Medical Group (Pasadena, California).
K_3PO_4 Normal ortho-potassium/ tribasic potassium phosphate.
KPP Kaolin-pectin preparation.
-KPP (Pri) Hypokalemic periodic paralysis (primary).
KPR Key pulse rate; Kuder Preference Record (psychology).
KPRO Kentucky Peer Review Organization.
KPS Karnofsky Performance Status.
KPs Keratic precipitates (in iritis).
KPSOS Kaiser Permanente Share OverSeas (program - Panaroma city, CA).
KPT Keratoplastic transplant; Kidney punch test.
KPTI Kunitz pancreatic trypsin inhibitor.
KPTT Kaolin partial thromboplastin time.
KPV Key process variable; Killed parenteral vaccine; Killed poliomyelitis vaccine (see PKV).
KQC Key quality characteristics.
KR Key ridge; Kopper Reppart (medium); Kussmaul's respiration (Air hunger) as seen in diabetic ketoacidosis.
Kr Krypton (Z = 36) (see Elements - Krypton).
kR kiloroentgen.
KRA Kappa-receptor agonist.
KRB Krebs-Ringer (bicarbonate) buffer.
KRBG Krebs-Ringer bicarbonate buffer with glucose.
KRBS Krebs-Ringer bicarbonate solution.
kreo- prefix meaning flesh (Gr. kreas) (see creo-).
KRI Kenny Rehabilitation Institute.
KRP Kolmer test with Reiter protein (antigen); Krebs-Ringer phosphate (intravenous solution).
KRRS Kinetic resonance Raman spectroscopy.
KRS Kerato-refractive surgery (LASIK; PKR; etc.); Knee rating system; Knee repair/ replacement surgery (Orthopedics).
krypto- prefix meaning hidden or secret (Gr. kryptos) (see crypto-).
KS Kallmann/ Kartagener/ Kawasaki syndrome; Kaposi's sarcoma; Keratan sulfate; Ketosteroid; Klinefelter's syndrome (a condition characterized by the presence of small testes, with fibrosis and hyalinization of the seminiferous tubules, associated with an abnormality of the sex chromosomes); Korsakoff's syndrome (thiamine deficiency); Kveim-Siltzbach (test); Kyphoscoliosis.
ks kilosecond (= 1000 seconds; 10^3 seconds).
17-KS 17-ketosteroids (see 17-K).
KSA Keratinocyte-specific antigen; Knowledge, skills, and abilities.
KSAHV Kaposi sarcoma-associated herpesvirus (Human herpesvirus 8) (see HHV8).
KSARV Kaposi's sarcoma-associated rhadinovirus (HHV8).
KSC Cathodal/ Kathodal shutting/ stopping contraction (see CCC).
KSCN Potassium thiocyanate (broth).
K+SD Potassium (Kalium)-sparing diuretic/ drug (see PSD).
K+SE Potassium-sparing effect (see K+SD).
KSHV/HHV8 Kaposi's sarcoma-associated herpesvirus (see HHV8).
KSL Knowledge Systems Laboratory (Stanford University, USA).

K_2SO_4 Potassium sulfate.
KS/OI Kaposi's sarcoma with opportunistic infection.
KSP Karolinska Scales of Personality; Kidney-specific protein.
K_{sp} Solubility product.
KSS Kearns-Sayre/ Kearns-Sayre-Shy syndrome.
KSs Koplik's spots (in the prodromal stage of measles).
KST Cathodal/ Kathodal shutting/ stopping tetanus (see CCT).
K stoff (Ger.) Chloromethyl chloroformate (a war gas).
KT Kahn test (see STS-KT); Kidney transplant(ation); Klatskin tumor (adenocarcinoma of junction of the hepatic ducts).
KTC Killer T-cell (killer WBC).
KTI Kallikrein-trypsin inhibitor.
KTN Kidney tubular necrosis (see RTN).
KTP Potassium (kalium), titanyl and phosphate (see LASER); Kidney transplant patient/ program (= RTP).
KTR Kidney-transplant recipient (= RTR).
KTSA Kahn test of symbol arrangement.
KTU Kidney transplant unit.
Kt/V Distribution volume.
KTVS Keystone Telebinocular Visual Survey.
KTW Klippel-Trenaunay-Weber (syndrome).
KTWS Klippel-Trenaunay-Weber syndrome.
KU Kallikrein/ Karmen/ Kienboeck/ Kimbel (transaminase level)/ Kunitz unit.
Ku Kurchatovium (Z = 104) (see Elements - Kurchatovium); Peltz factor.
KUB Kidneys and urinary bladder; Kidneys, ureter, and bladder (X-ray/ urology) (see KFT - KUB).
KUMC Kansas University Medical Center.
k-urane kilurane (= 1000 uranium units; 10^3 uranium units) - a unit of radioactivity.
KUS Kidney, ureter, and spleen.
KV Kanamycin and vancomycin; Killed vaccine.
kV; kv kilovolt (= 1000 volts; 10^3 volts) - a unit of electrical pressure or electromotive force.
kVA; kva kilovolt-ampere.
kvar kilovar (= kilovolt-ampere reactive).
KVBA Kanamycin-vancomycin blood agar.
kVcp; kvcp kilovolt constant potential.
KVD Kidney vascular disease (see RVD).
KVE Kaposi's varicelliform eruption.
KVLBA Kanamycin-vancomycin laked blood agar.
KVO Keep vein open (intravenous therapy).
kVp; kvp kilovolt peak (the maximum voltage being used by an X-ray machine).
KW Keith-Wagener (eyeground/ ophthalmoscopic finding); Kimmelstiel-Wilson (disease/ syndrome); Kugelberg-Welander (syndrome).
Kw Weighted kappa (see kappa).
kW; kw kilowatt (= 1000 watts; 10^3 watts) - a unit of electric power.
K_w Dissociation constant of water.
KWB Keith, Wagener, and Barker (classification of ophthalmoscopic findings in hypertension).
KWD Kugelberg-Welander disease (chronic childhood spinal muscular atrophy) (see KW).
K+WD Potassium-wasting diuretic.
KWF Kirschner wire fixation (Orthopedics).
KWH; kWh; kwh; kW-h; kw-h; kW-hr; kw-hr; kW/hr; kw/hr kilowatt-hour (a unit of electrical energy or work, equal to that done by 1 kilowatt in 1 hour).
KWIC Key-word-in-context (index) (JCPDS).
K wire Kirschner wire.
KWOC Key-word-out-of-context (index).
KWT Kepler water test (for measuring water or urine concentration in diabetes mellitus); Kruskal-Wallis test (for continuous variables in statistical analysis) (see CST).
kX kilo X-ray (unit) (= 1.002063×10^{-10} meter).
KY A sterile lubricating jelly (see K-Y Jelly); US Public Health Service (Narcotics) Hospital in Lexington, Kentucky.
K-Y Jelly A sterile non-greasy lubricating jelly, used in medicine and surgery; contains gum tragacanth (trade name: KY).
kysth- prefix meaning vagina (obsolete; Gr. kysthos).
kyto- prefix meaning cell or hollow (Gr. kytos) (see cyto-).
Kα X-rays ($n = 2 \rightarrow 1$ transitions).
Kβ X-rays ($n > 2 \rightarrow 1$ transitions).
KZ Ketoconazole.

L

L Angular momentum; Boundary (L. limes); Coefficient of induction (Avogadro's constant); Diffusion length; Fifty (see Symbols - 6); Heat labile component of protein antigen of vaccine and variola viruses; Inductance; Labile; Lactobacillus; Lacuna; Lambda; Lambert (a unit of light) (= La) - the centimeter-gram-second (cgs) unit of brightness or light, equal to that of a perfectly diffusing surface when it reflects or emits 1 lumen per square centimeter; Lancet (UK journal); Lancet coefficient (a number representing the disinfecting value of a substance as compared with carbolic acid); Latent heat; Latex; Latin; Leader sequence; Lederle (USA), Sandoz (USA), Merck Sharp & Dohme code for experimental substances; Left; Legionella; Leishmania; Length; Lente insulin; Lethal (L. letha) - Ehrlich's symbol for deadly, fatal; Leucine; Levo-; Lewisite (a war gas); Liber (L.) Book; Libra (L.) - Pound or Balance; Licensed (to practice); Lidocaine; Ligament; Light; Light (chain of protein molecules); Light sense (the faculty by which different degrees of brilliancy are distinguished); Lilac (an indicator color); Lime; Limes death; Line (L. linea), e.g. Hunter's Line = linea alba; Lingual; Listeria; Liter (Fr. litre) - the basic unit of capacity in the metric system (= l; lit); Liver; Low (especially when followed by another abbreviation, e.g. LBP = Low back pain); Lower; Lowest; Luer (tubing connector); Lumbar (pertaining to vertebral numbers); Luminance; Lung; Lying down; Lymph; Lymphocyte (= LY; Lym; Lymph); Lyosome; Outer membrane layer of cell wall of gram-negative bacteria (layer); Pound (L. libra); Radiance; Self-inductance; Syphilis (L. lues); Threshold (L. limen).

l azimuthal quantum number; laevorotatory (= levorotatory) (see L-); left; left eye; length; lethal; liter (= litre); long; longitudinal (with reference to sections); lumen; specific latent heat.

λ Lambda (the eleventh letter of the Greek alphabet) (= La); Craniometric point; Decay constant; Immunoglobin light chain; Mean free path; Microliter; Thermal conductivity; Wavelength.

Ⓛ Left.

L- Laevo-/Laevorotatory (= l; levo-; levorotatory) - counter clockwise/ in chemical formula.

L+ Ehrlich's symbol for limes death (L. limes tod), representing a toxin-antitoxin mixture containing one fatal dose in excess, and capable of killing the experimental animal.

Lo Ehrlich's symbol for limes zero (L. limes nul), representing a completely neutralized toxin-antitoxin mixture, and therefore non-fatal.

L1, L2, L3, .. First, Second, Third,... lumbar vertebra.

LI, LII, LIII First, Second, and Third stage of syphilis.

L/3 Lower third (with reference to long bones).

L-6 Upper left 6-year molar tooth.

l-6 Lower left 6-year molar tooth.

L 67 Prilocaine hydrochloride (= Propitocaine HCl) - a local anesthetic having a quicker and longer action than procaine and twice the potency.

L 395 Dimethoate (= Am Cyanamid 12880; Rogor; Dimethyl S-methylcarbamoylmethyl phosphorothiolothionate) - an organophosphorus insecticide.

L 2103 Hexapropymate (= Hexapropynate) - a non-barbituric hypnotic, having a rapid and fairly prolonged action.

L 2329 Benziodarone (= Ethofuriodone; Ethylbenziodone) - a coronary vasodilator, related to coumarin, but with no direct effect on blood circulation when given alone in normal dosage. Has been used in the prophylaxis of angina pectoris and after myocardial infarction.

L 3123 Puromycin (see CL 13900).

L-735,524 Original preclinical name for Indinavir, a PI anti-HIV drug, first employed in 1995 (see PI).

LA According to the art (see la); d-lysergic acid amide (see LSD); Hoffmann-La Roche code for experimental substances; Lab

Animal (journal); Laboratory Animals (UK journal); Lactic acid (laboratory/ chemistry); Lactic acidosis; Language age; Large amount; Late abortion/ antigen; Latex agglutination; Latin American; Left angle/ angulation (orthopedics); Left arm/ atrium/ auricle; Leucine aminopeptidase; Leukemia Abstracts (journal); Leukemia antigen; Leukoagglutination; Leuprolide acetate; Levator ani; Light accommodation; Linguoaxial; Linoleic acid; Lipoatrophy (see LAT); Lobuloalveolar; Local anesthesia; Long-acting (drug); Long arm; Low anxiety; Ludwig's angina; Lung assocation; Lupus anticoagulant; Lygranum antigen (= ML); Lyme arthritis; Lymphocyte antibody.

La Labial; Lactate (blood) (see Lact); Lactation (see Lact); Lambda (see λ); Lambert (see L); Lanthanum (Z = 57) (see Elements - Lanthanum).

la according to the art (L. lege artis) (= LA).

L&A Light and accommodation (pupil reaction); Living and active.

LA 50 Lethal area 50 (i.e. total body surface area of burn that will kill 50% of patients).

LA 111 Diazepam (= Ro 5-2807; Wy 3467; Valium (Hoffmann-La Roche) - a derivative of chlordiazepoxide (a benzodiazepine tranquillizing drug), used in the treatment of anxiety, agitated depression, and schizoaffective reactions.

LA 956 Pemoline (= PIO; Phenilone; 5-Phenylisohydantoin) - a stimulant of the central nervous system, used in the treatment of fatigue and reactive depression.

LA 6023 Metformin hydrochloride (= Dimethyldiguanide HCl; DMGG) - a diguanide derivative used in the treatment of diabetes mellitus. Known by the proprietary name Glucophage.

Lα; Lβ; Lγ X-rays (transitions to n = 2).

LAA Left atrial appendage; Legal Assistance Association; Leukemia-associated antigen; Leukocyte ascorbic acid; Lipid-altering agent; Long-acting agent (see LAD).

LAABNMS Latin American Association of Biological and Nuclear Medicine Societies.

LAAM l-α-acetylmethadol (an opioid methadone derivative).

LAAO L-amino acid oxidase.

LA/Ao Left atrial/aortic (ratio).

LAB Laboratory (see Lab).

Lab Laboratory (= LAB); Rennet (Ger).

LABAD Laboratory based automated diagnosis.

LABD Long-acting bronchodilator.

labi- prefix meaning lip (L. labium).

Lab proc Laboratory procedure.

LABS Laboratory Admission Baseline Studies.

LABV Left atrial ball valve.

LAC La Crosse (virus); Left atrial contraction; Linguoaxiocervical; Long-arm cast; Low-amplitude contraction; Lung adenocarcinoma cells; Lupus anticoagulant.

LaC Labiocervical.

Lac Laceration; Lactate/ation (see Lact); Lacuna (L.) - pit or hollow cavity (e.g. Lac urethralis, Lacunae u, or Lac of Morgagni = numerous small pits or depressions in the mucous membrane of the urethra); Lacus (L.) - lake (e.g. Lac lacrimalis = the triangular space at the medial angle of the eye, also known as the lacrimal lake).

LACH Latin American Congress on Hypertension.

LACIE Large Area Crop Inventory Experiment (NASA).

LACMA Los Angeles County Medical Association.

LACN Local area communications network.

lacr lacrimal.

LACT Long-acting corticosteroid therapy.

Lact Lactation (journal).

Lact; lact Lactate/ating/ation (= La; Lac); Lactic.

lact- combining form meaning milk (L. lactis).

LACT-ART Lactate arterial.

lact hyd lactalbumin hydrolysate (see LAH).

LAC-USC Los Angeles County - University of Southern California.

LAD Lactic acid dehydrogenase (see LADH); Large-artery disease (= LAL); Left anterior descending (coronary artery) (see LADCA); Left axis deviation; Leukocyte adhesion deficiency; Ligament augmentation device; Linoleic acid depression; Lipoamide dehydrogenase; Liver-assist device; Locally advanced disease (e.g. stage III in lung cancer); Long-acting drug (= LAA); Lymphocyte-activating determinant.

L-AD Liver alcohol dehydrogenase (see LADH).

LADA Laboratory animal dander allergy; Latent autoimmune diabetes in adults; Left acromio-dorso-anterior (position of fetus).

LADCA Left anterior descending coronary artery (= LAD).

LADD Lacrimo-auriculo-dento-digital (syndrome); Left anterior descending diagonal (coronary artery).

LADH Lactic acid dehydrogenase (= LAD); Liver alcohol dehydrogenase (= L-AD).

LAD-MIN Left axis deviation, minimal.

LADP Left acromio-dorso-posterior (position of fetus).

Lady Snow Cocaine (see Erythroxylum).

LAE Laboratory/ Local adverse effect(s)/ event(s)/ experience(s); Left atrial enlargement; Life-altering experience (such as inability to keep one's job, to maintain one's social life, to enjoy life in general, etc.); Long above elbow.

LAEDV Left atrial (in end diastole) volume.

LAEI Left atrial emptying index.

LAESV Left atrial (in end systole) volume.

Laetrile Laevo-mandelo-nitrile-beta-glucuronic acid (anti-cancer drug, banned in US and Canada).

laev left (L. laevus).

laeve- prefix meaning left or counterclockwise (L. laevus).

LAF Laminar air flow; Latin American female; Left-angle forceps; Leukocyte-/ Lymphocyte-activating factor; Limited ankle flexion; Low animal fat.

LAFB Left anterior fascicular block.

LAFR Laminar air flow room.

LAFU Laminar air flow unit.

LAG Linguo-axiogingival; Lymphangiogram.

LaG Labiogingival.

Lag; lag A flask or bottle (L. lagena).

la grippe (Fr.) 1. Influenza; 2. Any viral infection of the respiratory or gastrointestinal system (= flu; grippe).

LAH Lactalbumin hydrolysate (= lact hyd); Left anterior hemiblock (see LAHB); Left atrial hypertrophy; Licentiate of Apothecaries Hall (Dublin); Lithium, aluminium, hydroxide; Local Authority Home; Long-acting histamine; Lymphocytic adenohypophysitis (= LCH).

LAHA Long-acting histamine antagonist.

LAHB Left anterior hemiblock (ECG) (= LAH).

LAHC Low affinity-high capacity.

LAHSS Lactic acidosis/ hepatic steatosis syndrome.

LAHV Leukocyte-associated herpes virus.

LAI Latex (particle) agglutination inhibition (see LAIT); Left atrial isomerism (Polysplenia); Leukocyte adherence inhibition; Limited alcohol intake; Long-acting inhibitor/ insulin (see Insulin).

LaI Labioincisal.

LAID Locally advanced inoperable disease (e.g. stage IIIB in lung cancer).

LAIF Leukocyte adherence inhibition factor.

LAIR Letterman Army Institute of Research.

LAIT Latex agglutination inhibition test (for pregnancy - laboratory/ serology).

LAK Lymphokine-activated killer (cells).

LAL Large-artery lesion (see LAD); Left axillary line; Light-adjusting lens; Limulus (a Horseshoe King Crab) amebocyte lysate; Low-air-loss (bed); Lower age limit; Lysinoalanine; Lysosomal acid lipase.

LaL Labiolingual.

lal- combining form meaning talk (Gr. laleo).

LALA Long-acting local anesthesia/thetic (e.g. Bupivacaine).

LALI Lymphocyte antibody - lymphocytolytic interaction.

LALM *Limulus* amebocyte lysate method (see LAL).

LAM Lactational Amenorrhea Method (of contraception); Laminectomy (see Lam); Lamivudine; Late ambulatory monitoring; Latin American male; Left anterior measurement; Left atrial myxoma; Lower abdominal malignancy; Lymphangioleio-myomatosis.

LAm Left atrial mean (pressure) (see LAMP).

Lam; lam Laminectomy (= LAM).

La m Lamella medialis (thalamus).

LA Max Left atrial maximal (volume) (see LAMV).

Lambda See λ (after l).
LAMMA Laser microprobe mass analyzer.
LAMP Left atrial mean pressure (= LAm).
LAMPF Los Alamos Meson Physics Facility (Scientific Laboratory).
LAMV Left atrial maximal volume (= LA Max).
LAN Local area network; Long-acting narcotic/ nitrate/ neuroleptic (agent).
LANA Latency-associated/ Latent nuclear antigen (= LNA; LNP).
LANC Long-arm navicular cast.
Lancefield classification of hemolytic *Streptococci* based on the precipitation test (Rebecca C. Lancefield, New York bacteriologist), and whose natural habitat is as follows: Group A - Streptococci pathogenic for man; Group B - Especially pathogenic from patients with mastitis; Group C - From pathological conditions of lower animals; Group D - Isolated from cheese; Group E - Isolated from milk; Group F - Isolated from human throats; Group G - Isolated from man, dogs, and monkeys; Group H&K - Non-pathogenic streptococci isolated from nose and throat.
Lancet (UK journal).
LANV Left atrial neovascularization.
LAO Left anterior oblique; Left atrial overload(ing); Licentiate of the Art of Obstetrics; Lipophilic antioxidant; Long-acting opioid.
LAP Laparoscopy/ Laparotomy (see Lap; lap); Left arterial/ atrial pressure; Leucine aminopeptidase; Leukocyte alkaline phosphatase (activity or score - laboratory/ hematology); Lipoprotein-associated phospholipase (A2) = (platelet-activating enzyme/ factor, acetylhydrolase); Localized abdominal pain; Long-acting progestogen; Low allergenic potential; Low atmospheric pressure; Lower auditory pathway; Lymphadenopathy; Lympholized anterior pituitary (tissue).
Lap; lap Laparoscopy (procedure/ abdominal) (= LAP; Laparo); Laparotomy (operation/ abdominal) (= LAP).
lap- prefix meaning loin.
LAPA2 Lipoprotein-associated phospholipase A2 (an enzyme, also known as Platelet-activating factor acetylhydrolase).
Laparo Laparoscope/scopy (see Lap).
Lap chole Laparoscopic cholecystectomy (see LCC).
lapid of stone or stony (L. lapideum; lapideus).
LAPMS Long arm posterior molded splint.
LAPW Lateral aspect of the pharyngeal wall; Left atrial posterior wall.
LAQ Long arc quad.
LAR Laryngology (see Lar); Late asthmatic response; Late reaction; Left arm reclining/ recumbent (= Lar; lar); Liver allograft rejection; Local adverse reaction; Lower abdominal reflex.
Lar; lar Laryngologist/ogy (= LAR; Laryng; Laryngol); Laryngoscope/py (= LAR; Laryngos); Larynx (= LAR); Left arm reclining/ recumbent (see LAR).
LARAM Line-accessed random-accessed memory.
LARC Leukocyte Automatic Recognition Computer (Corning Glass Co/AHSC).
LARD Lacrimo-auriculo-radio-dental (syndrome).
Laryng Laryngologist/ogy (see Lar); Laryngoscope/py (see Lar); Laryngoscope (ALROS journal).
laryng- prefix meaning windpipe (Gr. larygx).
Laryngol Laryngologist/ogy (see Lar).
Laryngos Laryngoscope/py (see Lar).
LAS Laboratory automation system; Lateral amyotrophic sclerosis; Laxative abuse syndrome; Left anterior-superior; Leucine acetylsalicylate/ aminopeptidase; Linear alkylsulfonate; Live attenuated strain (bacteria/ vaccine); Local adaptation syndrome (stress); Long-acting sulphonylurea (e.g. chlorpropamide); Long arm splint; Loose anagen syndrome (Hair shaft irregularity - see HSA); Lower abdominal surgery; Lymphadenopathy syndrome; Lymphangioscintography.
LASA Lipid-associated sialic acid.
LASER Light amplification by stimulated emission of radiation. i. Argon laser - for cutting and vaporizing. ii. Candela laser (a tunable dye laser) - works best on red tissue. iii. CO_2 (dioxide) laser - good for cutting and vaporising. iv. KTP laser (potassium, titanyl and phosphate laser). v. YAG laser (yttrium, aluminium and garnet laser) - for coagulate

cuts and incisions.

LASH Left anterior superior hemiblock.

LASIK Laser in Situ Keratomileusis (a combination of laser and lamellar corneal surgery).

LASL Los Alamos Scientific Laboratory.

L-ASP L-asparaginase.

LASS Labile aggregation stimulating substance; Linguistic Analysis of Speech Samples.

LAT Language-associated thought; Lateral (see lat); Latex agglutination test; Left anterior thigh (injection site); Left atrial thrombosis; Linear array transducer (Ult S Sys); Lipoatrophy (= LA); Local antibiotic therapy; Lysolecithin acyltransferase.

Lat Latin.

lat latent; lateral (L. lateralis) (= LAT).

lat- combining form meaning carry (L. latus).

lat admov let it be applied to the side (L. lateri admoveatum).

lat bend lateral bending.

LATCH Literature attached to charts.

Lat Da St Latter-Day Saints (Mormon) church member.

lat dol to the painful side (L. lateri dolenti).

later- combining form meaning side (L. lateris).

l-atm liter atmosphere.

lat men lateral meniscus/ meniscectomy.

LATP Left atrial transmural pressure.

LATPT Left atrial transesophageal pacing test.

LATS Long-acting thyroid stimulation/ator.

LATSH Long-acting thyroid stimulating hormone (see LATS).

LATS-P Long-acting thyroid stimulator-protector.

LATT Lithium-associated thyrotoxicosis.

LATu Lobulo-alveolar tumor.

Laughing gas Nitrous oxide (see N_2O).

LAV Last annual visit; Leafhopper A virus; Live-attenuated vaccine/ virus; Lymphadenopathy-associated virus (= the AIDS virus) - for the swollen lymph nodes that are an early symptom of AIDS (see AIDS).

lav lavatory (L. lavare).

LAV/HTLV III The AIDS virus (see AIDS).

LAVV Left atrioventricular valve (= Bicuspid or Mitral v) (see BCV); Live attenuated virus vaccine (such as measles, mumps, rubella, polio; varicella-zoster, etc.) (= LAV).

LAW Left anterior/ atrial wall.

Lax; lax Laxative (medication order): i. Bulk forming (e.g. Plantago ovata, Psyllium), ii. Lubricant (e.g. Paraffin), iii. Osmotic (e.g. Lactulose, $MgSO_4$), and iv. Stimulant (e.g. Senna, Biscodyl); Laxity.

LB Laboratory data; Lamellar/ Lewy/ Lipid/ Loose bodies/dy; Large bowel; Left breast/ bundle/ buttock (injection site); Leiomyoblastoma; Live birth; Liver/ Lung biopsy; Low back (disorder/ pain/ syndrome) (see LBD; LBP; LBS).

LB# Long-bone fracture (see LBF).

Lb Pound force (= lbf).

lb pound (L. libra) (= lib).

L&B Left and below.

LBA Left basal artery.

LBB Left breast biopsy; Left bundle branch (heart); Low back bending; Low Boy bathtub (used for patients before exercising).

LBBB Left bundle branch block (ECG/ heart).

LBBsB Left bundle branch system block.

LBC Large bowl curet (Neurosurgery); Lidocaine blood concentration; Localized breast cancer/ carcinoma; Lymphadenosis benigna cutis.

LBCD Left border of cardiac dullness.

LBCF Laboratory Branch Complement Fixation (test).

LBD Large bile duct; large bowel diverticulitis; Left border of dullness (heart - to percussion); Lewy body dementia; Low back disorder (see LB); Low bone density; Low-bulk diet (see LFD).

LBE Lifeboat ethics (triage); Long below elbow.

LBF Lactobacillus bulgaricus factor (pantetheine); Limb/ Liver blood flow; Long-bone fracture (e.g. of the femur) (= LB#); Loose body forceps.

lbf pound force (see Lb).

lbf-ft pound force foot.

LBG Longitudinal bone growth (Orthopedics); Loss of bowel gas; Lysomal beta-glucosidase (a metabolic enzyme lacking in, and used in the treatment of Gaucher's disease).

LBGM Laboratory of Biochemical Genetics and Metabolism.

LBH Length, breadth, height.

LBI Live birth index; liveborn infant: Low back injury; Low (serum-)bound iron; Lymphoblastic infiltration.

lb/in² pounds per square inch.

LBJ Methyl-piperidyl-benzitate hydrochloride (= JB 336) (see JB).

LBL Labeled lymphoblast; Lawrence Berkeley Laboratory; Lipid blood level; Lymphoblastic leukemia/ lymphoma.

LBM Lean/ Low body mass; Loose bowel movement; Low bone mass; Lung basement membrane; Lytic bone metastases/sis.

LBN Large-bore needle; Liver biopsy needle (TruCut); Lymphoblastic neoplasm.

LBNP Lower-body negative pressure.

LBNPD Lower-body negative pressure device.

LBO Large bowel obstruction.

LBP Low back pain (see LB); Low blood pressure; Low body pain; Lying blood pressure.

LBPF Long bone or pelvic fracture.

LBPQ Long/ Low Back Pain Questionnaire.

LBRF Louse-borne relapsing fever.

LBS Louis-Bar syndrome (= Ataxia-telangiectasia); Low back syndrome (see LB); Lower blood sugar.

LBs Lewy bodies (cytoplasmic eosinophilic hyaline inclusions, found in Parkinson's disease) (see parkin gene).

LBSA Lipid-bound sialic acid.

LBT Louse-borne typhus (= Epidemic typhus - caused by *Rickettsia* prowazeki and usually transmitted by the human body louse, *Pediculus* humanus); Low back tenderness/ trouble; Lupus band test; Lymphoblastic tumor.

LBT# Long-bone-type fracture (see LBTF).

LBTF Long-bone-type fracture (of the spine, as seen in ankylosing spondylitis) (= LB#).

LBTI Lima bean trypsin inhibitor.

lb tr pound troy.

LBV Left brachial vein; Left bundle to ventricular (activation); Lung blood volume.

LBVAH Long Beach Veterans' Administration Hospital (California).

LBW Lean body weight; Low birth/ body weight.

LBWC Low birth weight child(ren).

LBWI Low-birth-weight infant.

LBWR Lung/body weight ratio.

LC Laennec's cirrhosis; Langerhans' cell; Large chromophobe; Late clamped (umbilical cord); Lecithin cholesterol (acyltransferase) (see LCAT); Left center/ coronary (artery) (see LCA); Leisure counseling; Lethal concentration; Leydig cell; Library of Congress; Life care/-cycle; Liga clip or Hemoclip (Neurosurgery); Light chain; Linguocervical; Lipid cytosomes; Liquid chromatography/ crystal (see LCD); Live clinic; Liver cirrhosis; Living children; Locus ceruleus/ coeruleus (L.) - the noradrenergic nucleus (= L. cinereus; L. ferrugineus. A pigmented eminence in the superior angle of the floor of the fourth ventricle); Long chain; Low calorie; Lung cancer/ cell.

lc lower case.

LC1 Lethal concentration for 1%.

LC_{50} Median lethal concentration.

LCA Leber's congenital amaurosis; Lecithin cholesterol acyltransferase (see LCAT); Left circumflex artery (coronary) (see LCCA); Left coronary artery (= LC); Leukocyte common antigen; Leydig cell adenoma; Light contact assist; Lithocholic acid; Lymphocyte chemotactic activity.

LCAO Linear combination of atomic orbitals.

LCAR Late cutaneous anaphylactic reaction.

LCAT Lecithin cholesterol acetyl/ acyl transferase (= LC; LCA).

LCB Laboratory of Cancer Biology; Left costal border; Lymphomatosis cutis benigna.

LCBF Local cerebral blood flow.

LCBS Large core bronchoscope; Low capacity binding site.

LCC Lactose coliform count; Laparoscopic cholecystectomy (= Lap chole); Large-cell carcinoma (lung, etc.); Left circumflex coronary (artery) (see LCCA); Left common carotid (artery) (see LCCA); Left coronary cusp; Leukemia cancer cell; Lipid-containing cell; Liver cell carcinoma; Lysis centrifugation culture (blood).

LCCA Late cortical cerebellar atrophy; Left circumflex coronary artery (= LCA; LCC; LCF; LCx); Left common carotid artery (= LCC); Leukoclastic/ cytoclastic angiitis.

LCCME Liaison Committee on Continuing Medical Education.

LCCP Lung cancer chemoprevention.

LCCS Low(er) cervical caesarean/ cesarean section.

LCCSCT Large-cell calcifying Sertoli cell tumor.

LCD Liquid crystal diode/ display; Liquor carbonis detergens (coal tar solution); Lobster-claw deformity (= Bidectyly, an abnormal condition in which the second, third, and fourth fingers of the same hand are missing); Localized collagen dystrophy; Low calcium/ calorie/ carbohydrate diet.

LCDB Library of Congress, Division for the Blind.

LCDC Laboratory Center for Disease Control (HPB).

LCDD Light chain deposition disease.

LCF Least common factor; Left cirmumflex (coronary artery) (see LCCA); Long-chain fat(s) - polyunsaturated (see LCFA); Lymphocyte culture fluid.

LCFA Long-chain fatty acid (= LCF).

LCFB Lahey Clinic Foundation Bulletin.

LCFM Left circumflex marginal.

LCFU Leukocyte colony-forming unit.

LCG Langerhans cell granule.

LCGL Large-cell granulocytic leukemia.

LCGME Liaison Committee on Graduate Medical Education.

LCGU Local cerebral glucose utilization.

LCH Langerhans cell histiocytosis; Leydig cell hyperplasia; Local city hospital; Lymphocytic hypophysitis (e.g. in Sjogren's syndrome see LAH).

LCh Licentiate in Surgery.

LCHA Lens culinaris hemagglutinin A.

L chain; Lambda chain LC Light chain - one of two major types of light (polypeptide) chains used in Immunology (see λ; H chain; kappa chain).

LCHB Lens culinaris hemagglutinin B.

LCHP Low carbohydrate, high protein (diet).

LCHTM London School of Hygiene and Tropical Medicine.

LCI Laboratory-confirmed influenza; Length-complexity index; Lung clearance index.

LCIS Lobular carcinoma in situ (= LCS).

LCL Large-cell lymphoma; Lateral collateral ligament (knee joint); Lens culinaris lectin; Levinthal-Coles-Lillie (bodies/dy) (bacteriology); Lower confidence limit; Lymphoblastoid/ Lymphoid cell line; Lymphocytic lymphosarcoma.

LCLC Large cell lung carcinoma.

LCLo Lowest published lethal concentration.

LCM Laboratory control microorganism; Latent cardiomyopathy; Least/ Lowest common multiple; Left costal margin; Leukocyte-conditioned medium; Lymphatic/ Lymphocytic choriomeningitis (disease/ virus) (see LCMV).

LCME Liaison Committee on Medical Education.

LCMG Long-chain monoglyceride.

L/cm H_2O Liters per centimeter of water.

LC/MS/MS assay Liquid chromatography, mass spectrometry, morphine sulfate assay (to quantify morphine concentration in plasma).

LCMV Lymphatic/ Lymphocytic choriomeningitis (disease/ virus) (= LCM).

LCN Lateral cervical nucleus; Lateral cutaneous nerve (of the thigh) (see MP); Left caudate nucleus.

LCO Low cardiac output.

LCOS Low cardiac output syndrome.

LCP Legg-Calvé-Perthes (disease) (see LCPD); Long chain poly saturated/ unsaturated (fatty acid) (see LCPS; LCPU; LCPUFA; LC PUFA; LC-PUFA); Lymphocytophoresis.

LCPD Legg-Calvé-Perthes disease (= LCP).

LCPS Legg-Calvé-Perthes' syndrome (see LCP; LCPD; LPC; LPD; OCD; ODJ); Licentiate of the College of Physicians and Surgeons; Long chain polysaturated (fatty acid) (= LCP); Lung Cancer Prevention Study (see ATBC) (NCI).

LCPU Long chain polyunsaturated (fatty acid) (= LCP) (see LCPUFA).

LCPUFA; LC PUFA; LC-PUFA Long-chain polyunsaturated fatty acid(s) (= LCP; LCPU).

LCR Late cortical response; Late cutaneous

reaction; Leurocrystine; Low cardiac reserve (see PCR); Lung-cancer risk.

LCS Cerebrospinal fluid (L. liquor cerebrospinalis) (see CSF); Left coronary sinus; Lesser curve of the stomach; Leydig cell stimulation; Life care service; Lobular carcinoma (in) situ (see LCIS); Low constant/ continuous suction; Lymphocyte culture supernatants.

LCSB Liaison Committee for Specialty Boards.

LCSG Lung Cancer Study Group (see CLGB; ECOG; NCCTG; RTOG; SWOG).

LCSS Lung Cancer Specific Symptoms (one of the seven subscales of the FACT-Lung questionnaire in the ECOG study) (see ECOG; FACT).

LCSW Licensed Clinical Social Worker.

LCT Liver cell tumor; Long-chain triglyceride; Low cervical transverse; Lymphocytotoxicity/cytotoxin (test).

LCTA Lymphocytotoxic antibody.

LCTD Low calcium test diet.

LCU Life change unit.

LCUME Liaison Committee on Undergraduate Medical Education.

LCV Lecithovitellin; Leucovorin (= LV; LVR); Leukocytoclastic vasculitis (causing necrosis of the small blood vessels); Liminocapsular vein (Orthopedics); Low cervical vertical.

LCVA Low-contrast visual acuity.

LCx Left circumflex artery (coronary) (see LCCA).

LCYH l-cystathionine.

LD Labor and delivery (see L&D); Laboratory data; Labyrinthine defect; Lactate/ Lactic dehydrogenase (see LDH); Laryngeal diphtheria; Last/ Loading/ Low dose; Learning disability/ disorder; Left deltoid (injection site); Legionnaires'/ Leigh's/ Limited/ Liver disease; Leishman-Donovan (body) (see L-D); Lethal dose (L. dosis lethalis) (= DL; FD; LD 100); Levodopa; Light-dark (cycle) (see L/D); Light difference (perception of) - the difference between the two eyes in their sensitiveness to light (eye examination); Light differentiation/ duty; Linear dichroism; Linguodistal; Lipodystrophy; Living donor; Local Dentist; Lombard-Dowell (agar); Longdwell; Longitudinal diameter; Loop diuretic (a diuretic which works in the loop of Henle); Low density; Lyme disease (an infective disease caused by the spirochaetal bacterium, *Borrelia* burgdorferi and transmitted primarily by the deer tick *Ixodes* dammini in NE and mid-W USA, I. pacificus in Western USA and I. ricinus in Europe); Lymphocyte-defined (antigen) (see LDA); Lymphocyte-dependent (antibody) (see LDA); Lymphocyte-deplete/tion; Lymphocyte-derived (chemotactic factor) (see LDCF); Lymphocyte determinant (see LD-7a).

Ld Leishmania donovani.

L-D Leishman-Donovan (body) (= LD); Light-dark (cycle) (see L/D).

L/D Light/dark(ness) (cycle or ratio) (= LD; L-D) (see LDD).

L&D Labor and delivery (= LD).

LD 1 Isoenzyme of lactate dehydrogenase found in the heart, erythrocytes, and kidneys.

LD 2 Isoenzyme of lactate dehydrogenase found in the lungs.

LD 3 Isoenzyme of lactate dehydrogenase found in the lungs.

LD 4 Isoenzyme of lactate dehydrogenase found in the liver.

LD 5 Isoenzyme of lactate dehydrogenase found in the liver and muscles.

LD_{50}; LD-50; LD 50 Median lethal dose - a dose which is lethal for 50% of the test subjects (see MLD).

$LD_{50/30}$; LD 50/30 A dose that is lethal for 50% of test subjects within 30 days.

LD 100 Lethal dose (in all exposed subjects) (see LD).

LDA Laser Doppler anemometry; Left dorsoanterior (position of fetus); Leucocyte differentiation antigen; Linear discriminant/ diplacement analysis; Lithium diisopropyl amide; Low-dose aspirin; Lymphocyte-defined antigen (locus test) (= LD); Lymphocyte-dependent antibody (= LD).

LD-7a Lymphocyte determinant (= LD).

LDAC Low-dose cytosine arabinoside.

LDAR Latex direct agglutination reaction.

LDB Large data base.

LDB; LDb Lamb dysentery bacillus;

Legionnaires' disease bacillus.

L-D bodies Leishman-Donovan bodies or amastigotes (seen in the reticulo-endothelial macrophages in Kala-azar) - round to oval organisms, the protozoal parasites (*Leishmania* donovani), 2-4 μm in size with a large nucleus and a rod-like kinetoplast, having no flagellum,and consisting of DNA material (cause of visceral leishmaniasis).

LDC Laboratory Data Control Co; Le Dain Commission (Canadian Commission on Non-Medical Use of Drugs 1970); Less-developed country; Lymphoid dendritic cell; Lysine decarboxylase.

LDCC Lectin-dependent cellular cytotoxicity.

LDCF Lymphocyte-derived chemotactic factor (for macrophages or monocytes, which it attracts to the sites of inflammation) (= LD).

LDCI Low-dose continuous infusion.

LDCT Late distal cortical tubule.

LDD Late dedifferentiation; Light-dark(ness) discrimination (eye examination); Lumbar disc disease; Lung dust disease (see Pneumoconiosis).

LDDS Licentiate Doctor of Dental Surgery.

LDE Lauric diethamide; Lifestyle-disease epidemic (e.g. Type-2 diabetes).

LDER Lateral-view dual-energy radiography.

LD-EYA Lombard-Dowell egg yolk agar.

LDF Laser Doppler flux(ometry); Limit dilution factor.

LDG Lactate/ctic dehydrogenase (see LDH); Liquid developmental groove; Low-dose group; Lumbar discography.

LDH Lactate/ Lactic dehydrogenase (= Lactic acid dehydrogenase; LD; LDG; LDL; LDP) (see LFT); Low-dose heparin; Lumbar disc herniation.

LDH-A Lactate/ Lactic dehydrogenase A.

LDH-B Lactate/ Lactic dehydrogenase B.

LDH-C Lactate/ Lactic dehydrogenase C.

LDHI Lactate dehydrogenase isoenzyme(s).

LDH-K Lactate/ Lactic dehydrogenase K.

LDH-P Lactate/ Lactic dehydrogenase P.

LDHS Lyon Diet Heart Study.

LDH-X Sperm lactate/ lactic dehydrogenase.

LDI Laboratory-documented infection.

LDIH Left direct inguinal hernia.

LDL Lactate/ Lactic dehydrogenase (see LDH); Loudness discomfort level; Low density lipoprotein (the principal cholesterol carrier in the blood (= LDLP).

LDLA Low density lipoprotein apheresis.

LDLC Low density lipoprotein cholesterol.

LDLL Low density lipoprotein lipid(s).

LDLLT Living-donor lobar lung-transplant (operation/ procedure).

LDLo Lowest published lethal dose.

LDLP Low density lipoprotein (see LDL).

LDLPS Low-density lipoprotein particle size.

LDLs Low density lipoproteins.

LDLT Living-donor lobar transplant (see LDLLT).

LDM Lactate dehydrogenase, muscle; Late diastolic murmur (of mitral stenosis) (see PSA); Latent diabetes mellitus.

LD-NEYA Lombard-Dowell neomycin egg yolk agar.

L-DOPA; L-Dopa; L-dopa Levodopa (= Levo-dihydroxyphenylalanine) (see DOPA).

LDP Lactate/ Lactic dehydrogenase (see LDH); Lateral decubitus position; Lateral disc protrusion; Left dorsoposterior (fetal position); Low dose pill; Lyme Disease Program (NEMC).

LDPE Low density polyethylene (medicine bottle).

LDR Labor, delivery, and recovery; Lethal dose range; Linear dose response; Linear dynamic range; Loading dose regimen; Low-dose radiation/ recipient/ regimen.

LDR/P Labor, delivery, recovery, and postpartum.

LDRR Linear dose response relationship.

LDRS Long-distance robotic surgery (= LDS).

LDRT Low-dose radiation therapy.

LDS Latter-Day Saints - Church member (Mormon)/ Hospital (Utah); Licentiate in Dental Surgery; Liposome delivery system; Long-distance surgery (see LDRS); Lumbar disc surgery.

LDSc Licentiate in Dental Science.

LDT Lactate dehydrogenase, total; 'Last ditch' therapy/ treatment; Left dorsotransverse (position of fetus); Lie detection technique/ technology; Lie detector test (= PGT); Living donor transplant.

LDUB Long double upright brace.

LDV Lactic dehydrogenase virus; Lamivudine (HIV reverse transcriptase inhibitor); Large dense-cored vesicle; Laser Doppler velocimetry; Lateral distant view; Lyme disease vaccine.

LDY Lipodystrophy (= LD).

LE Lambert-Eaton (syndrome) (see LES; MMS); Left ear/ eye; Lens extraction; Leukocyte elastase; Leukoerythrogenetic/nic; Live embryo; Long Evans (rat); Low exposure; Lower extremity (= L ext; L/ext); Lupus erythematosus.

Le Leonard (unit for cathode rays); Lewis (antigen).

LE 29060 Vinblastine sulfate (= NSC 49842; Vincaleucoblastine sulfate; Vincaleukoblastine sulfate) - an alkaloid extracted from VINCA rosea (family Apocynaceae), a cytotoxic agent, mainly used in the treatment of Hodgkin's disease and chorionepithelioma.

LEA Lower extremity amputation; Lower extremity, arterial; Lumbar epidural anesthesia.

LEAA Law Enforcement Assistance Administration (DOJ).

Leaper Amphetamine tablet (see Amphet).

LEb Lupus erythematosus body.

Lebanese Hashish (see Cannabis).

LEC Laboratory exclusion criteria; Laser Eye Center; Leukoencephalitis; Lower esophageal contractility.

LECA Left external carotid artery.

LECP Low-energy charged particle.

LECT Lupus erythematosus cell test.

Lect Lecturer.

LED Light-emitting diode; Lowest effective/ emitting dose; Lupus erythematosus disseminatus (see SLE).

LED; LEDOX Liposome-encapsulated doxorubicin (cancer therapy).

LEE Lower extremity edema.

LEED Low-energy electron diffraction.

LEEDS Low-energy electron diffraction spectroscopy.

LEEP Left end-expiratory pressure; Long established ethical principle(s).

LEF Leukokinesis-enhancing factor; Lupus erythematosus factor; Lupus Erythematosus Foundation (Inc).

leg legislate/tion; legal(ly).

leg com legally committed.

LEGJ Ligation of the esophagogastric junction (= LEJ).

LEGS Learning Experience Guides for Nursing Students (training materials); Legislative Effort Group System (AMA).

LEHPZ Lower esophageal high pressure zone.

LEI Liver enzyme induction.

LeIF Leukocyte interferon.

leio- prefix meaning smooth (Gr. leios).

leipo- prefix meaning fat (see lipo-).

LEIS Low-energy ion scattering.

Leishmaniasis Named after a Scottish army pathologist, Sir William B. Leishman, serving in British India in 1903: Visceral leishmaniasis: Dum dum fever; Kala azar. Cutaneous or Skin leishmaniasis (Old Word): Aleppo evil; Baghdad boil; Biskra button; Oriental sore. Cutaneous or Skin leishmaniasis (new World): Bay sore; Chiclero's ulcer; Forest yaws; Uta.

LEJ Ligation of the esophagogastric junction (see LEGJ).

LEL Lower exposure limit (of a gas mixture); Lowest effect level.

LEM Lateral eye movement; Leibovitz-Emory medium; Leukocyte/tic endogenous mediator; Light electron/ emission microscope/py; Liver enzyme monitoring; Lower-extremity muscle.

LEMO Lowest empty molecular orbital.

LEMS Lambert-Eaton myasthenic syndrome.

lenit gently/ lenitive (L. leniter).

lent- combining form meaning lentil (L. lentis).

LEOPARD Lentigines, EKG abnormalities, Ocular hypertelorism, Pulmonary stenosis, Abnormalities of genitalia, Retardation of growth, and Deafness (syndrome).

LEP Lethal effective phase; Lipoprotein electrophoresis; Localized epigastric pain; Low egg passage (virus strain); Lower esophageal pressure/ esophagus.

lep- combining form meaning seize or take (Gr.).

LEP 2 Leptospirosis 2.

L_{EPN}; L_{epn} Effective perceived noise level.
LEPRAN British Leprosy Relief Association News.
LE prep Lupus erythematosus preparation (laboratory/ hematology).
Lept Leptospira.
Leq Loudness equivalent.
LER Leading-edge research; Lysozomal enzyme release.
LERG Local electroretinogram.
L-ERX Leukoerythroblastic reaction.
LES Lambert-Eaton syndrome; Laser eye surgery; Lawrence Experimental Station (agar); Lingual epithelial surface; Local excitatory state; Locke egg serum (medium); Low excitatory state; Lower esophageal segment/ sphincter/ stricture (= LOS); Lupus erythematosus, systemic (see SLE).
les lesion.
LESP Lower esophageal sphincter pressure (= LOSP).
LESS Lateral electrical spine stimulation.
LET Leading-edge technology; Linear/ Low energy transfer; Local estrogen therapy (see TET); Low environmental temperature; Lower extremity trauma.
LETD Lowest effective toxic dose.
LETS Large external transformation-sensitive (protein).
LEU Leucine (see Leu); Leucovorin; Leukocyte equivalent unit.
Leu Leucine (= LEU); Leukocyte (= Leuc; Leuco; Leuk; Leuko) - any colorless ameboid cell mass (the name especially designates the white blood cells).
Leuco; leuco; Leuc; leuc; Leuko; leuko; Leuk; leuk Leukocyte (see Leu).
leuk-; leuc- prefix meaning white (Gr. leukos).
LEV Levator (muscle); Lipid-enveloped virus (e.g. hepatitis B, C; HIV); Lower extremity, venous.
Lev; lev Levarterenol (bitartrate); Light (L. levis).
levo- prefix meaning left or counterclockwise (L.).
LEW Lewis (rat).
L ext; L/ext Lower extremity (see LE).
LF Labile factor (= Proaccelerin) (see Factor - V); Lactoferrin (= lf; LFN); Laryngofissure; Lassa fever (a hemorrhagic fever caused by the arenavirus and transmitted by rodents); Latex fixation (test - laboratory/ serology) (see LFT; L-F test); Latex flocculation (test) (see LFT); Left foot/ forearm; Lethal/ Leukotactic factor; Lifeform (anatomical replica); Ligamentum flavum; Limit of flocculation (see Lf); Lipofuscin (= AS - Age spot, associated with senility); Liver function (test) (see LFT); Loudness function (test) (see LFT); Low fat (diet); Low forceps (delivery) (see FLD); Low frequency (see lf); Lupus Foundation; Lymphatic filariasis.
Lf Limit of flocculation (= LF).
lf lactoferrin (see LF); low frequency (= LF) (see LFT).
L_f Flocculation unit(s) (= L_f unit of toxin per ml).
LFA Left femoral artery; Left forearm; Left frontoanterior (fetal position - brow or face-chin presentation) (= LMA); Leukocyte/ Lymphocyte function-associated antigen; Leukotactic factor activity; Low-friction arthroplasty (see LFP).
LFA-1 Lymphocyte function associated antigen - 1 (a protein molecule involved in the adhesion of lymphocytes).
LFBD Lingual-facial-buccal dyskinesia (= TD - Tardive d).
LFC Lateral femoral condyle; Left frontal craniotomy; Living female child; Low fat and cholesterol (diet).
LFCT Leucovorin-fluorouracil chemotherapy.
LFD Lactose-free diet; Large for date (fetus); Late fetal death; Lateral facial dysplasia; Least fatal dose (of a drug/ toxin); Less frequent dosing; Low-fat/ fiber diet; Low forceps delivery.
LFER Linear free-energy relationship.
LFF Left fifth finger.
LFGA Large-for-gestational-age (infant).
LFH Left femoral hernia.
LFHFD Low-fat, high-fiber diet.
LFI Local fungal infection.
LFL Left frontolateral; Leukocyte feeder layer; Lower flammable limit.
LFM Less frequent monitoring.
LFMCS Line-focusing monochromator-spec-

trometer.

LFN Lactoferrin (see LF).

L-(form) A defective bacterial variant that can multiply on hypertonic medium.

LFP Laser fimbrioplasty; Left facial palsy; Left femoral pulse; Left frontoposterior (fetal position - brow or face-chin presentation) (= LMP); Low filling pressure (cardiac, etc.); Low-fric- tion prostheses/esis (Orthopedics - e.g. the Charnley device).

LFPPV Low-frequency positive pressure ventilation.

LFPS Licentiate of the Faculty of Physicians and Surgeons.

LFR Lymphoid follicular reticulosis.

LFS Lateral facet syndrome; Li-Fraumeni syndrome (a familial cancer syndrome, characterized by a familial clustering of pediatric sarcomas, breast cancer, leukemia, brain tumors, and adrenocortical carcinoma associated with germ-line mutations of the p53 tumor-suppressor gene); Limbic forebrain structure; Liver function series.

LFT Latex fixation test (= L-F test); Latex flocculation test; Left frontotransverse (fetal position/ brow or face-chin presentation) (= LMT); Liver function test(s); Loudness function test(s); Low-frequency tetanus; Low-frequency transduction (= lf); Low-frequency transfer; Lung function test(s) (see PFT).

LFT Liver function tests (= HFT or Hepatic function tests):
ASFT: Ammonium sulfate flocculation test.
BC: Blood cholesterol.
BSP: Bromsulfalein/ Bromsulphalein test.
CBr: Hepatic bilirubin clearance.
CCFT: Cephalin cholesterol flocculation test.
CGFT: Colloidal gold flocculation test.
CPG: Copper binding globulin (= Ceruloplasmin).
FBG: Fasting blood glucose (see FBS).
FBS: Fasting blood sugar (= FBG).
FU: Fecal urobilinogen (= Stercobilinogen).
GlTT: Glucose tolerance test (see GTT).
GST: Glycogen storage test.
GT: Glucagon test.
GTT: Galactose tolerance test; Glucose tolerance test (= GlTT).
HAET: Hippuric acid excretion test.
ICD: Isocitric dehydrogenase (= ICDH; IDH).
ICDH: Isocitric dehydrogenase (see ICD).
IDH: Isocitric dehydrogenase (see ICD).
II: Icterus index.
LD: Lactate/ Lactic dehydrogenase (see LDH).
LDG: Lactate/ Lactic dehydrogenase (see LDH).
LDH: Lactate/ Lactic dehydrogenase (= LD; LDG; LDL; LDP).
LDL: Lactate/ Lactic dehydrogenase (see LDH).
LDP: Lactate/ Lactic dehydrogenase (see LDH).
PT: Prothrombin time.
SAP: Serum alkaline phosphatase.
SB: Serum bilirubin (direct, indirect, and total).
SC: Serum cholinesterase.
SGOT: Serum glutamic oxalacetic transaminase.
SGPT: Serum glutamic pyruvic transaminase.
SP: Serum proteins (albumin, globulin, and albumin/ globulin ratio).
TFT: Thymol flocculation test.
TTT: Thymol turbidity test.
UB: Urine bilirubin.
UU: Urine urobilinogen.
VDB; VdB; vdB: van den Bergh (reaction/ test).
VDBR: Volume of distribution of bilirubin.
ZSFT: Zinc sulfate flocculation test.
ZTT: Zinc turbidity test.

L-F test Latex fixation test (see LFT).

LFU Laboratory follow-up (see CFU); Limit flocculation unit; Lipid fluidity unit.

LFV Lassa fever virus; Low-frequency ventilation (see LFPPV).

LFx Linear fracture.

LG Lactoglobulin; Lamellar granule; Langer-Giedion (syndrome) (see TRP Type II); Laryngectomy; Left gluteal/eus (injection site); Lennox-Gastaut (syndrome); Leucylglycine (= dileucylglycine); Linguogingival; Lipoglycopeptide; Liver graft; Lou Gehrig('s disease) (see ALS); Low glucose; Lymph(atic) gland.

lg large (= lge); leg.

LG 254 Pipazethate hydrochloride (= Piperstazine HCl) - an antitussive agent inhibiting the cough center, but having a depressive action on respiration.
LGA Large for gestational age; Left gastric artery; Limulus gelation assay (for endotoxin in the spinal fluid in cases of meningeal plague or plague meningitis).
LGB Landry-Guillain-Barré (syndrome); Lateral geniculate body.
LGBS Landry-Guillain-Barré-Strohl (syndrome); Landry-Guillain-Barré syndrome.
LGC Lab-grown cell; Low-grade carcinoma.
LGD Lacrimal gland disorder; Lethal genetic defect(s); Limb girdle dystrophy; Lou Gehrig's disease (see ALS).
LGE Langat encephalitis.
lge large (see lg).
LGEMTV Live gal-epimerase mutant typhoid vaccine.
LGF Lateral giant fiber; Local growth factor (Bone formation); Low grade fever.
LGFB Look good...feel better (ACS - American Cancer Society cosmetic and psychological program in women undergoing chemotherapy).
LGG *Lactobacillus* Gorbach Goldin (see L-GG).
L-GG *Lactobacillus* - GG strain (a probiotic used to treat diarrhea in infants) (see PB).
LGH Lactogenic hormone (see Hormones - LGH; LH i).
LGI Laparoscope-guided injection; Large glucagon immunoreactivity; Lower gastrointestinal (series).
5-LGI 5-Lipoxygenase inhibitor.
LGL Large granular leukocyte/ lymphocyte; Lown-Ganong-Levine (syndrome) - a pre-excitation syndrome with cardiac arrhythmia and tachycardia.
LGL-NK Large granular lymphocyte - natural killer.
LGM Lipoid granulomatosis (= Gaucher's disease) (Orthopedics); Low-grade malignancy.
LGMD Limb-girdle muscular dystrophy.
LGN Lateral geniculate nucleus; Lobular glomerulonephritis; Lown-Ganong-Levine (syndrome) (see ABT); Lupus glomerulonephritis.
LGO Lab-grown organ (for transplant).
LGP Low grade pyrexia (see LGF).
LGR Linear growth retardation.
LGS Lab-grown skin (for transplant); Langer-Giedion syndrome (= TRPS with exostosis) (see HDA; TRPS); Laparoscopic gallbladder surgery; Leaky-gut syndrome; Lennox-Gastaut syndrome; Limb girdle syndrome.
LGT Lab(oratory)-grown tissue(s); Late generalized tuberculosis; Lower genital tract.
LGTI Lower genital tract infection.
LGUT Lower genitourinary tract.
LGV Large granular vesicle; Low genetic vulnerability; Lymphogranuloma venereum.
LGVHD Lethal graft-versus-host disease.
LgX Lymphogranulomatosis X.
LH Lactogenic hormone (see Hormones - LH i); Langerhansian hormone (see Hormones - LH ii); Late healing; Lateral habenula/ hypothalamus/ hypothalamic (syndrome); Left hand/ heart/ hemisphere/ hyperphoria; Life and Health (journal, now Health for Life); Liver/ Lung homogenate; Living homograft (section of human tissue used as a graft); Local hormone (see Hormones - LH iii); Lower half; Lues hereditaria; Luteal hormone (see Hormones - LH iv); Luteinizing hormone (= ICSH) (see Hormones - LH v).
LH2 Luciferin.
LHA Lateral hypothalamic area; Left hepatic artery; Linear hearing aid.
LHA/D Liters of hyperalimentation (solution) per day.
LH2-AMP Luciferyl adenylate.
LHB Left heart border; Long-held belief.
LHBCEMR Lothian Health Board Committee on Ethics of Medical Research (NHS - UK).
LHBV Left heart blood volume.
LHC Langerhans cell histiocytosis; Left heart catheterization; Left hypochondrium; Light-harvesting complex; Local Health Council; Low hydrocarbon (compressed gas).
LHCP Less Hazardous Cigarette Program.
LHD Local Health Department.
LHE Live/ Living human embryo.
LHF Left heart failure/ function (= LVF).
LHFA Lung Hageman factor activator.
LH/FSH/RH Luteinizing hormone/ follicle-

stimulating hormone/ releasing hormone (see Hormones - LH/FSH/RH).

LHG Left hand grip; Localized hemolysis in gel.

LHH Left homonymous hemianopsia.

LHI Lipid hydrocarbon inclusion.

LHL Left hemisphere lesion(s); Left hepatic lobe; Long half-life.

LHLY l-hydroxylysine.

LHM Lysuride hydrogen maleate.

LHMP Life Health Monitoring Program.

LHN Lateral hypothalamic nucleus.

LHON Leber's hereditary optic neuropathy.

LHP Left hemiparesis/ hemiplegia.

LHPMG Lypholized human post-menopausal gonadotrophin (see HMG; PMG).

LHPR Laboratory for Human Performance Research.

LHPZ Low/ Lower (esophageal) high-pressure zone.

LHR Labor and Human Resources (Committee); Laser hair removal (Cosm. surgery); Leukocyte histamine release; Local hypersensitivity reaction(s).

l-hr lumen-hour.

LHRF Luteinizing hormone-releasing factor (see Hormones - LHRF).

LHRH; LH-RH Luteinizing hormone-releasing hormone (see Hormones - LH-RH).

LHS Left hand side; Left heart strain (= LVS); Left heelstrike; Long-handled shoehorn (Orthopedics); Lowest hemoglobin saturation (sleep apnea); Lymphatic/ hematopoietic system.

LHSC London Health Science Centre (Ontario, Canada).

LHT Left hypertrophy/ hypertropia; Lifestyle Heart Trial.

L-5 HTP L 5-Hydroxytryptophan (used in the treatment of myoclonus) (see HTP).

LHV Left ventricular hypertrophy (see LVH); Lymphotropic herpesvirus.

LI Labeling/ Lithogenic index; Laboratory of Immunodiagnosis (NCI); Laboratory Investigation (journal); Lactose intolerance; Lacunar infarct; Lamellar ichthyosis; Large intestine; Learning impaired; Lente insulin (see Insulin - IZS); Leptospira icterohaemorrhagica; Linguoincisal; Low impulsiveness.

Li A blood group system; Labrale inferius; Limitans; Lithium (Z = 3) (see Elements - Lithium).

L&I Liver and iron.

L I Lues I or Primary syphilis.

L II Lues II or Secondary syphilis.

L III Lues III or Tertiary syphilis.

LI-4 Acupuncture point (Hegu as in Sanyinjiao, and located between os metacarpals I and II Obs/Gyn) (see SP-6).

LIA Laser Institute of America; Leukemia-associated inhibitory activity; Line immunoassay; Liver infusion agar; Lock-in amplifier; Lymphocyte-induced angiogenesis; Lysine iron agar.

LIAFI Late infantile amaurotic familial/ family idiocy.

LIAs Low-impact aerobics.

LIB Left in bottle.

Lib Liberation; Librium.

lib a pound (L. libra) (see lb).

LIBC Latent iron-binding capacity.

LiBr Lithium bromide.

LIC Left iliac crest; Left internal carotid (artery); Leisure interest class; Limiting isorrheic concentration; Lithium-induced coma; Local intravascular coagulation.

Lic Licentiate.

LICA Left internal carotid artery.

LICD Lower intestinal Crohn's disease.

LICH Left intracerebral hemisphere.

LICM Left intercostal margin.

LicMed Licentiate in Medicine.

Li_2CO_3 Lithium carbonate.

LICS Left intercostal space.

LID Late(-onset) immunoglobulin deficiency; Latent iron deficiency; Levodopa-induced dyskinesia; Life insurance data; Lymphocytic infiltrative disease.

LIDC Low-intensity direct current.

Lido Lidocaine.

Lid pop Lid popper (amphetamine tablet) (see Amphet).

LIE Low-impact exercise.

lien- prefix meaning spleen (L.).

LIF Laser-induced fluorescence; Latency-intensity function (of the cochlear hearing mechanism); Left iliac fossa; Left index finger; Leukemia-inhibiting factor; Leukocyte/

Leucocyte inhibiting/ inhibitory factor - for leukocytes (= leucocytes; neutrophils), i.e. for migratory inhibition, keeping them at the sites of inflammation, or inhibiting migration of the leukocytes away from sites of inflammation (an esterase) (= LMI; LMIF); Leukocytosis-inducing factor (as above); Liver (migration) inhibitory factor; Low-iron formula (in infants) (see LIIF).

LIFA Latent immunofluorescence antigen.

LIFE Living Implants From Engineering (Tissue engineering project); Losartan intervention for endpoint (reduction) (hypertension study); Lung imaging fluorescence endoscope.

LIFO Last in, first out.

LIFT Lymphocyte immunofluorescence test.

Lig; lig Ligament (L. ligamentum) - a band of tissue connecting bones or supporting viscera; Ligation.

Ligand A drug or endogenous substance which binds to a receptor or specific, membrane-bound or intracellular, tissue protein) (e.g. histamine is a ligand at histamine receptors).

LIH Left inguinal hernia.

LIHA Low impulsiveness, high anxiety.

LIIF Low-iron infant formula (= LIF).

LIIS Lentovirus-induced immune suppression.

LIJH Long Island Jewish Hospital (New York).

LIJ-HMC Long Island Jewish - Hillside Medical Center (New York).

LILA Low impulsiveness, low anxiety.

Lilly Lilly Endowment, Inc.

LIM Line isolation monitor.

Lim; lim Limit(ed).

LIMA Left internal mammary artery.

Lin; lin; Linim Liniment (L. linimentum).

lin linear.

LINC Laboratory instrument computer.

Linct An electuary or linctus (L. linctus = a "licking").

Ling Lingual.

lingu- combining form meaning tongue (L. lingua).

LINH Lymphocytic infundibuloneurohypophysitis (a cause of central diabetes insipidus).

Linim Liniment (see Lin).

Linn Linnaean; Linnaeus.

LINT Levodopa-induced neurotoxicity.

Lint (L. linteum) - an absorbent dressing material.

LIO Left inferior oblique.

Li_2O Lithium oxide.

LiOH Lithium hydroxide.

LIP Lead-in period (in medication); Lithium-induced polydipsia/ polyuria; Lymphocytic/oid interstitial pneumonia/itis.

Lip Lipase; Lipid; Lipoate; Lipoic (acid).

lip- combining form meaning fat (Gr. lipos).

LiPA Line probe assay.

LIPID Long-term Intervention with Pravastatin in Ischemic Disease (study).

Lipids (journal).

LIPM Lister Institute of Preventive Medicine (London).

lipo- prefix meaning fat (Gr. lipos) (= leipo-).

LipoMM Lipomyelomeningocele.

LIPS Leiter International Performance Scale.

LIQ Low(er) inner quadrant.

Liq; liq Liquid/ Liquor (L. liquor) - a fluid.

liq dr liquid dram.

liq oz liquid ounce.

liq pt liquid pint.

liq qt liquid quart.

LIR Left iliac region; Left inferior rectus; Local(ized) immune reaction/ response; Local(ized) inflammatory reaction/ response.

LIRBM Liver, iron, red bone marrow.

LIS Laboratory information system; Lateral intercellular space; Left intercostal space; Lithium diiodosalicylate; Lobular in situ (mammary carcinoma); Locked-in syndrome; Low insulin sensitivity; Low intermittent suction; Low ionic strength; Lymphoid immune system.

LISA Library and Information Science Abstracts (journal).

LISP List Processing Language.

LISS Low-ionic-strength saline.

Lit Liter (see L. Liter).

lit literal(ly).

lith- combining form meaning stone (Gr. lithos).

LIV Law of initial value (Joseph Wilder); Left innominate vein; Liver battery test (dentistry).

liv live; living.

LIV-BP Leucine, isoleucine, and valine-binding protein.

LIVC Left inferior vena cava.

LIVEN Linear inflammatory verrucous epidermal nevus.

LivPro Liver profile.

LJ Lockjaw (or trismus, seen in tetanus).

L-J Löwenstein-Jensen (see L-J medium).

LJC Lion-jaw clamp (see BHF).

LJI List of Journals Indexed.

LJM Limited joint mobility; Löwenstein-Jensen medium (see L-J medium).

L-J medium Löwenstein-Jensen medium-used in the cultivation and differentiation of human and bovine types of the Tubercle Bacillus.

LJS Large joint synovitis.

LK Lamellar keratoplasty; Left kidney; Lichenoid keratosis; Lymphokine.

L-K Linguistic-kinesic (method).

LK+ Low potassium ion.

LKA Lazare-Klerman-Armour (Personality Inventory).

LKAL Leeds-Keio artificial ligament (artificial, prosthetic knee implant, made of Terylene, an open-chain polyester) (GPL; LKL).

LKKS Liver, kidneys, spleen.

LKL Leeds-Keio ligament (see LKAL).

LKM Liver-kidney microsomal (antibody).

LKP Lamellar keratoplasty; Leeds-Keio prosthesis (Intraarticular graft for reconstruction of the Anterior cruciate ligament) (Orthopedics) (= APT; LKAL; LKL; LKR).

LKPD Lillehei-Kaster pivoting disk (artificial cardiac valve).

LKPT Liver, kidney, and pancreas transplant(ation)/ plants.

LKQCPI Licentiate of the King and Queen's College of Physicians of Ireland.

LKR Leeds-Keio reconstruction (see LKP).

LKS Landau-Kleffner syndrome; Liver, kidney, spleen.

LKSB Liver, kidneys, spleen, bladder.

LKSnp Liver, kidneys, spleen non-palpable.

LKT Living kidney transplant(ation).

LKV Laked kanamycin vancomycin (agar).

LL Large lymphocyte; Lateral leminiscus; Lederle Laboratories Inc code for experimental substances; Left lateral (see L lat); Left leg/ limb/ lower/ lung; Lepromatous leprosy; Life and Lung (journal); Lipoprotein lipase; Loudness level; Low level (test); Lower (eye)lid/ lip/ lobe; Lumbar length; Lymphocytic leukemia (see LLC); Lymphoblastic/phocytic lymphoma; Lymphoid leukemia; Lysolecithin.

LL 2 Limb lead two (ECG).

LLA Lessened/ Limited/ Lowered locomotor activity (see DLA); Limulus lysate assay; Lipid-lowering agent (= LLD); Long-lasting antagonism (of actions, drugs, effects, etc.); Lower-limb amputation/ amputee/ ataxia; Lupus-like anticoagulant.

LLAD Linear log-analog-to-digital (converter).

L lat Left lateral (= LL).

LLB Left lateral border; Long-lasting binding; Long-leg brace (orthopedics).

LLBCD Left lower border of cardiac dullness.

LLC Lewis lung carcinoma; Liquid-liquid chromatography; Long-lasting channel (= L-type calcium channel in the voltage-dependent cardiac muscle) (see TC); Long-leg cast; Lymphocytic leukemia (= LL).

LLCC Long-leg cylinder cast.

LLCD Laser-luminescence cavity detector (Dentistry).

LLC-MK1 Rhesus monkey kidney cells.

LLC-MK2 Rhesus monkey kidney cells.

LLC-MK3 Circopithecus monkey kidney cells.

LLC-RK1 Rabbit kidney cells.

LLD Doctor of Law; Lactobacillus lactis Dorner (factor - vitamin B12); Left lateral decubitus (muscle); Leg length discrepancy; Life-long disease; Limb-length discrepancy; Lipid-lowering diet/ dose (see LAA)/ drug (see LLA); Long-lasting depolarization; Lower limb damage; Lymphoma-like disorder.

LLDH Liver lactate dehydrogenase.

LLE Left lower extremity; Localized lupus erythematosus; Long-lasting effect.

LLF Laki-Lóránd factor (= Fibrin stabilizing factor) (see Factor XII); Left lateral femoral

(site of injection)/ flexion.
LLFR Long-lived free radical(s).
LLG Lower leg/ limb gangrene; Lower limb girdle.
LL-GXT Low-level graded exercise test.
LLI Lupus-like illness.
LLJ Lower limb joint.
LLL La Leche League (International) (see LLLI); Left liver lobe; Left lower/ Lower left leg/ lid (eyelid)/ limb/ lobe (of lung); Lower limb lesion.
LLLE Lower lid, left eye (see LLOS).
LL leprosy Lepromatous leprosy (caused by *Mycobacterium* leprae); Lower limb.
LLLI La Leche League (International) (= LLL).
LLLM Low liquid level monitor.
LLLNR Left lower lobe no râles.
LLM Lipid-laden macrophage (= foam cell); Lipid-lowering medication; Localized leukocyte mobilization.
LLN Lower limit of normal.
LLO Legionella-like organism.
LLOD Lower lid, right eye (L. oculus dextra) (= LLRE).
LLOS Lower lid, left eye (L. oculus sinistra) (= LLLE).
LLP Late luteal phase; Log-linear portion (of AUC - plasma time concentration curve); Long-lasting potentiation.
LLQ Left lower quadrant (of abdomen).
LLR Large local reaction; Left lateral rectus (muscle); Left lumbar region; Lipid level reduction; Long-lasting reduction; Low-level release.
LLRE Lower lid, right eye (see LLOD).
LLS Lax ligamentous structure; Lazy leukocyte syndrome; Leukemia and Lymphoma Society (Ca., US); Leukemia/ Lymphoma syndrome; Lipid-lowering strategy; Long-leg splint; Lower limb surgery; Lupus-like syndrome.
LLSB Left lower scapular/ sternal border.
LLSC Long-leg spica cast (bilateral/ unilateral).
LLT Lateral left/ Left lateral thigh (injection site); Left lower thorax; Lipid-lowering therapy/ treatment (see LAA; LLA; LLD); Lock-layer transistor; Limulus lysate test (for endotoxin); Lysolecithin.
LLU Lower leg/ limb ulcer(ation).
LLUSM Loma Linda University School of Medicine.
LLV Lymphatic leukemia virus.
LLV-F Lymphatic leukemia virus, Friend associated.
LLVP Left lateral ventricular pre-excitation.
LLW Left lateral wall (of chest, etc.).
LLWC Long-leg walking cast.
LLX Left lower extremity.
LM Laboratory Management/ Medicine (journals); Lactic acid mineral (medium); Lactose malabsorption; Laryngeal/ Longitudinal muscle; Lateral malleolus; Laval Medical (journal, now VMCF); Left median/ middle; Legal medicine; Lemniscus medialis (thalamus) (= Lm); Licentiate in Medicine (= ML)/ Midwifery; Light microscope/py/ minimum; Lincomycin; Lingual margin (= ML); Linguomesial; Lipid mobilization; Lipid mobilizing (hormone) (see Hormones - LMH); Liquid membrane; Listeria monocytogenes (see Lm); Localized movement; Lower motor (neurone) (see LMN).
Lm Lemniscus medialis (see LM); Listeria monocytogenes (= LM).
lm lumen.
l/m liters per minute (see l/min).
LMA Left mentoanterior (position of fetus) (see LFA); Light microscopic analysis; Limbic midbrain area; Liver cell membrane autoantibody.
LMB Laboratory of Molecular Biology (MRC, England); Laurence-Moon-Biedl (syndrome); Leiomyoblastoma.
LMBB Laurence-Moon-Bardet-Biedl (syndrome).
LMBS Laurence-Moon-Biedl syndrome.
LMC Large motile cell; Lateral motor column; Left main coronary (artery); Left middle cerebral (artery); Leptomeningeal carcinoma(tosis); Living male child; Lymphocyte-mediated cytotoxicity; Lymphomyeloid complex.
LMCA Left main coronary artery; Left middle cerebral artery.
LMCAD Left main coronary artery disease.
LMCAT Left middle cerebral artery thrombo-

sis.

LMCC Licentiate of the Medical Council of Canada.

LMCL Left midclavicular line.

LMCN Laboratory of Molecular and Cellular Neuroscience.

LMD Lipid-moiety modified derivative; Local medical doctor; Low/ Lower/ Lowest maintenance dose; Low molecular weight dextran (intravenous solution) (= LMDX).

LMDX Low-molecular-weight dextran (see LMD).

LME Left mediolateral episiotomy; Leukocyte migration enhancement.

L Med Ch; LMed&Ch; L Med L Ch Licentiate in Medicine and Surgery.

LMEE Left middle ear exploration.

LMF Left middle finger; Lymphocyte mitogenic factor (stimulates B- and T-lymphocyte proliferation and B-Lymphocyte Ig production).

LMFBR Liquid metal fast breeder reactor.

LMFCC Licensed marriage, family and child counselor.

lm/ft² lumens per square foot.

LMG Labial minor (salivary) gland; Lethal midline granuloma.

LMH Lactose monohydrate (an inactive ingredient used in placebos); Lipid-mobilizing hormone (see Hormones - LMH).

lmh lumen hour.

LMI Leukocyte migration inhibition (see LIF).

LMIF Leukocyte migration inhibition factor (see LIF).

l/min liters per minute (= l/m; LPM; lpm).

LMJ Lawyer's Medical Journal.

LML Large and medium leukocytes; Left mediolateral (e.g. episiotomy incision - operation/ obstetrics); Left middle lobe; Lepromatous leprosy (see MBL; PBL; TCL).

LMLE Left mediolateral episiotomy.

LMM Lactobacillus maintenance medium; Lentigo maligna melanoma; Light meromyosin.

lm/m² lumens per square meter.

LMN Low molecular number (weight); Lower motor neurone (= LM).

LMND Lower motor neurone degeneration.

LMNFP Lower motor neurone facial palsy (= BP - Bell's palsy).

LMNL Lower motor neurone lesion.

LMNP Lower motor neurone palsy/ paralysis/ paresis/ pathology (= LMNL; LMNW).

LMNW Lower motor neurone weakness (see LMNP).

LMO Localized molecular orbital.

LMP Laboratory of Molecular Psychiatry (Yale Univ., US); Last menstrual period; Latent membrane potential; Left mentoposterior (position of fetus) (see LFP); Lumbar puncture (see LP).

LMR Left medial rectus (muscle); Low(er) mortality rate; Lymphocytic meningopolyradiculitis.

LMRCP Licentiate in Midwifery of the Royal College of Physicians.

LMS Lateral medullary syndrome; Leiomyosarcoma; Licentiate in Medicine and Surgery; Lingual-mucosa scraping; Liver microsomal stimulation; Locomotor system.

lms lumen-second.

LMSA Labor-Management Services Administration (DOL).

LMSSA Licentiate in Medicine and Surgery of the Society of Apothecaries (London).

LMSV Left maximal spatial voltage.

LMT Left main trunk; Left mentotransverse (position of fetus) (see LFT); Leukocyte migration technique; Lowenfeld Mosaic Test.

LMTA Language Modalities Test for Aphasia.

LMTH Luteomammotropic hormone (= Lactogenic h) (see Hormones - LH i).

LMV Larva migrans visceralis; Lowest minimal value/ volume.

LMW Low molecular weight.

lm/W lumens per watt (= l/m).

LMW-CSA Low molecular weight - colony-stimulating activity.

LMWD Low molecular weight dextran.

LMWH Low-molecular weight heparin (Dalteparin, Enoxaparin, etc.).

LMW-Ig Low molecular weight - immunoglobulin (= LMW-γM).

LMW-γM See LMW-Ig.

LN Lesch-Nyhan (syndrome) (see L-N); Lipoid nephrosis; Liquid nitrogen; Low necrosis; Lupus nephritis; Lymph node.

ln natural logarithm (base e).
L-N Lesch-Nyhan (disease/ syndrome) (= LN).
L/N Letter/numerical (system).
L&N Leeds and Northrup Co.
LN_2 Liquid nitrogen.
LNA Latent nuclear antigen (see LANA); α-Linolenic acid (= $C_{18}H_{30}O_2$) - an omega-3 polyunsaturated fatty acid, extracted from linseed oil.
LNAA Large neutral amino acid.
L-NAME N3-Nitro-L-Arginine methyl ester.
LNC Lymph node cell.
LND Lesch-Nyhan disease; Light-near dissociation; Lymph node disease/ dissection.
LNE Lymph node enlargement.
L-NE L-norepinephrine (= L-noradrenaline).
LNG Liquified natural gas.
LNH Large number hypothesis.
LNI Lymph-node infection/ involvement.
LNKS Low natural killer syndrome.
LNL Lymph node lymphocyte.
LNLS Linear-non-linear least squares.
LNM Lymph-node metastases/stasis.
L-NMMA N-monomethyl-L-arginine.
LNMP Last normal menstrual period.
LNNB Luria-Nebraska Neuropsychological Battery.
LNP Large neuronal polypeptide; Latent nuclear protein (see LANA).
LNPF Lymph node permeability factor.
LNS Lateral nuclear stratum; Lesch-Nyhan syndrome (Congenital absence of the enzyme HGPRT or Hypoxanthine-guanine phosphoribosyltransferase and associated with childhood gout, mental deficiency, tendency to self-mutilation and early death).
LO Lateral oblique (x-ray); Linguo-occlusal; Lomustine (see CCNU); Lumbar orthosis.
lo low.
LOA Leave of absence; Leber's optic atrophy; Left occipitoanterior (position of fetus, i.e. vertex presentation); Lysis of adhesions.
LOAD Late-onset Alzheimer's disease (assoc. with chromosomes 12 & 19).
LOC Laxative of choice; Level/ Loss of consciousness; Liquid organic compound; Locus of control.
LOC; LO_2C Lowered oxygen consumption (see ROC; RO_2C).
loc- prefix meaning place (L. locus).
lo cal low calorie (diet).
lo calc low calcium (diet).
loc cit in the place cited or previously quoted (L. loco citato).
loc dol to the painful area or spot (L. loco dolenti).
LOCF Last observation carried forward (analysis/ technique); Low output cardiac failure.
lo CHO low carbohydrate.
lo chol low cholesterol.
LOCM Low-osmolar contrast media/ium.
Loco Marijuana (see Cannabis).
LOCODOSA Computer program for calculating dose distribution of implanted radioactive wires.
LOD Late onset diabetes (= LODM).
LOD; LoD Life-or-death; Line of duty.
LODM Late onset diabetes mellitus (see LOD).
LOF Lofexidine.
log logarithm (common).
log- combining form meaning account for or speak (Gr.).
log_e logarithm to the base e.
log_{10} logarithm to the base 10.
-logist suffix meaning a scholar or specialist (Gr. log-).
logo- prefix meaning words or speech (Gr. logos).
-logy suffix meaning a field of study (Gr. log-).
LOH Loop of Henle (see LoH); Loss of heterozygosity.
LoH Loop of Henle (= LOH).
LOI Level of incompetence; Limit of impurities.
LOIH Left oblique inguinal hernia.
lo K; lo k low potassium.
LOL Languid/ Lean/ Left-handed/ Likeable/ Listless/ Little/ Lively/ Lonely/ Loopy/ Loquacious/ Lovely/ Ludicrous old lady; Left occipitolateral (position of fetus).
LoL Loss of libido.
LOM Laboratory of Oral Medicine (NIDR); Left otitis media; Limitation/ Loss of motion/ movement (see LoM); Low-osmolar (con-

trast) media/ium.

LoM Limitation/ Loss of motion/ movement (= LOM).

LOMPT Lincoln-Oseretsky Motor Performance Test.

LOMSA Left otitis media suppurativa acuta (suppurative, acute).

LOMSC; LOMSCh Left otitis media suppurativa chronica (suppuative, chronic).

lo Na low sodium.

long longitudinal.

LOP Leave on pass; Left occipitoposterior (position of fetus).

LOP (program) Leukeran, Oncovin and Prednisone (Chemotherapy).

LOPS Length of patient's stay (= LOS).

LOQ Lower outer quadrant.

LOR Long open reading (frame); Lorazepam; Loss of righting (reflex).

Lord Lordosis; Lordotic.

LORS-I Level of Rehabilitation Scale - I.

LOS Length of stay (see LOPS); Licentiate in Obstetrical Science; Lipo-oligosaccharide; Low (cardiac) output syndrome; Lower oesophageal segment/ sphincter/ stricture (see LES).

LOSP Lower oesophageal sphincter pressure (see LESP).

LOST Life-or-sight-threatening (disease).

LOT Lateral olfactory tract; Left occipito-transverse (position of fetus - vertex presentation); Lengthened off-time (test); Licensed Occupational Therapist; Low oxygen tension.

Lot; lot Lotion (L. lotio).

LOV Large opaque vesicle; Loss of vision.

LOWBI Low-birth-weight infant ("Low birth-weight infant"/ "Low weight, birth, infant").

LOX Liquid oxygen.

Loz Lozenge.

LP Labile peptide/ protein; Laboratory Practice (journal); Laboratory procedure; Lactic peroxidase; Lamina propria; Landry's paralysis; Laryngopharyngeal; Latent/ Latency period; Lateral plantar/ position/ posterior/ pylorus; Legionella pneumophila; Leukocyte-poor; Leukocytic pyrogen; Lichen planus; Light perception (eye examination); Linear programming; Lingua plicata; Linguopulpal; Lipid proteinosis; Lipoprotein (see Lp); Liver plasma (see L/P); Loss of privileges; Low position/ potency/ power/ pressure/ protein; Lumbar puncture (= LMP); Lumboperitoneal; Lung parenchyma; Lymphocyte predominant; Lymphoid plasma; Lymphomatoid papulosis.

Lp Lipoprotein (= LP); Sound pressure level.

L/P Lactate/pyruvate (ratio) (laboratory/ endocrinology); Liver plasma (concentration) (= LP); Lymph/plasma (ratio); Lymphocyte/polymorph (ratio).

LPA Latex particle agglutination; Lecithin palmitic acid (concentration in the amniotic fluid; it gives an accurate index of fetal pulmonary maturity); Left pulmonary artery; Lysophosphatidic acid.

LP-a; Lp-a Lipoprotein a (related to murine H2 antigen).

LPAM; L-PAM L-phenylalanine mustard.

LPB Low protein binding.

LPB; Lp-B Lipoprotein B.

LPBP Low-profile bioprosthesis.

LPC Laser photocoagulation; Late positive component; Legg-Perthes-Calvé (disease) (growth disturbances at the proximal end of the femur) (Orthopedics); Leukocyte-poor cells (leukocyte depleted); Lipophilic compound; Lipoprotein C (see Lp-C); Low platelet count; Lysophosphatidyl choline.

Lp-C Lipoprotein C (= LPC).

LPCM Low-placed conus medullaris.

LPcP Light perception with projection.

LPCS Light pen control system.

LPCT Late proximal cortical tubule.

LPD Legg-Perthes disease (see LCP; LCPD; LCPS; LPC; OCD; ODJ); Liquid protein diet; Liver parenchymal damage; Low-protein/ purine diet; Luteal phase defect; Lymphoproliferative disease (e.g. Lymphoma)/ disorder (of B cells, a specific subtype of Castleman's disease see CD; PEL).

LPDF Lipoprotein-deficient fraction.

LPE Linear polyethylene (high density); Lipoprotein electrophoresis (laboratory/ chemistry).

LPED Lowest possible effective dose.

LPF Leukocytosis-promoting (or Lymphocytosis-promoting)/ Leukopenia/

Lipopolysaccharide factor; Lipoprotein fraction; Liver plasma flow; Localized plaque formation; Lowpass filter (see LPFN); Low-power field (see lpf).
lpf low-power field (microscopy) (= LPF).
LPFB Left posterior fascicular block.
LPFN Low-pass filtered noise.
LPFS Low-pass filtered signal.
LPG Liquified petroleum gas; Lysophosphoglyceride.
LPH Left posterior hemiblock (ECG); Lipotropic pituitary hormone (see Hormones - LPH).
LPI Laser peripheral iridectomy; Left posterior-inferior; Leukotriene pathway inhibitor; Leukotriene production inhibitor (see LTPI); Lysinuric protein intolerance.
LPIFB Left posteroinferior fascicular block.
LPIH Left posteroinferior hemiblock.
LPK Liver pyruvate kinase.
LPL Lichen planus-like lesion; Lipoprotein lipase; Lysophospholipid.
LPLA Lipoprotein lipase activity.
LPLC Low pressure liquid chromatography.
LPM Lateral pterygoid muscle; Lines per minute (see lpm); Liver plasma membrane; Lymphoproliferative malignancy.
lpm lines per minute (printer) (= LPM); liters per minute (see l/min).
LPMT Life-preserving/ prolonging medical treatment (= LPT).
LPN Laboratory Primate Newsletter; Licensed Practical Nurse; Localized pressure necrosis.
LPNA Licensed Practical Nurse Association.
LPO Lateral preoptic (area); Left posterior oblique; Light perception only (eye examination); Lipid peroxidase (enzyme)/ peroxidation; Lipoperoxide; Lipophilic opioid.
Lpo Nucleus latero-polaris (of the thalamus).
LPP Lateral pterygoid plate; Lichen planopilaris; Lithium powered pacemaker; Low pharmacological potency.
LPPH Late postpartum hemorrhage.
LPPL Lipid peroxide plasma level.
LPPR Laboratory Product Problem Report (USP for FDA).
LPR Lactate-pyruvate ratio; Lead-pipe rigidity (in Parkinsonism); Lipoprotein receptor.
LPRA Low plasma renin activity (see PRA).
LPRBC Leukocyte-poor red blood cells.
LPS Levator palpebrae superioris (muscle); Linear profile scan; Linear programming system; Lipase; Lipopolysaccharide; Liquid protein supplement; Liters per second (see l/sec); "Little professor" syndrome (see GS; ORB; SMC); Low-pressure sodium (lamp).
lps liters per second (see l/sec).
LPSR Lipopolysaccharide receptor.
LPT Licensed Physical Therapist; Life-preserving/ prolonging therapy/ treatment (see LPMT); Lipotropin; Lymphocyte transfer (reaction).
LPV Left portal view; Left pulmonary vein.
LPVP Left posterior ventricular preexication.
LPW Lateral pharyngeal wall; Left posterior wall.
lpw lumens per watt.
LPX; LP-X; Lp-X Lipoprotein-X (abnormally low-density lipoprotein).
LQ Laterality/ Longevity/ Lordosis quotient; Linacre Quarterly; Lower quadrant.
LQTS Long QT syndrome.
LR Labeled release; Labor room; Laboratory reference(s)/ report; Lactated Ringer's (solution); Large reticulocyte; Laryngeal reconstruction; Latency reaction/ relaxation; Lateral rectus (muscle)/ retinaculum; Left rotation; Legislative Roundup (journal); Leprosy Review (journal); Light reaction/ reflex; Limb reduction (defect); Limit of reaction; Limited register (doctor/ medical practitioner - GMC, UK); Lip rehearsal; Logistic regression; Low renin; Lymphocyte recruitment.
Lr Lawrencium (Z = 103) - formerly Lw (see Elements - Lawrencium); Limes reacting dose of diphtheria toxin.
L/R Left-to-right (ratio).
L&R Left and right.
L→R Left to right.
LRA Leukotriene receptor antagonist (e.g. Montelukast) (see CLT; Cys LT1); Linear (drug assay)/ Logistic (see MVLRA) regression analysis; Low right atrium.
LRC Light-resistant container (for medicines); Lipid Research Clinic (NHLI); Lower rib cage; Lymphoreticular cancer/ carcinoma.
LRCP Licentiate of the Royal College of

Physicians; Lipid Research Clinical Program.
LRCPE Licentiate of the Royal College of Physicians, Edinburgh.
LRCPI Licentiate of the Royal College of Physicians, Ireland.
LRCP&SI Licentiate of the Royal College of Physicians and Surgeons in Ireland.
LRCS League of Red Cross Societies; Licentiate of the Royal College of Surgeons.
LRCSE Licentiate of the Royal College of Surgeons, Edinburgh.
LRCSI Licentiate of the Royal College of Surgeons, Ireland.
LRD Lipid-related discipline(s); Living related/ renal donor; Lowest recommended dose; Low residue diet.
LRDT Living related donor transplant.
LRE Lamina rara externa; Leukemic reticuloendotheliosis; Lymphoreticuloendothelial (see L-RE).
L-RE Lymphoreticuloendothelial (= LRE).
LREH Low renin essential hypertension.
LRF Latex and resorcinol formaldehyde; Left rectus femoris; Left ring finger; Leukoreduction filter (blood transfusion); Liver residue factor; Luteinizing hormone-releasing factor (see Hormones - LH-RH).
LRFPS Licentiate of the Royal Faculty of Physicians and Surgeons, Scotland.
LRG Low-risk group.
LRH Luteinizing hormone-releasing hormone (see Hormones - LH-RH).
LRHPB Long-Range Health Planning Branch (DNHW).
LRI Lamina rara interna; Ligand-receptor interaction(s) (see Ligand); Long-range implication; Lower respiratory (tract) illness/ infection; Lymphocyte reactivity index.
LRL Lunar Receiving Laboratory.
LRLT Living-related liver transplantation.
LRM Left radical mastectomy; Low-risk method.
LRMP Last regular menstrual period.
LRN Lateral reticular nucleus.
LRNA Low-renin, normal/ near-normal aldosterone.
LRND Left radical neck dissection.
LROP Lower radicular obstetrical paralysis.
LRP Laparoscopic radical prostatectomy (see LRPB); Lichen ruber planus; Long-range planning; Low density lipoprotein receptor-related protein; Low-risk pregnancy.
LRPB Laparoscopic radical prostatectomy and brachytherapy (= LRP; LSP) (see TUSRI).
L/RPLT Liver/related partial liver transplant.
LRQ Lower right quadrant.
LRR Labyrinthine righting reflex; Light reflection rheograph(y); Low(er) response rate; Lymph return rate.
LRS Lactated Ringer's solution (IV); Lateral recess syndrome; Lidge reducer sleeve (Arthroscopy); Low rate of stimulation; Lumboradicular syndrome; Lymphoreticular system (see RES).
LRSF Lactating rat serum factor; Liver regenerating serum factor.
LRSM Logistic regression survival model.
LRSP Long Range Systems Planning.
LRSS Late respiratory systemic syndrome.
LRT Living-related transplantation; Local radiation therapy; Log-rank test (in statistical analysis) (see M-C); Long terminal repeat; Lower respiratory tract.
LRTI Lower respiratory tract illness/ infection.
LRTKS Link rotating total knee system (Orthopedic implants).
LRV Lassa related virus; Left renal vein.
LRZ Lorazepam.
LS Lady snow (cocaine) (see Erythroxylum); Lambda sign (see TCPS); Lateral septal (nucleus) (see LSN); Lateral suspensor; Layman Speaks (journal); Left sacrum/ septum/ side; Legally separated; Leiomyosarcoma; Lenegre's syndrome (ICSD - Intrinsic conduction system disease); Length of stay; Leriche syndrome; Leukemia Society; Lev's syndrome (Pre-excitation in Idiopathic myocardial hypertrophy or IMH, with fibroelastosis of left ventricle and associated with Wolff-Parkinson-White syndrome); Licentiate in Surgery; Life Sciences (journal); Life-span; Life Suit (a respiratory support system or modern "iron lung"); Light sensitive; Light-sensitivity; Light sleep; Liminal sensation/ sensitivity; Linear scleroderma; Linnean Society; Lipid synthesis;

Liposuction; Liquid scintillation; Liver and spleen (see L&S); Liver scan; Long single (cone of eye) (see LSC); Long sleep; Low-salt/ sodium (diet) (see LSD); Lower strength; Lumbar spine/ sympathectomy; Lumbosacral (see L-S); Lung surfactant; Lymphosarcoma (= LSA).

LS; L/S Late-stage (disease/ disorder/ illness/ infection).

L-S Lumbosacral (= LS).

L/S Lactase/sucrase (ratio); Lecithin/sphingomyelin (ratio) (see L/S ratio); Lipid/saccharide (ratio).

l/s liters per second (see l/sec).

L&S Liver and spleen (= LS).

L5/S1; L5-S1 Lumbar fifth vertebra to sacral first vertebra.

LS 519 Pirenzepine (= Pir; PRZ) - a pyridobenzodiazepine, tricyclic, anti-muscarinic compound, used in the treatment of gastric and duodenal ulcer.

LSA D lysergic acid (see LSD); Large-segment allograft (orthopedic surgery); Latex slide agglutination (test); Left sacroanterior (position of fetus - breech or pelvic presentation); Left subclavian artery; Leukemia Society of America; Leukocyte-specific activity; Licentiate of the Society of Apothecaries (London); Lichen sclerosus et atrophicus (see LS&A); Lipid-bound sialic acid; Lipid-soluble agent (see LSD); Longitudinal Study on Aging (Baltimore); Low systemic activity; Lymphosarcoma (see LS).

LS&A Lichen sclerosus et atrophicus (= LSA).

LSAb Lispro-specific antibody (to Insulin).

LSANA Leukocyte-specific antinuclear antibody.

LSA/RCS Lymphosarcoma-reticulum cell sarcoma.

LSB Least significant bit; Left scapular/ sternal border; Long spike burst.

LS-BMD Lumbar spine bone mineral density.

LSBPS Laparoscopic bilateral partial salpingectomy.

LSC Laser Surgery Center; Late systolic click; Left side (colon) cancer (see LSCC); Lichen simplex chronicus; Life Safety Code; Light-sensing cell(s) (see PRC); Liquid scintillation counter/ting; Liquid-solid chromatography; Long single cone (eye) (= LS; LSG; LSR); Long-standing controversy; Lumbosacral canal/ corset.

LSc Local scleroderma.

LScA Left scapuloanterior (position of fetus - shoulder presentation).

LSCC Left side colon cancer (= LSC).

LSCL Lymphosarcoma cell leukemia.

LSCl Low systemic clearance (in l/min).

LScP Left scapuloposterior (position of fetus - shoulder presentation).

LSCS Lower segment cesarean section.

LSD League for Spiritual Discovery (now defunct); Least significant difference/ digit; Life-saving device; Life-saving/ supporting/ sustaining drug; 'Lifestyle' drug (such as Sildenafil [Viagra] for sexual dysfunction, Finasteride [Propecia] for hair loss, and Orlistat [Xenical] for obesity); Life-support device (see AED; ALSD); Limited susceptibility data; Lipid-soluble drug (= LSA); Long-standing depression/ diabetes/ disease; Low salt/ sodium diet (= LS); Lysergic acid diethylamide: (= $C_{20}H_{25}N_{30}$) - a very powerful psychotropic hallucinogenic compound derived from ergot, and used experimentally in psychotherapy. Extremely dangerous in untrained hands. Other names are: Acid; Beast; big D; Blue acid; Bol-148 (= d-z-bromolysergic acid); Chief; Cube (= LSD-25 on sugar); Deeda (= LSD-25); d-lysergic acid diethylamide ("Acid"); Frisco speedball (mixture of heroin, cocaine, and LSD-25); FS (= Frisco speedball); Ghost (= LSD-25); LSA (= D lysergic acid); LSD 25 (= Lysergide) (see LSD-25); LSH (= Lysergide) (see LSD-25); Lysergide; MGS (Morning glory seeds); Mike (a microgram of illicit LSD); Ticket; Twenty-five (= LSD 25) (see LSD-25); Wedge (a flat LSD-25 tablet - see LSD-25).

LSD-25 Lysergide (= Lysergic acid diethylamide-25; d-lysergic acid diethylamide tartrate-25) - named after the initial weekly dose of 25 μg (micrograms) used in analytical therapy (see LSD).

LSE Laboratory side effect(s); Libman-Sacks endocarditis; Life Support Equipment (Corp); Lipolytic sparing effect (of growth hormones, etc.); Local side effects; Low self-esteem; Low systemic exposure.

l/sec liters per second (= LPS; lps; l/s).

LSEP Left/ Lumbosacral somatosensory evoked potential; Long stay elderly patient.

LSF Line spread function; Low saturated fat; Lymphocyte-stimulating factor (see Hormones - LSH ii).

LSG Labial salivary gland; Long single (cone of eye), green (see LSC).

LSH Lutein-stimulating hormone (see Hormones - LSH i); Lymphocyte-stimulating hormone (see Hormones - LSH ii); Lysergide (see LSD).

LSHTM London School of Hygiene and Tropical Medicine.

LSI Large-scale integrated/ation (digital logic circuit); Local(ized) skin infection/ inflammation/ injury/ irritation; Lumbar spine index.

LSIEL Low-grade squamous intraepithelial lesion (Pap smear).

LSK Liver, spleen, kidneys.

LSKM Liver-spleen-kidney-megalia.

LSL Left sacrolateral (position of fetus - breech position); Left short leg; Lymphosarcoma (cell) leukemia.

LSLF Least squares linear fit (laser measurement).

LSM Late systolic murmur; Liposome - a microscopic phospholipid sac, similar to a cell membrane, used to deliver medicines to diseased tissues in high concentrations (see LUV; MLV; SUV); Life-saving measure(s); Long saltatory movement(s); Lymphocyte separation medium; Lysergic acid morpholide.

LSMS Louisiana State Medical Society.

LSN Latent spontaneous nystagmus; Lateral septal nucleus (= LS); Left substantia nigra.

LSND Long-standing nasal discomfort/ distress/ disturbance/ dryness.

LSO Lateral superior olive; Left salpingo-oophorectomy; Left superior oblique; Lumbosacral orthosis.

LSP Laparoscopic prostatectomy (see LRP; LRPB); Left sacroposterior (position of fetus - breech presentation); Life-saving procedure; Life-span perspective; Light-skinned people/ person; Limb-salvage/-sparing procedure (see LSS); Liver-specific protein; Lumbosacral plexus.

LSp Life span.

L-Spar Asparaginase (Elspar).

LSPN Lesser superficial petrosal nerve.

LSPR Lumbosacral polyradiculopathy (see LSPRP).

LSPRP Lumbosacral polyradiculopathy (= LSPR).

LSR Lanthanide shift reagent; Laser skin resurfacing (Cosm. surgery); Lecithin/sphingomyelin ratio (see L/S ratio); Left superior rectus (muscle); Local skin reaction(s) (such as edema, erosion, erythema, excoriation, flaking, induration, rash, redness, scabbing, ulceration, vesicles, etc.); Limb-sparing resection (see LSS) (Orthopedics); Long single (cone of eye), red (see LSC); Low success rate; Lumbar spinal root; Lumbosacral radiation (of low back pain); Lung scan report.

LSRA Longstanding rheumatoid arthritis; Low septal right atrium.

L/S ratio Lecithin/sphingomyelin ratio - the ratio of the lecithin and sphingomyelin concentration in the amniotic fluid: an index of fetal pulmonary maturity. A value greater than 2.0 is regarded as a sign of adequate production of the surfactant factor (= L/S; LSR).

LSRO Life Sciences Research Office (FASEB).

LSS Laparoscopic surgeon/ery; Lifesaving station; Life support station; Life Support System (see ELSS - Environmental LSS); Limbic system surgery; Limb-salvage/ sparing surgery (= LSP; LSR); Liver-spleen scan; Long scarf syndrome; Long-standing symptom(s); Lumbosacral spine.

LST Lateral spinothalamic tract; Latex slide test (for pregnancy); Left sacrotransverse (position of fetus - breech presentation); Left-sided thoracotomy; Lepromin skin test (for leprosy); Lifesaving therapy/ treatment; Life-Styles Tomorrow (journal); Life-sustaining treatment; Lowered seizure threshold.

LSTC Laparoscopic tubal coagulation.

LSTL Laparoscopic tubal ligation.

L's & T's Lines and tubes.

LSU Lactose-saccharose-urea (agar culture medium); Life support unit.
LSV Lateral sacral vein; Left subclavian vein.
LSVC Left superior vena cava.
LSW Long-stay ward.
LSWA Large amplitude slow wave activity.
LT Labial tumescence; Labile toxin (= Heat-labile bacterial enterotoxin); Laboratory technician; Laminar tomography; Left (see lt); Left thigh; Less than; Lethal time (see LT 50); Leukotriene(s) (e.g. LTA; LTB; LTB4; etc); Levin tube (for gastrointestinal suction); Levothyroxine (see Hormones - TH iiA; LT4); Light (see lt); Long-term; Low temperature/ tension (see lt); Lower tertile (level) (see LTL); Lues (syphilis) test(s) (see STS); Lumbar traction; Lundh test (see PEOT); Lymphocyte transformation; Lymphocytotoxin; Lymphotoxin.
L-T Lunotriquetral (dissociation - of the Lunate and Triquetrum carpal bones; similar to S-L dissociation, but traumatic in origin) (see S-L).
lt counterclockwise; left/ light/ low tension (= LT).
LT-1 Succinylcholine bromide.
LT3; L-T3 L-/Levo-triiodothyronine (see Hormones - TH iiA).
LT4; L-T4 L-/Levo-thyroxine (= LT) (see Hormones - TH iiA).
LT 50 Lethal time for 50% of the population.
LTA Late-term abortion; Lead tetra-acetate; Leukotriene A; Life-threatening arrhythmia; Lipoate transacetylase; Lipotechoic acid; Local tracheal anesthesia; Long-term administration/ approach.
LTAD Life-threatening/ Long-term arterial damage.
LTAE Life-threatening adverse effect(s).
LTAR Life-threatening adverse reaction.
LTAS Lead tetra-acetate Schiff.
LTAT Long-term antibiotic/ aspirin therapy/ treatment.
LTB Laparoscopic tubal banding; Laryngo-tracheo-bronchitis (croup); Leukotriene B/B4 (see LTB4); Long-term benefit(s).
LTB4 Leukotriene B4 (an inflammatory mediator, believed to participate in delayed allergic reponse).
LTC Laboratory Test Category; Large transformed cell; Lateral tibial condyle; Left to count; Less than carload; Leukotriene C/C4 (see LTC4); Lidocaine tissue concentration; Life-threatening cancer/ clot (arterial/ venous)/ complication(s)/ condition; Liver transplantation center; Long-term care/ commitment/ complication(s)/ consequence(s)/ control/ culture/ cure; Long Term Care (Division of - HSR); Loving tender care; Low therapeutic concentration(s).
LTC4 Leukotriene C4 (an inflammatory mediator and most potent bronchoconstricting agent).
LTCF Long-term care facility.
LTCPs L-tryptophan-containing products.
LTCS Low-transverse cesarean section.
LTCT Long term corticosteroid therapy.
LTD Largest tumor dimension; Laron-type dwarfism; Leukotriene D/D4 (see LTD4); Life-threatening danger/ diarrhea/ disease; Long-term data/ diabetes/ dialysis/ disability/ durability; Platinum resistance thermometer.
LtD Less-than-daily (dose).
Ltd Limited.
LTD4 Leukotriene D4 (a mediator with a most potent bronchoconstricting action).
LTDA Long-term drug abuse.
LTDC Long-term disease control/ dosing conditions.
LTDF Long-term differentiated function (of organ cells, such as liver cells, etc.).
LTDO Long-term developmental outcome.
LTDT Long-term drug therapy.
LTE Laryngo-tracheo-esophageal; Leukotriene E/E4 (see LTE4); Life-threatening emergency; Local thermodynamic equilibrium; London Total Elbow; Long-term effect(s)/ efficacy (of a drug/ medication)/ exercise.
LTE4 Leukotriene E4 (an inflammatory mediator: a product of the lipoxygenase pathway).
LT-ECG Long-term electrocardiography.
LTF Lactotransferrin; Lipotropic factor (= Prolactin; PRL) (see Hormones - LH i); Long-term fatigue/ function; Lymphocyte-transforming factor; Lymphocytic transfer factor.
LTFU Long-term follow-up.

LTG Long-term goal.

LTGA Left transposition of great artery.

LTGAs Levo-transposition of the great arteries.

LTH Lactogenic/ Luteotropic hormone (see Hormones - LH i); Life-threatening hemorrhage/ hypoxemia; Local tumor hyperthermia; Low temperature holding.

LTHA Lactose-tolerant healthy adult.

LTHP Long-term health problem.

LTHR Life-threatening hypersensitivity reaction.

LTI Life-threatening illness/ infection; Localized tissue irritation; Long-term illness/ immunity/ infection/ issue; Lupus-type inclusion(s).

LTL Laparoscopic tubal ligation; Left temporal lobe (see SPA); Life-threatening leucopenia; Long-term level; Lower tactile level (= LT).

LtL Layer-to-layer (suture).

lt lat left lateral.

LTM Leukotriene modifier (used in asthma therapy); Life-threatening malformations (Obstetrics); Long-term maintenance/ management/ measure/ memory/ monitor(ing)/ mortality.

LtM Low-to-moderate (dose).

LTMT Long-term maintenance therapy.

LTN Long-term nature.

LTNM Long-term neurologic morbidity/ mortality.

LTO Long-term outcome (of an illness).

LTOI ife-threatening opportunistic infection (see SOI).

LTOT Long-term oxygen therapy.

LTP Laboratory test parameter/ procedure; Laser trabeculoplasty; Last trimester of pregnancy (= TTP); Leukocyte thromboplastin; Liver transplant program; Long-term pain/ palsy/ paralysis/ phase/ planning/ potentiation/ prescribing/ problem/ procedure/ prognosis/ project/ prophylaxis/ prospect/ive/ protection; Long Term Preceptorship; L-tryptophan.

L-TP Lamivudine triphophate (see NSA).

LTPA Leisure-time physical activity.

LTPC Long-term patient compliance.

LTPE Life-threatening psychiatric event (such as attempted suicide, suicidal ideation, etc.).

LTPI Leukotriene production inhibitor (= LPI).

LTPP Lipothiamide pyrophosphate.

LTR Leukotriene receptor (see CLT; CysLT); Liver transplant recipient; Long terminal repeat; Long-term record(s)/ rehabilitation/ relief/ remission/ response/ result(s)/ risk; Low transmission rate.

LtR Left-to-right.

LTRA Leukotriene receptor antagonist.

LTRC Leukotriene receptor antagonist.

LTR gene. Long terminal redundancy gene, a regulatory gene, one of the two genes of the AIDS (HIV-1) genome that contain sequences giving promotor, enhancer and integration signals (see LTRs).

LTRs Long terminal redundancies - stretches of DNA (or DNA sequences) that have a role in controlling the expression of the AIDS virus (three retroviral AIDS genes) (see AIDS).

LTS Laparoscopic tubal sterilization; Leiden Thrombophilia Study; Life-threatening situation/ stress/ stroke; Light-touch sensation; Local tolerance study; Long-term safety (of a drug)/ sequelae/ smoker/ strategy/ stress/ study (of a disease)/ success (of treatment)/ supplementation/ survival/ survivor; Lung-thorax system.

LTSP Long-term strategic plan.

LTT Lactose/ Leucine tolerance test; Lateral tibial tubercle (= Gerdy's tubercle); Limited treadmill test; Long-term therapy/ tinnitus/ treatment/ trial; Lymphoblastic/ Lymphocyte transformation test.

LTTD Long-term tissue destruction (as in viral myocarditis, leading to dilated cardiomyopathy).

LTTS Long-term toxicity study.

LTU Long-term use.

LTV London television; Long-term ventilation; Low(er) tidal volume (ventilation in ALI and ARDS); Luche tumor virus; Lung thermal volume.

LTVA Life-threatening ventricular arrhythmia.

LTW Leydig-cell tumor in Wistar rat.

LU Left upper (limb); Living/ Loudness/ Lytic unit; Lowry unit (see L-unit).

Lu Lowry unit (see L-unit); Lung; Lutetium (Z = 71) (see Elements - Lutetium); Lutheran (blood group).

L&U Lower and upper.

LUA Left upper arm.

LUC Large unstained cell; Lean umbilical cord (area <10th centile Obstetrics).

Lucanth Hydrochlor Lucanthone hydrochloride (see BW 57-233; NSC 14574).

Lu_{creat} Urine creatinine concentration, left kidney (see KFT - Lu_{creat}).

LUE Left upper extremity; Low urinary excretion.

Lues I Primary syphilis (see L I).

Lues II Secondary syphilis (see L II).

Lues III Tertiary syphilis (see L III).

LUF Luteinized unruptured follicle (syndrome) (see LUFS).

LUFS Luteinized unruptured follicle syndrome.

LuH-6 Toxogonin - has been used as an antidote to poisoning by organophosphorus compounds by virtue of its cholinesterase reactivation properties.

Luic Luetic.

LUL Left upper lid (eyelid)/ limb/ lobe/ lung.

lumb lumbar.

lumb- combining form meaning loin (L. lumbus).

LUMD Lowest usual maintenace dose.

LUMO Lowest unoccupied molecular orbital.

LU_{Na} Urine sodium concentration, left kidney (see KFT - LU_{Na}).

L-unit Lowry unit (LU; Lu).

LUO Left ureteral orifice.

LUOB Left upper outer buttock.

LUOQ Left upper outer quadrant.

LUP Left upper pole (kidney); Left uteropelvic.

LUQ Left upper quadrant (abdomen).

LURD Living unrelated donor.

LUS Lower uterine segment.

LUSB Left upper scapular/ sternal border.

LUT Lower urinary tract.

Lut; lut Yellow (L. luteum).

lute- prefix meaning yellow (L. luteus).

Luth Lutheran (Church member).

LUV Large unilamellar vesicle.

LV Laryngeal vestibule; Lateral/ Left ventricle; Lecithovitellin; Left ventricular; Lepromatous variety; Leucovorin; Leukemia virus; Live vaccine/ virus; Low voltage/ volume; Lumbar vertebra; Lung volume.

Lv Brightness or luminance.

lv leave.

LVA Left ventricular aneurysm; Left vertebral artery.

LVAD Left ventricular assist device.

L-VAM Leuprolide acetate - vinblastine, Adriamycin (doxorubicin), and mitomycin.

LVAS Left ventricular assist system.

LVAT Left ventricular activation time.

LVBP Left ventricular bypass pump.

LVC Low-viscosity cement.

LVCS Low vertical cesarean section.

LVD Large vessel disease; Left ventricular dysfunction.

LVDd Left ventricular dimension in end-diastole.

LVDI Left ventricular dimension.

LVDP Left ventricular diastolic pressure.

$LV(dp/dt)_{max}$ Cardiac output.

LVDT Linear variable differential transformer.

LVDV Left ventricular diastolic volume.

LVE Left ventricular ejection/ enlargement.

LVED Left ventricular end-diastole (see LVEDP).

LVEDC Left ventricular end-diastolic circumference.

LVEDD Left ventricular end-diastolic diameter.

LVEDP Left ventricular end-diastolic pressure (= LVED; LVEP).

LVEDV Left ventricular end-diastolic volume.

LVEF Left ventricular ejection fraction.

LVEP Left ventricular end-diastolic pressure (see LVEDP).

LVES Low-vision enhancement system.

LVESD Left ventricular end-systolic dimension.

LVESP Left ventricular end-systolic pressure.

LVESV Left ventricular end-systolic volume.

LVESVI Left ventricular end-systolic volume index.

LVET Left ventricular ejection time.

LVETc Left ventricular ejection time corrected (for heart rate).

LVETI Left ventricular ejection time index.

LVF Left ventricular failure/ function (see LHF); Left visual field; Low voltage fast/ foci.

LVFP Left ventricular filling pressure.

LVG Left ventriculography; Left ventrogluteal; Lymphogranuloma venereum group.

LVH Large vessel hematocrit; Left ventricular hypertrophy.

LVI Left ventricular insufficiency/ ischemia.

LVID Left ventricular internal diameter/ dimension.

LVIDd Left ventricle/cular internal diameter/ dimension diastole.

LVIDP Left ventricular initial diastolic pressure.

LVIDs Left ventricle/cular internal diameter/ dimension systole.

LVIV Left ventricular infarct volume.

LVL Left vastus lateralis; Lennert's variant lymphoma (diffuse, mixed type, malignant lymphoma).

LVLG Left ventrolateral gluteal (site of injection).

LVM Left ventricular mass.

LVMF Left ventricular minute flow.

LVMI Low-velocity-missile injury.

LVMM Left ventricular muscle mass.

LVN Lateral ventricular nerve; Lateral vestibular nucleus; Licensed Visiting/ Vocational Nurse.

LVO Left ventricular obstruction/ outflow.

LVOP Left ventricular outflow pressure.

LVOT Left ventricular outflow tract.

LVP Large volume parenteral (infusion)/ purge; Left ventricular performance/ pressure; Levator veli palatini; Low-vulnerable person; Lysine-vasopressin.

LVPF Left ventricular power failure.

LVPFR Left ventricular peak filling rate.

LVPSF Left ventricular peak systolic pressure.

LVPW Left ventricular posterior wall.

LVR Leucovorin (see LCV); Limb vascular resistance.

LVS Left ventricular strain (see LHS).

LVSD Left-ventricular systolic dysfunction.

LVSEMI Left ventricular subendocardial myocardial ischemia.

LVSF Left-ventricular systolic function.

LVSI Left ventricular systolic index.

LVSO Left ventricular systolic output.

LVSP Left ventricular stroke/ systolic pressure.

LVST Lateral vestibulospinal tract.

LVSV Left ventricular stroke volume (= LVV).

LVSW Left ventricular stroke work (= LVSW).

LVSWI Left ventricular stroke work index (= LVWI).

LVT Left ventricular tension; Lysine vasotonin.

LVV Left ventricular volume (see LVSV); Le Veen valve; Live varicella vaccine/ virus; Live vector/ virus vaccine.

LVW Lateral vaginal wall; Left ventricular wall/ work (see LVSW).

LVWI Left ventricular work index (see LVSWI).

LVWM Left ventricular wall motion.

LVWMI Left ventricular wall motion index.

LVWT Left ventricular wall thickness.

LW Lacerating wound; Lateral wall; Lee-White (method) (see L-W).

Lw Lawrencium (Z = 103) (now Lr) (see Elements - Lawrencium).

L/W; L&W Living and well.

L-W Lee-White (method) (clotting time - see LWCT).

l/w lumens per watt (see lm/W).

L-10-W Levulose 10% in water.

LWBR Light-water breeder reactor.

LWBS Left without being seen.

LWC Leave/ Left without consent.

LWCT Lee-White clotting time (= LW; L-W).

LWK Large white kidney.

LWMEL Leonard Wood Memorial for the Eradication of Leprosy.

LWP Large whirlpool; Lateral wall pressure.

LWR Light-water reactor.

LWT London weekend television.

LX Local irradiation; Lower extremity (see lx).

Lx Latex.

lx larynx; lower extremity (= LX); lux.

LXC Laxative of choice.

LXS Late xerostoma (in head and neck cancer).

LXT Left exotropia.
LY Lactalbumin-yeastolate (culture medium); Lymphocyte (see L.).
Ly Langley (unit of sun's heat); T-cell antigen used for grouping T-lymphocytes into different classes.
ly- combining form meaning loose or soluble (Gr. lyo).
LYDMA Lymphocyte-detected membrane antigen.
LYES Liver yang exuberance syndrome.
LYG Lymphomatoid granulomatosis.
Lym; lym Lymphocyte/tic (see L.).
Lymph Lymphocyte (see L.); Lymphology (ISL journal).
lymph- prefix meaning water (L. lympha).
Lymphos; Lymphs Lymphocytes.
LyNeF Lytic nephritic factor.
lyo lyophilized.
LYP Lactose, yeast, and peptone (agar medium); Lower yield point.
LYS; Lys Lysine; Lytes electrolytes.
-lysis suffix meaning breaking up or dissolving.
LySLk Lymphoma syndrome leukemia.
LysOH Hydroxy-lysine (= Lysine hydroxide).
lytes electrolytes (laboratory/ chemistry).
LZM; Lzm Lysozyme.

M

M Blood factor in the MNS blood group system; Chin (L. mentum); Concentration in moles per liter; Death (L. mors); Dullness (of sound) (L. mutitas); Handful (L. manipulus); J.F. Macfarlan & Co. (Scotland), Reckitt & Sons Ltd. (England) code for experimental substances; Macerate(d)/tion (L. macerare - see mac); Macrocyte (= Gigantocyte/ Megalocyte) - an abnormally large erythrocyte (10^{-12} μ in diameter); Macroglobulin; Magnetization; Male (see Symbols); Malignant (with reference to tumors); Mammillary (nucleus); Manipulus (L.) - a handful; Marital; Married; Masculine; Mass (L. massa); Massage; Maternal (contribution); Matrix; Mature; Maximal/mum; Mean; Meatus; Median; Mediator (chemical/ released in tissues); Medical; Medicine, e.g. Forensic M. (= Legal M) (the application of medical knowledge to questions of law; medical jurisprudence); Medium; Mega (Gr. megas = big or great) - metric prefix for 10^6; million (= mega-), e.g. Mv. = 10^6 volts; Megavolt; A million volts; Megalocyte; Megohm; Membrane; Memory (associative); Mental; Mesial; Metabolite; Metanephrine; Metastasis(es); Meter (= m; Metre) - i. The basic unit of linear measure in the metric system = 39.37 in (approx.) - ii. An apparatus measuring the quantity of anything (electric current, gas, light, etc.), passing through it, e.g. Light M. (an instrument for measuring light in foot candles); Methionine; Methotrexate; Micrococcus; Microfilaria; Microspira; Microspironema; Microsporon; Microsporum; Mil (L.)/ Mille (L.) - Thousand; Milli- (metric prefix for 1/1000) (see m); Million; Minim (L.) - minimum (see Symbols). A unit of capacity (liquid measure = 0.0616 ml); Minute (a unit of time = 60 seconds); Mitochondria; Mitosis; Mix (L. misce); Mixed; Mixture (L. mistura); Mol (see M. Mole); Molar - i. Permanent tooth (see m. molar); ii. Solution/ Pertaining to a mass (L. moles) (not molecular; molar concentration/ weight), e.g. M/10 = tenth molar (strength of a solution in comparison with the molar); Molarity; Mole (= Mol) - that amount of a chemical compound whose mass in grams is equivalent to its formula mass/ concentration of moles per liter (mol/l), e.g. 1 μM = 1 μmol/l; Molecular weight; Moment of force; Monday; Monkey; Monocyte - a large leukocyte (diameter 9-12 μ); Month; Morgan; Morning; Morphine; Mother; Motile; Mouse; Mu (see μ - the twelfth letter of the Greek alphabet; Mucoid (colony/ bacteria) - a group of mucus-like conjugated proteins of animal origin; they include colloid and ovomucoid (also called mucinoid); Mucosa; Mucous; Multipara; Murmur (cardiac); Muscle (L. musculus); Muscular response (wave) to an electrical stimulation of a motor nerve; Mycobacterium; Mycocandida; Mycoplasma; Myeloma/ Macroglobulinemia (component); Myopia (error of refraction); Strength of pole; Thousand (L. mil; mille).

m electron rest mass; electromagnetic moment; magnetic moment/ quantum number; mane (L.) - in the morning; manipulus (L.) - a handful; mass; married; medial/ian; melting (temperature); melts (at) (when followed by a figure denoting temperature); meso-; meta- (Gr.) - after, beyond, or over (see m-) i. change, exchange, transformation; ii. after, next; iii. the 1,3 position in derivatives of benzene, e.g. m-chemical (= metachemical) - beyond the bounds of chemistry; metal (chemistry); metastable (state); meter (Gr. metron; Fr. mètre; Eng. metre) - i. The basic unit of linear measure in the metric system = the distance light travels through space in 1/299,792,458 of a second; ii. An apparatus designed to measure the quantity of anything passing through it, such as gas, electricity, light, etc. (see M. Meter); micro (millionth) = 10^{-6}; μ; 1/1,000,000 (see μ); milk; milli- (metric prefix for 1/1000; 10^{-3}) (= M; mill-; milli-) (L. mille), e.g. mg (= mgm; milligram; 10^{-3} gm; one-thousandth of a gram); minim (= 1/60 of a dram; one drop) (see Symbols); minimum; minute (see M. Minute); misce (L.) mix (see M. Mix); mistura (L.) a mixture (see Mixture); mitte (L.) send; molality; molar (deciduous tooth) (see M. Molar i.); mouth (by) (L. per os); murmur (heart); send (L. mitte).

μ Greek letter mu - the twelfth letter of the Greek alphabet (= M; mu); chemical potential; electrophoretic mobility; heavy chain of immunoglobulin M; linear attenuation coefficient; magnetic moment; mean; micro (prefix) - 10^{-6}; mu (e.g. μg = microgram = 10^{-6} gram); micron (Gr. mikros) small - A unit of linear measure in the metric system (= μm; 10^{-6} meter; 10^{-3} millimeter; micrometer; mu); Microne - A mass of extremely small size visible only with a microscope (= mu); mutation rate; permeability.

♏ minim (L). minimum or least (= m) - a unit of capacity or liquid measure = one drop = 1/60 of a dram (drachm) = 0.0616 milliliter.

m- meta- (in chemical formulas) (see m. meta-); prefix denoting meso-position (see m. meso-).

M_l Left mastoid.

M_1 Mitral first (heart sound); Myeloblast; Slight dullness (auscultation).

M-I First meiotic metaphase.

M2 Right mastoid.

M_2 Dose per square meter of body surface; Marked dullness (auscultation); Mitral second (heart sound); Promyelocyte.

M-2 Vincristine, carmustine, cyclophosphamide, melphalan, and prednisone.

M-II Second meiotic metaphase.

M^2; m^2 Square meter (of body surface) (see sq m).

2-M 2-Microglobulin.

M_3 Absolute dullness (auscultation); Myelocyte at the third stage of maturation.

M^3; m^3 Cubic meter (see cu m).

M/3 Middle third (long bones).

3-M Miller, McKusick, and Malvaux (syndrome) - who first described it.

M_4 Myelocyte at the fourth stage of maturation.

M_5 Metamyelocyte.

M_6 Band form in the sixth stage of myelocyte maturation.

M_7 Polymorphonuclear neutrophil.

m_8 spin quantum number

M/10 Tenth molar solution.

M 81 Thiometon (= Dithiometon) - an organophosphorus insecticide.

M 99 Etorphine hydrochloride - a morphine derivative; highly potent analgesic and a narcotic. Has been tried as a sedative to control large animals.

M/100 Hundredth molar solution.

M 183 Acetorphine hydrochloride - a morphine derivative; highly potent analgesic and narcotic. Same uses as M 99.

M 285 Cyprenorphine hydrochloride - a highly potent narcotic antagonist with actions similar to those of nalorphine. Has been used to antagonize the effects of etorphine (M 99) and acetorphine (M 183).

M - 1960 An insect repellent containing butylethylpropanediol 30%, butylacetanilide 30%, benzyl benzoate 30%, and an emulsifier 10% - used by the US Army for impregnating clothing.

M 4943 Chlorproguanil hydrochloride - an antimalarial drug with a similar action to that of proguanil.

M 5050 Diprinorphine.

MA Machine; Macrolide antibiotic (Azithromycin; Clarithromycin; Erythromycin; etc); Mafenide/ Megestrol acetate; Malignant arrhythmia; Management audit (Branch); Mandelic acid; Manpower Administration (Dept. of Labor); Masseter; Master of Arts (= AM); Mean arterial (blood pressure); Mechanical axis (a line which passes through the femoral head and the center of the ankle); Medical Affairs (journal, now Health Affairs); Medical assistance/ audit/ authorization; Mega-ampere; Megaloblastic anemia; Membrane antigen (cell); Menstrual/ mental age; Mentum anterior (fetal position); Metabolic acidemia/dosis / alkalemia/kalosis; Metatarsus adductus; Meter angle (= ma); Mexican American; Microadenoma; Micro/ Microscopic/ Mixed agglutination; Microaneurysm; Miles Laboratories Inc. (USA) code for experimental substances; Miller-Abbott (tube) - for gastrointestinal suction; Milliampere; Mitochondrial/ Monoclonal antibody; Mitogen activation; Mitotic apparatus;

Moderately advanced; Monoamine; Mothers Anonymous (now Parents Anonymous); Motor/ Motorcycle (see MCA) accident; Multiple action; Mutagenic activity; Myelinated axon.

Ma Mass of atom; Massurium (now Technetium - Tc; Z = 43) (see Elements - Technetium).

mA; ma meter-angle (see MA); milliampere (electrical measurement).

mÅ milliångström.

M/A Male, altered (animal); Mood and/or affect.

μA microampere.

MA-1 A type of respirator.

MA-104 Embryonic rhesus monkey kidney cells.

MA 110 Ectylurea (= Ectylcarbamide; N-2-Ethylcrotonurea) - has been used as a sedative in anxiety and tension states. May cause jaundice, and is contra-indicated in hepatic disease.

MA-111 Embryonic rabbit kidney cells.

MA-163 Human embryonic thymus cells.

MA-184 Newborn human foreskin cells.

MAA Macroaggregated albumin; Maternal-age-associated (disease, infertility, etc.); Medical Alumni Association (US); Medical Assistance for/to the Aged; Melanoma-associated antigen; Moderate aplastic anemia; Modulating-antibody assay (measures the degradation of the acetylcholine receptor) (see SARAA); Monoarticular arthritis; Motility-altering agent (= MAD).

MAAC Medical Assistance/ Assistants' Advisory Council.

MAACL Multiple Affect Adjective Check List.

MAAGB Medical Artists Association of Great Britain.

MAA ^{131}I Macroaggregates of radioactive iodine.

MAAS Multicenter Anti-Atheroma Study.

MAB Man and Biosphere (program - UNESCO); Mean absolute bioavailability; Medical Advisory Board; Metropolitan Asylums Board (GB); Monoclonal antibody (see MAb).

MAb Monoclonal antibody (= MAB; MCA; MCAB).

m-AB m-Aminobenzamide.

MABA Mean absolute bioavailability (see ABA_m).

MABD Metabolic acid-base disorder/ disturbance.

MABP Mean arterial (systemic) blood pressure.

Mabs Monoclonal antibodies.

MAC MacConkey's (broth); Macrocytic (erythrocyte); Macula; Malignancy-associated changes; Malignant astrocytoma; Maximum acceptable/ allowable concentration (of poisons encountered in industry - now TLV); Maximum allowable cost (of a drug, HEW); Mechanical axis cord (Orthopedic implant); Medical Advisory Committee; Medical alert center; Membrane attack complex; Methacrylic acid copolymer; Methotrexate, Actinomycin D (dactinomycin), and cyclophosphamide; Midarm circumference; Military Air Command; Minimum alveolar (see PFT - MAC)/ antibiotic concentration; Mitral annular calcium; Modulator of adenylate cyclase; Monitored anesthesia care; Multiple arthrocenteses (Orthopedics); Mycobacterium avium complex.

mac macerate(d)/tion (L. macerare) (= M; macer).

MACC Methotrexate, Adriamycin (doxorubicin), cyclophosphamide, and CCNU (lomustine).

m accur mix intimately/ very accurately (L. misce accuratissime).

MACD Monoclonal-antibody cancer drug (e.g. Rituximab [Rituxan]) (= MAB; MAb; MCA; MCAB); Mood, Anxiety, and Cognitive Disorders.

MACDP Metropolitan Atlanta Congenital Defects Program.

MACE Methylchloroform chloroacetophenone.

Mace (L. macis) the arillode or dried aril of the seed of the nutmeg tree, Myristica fragrans (family Myristicaceae); it contains a volatile oil, macene - used as a flavoring agent, but in large doses may cause epileptiform convulsions.

macer macerate(d)/tion (L. macerare) (see

mac).

MACH 1 Metronidazole, Amoxycillin, Clarithromycin, Helicobacter pylori 1 week (study/ therapy).

MACHPA Mid-America Comprehensive Health Planning Agency (Kansas City).

mAChR Muscarinic acetylcholine receptor.

Macon Cannabis (see Cannabis).

MACOP-B Methotrexate, Adriamycin (doxorubicin), cyclophosphamide, Oncovin (vincristine), prednisone, and bleomycin.

MACR Mean axillary count rate.

macr- prefix meaning large (Gr. makros).

MACR-2 Muscarinic acetylcholine receptor - 2 (in IDC - Idiopathic dilated cardiomyopathy).

Macro Macromolecules (journal).

macro macrocyte/tic; macroscopic.

MACS Multicenter AIDS Cohort Study.

MACT Myeloablative chemotherapy (= MAT).

MAD Major affective disorder; Malabsorption disorder (= MD); Matched allogeneic donor; Maximum allowable dose; Mean accumulated dose (radiation); Methadone-assisted detoxification; Methandriol; Methylandrostenediol; Mind-altering drug; Minimum average dose; Motility-altering drug (see MAA); Myoadenylate deaminase; Myriad anxiety disorders.

mAD; MADA Muscle adenylate deaminase.

'Mad apple' The English street name for preparations made from *Datura* stramonium and used by drug addicts (see 'Jimson weed').

MADD Mothers Against Drunk Drivers (Inc); Multiple acyl-CoA dehydrogenase deficiency.

MADDS Monoacetyl dapsone (see DADPS; DDS).

MADP Most appropriate diagnostic procedure.

MADRS Montgomery Asberg Depression Rating Scale.

MADU Methyl-amino-deoxy-uridine.

MAE Major/ Minor/ Moderate adverse effect(s); Medical air evacuation; Mind-altering effect (of serotonin-boosters such as MDMA or "Ecstasy", Fluoxetine or "Prozac", Paroxetine or "Seroxat", etc.) (see MAD; SND); Moves all extremities.

MAEDC Michigan Association for Emotionally Disturbed Children.

MAEEW Moves all extremities equally well.

MAEW Moves all extremities well.

MAF Macrophage activating/ activation/ agglutinating/ arming factor (promotes macrophage bactericidal and tumorocidal activity); Maximum atrial fragmentation; Medic Alert Foundation; Minimum audible field; Ministry of Agriculture, Fisheries and Food (UK); Mouse amniotic fluid.

MAFH Macroaggregated ferrous hydroxide.

MAFI Medic Alert Foundation International.

MAFMs Multiple affected family members.

MAFP Michigan Academy of Family Physicians.

MAFs Movement-associated fetal (heart rate) accelerations.

MAG Antiglobulin (to cultured human lymphocytes); Myelin-associated glycoprotein.

Mag Large/ Magnification (see mag); Magnesium (see Mg; Elements - Magnesium).

mag large/ magnification (L. magnus) (= Mag; magn; magnif).

MAGA Male androgenetic alopecia (see MPAGA).

mag cit magnesium citrate (a laxative).

MAGE Mean amplitude of glycemic excursions.

MAGF Male accessory gland fluid.

MAGG Microagglutination (test).

MAggF Macrophage agglutination factor.

MAGIC Microprobe analysis generalized intensity correction(s).

'Magic mushroom' The Liberty cap or *Psilocybe* semilanceata, a species of Gill Fungi of the family *Agaricaceae*, known as such in the UK. It distorts reality and induces hallucination, due to the psychotomimetic alkaloid it contains, Psilocybin (= 4-Phosphoryloxy-NN-dimethyltryptamine).

magn; magnif large/ magnification (see mag).

mag sulf magnesium sulfate (a laxative).

mAH; mA-h milliampere-hours.

MAHA Microangiopathic hemolytic anemia.

mAHA Medial anterior hypothalamic area.

MAHCH Magnesium aluminium hydroxide

carbonate hydrate (monosubstance hydrotalcite) - a non-systemic antacid.

MAHH Malignancy-associated humoral hypercalcemia.

MAHL Mid-area hair loss.

MAHS Medical Aspects of Human Sexuality (journal).

MAI Massive allograph implantation; Maximal/ Microscopic aggregation index; Mild aortic insufficiency; Minor acute illness; Moderate alcohol intake; Movement assessment of infants; Mycobacterium avium intracellulare.

MAIDS Mouse acquired immunodeficiency syndrome.

mAIMS Modified version of the Abnormal Involuntary Movement Scale (in the assessment of tardive dyskinesia & other extrapyramidal disorders).

Maint Maintenance.

MAJ Multiaxial joint (= Articulatio spheroidea) (see BASJ).

Majoon Candy containing hashish or cannabis (see Cannabis).

MAK Methylated-albumin-kieselguhr.

MAKA Major karyotypic abnormality.

MAL Midaxillary line; Mild airflow limitation (in Pulmonary function tests) (see PFT).

Mal Malate; Malfunction; Malignancy.

mal malaise; malposition.

mal- prefix meaning bad, disordered, ill or poor (L. malus).

malac- combining form meaning abnormally soft (Gr. malakos).

maladie-de-Roger Roger's disease, a congenital heart defect (pronounced "ro-zha").

Mal-BSA Maleated bovine serum albumin.

MALG Minnesota antilymphoblast globulin.

Mal Hyp Malignant hypertension.

malig malignant.

MALiMET Master List of Medical Indexing Terms.

Mallory PTAH Mallory phosphotungstic acid-hematoxylin.

MALT Male, altered (animal); Mucosa-associated lymphoid tissue; Munich Alcoholism Test.

MAM Major active metabolite; Medical Aspects of Medicine (journal); Menstrually associated migraine; Methyl-azoxy-methanol (= Methylazomethanol); Middle-aged man/ men.

Mam Mammal.

maM milliampere-minute. A unit of electrical quantity equivalent to that delivered by one milliampere in one minute (= mam; ma-min; m ampmin).

mam milliampere-minute (see maM); myriameter.

M + Am Compound myopic astigmatism (see M + As).

MAMA Mobile automatic metabolic analyzer (see MSFC); Monoclonal antimalignin antibody.

MAM Ac Methylazoxymethanol acetate.

MAMC Mean arm/ Mid-arm muscle circumference.

ma-min milliampere-minute (see maM).

mamm- combining form meaning breast (L. mamma) (see mazo-).

Mammo Mammography.

MAMP Monoamniotic multiple pregnancy.

m amp milliampere. One thousandth part of an ampere.

m amp-min milliampere-minute (see maM).

MAMs Multiple affected members (see MAFMs).

m-AMSA Amsacrine (= Acridinyl anisidide) (see AMSA).

MAN Mannose (see Man); Medial articular nerve; Medic Alert Newsletter; Molecular anatomy (program/ laboratory).

Man Mannose (= MAN); Mantra (TM or Transcendental meditation).

man a handful or manipulate/tion (see manip); morning (L. mane).

man- combining form meaning hand (L. manus).

mand mandible/ mandibular.

mani- combining form meaning mental aberration (Gr. mania).

mania *Form I.* A form of mental disorder characterized by elation, hyper-emotion, hyperirritability, and increased motor activity: Acute hallucinatory mania (= Ganser's syndrome - amnesia, disturbance and hallucinations); Akinetic mania - marked emotional exaltation with decreased psychomotor activity; mania A po'tu - delirium tremens (see under Form II - Potomania); Bell's mania - acute maniacal excitement often leading to fatal exhaustion; Dancing mania - a mental disorder characterized by uncontrolled dancing; Doubting mania (Folie de/ du doute) - pathologic inability to make even the most trifling decisions; emotional mania - a Monomania for one or a few related emotions; Homicidal mania (see under Form II - Phonomania; hanatomania); Hysterical mania - as one of the forms of hysteria; Intellectual mania - a Monomania with one or a few related delusions; mania. Mitis - the mildest form of mania; Periodical mania - of varying duration, at more or less regular intervals; Puerperal mania - following childbirth (see under Form II - Maieusiomania; Tocomania); Ray's mania - so-called moral insanity; Reasoning mania - with perverted ideation; Religious mania - with abnormal/ perverted religious impulses (see under Form II - Hieromania; Theomania); mania Secandi - with undue haste to perform unnecessary surgical procedures (see under Form II - Ergomania); Suicidal mania (see under Form II - Thanatomania); Transitory mania - severe frenzied attacks of short duration; Unproductive mania - maniacal behavior, but the patient's thinking and speech are repressed.

Form II. As a combining form, signifying abnormal and/or obsessive preoccupation with something: Ablutomania - abnormal interest in washing or bathing; Aboulomania (see Abulomania); Abulomania (= Aboulomania) - characterized by emotional weakness or indecision of character; Acromania - marked by great motor activity; Agromania - with inane passion for solitude in or outdoors; Aidoiomania - abnormal sexual desire; Alcoholomania - with maniacal craving for intoxication by alcoholic beverages (see Dipsomania); Amenomania (= Habromania) - insanity with agreeable halucinations; Andromania (= Nymphomania) - exaggerated sexual desire for/in males; Androphonomania - Homicidal insanity; Antipyrinomania - insanity from excessive use of/ maniacal addiction to antipyrine; Bruxomania - neurotic teeth grinding in the waking state; Brychomania (= Bruxomania) - gnashing of teeth; Cacodemonomania - a condition marked by delusions of being possessed by evil spirits; Callomania - a condition marked by delusions of personal beauty; Cheromania - mania characterized by cheerfulness and exaltation; Choleromania - mania seen sometimes in cholera; Choreomania (= Choromania; Dinomania) - Dancing mania; Choromania - a morbid desire to dance (see Choreomania); Cleptomania - an uncontrollable impulse to steal (see Kleptomania); Clitoromania (see Nymphomania); Dacnomania - a morbid impulse to kill; Demonomania - a monomania, in which the patient considers her/him self possessed of devils; Dinomania - Dancing mania (see Choreomania); Dipsomania (= Alcoholomania; Enomania; Methomania; Posiomania; Potomania) - an uncontrollable desire for alcohol and/or other spirituous liquor; Doromania - a morbid desire to give presents; Drapetomania - the insane desire to wander away from home; Dromomania - a mania for roaming (see Ecdemomania); Ecdemomania (= Dromomania; Poriomania) - an insane desire to wander away from home; Ecomania (= Oikomania) - domination towards family members, but humility to those in authority; Eleutheromania - abnormal enthusiasm for freedom; Enomania - i) a periodical or maniacal craving for strong drink (see Dipsomania), ii) Delirium tremens (see Potomania); Enosimania - insanity characterized by extreme terror; Ergasiomania - insane urge to keep on operating/ working (see Ergomania); Ergomania (= Ergasiomania) - i) An insane desire to be continually at work, ii) Undue eargerness to perform surgical operations (= Mania Secandi) (see Tomomania); Eroticomania - an insane interest in the other sex (see Erotomania); Erotographomania - morbid interest in writing love letters; Erotomania (= Eroticomania) - a Sexomaniac, with a morbid exaggeration of/ interest in sexual behavior or reaction; Erythromania - excessive/ uncontrollable blushing;

Esthesiomania - insanity with perversion of the senses; Gamomania - a morbid desire to marry; Graphomania (= Graphorrhea; Scribomania) - an obsessive desire or urge to write; Gynecomania (= Satyriasis) - an excessive venereal impulse in the male; Habromania - an insane gaity or cheerfulness (see Amenomania); Hieromania - a Religious mania with theologic insanity or frenzy (see Theomania); Hydromania - a mental disorder marked by a tendency to commit suicide by drowning; Hypermania - intense mania with overwelming tensions and marked disorientation; Hypomania (= Submania) - a moderate form of mania; Hysteromania - i) Hysterical mania, ii) Nymphomania; Iconomania - morbid interest in images, real or symbolic; Kleptomania (= Cleptomania) - an uncontrollable impulse to steal; Krauomania - a tic marked by rhythmic movements, such as balancing, rotating the head, etc.; Letheomania - narcotic addiction; Logomania - i) Overtalkativeness, ii) Aphasia; Lycomania (= Lycanthropy) - a delusion in which the patient believes her/him self a wolf; Lypemania - a state of morbid depression; Macromania - i) a delusive belief that external objects or one's own possessions are larger than they really are, ii) Delusions of grandeur (see Megalomania); Maieusiomania - Puerperal mania (see Tocomania); Megalomania (= Macromania) - delusions of grandeur; Melomania - an obsessive fondness for music; Mentulomania - Masturbation; Methomania - insanity caused by habitual misuse of alcoholic drinks (see Dipsomania; Potomania); Metromania - i) Nymphomania, and/or ii) a mania for writing verse; Micromania - a delusional belief of self-reduction in importance, personality, size, etc.; Monomania - insanity on a single subject or class of subjects: includes Emotional and Intellectual mania, etc.; Morphinomania (= Morphiomania) - i) A morbid and habitual craving for morphine, ii) Insanity due to the misuse of morphine; Morphiomania (see Morphinomania); Musicomania (= Musomania) - insane fondness for music; Musomania (see Musicomania); Narcomania - i) An insane desire for narcotics (= Narcosomania), ii) Alcoholic insanity; Narcosomania - an insane or pathologic craving for narcotics (see Narcomania); Necromania - a morbid or insane preoccupation with death or dead persons; Nosomania - incorrect or insane belief of having some special disease; Nostomania - Intense or insane nostalgia; Nudomania - an abnormal devotion of/ or urge to, going naked; Nymphomania - exaggerated sexual desire in a female (includes Andromania, Clitoromania, Hysteromania, Metromania, Uteromania); Oikomania - familial domination, but humility to outside authority (see Ecomania); Oligomania - insanity/ mental impairment concerning a few subjects or faculties; Oniomania - a morbid desire to make purchases; Onomatomania - Mental derangement with regard to names or words; Onychotillomania - Neurotic picking at the nails; Opiomania - an insane craving for opium; Opsomania - a craving for some special food; Oreximania - enormous increase in appetite and food intake due to fear of becoming thin; Paramania (= Parathymia) - a perverted, contrary, emotional state with manifestation of joy by complaining; Pathomania - moral insanity; Peotillomania (= Pseudomasturbation) - a ticlike movement consisting of pulling at the penis; Phagomania - an insatiable craving for food (see Sitomania); Phaneromania - an obsession of abnormal and persistent attention to some exterior growth, such as a pimple, wart, etc.); Pharmacomania - an uncontrollable desire to take or administer medicines; Philopatridomania - Uncontrollable desire to return to one's native land; Phonomania - maniacal tendency to commit murder (see Thanatomania); Photomania - maniacal symptoms developing under the influence of light; Phthisiomania (= Tuberculomania) - a morbid belief that one has tuberculosis; Poriomania (= Ambulatory automatism) - an impulsive tendency to wander away from home (see Ecdemomania); Pornographomania - Morbid impulse toward obscene writing; Posiomania (see

Dipsomania; Potomania); Potomania (= Alcoholomania; Dipsomania; Enomania; Mania a po'tu; Posiomania; Tromomania) - i) An abnormal desire to drink, ii) Delirium tremens; Premaniacal - preceding an attack of mania; Pseudomania - i) false or pretended mental disorder, ii) pathologic hypocracy or lying; Pyromania - an obsessive preoccupation with fires; also incendiarism; Scribomania - an obsessive urge or desire to write (see Graphomania); Sebastomania - Religious insanity; Sexomaniac - a person predominantly male, with an abnormal attraction towards the opposite sex (see Eroticomania; Erotomania); Sitomania (= Phagomania) - i) excessive hunger, or insane craving for food, ii) Periodic bulimia; Sophomania - an intense belief in one's own great wisdom. Submania (see Hypomania); Symmetromania - an insane tendency to make symmetrical motions or movements, as of both arms instead of one; Syphilomania (= Syphilophobia) - a delusion or morbid fear of being infected with syphilis; Thanatomania - i) Homicidal mania (= Phonomania) - maniacal tendency to commit murder, or ii) Suicidal mania; Theomania (= Hieromania) - religious insanity, in which the patient believes her/him self inspired by or possessed of divinity; Thyroidomania - a mental disorder associated with hyperthyroidism; Tocomania - Puerperal mania, following childbirth (see Maieusiomania); Tomomania - i) Undue eagerness to perform surgical operations (see Ergomania), ii) An hysterical desire to be operated upon surgically; Toxicomania - an intense desire for poisons, intoxicants, or narcotic drugs; Trichokryptomania (see Trichorrhexomania); Trichomania (see Trichotillomania); Trichorrhexomania (= Trichokryptomania) - a morbid tendency to break off the hair by pinching it with the fingernail; Trichotillomania (= Trichomania) - a morbid impulse to pull out one's own hair; Tristimania (= Melancholia) - a depressed and unhappy emotional state with abnormal inhibition of mental and bodily activity; Tromomania (= Delirium tremens) (see Potomania); Tuberculomania - a morbid fear of tuberculosis (see Phthisiomania); Typhomania - the state of muttering delirium accompanying typhus or typhoid fever, and characteristic of the typhoid state; Uteromania (see Nymphomania); Zoomania - a morbid love of animals.

manifest manifestation.

manip a handful or manipulate/tion (L. manipulus) (= man).

MANOVA Multivariate analysis of variance.

man pr; man prim early in the morning (L. mane primo).

MANT Monoamine neurotransmission/mitter.

MANTA Middle Atlantic Neutron Therapy Association.

MANTRA Monitoring and Actualization of Noetic Training in Cardiovascular Medicine (Noetic therapy does not use drugs, devices, or surgery - but does employ relaxed breathing, yoga exercises, music, prayer, "hands-on"/ "healing touch" procedures, etc., in reducing stress.

manuf manufacture.

MANZ Medical Association of New Zealand.

MAO Massive accidental overdosage/dose; Master of the Art of Obstetrics; Maximal/imum acid output; Minneapolis Age and Opportunity (Center); Mitochondrial antioxidant (e.g. Lipoic acid); Monoamine oxidase.

MAOA Methaqualone; Monoamine oxidase A (an enzyme that breaks down three important neurotransmitters or chemicals in the brain: dopamine, norepinephrine, and serotonin.

MAOB Monoamine oxidase B.

MAOGP Michigan Association of Osteopathic General Practitioners.

MAOI Monoamine oxidase inhibitor.

MAOP Michigan Association of Osteopathic Physicians.

MAOT Member of the Association of Occupational Therapists.

MAP Macro/Micro angiopathy; Malignant atrophic papulosis; Maximal aerobic power; Mean airway/ aortic/ arterial pressure; Measurement assurance program (NBS); Mediastinal adenopathy; Medical Art Program (MCRM - UCLA); Medical assistance program (AID); Medical Assistance

Programs, Inc.; Medical Audit Program (utilization review); Megaloblastic anemia of pregnancy; Mercapturic acid pathway; Methyl acceptor protein; Methylacetoxyprogesterone; Methyl alcohol poisoning; Methylaminopurine; Microtubule-associated protein; Middle-aged patient; Mildly asthmatic patient; Minimum audible pressure; Mitogen-activated protein (kinase); Mitomycin, Adriamycin (doxorubicin), and Platino (cisplatin); Mitral anuloplasty; Modular assembly protheses; Monoamniotic pregnancy (Obstetrics); Monophase/ Motor (nerve)/ Muscle action potential; 'Morning after' pill (contraceptive, within 72 hours of unprotected coitus); Mouse antibody production.

MAPA Medical Alliance for Political Action; Muscle adenosine phosphoric acid.

MAPC Migrating action potential complex.

MAPF Microatomized protein food.

MAPI Microbial alkaline protease inhibitor; Millon Adolescent Personality Inventory.

MAPJ Metal-and-plastic joint (JRS - Joint replacement surgery).

MAPL Micro-Aire Pulse Lavage (Orthopedics).

MAPLS Maternal antiphospholipid syndrome (found in Neonatal lupus with CCHB or Congenital complex block in the fetus).

MAPP French - Marche à petit pas: small dance steps i.e. shuffling short steps, as in senile gait syndrome (see SGS).

MAPPCOM Mountains and Plains Perinatal Communications.

MAPPS Matrix Print/ Plot System.

MAPRL Memory, attention, praxis, reason, and language (psychometric assessment score).

MAPS Make a Picture Story (psychology test).

MAPWP Medical Association for the Prevention of War Proceedings.

MAR Main admissions room; Marasmus; Marrow; Maximal aggregation ratio; Medication administration record; Mild allergic reaction; Mineral apposition rate (of cancellous bone at implantation site); Minimal angle resolution; Mixed antiglobulin reaction; Muscarinic acetylcholine receptor.

Mar March.

mar margin; marker (chromosome).

MARC Multifocal and recurrent choroidopathy.

MARCER Mid-America Regional Council Emergency Rescue.

marche à petit pas French - small dance steps (see MAPP; SGS).

MARCO Medical Amateur Radio Concil.

MARCOM Mid-Atlantic Regional Conference in Occupational Medicine.

MARGMNP Medicine: Analytical Reviews of General Medicine, Neurology, and Pediatrics.

MARGO Lung margin.

MARP Medically assisted reproduction program.

MARS Mouse anti-rat serum.

MARU Middle America Research Unit.

Mary Morphine (see Papaver).

Mary Ann Marijuana (see Cannabis).

Mary Jane Marijuana (see Cannabis).

MAS Malabsorption syndrome; Male Aging Study (Massachusetts, US); Manifest Anxiety Scale (Taylor); Managed appraisal system (GMP, GMC, UK); Masters-Allen syndrome (see AMS; UJC); Maternal antiphospholipid syndrome (see APLS; MAPLS); McCune-Albright syndrome; Mean after-survival (time) - radiation; Mean Arthritic Score; Meconium aspiration syndrome; Medical advisory service; Medical Aid Schemes (South Africa); Mesoatrial shunt; Microassay scanner (such as nucleic acid); Milk-alkali syndrome; Milliampere-second (see MaS); Minor axis shortening; Mobile arm support; Monkeberg's arteriosclerosis (a form of arteriosclerosis in which many calcium deposits are found in the artery lining) (= Medical AS); Monoclonal antibodies (= MCABs); Morgagni-Adams-Stokes (syndrome); Motion analysis system; Mullerian adenosarcoma (uterus); Multiple animal/ application studies/dy; Multisite agent-specific (anesthetics).

MASCC Multinational Association of Supportive Care in Cancer.

MaS; mA-s; ma-s Milliampere-second - Unit of X-ray exposure (= MAS; mas).

mas masculine (see masc); milliampere-second (see MaS); milliarcsecond.
M + As Compound myopic astigmatism (= A + Am).
MASA Medical Association of South Africa/ the State of Alabama.
masc masculine (= mas); mass concentration (= massc).
MASER Microwave amplification by stimulated emission of radiation (radiation therapy).
MASH Male Anglo-Saxon Heterosexual; Members of Arthritics for Self-Help; Mobile Army Surgical Hospital; Mobilization for Adolescent Student Health (New York); Multiple automated sample harvester.
Mash Allah Opium (see Papaver).
mas pil pill mass (L. massa pilularum).
mass massage.
massc mass concentration (see masc).
MAST Michigan Alcoholism Screening Test; Military antishock trousers; Military Assistance to Safety and Traffic.
mast mastectomy; mastoid.
mast- combining form meaning breast (Gr. mastos).
MASTA Medical Advisory Service for Travellers Abroad.
MASU Mobile Army Surgical Unit.
MAT Manual arts therapist; Master of Arts in Teaching; Mean absorption time; Medical assistance (emergency) team; Medication administration team; Mental Abilities Test (assesses intellectual functioning); Methionine adenosyltransferase; Metropolitan Achievement Test; Microagglutination test; Microarray analytical technique; Miller Abbot tube (General Surgery); Miller Analogy Test; Monoamniotic twin (Obstetrics); Monoclonal-antibody therapy (for cancer) (see MCAB); Motivation Analysis Test; Multifocal atrial tachycardia; Multiple agent therapy; Myeloablative therapy (see MACT).
Mat; mat Maternal (origin); Maternity; Mature.
mat gf maternal grandfather.
mat gm maternal grandmother.
math mathematical/cs.
Mat med Materia medica. That branch of medical study dealing with drugs, their properties, sources and uses.
Mat Med Pur Materia Medica Pura - Samuel Hahnemann's work on 61 drugs, forming the basis of the Homeopathic materia medica.
MATSA Marek-associated tumor-specific antigen.
matut in the morning (L. matutinus).
MAV Mean apparent volume; Mechanical auditory ventricle; Mild/ Moderate acne vulgaris; Minimum apparent viscosity; Movement arm vector; Myeloblastosis-associated virus.
MAVIS Mobile artery and vein imaging system.
MAVR Mitral and aortic valve replacement.
MAW Middle-aged woman/ women.
max maxilla(ry); maximal/imum.
MaxEP Maximum esophageal pressure.
MAYDAY Cardiopulmonary resuscitation (or other heroic measures).
mazo- prefix meaning breast (Gr. mazos) (see mamm-).
MB Bachelor of Medicine (L. Medicinae Baccalaureus) (= BM); Buccal margin (see BM); Isoenzyme of creatine kinase containing M and B subunits (see MB-CK); Mallory/ Mammillary body; Manipulative behavior; Mansfield balloon (Coronary angioplasty); Marsh-Bender (factor) - an ATP inhibitor in muscle tissue (see MBF); Maximum breathing; May and Baker Ltd (England) code for experimental substances (see M&B); Medicus bed (for decubitus care); Medulloblastoma; Megabyte; Membrane Biology (journal); Mesiobuccal; Methyl bromide; Methylene blue (see MeB); Microbiological assay; Million barrels (of oil); Muscle balance; Muscle biopsy; Muscle brain (hybrid CPK isoenzyme, also known as CPK-2, found in blood after myocardial infarction, see CPK-2); Myocardial band.
Mb Megabase (= 10,000,000 base pairs) (see bp); Megabit (10^6 bits of computer memory); Mouse brain; Myoglobin.
mb millibar (= mbar); mix well (L. misce bene).
μb microbar (= μbar).
μ_B Bohr magneton.

M&B May and Baker Ltd (England) code for experimental substances, some commonly incorporated as trade names for various drugs (= MB).
M&B 693 Sulphapyridine (= Sulfapyridine; Sulphapyrid) - one of the original sulphonamides, now superceded by less toxic chemotherapeutic agents, such as sulfadiazine and sulfamethoxazole.
M&B 693 Soluble Sulfapyridine Sodium (= Soluble Sulphapyridine; Sulphapyridinum Natrium) - a form of sulfapyridine suitable for the preparation of solutions for intravenous injection.
M&B 744 Stilbamidine Isethionate - an antiprotozoal and antifungal drug, now superceded by pentamidine (see M&B 800) in the treatment of trypanosomiasis, blastomycosis and kala-azar, because of the occurrence of trigeminal neuropathy. The effect of stilbamidine on the trigeminal nerve has been utilized to relieve tic douloureux.
M&B 760 Sulfathiazole (= Norsulfazol; Sulfanilamidothiazolum; Sulfathiazolum; Sulfonazolum; Sulphathiaz; Sulphathiazole) - a chemotherapeutic sulfa drug, rapidly absorbed when given by mouth, and more rapidly excreted than sulfanilamide, sulfadimidine, and sulfadiazine, a single dose being almost completely excreted in 24 hours.
M&B 800 Pentamidine Isethionate (= Pentamid Isethion; Pentamidini Isethionas) - effective in the treatment of early cases of African trypanosomiasis; also used in the treatment of leishmaniasis.
M&B 2050 A Pentolinium Tartrate (= Pentolin Tart; Tartrate de Pyrroplegium; Pentapyrrolidinium Bitartrate) - a ganglion-blocking agent used in the treatment of moderately severe to malignant hypertension.
M&B 2948 A Amphotalide (= RP 6171) - used in the treatment of schistosomiasis, especially in Schistosoma hematobium infections.
M&B 4180 A Isometamidium Hydrochloride - a trypanocide used in veterinary medicine.
M&B 4438 Sulfasomizole (= Sulphasomizole; TH 2132) - a sulfonamide compound used in the treatment of throat and urinary infections.
M&B 5062 A Amicarbalide Isethionate - a drug used in veterinary medicine for the treatment of bovine babesiasis.
M&B 8430 Clorexolone (= 5-Chloro-2-cyclohexyl-1-oxo-6-sulphamoyl-isoindoline: $C_{14}H_{17}ClN_2O_3S$) - a diuretic used in the treatment of hypertension, as an adjuvant to other antihypertensive agents.
MBA Mallory body antigen; Master of Business Administration; Mechlorethamine (a war gas); Methods of Biochemical Analysis (journal); Methylbenzyl alcohol; Methyl bovine albumin; Mind-body approach (to enhance healing) (see SRT).
MBAC Member of the British Association of Chemists.
M-BACOD Methotrexate, (Calcium Folinate/ Leucovorin or CF - Citrovorum factor/ Folinic acid), bleomycin, Adriamycin (doxorubicin), cyclophosphamide, Oncovin (vincristine), and dexamethasone.
MBAR Myocardial beta adrenergic receptor.
mbar millibar (see mb).
μbar microbar (see μb).
6MB Six meal bland (diet) (diet order).
MBAS Methylene blue active substance.
MBB Modified barbiturate buffer; Mucus-bicarbonate buffer.
MBC Male breast cancer; Mature blood cell; Maximal/mum bladder capacity; Maximal/mum breathing capacity (now MVVF) (see PFT - MBC; MVVF); Metastatic bladder/ bone/ brain/ breast cancer; Methotrexate, bleomycin, and cisplatin; Methylthymol blue complex; Microcrystalline bovine collagen; Minimum bactericidal concentration.
MB-CK Isoenzyme of creatine kinase containing M and B subunits.
MBCL Monocytoid B-cell lymphoma.
MbCO Carbon monoxide myoglobin.
MBD Malignant breast disease; Marchiafava-Bignami disease; Maximal bone density; Maximum bactericidal dilution; Mental Deterioration Battery; Metabolic bone disease; Methoxybenzylamino nitrobenzoxadiazole; Methylene blue dye; Minimal/ Minor brain damage/ dysfunction; Morquio-

Brailsford disease; Mosquito-borne disease (such as dengue or breakbone fever, malaria, West Nile fever, yellow fever, etc.); Multibacillary disease (as in leprosy).

MBDG Mesiobuccal developmental groove.

MBE Medical and Biological Engineering (IFMBE journal); Medium below elbow.

MBEH Monobenzyl ether of hydroquinone (= Monobenzone; p-Benzyloxyphenol) - an ointment prepared by the Royal Free Hospital, London and used locally as a depigmenting agent in Addison's disease and pregnancy.

MBEST Modulus blipped echo-planar single-pulse technique.

MBF Marsh-Bender factor (= MB factor) - an ATP inhibitor in muscle tissue; Mean/ Medullary/ Muscle/ Myocardial blood flow; Meat base formula.

MBFC Medial branch fascial compartment.

MBFLB Monaural bifrequency loudness balance.

MBG Mean blood glucose; Medicine Book Guide (journal); Morphine-benzedrine group (scale).

MBH Medial basal hypothalamus.

MBH_2 Reduced methylene blue.

MBI Marine Biomedical Institute; Maslach Burnout Inventory; Maximum blink index; Metabolism-based interaction; Methylene blue installation; Minor bronchial irritation.

M-BIC Minorities-Barriers Identification Contract (ASAHP).

MBK Methyl-n-butyl ketone (industrial poison).

MBL Major/ Massive/ Menstrual/ Minimal/ Minor blood loss; Marine Biological Laboratory (Woods Hole, Massachusetts); Metallo-beta-lactamase; Minimal/mum bactericidal level; Multibacillary leprosy (the more severe form of Hansen's disease or Leprosy, with six or more skin patches, and cured with a combination of the rifamycin antibiotic, Rifampicin and other antibacterial agents, such as Clofazimine, Minocycline, and/or the fluoroquinolone antibiotic Moxifloxacin, within twelve months see PBL).

MBLA Methylbenzyl linoleic acid; Mouse-specific bone-marrow-derived lymphocyte antigen.

MBM Magnetic bubble memory; Mechanism-based model; Mind-Body Medicine; Mineral basal medium; Mother's breast milk; Mouse bone marrow.

MbM Meal-by-meal (glycemic control therapy in diabetics).

MBMCA Mouse bone marrow clastogenic assay.

MBMI Mean body mass index (kg/m^2).

MBMMA Mouse Bone Marrow Micronucleus assay.

MBN Medical benefits notice (Medicare).

MBNOA Member of the British Naturopathic and Osteopathic Association.

MBNW Multiple-breath nitrogen washout.

MBO Male body obsession (or the Adonis complex); Management by objective; Mesiobucco-occlusal.

MBO_2 Oxymyoglobin.

MBP Major basic protein (an eosinophil protein produced as a delayed response in bronchial asthma); Male breast pain; Maltose-binding protein; Maternal/ Mean blood pressure; Mechanical (non-specific) back pain (see MLBP); Melitensis, bovine, porcine (antigen) - an antigen prepared from Brucella melitensis, B. bovis, and B. suis, for use in the treatment of brucellosis; Mesiobuccopulpal; Metastatic bone pain; Myelin basic protein.

MBPD Medical and Biological Physics Division (CAP - Canadian Association of Physicists).

MBPS Multigated blood pool scanning.

Mbps Megabit per second (see Mb/s).

MBq Megabecquerel.

MBR Methylene blue, reduced.

MBR 4197 Flucrylate (tissue adhesive).

MBRT Methylene blue reaction/ reduction time.

MBS Martin-Bell syndrome; Maximal bone strength; Mindblindness syndrome (= autism) (see PDD); Monobromo-salicylanilide.

Mb/s Megabit per second (computer data rate) (= Mbps) (see Mb).

MBSA Methylated bovine serum albumin.

MBSC MindBodySpirit Connection.

MBT Malignant bone/ brain tumor; Manual Bulletin Transmitted; Medical Bulletin on

Tobacco; Mercaptobenzothiazole; Mind-body technique; Mixed bacterial toxin; Molecular biological technique.

MBTE Meningeal tick-borne encephalitis.

MBTFA Methyl-bis-trifluoro-acetamide.

MBTH 3-Methyl-2-benzothiazoline hydrazone.

MBTS Dithio-bis-benzothiazole.

MBVA Medical Bulletin of the Veterans' Administration.

MBVG Methylene blue 5%, Gentian violet 5%.

MC Magic Carpet (DDA journal); Malpractice Commission (HEW); Mary Caterall (mask) (see MC mask); Mass casualties; Mast cell (on blood smear); Master of Surgery (L. Magister Chirurgiae) (see MCh); Maximum concentration; Mayo Clinic; Medicaid; Medical Care (APHA journal); Medical Center/ Corps; Medical Chronicle/ Counterpoint (journals); Medical Communications (AMWA journal); Medicare; Medium chain; Medullary cavity/ cyst; Megacolon; Megacoulomb; Melanoma/ Merkel's/ Monkey/ Mononuclear/ Mucous cell Menstrual/ Mitotic cycle; Mercy Corps (see MCI); Mesiocervical; Mesocaval (shunt); Metacarpal (joint); Metatarso-cuneiform; Metcoff count (method of assay of urinary creatinine); Methyl cellulose; Microcephaly; Microcirculation; Midcapillary; Midwives Chronicle (RCM journal); Millicurie (see mC); Mineralo-corticoid (see M-C); Minimal change; Mitomycin C; Mitoxantrone and cytarabine; Mitral commissurotomy; Mixed cellularity/ cryoglobulinemia; Molluscum contagiosum; Monochrometer; Monocomponent (highly purified pork insulin) (see MCI; Insulin - MC); Mouth care; Mychosis coli (= Spastic colon diverticulosis); Mylar catheter (used in coronary angiography); Myocarditis; Myotonia congenita.

Mc Megacurie (= 10^6 curies; one million curies); Megacycle (= 10^6 cycles per second) now Mhz (see Mhz).

mC millicoulomb; millicurie (= 10^{-3} curie; MC; mC; mc; MCU; one thousandth of a curie) (radioactivity measurement).

mc millicurie (see mC).

μc microcurie (= 10^{-6} curie; one millionth of a curie) (= μCi).

μC microcoulomb (= μcoul).

M/C Male, castrated (animal).

M-C Magovern-Cromie (prothesis) (see M-CP); Mantel-Cox (log-rank test) (for drug mean retention time); Medico-Chirurgical; Mineralocorticoid (with reference to the adrenal cortical hormones) (= MC).

M&C Morphine and cocaine (drug addiction) (see Erythroxylum; Papaver).

MCA Major coronary artery; Manufacturing Chemists Association; Marrow-containing autograft; Maternity Center Association; Medical care administration; Medical Correctional Association; Medicines Control Agency (GMC, Brit); Megestrol, cyclophosphamide, and Adriamycin (doxorubicin); Methylchloroanthrene; Methylcholanthrene; Metric Conversion Act (of 1975); Middle cerebral aneurysm/ artery; Monoclonal antibiotic (e.g. Muromonab)/ antibody (see MAb); Motion capture analysis; Motorcycle accident (= MA); Multichannel analyzer; Multiple congenital abnormalities/ anomalies.

MCA-10 Methylchloroanthrene-induced fibrosarcoma.

MCAAP Medical College Admissions Assessment Program (AAMC).

MCAB Monoclonal antibody (see MAb).

MCABs Monoclonal antibodies (see MAS).

MCAD Mast cell activation disorder (= MCD); Medium chain acyl-CoA dehydrogenase.

MCAE Most common adverse event.

MCA/MR Multiple congenital anomalies/ mental retardation (syndrome).

MCAO Middle cerebral artery occlusion.

MCAR Mixed cell agglutination reaction.

MCAS Medical College Application Service; Middle cerebral artery syndrome.

MCAs Multiple congenital anomalies (such as Ectopic bone formation, Microdactyly of the thumbs and big toes, Hypospadias, Bilateral ectopic testes, Myositis ossificans progressiva, Fusion of cervical vertebrae, Secxual infantilism, etc.) (Orthopedics).

MCAT Mammalian chromosome aberration

test; Mean corpuscular average thickness; Medical College Admission/ Aptitude Test; Middle cerebral artery thrombosis.

m caute mix cautiously/ with caution (L. misce caute).

MCB Major cognitive breakthrough; Mason/ Menninger Clinic Bulletin; Membranous cytoplasmic bodies/ body; Molecular and Cellular Biochemistry (journal); Mutant cell bank (NIA).

McB McBurney's (point) (see McB pt).

MCBC Metropolitan Chicago/ Michigan Community Blood Center; Multicenter baseline-controlled (see MCBCS).

MCBCS Multicenter baseline-controlled study.

mCBF Mean cerebral blood flow.

MCBM Muscle capillary basement membrane.

MCBO Multiple-coronary-bypass operation.

McB pt McBurney's point (= McB).

MCBR Minimum concentration of bilirubin.

MCC Macrophage/ Monocyte cell culture; Mammalian cell culture (medium); Marked cocontraction; Mean corpuscular (hemoglobin) concentration (see MCHC); Medial cell column; Meta-cerebral cell; Metastatic colorectal cancer; Metastatic cord compression; Microcrystalline collagen; Midstream clean-catch (urine sample); Minimum complete-killing concentration; Most common cause; Mucociliary clearance; Mucocutaneous candidiasis.

MCc Limiting living concentration/ population-density of microorganisms possible in any fluid culture medium (see C. Concentration).

McC McCarthy (panendoscope) - a foroblique cystoscope which gives a wide view of the urinary bladder.

MCCD Minimum cumulative cardiotoxic dose; Modern Concepts of Cardiovascular Disease (AHA journal); Multicentric Castleman's disease (e.g. of the plasma-cell type).

MCCHA Multi-channel compression hearing aid.

MCCNU Methyl CCNU or Semustine (see Methyl CCNU).

MCCT Multicenter clinical/ controlled clinical trial.

MCCU Mobile coronary care unit.

MCD Mad Cow Disease (see CJD); Magnetic circular dichroism; Managed-care doctor (= MCP); Mast-cell degranulation/ disorder (see MCAD); Mean cell/ corpuscular diameter; Mean claudication distance; Mean of consecutive differences; Median control death; Medullary collecting duct; Medullary cystic disease; Metabolically-induced coronary (vaso)dilatation; Metacarpal cortical density; Microzone computing densitometer; Minimal cerebral dysfunction; Minimal change disease; Mitchondrial disease/ disorder; Multicentric Castleman's disease; Multiple carboxylase deficiency; Muscle carnitine deficiency; Muscle cell disease; Myocardial-cell damage.

mCd; mcd millicurie-destroyed.

MC-DA Monochorionic-diamniotic (gestation, in multifetal pregnancy).

MCDH Municipal Contagious Disease Hospital.

MCDI Minnesota Child Development Inventory.

MCDK Multicystic dysplastic kidney.

MCDP Memphis Chronic/ Methadone Chest Disease Program.

MCDT Mast cell degranulation test.

MCE Major cardiac/ coronary event; Manual core endarterectomy; Manually Coded English; Mean color energy (Ultrasound see ICE); Medical care evaluation; Metabolism, Clinical and Experimental (journal); Metacarpal echindromata (Orthopedics); Multicystic encephalopathy; Multiple cartilaginous exostosis.

MCEI Minnesota Committee for Environmental Information.

M cell Microfold cell (an antigen presenting cell in the dome of a Peyer's patch).

MCES Multiple cholesterol emboli syndrome.

MCF Macrophage chemotactic factor; Managed-care facility; Median cleft face; Medical Care Foundation; Medium corpuscular fragility; Mega/ Million cubic feet (of gas); Microcomplement fixation; Minicentrifuge; Mitochondrial function;

Moderate cardiac failure; Mononuclear cell factor; Most comfortable frequency (of phonation); Motor control function; Myocardial contractile/ion force; Thousand cubic feet of gas (kCF preferred).

MCFA Medium-chain fatty acid; Miniature centrifugal fast analyzer.

MCFP Mean circulating filling pressure.

MCG Magnetocardiogram; Medical College of Georgia; Membrane coating granule; Monoclonal gammopathy.

mcg; mcgm microgram (see μg) (after mg; mγ).

MCGC Metacerebral giant cell.

MCGCA Mitotic Crossover and Gene Conversion Assay (*Saccharomyces* cerevisiae).

MCGF Mast cell growth factor.

MCGH Milwaukee County General Hospital.

MCGN Mesangiocapillary/ Minimal change/ Mixed cryoglobulinemia with - glomerulonephritis.

MCGs Membrane-coating granules.

MCH Marrow-containing homograft (Orthopedics); Maternal and Child Health; Mean corpuscular hemoglobin (= MCHb; MCHg; MCHgb); Milwaukee County Hospital; Muscle contraction headache; Myocardial hypoxia.

MCh Master of Surgery (L. Magister Chirurgiae) (= MC; MChir; MS; MSurg).

mCh millicurie-hour. A unit of dose equivalent to that obtained by exposure for one hour to radioactive material, disintegrating at the rate of 3.7 x 10^7 atoms per second (= mch; μch; mc-h; mchr; mc-hr; MCi-hr).

mch; μch; mc-h millicurie-hour (see mCh) (= μC-hr; μCi-hr).

MCHB Maternal and Child Health Bureau (CoN).

MCHb Mean corpuscular hemoglobin (see MCH).

MCHC Maternal and child health care; Mean corpuscular hemoglobin concentration (= HbE - Hemoglobin entity; MCC)/ count; Microhematocrit (test).

MChD Master of Dental Surgery (= MDS).

MCHg; MCHgb Mean corpuscular hemoglobin.

MChir Master of/in Surgery (see MCh).

MCHN Maternal and child health nursing.

MChOrth Master of Orthopaedic Surgery.

MChOtol Master of Otology.

MCHP Medcenter Health Plan.

MCHR Medical Committee for/on Human Rights.

mchr; mc-hr millicurie-hour (see mCh).

μC-hr microcurie-hour (see μch).

MCHS Maternal and Child Health Service(s).

MChS Member of the Society of Chiropodists.

MCI Major/ Minor clinical importance; Mean cardiac index; Medical contraindication; Mercy Corps International (UN); Methicillin; Mild cognitive impairment (early/ preclinical Alzheimer's disease); Monocomponent insulin (= MC insulin; see Insulin - MCI); Mucociliary insufficiency; Multicenter investigation.

MCi Megacurie (= 10^6 curies).

mCi millicurie (= 10^{-3} curie) (see mC).

μCi microcurie (see μc).

MCIC Medical Care Insurance Commission; Metals and Ceramics Information Center (Columbus, Ohio, USA).

MCICU Medical coronary intensive care unit.

MCi-hr millicurie-hour (see mCh).

μCi-hr microcurie-hour (see μch).

MCINS Minimal change idiopathic nephrotic syndrome.

MC insulin see MCI; Insulin - MCI.

MCJ Metacarpal/ Metacarpocarpal joint (see CMJ); Midcarpal joint (= Articulatio mediocarpea); Mucocutaneous junction.

MCK Multicystic kidney (see UMK).

MCKD Multicystic kidney disease.

MCL Macrocyclic lactone (an ISA or Immunosuppressive agent such as Rapamycin or Sirolimus, with the molecular formula $C_{51}H_{79}NO_{13}$, and produced by *Streptomyces* hygroscopicus); Maximum containment laboratory; Medial collateral ligament; Midclavicular/ Midcostal line; Minimal change lesion; Mixed cell lymphoma (see MCTL); Mixed culture, leucocyte (see MLC); Modified chest lead (ECG); Most comfortable (listening/ loudness) level; Mucocutaneous leishmaniasis (= American l.;

Chiclero's ulcer; Espundia; Forest yaws; New World leishmaniasis; Uta); Myelomonocytic chronic leukemia (= MLC).
mcl microliter (see ìl).
MCLD Metachromatic leucodystrophy.
MCLNS; MCLS Mucocutaneous lymph node syndrome (= KD - Kawasaki's d; MLNS).
MClSci Master of Clinical Science.
MCM Major circulating metabolite; Major congenital malformation; Miniature continuous monitor; Minimum capacitation medium; Mitochondrial myopathy; Monte Carlo method; Multiple concomitant medication(s).
MCMA Mammalian cell mutagenesis assay (in vitro assay) (see CAA).
MC-MA Monochorionic-monoamniotic (gestation, in multifetal pregnancy).
MC Mask Mary Caterall mask (for oxygen administration) (= MC).
MCMI Millon Clinical Multiaxial Inventory.
MCMM Mucocutaneous myeloid metaplasia (see PPMM).
mcmol micromole(s).
MCMS Multnomah County Medical Society.
MCMV Murine cytomegalovirus.
MCN Minimal change nephropathy; Mixed cell nodular (lymphoma).
McN McNeil Laboratories Inc (USA) code for experimental substances.
MCNA The Medical Clinics of North America (journal).
McN-JR McNeil Laboratories Inc (USA) code for experimental substances.
McN-JR 3345 Dipiperon (= Floropipamide; R 3345) - a tranquillizing drug, used in the treatment of chronic schizophrenia.
McN-JR 8299 Tetramisole hydrochloride (see ICI 50,627).
MCNP Multiple cranial-nerve palsies/ palsy.
MCNS Minimal change nephrotic syndrome.
MCO Managed/ Medical care organization; Multicystic ovary.
MCOM Michigan College of Osteopathic Medicine.
MCommH Master of Community Health.
MCOP Managed Care Outcomes Project.
mcoul millicoulomb. A unit of quantity of current electricity, being one-thousandth (10^{-3}; 1/1000) of a coulomb.
µcoul microcoulomb (= 10^{-6} coulomb) (see µC).
MCP Magnocellular or (m) pathway (the faster light transmission awareness/ response to a moving object) (see PCP; LED); Managed-care physician (see MCD)/ plan (= POS); Maximum closure pressure; Maximum contraction pattern; Mayo Clinic Proceedings (journal); Medical Care Program; Medical College of Pennsylvania; Melphalan, cyclophosphamide and prednisone; Metacarpophalangeal (joint) (= MCPH); Metoclopramide (an anti-emetic drug); Methylchloro-phenoxyacetic acid (see MCPA); Mitotic-control protein; Monochorionic placenta/ pregnancy; Mucin clot prevention; Mucosal cell proliferation.
M-CP Magovern-Cromie prothesis (= M-C).
MCP 875 Dextromoramide (= Dextrodiphenopyrine; D-Moramid; Jetrium; Palfium; Pyrrolamidol; R 875; SKF 5137) - an analgesic used in the treatment of severe pain; may cause addiction.
MCPA Member of the College of Pathologists, Australasia (= MCPa); Methylchloro-phenoxy-acetic acid - a plant hormone used as a selective herbicide for broad-leaved plants.
MCPa Member of the College of Pathologists, Australasia (see MCPA).
MCPAHS Massachusetts College of Pharmacy and Allied Health Sciences.
MCPBCCS Multicenter population-based case-control study (e.g. IAAAS).
MCPC-603 McIntire plasmacytoma.
MCPH Metacarpophalangeal (see MCP).
MCPP Metacarpophalangeal pattern profile; Meta-chlorophenylpiperazine.
MCPPP Metacarpophalangeal pattern profile plot.
MCPR Manual cardiopulmonary resuscitation.
MCPS Manitoba College of Physicians and Surgeons; Member of the College of Physicians and Surgeons.
Mcps Megacycles per second (see Mhz).
MCQ Multiple-choice question.
MCR Medical Corps Reserve; Medullary chemoreceptor(s) (see CCR); Message com-

petition ratio; Metabolic clearance rate/ ratio; Monocyte cytokine release; Morphine, controlled-release (tablets); Mother-child relationship; Multicenter comparison.

MCRA Member of the College of Radiologists, Australasia.

MCRC Medical Computing Resources Center (UTHSCD); Metastatic colorectal cancer.

MCRE Mother-child relationship evaluation.

MCRG Multiple chemoresistance/ant gene.

MCRH Multicentric reticulohistiocytosis.

MCRI Multifactorial Cardiac Risk Index.

MCRM Medical Center Replacement Hospital (UCLA).

MCS Male climacteric syndrome; Malignant carcinoid syndrome; Managed/ Medical care system; Massage of the carotid sinus; Mast cell stabilizer; Maternal clinical status; Medicare-covered service(s) (US); Mesenchymal/ Metastatic chondrosarcoma; Mesocaval shunt; Methylcholanthrene sarcoma (induced); Microcrystal suspension; Microculture and sensitivity; Mild chromic suture (see Sutures); Mineralo-corticosteroid (see GMC); Minimally conscious state; Modular cooling system; Moisture-control system; Monocyte complement stimulator. Promotes the differentiation of monocytes into complement (C2), producing macrophages; Multicenter study/ survey; Multichannel scaler; Multiple chemical sensitivities/vity (= CHS; CSD; EI; TAS); Multiple combined sclerosis; Myocardial contraction state.

Mc/s; mc/s Megacycles per second (see Mhz).

MCSA Medical Computer Services Association; Minimal cross-sectional area; Moloney cell surface antigen.

MCSB Major conceptual scientific breakthrough.

MCSC Macromolecular and Cellular Structure and Chemistry (Program) (TSRI, La Jolla, CA).

MCSDA Mentored Clinical Scientist Development Award (NHLBI).

MCSDS Marlowe-Crowne Social Desirability Scale.

MCSF; M-CSF Macrophage colony-stimulating factor (see Hormones - HGF; M-CSF).

MCSN Medical Computer Services Newsletter.

MCSP Member of the Chartered Society of Physiotherapists/ Psychotherapy.

MCT Manual cervical traction; Mature connective tissue; Mean cell/ corpuscular thickness; Mean cell threshold; Mean circulation time; Median chain triglyceride (oil); Medium-chain triglyceride(s); Medullary carcinoma of the thyroid; Medullary collecting tubule; Microcentrifuge tube; Microtoxicity test; Midline cerebellar tumor; Minimal cognitive testing; Monochemotherapy; Monochorionic twin; Mucociliary transport; Multicenter clinical trial/ trial; Multiple compressed tablet; Multiple cycle treatment.

MCTC Metrizamide computed tomography cisternography.

MCTD Mixed connective tissue disease.

MCTF Mononuclear cell tissue factor.

MCTL Mixed cell type lymphoma.

MCTP Monochorionic twin pregnancy.

MCTR . Multiplecycle treatment regimen.

MCU Malaria control unit; Maximum/ Medical care unit; Medical check-up; Micturating cystourethrogram/graphy (= MCUG); Millicurie (see mC); Motor cortex unit.

MCUG Micturating cystourethrogram/graph (see MCU).

MCV Maximum/ Minimum calibrated volume; Mean/ Median cell/ corpuscular volume (in μm^3; cubic microns; fl; femtoliters; 10^{-15} liter) = Packed cell volume or hematocrit, multiplied by ten, and divided by the total RBC count (in millions) = PCV x 10 / RBC count; Mean clinical value (total clinical response numerically added, and divided by the number of patients treated); Medical College of Virginia; Motor conduction velocity.

MCVE Major cardiovascular (e.g. MI, Stroke, CV death, etc.)/ cerebrovascular (e.g. CVA, CV death, etc.) event.

MCW Medical College of Wisconsin.

MCWA Malaria Control in War Areas (now included in the agency CDC - Centers for Disease Control).

MCZ Museum of Comparative Zoology

(Harvard Univ).

MD Doctor of Medicine (L. Medicinae Doctor) (= DM; Dr Med); Macular degeneration; Magnesium/ Mental/ Multiple deficiency; Main duct; Maintenance dialysis/ dose; Major/ Mental depression; Malabsorption disorder (see MAD); Malate/ Malic dehydrogenase; Malignant/ Marek's/ Mediastinal/ Meniere's/ Minamata's/ Mitral/ Myocardial disease; Malrotation of duodenum; Mammary dysplasia; Manic-depressive; Mantoux diameter; March of Dimes; Maternal deprivation; Maximum/ Medium/ Minimum dosage/ dose; Mean deviation; Meckel's diverticulum (see Md); Medical Department; Medical Design (brace); Medical Digest (journals in UK, India); Medical Dimensions (journal); Medical director; Medical Doctor (see MD - Doctor of Medicine); Medicine Digest (journal); Mediodorsal; Mentally deficient/ depressed; Mesiodistal; Metered-dose; Microdensitometer; Mixed diet; Moderate disability; Monocular deprivation; Movement disorder; Multiple-dose (study/ therapy/ treatment/ trial); Muscular/ Myotonic dystrophy; Myelodysplasia; Myocardial damage.

Md Meckel's diverticulum (= MD); Mendelevium (Z = 101) (= Mv) (see Elements - Mendelevium).

md median (see mdn); with the right hand (Ital. mano destra).

516 MD Cinnarizine (= R 516; R 1575). An histamine drug used in various allergic disorders, vertigo and Meniere's disease.

MD 2028 Haloanisone (= Fluanisone). A rapidly acting tranquillizer chemically related to haloperidol.

MDA Malondialdehyde; Malonyldialdehyde; Manual dilatation/ dilation of the anus; Medical Devices Agency (GMC, Brit); Medical Division Approval; Mentodextra anterior (right mento-anterior - position of fetus); 3,4-Methylene dioxyamphetamine (hallucinogen); Michigan Dental Association; Microdermabrasion (with Al2O3 - Cosm. surgery); Minimal deviation adenocarcinoma; Minimum detectable amount; Mixed dentition analysis; Monodehydroascorbate; Motor discrimination/tive acuity; Muscular Dystrophy Association; Multidisciplinary approach; Multidrug abuse(r); Multiple-dose administration; Multivariant discriminant analysis; Red Shield of David (Society) (Heb. Magen David Adom - equivalent to the Red Cross, in Israel); Right mento-anterior (fetal position) (L. mento-dextra anterior).

MDa Megadalton.

MDAA Muscular Dystrophy Association of America.

MDAB Medical Devices Applications Branch.

MDAC Multiplying digital-to-analog converter.

MDAD Mineral dust airway disease.

MDAP Machover Draw-A-Person (test); Medical Devices Applications Program.

MDAR Minimum daily adult requirement (now RDA) (see RDA).

MDAU Medical Data Acquisitions Unit.

MDB Marked dropping bottle; Medical defence body; Methylene-dioxybenzene; Minimally distant border (vision); Molecular Disease Branch (NHI).

MDBDF March of Dimes Birth Defect Foundation.

MDBK Madin-Darby bovine kidney (cell).

MDC Macular Degeneration Center; Major diagnostic categories; Mean daily cost; MD of Canada (journal); Medial dorsal cutaneous (nerve); Mental Development Center; Microdrip chamber (intravenous); Minimum detectable concentration; Monocyte-depleted mononuclear cell; Multidose container.

MDCK Madin-Darby canine kidney (cell line).

MDCR Multidisciplinary clinical review.

MDCT Multiple dose clinical trial.

MDD Doctor in Dental Medicine (see DDM); Maintenance/ Maximum/ Mean daily dose; Major/ Manic/ Mixed depressive disorder; Malondialdehyde; Marked drug dependence; Myelodysplastic disorder (see UHD).

MDDS Multi-dose delivery system.

MDDUS Medical Defense Union of Scotland (malpractice protective union).

MDE Major depressive episode; Modern Drug Encyclopedia; Motility disorders of the esophagus (= MDO).

MDEBP Mean daily erect blood pressure.

MDentSc Master of Dental Science.

MDER Multidisciplinary ethical review.

MDF Mean dominant frequency; Methylene diphosphate/sphonate (see MDP); Myocardial depressant factor.

MDFC Macrophage-derived foam cell.

MDG Manic-depressive gene; Mean diastolic gradient.

MDGF Macrophage-derived growth factor.

MDGGB Muscular Dystrophy Group of Great Britain.

MDH Malate/ Malic dehydrogenase; Medullary dorsal horn.

MDHR Maximum determined heart rate.

MDHV Marek's disease herpes virus.

MDI Diphenylmethane di-isocyanate; Magnesium deficiency-induced (cerebral vascular damage, myocardial injury, etc.); Major/ Manic depressive illness; Maximum/ Mininum daily intake; Maximum/ Mean/ Minimum/ Missed dose intake; Mean/ Median duration of illness; Mental deterioration index (Wechsler); Metered-dose inhaler; Methylenedioxyindene(s); Mild/ Moderate depressive illness; Multiple daily injection; Multiple dosage insulin; Multiple drug ingestion/ involvement; Multiscore Depression Inventory.

MDi-193 Cyclothiazide. A diuretic, more potent than chlorothiazide, acting by reducing the resorption of electrolytes from the proximal renal tubules, thereby increasing the excretion of sodium, potassium, and chloride ions, and consequently of water.

MDIA Mental Development Index, Adjusted.

m dict as directed (L. more dicto); in the manner directed (L. modo dictu).

MDII Multiple daily insulin injection.

MDIPT Multicenter Diltiazem Postinfarction Trial.

MDIT Mean disintegration time.

MDL Mixed dyslipidemia (Frederickson Types IIa and IIb).

MDLP Macrodystrophia lipomatosa progressiva (= MLP).

MDM Maternal diabetes mellitus; Medical decision making; Mid-diastolic murmur; Minor determinant mix(ture) (test for penicillin sensitivity); Mitochondrial-dysfunction method; Mucosal defence mechanism; Multidisciplinary management (of patients).

MDMA 3,4-Methylene-dioxy-methamphetamine (= 3-methylfentanyl). The "ecstasy" drug; a derivative of Oil of Sassafras or Oil of Nutmeg (see Amphet - MDMA).

MDMH Hydroxymethyl-dimethylhydantoin.

MDMNM MD Medical News Magazine.

MDN Metered-dose nebulizer; Mood-disorder nosology; Muscular Dystrophy News (MDA journal).

mdn median (= md).

MDNARST Mammalian DNA repair synthesis test.

MDNB Mean daily nitrogen balance; Metadinitrobenzene.

Mdnt Midnight (= Midnoc).

MDO Manual dilatation/ dilation of the os; Motility disorders of the oesophagus (see MDE); Multiple drug overdosage/ dose.

MDOP; mdop Methyldopa.

MDP Mania, depression and psychosis (see SAD); Manic-depressive psychosis; Maximum digital pulse; Mento-dextra posterior (L.) (right mentoposterior - position of fetus); Methylene diphosphate/sphonate (= MDF); Multiple-dose protocol; Muramyldipeptide; Muscular dystrophy, progressive; Right mentoposterior (fetal position) (L. mento-dextra posterior).

MDPD Maximum daily permissible dose.

MDPI Maximum daily permissible intake.

MDPKS Multiple-dose pharmacokinetic study.

MDPNC Multidisciplinary prenatal care (see MPC).

MDQ Memory deviation quotient (and freedom from distractibility); Menstrual Distress Questionnaire; Minimum detectable quantity.

MDR Maladie-de-Roger (Roger's disease; a congenital heart defect); Maternal death rate (= MMR); Median duration of response; Medical device reporting; Medical Doctors Research (Group); Minimum daily requirement (food, now RDA) (see RDA); Multidrug resistance (protein)/ resistant (bacteria).

MDR1 Multidrug resistance (gene) (a negative prognostic factor [NPF] in Acute myelocytic leukemia [AML]).

MDRD Modification of Diet in Renal Disease.

MDRP Mood Disorders Research Program (UCLA); Multi-drug resistant pneumonia.

MDRS Mattis Dementia Rating Scale; Multidrug-resistant strain (bacterial).

MDR TB Multidrug-resistant tuberculosis.

MDS Manic-depressive syndrome; Master of Dental Surgery (see MChD); Materials Distribution System; Maternal deprivation syndrome; Maximal/ Minimal/ Modified dose schedule; Medical data screen(ing)/ system(s); Mesonephric duct system; Metered dose spray; Microdilution system; Mid-dorsal spine (see MTS); Milk drinker's syndrome; Miller-Dieker syndrome; Multiple-dose study; Multivitamin-deficiency state; Myelodysplastic syndrome; Myocardial depressant substance.

MDSBP Mean daily supine blood pressure.

MDSG Mood Disorders Support Group (Inc. - NY).

MDSO Mentally deranged/ disturbed sex offender.

MD's Wife (journal).

MDT Mast (cell) degeneration test; Mean dissolution time; Median detection threshold; Multidisciplinary team; Multiple dose/ drug therapy/ treatment; Right mentotransverse (fetal position) (L. mento-dextra transversa).

MDTM Multidisciplinary team meeting.

MDTP Multidisciplinary treatment plan.

MDTR Mean diameter/thickness ratio.

MDTS Multidose titration study.

MDU Medical Defence Union (Br.); Multidisciplinary use; To be used as directed (L. more dicto utendum).

MDUO Myocardial disease of unknown origin.

MDV Marek/ Mucosal disease virus; Mean dye velocity (bolus); Merrieux Diploid Vaccine (used for immunization in rabies); Multi-dose vaccine; Multiple dose vial (prescriptions).

MDY Month, date/ day, year.

Mdyn Megadyne.

ME Excitatory sympathin E; Macular edema; Malic enzyme; Manic episode; Maximum effort; Median eminence (of hypothalamus); Medical Economics (journal); Medical education; Medical Equipment (journal); Medical examination/ examiner; Megaesophagus; Meningoencephalitis; Mercaptoethanol; Metabolic/izable energy; Metabolism; Methamphetamine hydrochloride (see Amphet - ME); Methods in Enzymology (journal); Microembolism; Middle ear; Moessbauer effect; Mouse embryo; Mouse epithelial (cell); Myalgic encephalomyelitis; Myoepithelial.

Me Menton; Methyl group (CH_3-).

M/E; M:E Myeloid/Erythrocyte (ratio); Myeloid/Erythroid (ratio); Myelocytes:eosinophils (bone marrow).

m/e mass/charge (ratio in spectrometer).

2-ME 2-mercaptoethanol.

MEA Medical Exhibition/tor's Association; Mercaptoethyl amine (= Cysteamine; Mercamine; Mercaptamine; 2-Mercaptoethylamine) - has been used particularly in Russia, for the prevention and treatment of radiation sickness); Microsomal enzyme activation (see MEAS); Moisture evolution analyzer; Monoethanolamine; Most effective approach (to prevention of infective disease[s]); Multiple endocrine adenomas/matosis.

MEA I; MEA 1 Multiple endocrine adenomatosis, type I or 1.

MEA II; MEA 2 Multiple endocrine adenomatosis, type II or 2.

mEAD Monophasic action potential early afterdepolarization.

MEAS Microsomal enzyme activation system.

meas measure(d)/ment.

MEB Medical Evaluation Board; Muscle-eye-brain (disease).

MeB Methyl/ Methylene blue (= MB).

ME-BH Medial eminence of basal hypothalamus.

MeBSA Methylated bovine serum albumin.

MEC Median/ Minimum effective concentration; Middle ear canal/ cell; Moderately emetogenic chemotherapy; Mucosal epithelial cell; Multiethnic Cohort (Study Hawaii/ Los Angeles).

mec meconium.

MECA Monocyte-endothelial cell adhesion.
Mecano Mechanotherapy.
MECCA Minnesota Environmental Control Citizens Association.
MECCNU Semustine (= Methyl-1-[2-chloroethyl]3-4-methyl cyclohexyl-1-nitrosurea).
MECG Maternal electrocardiogram; Mixed essential cryoglobulinemia.
mech mechanical/ics.
MECO Medical Education Community Orientation (program).
MeCP Methyl-CCNU (MCCNU or semustine), cyclophosphamide, and prednisone.
MECT Maximum extrapolated clotting time.
MECTA Mobile electroconvulsive therapy apparatus.
MECY Methotrexate and cyclophosphamide.
MED Median erythrocyte diameter; Medical/ication/icine (see Med; med); Medical Electronics & Data (journal); Medical Electronics Division (HP); Medicine (London, MEI journal); Medium erythema dose (X-ray therapy); Menopausal estrogen deficiency; Minimal/imum effective/ erythema/ erythematous dose; Multi-exponential decline/ degeneration (see MEE); Multiple endocrine deficiency; Multiple epiphyseal dysplasia.
Med; med Medial/ian(al)/ium; Medical/ication/icine (= MED).
MEDAC Multiple endocrine deficiency, Addison's disease and candidiasis (syndrome).
MED-ART Medical Automated Records Technology.
MEDCATE Medical College Admissions Test.
MEDCOMP International Congress on Computing Medicine.
MEDEX Médecin extension (Fr.) - extension of the physician (with reference to recruitment program).
Medi Medicare.
medi- combining form meaning middle (L. medius).
MEDIAN Medical information access network.
MEDIC Medical Education Development In Communities; Monthly Ethical Drug Indexed Compilation.
Medic; medic Military medical corpsman (L. medicus).
MediCARxES Medicare Choice and Access to Prescription Drugs for Every Senior (citizen).
MEDICO Medical International Corporation.
MEDIHC Military Experience Directed Into Health Careers (HEW, DoD).
MEDLARS Medical Literature Analysis and Retrieval System (NLM).
MEDLINE An on-line segment of MEDLARS (MEDLARS on-line interactive bibliographic searching systems - NLM). National Institutes of Health (HEW).
MED-MAR Medical Minority Applicant Registry (AAMCOMA).
Med N Median nerve.
MEDPAR Medical Provider Analysis and Review.
MED-PED-FH Making early diagnosis to prevent early deaths (in medical pedigrees) with familial hypercholesterolemia.
MEdREP Medical Education Reinforcement and Enrichment Program.
meds medications; medicines.
MEDScD Doctor of Medical Science (see DMSc).
MEDSOC Medical Socioeconomic (Research Sources).
MedSTAR Medical Shock Trauma Acute Resuscitation (Unit).
Med-surg Medicine and surgery.
Med Tech Medical technician/nologist(/gy).
MEE Measured energy expenditure; Methylethyl ether; Middle ear effusion; Multiexponential elimination (of a drug) (see MED).
MEEI Massachusetts Eye and Ear Infirmary.
MEEN Medical Electronics and Equipment News.
MEET Multistage exercise electrocardiographics test.
MEF Major etiological factor; Maximal/imum expiratory flow (see PFT - FEF); Middle ear fluid; Midexpiratory flow; Migration enhancement factor; Mouse embryo fibroblast.

MEF_{50} Mean maximal/imum expiratory flow (see PFT - MEF_{50}).
MEFR Maximal/imum expiratory flow rate (see PFT - FEF); Mid-expiratory flow rate.
MEFV Maximal/imum expiratory flow volume (see PFT - FEF).
MEG Magnetoencephalogram/raphy; Megakaryocyte (see meg); Mercaptoethylguanidine; Multifocal eosinophilic granuloma.
meg megacycle (unit of frequency equal to 1 million cycles per second); megakaryocyte (= MEG); megaloblast; megohm (a million ohms).
meg-; mega- metric prefix for 10^6 or 1 million (Gr. megas) (see M. Mega-); prefix meaning very large.
Megace Megestrol acetate (hormone - used in cancer therapy).
megal- combining form meaning large (Gr. megas).
MEGD Minimal euthyroid Graves' disease.
mEGF Mouse epidermal growth factor.
MEGX Monoethylglycinexylidide.
MeH Methyl-histidine.
MeHg Methyl mercury.
MEHS Multiple eyelid hidrocystoma syndrome (marked hypotrichosis of scalp, hypodontia, dystrophic nails and cysts of eyelid margins - an autosomal recessive, ectodermal dysplasia) (= SS - Schopf syndrome).
MEI Medical Education International (journal, UK); Microsomal enzyme induction.
MEIA Microparticle enzyme immunoassay.
MEIN Medium energy intense neutron (facility, BNL).
meio- prefix meaning smaller (Gr. meion).
MEK Methylethylketone.
MEL Metabolic equivalent level; Mouse/ Murine erythroleukemia.
mel melena; melanoma.
mel- combining form meaning limb or member (Gr. melos).
melan- combining form meaning black (Gr. melas).
MELAS Mitochondrial encephalomyopathy - lactic acidosis - and stroke-like symptoms (syndrome).
Mel B; MEL B Melarsoprol (= Arsobal; Melarsen Oxide - BAL; RP 3854) - an organic arsenic trypanocide used in the treatment of advanced sleeping-sickness caused by Trypanosoma rhodiense and T. gambiense, in which the parasites have invaded the central nervous system.
MELC Mouse/ Murine erythroleukemia cell.
MELD Minnesota Early Learning Design (parenting and child development).
meli- prefix meaning sweet (from the Greek word for honey).
Mel W Melarsonyl potassium (= Melarsenoxide potassium dimercaptosuccinate; Pentylthiarsphenylmelamine; RP 9955) - a water-soluble derivative of melarsoprol (see Mel B), used in the treatment of advanced trypanosomiasis.
MEM Macrophage electrophoretic mobility; Malic enzyme, mitochondrial; Middle-ear muscle; Minimal/imum essential medium; Morpholinyl-ethyl-morphine (= Pholcod; Pholcodine; Pholcodinum) - resembles codeine in suppressing cough, but is less toxic and more effective in smaller doses; Myalgic encephalomyelitis; Myxedema(tous) madness (in severe hypothyroidism) (= MOM).
Mem Member.
MEMA Methyl methacrylate.
memb membrane/nous.
MEMR Multiple esostoses - mental retardation (syndrome).
MEN Multiple endocrine neoplasia/sm.
men meningeal/ges/gitis; meniscus; menstruation.
men- combining form meaning month (Gr. men).
MEN-I Multiple endocrine neoplasia/sm - type I.
MEN-2 Multiple endocrine neoplasia/sm - type 2.
MEND Medical Education for National Defence.
mening- combining form meaning membrane (Gr. meningos).
Menn Menninger; Mennonite (religion).
ment mental(ity).
ment- combining form meaning mind (L. mens; mentis) or chin (L. mentum).

MEO Malignant external otitis.

5-MeODMT 5-Methoxy-N,N-dimethyltryptamine.

MeOH Methyl alcohol (see CH_3OH).

MEOS Microsomal ethanol oxidizing system.

MEP Marrow-extraction process (prior to chemotherapy in cancer patients); Maximal/imum expiratory pressure (see PFT - MEP); Mean effective pressure; Meperidine (see Mep); Meprobamate (proprietary name for) - a tranquillizer (= Mep; mep; MPB); Microbiologically evaluable population; Mitrochondrial encephalopathy; Motor-end plate.

Mep; mep Meperidine (Trade name: Demerol) (= MEP); Meprobamate (see MEP).

MEPC Miniature end-plate current.

MEPP Miniature end-plate potential.

mEq; mEQ; meq milliequivalent (= 10^{-3} Eq).

mEq/24 H milliequivalents per 24 hours.

mEq/l; mEQ/l; meq/l milliequivalents per liter.

MER Ethamoxytriphetol (an anti-estrogen); Man-environmental relations; Mean ejection rate; Median evoked response; Methanol extraction/truded residue (of BCG); Wm S Merrel Co (USA) code for experimental substances.

mer- combining form meaning member or part of a group (Gr. meros).

MER-17 Azacyclonal hydrochloride - a tranquillizer used in the treatment of schizophrenia.

MER-29 Triparanol - a chlorophenyl tolylethanol compound, an inhibitor of the biosynthesis of cholesterol from its immediate precursor, desmosterol (= 24-dehydrocholesterol). A toxic drug, formerly used to reduce the blood-cholesterol level, particularly in atherosclerosis.

M/E ratio; M:E ratio Ratio of myeloid to erythroid cells in bone marrow.

MERB Medical Examination and Review Board.

MERC Medical Education Resource Center.

MERES Matrix of Environmental Residues for Energy Systems (BNL).

MERG Macular electroretinogram.

MERLIN Multi-Element Radio Link Interferometer.

Merm Male hermaphrodite (see Ferm; Herm).

MERMLS Mideastern Regional Medical Library Service.

MERRF Myoclonic/nus epilepsy and/with ragged red fibers (disease/ syndrome).

MeRS Methicillin-resistant staphylococcus.

MES Maintenance electrolyte solution; Maximal electroshock; Maximal electroshock seizure(s); Medical emergency service; Monroe Efficacy Study (in vaccine therapy); Morpholino-ethane sulfonic acid (buffer used in staining mixtures); Multiple endocrine syndrome; Myoelectric signal.

Mes Mesencephalic/lon.

MESA Marine Ecosystems Analysis (program - NOAA); Medical Emergency Service Associates; Mining Enforcement and Safety Administration (USDI); Myoepithelial sialadenitis.

MESBC Metastasizing estrogen-sensitive breast cancer (in post menopausal or oophorectomised women).

Mesc Mescaline - other names are: Big Chief; Cactus; Mescal (peyote); Peyote ("Moon"); Peyotl.

Mescal Mescaline or Peyote (see Mesc).

MESCH Multi-Environment Scheme.

MeSH Medical Subject Headings (List - NLM).

MESPGN Mesangial/gio proliferative glomerular nephritis (see PGN).

MesPGN Mesangial proliferative glomerulonephritis.

MET Medical emergency technician/ treatment; MET Electrical Testing Co; Metabolic equivalent of the task; Metastasis/static (see Metas); Methionine (see Met); Midexpiratory time (see PFT - MET); Minimal endometrial thickness (for pregnancy) - 6 to 7 mm; Multistage exercise test; Oxygen expenditure at rest, equivalent to 3.5 ml of oxygen per kilogram of body weight per minute.

Met Metabolic; Metamyelocyte(s) (see Meta); Metaramicol; Methionine (= MET; Meth).

met metallic (with reference to chest sounds); metallurgy (see Metall; metastasis (see Metas).

met- prefix meaning after, accompanying, or

changing (Gr. meta) (see meta-).
MET-501 MET Electrical Testing Co medical equipment evaluation and labeling standard (see APE; OEE; OER).
Meta Metamyelocyte(s) (= Met).
meta- prefix meaning after, accompanying, or changing (Gr. & L.) (see met-).
Metab Metabolic/ism; Metabolism: Clinical and Experimental (journal).
Metall Metallurgy (= met).
Metaph Metaphysics.
Metas Metastases/ Metastasis/ Metastasize/ Metastatic (= MET; met; mets).
Met-Enk Methionine-enkephaline.
Meteor Meteorology.
2-me test 2-mercaptoethanol test (serological test for brucellosis).
METH Methicillin.
Meth Methadone; Methedrine (see Amphet); Methionine (see Met); Methodist (church member).
meth methyl group (CH_3-).
Met Hb; Met-Hb Methemoglobin.
MeThCh Methylthiocholine.
MeTHF Methyltetrahydrofolic acid.
Methotrex Methotrexate (= Aminomethyl pteroylglutamic acid) - therapy for cancer.
Methyl CCNU Semustine (= MCCNU).
Methyl G Mitroguazone dihydrochloride (= Methyl GAG).
Methyl GAG Methylglyoxal-bis-guanylhydrazone. A drug used in the treatment of leukemia.
MetMb Metmyoglobin.
m et n morning and night (L. mane et nocte) (see M&N).
Metopon Methyldihydro-morphinone (see Papaver).
Metp Methylprednisolone.
metr- combining form meaning measure (Gr. metron) or womb (Gr. metra).
METS Masters Exercise Test; Metabolic equivalents (of oxygen consumption).
mets metastases (see Metas).
met series metastatic series (X-ray chest, bones, skull).
M et sig; m et sig mix and (write a) label (L. misce et signa).
METT Maximum exercise tolerance test.
MEU Maximum expected utility.
MEV Maximum exercise ventilation; Murine erythroblastosis virus; Myalgic encephalomyelitis virus.
MeV; mev; 10^6 eV; 1 6 x 10^{-6} ergs. Mega (million) electron volt(s).
MEW Moderately exuding wound.
MEWD Multiple evanescent white dot (syndrome) (see MEWDS).
MEWDS Multiple evanescent white dot syndrome.
MEX Mexican.
Mexican brown Marijuana (see Cannabis).
Mexican green Marijuana (see Cannabis).
Mexican red Sodium secobarbital (see Barb).
Mex. P Mexican Pharmacopoeia (Farmacopea Nacional de los Estados Unidos Mexicanos).
MF Malassezia furfur; Mass fragmentography; Mayo/ Menninger Foundation; Meat free (diet); Medium/ Mutation frequency; Megafarad; Membrane filter; Merthiolate-formaldehyde (solution); Methotrexate, fluorouracil (and calcium leucovorin); Methoxyflurane; Microfibril; Microfiche; Microfilament; Microfilia; Microflocculation; Microscopic/ Mitogenic/ Multiplication/(plying) factor; Midcavity forceps; Millipore filter (for IV therapy - see MF method); Mitochondrial fragments; Mitomycin-fluorouracil; Mitotic/ Myelin figure; Mucosal fluid; Multifactorial; Muscle feedback; Mycosis fungoides; Myelofibrosis; Myocardial fibrosis; Myofibrillar.
Mf Maxillofrontale; Microfilaria.
mF millifarad (= mf; 10^{-3} farad) - electrical measurement.
mf microfilaria; millifarad (see mF).
µf; µF microfarad (= mfd; µfd; 10^{-6} farad) - electrical measurement.
M/F Male/female (ratio); Masculinity/feminity.
M&F Male and female; Mother and father.
MFA Methyl/ Mono fluoroacetate; Multifactorial analysis; Multifocal functional autonomy; Multiple factor analysis; Muscle fiber atrophy.
MFAT Multifocal atrial tachycardia.
MFB Medial forebrain bundle; Metallic foreign body.

MFBAT Multofocal bronchoalveolar tumor (in NSCLC - Non-small-cell lung cancer).

MFC Management flow chart; Man-fly contact; Marriage and family counselor; Master facility census; Maternal-fetal clinic; Médecin de Famille Canadien (journal) (Canadian Family Physician); Medial femoral condyle; Minimal fungicidal concentration; Multifaceted challenge.

MFCM Master, Faculty of Community Medicine.

MFCT Maternofetal cell transfer (causing GVHR).

MFCV Muscle fiber conduction velocity.

MFD "Mad fish" disease - a virulent, necrotizing fasciitis or toxic pharyngitis, the so-called "flesh-eating" disease, caused by Streptococcus iniae (of the group A Streptococcus family, i.e. Streptococcus A), found in fresh water and transferred to humans by the dermal route (i.e. through broken skin); Mandibulofacial dysostosis; Memory-for-Designs (test); Midforceps delivery; Milk-free diet; Minimum fatal dose; Mitochondria-focused drug; Modified fat diet; Multifactorial disease/ family disease; Multifollicular development (IVF).

mfd; μfd microfarad (see μf).

MFE Myrcene, racemic frontalin, and racemic exo-brevicomin pheromone (mixture).

MFED Mercury-filled esophageal dilator (Maloney).

MFEM Maximal forced expiratory maneuver.

MFES Modified functional evaluation system (Enneking's) (Orthopedics).

MFF Matching Familiar Figures (test in psychology).

MFG Modified heat-degraded gelatin (a plasma extender); Multifetal gestation (see MFP).

mfg manufacture(d)/ring.

MFH Malignant fibrous histiocytoma; Marrow-free homograft (see MCA; MCH); Mild/ Moderate fetal hydronephrosis (Obstetrics).

MFHom Member of the Faculty of Homeopathy.

MFI Master facilities inventory; Maternal-fetal interaction; Maxillofacial injuries/ry; Mild febrile illness.

MFID Multi-electrode flame ionization detector.

MFL Master facilities list.

M flac Tympanic membrane (L. membrana flaccida) (= Pars flaccida membranae tympani - Nomina Anatomica; Shrapnell's membrane).

MFM Muscle fiber membrane.

MF method Membrane or millipore filter method (bacteriology).

MFMPP Maternal-Fetal Medicine Principles and Practice (journal, Phil).

MFMT Mammalian forward mutation test.

MFO Mixed function oxidase/ oxygenase.

MFOM Master, Faculty of Occupational Medicine.

MFP Method(s) of family planning (see NFPM); Mono-fluorophosphate (sodium); Multifetal pregnancy (= MFG); Myofacial/ Myofascial pain.

MFR Macula flava retinae (= MR - Macula retinae); Maternal-fetal relationship; Mean/ Mucus flow rate; Mid-forceps rotation; Multifunctional receptor.

mfr manufacturer.

MFRS Maxillofacial reconstructive surgery.

MFS Malformation syndrome (see DMS); Marrow failure state (aplastic anemia, myelodysplasia, etc.); Maxillo-facial surgeon/ery; Mean fixed stiffness (by fixation device) (see AFS; MIS); Medical fee schedule; Miller Fisher syndrome (a variant of GBS or Guillain-Barré syndrome, with an acute onset of ophthalmoplegia, ataxia and areflexia); Mono/Multi filament suture (see Sut); Multifollicular stimulation (Gyn & Obst).

MF sol Merthiolate-formaldehyde (stock) solution (see MIF).

MFSS Medical Field Service School.

MFST Medical Field Service Technician.

MFT Materno-fetal transmission (see HT; VT); Microfoam tape; Multifocal (atrial) tachycardia; Muscle function test (procedure/ physical medicine).

M ft; m ft Let a mixture be made/ Make a mixture (L. mistura fiat); Mix to make (L. misce fiat).

M ft mist Mix to make a mixture (L. misce

fiat mistura).

MFV Metal fume fever (= Brassfounder's ague; Zinc chill).

MFVNS Middle fossa vestibular nerve section.

MFVPT Motor Free Visual Perception Test.

MFW Multiple fragment wounds.

MG Mandril graft (used in vascular surgery); Marcus Gunn (pupil); Margin; Medial gastrocnemius (muscle); Membranous glomerulonephritis; Menopausal gonadotrophin/tropin (see Hormones - MG; HMG); Mesiogingival; Methyl glucoside/ guanidine; Monoclonal gammopathy; Monoglyceride; Mucus granule; Muscle group; Myasthenia gravis; Myoglobin (= Mg; Mgl).

Mg Magnesium (Z = 12) (see Elements - Magnesium) (= Mag); Myoglobin (see MG).

mg milligram (= mgm; mgr; 0.001 gram; 10^{-3} gram; 10^{-3} g; 10^{-3} gm; 10^{-3} G).

mγ milligamma (= mμg; millimicrogram; 10^{-9} gram; ng; nanogram).

μg microgram (= μgm; μgr; mcg; mcgm; 10^{-6} gram; gam; one millionth of a gram).

μγ microgamma (= μμg; micromicrogram; 10^{-12} gram; pg; picogram).

μg/kg micrograms per kilogram.

μg/l micrograms per liter.

μGy microgray.

mg% milligrams per cent (= milligrams per 100 ml/100 cc; milligrams per hundred milliliters).

M3G Morphine-3-glucuronide.

m^{7}G 7-Methylguanosine.

MGA Macroglobulinaemia; Mean gestational age (Obstetrics); Medical gas analyzer; Melengestrol acetate (a progestin).

MGAC Mammary gland adenocarcinoma.

MGAS Medical Gynaecology, Andrology and Sociology (UK journal, formerly GS - Gynaecology and Sociology).

MgATP Magnesium adenosine triphosphate.

MGB Medial geniculate body; Myelographic block (see PMB).

MGBG Methylglyoxal-bis-(guanylhydrazone).

MGC Maternal glycemic control (of fetal development); Maternity and gynecologic care; Minimal glomerular change; M(yasthenia) G(ravis) Conquest (journal); Multinuclear/ated giant cell.

MgC Magnocellular neuroendocrine cell.

MGCE Multifocal giant cell encephalitis.

$MgCl_2$ Magnesium chloride.

$MgCO_3$ Magnesium carbonate.

MGD Maximal glucose disposal; Mixed gonadal dysgenesis.

mgd million gallons per day.

mg/dl milligrams per deciliter.

MGDS Magnesium-depletion study; Member in General Dental Surgery.

MGE Molecular genetic evaluation (Obstetrics).

mg-el milligram element.

MGES Multiple gated equilibrium scintigraphy.

MGF Macrophage growth factor; Maternal grandfather; Myasthenia Gravis Foundation (Canada).

MGFN Myasthenia Gravis Foundation Newsletter.

MGG May-Grunwald-Giemsa (stain); Molecular and General Genetics (journal); Mouse gamma globulin.

MGGH Methylglyoxal guanylhydrazone.

MGH Massuchusetts General Hospital; Monoglyceride hydrolase.

mgh milligram-hour (the radium dose obtained by the application of one milligram of radium element for one hour).

MGI Maximal/ Minimal/ Moderate growth inhibition (cancer therapy).

MGJ Manubrio-gladiolar junction (= Synchondrosis sternalis); Mucogingival junction.

mg/kg milligrams per kilogram.

mg/kg/d milligrams per kilogram per day.

mg/kg/hr milligrams per kilogram per hour.

MGL Minor glomerular lesion.

Mgl Myoglobin (see MG).

mg/l milligrams per liter.

MGM Maternal grandmother; Medical Group Management (journal).

mgm milligram (see mg).

μgm microgram (see μg).

MGMA Medical Group Management Association.

MGMP Maintaining Good Medical Practice

(UK booklet - GMC).

MGMT O -Methylguanine-DNA methyltransferase (DNA-repair enzyme/ gene).

MGN Mammary gland neoplasm; Medial geniculate nucleus; Membranous glomerulonephritis.

MgO Magnesium oxide.

MGP Marcus-Gunn pupil; Marginal granulocyte pool; Membranous glomerulonephropathy; Methyl green pyronine; Minimal-genome project (Study of the 470 genes of *Mycoplasma* genitalium, a miniscule microorganism, just 0.3-0.9 μm in diameter. E. coli is 9 times larger); Mucin glycoprotein; Multicor Gamma pacemaker; Multiple gestation pregnancy (Obstetrics); Mutagenic potential; Myasthenia gravis pseudoparalytica (name given by Jolly in 1895, now called Myasthenia gravis and treated by RNS or repeated nerve stimulation).

MgPP Magnesium protoporphyria.

MGR Modified gain ratio; Multiple gas rebreathing.

MGR; μGR Microgravity research.

mgr milligram (see mg).

μgr microgram (see μg).

MGS Mediastinal granulocytic sarcoma; Metric gravitational system; Morning glory seeds (a hallucinogen) (see LSD); Motor grading system (BMRC) (Orthopedics): Grade Muscle Response: 0. No muscle contraction; 1. Flickeror trace of contraction (no joint motion); 2. Active movement with gravity eliminated; 3. Active antigravity movement; 4. Active movement against gravity and some resistance; 5. Normal muscle strength; Multigenerational study.

MGSD Mediterranean Group for the Study of Diabetes (Israel).

$MGSO_4$ Magnesium sulfate.

MGSP Malaria Genome Sequencing Project.

MGT Male genital tract; Metaplastic gastric tissue; Modified grid treatment (laser technique in photocoagulation of the retina); Multiple glomus tumors.

Mgtis Meningitis.

MGUS Monoclonal gammopathies of undetermined significance.

MGV Mid-gut volvulus.

MGW Magnesium sulfate, glycerine, and water (enema); Montanglycol wax (an inactive ingredient used in placebos) (= Wax E).

M-GXT Multi-stage graded exercise test.

mGy milligray.

MH D-mannoheptulose; Maleic hydrazide; Malignant histiocytosis/ hyperpyrexia/ hypertension/ hyperthermia; Mammotropic hormone (see Hormones - LH; MH i; MTH); Marital/ Medical/ Menstrual history; Mass hysteria; Medial hypothalamic (lesion)/mus; Medical History/ Hypotheses (journals); Melanophore(-stimulating) hormone (see Hormones - MH ii; MSH ii); Mental health/ hygiene; Mental Hygiene (NAMH journal); Merphyrin; Migraine headache; Ministry of Health (UK); Modern Healthcare (journal); Moist heat; Monosymptomatic hypochondriasis; Mouse/ Murine hepatitis (virus - see MHV); Mutant hybrid; Myohyoid.

mH; mh millihenry.

M-H McGraw-Hill (publisher); Meuller-Hinton (agar/ base/ broth) (see MHB).

MH 532 Phenprobamate (= Proformiphen; 3-Phenylpropyl carbamate) - a muscle relaxant anticonvulsant and tranquillizer.

μH microhenry.

MHA Major histocompatibility antigen; Maryland/ Massachusetts Hospital Association; Master of Hospital Administration; May-Hegglin anomaly; Mental Health Administration/ Assistant/ Association/ in Australia (ANAMH); Methemalbumin; Microangiopathic hemolytic anemia; Microhemagglutination; Middle hepatic artery; Mild heart attack; Minnesota Heart Association; Mixed hemadsorption; Mueller-Hinton agar (see MHB).

MHAQ Modified Health Assessment Questionnaire.

MHATP; MHA-TP Microhemagglutination/tinin assay for Treponema pallidum (antibodies) (see STS).

MHB Maximum hospital benefit; Mental-health benchmark (see MPI); Molecular Hematology Branch (NHLI); Mueller-Hinton base; Mueller-Hinton broth (agar, culture, medium) (see MHA).

MHb Methemoglobin; Myohemoglobin.

MHBSS Modified Hank's balanced salt solution.
MHC Macrocytic hyperchromatism; Major (C)/ Mild (A)/ Minimal (A)/ Minor (A)/ Moderate (B) hepatic cirrhosis (Child-Pugh A, B, and C); Major-histocompatibility-complex (see MHCD); Malignant hypercalcemia; Managed Health Care; Maternal health care/ center/ clinic/ counselor; Mental health care (see MHCU)/ center/ clinic/ counselor; Multiphasic health checkup.
MHCAD Memorial Hospital for Cancer and Allied Diseases.
MHCD Major-histocompatibility-complex deficiency; Mental Health Career Development (program).
MHCF Mental health care facility.
MHCG Mu heavy-chain gene (mutated in agammaglobulinemia).
MHCP Mean horizontal candlepower.
MHCS Mental Hygiene Consultation Service; Multicenter Hemophilia Cohort Study (of late-stage HIV disease).
MHCT Microhematocrit centrifugation technique (laboratory procedure).
M/hct Microhematocrit (laboratory/ hematology).
MHCU Mental health care unit.
MHD Magneto-hydrodynamics; Maintenance hemodialysis; Male hypogonadal disorder; Maximum human dose (mg/day on a mg/m^2 basis); Mean/ Minimum hemolytic dilution/ dose; Mediastinal Hodgkin's disease; Mental health department; Mental Health Digest (defunct journal); Mild/ Minimal/ Moderate hepatic dysfunction (= MLD); Mild/ Moderate hepatic disease; Moving-head disk (computer memory).
MHDPS Mental Health Demographic Profile System.
MHE Malignant hemangioendothelioma (including VAS); Maximal/ Maximum hypotensive effect (of a drug); Maximum/ Medium/ Mild/ Minimum human exposure (to cold, disease, drugs, heat, sunlight, etc.); Mild/ Moderate hypoglycemic episode Multiphasic health examination.
MHEC Multiphasic health examination clinic.
MHF Marburg hemorrhagic fever (caused by the filovirus, a filamentous mammalian virus found in African green monkeys); Mental-health facility; Mental Health Foundation (UK); Mild/ Moderate heart failure.
MHG Maternal hyperglycemia.
mHg millimeter(s) of mercury.
μHg micron of mercury.
MHH Male hypothalamic hypogonadism.
MHHC Mouse-human hybrid cell.
MHI Malignant histiocytosis of the intestine; Mental Health Index; Mild/ Moderate hepatic impairment/ insufficiency; Montreal Heart Institute.
MHL Medial hypothalamic lesion; Mental health legislation; Metabolic half-life (see BHL; Half-life); Mixed hyperlipidemia.
MHLC Multidimensional Health Locus of Control.
MHLP Mental Health Law Project (ACLU).
MHLS Metabolic heat load stimulator.
MHM Major human metabolite; Modern Herbal Medicine.
MHMC Mental Health Materials Center.
MHMR Mental Health, Mental Retardation (journal) (see USC:MHMR).
MH/MR Mental health and mental retardation.
MHN Massive hepatic necrosis; Mental health nurse; Mohs hardness number; Morbus hemolyticus neonatorum.
MHO Microsomal heme oxygenase.
mho A unit of electric conductivity (reciprocal ohm, siemens unit - ohm spelled backwards).
MHOs Multiple health outcomes.
MHP Major/ Mental/ Minor health problem; Malignant hyperpyrexia; Maternal/ Mental/ Migrant health program; 1-Mercury-2-hydroxy-propane; Metatarsal head prolapse (Orthopedics); Monosymptomatic hypochondriacal psychosis.
MHPA Mild hyperphenyl-alaninemia.
MHPC Methyhydroxypropylcellulose.
MHPG Methoxy-hydroxyphenyl-glycol (= 3-Methoxy-4-hydroxyphenylethyleneglycol) - a metabolite of norepinephrine.
MHR Major histocompatibility region; Major/ Mild/ Moderate hypersensitivity reaction(s); Malignant hyperthermia resistance; Maternal/ Maximal heart rate; Meta carpal/ tarsal head

resection (Orthopedics); Methemoglobin reductase (activity); Multipoise head rest (Neurosurgery); Multitest Health Review (journal).

MHRD Maximum human recommended dose (see MRHD).

MHRI Mental Health Research Institute (University of Michigan).

MHS Major histocompatibility system; Male healthy subject; Malignant hyperthermia in swine/ syndrome; Malignant hyperthermia/ hypothermia susceptibility; Mental health status; Mucus hypersecretion; Multiple health screening.

MHSA Microaggregated human serum albumin.

MHSC Male homosexual couple.

MHT Malignant hepatic tumor (= MLT); Malignant hyperthermia; Mantel-Haenszel x 2 (statistical analysis) test; Mental-health therapy/ treatment (e.g. Arica therapy, a treatment that focuses on altered states of consciousness) (see AGT); Mild/ Moderate hyperthyroidism; Mixed hemagglutination test; Multiphase health testing.

MHTN Malignant hypertension.

MHTS Multiphasic Health Testing Services.

MHV Magnetic heart vector; Mouse/ Murine hepatitis virus.

MHVCN Midwife, Health Visitor and Community Nurse (UK journal).

MHW Medial heel wedge; Mental health worker.

MHx Medical history.

MHyg Master of Hygiene.

MHz; Mhz Megahertz (= Mc; Mcps; Mc/s; mc/s; 10^6 cycles/sec; a million cycles per second).

MI Maturation/ Melanophore/ Merck/ Metabolic/ Migration/ Mitotic/ Morphology/ Motility/ Mucoprotective index; Medical inspection/ insurance; Medical Instrumentation (journal); Membrane(s) intact; Menstruation induction; Mental illness/ institution; Mercaptoimidazole; Mesioincisal; Midwinter insomnia (north of the Arctic circle); Migration inhibition; Mild irritant; Minimally invasive (see MIBS; MICABG; MIHS; MIS; MIST; MIT; MIVS); Mitral incompetence/ insufficiency; Mononucleosis infectiosa (see IM); Myocardial infarct(ion)/ ischemia; Myoinositol.

mi mile; mitochondrium; mix.

MI 5 (Br). the section of Military Intelligence concerned with the security of the State.

MI 217 Ecothiopate iodide (= Echothiopate iodide; Ecothiophate iodide; Ecostigmine iodide) - an anticholinergic drug, acting like physostigmine and neostigmine. Used as eyedrops in glaucoma.

MIA Medically indigent adult; Mean interday accuracy (drug assay); Mild/ Moderate intermittent asthma; Missing in action.

MIAP Modified innervated antral pouch.

MIAs Multi-institutional arrangements; Medically indigent adults.

MIB Medical Impairment Bureau; Medical Information Bureau (association of life insurance companies); Mother-infant bond(ing).

MIBC Mean insulin binding capacity (= IBC) (Normal = 4 to 5 μg/l).

MIBG Meta-iodobenzyl-guanidine.

MIBiol Member of the Institute of Biology.

MIBK Methyl-isobutyl ketone.

MIBS Minimally invasive bypass surgery (see MIHS; MIS; MIST).

MIBT Methyl isatin-beta-thiosemicarbazone.

MIC Maternal and Infant Care; Maternity and infant care; Medical intensive care; Medical Interfraternity Conference; Microscopy; Minimal/mum inhibitory concentration (of the antibiotic for the infecting organism); Minimal isorrheic concentration; Minocycline; Model immune complex; Monolithic integrated circuit; Mononuclear inflammatory cell.

mic microcyte/ microscope (see micro).

MICABG Minimally invasive coronary artery bypass graft(ing).

MICC Metastatic islet cell carcinoma (of the pancreas) (see ICC); Mitogen-induced cellular cytotoxicity.

MICG Macromolecular insoluble cold globulin.

Mickey Finn Chloral hydrate (see Chloral hydrate).

MICN Mobile intensive care nurse.

MICP Maternity and Infant Care Project.
mic pan Bread crumb (L. mica panis).
MICR Magnetic ink chamber recognition; Metacholine inhalation challenge response.
micro microbiology (= microbiol); microcyte/tic; microscope/pic/py (= mic).
micro-; micr- metric prefix for 10^{-6} (Gr. mikros = small); prefix meaning small (= mikro-).
Microbios (journal).
microbiol microbiology (see micro).
MICRO-HOPE Microvascular Heart Outcomes Prevention Evaluation (substudy) (in people with diabetes mellitus) (see HOPE).
MICS Medical Instrument Calibration System.
mict dis micturition disorder.
MICU Medical/ Mobile intensive care unit.
MID Maintenance infusion dosage/dose; Manifest iron deficiency; Maximal/(imum)/Minimal/(imum) inhibiting/tory dilution; Medical index data; Medium infective dose (= DIM); Mesioincisodistal; Middle-aged patient; Minimal/imum infective/ inhibitory/ irradiation dose; Multi-infarct dementia; Multiple ion detection.
mid middle.
MIDAS Multicenter Isradipine Diuretic Arterio/ Athero sclerosis Study.
MIDCAB Minimally invasive direct coronary artery bypass (= BHB; KHB).
Mid I Middle insomnia.
Midnoc Midnight (see Midnt).
MIDS Management Information Decision System.
midsag midsagittal.
MIEC Medical Insurance Exchange of California.
MIF Macrophage inhibiting/tory factor (migration inhibition or inhibitory factor for macrophages at the sites of inflammation, or inhibiting migration of macrophages away from sites of inflammation); Maximum inspiratory flow (now FIF; see PFT - MIF); Melanocyte(-stimulating hormone) inhibiting factor (see Hormones - MIF); Melanotropin(-release) inhibiting factor (see Hormones - MIF); Merthiolate-iodine-formaldehyde (method or technique for fecal examination); Microimmuno-fluorescence; Mid-inspiratory flow; Migration inhibiting/tory factor (for macrophages as above); Mixed immunofluorescence; Müllerian inhibiting factor.
MIFC Merthiolate-iodine-formaldehyde concentration.
MIFR Maximal/imum inspiratory/ired flow rate (now FIFR; see PFT - MIFR).
MIG Measles immune globulin; Medicare Insured Groups; Mental-illness gene
MIg Malaria/ Measles/ Membrane immunoglobulin.
MIgAN Mesangial IgA nephropathy (or Berger's disease).
MIGT Multiple inert gas (elimination) technique.
MIGW Maximal/imum increase/ increment in growth and weight.
MIH Master of Industrial Health; Methylhydrazine (= Procarbazine) (see NSC-77213); Migraine with interparoxysmal/terval headache; Minimal intermittent heparin (dose).
MIHA Minor histocompatibility antigen.
MIHS Minimally invasive heart surgery (see MIBS; MIS; MIST).
MII Medicine-induced injury; Multi-item inventory.
MIJ Medical Instrumentation Journal (AAMI, formerly JAAMI).
MIKA Minor karyotype abnormalities.
MIKE Mass-analyzed ion kinetic energy.
Mike A microgram of illicit LSD (see LSD - Mike).
mikro- alternate spelling of micro- (see micro-).
MIL Mental Illness Lite (see MMI); Morphologically immature lung(s) (Obstetrics); Mother-in-law.
mil military; milliliter (see ml).
milieu French - environment/ middle course/ surroundings.
mill-; milli- metric prefix for 1/1000; 10^{-3} (L. mille) (see m).
millisec millisecond.
Mil Med Military Medicine (journal).
MILP Mitogen-induced lymphocyte prolifera-

tion.
MILS Medication information leaflet for seniors.
MIL-STD Military standard (purchase specification).
MIM Methods and Information in Medicine (journal).
MIMR Minimal inhibitor mole ratio.
MIMS Medical information/ inventory management system; Monthly Index of Medical Specialities (journal); Minimally invasive microsurgery.
MIMs Multiple immune mechanisms; Multiple inefficaceous medications.
MIN Medial interlaminar nucleus.
min mineral; minim (L. minimum) (= m; m.; a unit of capacity or liquid measure - see M. minim); minimal/imum - the smallest amount or lowest limit); minor; minute (= 60 seconds) - a unit of time.
ìin microinch.
MINA Mono-isonitroso-acetone.
min Br British imperial minim.
MIND National Association for Mental Health (UK).
MINE Mesna uroprotection, ifosfamide, Novantrone (mitoxantrone), and etoposide; Medical improvement not expected.
Mineral Mineralogy.
MINIA Monkey intranuclear inclusion agent.
M-in-L Mother-in-law.
Mino Minocycline (hydrochloride).
MInstSP Member of the Institution of Sewage Purification (= MISP).
min US United States minim.
MIO Minimal/imum identifiable odor; Minimally invasive operation (see MIST).
MiO Microorchidism.
mio- prefix meaning smaller (Gr. meion).
MIP Maximal/imum inspiratory pressure (see PFT - MIP); Mean/ Median incubation period; Mean intravascular pressure; Median/ Mild/ Moderate interstitial plasmacytosis (see PTPP); Medical improvement possible; Medical insurance program; Metabolically invasive procedure; Middle interphalangeal (joint); Minimal/imum inspiratory pressure; Minimally invasive procedure (see MIT); Missouri Institute of Psychiatry.
MIPI Medicine in the Public Interest.
MIR Maintenance infusion rate; Medical Instrument Reports (journal); Metabolic insulin resistance (see IIR); Micro-infrared (analyzer); Mild infusion reaction; Misguided immune response (as in Autoimmune diseases); Morphine (sulphate) immediate release (tablet); Multiple immune response(s); Multiple injection regimen (e.g. Insulin therapy in IDDM); Multiple isomorphous replacement.
MIRC Microtubuloreticular complex.
MIRD Medical internal radiation dose.
MIRP Myocardial infarction rehabilitation program.
MIRU Myocardial infarction research unit (NHLI).
MIS Management information system; Mean intact stiffness (by fixation device) (see AFS; MFS); Medical imaging system (e.g. MRI); Medical information service; Meiosis-inducing substance; Memory Impaiment Study (NIA); Minimally invasive surgery; Mitral insufficiency; Mucosal immune system; Müllerian inhibiting substance.
misc miscarriage; miscellaneous; miscible.
MISG Modified immune serum globulin.
MISHAP Microcephalus-imperforate anus-syndactyly-hamartoblastoma-abnormal lung lobulation-polydactyly (syndrome).
MISO Misonidazole.
MISP Member of the Institution of Sewage Purification (see MInstSP).
MISS Modified Injury Severity Scale/ Score.
miss- combining form meaning send (L. mitto).
MIST Management of Influenza in the Southern Hemisphere Trialists (Study Group); Medical Information Service by/via Telephone (Alabama); Minimally invasive surgical technique (= MIBS; MIHS; MIS; MIT).
mist a mixture (L. mistura) (= mix; mixt).
mistrans mistranslation.
MIT Male impotence test; Marrow iron turnover; Massachusetts Institute of Technology; Meconium in trachea; Melodic intonation therapy; Metabolism inhibition test; Migration inhibition test; Minimally

invasive technique (see MIST)/ therapy/ treatment; Miracidial immobilization test; Mitochondria; Mitomycin; Modern imaging technique/nology; Monoiodotyrosine (= 3-Iodo-L-tyrosine).

mit mitral; send (L. mitte) (= mitt).

MITC Methyl-isothiocyanate.

mit insuf mitral insufficiency.

mito- prefix meaning thread (Gr. mitos).

Mito C Mitomycin (= Mutamycin).

mit sang; mitt sang bleed (L. mitte sanguinem).

mitt send (see mit).

mit tal; mitt tal send such (L. mitte tales).

-mittent suffix meaning send (L. mittentis).

MITU Mobile inflatable treatment unit.

MIU Milli-International unit (see mIU); Million international unit(s); Myocardial Infarction Unit (Research Unit - NHLI).

mIU milli-International unit (= 1/1000 International unit; 10^{-3} IU).

μIU one-millionth of an International Unit.

MIV Mammographic image visualization.

MIVS Minimally invasive valve surgery.

mix mixture (see mist).

mix mon mixed monitor.

mixt mixture (see mist).

MJ Machado-Joseph (disease); Marijuana or Mary Jane (see Cannabis); Mead Johnson & Co (USA) code for experimental substances; Megajoule; Sotalol (a beta-blocker).

Mj Mary Jane (marijuana) (see Cannabis).

mJ; mj millijoule.

μj microjoule (= microule; 10^{-6} joule).

M-J Mowlem-Jackson (technique).

MJA Mechanical joint apparatus; Medical Journal of Australia.

MJAD Machado-Joseph Azorean disease.

MJC Medial joint compartment (knee).

MJD Machado-Joseph disease; Mseleni joint disease.

MJRC Mead Johnson Research Center.

MJRT Maximum junctional recovery time.

MJS Maximum/ Medium/ Minimum joint stability.

MJT Mead Johnson tube.

MK Megakaryocyte; Member of the Kenesset (Israel's Parliament); Merck and Co (USA) code for experimental substances; Monkey kidney (= MkK); Monkey (lung culture) (see MKLC); Myokinase.

Mk Mark (model); Monkey (= Mky).

MK 135 Cholestyramine - used in the treatment of hypercholesterolemia; also in biliary cirrhosis and pruritus.

MK 240 Protriptyline hydrochloride - an antidepressant drug with actions similar to those of amitriptyline.

MK 250 Emylcamate - a tranquillizer (see KABI 925).

MK 351 Methyldopa (= Alpha-methyldopa) - a hypotensive agent acting by interfering with the formation of noradrenaline at the sympathetic nerve endings, by inhibiting the conversion of dopa to dopamine, as a result of competition for the enzyme dopa decarboxylase.

MK 360 Thiabendazole (= Tiabendazole) - a veterinary anthelmintic used in nematode infestation. In humans it is especially effective against strongyloid worms, roundworms, threadworms and hookworms.

MK 485 Alpha methyldopa hydrazine - a peripheral carboxylase inhibitor.

MK 486 Alpha methyldopa hydrazine - a peripheral carboxylase inhibitor.

MK 595 Ethacrynic acid (= Etacrynic acid; Methylene-butyl phenoxyacetic acid) - a powerful diuretic, more potent than the thiazides, acting on the kidney nephron.

MK 870 Amiloride - a diuretic.

MKA Mucokinetic agent (e.g. bromhexine).

MKAB May keep at bedside.

mkat millikatal.

μkat microkatal.

mkat/l millikatals per liter.

MKB Megakaryoblast.

MKBs Meyers-Kouwenaar bodies (found in the lymph nodes, lungs, spleen and liver in patients with occult filariasis).

MKC Monkey kidney cell.

MK-CSF Megakaryocyte colony stimulating-factor.

MKD Mild/ Minimal/ Moderate kidney dysfunction (see MRD).

mkg; m-kg meter-kilogram.

MKHS Menkes' kinky hair syndrome.

MkK Monkey kidney (see MK).

MkL Megakaryoblastic leukemia.
MKLC Monkey kidney lung culture (= MK).
MKP Monobasic potassium phosphate.
MKS Meter-kilogram-second (see mks).
mks meter-kilogram-second. A system of measurements or units based on the meter as the unit of length, the kilogram as the unit of mass, and the second as the unit of time (= MKS).
MKSAP Medical Knowledge Self-Assessment Program.
MKTC Monkey kidney tissue culture.
MKV Measles, killed vaccine.
Mky Monkey (see Mk).
ML Licentiate in Medicine/ Midwifery (see LM); Lingual margin (see LM); Lygranum antigen (see LA); Malignant lymphoma; Marked latency; Maximum likelihood; Medial leminiscus; Medical Lab (journal); Mesiolingual; Middle lobe (of right lung); Midline; Molecular/ Muscular layer; Motor latency; Mucolipidosis; Multiple lentiginosis; Myeloid leukemia.
mL millilambert (= 1/1000 of a lambert; 10^{-3} L; mLa) (see L. Lambert).
ml; mL; Ml milliliter (= cc; cubic centimeter; 1/1000 of a liter; 10^{-3} l; mil; Ml).
μl; μL microliter (= 10^{-6} l; cu mm; cubic millimeter).
M/L Monocyte/lymphocyte (ratio); Mother-in-law.
M-L Martin-Lewis (medium).
ML I, II, III, IV Mucolipidosis I, II, III, IV.
MLA Medical Laboratory Automation, Inc; Medical Library Association; Medical Licensing Authorities (see IAMLA); Medical-licensing authority; Mento-laeva anterior (L.) (Left mento-anterior/ position of fetus); Mesiolabial (see MLa); Middle lobe atelectasis (MLS/ Middle-lobe syndrome) - right lung; Modern Language Association; Modern Learning Aids; Monocytic leukemia, acute; Motion-limiting adhesion(s) (Orthopedics); Mouse Lymphoma Assay; Mucolytic agent.
MLa; Mla Mesiolabial (= MLA).
mLa millilambert (see mL).
MLAB Medical Library Association Bulletin; Multilingual Aphasia Battery.
MLaI; Mlai Mesiolabioincisal.
MLAP Mean left atrial pressure.
MLaP; Mlap Mesiolabiopulpal.
MLB Monoaural loudness balance (test).
MLb Macrolymphoblast.
MLBP Mechanical low back pain.
MLC Medical Liability Commission; Metastatic liver/ lung cancer; Minimal/imum lethal concentration; Mixed leukocyte culture (= MCL); Mixed ligand chelate; Mixed lymphocyte concentration/ culture; Morphine-like compound; Multilamellar cytosome; Multi-level care; Multi-lumen catheter; Myelomonocytic leukemia, chronic (see MCL); Myosin light chain.
MLCFMA Mouse Lymphoma Cell Forward Mutation Assay.
MLCK Myosin light chain kinase.
MLCO Member of the London College of Osteopathy.
MLCP Myosin light chain phosphatase.
MLCR Mixed lymphocytic culture reaction.
MLCT Metal-to-ligand charge transfer.
MLD Masking-level difference; Mean/ Minimum lumen diameter; Mean lung deposition (of an inhaled drug); Median lethal dose (radiation) - a dose which is lethal for 50% of the test subjects (= LD_{50}; LD-50; MLD-50); Metachromatic leukodystrophy (sulfatase); Mild/ Moderate liver disease/ dysfunction (see MHD); Minimal lesion disease; Minimum lethal dose - the minimum dose of a drug or organism (in culture), which can kill a particular species of animal; Morphine-like drug (see ODD).
MLD_{50}; MLD-50 Median lethal dose (see MLD).
ml/dl milliliters per deciliter.
MLDT Medical Letter on Drugs and Therapeutics.
MLE Maximum likelihood estimation; Midline episiotomy; Morphinelike endorphin(s).
MLES Microsomal liver enzyme system.
MLF Medial longitudinal fasciculus; Morphine-like factor.
MLG Mesiolingual groove; Mid-late gestation; Mitochondrial lipid glycogen.
MLGN Minimal lesion glomerulonephritis.
ML-H Malignant lymphoma, histiocytic.

MLI Major/ Mild/ Minor/ Moderate liver impairment; Mesiolinguoincisal; Mixed lymphocyte interaction.

MLIVD Minimum lethal intravenous dose (in laboratory animals).

MLJ Medico-Legal Journal.

MLK 3 series of X-ray lines.

MLL Mediastinal lymphoblastic lymphoma.

ml/l milliliters per liter.

MLMA Mouse lymphoma mutation assay.

MLMIC Medical Liability Mutual Insurance Company (New York).

ml/min/m^2 milliliters per minute per square meter.

MLN Manifest latent nystagmus; Mediastinal lymph node (or IMLN - Ipsilateral MLN) (highest mediastinal, upper paratracheal, pretracheal, retrotracheal, lower paratracheal, subaortic, para-aortic, subcarinal, paraesophageal, and pulmonary ligament lymph nodes); Membranous lupus nephropathy; Mesenteric/ Metastatic lymph node.

MLNS Minimal lesion nephrotic syndrome; Mucocutaneous lymph node syndrome (= KD; MCLNS; MCLS).

MLO Medical Laboratory Observer (journal); Mediolateral oblique (view - X-ray); Mesiolinguo-occlusal; Mycoplasma-like organism.

MLP Macrodystrophia lipomatosa progressiva (see MDLP); Mento-laeva posterior (L.) - left mentoposterior fetal position; Mesiolinguopulpal; Microsomal lipoprotein; Multiple lipid parameters (HDL-C; LDL-C; Triglycerides).

ML-PDL Malignant lymphoma, poorly differentiated lymphocyte.

MLR Macula lutea retinae (= MR - Macula retinae); Major/ Minimal liver/ lung resection; Mean length of response; Middle latency response; Mixed leukocyte/ lymphocyte reaction/ response; Morbilliform-like rash (see MLSR); Multiple linear regression (e.g. of energy-adjusted nutrients, age, and smoking - in the Edinburg Artery Study); Multiple logistic regression.

MLRA Multivariate logistic regression analysis.

MLS Maximum length sequence(s); Mean/ Median/ Medium life span; Median longitudinal section; Medico-Legal Society (UK); Microlaryngoscope/py; Middle lobe syndrome; Mild/ Minimal luminal stenosis (e.g. CAS - Coronary artery stenosis); Mouse/ Murine leukemia virus; Myelomonocytic leukemia, subacute (= MSL).

MLSB Migrating long spike burst.

MLSP Multilinear solvent programmer.

MLSR Morbilliform-like skin rash.

MLT Malignant liver tumor (see MHT); Mean latency time; Median lethal time; Medical Laboratory Technician/nologist (ASCP); Mento-laeva transversa (L.) - left mentotransverse position of fetus; Mucolytic therapy/ treatment.

MLT(ASCP) Medical Laboratory Technician certified by the American Society of Clinical Pathologists.

MLTC Mixed leukocyte-trophoblast culture; Mixed lymphocyte tumor cell.

MLTI Mixed lymphocyte target interaction.

MLU Mean length of utterance.

MLV Moloney's leukemogenic virus; Monitored live voice; Mouse/ Murine leukemia virus; Multilamellar/laminar vesicle (Liposome) (see LSM).

MLVDP Maximum left ventricular developed pressure.

mlx millilux.

MM Macromolecule; Magnetic monopole; Main memory (computer); Major Medical (insurance); Malignant/ Metastatic melanoma; Manubrium to malleus; Marshall-Marchetti; Master of Management; Medial malleolus; Medicaid "mill"; Megamitochondria; Melanoma metastasis; Meningococcal meningitis; Menstrually-related migraine; Mercaptopurine and methotrexate; Methacryl methylate; Methadone maintenance; Michaelis-Menten (constant/ equation); Million (= 10^6; a thousand thousand); Military Medicine (AMSUS journal); Minimal medium; Mismatched; Modern Medicine (journal); Montreal Medical (journnal, now QM); Morbidity and mortality (see M&M); Motor meal; Mucous membrane (see mm); Multiple myeloma (tosis); Muscle CPK isoenzyme (see CPK-3); Muscularis mucosae; Myeloid metaplasia; Myelomeningocele; Two thousand (Roman numeral for) (see Symbols - 6).

mM millimol(e)/ar-solution - electrolyte measurement (= 10^{-3} mol/mole; mmol). A mol or mole is a unit of mass in grams, equivalent to its formula or molecular mass.

mm methylmalonyl; millimeter (= 10^{-3} m; 10^{-3} meter); mucous membrane (= MM); muscles.

mμ millimicron (= 10^{-9} M or 10^{-9} meter; 10^{-3} μ or 10^{-3} micron; 10^{-6} mm or 10^{-6} millimeter; mmu or millimu; mmm; nM, now nm or nanometer).

μm micrometer (= 10^{-6} meter); micromilli-.

μM; μm micromole (see mM - millimole); micromolar.

μμ micromicron (= 10^{-12} M or 10^{-12} meter; μμm or micromicrometer; 10^{-9} mm or 10^{-9} millimeter; nmm or nanomillimeter; pM or picometer; 10^{-6} μ or one millionth of a micron).

M&M Milk and molasses (enema); Morbidity and mortality (= MM).

mm² square millimeter (see sq mm).

mm³ cubic millimeter (see cu mm).

μm³ cubic micrometer (see μm).

MMA Mastitis-metritis-agalactia (syndrome); Maternal measles antibody; Medical materials account; Methylmanonic acid; Methylmethacrylate (see PMMA); Microbial mutagenesis assay (in vitro assay) (see CAA); Minor morphologic aberration; Monomer methyl methacrylate (liquid); Monomethyl adenosine; Montana Medical Association; Mouse micronucleus assay; Multiple migraine attack(s).

MMAb Maternal measles antibody (= MMA); Mouse monoclonal antibody.

MMAD Mass median aerodynamic diameter.

MMATP Methadone maintenance and aftercare treatment program.

MMB/d Million barrels (of oil) per day.

MMC Mainstream medical care; Malignant myeloma cell; Médecine Moderne du Canada/ Modern Medicine of Canada (journal); Megamitochondrion; Meningomyelocele; Metropolitan Medical Center (New York City); Methyl methacrylate (plastic material used in cranioplasty and arthroplasty); Migrating myoelectric complex; Minimal/imum medullary concentration; Mitomycin C; Monmouth Medical Center (New Jersey); Mucosal mast cell; Myelomeningocele (see SBC).

mμc millimicrocurie (= 10^{-9} c or 10^{-9} curie; 10^{-3} μc or 10^{-3} microcurie; mμCi; nc, nCi, or nanocurie.

μμc; μμC micromicrocurie (= 10^{-12} c or 10^{-12} curie; pc or picocurie).

mμCi millimicrocurie - now nCi (see mμc).

MMD Malignant myeloid disease; Mass median diameter (of particles); Menstrual mood disorder; Methyl-mercury dicyanimide; Micrometastatic disease (e.g. lung cancer); Minimum morbidostatic dose; Mitochondrial malate dehydrogenase (= MMDH); Moyamoya disease; Mucus-modifying drug (e.g. acetylcysteine, bromhexine, etc.) (see BSL); Multi-metabolic disease/ disorder; Multiple-memory device (= MMHA); Myotonic muscular dystrophy.

MMDA Methoxymethylene dioxyamphetamine (= trimethoxyamphetamine) (see Amphet - MMDA).

MMDH Mitochondrial malate dehydrogenase (see MMD).

MME Master of Medical Education (Univ. of Bern, Switzerland); M-mode echocardiography; Mouse mammary epithelium.

MMECT Multiple monitor electroconvulsive therapy.

MMED; M Med Master of Medicine.

MMEF Maximum midexpiratory flow (see PFT - $FEF_{25\text{-}75\%}$) (= MMF); Mean midexpiratory flow.

MMEFR Maximum midexpiratory flow rate (see PFT - $FEF_{25\text{-}75\%}$) (= MMFR).

MMF Magnetomotive force; Maximum midexpiratory flow (see MMEF); Mean maximum flow; Member of the Medical Faculty; Molecular mechanisms of fever; Mycophenolate mofetil (an immunosuppressant [2-morpholinoethyl] ester of MPA or mycophenolic acid; an IMPDH inhibitor) (see IMPDH).

μμF micromicrofarad (picofarad).

MMFR Maximum midexpiratory flow rate

(see MMEFR); Maximal midflow rate.

MMFV Maximal midexpiratory flow volume (see PFT - $FEF_{25-75\%}$).

MMG Manchester Medical Gazette (UK); Mean maternal glucose.

mμg millimicrogram (= mμgm, 10^{-3} μg, or 10^{-3} microgram; 10^{-9} g or 10^{-9} gram); μmg, μmgm, 10^{-6} mg, 10^{-6} milligram, or micromilligram; mγ or milligamma; 10^{-9} g, ng, or nanogram).

μmg micromilligram (nanogram) (see mμg).

μμg micromicrogram (= μμgm, 10^{-12} g, or 10^{-12} gram; pg or picogram).

MMGB Modern Medicine of Great Britain (journal).

mμgm millimicrogram (see mμg).

μmgm micromilligram (see mμg).

μμgm micromicrogram (see μμg).

MMH Monomethylhydrazine.

MMHA Multiple-memory hearing aid (see MMD).

mmHg millimeters of mercury (pressure unit).

μmHg micrometer of mercury.

mmH_20 millimeters of water (pressure unit).

MMI Macrophage migration inhibition; Male menopausal impotence; Methylmercapto-imidazole; Midland Medical Institute (UK); Mild mental illness (= MIL); Mucous membrane irritation.

MMIHS Megacystis-microcolon-intestinal hypoperistalsis syndrome.

MMIP Medical Malpractice Insurance Policy.

MMIS Medicaid/ Medical Management and Information System (HEW).

MMK Marshall-Marchetti-Krantz (cystourethroplexy).

MMK; μMK Micromegakaryocyte.

MML Moloney mouse/ murine leukemia; Monomethyl lysine; Myelomonocytic leukemia.

mM/l millimoles per liter.

MMLS Measuring for Medicine and the Life Sciences (journal).

MMLV Moloney murine leukemia virus.

MMM 3-M or Miller, McKusick, and Malvaux (syndrome) - who first described it; Medical Marketing and Media (journal, formerly PMM); Malignant mediastinal mass; Microsome-mediated mutagenesis; Minnesota Mining and Manufacturing Co (3M); Modern Medical Methods Inc; Myelofibrosis/ Myelosclerosis and/with myeloid metaplasia; Myeloid metaplasia and/with myelofibrosis.

mmm millimicron (see mμ).

μmm micromillimeter (nanometer).

μmμ meson.

MMMF Man-made mineral fibers.

MMMSD Multi-metabolic multi-system disease/ disorder.

MMMT Malignant mixed müllerian tumor.

MMN Medical Moral Newsletter (formerly MNR); Morbus maculosus neonatorum; Multiple mucosal neuroma.

MMNA Mouse micronucleus assay.

MMNC Marrow mononuclear cell.

MMNZ Modern Medicine of New Zealand (journal).

MMO Methane mono-oxygenase.

MMOA Maxillary mandibular odontectomy alveolectomy.

MMoL Myelomonoblastic leukemia.

mmol millimol(e) (see mM).

μmol micromol(e) (= 10^{-6} mole; 10^{-6} M; 10^{-6} mol).

mmol/L; mmol/l millimoles per liter or millimolar.

MMP Male menopause (= Andropause); Maternal medical problem; Monomorphous population (of cell types, etc.); Myeloid metaplasia (see MCMM; PPMM).

MMPB Michigan Medical Practice Board.

MMPI Minnesota Multiphasic Personality Inventory (psychological test).

MMPI-Ds Minnesota Multiphasic Personality Inventory - Depression scale.

MMPI Ps Minnesota Multiphasic Personality Inventory - Propensity scale.

MMPNC Medical Maternal Program for Nuclear Casualties.

mmpp millimeter of mercury partial pressure; millimeters partial pressure, i.e. partial pressure expressed in millimeters of mercury (mms Hg).

MMPR Methylmercaptopurine riboside.

MMPs Matrix metalloproteinases (protease enzymes); Multiple medical problems.

MMPW Matched mean percentage weight.

MMQ Moos Menstrual Questionnaire.

MMR Mass miniature radiography; Maternal mortality rate; Meaningful migraine relief; Measles-mumps-rubella (vaccine); Midland Medical Review (UK journal); Midline malignant reticulosis; Mismatch repair (gene); Mobile mass radiography; Mono-methylol-rutin; Mouth-to-mouth resuscitation; Myocardial metabolic rate.

MMS Male menopausal syndrome; Massachusetts Medical Society; Master of Medical Science (= MMSc; MScMed); Medical Mission Sisters; Methyl methanesulfonate; Military Medical Services; Mini-Mental Status (test); Modern Maturity Study/ Survey (see MMSS); Multiple 'mini-stroke(s)'; Myasthenic-myopathic syndrome (an autoimmune disorder).

MMSA Master of Midwifery, Society of Apothecaries.

MMSc Master of Medical Science (see MMS).

MMSE Mini-Mental State Exam.

mμs millimicrosecond.

mm/sec millimeters per second.

MMSS Modern Maturity Sexuality Study (AARP) (= MMS).

mm st muscle strength.

MMT Manual muscle test; α-Methyl-m-tyrosine; Mini Mental Test; Mouse mammary tumor; Mouse micronucleus test.

MMTA Methylmetatyramine.

MMTLV Mouse-mammary tumor-like virus (see MMTV; MTV).

MMTP Methadone Maintenance Treatment Program.

MMTS Methyl-methyl-thiomethyl sulfoxide (= FAMSO).

MMTV Mouse mammary tumor virus (= MTV).

MMU Medical maintenance unit; Mercaptomethyl uracil.

mmu millimass unit; millimicron or millimu (see mμ).

MMuLV Moloney murine leukemia virus.

MMV Mandatory minute volume.

MMVD Mixed mitral-valve disease.

MMVR Medicine Meets Virtual Reality (conference).

MMWR Morbidity and Mortality Weekly Report.

MN A blood group in the MNS blood group system (see MNS); Malignant nephrosclerosis; Master of Nursing; Medical News (journal, formerly MN-T); Medicolegal News (ASLM journal); Mega-newton; Melena neonatorum; Melanocytic nevus; Membranous nephropathy/ neuropathy; Mesenteric node; Metanephrine; Midnight (see M/N); Migraine News (UK journal); Migrainous neuralgia (see CH - Cluster headache); Mononuclear (leukocyte); Motoneuron; Motor neuron(e); Multinodular; Myoneural.

Mn Manganese (Z = 25) (see Elements - Manganese).

mN micronewton; millinormal (= 10^{-3} N; 1/1000 of Normal).

mn modal number.

μN nuclear magneton.

MN# Medial neck fracture (of femur).

M&N; m&n Morning and night (L. mane et nocte) (= m et n).

MNA Maximum noise area; Maximum/ Minimal/ Moderate neurological abnormalities/ty; Medical Nobel Assembly; Medical nurse associate; Micronucleus assay (for mutagenicity - experiment on rats, etc.).

MNAP Mixed nerve action potential.

MNB Murine neuroblastoma; Muscle needle biopsy.

5-MNBA 5-Mercapto-2-nitrobenzoic acid.

MNBCCS Multiple nevoid basal-cell carcinoma syndrome.

MNC Macronodular cirrhosis (of the liver) with leuconychia, pink palms, spider nevi, telangiectasia and testicular atrophy); Median nerve compression; Mononuclear cell (leukocyte); Motor nerve conduction; Motor nuclear cell.

MNCV Mean/ Motor nerve conduction velocity (procedure/ physical medicine).

MND Metabolic and nutritional disorder; Metastatic neoplastic disease; Micronutrient deficiencies/ncy; Minimum necrosing dose; Minor neurological dysfunction; Modified neck dissection; Motor neuron/ neurone disease; Multiple nutritional deficiencies.

MND/ALS Motor neurone disease/

Amyotrophic lateral sclerosis (= Lou Gehrig's disease).

MNE Malignant neoplasm of the endometrium.

mne- combining form meaning remember (Gr.).

MNF Motor neurone function; Multiple neurofibromatosis (= VRD).

MNG Multinodular goiter.

mng morning.

MNGC Multinucleated giant cell.

MNGIE Myo-, neuro-, gastrointestinal encephalopathy.

MNI Montreal Neurological Institute.

MNJ Myoneural junction.

MNL Marked neutrophilic leukocytosis; Maximum number of lamellae; Mononuclear leukocyte.

MNM Mononeuritis multiplex; Myokymia neuromyotonia (= SMS or Stiff-man syndrome).

MN/m² Meganewtons per square meter.

MNMS Myonephropathic metabolic syndrome.

MNN Median nerve neuropathy.

MNNG N-methyl N'-nitro-N-nitrosoguanidine.

MNO complex Contraction of sinus venosus.

MNOS Metal-nitride-oxide semiconductor.

MNP Medical nurse practitioner; Mononuclear phagocyte; Motor neuropathy.

MNP Mononeuropathy.

MNR Marrow neutrophil reserve; Medical Newsletter for Religions (now MMN).

MNS Medial nuclear stratum; Melnick-Needles syndrome; MN system (blood group antigens) (see MNSs); Multinational study.

Mn-SOD Manganese-superoxide dismutase.

MNSs A blood group system consisting of groups M, N, and MN.

MnSSEPs Median nerve somato-sensory evoked potentials.

MNT Micronucleus Test (on laboratory animals).

MN-T Medical News-Tribune (now MN).

MNTB Medial nucleus of the trapezoid body.

MNU Methylnitrosourea (= 1-methyl-1-nitroso urea; N-methyl-N-nitrosourea).

MNWLT Modified New World Learning Test (Walton-Black).

MO Abbot Laboratories (USA) code for experimental substances; Macroorchidism; Manual of operation; Manually operated; Master of Obstetrics/ Osteopathy; Medial oblique (x-ray); Medical Officer; Mesio-occlusal; Metastases, zero; Mineral oil; Minute output (of heart); Modus operandi (L.) - method of performing an action/ operation/ procedure; Molecular orbit(al) (contour); Mono-oxygenase; Months old; Morbid obesity.

Mo Mode (see mo); Moloney (strain); Molybdenum (Z = 42) (see Elements - Molybdenum); Monoclonal; Month (see Mth); Mother; Mouth (see mo).

mo mode (= Mo); month (see Mth); morgan; mouth (= Mo; Mth); reciprocal of the ohm (see mho).

μ_0 permeability of a vacuum.

MΩ Megohm (= 10^6 ohms).

mΩ milliohm (= 10^{-3} ohm).

μΩ microhm (= 10^{-6} ohm).

MO_2 Myocardial oxygen (utilization).

MO 911 Pargyline hydrochloride - a hypotensive monoamine oxidase inhibitor (see A 19120).

MoA Mechanism/Mode of action; Muscle(s) of accommodation (see BV; PMA).

MoAb Monoclonal antibody.

MOB Medical office building; Medicinal oil bath; Myocardial oxygen balance.

mob; mobil mobile/lity/lization.

MOBl Mitomycin-C, Oncovin and Bleomycin (Chemotherapy).

MOB-PT Mitomycin, Oncovin (vincristine), bleomycin, and Platinum compd (cisplatin).

MOC Maximum oxygen consumption; Monophasic oral contraceptive; Mother of child; Multiple ocular coloboma; Myocardial oxygen consumption; Myositis ossificans circumscripta.

MOD Macula-off detachment (retinal detachment involving the macula); Magnetico-optical disk; Maturity onset diabetes; Medical Officer of the Day; Medicine, Osteopathy, and Dentistry; Mesio-occlusodistal; Multiple oral dose/ dosing; Myocardial oxygen demand.

MoD March of Dimes.
Mod; mod Moderate/tion; Modern; Modification/fied; Modulate/tion/tor.
modem modulator/ demodulator.
MODM Maturity-onset diabetes mellitus.
mod praes(c) as/in the manner or way directed/ prescribed (L. modo praescripto).
MODS Medically Oriented Data System (FDA).
MODY Maturity-onset diabetes of the young.
MOEH Medical Officer for Environmental Health.
MOF Marine oxidation/ fermentation (medium); Methotrexate, Oncovin, and fluorouracil; Methoxy-flurane; Multiple organ failure.
MOFD Mandibulo-oculo-facial dyscephaly (beaked nose, bird-like mandible with ocular and dental defects, brittle and sparse hair following cranial sutures - a hereditary hypotrichosis syndrome) (= HSS; PAS).
MOFS Multiple organ failure syndrome (see MOSF).
MO&G Master of Obstetrics and Gynaecology.
mogi- prefix meaning difficult (Gr. mogis).
MOH Maternal oligohydramnios; Medical Officer of Health; Ministry of Health.
MOHSA Ministry of Health and Social Affairs (UK).
MOI Major/ Multiple opportunistic infection(s); Maximum oxygen intake (see PFT - MOI); Mild ocular irrigation/ irritation; Mineralized osseous implant (Orthopedics); Multiple organ implant/ involvement; Multiplicity of infection.
MOIVC Membranous obstruction of the inferior vena cava (= MOVC).
MOJAC Mood orientation, judgement, affect, and content.
Mojo Morphine, heroin or cocaine (see Papaver, Diamorph, Erythroxylum).
MOL Molecular/ule (see mol).
mol mole (= gram-molecule; unit of mass in grams, equivalent to its formula or molecular mass); molecular/ule (= MOL); soft (see moll).
molc molecular concentration.
MolFm Molecular formula.
molfr molecular fraction.
mol/kg moles per kilogram.
mol/L molecules per liter or molar (= mol/l).
moll soft (L. mollis) (= mol).
mol/l molecules per liter.
mol/m^3 moles per cubic meter.
mol/s moles per second.
mol wt molecular weight (= MW).
MOM Main outcome measure(s); Milk of magnesia (see MoM); Mucoid otitis media; Myxoedema(tous) madness (see MEM).
MoM Milk of magnesia (see MOM); Multiples of the median.
MOMA Methylhydroxymandelic acid (= Methoxy-hydroxy-mandelic acid).
MO-MOM Mineral oil and milk of magnesia.
MOMS Mothers Organized for Moral Stability; Multiple organ malrotation syndrome.
Mo-MS Moloney murine sarcoma (= MOS).
Mo-MSV Moloney murine sarcoma virus.
MOMX Macroorchidism-marker X chromosome (syndrome).
MON Mongolian (gerbil/ burrowing rodent).
Mon Monday; Monocyte (see mono).
mon monitor; monocyte (see mono).
mon- prefix meaning one or only (Gr. monos).
MONICA Multinational monitoring of trends and determinants in cardiovascular disease (project - WHO).
Mono Mononucleosis (Infectious) (see IM).
mono monocyte (= Mon; mon); monospot.
mono- prefix meaning one (Gr. monos).
MOO Multifocal osteoid osteoma (see BOB; COB; MSO; POB).
Moon Hashish/ Peyote (see Cannabis; Mesc).
Moota Marijuana (see Cannabis).
MOOW Medical Officer of the Watch.
MOP Major organ profile; Medical outpatient; Methoxy-psoralen (see 8-MOP); Moderately/ Morbidly obese patient; Mustarde otoplasty (correction of prominent ear due to absent antihelix); Myositis ossificans progressiva (or Fibrositis progressiva) (see MCAs).
μOP Mu opiate receptor.
8-MOP 8-Methoxypsoralen (= MOP; MP).
MOPEG 3-Methoxy-4-hydroxyphenyl-ethyleneglycol.

MOPP Mechlorethamine hydrochloride (= Mustine HCl; Nitrogen Mustard), Oncovin (= Vincristine sulfate), Procarbazine hydrochoride (Matulane), and Prednisone (a group of four drugs used in the chemotherapeutic treatment of cancer and Hodgkin's disease).
MOPP-LO-BLEO Mustine, Oncovin, Procarbazine, Prednisone, Lomustine, & Bleomycin (Chemotherapy).
MOPV Monovalent oral poliovirus vaccine.
MOR Medical Opinion and Review (journal); Mu-opioid receptor (CNS).
Mor; mor Morphine (see Morph).
Morav Moravian (church member).
MORC Medical Officers Reserve Corps.
MORD Magnetic optical rotatory dispersion.
mor dict in the manner directed (L. more dicto).
MORE Multiple Outcomes of Raloxifene Evaluation (trial, in cancer therapy).
Morgenstrasse German - "morning walk" - refers to the middle part of the greater curvature of the stomach, "where the food goes through".
Morm Mormon (church member).
Morph Morphine (= Mor; mor) (see Papaver); Morphology (see morph).
morph; morphol morphological/gy.
morph- combining form meaning form or shape (Gr. morphe).
mor sol in the usual manner or way (L. more solito).
mort; mortal mortal(ity).
MOS Medial orbital sulcus; Median overall status/ survival; Medical Outcome Study; Metal oxide semiconductor; Microsomal (ethanol-) oxidizing system; Mirror optical system; Molonoy (murine) sarcoma (see Mo-MS); Myelofibrosis osteosclerosis.
Mos Moslem (religion) (= Mus).
mOs milliosmol(e) (see mOsm).
mos months (see Mths).
MOSAIC Medical Outpatient Services Adapted In Child Care.
MOSF Multiple organ system failure (see MOFS).
MOSFET Metal oxide semiconductor field effect transistor (see MOST).
MOsm Milliosmol(e) (see mOsm).
mOsm milliosmol(e) (= mOs; MOsm; mOsmol; 10^{-3} Osm; 10^{-3} Osmol; 10^{-3} Osmole; 1/1000 Osm). A unit of osmotic pressure.
μOsm micro-osmolar.
mOsm/kg milliosmoles/osmols/osmolars per kilogram.
mOsm/l milliosmoles/osmols/osmolars per liter.
mOsmol milliosmol(e) (see mOsm).
MOSS Myelofibrosis-osteosclerosis syndrome.
MOSST Ministry of State for Science and Technology (Canada).
MOST Mercy Outreach Surgical Team (at Scripps Mercy Hospital, CA); Metal oxide semiconductor transistor (see MOSFET); Mothers of Supertwins.
MOT Mouse ovarian tumor; Multiorgan transplant.
MoT Mode of transmission (of a disease).
Mot; mot Motor.
mot- combining form meaning move (L. motus).
Mota Marijuana (see Cannabis).
MOTR Medical Oncology and Therapeutics Research (COH).
MOTs Metastatic ovarian tumors.
MOTT Mycobacteria other than the tubercle (bacilli)/ tuberculosis.
MOUS Multiple occurrence of unexplained symptoms.
MOV Multiple oral vitamin (tablet)/ vitamins.
MOVC Membranous obstruction (of the inferior) vena cava (see MOIVC).
MOVT Miller Object Visualization Test.
MoW Meals on wheels.
MOX Moxalactam.
MP A pill mass (L. massa pilularis); As directed (or in the manner prescribed) (see mp); Macrophage; Mallinckrodt Chemical Works (USA) code for experimental substances; Matrix protein; Mean pressure; Medical Pharmacy/ Post (journals); Medical Physics (AAPM journal); Medical Practitioner; Medicare Program; Medroxyprogesterone (acetate) (see MPA); Melphalan and prednisone; Melting point (see mp); Membrane/ Muscle potential; Menninger Perspective

(journal); Menstrual period; Mentum posterior; Meralgia paraesthetica (numbness on the lateral aspect of the thigh) (see LCN); Mercaptopurine (see 6-MP); Mesial pit; Mesiopulpal; Meta/ Metacarpo/ Metatarso phalangeal (joint) (see MPJ); Methoxypsoralen (see 8-MOP); Methylprednisolone; Methylpsoralen (see 8-MP); Mibelli's porokeratosis; Middle phalanx; Millard procedure (repair of cleft lip); Mitchell procedure (type of bunionectomy); Moist pack; Molecular Pharmacology (journal); Monophosphate; Mouth piece; Mucopolysaccharide; Multiparous; Multiprogrammable pacemaker; Mustard procedure (for correction of complete transposition of the great vessels of the heart); Mycoplasmal pneumonia; Myopotential (muscle electric charge); Myrhaug procedure (correction of recurrent jaw dislocation); Myringoplasty (Otolaryngology).

mp as directed or in the manner prescribed (L. modo prescripto) (= MP); melting point (= MP); millipond.

M/P Milk/plasma (ratio) (= M/PR); Most probable/ly.

μP microprocessor.

4MP4 Methylpyrazole.

6-MP 6-Mercaptopurine (an anti-cancer agent) (= MP).

8-MP 8-Methylpsoralen (= MP).

MPA Acid polymucosaccharide(s); Main pulmonary artery; Major/ Minor/ Moderate physical activity; Male-pattern alopecia (see MPAGA); Medial preoptic area; Medical Practice Act (Michigan); Medical Procurement Agency; Medroxyprogesterone/ Methylprednisolone acetate; Methylphosphonic/ Mycophenolic acid; Microscopic polyarteritis; Migratory polyarthropathy; Minor physical anomaly; Moderate persistent asthma.

MPa Megapascal.

μPa micropascal.

MPAb Murine parent antibody (in breast cancer therapy).

MPAD Maximum possible annual dose (radiation).

MPAG Mycophenolic acid glucuronide.

MPAGA Male-pattern androgenetic alopecia (= MAGA; MPA).

MPAP Mean pulmonary arterial/ artery pressure (in mms Hg).

MPAQ McGill Pain Assessment Questionnaire.

MPAS Mild perioxic acid Schiff (reaction).

MPB Male pattern baldness; Meprobamate (see MEP).

MPBB Maximum possible body burden (radionucleotides).

MPBT Malignant primary bone tumor.

MPC Marine protein concentrate; Maximum permissable concentration; Mean percentage change; Mean plasma concentration; Median prefrontal cortex; Medical Policy Committee (UMS); Meperidine, promethazine, and chlorpromazine; Metallophthalocyanine; Metastatic plasma/ prostate/atic cancer/ carcinoma; Miner's pneumoconiosis (= Anthracosis; Black lung; CWP or Coalworker's pneumoconiosis) (see IOD - Inorganic dust); Minimum mycoplasmacidal concentration; Minimum platelet count; Mucopurulent cervicitis; Multidisciplinary pain center; Multidisciplinary prenatal care (= MDPNC); Multiplacement calcium hydroxide (dentistry); Multiple polyposis coli (= FAP); Multipurpose catheter (= Bypass-type/ King catheter).

MPCE Maculopapular cutaneous eruption (see MPECE).

MPCH Morton Prince Clinic for Hypnotherapy.

MPCKS Microloc Porous Coated Knee System (Orthopedic Implants).

MPCN Microscopically positive but culturally negative.

MPCO Micropolycystic ovary syndrome.

MPCP Major Problems in Clinical Pediatrics (journal).

MPCU Maximum permissable concentration of unidentified (radionucleotides) (see MPCUR).

MPCUR Maximum permissable concentration of unidentified radionucleotides (in water) (= MPCU).

MPCWP Mean pulmonary capillary wedge pressure (in mms Hg).

MPD Macho Personality Disorder (see DDPD); Main pancreatic duct; Masticatory pain dysfunction; Maximum permissable dose (of radiation) - that amount of ionizing radiation allowed, that is not expected to lead to bodily harm (= MPE; MPL); Mean population doubling; Medical Products Digest (journal); Membrane potential difference; Minimal perceptible difference; Minimal phototoxic dose; Multiple personality disorder; Myeloproliferative disease; Myofascial pain dysfunction (see MPDS).

MPDC Mechanical Properties Data Center (Traverse City, Michigan).

MPDDS Multiparticulate drug delivery system (see SODAS).

MPDS Mandibular/ Myofascial pain dysfunction syndrome.

MPDW Mean percent desirable weight.

MPE Maculopapular erythema/ erythrodermia/ exanthema; Massive pulmonary; Maximum permissible exposure (see MPD); Maximum possible error.

MPEC Monopolar electrocoagulation.

MPECE Maculopapular erythematous cutaneous eruption.

MPED Minimum phototoxic erythema dose.

mPEG Monomethoxy-polyethylene glycol (see PEGs).

MPEH Methyl-phenyl-ethyl-hydantoin.

MPF Maturation-promoting factor; Mean power frequency; Measured physical fitness; Mucoprotein fiber.

MPFL Metropolitan Police Forensic Laboratory (London).

MPFS Median progression-free survival.

MPG Magnetopneumography; Mean plasma glucose; Membranoproliferative glomerulonephritis (see MPGN); Mercapto-propionyl-glycine; Methyl green pyronine.

MPGM Monophosphoglycerate mutase.

MPGN Membranoproliferative glomerulonephritis (= MPG).

MPH Male pseudohermaphroditism; Master of Public Health; Methylphenidate; Milk protein hydrolysate.

MPh Macrophage.

mph miles per hour.

MPharm Master in/of Pharmacy.

MPHBIM Methyl-p-hydroxy-benzimidate.

MPHD Multiple pituitary hormone deficiencies.

MPHL Male pattern hair loss (= AA - Androgenetic alopecia; MPB) - caused by Type II 5α-reductase in the hair follicles, an intracellular enzyme that metabolizes the androgen testosterone into DHT - Dihydrotestosterone.

mphot milliphot.

MPhysA Member of the Physiotherapists' Association (GB).

MPI Mannose phosphate isomerase; Master patient index; Maudsley Personality Inventory; Max Planck Institute; Maximum permitted intake; Maximum point of impulse; Mean percentage increase; Membrane pump inhibitor; Multiphasic Personality Inventory (psychological test); Myocardial perfusion imaging.

MPJ Meta/ Metacarpo/ Metatarso phalangeal joint; Multiprofessional journal.

mpk milligrams per kilogram.

MPL Maximum permissible level (see MPD); Melphalan; Mesiopulpolingual; Myophosphorylase (deficiency = McArdle's disease).

MPLa Mesiopulpolabial.

MPLB Maximum permissible lung burden (radiation).

MPM Malignant papillary mesothelioma; Medial pterygoid muscle; Miniphotometer; Minor psychiatric morbidity; Mortality Prediction Model; Movements per minute; Multiple peak monitor; Multiple primary malignancy; Multipurpose meal; Mycophenolate mofetil.

mpm miles per minute.

MPMD Manic phase manic depression.

MPME (5R,8R)-8-(4-p-methoxyphenyl)-1-piperazinylmethyl-6-methylergolene.

MPMP Methyl-piperidyl-methyl-phenothiazine (= 10[{1-methyl-3-piperidinyl}-methyl]-1OH-phenothiazine.

MPMT Murphy punch maneuver test.

MPMV Mason-Pfizer monkey virus.

MPN Most probable number.

MPO Maximum power output; Medical and Pediatric Oncology (journal); Minimal perceptible odor; Myeloperoxidase.

MPOA; mPOA Medial preoptic area.

MPOD Myeloperoxidase deficiency.

MPP Massive peritoneal proliferation; Maximum perfusion pressure; Mean pharmacokinetic parameter; Medical personnel planning/ pool; Mercaptopyrazido-pyrimidine; Metacarpophalangeal profile; Multiprogrammable pacemaker; Myocardial perfusion pressure (see CPP).

M(PP)A Medical (Professional Performance) Act of 1995 (UK).

MPPC Mean peak plasma concentration.

MPPCF; mppcf Millions of particles per cubic foot (of air), i.e. dust particles.

MPPEC Mean peak plasma ethanol concentration.

MPPG Microphotoelectric plethysmography.

MPPH Methyl-phenyl-phenyl-hydantoin (= Methyl-p-tolylphenylhydantoin).

MPPN Malignant persistent positional nystagmus.

MPPT Methylprednisolone pulse therapy.

MPPV Mechanical positive pressure ventilation.

MPQ McGill Pain/ Multidimensional Personality Questionnaire.

MPR Maculopapular rash; Marrow production rate; Massive preretinal retraction; Maximum possible response (of a drug); Maximum pulse rate; Myeloproliferative reaction.

M/PR Milk/plasma ratio (see M/P).

MPS Management planning system; Meconium plug syndrome; Medical Products Salesman (journal); Medical Protection Society (UK); Member of the Pharmaceutical Society; Microbial profile system; Microbial protein synthesis; Moderately potent/ powerful steroid (e.g. Clobetasone, Desoximetasone, Panthenol, etc.); Mononuclear phagocyte system; Montreal platelet syndrome; Movement-produced stimuli/lus; Mucopolysaccharide; Mucopolysaccharidosis (syndrome) (= MPSoSIS); Multiphasic screening; Multiple personality syndrome (see MPD); Muscle-pain-spasm (syndrome) (see MPSS); Myocardial perfusion scintigraphy; Myofascial pain syndrome.

mps meters/ miles per second.

MPS I Mucopolysaccharidosis (Hurler's syndrome).

MPS II Mucopolysaccharidosis (Hunter's syndrome).

MPS III Mucopolysaccharidosis (Sanfilippo's syndrome).

MPS IV Mucopolysaccharidosis (Morquio-Ullrich syndrome).

MPS V Mucopolysaccharidosis (Scheie's syndrome).

MPSoSIS Mucopolysaccharidosis (see MPS).

MPSS Methylprednisolone sodium succinate; Muscle-pain-spasm syndrome.

MPSV Myeloproliferative sarcoma virus.

MPsyMed Master of Psychological Medicine.

MPT Maximum phonation time (predicted); Methyl-p-tyrosine (see α-MPT); Michigan Picture Test; Monthly pregnancy test; Mouse protection test (of immunity) - used on mice in yellow fever districts; Multiparticulate technology.

α-MPT Alpha-methyl-p-tyrosine (= α-methyl-p-tyrosine) - an inhibitor of the enzyme, tyrosine hydroxylase, and consequently of catecholamine synthesis. Used in the treatment of hypertension, especially in phaeochromocytoma.

MPTP 1-Methyl-4-phenyl-1,2,3,6-tetrahydropyridine.

MPT-R Michigan Picture Test, Revised.

MPTRD Motor, pain, touch, reflex, and deficit.

MPU Medical Practitioners Union (GB); Medical Protection Union (British malpractice union); Microprocessing unit.

MPV Mean/ Median plasma volume; Mean platelet volume; Mitral valve prolapse.

MPVs Multiple psychological variables (anxiety, depression, hostility, multidimensional stress, and somatization).

mpz millipièze.

MQ Memory quotient.

MQC Microbiologic quality control.

MQL Medical Query Language (computer).

MR Macula retinae (see MFR; MLR); Maddox rods; Magnetic resistance/ resonance; Major/ Maximal/ Median/ Minimal/ Minor response; Mandibular reflex;

Mannose-resistant; May repeat; Measles and rubella; Medial raphe; Medial rectus (muscle); Medical Record (journal); Medical record/ rehabilitation/ release/ resident; Medical Reviews (see BMR); Medicare/ Merck Report (journals); Medium range; Megaroentgen; Meniscus retractor (Arthroscopy); Menstrual regulation; Mental Retardation (AAMD and CAMR journals); Mental retardation; Mentally retarded; Metabolic rate; Methemoglobin reductase; Methyl red (as indicator); Microvascular/ Mutation Research (journals); Mitochondria-rich (cell); Mitral reflux/ regurgitation; Moderate resistance; Modulation rate; Mortality rate/ ratio; Müllerian regression (factor) (see MRF); Multicentric reticulohistiocytosis; Multiple risk (factor) (see MRF); Muscle receptor/ relaxant.

Mr Mega rad (see Mrad).

M_r Relative mollecular mass (weight).

mR; mr millirad (see mrad); milliroentgen - a unit of dose equal to 1/1000 (= 10^{-3}) roentgen (measurement of radiation).

m_r relative migration value of agarose.

μR; μr microroentgen (= 10^{-6} roentgen).

μ/ρ mass attenuation coefficient.

M/R Myeloid/Nucleated (red cell ratio).

M&R Measure and record.

MR x 1,2,3, etc May repeat 1,2,3, etc. times.

MRA Magnetic resonance angiography; Main renal artery; Marrow repopulation activity; Medical records administrator; Medical regulatory authorities/ity (see IAMRA); Membrane reactive antibody; Mental Retardation Abstracts (journal); Mid-right atrium; Mucoregulatory action (see MRE); Multivariate regression analysis; Mu-receptor agonist; Muscarinic receptor antagonist (e.g. tolterodine).

MRAC Modal reference adaptive control.

MRACP Member of the Royal Australasian College of Physicians.

MRad Master of Radiology.

Mrad Mega rad (= Mr; 10^{-6} rad; one million rads).

mrad millirad (= mR; mr; 10^{-3} rad; one thousandth of a rad) - a unit of absorbed radiation dose.

MRAN Medical resident admitting note.

MRAP Maximal/mum resting anal pressure; Mean right atrial pressure (in mm Hg).

MRAS Main renal artery stenosis.

MRB Medical Research Bulletin (Australia).

MRBC Monkey/ Mouse red blood cell(s).

MRBF Mean renal blood flow.

MRC Mature red cell; Maximum recycling capacity; Medical Registration Council; Medical Research Council (Canada; UK; WHO); Medical Reserve Corps; Medullary respiratory center; Metastatic renal cancer (see RCC); Methylrosaniline chloride.

MRCC Metastatic renal cell carcinoma (= RRCC).

MRCD Maximum recommended clinical dose (see MRD).

MRCGP Member of the Royal College of General Practitioners (UK).

MRCI Medical Registration Council, Ireland; Medical Research Coucil of Ireland.

MRCN Medical Research Council Newsletter (Canada; also CRMA).

MRCNP Medical Research Council Neuroimmunology Project (in London).

MRCOG Member of the Royal College of Obstetricians and Gynaecologists.

MRCP Member of the Royal College of Physicians.

MRCPath Member of the Royal College of Pathology.

MRCPE Member of the Royal College of Physicians of Edinburgh.

MRCP (Glasg) Member of the Royal College of Physicians and Surgeons of Glasgow. qua Physician.

MRCPI Member of the Royal College of Physicians of Ireland.

MRCS Member of the Royal College of Surgeons.

MRCs Medical Royal Colleges (UK).

MRCSE Member of the Royal College of Surgeons of Edinburgh.

MRCSI Member of the Royal College of Surgeons in Ireland.

MRCVS Member of the Royal College of Veterinary Surgeons.

MRD Male reproductive disorder (ejaculation failure, erectile dysfunction, sterility, etc.);

Margin reflex distance; Maximum rate of depolarization; Maximum recommended dose (= MRCD; MRDD; MRDI); Measles-rinden-pest-distemper (virus group); Median response duration (see MRD; MR); Medical records department; Microscopic residual disease; Mild/ Minimal/ Major/ Moderate renal dysfunction (= MKD); Mild/ Minimal/ Major/ Moderate restrictive defect; Minimal/mum reacting/ive dose; Minimal renal/ residual disease.

mrd millirutherford.

MRDC Medical Research and Development Council (US Army).

MRDD Maximum recommended daily dose (see MRD); Mental Retardation and Developmental Disabilities.

MRDI Maximum recommended daily intake (see MRD).

MRDM Malnutrition-related diabetes mellitus.

MR-DWI Magnetic resonance diffusion-weighted imaging.

MRE Major/ Minor rejection episode (in organ transplantation); Manual resistance exercise; Maximal resistive exercise; Maximal respiratory effectiveness; Maximum respiratory excursion (see PFT - MRE); Medical Research Engineering (journal); Milligrams of radium equivalent; Mucoregulatory effect (= MRA).

MREE Measuring resting energy expenditure.

MREI Mean rate ejection index.

mrem millirem (= milliroentgen-equivalent-man) - the quantity of any ionizing radiation which has the same biological effectiveness as one millirad of X-rays. 1 millirem = 1 millirad x RBE (relative biological effectiveness).

mrep milliroentgen equivalent physical.

MRF Major/ Metabolic/ Minor/ Modifiable risk factor; Medical record file/ form; Medical Research Foundation (Palo Alto); Melanocyte-(stimulating hormone)-releasing factor (see Hormones - MSH ii); Mesencephalic/ Midbrain reticular formation; Mild/ Moderate renal failure; Mitral regurgitant/ation flow; Monoclonal rheumatoid factor (see mRF); MSH-releasing factor (see Hormones - MSH ii); Müllerian regression factor (= MR factor); Multiple risk factor (= MR factor).

mRF Monoclonal rheumatoid factor (= MRF).

MRFC Mouse rosette-forming cell.

MRFIT Multiple Risk Factor Intervention Trial (NHLI).

MRFT Modified rapid fermentation test.

MRG Murmurs, rubs, and gallops.

MRH Maddox rod hyperphoria; Meigs radical hysterectomy (in Stage IB and IIA carcinoma of the cervix); Melanocyte-stimulating hormone (MSH) - releasing hormone (see Hormones - MSH ii); Multicentric reticulohistiocytosis.

MRHA Mannose-resistant hemagglutination.

MRHD Maximum recommended human dose.

mrhm milliroentgens per hour at one meter.

MRHOD Maximum recommended human oral dose.

MRHT Modified rhyme hearing test.

MRI Machine-readable identifier; Magnetic resonance imaging (= NMR); Medical records information; Medical Research Institute; Member of the Royal Institution (UK); Membrane reactive immunity; Mental Research Institute (MRF); Midwest Research Institute; Mild/ Minimal/ Moderate renal impairment; Mild/ Minimal/ Moderate renal insufficiency.

MRIF Melanocyte(-stimulating hormone) release-inhibiting factor.

MRI.GSC.IPD Magnetic Resonance Image-Guided Stereotactic Cingulotomy for Intractable Psychiatric Disease.

MRIH Melanocyte(-stimulating hormone) release-inhibiting hormone.

MRIID Medical Research Institute of Infectious Diseases (US Army).

M&RI&O Measure and record intake and output (of fluids).

MRIPHH Member of the Royal Institute of Public Health and Hygiene (UK).

MRK Mayer-Rokitansky-Küster (syndrome).

MRL Magnetic Resonance Laboratory; Medical records librarian; Medical Research Laboratory; Wm S Merrell Co (USA) code for experimental substances; Merck Research Laboratories.

MRL 41 Clomiphene citrate (= Clomifene citrate; Chloramiphene citrate; NSC 35770) - a synthetic non-steroidal estrogen chemically related to chlorotrianisene; it stimulates the production of pituitary gonadotropic hormones, particularly the luteinizing hormone.
MRM Metabolic rate monitor (oxygen consumption); Modified radical mastectomy; Multiple regression method.
MRMC Michael Reese Medical Center.
MRMS Metastatic rhabdomyosarcoma.
MRN Malignant renal neoplasm; Medical Record News (AMRA).
mRNA messenger ribonucleic acid (= messenger RNA).
mRNP messenger ribonucleoprotein.
MRO Minimal recognizable odor; Multiresistant organism(s); Muscle receptor organ.
MROD Medical Research and Operations Directorate.
MRP Mean resisting potential; Mechanical robotic pattern(s) (of movement, speech, etc., as in Asperger syndrome - see AMS; GS; ORP; PDD; SMC); Medical Radiography and Photography (journal); Medical Rehabilitation Program (New York); Medical reimbursement plan; Medical Retirement Plan (AMA); Myocardial revascularization procedure (= CABA; CABG; PTCA).
MRPMD Menstruation-related periodic mood disorder (= PMD).
MRR Marrow release rate; Maximum relation rate.
M/R ratio Relation between myeloid and nucleated red cells (see M/R).
MRS Magnetic resonance scanner/ spectroscopy/ study; Male reproductive system; Mania Rating Scale; Medical receiving station; Median-range score; Melkersson-Rosenthal syndrome; Multicenter randomized study; Multiresistant strain (bacterial/ pathogenic/ viral); Muscarinic receptor stimulation (at the parasympathetic, cholinergic nerve terminal).
MRSA Methicillin/ Multiresistant *Staphylococcus* aureus.
MRSE Methicillin-resistant Staphylococcus epidermitis.
MRSH Member of the Royal Society of Health (UK).
MRT Magnetic resonance technique/ tomography; Major role therapy (psychiatry); Maximum relaxation time; Median range score; Median reaction/ relapse time; Median recognition threshold; Medical records technition/nology; Milk ring test; Muscle response test.
MRTDD Maximum recommended total daily dose.
MRTI Medical Radio and Television Institute.
MRTV Muscle relaxation, tracheostomy, and ventilation (treatment for neonatal tetanus) (see PTV).
MRU Mass Radiography Unit; Medical Resistance Union; Minimal reproductive unit(s) (bacteriology).
MRUS Maximal rate of urea synthesis.
MRV Minirotavirus; Minute respiratory volume; Mixed respiratory vaccine.
MRVI Mixed respiratory virus infection(s) (see MVRI).
MRVP Mean right ventricular pressure; Methyl red, Voges-Proskauer (medium).
MR_{X1} May repeat once/ one time (medication order).
MS Complex of substrate and activating metal ion; Maffuci/ Marfan/ Meckel/ Ménière's (= ELS; Labyrinthine hydrops)/ Menkes/ Menopausal/ Meretoja syndrome; Main Scale (psychology); Maladjustment/ Mean score; Marie-Strumpell (disease/ syndrome); Mass spectrometer/etry/roscopy; Master of Science (see MSc); Master of Surgery (see MCh); Mean square (statistics); Mechanical stimulation; Median sternotomy (see OCS - Open-chest surgery); Mediastinal shift; Medical services/ student/ supplies/ survey; Mental status; Methionine synthase; Methyl silicone; Meyerson sign (Ophthalmology); Microscope slide; Military Surgeon (journal); Milk shake; Minimal support; Mitral sounds/ stenosis; Mobile surgical (unit); Modal sensitivity; Moderately susceptible; Molar solution; Molder's sign (a positive sign for Morton's neuroma); Moleskin (skin wrap, especially under casts - Orthopedics); Moles of substitution; Mongolian spot; Monospecies (insulin)

(see MS insulin; Insulin - MSI); Morning sickness/ stiffness; Morphine sulfate (see ms; Papaver); Motile sperm; Moynahan syndrome (see AEOS); Mucosubstance; Multiple sclerosis (= DS; IS); Munchausen syndrome - after Baron Karl F.H. (Friedrich Hieronymus) von Munchausen (1720-1797), the 18th century cavalry officer who returned home from the war against the Turks and told fantastic and embellished tales of his so-called adventures, thus giving name to a condition characterized by habitual presentation for hospital treatment of an apparent acute illness, the patient giving a plausible and dramatic history, all of which is entirely fictitious; Muscle shortening/ spindle/ strength; Musculoactive substance; Musculo-skeletal; Myasthenic syndrome (see E-L or Eaton-Lambert; ELS).

M-S Medi-Strumpf (elastic stockings for venous thrombosis).

Ms Manuscript; Masrium (chemical symbol); Morgenstrasse (German) - "morning walk" - refers to the middle part of the greater curvature of the stomach; Murmurs.

ms millisecond (= msec; 1/1000 sec; 10^{-3} s); morphine sulfate (see Papaver); with the left hand (Ital. mano sinistra).

μs microsecond (= μsec; 10^{-6} s).

M&S Microculture and sensitivity.

M/S Medical - surgical.

m/s meters per second.

m/s^2 meters per second squared.

MS I, II, III, IV Medical student - first, second, third, and fourth year.

MS-222 Tricaine methane sulfonate.

MSA Major serologic antigen; Male-specific antigen; Mannitol salt agar (culture plate); Maritime Safety Act; Medical Services Administration (HEW; SRS); Medical Staff in Action (AMA journal); Membrane stabilizing action/ activity; Metropolitan statistical area; Mild superficial acne; Mine Safety Appliances Co; Mouse serum albumin; Movement, Strength and Alternate activity (treatment of Sprains); Multiple system atrophy; Multisystem abnormality; Muscle sympathetic activity; Myelosuppressive agent.

MSAA Multiple sclerosis - associated agent.

MSAD McEwen-Streitwieser-Applequist-Dessy (pK_a scale).

MSAF Meconium-stained amniotic fluid Obstetrics).

MSAFP; MS-AFP Maternal serum alpha-fetoprotein.

MSAN Medical student's admission note.

MSAP Mean systemic arterial pressure.

MSAT Medical School Aptitude Test.

MSB Macrosomic (big, fat, heavy and long)/ Microsomic (small, thin, light and short) baby (i.e. Macrosomia/ Microsomia); Major scientific breakthrough; Master of Science in Bacteriology; Meaningful survival benefit (e.g. from chemotherapy in lung cancer); Medical Sciences Bulletin; Medical Services Branch (DNHW); Methylstyryl benzene (scintillator); Mid-small bowel; Moist-sounding breathing (as in Bronchiectasis); Most significant bit; Mucin synthesis balance; Multiple Sclerosis (MS) Briefs (journal).

MSBC Maximum specific binding capacity.

MSBLA Mouse-specific B lymphocyte antigen.

MSBOS Maximum surgical blood order schedule.

MSBP Maximum systolic blood pressure; Mean seated/ standing/ supine blood pressure; Munchausen syndrome by proxy - a mental illness in which (mostly) parents hurt their children in order to gain sympathy or attention (= MSP) (see MS).

MSC Marrow/ Myogenic stem cell; Marrow stromal cell; Mature/ Mesenchymal stem cell; Medical school curricula/lum; Medical Service/ Staff Corps; Medical Social Coordinator; Medical speciality choice; Mental Self-Care; Mucus-secreting cell; Multispeciality challenge; Multistage carcinogenesis/oma; Myelosuppressive chemotherapy (see MSCT).

MSc Master of Science (= MS).

MSCA McCarthy Scales of Children's Abilities.

MScD Doctor of Medical Science (see DMSc); Master of Dental Science.

MSCET Mammalian sister chromatid exchange test; Myelosuppressive chemotherapy (= MSC).

MScMed Master of Science in Medicine (= M

of Medical Science) (see MMS).
MScN Master of Science in Nursing.
MSCP; mscp Mean spherical candle power.
MSCU Medical special care unit.
MSCWP Musculoskeletal chest wall pain.
MSD Doctor of Medical Science (see DMSc); Male sexual desire/ disease/ disorder/ disturbance/ dysfunction; Maple syrup disease; Marie-Strümpell disease (= Ankylosing spondylitis; Bamboo spine; Poker spine); Master of Science in Dentistry (see MSDent); Maxillary sinus disease; Maximum safe/ single/ starting dose; Mean square deviation; Merck, Sharpe and Dohme (Br. pharmaceutical firm); Metabolic screening disorder(s); Microsurgical dissectomy; Mid-sleep disturbance; Mild sickle-cell disease; Minor skin disease/ disorder; Moderately severe depression; Mood-stabilizing drug; Most significant digit; Motor system disease (see MND); Multiple sulfatase deficiency; Multisystem/ Musculoskeletal disability/ disease/ disorder; Myelosuppressive disorder/ drug (see MSS).
MsD Doctor of Metaphysics (see DMs).
MSDC Mass Spectrometry Data Center (UK); Medical Society of the District of Columbia.
MSDent Master of Science in Dentistry (= MSD).
MSDI Martin Suicide Depression Inventory.
MSD-MLD Multiple sulfatase deficiency form of metachromatic leukodystrophy.
MSDS Material safety data sheet.
MSE Major/ Maximal/ Minimal/ Minor/ Moderate side effect(s); Master of Science in Engineering; Medical support equipment; Membrane stabilizing effect (Class I antiarrhythmias); Mental status examination; Microscopic susceptibility effect(s) (e.g. distortion of local magnetic field of drugs); Mild side effect(s); Moderately severe episode; M-scan echocardiogram; Muscle-specific enolase; Myelosuppressive effect (chemotherapy).
mse mean square error.
MSEA Medical Society Executives Association.
MSEC Master of Science in Economic Aspects of Chemistry.
msec millisecond (see ms).
μsec microsecond (see ìs).
m/sec meters per second.
MSEL Myasthenic syndrome of Eaton-Lambert.
MSEnt Master of Science in Entomology.
MSER Mean systolic ejection rate; Mental Status Examination Record/ Report.
M-series X-radiation (transitions to n = 3).
MSES Medical school environmental stress.
MSF Macrophage slowing/ spreading factor; Meconium-stained fluid; Médecins Sans Frontières (= DWB - Doctors Without Borders) - an international relief organization; Mediterranean spotted fever; Megakaryocyte/ Melanocyte stimulating factor; Microspectrofluorometer; Modified sham-feeding.
MSFC Marshall Space Flight Center (Alabama).
MSG Medical-school graduate; Meleney's synergistic gangrene (of skin and subcutaneous tissues, usually following surgery); Methysergide; Monosialoganglioside (Gm1 - successfully binds cholera toxin or the heat-labile enterotoxin of E. coli in vitro/ in animal experiments); Monosodium glutamate (= Chinese Seasoning; Sodium L-glutamate) (used widely as a seasoning and flavoring agent; also used intravenously in the symptomatic treatment of hepatic coma); Mycoses Study Group (NIAID).
MSGV Mouse salivary gland virus.
MSH Marked sphincter hypertonia; Medical self-help; Melanin/ Melanocyte/ Melanophore - stimulating hormone (see Hormones - MSH ii); Moderately severe hyper/ hypoglycemia.
MSHA Mannose-sensitive hemagglutination; Master of Science in Hospital Administration; Mine Safety and Health Administration.
MSHF Moderately severe hepatic failure.
MSHFA Multiservice Health Facility Administration.
MSHIF Melanocyte-stimulating hormone-inhibiting factor (see Hormones - MSHIF).
MSHL Minimal sensorineural hearing level/ loss.
MSHRF Melanocyte-stimulating hormone-releasing factor (see Hormones - MSHRF).

MSHRH Melanocyte-stimulating hormone-releasing hormone (see Hormones - MSHRH).

MSHSC Multiple self-healing squamous carcinoma.

MSHyg Master of Science in Hygiene.

MSI Magnetic source imaging; Medium-scale integration (circuits); Mild/ Mycotic skin infection; Minor skin irritation; Monospecies insulin (see MS insulin; Insulin - MSI); Musculoskeletal impairment (Orthopedics).

MSIA Multiple Sclerosis Indicative Abstracts (journal).

MSID Multiple specific ion detection.

MSIE Medical Sciences Information Exchange (now SSIE).

MS insulin Monospecies insulin (= MS; MSI) (see Insulin - MSI).

MSIR Morphine sulphate immediate release (tablet).

MSIS Multi-State Information System (EDP).

MSK Medullary sponge kidney; Multiple Sclerosis Keynotes (journal) (= MS Keynotes).

MSk Musculoskeletal.

MSKCC Memorial Sloan-Kettering Cancer Center (NYC).

MSKCH Memorial Sloan-Kettering Cancer Hospital.

MSKF Moderately severe kidney failure (see MSRF).

MSKP Medical Sciences Knowledge Profile.

MSK (program) Memorial Sloan-Kettering (Doxorubinin, Vincristine, Procarbazine, Prednisone and Cyclophosphamide (Chemotherapy program for treatment of Hodgkin's disease).

MSL Medical Skills Library (ACP); Medicine, Science and the Law (BAFS journal); Midsternal line; Miles above sea level; Multiple symmetric lipomatosis; Myelomonocytic subacute leukemia (see MLS).

MSLA Mouse-specific lymphocyte antigen.

MSLC Medium-sized lymphoid cell.

MSLR Mixed skin (cell-)leukocyte reaction.

MSLT Multiple Sleep Latency Test.

MSM Mammalian striped muscle (Orthopedics); Maxon suture material (see Sutures); Medium-size molecule; Methyl-sulfonyl-methane; Mineral salts medium; Mitogenic signal mechanism; Multiple-step mutation.

MSMA Minnesota/ Missouri State Medical Association.

MSMC Mount Sinai Medical Center (NYC).

MSMS Michigan State Medical Society; Mount Sinai Medical School (New York, USA).

MSN Main sensory nucleus; Master of Science in Nursing; Medial septal nucleus (of the brain); Medical-surgical-neurological or Medico-surgico-neurological; Mildly subnormal; Multiple Sclerosis Newsletter (IFMSS).

MSNA Multi-symptom nasal allergy.

MSO Medial superior olive; Multifocal sclerosing osteoblastoma (= MOO) (Orthopedics); Musculoskeletal oncology.

MSO_4 Morphine sulfate.

MSOF Multiple systems organ failure.

MSP Malaria (parasite) surface protein (MSP-1 - a protein displayed on the surface of the malarial parasite and newly used as a "transgenic" oral vaccine in goats' milk for protection against malaria); Male sex(ual) partner/ problem; Maximum squeeze pressure; Mediterranean spotted fever (a rickettsial tick-borne disease) (see SF - Spotted fever; TT - Tick typhus); Metabolic stressed patient; Microspectrophotometry; Mid-sagittal plane; Morphine sulphate (tablet); Munchausen syndrome by proxy (see MSBP); Musculoskeletal pain.

msp muscle spasm.

MSPGN Mesangial proliferative glomerulonephritis.

MSPH Master of Science in Public Health.

MSPhar Master of Science in Pharmacy.

MSPHE Master of Science in Public Health Engineering.

MSPHEd Master of Science in Public Health Education.

MSPN Medical student's progress note.

MSPNG Medical Society of Papua, New Guinea.

MSPQ Modified Somatic Perception Questionnaire.

MSPS Myocardial stress perfusion scintigra-

phy.
MSPs Multiple sex partners.
MSPSN Multiple Sclerosis (MS) Patient Service News.
MSPU Medical short procedure unit.
MSQ Mental status questionnaire.
MSQoL Migraine-Specific Quality of Life.
MSR Manual of Statistical Requirements; Maternal serum relaxin (Obstetrics); Member of the Society of Radiographers; Monosynaptic reflex; Muscle/ Myotatic stretch reflex.
MSRC Medical Society Reference Committee.
MSRF Moderately severe renal failure (= MSKF).
MSRG Member of the Society for Remedial Gymnasts.
MSRPP Multidimensional Scale for Rating Psychiatric Patients.
MSRS Medical Socioeconomic Research Sources (abstracts).
MSR's Muscles, strength, reflexes.
MSRT Minnesota Spatial Relations Test.
MSS Manuscripts (see Mss); Marital Satisfaction Scale; Marshall-Smith syndrome; Massage (see Mss); Maternal serum screening; Medical Superintendents' Society; Medicare Statistical System; Medicine and Science in Sports (ACSM journal); Mental status schedule; Miniature short single (cone) (i.e. of the eye); Minor surgery suite; Modular spacer system (orthopedic surgery); Motion sickness susceptibility; Mucus-secreting structure; Mucus-stimulating substance; Multiple Sclerosis Society (UK); Multiple sclerosis susceptibility; Musculoskeletal sarcoma/ stiffness/ symptoms/ system; Muscular subaortic stenosis; Myelosuppression syndrome (including anemia, leukopenia, pancytopenia, and thrombocytopenia).
Mss; mss Massage (= MSS); Manuscripts (= MSS).
MSSc Master of Sanitary Science.
MSSD Model Secondary School for the Deaf; Musculoskeletal system disease/ disorder (Arthropathy, Involuntary muscle contractions, leg cramps, etc.) (see IMC).
MSSE Master of Science in Sanitary Engineering.
MSSG Multiple sclerosis susceptibility gene.
MSSM Mount Sinai School of Medicine (NYC).
MSSNY Medical Society of the State of New York.
MSSS Mass Spectral Search System (EPA + NIH).
MSSST Meeting Street School Screening Test.
MSSV Mean steady state volume (see MSSVD).
MSSVD Mean steady state volume of distribution (of a drug in the body tissues); Medical Society for the Study of Venereal Diseases (UK).
MST Manufacturer-supported trial (see IFDT); Mean skin temperature; Mean/ Median survival time; Mean swell time; Medical scanning technology; Metastatic tumor; Minor sore throat; Mitogenic signal transduction (in IDD - Immunodeficiency disease); Monospot test (for glandular fever = infectious mononucleosis); Mountain standard time; Musculoskeletal trauma; Myelosuppressive therapy.
MSTA Mumps skin test antigen.
MSTD Marine Safety Technology Division (US Coast Guard).
MSTFA Methyltrimethyl-silyl-tri-fluoroacetamide.
MSTh; Ms-Th Mesothorium (now radium and actinium, Z = 88.89) (see Elements - Mesothorium).
MSTI Multiple soft tissue injuries.
M-Strep Microacrophilic Streptococcus.
MSTS Musculoskeletal Tumor Society/ System.
MSU Maple sugar/ syrup urine; Medical Statistics Unit; Medical studies unit; Midstream urine; Mid-stream specimen of urine (procedure/ urine culture); Monosodium urate; Mosley stone crusher (Urology); Myocardial substrate uptake.
M substance Acid-soluble protein of the Streptococcus.
MSUD Maple syrup urine disease (an inherited metabolic disorder caused by the lack of an enzyme needed to process three

aminoacids - valine, leucine and isoleucine) (also called BCKA or Branched chain ketoaciduria).

MSurg Master of Surgery (see MCh).

MSV Maximum sustained (level of) ventilation; Mean scale value; Mean sputum volume; Medical Society of Virginia; Moloney/ Murine sarcoma virus.

MSVC Maximum sustained ventilatory capacity.

MSV maneuver Mauriceau-Smellie-Veit maneuver (flexion of the baby's head during breech delivery).

MSW Master of Social Welfare/ Work; Medical social worker; Multiple stab wounds.

MSWYE Modified sea water yeast extract.

MT Empty; Maintenance/ Malaria/ Maximal/ Maximum/ Medical/ Milieu/ Music therapy; Malignant teratoma; Malpighian tubule; Mammary tumor; Mammilothalamic tract; Manual traction; Martin-Thayer (medium/ plate); Mastoid tip; Medial thalamus/ thickness; Medical Technologist (ASCP journal; UK journal, formerly Medical Technician); Medical technologist/ transcriptionist; Medical Times/ Tribune (journals); Meditsinskaya Tekhnika (former USSR, now Russian journal); Melatonin; Membrana tympani; Mercaptomerin (see MT 6); Mesangial thickening; Metallothionein; Metatarsal (joint); Methoxytryptamine; Methoxytyramine (see 3-MT); Methyltestosterone; Methyltyrosine; Microtome; Microtubule (filament along which the chromosome travels to the opposite side of the cell) (see Mt); Mid-trachea; Migraine Trust (UK); Minimum threshold; Modern Treatment (journal); Minnesota tube (for treatment of esophageal varices); Monroe tidal (drainage); More than; Movement time; Multiple tics; Muir-Torre (syndrome); Mullerian tumor (sarcoma of uterine glands and stroma); Multitest (plate); Murine typhus (= Epidemic, shop or urban typhus - caused by *Rickettsia* typhi and transmitted principally by the tropical rat flea, *Xenopsylla* cheopis); Muscle test; Muscles and tendons; Tympanic membrane (see Mt).

mt mitochondria(l) (= Mt); send of such (L. mittere talis).

Mt Megatonne; Microtubule (= MT); Mitochondria (see mt); Mount(ain); Mycobacterium tuberculosis (see M tuberc); Tympanic membrane (L. membrana tympani) (= Eardrum; MT).

M/T Masses of tenderness; Myringotomy with tubes.

M-T Macroglobulin-trypsin.

M&T Monilia and Trichomonas; Myringotomy and tubes.

3-MT 3-Methoxytyramine (= MT).

MT 6 Mercaptomerin (= MT; Thiomerin) - a diuretic.

MTA Malignant teratoma, anaplastic; Medical Technical Assistant; Medical technologist, assistant; Metatarsus adductus; Mid-trimester amniocentesis (Obstetrics); Myoclonic twitch activity.

mTA Meta-tyramine.

MTAC Mass transfer area coefficient.

MTAD Membrana tympana auris dextrae (L.) - Tympanic membrane of the right ear.

MTAL Medullary thick ascending limb.

MTAS Membrana tympana auris sinistrae (L.) - Tympanic membrane of the left ear.

MTAs Multiple toxic agents.

MT(ASCP) Medical Technologist (Registered, and certified by the) American Society of Clinical Pathologists.

MTAU Membranae tympanae aurae uterque (L) - Tympanic membranes of both ears.

MTB Materials Transportation Bureau (DOT); Methylthymol blue; Mycobacterium tuberculosis.

MTb; Mtb Mycobacterium tuberculosis (see M tuberc).

MTBE Meningeal tick-borne encephalitis; Methyl tert-butyl ester/ ether.

MTBF Mean time before/between failures.

MTC Mass transfer coefficient; Maximum tolerated/ toxic concentration; Medical tibial condyle; Medical test cabinet; Medullary thyroid carcinoma; Methacycline (hydrochloride); Mitomycin C; Monopolar thermocoagulation (of the umbilical cord) (Obstetrics); Mother-to-child (transmission of disease - in utero or at birth, as in AIDS); Multiple treatment cycle (Ovulation) (Gyn/Obs).

99mTc Radioisotope of technetium Tc 99m (see 99 Tc).
MTCp; MTC$_p$ Mean total plasma clearance.
MTCT Mother-to-child transmission (e.g. HIV, etc.).
MTD Diploma in Medical Technology (see DMT); Maximum tolerance/rated dose; Maximum/ Mean/ Minimum treatment difference; Mean total dose; Metastatic trophoblastic disease; Metatarsal-tarsal dislocation; Midwife Teacher's Diploma; Monroe tidal drainage; Multiple tic disorder; Multiple topical dose(s).
mtd send such doses (L. mitte tales doses).
MTDDA Minnesota Test for Differential Diagnosis of Aphasia.
MTDI Maximum tolerable daily intake.
MT-DN Multitest, dermatophtes and Nocardia (plate).
MtDNA; mtDNA Mitrochondrial deoxyribonucleic acid.
MTDT Modified tone decay test.
MTE Major/ Minor traumatic episode; Marked transaminase elevation (SGOT, SGPT, etc.); Maximal/ Maximum/ Mild/ Minimal/ Minimum therapeutic effect; Medical teaching exercise.
MTET Modified treadmill exercise test.
MTF Maximum terminal flow; Medical treatment facility; Modulation transfer function (image intensifier); Mountain tick fever or Mountain/ Spotted fever (Rickettsia or viral infection carried to humans by the bite of a tick) (see AMF or American mountain fever, CTF or Colorado tick fever, RMSF or Rocky Mountain spotted fever, etc.).
MtF Male-to-female (transmission of disease, esp. STD, as in AIDS).
MTG Mid-thigh girth.
MTg Mouse thyroglobulin.
MTH Methyl-thio-hydantoin; Migraine/noustype headache; Mithramycin.
Mth; mth Month (= Mo; mo); Mouth (see mo).
m-th mamillothalamic (tract).
MTHF Methylenetetrahydrofolate.
5-MTHF 5-Methyl-tetrahydro-folate/folic acid.
MTHFR 5,10-Methylenetetrahydrofolate reductase.
Mths; mths Months (= mos).
MTI Malignant teratoma, intermediate; Medical treatment index/indices; Midtrimester abortion; Mild transient increase (e.g. in blood pressure, etc.); Minimum time interval; Moving target indicator.
MTIC Monomethyl triazenoimidazole carboxamide (antineoplastic agent); Mouse/ Mice tick infection cycle.
MTJ Metatarsal-tarsal joint (see TMJ); Musculotendinous junction.
MTL Morse taper lock (orthopedics - conical coupling joint with a self -locking feature).
MTLP Malignant toxemia of late pregnancy.
MTM Manual of Tropical Medicine; Thayer-Martin, modified (agar/ medium) (= Modified Thayer-Martin).
MT-M Multitest, mycology (plate).
MtM Made-to-measure; Male-to-male (transmission of disease in homosexuals, as in AIDS); Man-to-man (spread of infection); Mild-to-moderate; Moment-to-moment; Mouth-to-mouth (assisted ventilation, in CPR) (see PRFCC).
MTMAV Mouth-to-mouth assisted ventilation (see MtM).
MTMV Mouth-to-mouth ventilation (see MtM).
MTN Medical Television Network.
Mtn(s) Mountain(s).
MTO Main target organ; Medical Transport Officer; Methoxyhydroxy-phenylalanine.
MtO Made-to-order (medicine, etc.).
MTOC Microtubule/ Mitotic organizing center.
MTOP Maximal/mum time to open.
mTOR Mammalian Target Of Rapamycin (a key regulatory kinase) (see MCL).
MTOV Metatarsus omnis varus (angle) (Orthopedics).
MTP Marrow-transplantation program; Massive Transfusion Protocol (followed in bleeding patients in ER); Master treatment plan; Maximum tolerated pressure; Medial tibial plateau; Median time to progression; Medical termination of pregnancy; Metatarsophalangeal (joint); Microtubule protein; Midtrimester of pregnancy; Migratory

thrombophlebitis; Multiple- testing procedure.

MTPJ Metatarsophalangeal joint.

MTPV Metatarsus primus varus (angle) (Orthopedics).

MTQ Methaqualone.

MTR Maximum therapeutic response; Mean time to repair; Meincke turbidity reaction (for syphilis) (see STS-MTR); 5-Methylthioribose.

MTR-O No masses, tenderness, or rebound (abdomen).

MTRS Master Therapeutic Recreation Specialist (Licensed).

MTRX Methotrexate (see MTX).

MTS Marine Technology Society (IEEE); Maximum tensile strength (of sutures) (Surgery/ Orthopedics); Metastatic testicular seminoma; Mid-thoracic spine (= MDS); Miniature tubing system; Mono/Multitherapy study (see MTT); Multicellular tumor spheroid; Musculoskeletal Tumor Society

MtS Moderate-to-severe (pain).

MTS 1 Multiple tumor-suppressor (gene) 1 (defects in this gene can cause many kinds of cancer, including melanoma, lung, breast, and brain tumors) = p 16 (a tumor-suppressor gene, with molecular weight 16).

MTSAb Maternal thyroid-stimulating antibody.

MTST Maximal treadmill stress test (= MTT).

MTT Malignant teratoma, trophoblastic (= M. trophoblastic teratoma); Maximal treadmill test (see MTST); Meal tolerance test; Mean transit time (of blood through heart and lungs) (= TT); Metastatic testicular tumor; Modified treadmill test (Sheffield technique); Monotetrazolium; Mono/Multitherapy trial (see MTS); Myocarditis Treatment Trial (Mason et al. - 1986-1989, US).

MTTF Mean time to failure.

MTTFF Mean time to first failure.

MTTs Metastatic testicular tumors.

MTU Malignant teratoma, undifferentiated; Medical therapy unit; Methyl-thiouracil (= Methyl thiour) - formerly used in the treatment of thyrotoxicosis. Has been largely replaced by carbimazole.

M tuberc Mycobacterium tuberculosis (= Mt; MTb; Mtb).

MTV Mammary tumor virus; Metatarsus varus; Mouse mammary tumor virus (see MMTV).

MTX Methotrexate (= Mtx) - chemotherapy in cancer (see NSC 740).

Mtx Methotrexate (see MTX).

MTX's Methotrexate (see MTX).

MT-Y Multitest yeast (plate).

MTZ Mitoxantrone.

MU Mache unit (see Mu); Megaunit; Mescaline/ Monitor/ Montevideo/ Motor unit; Methyluric (acid); Million units; Mouse unit (see Mu); Myomata uteri.

Mu Mache unit (a German measure or unit expressing the concentration of radium emanation in solution; equals 3.64 eman) (= MU); Marijuana (see Cannabis); Mouse unit (the least amount of gonadotropin or estrus-producing hormone which will cause in a sprayed mouse, a characteristic change in the vaginal epithelium) (= MU; mu).

mU milliunit (10^{-3} or one thousandth of a standard unit).

mu micron (= μ; 10^{-6} meter) (see μ {after m}); mouse unit (see Mu).

μU microunit (10^{-6} or one millionth of a standard unit).

MUA Middle uterine artery; Motor unit activity.

MuA Mu-agonist (e.g. morphine).

MUAC Mean/ Mid/ Middle upper arm circumference.

MUAP Motor unit action potential.

MUC Maximum urinary concentration; Mucilage (see muc); Mucosal ulcerative colitis.

muc mucilage (L. mucilago) (= MUC); mucous; mucus.

muco- prefix meaning mucus (Gr).

MUCs Multiple underlying conditions.

MUD Minimal/mum urticarial dose (reaction-producing).

MUDR 5-Mercapto,2-deoxyuridine.

MUE Motor unit estimated.

MUF (Nuclear) material unaccounted for; Mono-unsaturated fat (found especially in olive oil).

MUFA Monounsaturated (free) fatty acid (see

MUF).

MUG MUMPS (Massachusetts General Hospital Utility Multi-Programming System) Users' Group.

MUGA Multiple gated acquisition (blood pool scan).

MUGEx Multigated (blood pool image during) exercise.

Muggle Marijuana cigarette (see Cannabis).

MUGR Multigated (blood pool image at) rest.

MUGX Multiple gated acquisition exercise.

MUH Menopausal urine hormone (see Hormones - HMG).

MUI Mild urge incontinence (urinary bladder) (see DHR; OAB).

mult multiple.

multi- prefix meaning many (L. multus).

multip multiparous.

multivits multivitamins (medication order/ prescription).

MuLV; MuLv Murine leukemia virus.

MumAB Murine monoclonal antibody (such as MumAB4D5, used in cancer therapy).

MUMPS Massachusetts General Hospital Utility Multi-Programming System.

MuMTV; MuMTv Murine mammary tumor virus.

MUN(WI) Münich Wistar (rat).

MUO Maximal urinary osmolality; Myocardiopathy of unknown origin.

MUP Major urinary protein; Maximal urethral pressure; Methyl-umbelliferyl phosphate; Monitor/ Motor unit potential.

MuR Mu receptor (see MOR).

MuRA Mu-receptor agonist.

MURC Measurable undesirable respiratory contaminants.

MurNAc N-acetylmuramate.

MURP Master of Urban and Regional Planning.

MUS Major/ Minor uterine surgery; Marie Unna syndrome (see HH - Hereditary hypotrichosis); Morquio-Ullrich's syndrome (Orthopedics); Mouse urologic syndrome.

Mus Mouse; Music; Muslim (religion) (see Mos).

MUSC Medical University of South Carolina.

musc muscle/cular/culature.

muscae volitantes (L.) small dark particles or floaters in the vitreous of the eye.

MUSE Minimum Uniform Standards for Education.

mus-lig musculoligamentous.

MUST Medical unit, self-contained and transportable.

MUT; mut Mutagen(ic).

Muta Marijuana (see Cannabis).

MUU Mouse uterine unit.

MUW Mouse uterine weight.

MUWU Mouse uterine weight unit.

MV Macro/ Microvascular; Mean variation; Measles virus; Mechanical ventilation; Megavolt; Microvilli/llus; Microwave (see MW); Minute ventilation/ volume (see PFT - MV); Mitoxantrone and etoposide; Mitral valve; Mixed venous (blood); Multivesicular (body) (see MVB); Multivessel; Veterinary physician (L. Medicus Veterinarius).

Mv Mendelevium (Z = 101) (= Md) (see Elements - Mendelevium).

mV; mv millivolt (= 10^{-3} V; 10^{-3} volt; one thousandth of a Volt).

μV; μv microvolt (= 10^{-6} V; 10^{-6} volt; one millionth of a Volt).

MVA Malignant ventricular arrhythmia; Mechanical ventricular assistance; Mevalonic acid; Mitral valve area; Modified vaccinia (virus-strain) Ankara; Motor vehicle accident; Multivariant approach; Multivariable/riate analysis (statistical).

MV-A Megavolt-ampere.

mV-A millivolt-ampere.

MVAC; M-VAC Methotrexate, vinblastine, Adriamycin (doxorubicin), and cisplatin.

mval millival.

MVB Mixed venous blood; Multivesicular body; Multivessel bypass.

MVC Maximal/mum voluntary contraction; Medullary vomiting center; Mitral-valve calcification; Myocardial vascular capacity.

MVD Doctor of Veterinary Medicine; Macro/ Micro vascular disease; Microvascular decompression; Millimeter-wave detector; Mitral valve disease; Multivessel coronary disease.

MVDD Millimeter-wave-detection device.

MVE Major/ Minor vascular event; Mitral valve echogram/ excursion; Murray Valley encephalitis.

MVH Massive vitreous hemorrhage.

MVI Mitral valve incompetence (see MVR); Multi(ple) vitamin infusion/ injection; Multivalvular involvement.

MVIC Maximal venous incremental capacitance (see MVIV).

MVII Minnesota Vocational Interest Inventory.

MVIV Maximal venous incremental volume (= MVIC).

MVL Maxi-vessel loop (Vascular surgery); Mesovarial leiomyoma (a benign neoplasm found in laboratory rats, treated with high doses of 2-adrenergic drugs); Mitral valve leaflet.

MVLRA Multivariate logistic-regression analysis.

MVLS Mandibular vestibulolingual sulcoplasty.

MVM Macrovascular morbidity (as in IGT or impaired glucose tolerance); Microvillose/llus membrane; Minute virus of mice; Multivariate model.

MVMT Movement (see mvt).

MVN Medial ventromedial nucleus.

MVO Maximal/mum venous outflow.

MVO_2; MV_{O2} Myocardial oxygen consumption.

mVO_2 Minute venous oxygen consumption.

MVOA Mitral valve orifice area.

MVOS Mixed venous oxygen saturation.

MVP Malaria vaccine program; Maximum vertical pocket (in cm - Doppler findings in oligo/ polyhydramnios) (Obstetrics) (see OPS); Mean venous/ Microvascular pressure; Mitral valve prolapse/ prosthesis; Modern Veterinary Practice (journal).

Mvp; mvp Million volts peak.

MVPP Mustine, vinblastine, procarbazine, and prednisone.

MVPS Medicare Volume Performance Standards; Mitral valve prolapse syndrome.

MVP-SC Mitral valve prolapse - systolic click (syndrome).

MVPT Motor-Free Visual Perception Test.

MVR Massive vitreous reaction/ retraction; Micro-vitreo-retinal; Minimal vascular resistance; Mitral valve regurgitation/ repair/ replacement.

MVRI Mixed virus respiratory infection(s) (= MRVI).

MVRR Multivariate relative risk.

MVS Major vascular/ Microvascular surgery; Microvideo system; Mitral valve stenosis/ surgery; Motor, vascular, and sensory.

mV-s millivolt-second.

mv's muscae volitantes (small dark patches in the vitreous of the eye; also known as "floaters").

MVT Microvascular thrombosis.

mvt movement (= MVMT).

MVV Maximum voluntary ventilation (see PFT - MVV); Mixed vespid venom; Monovalent vaccine.

MVVF Maximum voluntary ventilation, free (formerly MBC; see PFT - MVVF).

MW Mallory-Weiss (syndrome); Mean weight; Medical World (ASTMS journal); Megawatt (see Mw); Microwave (= MV); Minot-von Willebrand (syndrome); Molecular weight (see mol wt).

Mw Megawatt (= MW; 10^3 watts; 1000 watts).

mW; mw milliwatt (10^{-3} w; 10^{-3} watt).

μW; μw microwatt (= 10^{-6} w; 10^{-6} watt).

MW 343 Nifedipine (see BAY a 1040).

MV 450 Dilitiazem (see CRD 401).

MW 455 Verapamil (see D 365).

mWb milliweber.

MWCO Molecular weight cutoff (filter paper).

MWD Microwave diathermy; Molecular weight distribution; Multiple weekly dosage/ dose.

MWE Megawatt electrical (unit of power plant output).

MWI Medical Walk-In (Clinic).

MWIA Medical Women's International Association (CIOMS).

M width Medullary width.

MWL Maternal/ Maximal/ Minimal weight loss.

MWLT Modified Word Learning Test.

MWM Molecular-weight marker.

MWMT Monotonic Word Memory Test.

MWN Medical World News (journal).

MWP Mean wedge pressure.

MWS Mallory-Weiss syndrome (bleeding caused by ruptured varices and mucosal tears of the esophagus); Marden-Walker/ Mickety-Wilson/ Moersch-Woltman syndrome.

MWT Malpositioned wisdom teeth/ tooth; Mann-Whitney test (non-parametric t. on absolute nutrient intake); Maximum walking time (on treadmill); Myocardial wall tension/ thickness.

MX Matrix; Medix (= Mx); Methylxanthine; Microcrystalline.

Mx Maxwell; MEDEX (see MEDEX); Medix (see MX); Myringotomy.

MXE Excision of myoma.

M_{xy} Transverse magnetization.

My Mayer (see my); Myopia; Myxedema.

my mayer (a unit of heat capacity) - the capacity of a body warmed one degree centigrade by one joule (= My).

my- myria (metric prefix for 10,000); prefix meaning muscle (Gr. myos).

MYA Million years ago.

Myc Mycology (see Mycol).

myc- prefix meaning fungus (Gr. mykes) (= myk-).

-myces suffix meaning fungus (Gr. mykes).

mycet- combining form meaning fungus (Gr. myketos).

Myco Mycobacterium.

Mycol Mycologist/gy (= Myc).

MyD Myotonic dystrophy.

Myd Mydriatic.

MYEL; myelo Myelogram.

Myel; Myelo Myelocyte.

myel myelin(ated).

myel- prefix meaning spinal cord marrow (Gr. myelos).

MyG Myasthenia gravis.

Myg Myriagram.

myk- prefix meaning fungus (Gr. mykes) (see myc-).

Myl Myrialiter.

Mym Myriameter.

MyMD Myotonic muscular dystrophy.

MYO Myoglobin.

myo- prefix meaning muscle.

MYRTPHOS Cis-myrtanyl-diphenyl-phosphine.

Mythol Mythology.

MYX; Myx Myxedema; Myxoma.

myx- prefix meaning mucus or slime (Gr. myxa).

MZ Mantle zone; Meziocillin; Monozygote/tic (identical twin).

M_z Free moment; Longitudinal magnetization.

m/z mass-to-charge ratio.

MZA Monozygotic twins (raised/ reared) apart.

MZE Microzone electrophoresis.

MZL Marginal zone lymphocyte.

MZMG Monozygotic multiple gestation (Obstetrics).

MZP Monozygotic pregnancy.

MZT Monozygotic twins (raised/ reared) together (also called Enzygotic twins, Identical twins, True twins, Uniovular twins).

N

N Asparagine; Avogadro's number; Blood factor in the MNS blood group system; Born (L. natus); Cementex (USA) and Stauffer Chemical Co code for experimental substances; Index of refraction; Loudness; Nasal (L. nasalis) - pertaining to the nose; Nasion; Nature (journal); Negative (-); Negro; Neomycin; Neper; Nephron (journal); Nerve (L. nervus; Gr. neuron) (= n); Neuraminidase; Neurologist/gy; Neuropathy; Neuter; Neutral; Neutron number; Neutrophil (A polymorphonuclear neutrophilic leukocyte - stainable by neutral dyes); Never; Newton (= n; Newt; $kgms^{-2}$; kg/s^2) (the MKS or Meter-kilogram-second unit of force, which when acting continuously upon a mass of one kilogram, will impart to it an acceleration of one meter per second per second); Nicotinamide; Nifedipine; Nitrogen (Z = 7) (see Elements - Nitrogen); No; Node(s); Nodule; None; Non-malignant (with reference to tumors); Nonne (globulin test); Normal i) chemical symbol for normal (solution - containing in each 1000 mil, 1 gram equivalent weight of the active substance), e.g. 2N = twice normal or twice the strength of a solution in comparison with the normal, N/2 = 0.5 N = one-half normal, 0.1 N = one tenth normal, etc. ii) with reference to structure and functioning of organs (= nor; norm); North; Nostril (L. naris); Not; Noun; NPH insulin; Nucleoside; Nucleus; Number (= n; No) (in sample; of molecules/ of molecular density; of neutrons in an atomic nucleus); Population size; Radiance; Refractive index; Spin density.

n amount of substance expressed in moles; born (L. natus); haploid chromosome number; index of refraction or refractive index; name; nano (prefix for 10^{-9}) (see nano-); nasal; nerve; neuter; neutral; neutron; neutron number density/ dosage (unit of - corresponding to the roentgen); newton (see N); noon; normal (see N); nostril (L. naris); number (see N); principle quantum number; refractive index; rotational frequency; sample size.

ν nu. the 13th letter of the Greek alphabet; degrees of freedom; frequency; kinematic velocity; neutrino.

N- a symbol prefixed to a radical to show that it is attached to a nitrogen atom (chemistry).

0.02N fiftieth-normal (solution) (see N/50).

0.1N tenth-normal (solution) (see N/10).

0.5N half-normal (solution) (see N/2).

NI, NII, NIII, ... NXII First, Second, Third, ... to Twelfth cranial nerves.

2N double normal solution.

2n diploid; diploid (haploid chromosome) number.

N_2 Neuraminidase enzyme; Nitrogen.

N/2 half normal (solution) (= 0.5N).

3n triploid.

N-3 Methetoin (= 5-Ethyl-1-methyl-5-phenylhydantoin) - an anticonvulsant used in the treatment of epilepsy.

4n tetraploid.

5'-N 5'-Nucleotidase.

N/10 tenth-normal (solution) (= 0.1N).

^{15}N Radioactive nitrogen.

N/50 fiftieth-normal (solution) (= 0.02N).

N 714 Chlorprothixene (= Chlorprothixan; Ro 4-0403) - a prothiazine compound having sedative, antiemetic, antihistamine, adrenolytic and parasympatholytic properties. Used in the treatment of agitation, mania and delirium tremens.

NA Nalidixic/ Nicotinic/ Nitric/ Nucleic acid; Naphthylamine (a carcinogen); Narcotic analgesic (such as codeine, dextropropoxyphene, diamorphine or heroin, dihydrocodeine, methadone, morphine and pethidine; Narcotics Anonymous; Native American; Negro adult; Network administrator; Neuraminidase; Neurologic age; Neutralizing/ Neutrophil/ Nuclear antibody; No action (see N/A); Nomina Anatomica; Non-adherent; Noradrenalin(e); Norwalk agent (a type of virus); Not admitted/ answered/ applicable/ attempted/ available (see N/A); Nucleoside analogue (see NSA); Nucleus ambiguus; Numerical aperture; Nurse Anesthetist; Nurse assistant/ associate; Nurse's aid; Nursing assistant/ auxiliary; Organon Inc (USA) code for experimental substances.

Na Avogadro's number; Sodium (L. natrium) (= Sod; natr. Z = 11, see Elements - Sodium).
nA nanoampere.
N/A No action (= NA); Not admitted/ answered/ applicable/ attempted/ available (= NA).
N&A Normal and active.
NA1 Neutrophil-specific antigen.
^{24}Na Radioactive sodium.
NAA Naphthalene-acetic acid; National Arthritis Act (1974); National Ash Association; Neutral aminoacid; Neutron activation analysis; Neutrophil aggregation activity; Nicotinic acid amide/ analogue; No apparent abnormalities/ty; Nocturnal apnoeic attack; Non-African American.
NAAA Non-antibiotic antimicrobial agent.
NAAC No apparant anesthetic complications.
NAACLS National Accrediting Agency for Clinical Laboratory Sciences.
NAACOG Nurses Association of the American College of Obstetricians and Gynecologists.
NAACOGBN Nurses Association of the American College of Obstetricians and Gynecologists Bulletin News.
NAACP National Association for the Advancement of Colored People.
NAAFA National Association to Aid Fat Americans.
NAAP N-acetyl-4-amino-phenazone.
NAAQS National Ambient Air Quality Standards (EPA).
NAAR National Alliance for Autism Research.
NAASO North American Association for the Study of Obesity.
NAB National Association of Bioengineers/ Broadcasters; Novarsenobenzene/zol (see NAB 914).
NAb Neutralizing antibody (see IANA; NMAb).
NAB 914 Neoarsphenamine (= NAB; Neo; Neoarsaminol; Neoarsphen; Neoarsphenolamine; Neosulvarsan; Ninefourteen; 914; Novarsenobenzine; Novarsenobenzol; Novarsenol). Before the age of antibiotics, neoarsphenamine was once the treatment of choice in syphilitic infections. It has now been almost entirely replaced by penicillin.
NABCO National Alliance of Breast Cancer Organizations.
$Na_2B_4O_7 + 10H_2O$ Borax.
NABP National Association of Boards of Pharmacy.
NABPLEX National Association of Boards of Pharmacy Licensing Examination.
NaBr Sodium bromide.
NABS Normoactive bowel sounds.
NABSP National Association of Blue Shield Plans.
NABT National Association of Biology Teachers.
NABVH National Accreditation of the Blind and Visually Handicapped.
NAC Acetylcysteine (= N-acetyl-L-cysteine) - used as the sodium salt solution, by direct inhalation or nebulization, to reduce the viscid pulmonary secretions in cystic fibrosis of the pancreas, and other disorders where mucolytic therapy is indicated, such as chronic bronchitis and COLD/COPD, etc. Also being tried in the treatment of AIDS; National Association for Continence; National Asthma Campaign (UK); National Asthma Center; Native American Church (uses peyote ceremoniously); Noise Advisory Council; Nucleus accombens (= Nucleus acusticus or nucleus of the acoustic nerve; Nucleus nervi vestibulocochlearis) - one of the nuclei of the sensory fibers of the vestibular and cochlear divisions of the eighth cranial nerve.
NACA National Agricultural Chemists Association.
NACBT National Association of Cognitive-Behavioral Therapists.
NACC National Advisory Cancer Council.
NACCRRA National Association of Child Care Resource and Referral Agencies.
NACDE National Action Committee for Drug Education (USOE).
NACDL National Association of Certified Dental Laboratories, Inc.
NACDS North American Clinical Dermatological Society.
NACE National Association to Control Epilepsy, Inc.

NACED National Advisory Council on the Employment of the Disabled.
NAC-EDTA N-acetylcysteine EDTA.
NACGN National Association of Colored Graduate Nurses (dissolved in 1951).
NACHM National Advisory Commission on Health Manpower.
nAChR Nicotinic acetylcholine receptor.
NACI National Advisory Committee on Immunization.
NaCl Sodium chloride.
NaClO Sodium hypochlorite.
$NaClO_3$ Sodium chlorate.
NACO National Association of Counties.
Na_2CO_3 Sodium carbonate (= Soda; Washing soda).
NACOA National Advisory Committee on Oceans and Atmosphere.
NACOR National Advisory Committee on Radiation; National Committee relating to Organ Retention (UK).
NACP Nordic Association of Clinical Physics.
NACS National Ambulatory Care Survey (NCHS).
NACSAP National Alliance Concerned with School-Age Parents.
NACT Neoadjuvant chemotherapy.
NAD National Association for/of the Deaf; National Association of Druggists; New antigenic determinant; Nicotinamide-adenine dinucleotide (= Nad; Nadide) (formerly DPN - see Co-1); Nicotinic acid dehydrogenase; No abnormal discovery; No active/ appreciable disease; No acute/ apparent distress; No adequate data; Non-adrenal disorder (such as allergic, arthritic, collagen, hematological, inflammatory bowel, etc. disorders); Normal axis deviation; Nothing abnormal detected.
NaD Sodium dialysate.
Nad Nadide (= Nicotinamide-adenine dinucleotide) (see NAD).
NAD+ Oxidized form of NAD (= Oxidized nadide).
NADA New Animal Drug Application.
NADABA N-adenoxyl-diamino-butyric acid.
NADB National Aerometric Data Bank (EPA).
NADG Nicotinamide-adenine dinucleotide glycohydrolase; North American Dermatitis Group.
NADH Nicotinamide-adenine dihydronucleotide (= Reduced form of nicotinamide-adenine dinucleotide - see DPNH).
NADL National Association of Dental Laboratories.
NADLJ National Association of Dental Laboratories Journal.
$NaDodSO_4$ Sodium dedecyl sulfate.
NADP Nicotinamide-adenine dinucleotide phosphate (formerly TPN - see Co-2).
NADP+ Oxidized form of NADP (= Oxidized nadide phosphate).
NADPH Nicotinamide-adenine dihydronucleotide phosphate (= Dihydronicotinamide adenosine dinucleotide phosphate; Nicotinamide-adenine dinucleotide phosphate hydrogenase; Reduced form of nicotinamide-adenine dinucleotide phophate; Reduced nadide phosphate; TPNH).
NADPH-d NADPH-diaphorase (a brain enzyme).
NaDS Sodium (L. Natrium) depletion state (see EIS).
NADSIC No apparant disease seen in chest.
NADSP National Association of Dental Service Plans.
NADT3 Sodium dextro-triiodothyronine.
NAE National Academy of Engineering; Net acid excretion; No adverse effect(s).
NA^E; NA_e; NaE; Na_e Exchangeable body sodium.
NAEC National Advisory Eye Council (NIH).
NAEL National Association of Earmold Laboratories.
NAEMT National Association of Emergency Medical Technicians.
NAEP National Assessment of Educational Progress; National Asthma Education Program.
NaERC Sodium efflux rate constant.
NAF Nafcillin; Nasal airflow; National Alcoholism Forum; National Amputation/ Ataxia Foundation; Negro adult female; Net acid flux.
NaF Sodium fluoride.
NAFFP National Association of Frozen Food Packers.
NAFLD Non-alcoholic fatty liver disease.
NAFPD National Association of Family

Planning Doctors.

NAG N-acetyl-D-glucosaminidase; Narrow-angle glaucoma; Non-agglutinable/nating.

NAGO Neuraminidase and galactose oxidase.

NAG v's Non-agglutinating vibrios (i.e. Vibrio cholerae).

NAH 2-hydroxy-3-naphthoic acid hydrazide; Nitrosamine hypothesis (or theory = NAT) (see NNC): Stomach bacteria, including *Helicobacter* pyloriv. Dietary nitrate → Nitrite. Low pH → ← Bacteria v. N-nitrosamine.

NAHA National Association of Health Authorities;

NaHA Sodium hyaluronate (see HUA).

NAHB National Association of Home Builders.

NAHC National Advisory Heart Council; National Association for Home Care.

$NAHCO_3$ Sodium bicarbonate (= Soda bicarb; Baking soda).

NAHCS National Association of Health Center Schools.

NAHD National Association for Hospital Development.

NAHG National Association of Humanistic Gerontology.

NAHI National Athletic Health Institute.

NAHMOR National Association of Health Maintenance Organization Regulators.

NAHPA National Association of Hospital Purchasing Agents.

NaH_2PO_4 Monosodium acid phosphate (= Sodium biphosphate).

Na_2HPO_4 Disodium acid phosphate (= Sodium phosphate).

NAHSA National Association for Hearing and Speech Action; National Association of Hearing and Speech Agencies (formerly AHS).

NAHSE National Association of Health Services Executives.

NAHU National Association of Health Underwriters.

NAHUC National Association of Health Unit Clerks/ Coordinators.

NAHW Non-active hairy wart.

NAI Native American Indian; Naturally acquired immunity (e.g. of the fetus, from its mother during pregnancy); Net acid input (urinary - see KFT - NAI); Neuraminidase inhibitor; No/Non-accidental injury; No acute inflammation; Non-adherence index; Nosocomially acquired infection.

NaI Sodium iodide.

NAIC National Association of Insurance Commissioners.

NaIC Sodium iodide cotransporter (high serum concentration in thyroid disease).

NAIR Non-adrenergic inhibitory response.

NaK Sodium-potassium eutectic.

Na-K-ATPase Sodium-potassium-adenosine-triphosphatase ("sodium" pump).

Na + K-ATPase Sodium-potassium-activated adenosine-triphosphatase (pump).

NAL National Acoustic Laboratories; Non-adherent leukocyte; Normal active life(style).

NALD Neonatal adrenoleukodystrophy.

NALS Normal active lifestyle (see NAL).

$NaLSO_4$ Sodium lauryl sulfate.

NAM National Association of Manufacturers (now merged into the Assoc. of Commerce and Industry); Natural actomyosin; Negro adult male; Non-active metabolite; Nucleic acid metabolism.

NAMC Naval Aerospace Medical Center.

NAMCA Norfolk Area Medical Center Authority.

NAMCS National Ambulatory Medical Care Survey.

NAME National Association of Medical Examiners; Nevi, atrial myoxma, myxoid neurofibroma, and ephelides (syndrome); Nitro-arginine methyl ester (see L-NAME).

NAMH National Association for Mental Health (UK/USA).

NaMH Sodium methohexital (IV general anesthetic).

NAMI National Alliance for the Mentally Ill.

NAMIRL Naval Aerospace Medical Institute and Research Laboratory.

NAMN Nicotinic acid mononucleotide.

NAMRL Naval Aerospace Medical Research Laboratory.

NAMRU Navy Aerospace Medical Research Unit.

NAMS N-methane-sulfonoxy-ethyl-p-nitrosoaniline.

NAMs Neural axis malformations (such as Acrania, Anencephaly, Arrhinoencephaly; Holoprosencephaly, Meningocele, Meningomyelocele, and Microcephaly) (see DRMs).

NAMSA National Ambulance Medical Suppliers Association.

NAMT The National Association for Music Therapy, Inc.

NAN; NANA N-acetyl neuraminic acid.

NaN_3 Sodium azide.

NANB Non-A, non-B (hepatitis).

NANB/C Non-A, Non-B/C (Chronic hepatitis).

NANBH Non-A, non-B hepatitis.

NANC Non-adrenergic non-cholinergic (nervous mechanism/ system).

NAND Not-and.

NANHC National Association of Neighborhood Health Centers.

NANM N-allylnor-morphine.

nano- metric prefix meaning 10^{-9} (symbol: n) (Gr. nanos, L. nanus = dwarf), e.g. ng = nanogram.

$NaNO_2$ Sodium nitrite.

$NaNO_3$ Sodium nitrate (= Chile saltpeter).

Na_2O_2 Sodium peroxide.

NaOH Sodium hydroxide (= Caustic soda).

NAOO National Association of Optometrists and Opticians.

NAOP National Alliance for Optional Parenthood.

NAP Narrative, assessment, and plan; Nasal air pressure; Nasion, point A, and pogonion (angle of concavity/ convexity of the facial profile); Nerve action potential; Neutrophil alkaline phosphate/tase; Nodular adrenocortical pathology; Nomina Anatomica Parisiensia; Non-accidental poisoning; Non-ambulatory patient; Nucleic acid phosphatase/ phosphate/ phosphorus.

NAPA N-acetyl-p-aminophenol; N-acetyl procainamide; Network Against Psychiatric Assault.

NAPAN National Association for the Prevention of Addiction to Narcotics.

NAPCA National Air Pollution Control Administration.

NAPCC National Association for Poison Control Centers.

NAPD No active pulmonary disease.

Na Pent Pentothal Sodium.

NaPG Sodium pregnanediol glucoronide.

NAPH Naphthyl; Nicotinamide adenine dinucleotide phosphate.

Naph Naphthalene (scintillator).

NAPHT National Association of Patients on Hemodialysis and Transplantation, Inc.

NAPM National Association of Pharmaceutical Manufacturers/ Purchasing Management.

NAPN National Association of Physicians' Nurses.

NAPNAP National Association of Pediatric Nurse Associates and Practitioners.

NAPNES National Association for Practical Nurse Education and Services.

NAPPH National Association of Private Psychiatric Hospitals.

NAPPHJ National Association of Private Psychiatric Hospitals Journal.

NAPPHN National Association of Private Psychiatric Hospitals Newsletter.

NAPS National Auxillary Publications Service.

NAPT National Association for the Prevention of Tuberculosis.

NAR Nasal airway resistance; National Amniocentesis Registry; National Association for Retarded (Children/ Citizens); Neurological adverse reaction(s); No action required; Normal auditory reflex; Not at risk; Nucleic Acids Research (journal).

NARA Narcotics Addict Rehabilitation Act; National Association of Recovered Alcoholics.

NARAL National Abortion Rights Action League.

NARC Narcotic (see Narc); Narcotics Addiction Rehabiltation Center; Narcotics officer (see Narco); Nasal Airway Resistance Computer; National Association for Retarded Children/ Citizens; Non-articular rheumatic condition; Nucleus arcuatus.

Narc Narcotic (= NARC); Narcotics officer (see Narco).

narc- combining form meaning numb (Gr. narke).

Narco Narcotics hospital; Narcotics officer (= Narcotic, narcotic addict, and/or drug enforcement agent) (= NARC; Narc); Narcotics treatment center.

narco- prefix meaning stupor (Gr. narke).

NARD National Association of Retail Druggists.

NARES Non-allergic rhinitis - eosinophilia syndrome.

NARF National Association of Rehabilitation Facilities.

NARI National Association of Residents and Interns.

NARMC Naval Aerospace and Regional Medical Center.

NARMH National Association for Rural Mental Health.

NARS National Acupuncture Research Society.

NART National Association of Recreational Therapists, Inc.

NARTI Nucleoside analogue reverse transcriptase inhibitor (see NRTIs).

NAS Nasal (see Nas); National Academy of Sciences; National Association of Sanitarians; National Audubon Society; Neonatal abstinence/ air-leak syndrome; Neonatal adrenal suppression; Nephro arterio(lar)/athero sclerosis; Neuroallergic syndrome; No added salt; Non-aqueous solution; Non-automated syringe (standard); Nucleic acid synthesis; Nutrient Analysis System.

Nas Nasal (= NAS).

NASA National Aeronautics and Space Administration; North American Student Association.

NASAHP National Association of Schools of Allied Health Professions.

NASBM National Academy of Sciences Board of Medicine.

NASCD National Association for Sickle Cell Disease.

NASCET North American Symptomatic Carotid Endarterectomy Trial.

NASDAD National Association of Seventh Day Adventist Dentists.

NASE National Association for the Study of Epilepsy; Neuraminidase (= N).

NASEAN National Association for State Enrolled Assistant Nurses.

NASH Non-alcoholic steatohepatitis.

NASIM National Academy of Sciences' Institute of Medicine.

NASJ National Analgesia Society Journal.

NASM Naval Aviation School of Medicine.

NASMHPD National Association of State Mental Health Program Directors.

NASMV National Association on Standard Medical Vocabulary.

NAS-NRC National Academy of Sciences - National Research Council.

Na_2SO_4 Sodium sulfate (= Disodic sulfate).

$Na_2S_2O_3$ Sodium thiosulfate.

NASPE North American Society of Pacing and Electrophysiology.

NASS National Ankylosing Spondylitis Society (UK).

NAST Non-adhesive skin traction.

NASUP National Association on Service to Unmarried Parents.

NASW National Association of Science Writers/ Social Workers.

NAT N-acetyltransferase; Natal; National Drug Co (USA) code for experimental substances; Neoadjuvant therapy (e.g. chemotherapy before surgery in advanced breast cancer); Neonatal alloimmune thrombocytopenia; Neuralgic amyotrophy (see BN - Brachial neuralgia); New applanation tonometer; Nitrosamine theory (see NAH); No action taken; No-active-treatment; Non-accidental trauma.

NaT Sodium tartrate.

Nat National/ Native/ Natural (see nat); Nature (journal).

nat national/ native/ natural (= Nat).

NATA National Athletic Trainer Association.

NATAS North American Thermal Analysis Society.

NATC Neonatal alloimmune thrombocytopenia.

NATCO North American Transplant Coordinator Organization.

NATFU No-active treatment folow-up.

NATNN National Association of Theatre Nurses News (UK).

NAT-OJT National On-the-Job Training (Program).

NATP Neonatal autoimmune thrombocytopenic purpura.
Natr; natr Sodium (L. natrium) (see Na).
-natremia suffix meaning blood sodium.
Naturwis Naturwissenschaften (journal).
NAUI National Association of Underwater Instructors.
Naut Nautical.
NAV Association of Private Practitioners of Germany; The North American Veterinarian (journal).
NAVC National Audiovisual Center (GSA).
NAWF North American Wildlife Foundation.
Naz Nazarene (church member).
NB Nail bed; Needle biopsy; Negri bodies; Nerve biopsy; Neuro-Behçet (syndrome); Neuroblastoma; Neurometric battery; Newborn (= nb); Nitrogen balance; Nitrous (oxide) barbiturate (see Barb); Normoblast (see Nbl); Note well/ take notice (L. nota bene) (= nb); Nutrient broth.
Nb Niobium (Z = 41, formerly Columbium - Cb) (see Elements - Niobium).
nb new born (see NB); note well (see NB).
NB_1 Neutrophil specific antigen.
^{95}NB Radioactive niobium.
NBA Nail-bed ablasion; National Boxing Association; Neuron-binding activity; Neuron-blocking antihypertensive; Nitrobenzene poisoning.
NBAAD Non-bronchodilator anti-asthmatic drug(s).
NBAC National Bioethics Advisory Commission.
NBAS Neonatal Behavioral Assessment Scale.
NBB Negative bone balance.
NBBB National Better Business Bureau.
NBBP National Blood Bank Program.
NBC Neoplastic blast cell; Non-battle casualty; Non-bed care; Normal baseline cognition (in the elderly); Nursing-bottle caries (= BMS or Bottle-mouth syndrome).
NBCC National Breast Cancer Coalition; Nevoid basal cell carcinoma.
NBCCS Nevoid basal cell carcinoma syndrome.
NBCIE Non-bullous congenital icthyosiform erythroderma.
NBD Neurogenic/ Neurologic bladder dysfunction; No brain damage; Non-bloody diarrhea.
NBD chloride Chloro-nitrobenzo-oxadiazole.
NBDE National Board of Dental Examiners (ADA).
NBDHE National Board Dental Hygiene Examination (ADA).
NBDRC National Blood Data Resource Cemter (Bethesda, Md).
NBE National Board Examiner (journal).
NBEO National Board of Examiners in Optometry.
NBF New bone formation; No breast feeding; Normal bacterial flora; Not breast fed.
NBFC New bone-forming capacity (Orthopedics).
NBFW Non-breast-feeding woman/women.
NBF; -veBF Negative biopsy finding(s).
NBFW Non-breast-feeding woman/ women.
NBH Normal baseline hemoglobin; Normal bowel habit(s).
NBHH Newborn helpful hints.
NBI Neutrophil bactericidal index; No bodily/ body/ bone/ bony injury; Non-battle injury.
NBICU Newborn intensive care unit.
NBIE National Burn Information Exchange.
NBIL; NBil Neonatal bilirubin.
NBIMC Newark Beth Israel Medical Center.
NBL Necrobiosis lipoidica; Net bone loss.
Nbl Normoblast (on hematology reports) (= NB).
NBM No/ Normal bowel movement; Normal bone marrow; Nothing by mouth; Nylen-Barany maneuver (see DHM).
nbM Newborn mouse.
nbMb Newborn mouse brain.
NBME National Board of Medical Examiners; Normal bone marrow extract.
NBMR National Bone Marrow Registry.
NBN Narrow-band noise; Newborn nursery.
NBO Non-bed occupancy.
NBP National blood policy; National Board of Podiatry; Needle biopsy of prostate; Neonatal/ Normal blood pressure; Neoplastic brachial plexopathy; Neuroscience and Behavioral Physiology (journal); Non-black patient/ person.
NBPK Narcotic-based painkiller (= NPR).
NBQC Narrow base quad cane.

NBR Natural bone regeneration.
NBRA National Biomedical Research Association.
NBRF National Biomedical Research Foundation; Navy Bioengineering Research Facility.
NBRP National Blood Research Program.
NBRT National Board for Respiratory Therapy, Inc.
NBS National Bureau of Standards; N-bromosuccinimide; Neurobiology of suicide; Nevoid basal (cell carcinoma) syndrome; New Brunswick (NJ) Scientific Co.; Newborn screen (serum thyroxine and phenylketonuria); Nijmegen breakage syndrome; No bacteria seen (microscopy); No/ Normal bowel sounds; Normal blood sugar; Normal brain stem; Normal burro serum; Nystagmus blockage syndrome.
NBSS Newsletter of Biomedical Safety and Standards.
NBT Nitroblue tetrazolium (dye - histochemical staining technique); Non-tumor-bearing; Normal blood test; Normal breast tissue.
NBT-DF Nitroblue tetrazolium (chloride) diformazan.
NBTE Non-bacterial thrombotic endocarditis.
NBTGN P-nitrobenzyl-thioguanosine.
NBTNF Newborn, term, normal, female.
NBTNM Newborn, term, normal, male.
NBT-PABA N-benzoyl-L-tyrosyl para-aminobenzoic acid.
NBTS National Blood Transfusion Service.
n-Bu n-butyl.
NBVP Non-bacterial vaginosis/ vulvovaginosis pathogen (such as *Candida* (*Monilia*) albicans, Herpes simplex virus, *Trichomonas* vaginalis, etc.) (see BVP).
NBW Normal birth/ body weight.
NC Nasal cannula/ clearance; Nature Conservancy; Neck complaint; Negro child; Neonatal cholestasis; Nerve conduction; Neural crest; Neurologic(al) check/ controls; Neutralization capacity (antivenom); Nevus comedonicus; Night call; Nitrocellulose; No casualty/ change/ charge/ complaint(s) (see N/C); Noise criterion; Non-cirrhotic; Non-contributory (see N/C); Non-coronary; Normally closed (switch); Normocephalic; Nose clips/ cone; Not classified/ completed/ counted/ cultured (= nc); Nucleocapsid; Nurse clinician; Nurse Corps; Nursing Care (NFLPN journal); Nursing coordinator; Sandoz (USA), and Warner-Lambert Pharmaceutical code for experimental substances.
nC nanocoulomb.
nc nanocurie (= 10^{-9} curie; 10^{-9} c; millimicrocurie; mμc; 10^{-3} microcurie; 10^{-3} μc; nCi) - measurement of radioactivity; not classified/ completed/ counted/ cultured (see NC).
N/C No casualty/ change/ charge/ complaint(s) (= NC); Non-contributory (= NC).
N:C Nuclear-cytoplasmic ratio.
NCA Narcotics Control Act (Canada); National Cancer Act; National Certification Agency; National Clearing-house/ Council on Alcoholism; National Commission on Accrediting; National Council on Aging; N-carboxyaminoacid; Neurocirculatory asthenia (a symptom-complex characterized by breathlessness, giddiness, chest pains, palpitations, fatigue, etc. Also called Anxiety neurosis, Cardiac neurosis, DaCosta's syndrome, DAH or Disordered action of the heart, Effort syndrome, Hypochondriac syndrome or Hypochondriasis, Irritable heart, Pschosomatic syndrome, Soldier's heart, etc.); Neutrophil chemotactic activity; New Communities Administration; No congenital abnormalities; Nodulocystic acne; Non-compartmental analysis; Non-contractile area; Non-specific cross-reacting antigen; Normo chromic/cytic anemia; Nuclear cerebral angiogram/graphy; Nucleic acid.
NCAA National Clinical Assessment Authority (GMC, UK).
NCAB National Cancer Advisory Board (NCI).
n-CAD Negative coronoradiographic documentation.
NCAE National Council for Alcohol Education.
NCAH National Child Abuse Hot-line.
NCAHF National Council Against Health Fraud.
NCAMI National Committee Against Mental

Illness.

NCAMLP National Certification Agency for Medical Laboratory Personnel.

NcAMP Nephrogenous cyclic adenosine monophosphate.

N-CAP Nurses Coalition for Action in Politics.

NCAR National Center for Atmospheric Research (Boulder, Colorado).

NCARMD National Commission on Arthritis and Related Musculoskeletal Diseases.

NCAS Neocarzinostatin.

NCASA National Cancer Association of South Africa.

NC/AT Normal cephalic atraumatic; Normocephalic/ Atraumatic (used in HEENT examination) (see HEENT).

NCB Narcotics Control Board; Needle core biopsy; No code blue; Nuffield Council on Bioethics (UK).

NCBA National Caucus on the Black Aged.

NCBI National Center for Biotechnology Information.

NCBP Non-cyclical breast pain.

NCC Narrow cervical canal (c/cout quadriplegia); Nested case-control; Neurochemical change(s) (in the brain); Neurocysticercosis (as in *Taenia* solium infestation); No clinical consequence; No concentrated carbohydrates; Non-conception cycle (e.g. in embryo transfer, IVF, etc.) (= NPC); Non-coronary cusp; Nursing care continuity; Nursing clerical coordinator.

NCCAN National Center on Child Abuse and Neglect (HEW).

NCCC National Cancer Cytology Center.

NCCCSA National Council for the Care of Cripples in South Africa.

NCCDC National Center for Chronic Disease Control.

NCCEA Neurosensory Center Comprehensive Examination for Aphasia.

NCCF National Childhood Cancer Foundation.

NCCHS National Commission on Community Health Services.

NCCIP National Center for Clinical Infant Program.

NCCLS National Committee for Clinical Laboratory Standards.

NCCLVP National Coordinating Committee on Large Volume Parenterals.

NCCMHC National Council for Community Mental Health Centers.

NCCML National Committee for Careers in the Medical Laboratory.

NCCN National Comprehensive Cancer Network (US).

NCCPA National Commission on Certification of Physician Assistants.

NCCS National Coalition for Cancer Survivorship.

NCCTG North Central Cancer Treatment Group (see ECOG).

NCCU Newborn convalescent care unit.

NCD Nanocephalic dwarf (or Bird-headed dwarf) (see BHD); National Commission on Diabetes; National Council on Drugs; Natural cell death (= Apoptosis); Nerve cell death/ degeneration (as in Alzheimer's disease, etc.); Nerve compression disorder; Net- connected doctor (Web site, e-mail); Neurocirculatory dystonia; Night Care doctor/ dose; Nitrogen clearance delay; Normal childhood disease(s)/ disorder(s); Not considered disabling.

NCDA Nationa Council on Drug Abuse.

NCDAI National Clearinghouse for Drug Abuse Information.

NCDB National Center for Drugs and Biologics (FDA).

NCDC National Communicable Disease Center (Atlanta).

NCDHW National Children's Dental Health Week.

NCDV Nebraska calf diarrhea virus.

NCE Negative contrast echocardiogram/graphy; Negative cumulative effect; New chemical entity; Newly conceived embryo (= JCE); No clinical experience; Non-convulsive epilepsy; Normal chick embryo.

NCEC National Clearinghouse on Environmental Carcinogenesis (NCI).

NCECC National Committee for/on Early/ Emergency Coronary Care.

NCEP National Cholesterol Education Program (US).

NCEP-ATP National Cholesterol Education Program - Adult Treatment Panel (US).

NCF National Cancer Foundation; Neutrophil chemotactic factor (see NCF-A).
NCFA Narcolepsy and Catalepsy Foundation of America.
NCF-A Neutrophil chemotactic factor of anaphylaxis.
NCF-C; NCF(C) Neutrophil chemotactic factor (complement).
NCFF National Cystic Fibrosis Foundation.
NCFM National Center of Forensic Medicine (Israel).
NCFNB National Cystic Fibrosis News Bulletin.
NCFP National Center for Family Planning (HSMHA).
NCFR National Council on Family Relations.
NCFRF National Cystic Fibrosis Research Foundation.
NCFS Non-contingent footshock.
NCG National curricular guideline(s); National cylinder gas; Nerve cell/ Non-cancerous growth.
NCGS National Cooperative Gallstone Study.
NCH National Council on the Humanities (NEH); Northwest Community Hospital (Des Moines, Iowa).
NCHC National Council of Health Centers.
NCHCA National Commission for Health Certifying Agencies.
NCHCS National Council of Health Care Services.
NCHCT National Center for Health Care Technology.
NCHD Normal childhood diseases.
NCHE National Center for Health Education.
NCHF National Council against Health Fraud (NY).
NCHGR National Center for Human Genome Research.
NCHHHAS National Council for Homemaker-Home Health Aid Services, Inc.
NCHLS National Council of Health Laboratory Services.
NCHM National Council on Hunger and Malnutrition.
NCHPD National Council on Health Planning and Development.
NCHS National Center for Health Statistics (HRA).
NCHSPCS National Council for Hospices and Specialist Palliative Care Services (UK).
NCHSR National Center for Health Services Research.
NCHSRD National Center for Health Services Research and Development.
NCI Naphthalene, creosote, iodoform (powder) - treatment for pediculosis; National Cancer Institute (Canada; NIH; PHS); No clinical information; Non-criterion ischemic (animal); Nosocomial infection (= HAI); Nuclear contour index; Nursing care integration.
nCi nanocurie (see nc).
NCIA Non-corticosteroid immunosuppressant agent.
NCIB National Collection of Industrial Bacteria.
NCIB 8710 A certain strain of the slime-forming saprophytic bacterium, Leuconostoc mesenteroides, found in milk and fruit juices and used in the fermentation of sucrose, producing degraded dextrans or glucose polymers, from which is prepared dextran injections.
NCIC National Cancer Institute of Canada; National Crime Information Center (FBI).
NCICAS National Cooperative Inner-City Asthma Study (US).
NCID National Center for Infectious Diseases.
NCIF National Center for Infectious Diseases (CDC).
NCIH National Council for International Health.
NCIJ National Cancer Institute Journal.
NCIPC National Center for Injury Prevention and Control (US).
NCJ Needle catheter jejunostomy.
NCJISS National Criminal Justice Information and Statistics Service.
NCL National Chemical Laboratory; Neural cell line (see DSNCL); Neuronal cell loss; Neuronal ceroid lipofuscinosis; Nuclear cardiology laboratory.
NCLEX-RN National Council Licensure Examination for Registered Nurses.
NCLIS National Commission on Libraries and Information Science.

NCM Nailfold capillary microscope; Non-cytokine marker (e.g. C-reactive protein [CRP]; Serum Ferritin; etc.).
ncm non compos mentis (L.) - not of sound mind.
N/cm^2 Newtons per square centimeter.
NCMC Nassau County Medical Center (Long Island, New York); Natural cell-mediated cytotoxicity.
NCMDA National Commission on Marijuana and Drug Abuse.
NCME Network for Continuing Medical Education.
NCMH National Committee for Mental Health.
NCMHI National Clearinghouse for Mental Health Information (HEW).
NCMI National Committee against Mental Illness.
NCMM National Council on Medical Malpractice.
NCMS North Carolina Medical Society.
NCMTD Neuronal Charcot-Marie-Tooth disease (= HMSN Type II) (see HMSN).
NCMTE National Council on Medical Technology Education.
NCN National Council of Nurses.
NCNA Nursing Clinics of North America (journal).
NCNC Normochromic normocytic.
NCNR Natural Center for Nursing Research.
NCO No complaints offered; Non-commissioned officer.
NCOD National Center on Deafness (CSUN).
NCOL National Council on Occupational Licensing.
NCP National Cancer Program; Neomycin, chlorhexidine, and polymyxin B (cream) - a prophylactic cream for the treatment of burns; Nitrogen-containing compound (amino, pyridinyl, etc.); No consistent pattern; Non-carrier patient; Non-collagen protein; Non-compliant participant/ patient; Nursing care plan.
n-CPAP Nasal continuous positive airway pressure.
NCPAS National Computer Program Abstract Service.
NCPAT National Council for the Public Assessment of Technology.
NCPCA National Committee to Prevent Child Abuse.
NCPCC National Clearinghouse for Poison Control Centers (see NCPIC).
NCPCR National Center for the Prevention and Control of Rape (NIMH).
NCP cream See NCP.
NCPD Non-cardiogenic pulmonary edema.
NCPE Non-cardiac pulmonary edema.
NCPHS National Commission for the Protection of Human Subjects of Biomedical and Behavioral Research (HEW).
NCPIC National Clearinghouse for Poison Information Centers (NCPCC).
NCP-NIDR National Caries Program of the National Institute of Dental Research.
NCPIE National Council on Patient Information and Education.
NCPP National Cancer Program Plan (NCI).
NCPPB National Collection of Plant Pathogenic Bacteria.
NCPR No cardiopulmonary resuscitation.
NCPS National Commission on Product Safety.
NCPT National Congress of Parents and Teachers.
NCQA National Committee for Quality Assurance (Health Plan, US).
NCR National Cancer Registry; National Council on Rehabilitation; National Council for Research (see NRC); Nerve cell receptor; No clinical relevance/ response; Nuclear/ cytoplasmic ratio.
NCRC Non-child resistant container.
NCRE Non-cephalic reference electrode.
NCRH National Center for Radiological Health; National Conference on Rural Health.
NCRHI National Council for Reliable Health Information.
NCRND National Committee for Research in Neurological Diseases/ Disorders.
NCRP National Council on Radiation Protection (NBS).
NCRPM National Council on Radiation Protection and Measurements (NBS).
NCRR National Center of Research Resources (NIH).
NCRS National Committee for Radiation

Safety.

NCRV National Committee for Radiation Victims.

NCS National Cancer Survey; National Collaborative Study; N-chlorosuccinimide; Neocarcinostatin; Nerve conduction study; Newborn calf serum; No clinically significant (action, change, interaction, result); No concentrated sweets; Non-circumferential stenosis; Non-clinical study; Nutcracker's syndrome (of occlusion of superior mesenteric artery); Nystagmus concentration syndrome.

NCSBB Non-cardioselective â-blocker (= NSBAB; NSBB).

NCSC National Care Standards Commission (GMC, UK); National Council of Senior Citizens.

NCSCS Non-compressive spinal cord syndrome.

NCSD No clinically significant difference(s).

NCSH National Clearinghouse on Smoking and Health (HEW).

NCSN National Council for School Nurses.

NCSR National Center for Scientific Research.

NCSS National Center for Social Statistics.

NCST National Council of Science and Technology; Non-compensatory sinus tachycardia.

NCT Narcan challenge test (for opioid dependency); National Center for Toxicogenomics (NIEHS); National Childbirth Trust (UK); National clinical trial; Neural crest tumor; Neutron capture therapy; New cancer therapy/ treatment; Non-cancerous tissue/ tumor; Non-clinical/-comparative trial; Non-contact tonometry.

NCTC National Cancer Tissue Culture; National Collection of Type Cultures.

NCTR National Center for Toxicological Research (FDA).

NCTT Non-contact therapeutic touch.

NCU Normal clinical use.

NCV Nerve conduction velocity; Non-cholera vibrio.

NCVS National Center for Vital Statistics/ Voice and Speech; Nerve conduction velocity study.

NCWQ National Commission on Water Quality.

NCYC National Collection of Yeast Cultures.

ND Doctor of Naturopathy (see DN); Nasal deformity; Natural/ Neonatal death; Naval Dispensary; Neoplastic/ Newcastle/ Norrie disease; Neurological development; Neurological Disorder (journal); Neuropsychological deficit; Neurotic depression; Neutral density; New drug; New Drugs (book); News in Dentistry (journal); No data/date/ disease; No defects (see N/D); Non-dectectable; Non-diabetic; Non-disabling; None/ Not detectable; Normal delivery/ development; Nose drops; Not detected/ determined/ diabetic/ diagnosed; Not(hing) done (see N/D); Nurse's diagnosis; Nursing Digest (journal); Nutritionally deprived.

Nd Neodymium (Z = 60) (see Elements - Neodymium); Number of dissimilar (matches/ pairs).

N_D; N_d; n_D; n_d Refractive index (eye examination).

N/D No defects (= ND); Not(hing) done (= ND).

N&D Nodular and diffuse.

NDA National Dental Association; New Drug Application (FDA); No data available; No demonstrable/ detectable activity/ antibody; No dose adjustment; Non-deforming arthritis; Non-dominant arm; Normal daily activity.

NDAA Non-dopamine-agonist agent.

NDAC National Drug Abuse Council.

NDAQ National Dental Association Quarterly.

NDB Nucleus of the diagonal band (of the brain).

NDC National Dairy Council; National Data Communications; National Drug Code; Naval Dental Clinic; Non-differentiated cell.

NDCD National Drug Code Directory (FDA).

NDCP National Drug Control Policy (Washington, DC).

NDD Neurodegenerative disease/ disorder; Neurodevelopmental disease/ disorder; No dialysis days.

NDDF National Digestive Disease Foundation.

NDDG National Diabetes Data Group.

NDDI Non-delusional depressive illness.

NDDIC National Digestive Diseases

Information Clearinghouse (NIH).
NDDS Nanoscale drug-delivery system.
NDE Near-death experience; Need for Drug Elimination; Non-diabetic extremity.
NDF Neutrophil diffraction factor; New dosage/ dose form; Non-disease factor.
NDFDA Nonadecafluoro-n-decanoic acid.
NDGA Nordihydro-guaiaretic acid. Used as an effective antioxidant for oils and fats.
NDGC Non-directive genetic counselling.
NDH Natural disaster hospital.
NDHS National Diet Heart Study.
NDI National Death Index; Naylor Dana Institute (AHF); Nephrogenic diabetes insipidus.
NDIDP Naylor Dana Institute for Disease Prevention.
NDIR Non-dispersive infrared (analyzer).
NDL No definitive link.
NDLI Neutrophil-dependent lung injury (see NMLI).
NDM N-desmethyl-methsuximide; No dose modification; Non-diabetic mother.
NDMA Nitroso-dimethyl-amine/-aniline; Non-fat Dry Milk Act (1956).
NDMDA National Depressive and Manic Depressive Association.
NDMHA Non-directional microphone hearing aid.
NDMR Non-depolarizing muscle relaxant (see NDNMA).
NDMREA National Diabetes Mellitus Research and Education Act (1974) (= NDREA).
NDMS National Drug Monitoring System (FDA).
NDN Non-invasive Diagnostics Newsletter (journal).
NDNA; nDNA Native (double-strand) deoxyribonucleic acid.
NDNAV Naked DNA vaccine (see DNA).
NDNMA Non-depolarizing neuromuscular agent (e.g. Atracurium, Miracurium, Roruronium, Vecuronium, etc.) (= NDMR; NMA).
Nd/Nt Non-distended, non-tender.
NDO National diabetic organization; Neurodevelopmental observation/ outcome (e.g. in full-term infants); Non-digestible oligosaccharides.
NDP Generic designation for series of nucleoside 5'-diphosphoric acids; Net/ No dietary protein; No drug problem; Non-diabetic population; Nucleoside diphosphate.
NDPW Non-diabetic pregnant woman/ women.
NDR National Dialysis Registry; National Drug Co code for experimental substances; Neonatal death rate; Neurotic depressive reaction; Normal detrusor reflex.
NDR 5061 A Aletamine hydrochloride (= alpha-allyl-phenethylamine hydrochloride) - an analgesic.
NDREA National Diabetic Research and Education Act (see NDMREA).
NDRI Noradrenaline and dopamine reuptake inhibitor (e.g. Bupropion).
NDS National Delphi Survey (named after the Delphi Oracle); Naval Dental School; New drug submission; Non-disabling stroke (see TIA); Normal dog serum.
NDSB Narcotic Drugs Supervisory Board.
NDSMR Non-depolarizing skeletal muscle relaxant (e.g. tubocurarine).
NDT Nephrology Dialysis Transplantation (journal, US); Noise detection threshold; Non-destructive test; Non-destructive Testing (journal); Non-developmental treatment; Non-drug therapy.
NDTDSC Non-destructive Testing Data Support Center (San Antonio, Texas).
NDTI National Disease and Therapeutic Index.
NDTIR National Disease and Therapeutic Index Review (journal).
NDTN Non-dystrophic toenail.
NDU Non-diabetic ulcer.
NDV Newcastle disease virus.
NDV_{uv} Ultraviolet-irradiated Newcastle disease virus.
NDW Number of different words.
NDX Non-dispersive X-ray spectroscopy.
NDY Not Dead Yet (lobby group, Ohio).
Nd/YAG Neodymium/yttrium-aluminum-garnet (laser).
NE Narcotics Education (journal); National Emergency; Necrotic enteritis; Neomycin (on culture and sensitivity reports - see NM);

Nephropathia epidemica; Nerve ending/ excitability (test)/ excitation; Neuroendocrinology; Neuroepithelium; Neurological examination; Neutrophil elastase; Never exposed; No effect/ enlargement/ expense/ exposure; Nocturnal exacerbation/ erection; Non-elastic; Non-endogenous; Non-invasive evaluation; Norepinephrine (= 3h-norepinephrine; noradrenaline); Not elevated/ enlarged/ equal/ evaluated/ examined; Nutcracker esophagus.

Ne Neon (Z = 10) (see Elements - Neon).

ne- combining form meaning new or young (Gr. neos).

NEA National Education Association; National Endowment for the Arts; Neoplasm embryonic antigen; Neuroexcitatory activity; Newspapers Enterprise Association; No essential abnormality; No evidence of abnormality; Nuclear Energy Agency (OECD).

NEAA Non-essential aminoacid(s) (9 acids - see EAA): Alanine, Arginine, Aspartic acid, Cystine, Glutamic acid, Glycine, Proline, Serine, and Tyrosine.

NEB Neuroendocrine body.

Neb Nebulizer.

neb; nebul a spray (L. nebula).

Nebbie Nembutal capsule (Pentobarbitone) (see Barb).

NEC National Electrical Code (NFPA); National Engineering Consortium, Inc; Necrotizing enterocolitis; Neurenteric canal (a passage in the embryo from the posterior part of the neural tube into the archenteron) (= Braun's canal; Kovalevsky's canal); Neuroendocrine cell/ change(s) (brain); Neutropenic enterocolitis (typhlitis); No essential changes; Non-esterified cholesterol; Not else(where) classifiable/fied; Nuclear Energy Committee (International).

NECA National Electrical Contracters Association.

NECAHP National Economic Council of Associations of Health Professions.

NECHI Northeastern Consortium for Health Information.

NECO New England Council of Optometrists.

necr- prefix meaning corpse or death (Gr. nekros).

NED No-effect dose; No evidence of disease; No expiration date; Normal equivalent deviation.

NEDA National Electronic Distributors Association.

NEDC National Economic Development Council (UK).

NEDH New England Deaconess Hospital.

NEDL No effect dose level (see NOED).

NEDNA National Emergency Department Nurses Association.

NEE Needle electrode examination; Norethindrone enanthate.

NEEE Near East equine encephalomyelitis.

NEEP Negative end-expiratory pressure (see PFT - NEEP).

NEF Negative expiratory force; Nephritic factor.

NEFA Non-essential/ Non-esterified fatty acid.

NEG Non-enzymatic glycosylation (of structural proteins, an etiological factor in the development of diabetic retinopathy and nephropathy).

neg negative (symbol: - ; N) (see Symbols - Calculation); neglect; negro.

NEGRO National Economic Growth and Reconstruction Organization.

NEH National Endowment for the Humanities (NFAH).

NEHA National Environmental Health Association; National Executive Housekeepers Association, Inc.

NEHE Nurses fo Environmental Health Education.

NEI National Eye Institute (NIH; HEW).

NEIB Neuroendocrine immune basis (e.g. of the Rheumatic diseases).

NEIC National Earthquake Information Center (now NEIS).

NEIS National Earthquake Information Service (USGS).

NEISS National Electronic Injury Surveillance System (CPSC).

NEJ Neuroeffector junction.

NEJM New England Journal of Medicine (formerly BMSJ).

NEJO New England Journal of Optometry (NECO).

NEL National Epilepsy League, Inc; Naval Electronics Laboratory; No-effect level (mg/kg/day of a drug).

NEM N-ethylmaleimide; No evidence of malignancy.

nem nutritional milk unit (acronym for the German: Nahrungs-Einheit-Milch; Nahrungst-Einheit-Milch - "nutritional unit milk") - the unit of nutrition (Pirquet's system of feeding), equivalent to the nutritive value of 1 Gram of breast milk.

NEMA National Eclectic Medical Association; National Electrical Manufacturers Association.

Nema; nema Nematode (threadworm).

NEMC New England Medical Center (Boston, Mass).

NEMCH New England Medical Center Hospitals.

NEMD Non-specific esophageal motility disorder/ motor dysfunction.

Nemish Nembutal capsule (see Barb).

Nemmie Nembutal capsule (see Barb).

NEN New England Nuclear Co.

NENA Northeast Neighborhood Association.

Ne/Nγ Internal conversion coefficient. A measure of the relative numbers of conversion electrons and gamma-rays emitted in a given transition (see IC - Internal Conversion).

NEO A standard personality inventory test (see NEOAC).

Neo; neo Neoarsphenamine (see NAB 914); Neomycin; Neoplasm/stic.

NEOAC Neuroticism, extroversion, openness, agreeableness and conscientiousness (five broad scales in the personality inventory test (= NEO).

NEOH Neonatal high (risk).

NEOM Neonatal medium (risk).

Neonat Neonatal/tology.

NEP Negative esophageal pressure (increased in snoring and upper-airway resistance); Negative expiratory pressure; Nephrectomy/rology/ron (see Neph); Neuroendocrine pathway; Neutral endopeptidase; No evidence of pathology; Non-emergency patient; Non-enzymatic process.

Nep; nep Nephrectomy/rology/ron (see Neph).

NEPA National Environmental Policy/ Protection Act (1970).

Neph Nephrectomy/rology/ron (= NEP; Nep; nep).

nephelo- prefix meaning cloudy (Gr. nephele).

NEPHGE Non-equilibrated pH gradient electrophoresis.

nephr- combining form meaning kidney (Gr. nephros).

NEPHRO Nephrogram.

NER Nodal escape rhythm; No evidence of recurrence.

ner nervous (= nerv).

NERAC New England Research Application Center.

NERB North East Regional Boards.

NERD No evidence of recurrent disease.

NERF National Eye Research Foundation.

NERO Non-invasive evaluation of radiation output.

nerv nervous (see ner).

NES Neuroelectric Society; Not elsewhere specified.

NESC Neural epithelial stem cell.

NESO Northeastern Society of Orthodontists.

NESP Nurse Education Support Program.

NESSCCA National Easter Seal Society for Crippled Children and Adults.

NET Nasoendotrachial tube; Nerve excitability test; Neuroendocrine tumor.

Neth. P Netherlands Pharmacopoeia (Nederlandse Pharmacopee).

Neti Nuclear embryo transfer infant (acronym for one of two cloned, rhesus monkeys, the other named Ditto, given by Don Wolf, a senior scientist at the Oregon Regional Primate Research Center in Beaverton, Oregon, using a technique similar to the one used to make Dolly, the world's first cloned sheep).

n et m night and morning (i.e day) (L. nocte et mane).

NETT Nasal endotracheal tube.

ne tr s num do not deliver unless paid (L. ne tradas sine nummo).

Neu Neuraminidase.

neu neurilemma.

NEUP Noepinephrine-uptake transporter (in adrenergic tissue) (= NEP).

Neur; neur; Neuro; neuro; Neurol; neurol neurological/gist/gy.
neur- combining form meaning nerve (Gr. neuron).
Neuroend Neuroendocrinology (journal).
Neurol Neurology (see Neur); Neurology (AAN journal).
Neuropath Neuropathologist/gy.
Neuropharm Neuropharmacology (journal).
Neuropsy Neuropsychologica (journal).
Neurorad Neuroradiology (ESN journal).
Neurosc Neuroscience (journal).
Neuro-Surg Neurosurgeon/gery.
Neut; neut Neuter; Neutral; Neutralizing (antibody); Neutrophil (see Neutro).
Neutr Neutrophil (see Neutro).
Neutro Neutrophil (= Neut; neut; Neutr).
NEV Non-enveloped virus (e.g. hepatitis A).
Newt Newton (a unit of force) (see N. Newton).
NEX Nose to ear to xiphoid.
NEXT Nationwide Evaluation of X-ray Trends (FDA).
NEY Neomycin egg yolk (agar).
NEYA Neomycin egg yolk agar.
NF Eaton Laboratories Inc (USA) code for experimental substances; Nafcillin (on culture and sensitivity reports); National Formulary (drugs - ADHA); National Foundation (The) (formerly NFIP); Negro female; Nephritic/ Noise factor; Neurofibromatosis; Neurofilament; Neutral fraction; New Formula; Nitrofurantoin; Noise figure; None/ Not found; Non-fatal; Non-function (transplanted organ); Normal flow; Not filtered; Nursed fair; Nursing Forum (journal); Nutrition Foundation.
nF nanofarad.
NFA Neutralizing factor assay (an antibody a.ssay).
NFAC National Foundation for Asthmatic Children.
NFAH National Foundation on the Arts and the Humanities.
NFAIS National Federation of Abstracting and Indexing Services.
NFAT Nuclear factor of activated T cells.
NF-AT Nuclear factor of activated T (leukocytes).
NFB National Federation of/ Foundation for the Blind; Neurofeedback; Newly formed bone; Non-fermenting bacteria.
NFC National Fertility Center; Non-fatal condition; Not favorably considered.
NFCF National Foundation for Cystic Fibrosis.
NFCPG National Federation of Catholic Physicians Guild.
NFCR National Foundation for Cancer Research.
NFD Neurofibrillary degeneration; No family doctor; Non-febrile disease.
NFDI National Foundation for Depressive Illness.
NFDM Non-fat dried milk.
NFDR Neurofaciodigitorenal (syndrome).
NFE Non-fatal event; Non-ferrous extract.
NFGND National Foundation for Genetics and Neuromuscular Diseases.
NFH Negative family history (see -veFH); Non-familial hematuria/ hypercholesterolemia.
NFHA National Funeral Home Association.
NFI Normal food intake.
NFIC National Foundation for Ileitis and Colitis.
NFID National Foundation for Infectious Diseases.
NFIP National Flood Insurance Program; National Foundation for Infantile Paralysis (now NF).
NFK Non-functional/oning kidney(s).
NF-kB Nuclear factor Kappa B (a cellular gene which regulates and activates many kinds of cells).
NFL Nerve fiber layer.
NFLB National Federation of Licensing Bodies.
NFLD Nerve fiber layer defect.
NFLPN National Federation of Licensed Practical Nurses, Inc.
NFM Neurofibromatosis; Nikon fluorescent microscope (Nikon, Garden City, New York).
NFMD National Foundation for Muscular Dystrophy; National Foundation - March of Dimes.
NFMDN National Foundation - March of Dimes News.

NFME National Fund for Medical Education.
NFMI Non-fatal myocardial infarction.
NFND National Foundation for Neuromuscular Diseases (see NFNMD).
NFNHS Non-fatal non-hemorrhagic stroke.
NFNID National Foundation for Non-Invasive Diagnostics.
NFNMD National Foundation for Neuromuscular Diseases, Inc (= NFND).
NFO Negative fetal outcome (Obstetrics).
NFOF New Face of Fitness (an exercise program).
NFP No family physician; Non-fatal pancreatitis; Nortestosterone-furyl-propionate.
NFPA National Fire Protection Association.
NFPCA National Fire Prevention and Control Administration (Dept. of Commerce).
NFPM Natural family planning method (any method of family planning that does not require a drug or a device to avoid pregnancy, such as):
BBTMFP - Basal body temperature method of family planning.
CMFP - Calendar method of family planning (= Rhythm method).
OMFP - Ovulation method of family planning.
RMFP - Rhythm method of family planning or Rhythm method (see CMFP).
STMFP - Symptothermal method of family planning.
NFR Normal fasting range (of blood sugar).
NFS National Fertility Study; Non-fatal stroke (see NFNHS).
NFSID National Foundation for Sudden Infant Death.
NFT Neurofibrillary tangle.
NFTC National Foreign Trade Council.
NFTD Normal full term delivery.
NFTSD Normal full-term spontaneous delivery.
NFTT Non-organic failure to thrive.
NFU National Formulary Unit(s).
NFV Nelfinavir.
NFW Normal fertile woman/ women; Nursed fairly well.
NG Nasogastric (tube); New/ No growth; Nitroglycerin(e); No good (see N/G); Nodose ganglion; Non-groupable (meningococci); Not given.
ng nanogram (= 10^{-9} g; 10^{-9} gram; mμg; ngm; 10^{-3} μg; 10^{-3} microgram; millimicrogram; mγ; milligamma) (see mμg); no good (see N/G).
N/G No good (= NG; ng).
NGA Nutrient gelatin agar.
NGB Neurogenic bladder.
NGC Narrow guage catheter; Nucleus reticularis gigantocellularis.
NGD Nasogastric drainage.
NGE Non-gonadal endocrinopathy (e.g. adrenal, pituitary, or thyroid disorders).
NGEF Nasogastric enteral feeding.
NGEW Nurses Guild of England and Wales.
NGF Nasogastric feeding; National Genetics Foundation; Nerve growth factor; Neutrophil growth factor (= Filgrastim; G-CSF).
NGGR Non-glucogenic/ Glucogenic ratio.
NGH Normal glucose homeostasis; Normogonadotrophic hypogonadism.
NGI Nuclear globulin inclusions; Nuremberg Geriatric Inventory.
n giv not given.
NGL Natural gas liquids; Neutral glycolipid.
ngm nanogram (see ng).
NGNV No-glasses-needed vision (Ophthalmic surgery) (see KRS).
NGO Non-government observer; Non-governmental organization.
NGOI Normogonadotrophic ovarian insufficiency.
NGP Normal genetic predisposition.
NGR Narrow guaze roll; Nasogastric replacement.
NGRF Non-glycemic risk factor (Hypolipidemia, hypertension, smoking) - in the treatment of NIDDM.
NGRI Not guilty by reason of insanity.
NGS Nasogastric suction; National Geographic Society; Normal goat serum.
NGSA Nerve growth stimulating activity.
NGSF Non-genital skin fibroblast.
NGT Nasogastric tube; Normal glucose tolerance.
NGU Non-gonococcal urethritis.
NGVL National Gene Vector Laboratory (COH).
NH Natriuretic hormone; Naval Hospital;

Neonatal hepatitis; Neurologically handicapped; New Health (journal); Nocturnal hypoventilation; Non-human; Nursing home; Nursing Homes (journal).
N(H) Proton density.
N-H Norwood-Hamilton (classification/ scale of hair loss in androgenetic alopecia - AA).
-NH_2 Amino group.
NH_3 Ammonia.
$^{13}NH_3$ Radioactive ammonia.
NHA National Health/ Hearing/ Hemophilia Association; National Heart Act; Non-specific hepatocellular abnormality.
NHANES National Health and Nutrition Examination Survey.
NHAS National Hearing Aid Society.
NHBCL Non-Hodgkin's β-cell lymphoma (= NHL).
NHBPCC National High Blood Pressure Coordinating Committee.
NHBPEP National High Blood Pressure Education Program.
NH_4Br Ammonium bromide.
NHBS Formerly "The National History Book Service", now "NHBS Mailorder Bookstore" (UK); National Horticultural and Biological Society.
NHC National Headache Consortium; National Health Council; Neighborhood Health Center; Neonatal hypocalcemia; Non-histone chromosomal (protein) (see NHCP); Non-hormonal contraception/ceptive (= NHCM; NHCP); Nursing home care.
NH_4Cl Ammonium chloride.
NHCM on-hormonal contraceptive method (see NHC).
NH_4CNO Ammonium cyanate.
$(NH_2)_2CO$ Urea.
$(NH_4)_2CO_3$ Ammonium carbonate.
$NH_4.CO.NH_2$ Ammonium carbamate.
NHCP Non-histone chromosomal protein; Non-hormonal contraceptive precaution (see NHC).
NHCS National health care system (= UHCC).
NHCU Nursing home care unit.
NHD Normal hair distribution.
NHDC National Hansen's Disease Center.
NHDF Normal human diploid fibroblast.
NHDL Non-high-density lipoprotein.
NHDR National Hospital Discharge Register.
NHDS National Hospital Discharge Survey.
NHDU National Hospital Doctors Union.
NHES National Health Examination Survey.
NHF National Headache/ Hemophilia Foundation; National Health Federation; Non-immune hydrops fetalis; Normal heart/ hepatic function (see NLF).
NHFRA National Hay Fever Relief Association.
NHG Normal human globulin/ growth.
NHGD Normal human growth and development.
NHGJ Normal human gastric juice.
NHGRI National Human Genome Research Institute (NIH).
NHH Neurohypophyseal hormone.
NH_2Hg2NO_3 Mercuro-amido-nitrate.
$(NH_4)HS$ Ammonium hydrosulfide.
NHI National Health Institute/ Insurance (UK); National Heart Initiative (US)/ Institute.
NHIBAC National Health Insurance Benefits Advisory Council (= NIBAC).
NHIF National Head Injury Foundation.
NHIP National Health Insurance Plan.
NHIS National Health Interview Survey.
NHK Normal human kidney.
NHL Nodular histiocytic lymphoma; Non-Hodgkin's lymphoma.
nHL Normalized hearing level.
NHLBI National Heart, Lung, and Blood Institute.
NHLI National Heart and Lung Institute (NIH - see NHLBI).
NHML Non-Hodgkin's malignant lymphoma.
NHMRC National Health and Medical Research Council.
NHNES National Health and Nutrition Examination Survey (US).
NH_4NO_3 Ammonium nitrate.
NH_4OH Ammonium hydroxide.
NHP National Health Plan (UK); National health problem; Neurohormonal profile; Neurohypophysis; Non-health practitioner; Non-hemoglobin/ Non-histone (acidic) protein; Non-human primate; Nottingham Health Profile; Normal human pooled (plasma) (see

NHPP); Nursing home placement; Nursing Home Practice.
NHPC National Health Planning Council.
NHPF National Health Policy Forum.
NHPIC National Health Planning Information Center.
NHPO National Health Program for Orthopaedics (AAOS).
NHPP National human pooled plasma (= NHP); National Human Pituitary Program.
NHPPN National Health Professions Placement Network.
NHPRDA National Health Planning and Resources Development Act of 1974.
NHR Net histocompatibility ratio.
NHRC National Health Research Center.
NHRIC National Health Related Items Code (other than drugs).
NHRPAC National Human Research Protection Advisory Committee (NIH).
NHS Nance-Horan syndrome; National Health Service (GB); National Health Survey; N-hydroxy-succinimide; Neurohypophyseal system; Non-hemorrhagic stroke (see NFNHS); Non-hospital setting; Normal healthy subject; Normal horse/ human serum; Nurses' Health Study; Scarlet hemolytic streptococcus.
NHSA National House Staff Association.
NHSAS National Health Service Audit Staff.
NHSLS National Health and Social Life Survey (Univ. of Chicago).
NHSB National Highway Safety Bureau (DoT); Normal human social behavior.
NHSC National Health Service Corps (PHS).
NHSD National Health Survey Division (NCHS).
NHSO National House Staff Organization.
$(NH_4)_2SO_4$ Ammonium sulfate.
NHSPC Non-hormone-sensitive prostatic cancer.
NHSR National Hospital Service Reserve.
NHSREC National Health Service Research Ethics Committee (UK) (see COREC; GafREC).
NHT Neonatal hyperthyroidism; Non-penetrating head trauma.
NHTHN Non-hypotonic hyponatremia.
NHTR Non-hemolytic transfusion reaction.
NHTSA National Highway Traffic Safety Administration.
NHV Normal healthy volunteer.
NHVT Non-hormonal vaginal therapy.
NHW National Health and Welfare (Canada); Non-healing wound.
NI Nerve impulse; Neuraminidase inhibition; Neurological improvement; Neutralization/ Noise index; No information; Non-invasive; Not identified/ isolated; Nucleus intercalatus; Nutrition Institute (USDA).
Ni Nickel (Z = 28) (see Elements - Nickel).
NIA National Institute of Allergy/ on Aging (HEW; NICHHD); Nephelometric inhibition assay; Neuraminidase-inhibition (gene) assay; Niacin (see nia); No information available; Nutritional Institute of America.
nia niacin (= NIA).
NIAAA National Institute on Alcohol Abuse and Alcoholism (ADAMHA).
NIAB National Institute of Agricultural Botany.
NIADDK National Institute of Arthritis, Diabetes, Digestive and Kidney Diseases.
NIAID National Institute of Allergy and Infectious Diseases.
NIAL Not in active labor.
NIAMCB National Institute of Aging Mutant Cell Bank.
NIAMD National Institute of Arthritis and Metabolic Diseases.
NIAMDD National Institute of Arthritis, Metabolism, and Digestive Diseases (NIH).
NIAMHN Northern Island Association for Mental Health Newsletter.
NIB National Institute for the Blind; Negative iron balance; Normal intact brain.
NIBAC National (Health) Insurance Benefits Advisory Council (see NHIBAC).
NIBP Non-invasive blood pressure.
NIBSC National Institute for Biological Standards and Control.
NIC National immunization campaign; National Inventors Council; Neonatal intensive care (see ICN); Neurogenic intermittent claudication; New International Clinics (journal); Numerical interactive controller; Nurse/ Nursing interim care.
Nic Nicotinyl.
Ni-Cad Nickel-cadmium (battery).

NICB National Industrial Conference Board.
NICC Neonatal intensive care center.
NICE National Institute for Clinical Excellence (GMC, UK).
NICH Northern Ireland Committee for the Handicapped.
NICHD National Institute of Child Health and Development (see NICHHD).
NICHHD National Institute of Child Health and Human Development (NIH) (= NICHD).
NICM Non-ionic contrast medium; Non-ischemic cardiomyopathy; Nuffield Institute of Comparative Medicine.
Nicotine Named after the 16th century Frenchman, Jean Nicot, one-time French ambassador to Portugal, who sent some snuff he secured from the tobacco plant of a botanist friend, to the queen of France, where it was dubbed "the queen's herb", after it had supposedly cured her of her headaches.
NICP Non-immunocompromised patient.
NICU Neonatal/ Neurological/ Neurosurgical/ Newborn Intensive Care Unit; Non-immunologic contact urticaria.
NID Nitrate-induced dilation; Nitroglycerin-induced (vaso)dilation (see NMD); Non-immunological disease; Non-invasive diagnostics.
NIDA National Institute of/on Drug Abuse (ADAMHA; HEW).
NIDD Non-insulin-dependent diabetes.
NIDDKD National Institute of Diabetes, Digestive and Kidney Diseases.
NIDDM Non-insulin-dependent diabetes mellitus.
NIDDY Non-insulin-dependent diabetes in the young.
NIDM National Institute for Disaster Mobilization.
NIDR National Institute of Dental Research (NIH).
NIDS Non-ionic detergent soluble.
NIE National Institute of Education (HEW); Negative inotropic effect; Not intractable epilepsy.
NIEF Non-infectious environmental factor (e.g. diet, smoking, etc.).
NIEHS National Institutes of Environmental Health Sciences/ Services (NIH).
NIF Negative inspiratory force; Neuro-ischemic foot (Diabetic); Neutrophil immobilizing factor; Non-intestinal fibroblast; Not in file.
NIG NSAIA induced gastropathy (see NSAIA).
NIg; Nig Non-immunoglobulin.
nig black (L. niger).
NIGEMS See NIGMS.
NIGMS National Institute of General Medical Sciences (NIH) (= NIGEMS).
NIGMSGMCR National Institute of General Medical Sciences Genetic Mutant Cell Repository.
NIGT Non-invasive genetic testing (Obstetrics/ Gynecology).
NIH Hoffman-La Roche (USA) code for experimental substances; National Institutes of Health (Bethesda, Md; HEW); Neointimal hyperplasia; Nitrate-induced headache; Not invented here.
NIH 204 Tetrahydroxy-phenanthrene hydrochloride compound (= 9-2-diamylamino-1-hydroxyethyl-1,2,3,4-tetrahydroxyphenanthrene hydrochloride) - an antimalarial drug with action similar to that of mepacrine (atebrine).
NIH 7519 Phenazocine hydrobromide (= Phenethylazocine bromide) - a narcotic analgesic with actions and uses similar to morphine, but more effective in smaller doses, acting more quickly and lasting longer.
NIH 7958 Pentazocine (= Win 20,228) - a narcotic analgesic with actions and uses similar to morphine. Used as an alternative to pethidine and morphine.
NIHCC National Institute of Health Clinical Center.
NIHCD National Institute of Health Care Delivery.
NIHF Non-immune hydrops fetalis (Obstetrics).
NIHL Noise-induced hearing loss.
NIHPC National Institute of Health Plateletpheresis Center.
NIHPHSR National Institute for Health Policy and Health Services Research (Israel).
NIHR National Institute of Handicapped/ Healthcare Research.

NIHS National Institute of Hypertension Studies.
NII Neutral insulin injection (see Insulin - NII); No increased incidence; Non-infective inflammation.
NIIA Non-immunological inflammatory reaction.
NIIC National Injury Information Clearinghouse.
NIIP National Institute of Industrial Psychology.
NIIS National Institute of Infant Services.
NIL Noise interference level; Not in labor; Nothing in light (microscope).
nil none (L. nihil).
NILECJ National Institute of Law Enforcement and Criminal Justice.
NILS National Institute of Longevity Sciences (Japan).
NIM National Institute of Medicine; National Instrumentation Methods (Committee); Neuroimmunomodulation; Not intractable migraine; Nuclear instrument module; Nuclear Instruments and Methods (Netherlands journal).
NIMAJ National Integrated Medical Association Journal.
NIMBY Not in my back yard.
Nimby Nembutal capsule (see Barb - Nimby).
NIMD Non-invasive method(s) of diagnosis.
NIMH National Institute of Mental Health (ADAMHA).
NIMHDIS National Institute for Mental Health Diagnostic Interview Schedule.
NIMP National Intern Matching Program.
NIMR National Institute for Medical Research (London).
NIMS National Infant Mortality Surveillance.
NINCDS National Institute of Neurological and Communictive Disorders and Stroke (NIH; formerly NIND, NINDB and NINDS).
NIND National Institute of Neurological Diseases (NIH; now NINCDS).
NINDB National Institute of Neurological Diseases and Blindness (NIH; now NINCDS).
NINDS National Institute of Neurological Diseases and Stroke (NIH; now NINCDS).
Nine-fourteen (914) Neoarsphenamine (see NAB 914).
NINT Non-invasive neurological testing.
NINU Neuro-intermediate nursing unit.
NINVS Non-invasive neurovascular studies.
NIOE Non-infective otitis externa.
NIOSH National Institute for Occupational Safety and Health (PHS).
NIP National Immunization Program (CDC, DHHS, US); Nipple (see Nip); Nitro-iodophenyl (= Mono-nitroiodophenyl); No infection/ inflammation present; Non-invasive procedure (see NIT).
Nip Nipple (= NIP).
NIPH National Institute for/of Public Health.
NIPS Neuroleptic-induced Parkinson syndrome.
NIPT Non-interventional pain treatment.
NIPTS Noise-induced permanent threshold shift.
NIR Near infrared.
nIR Non-insulin-resistance.
NIRA Near infra-red analysis; Nitrite reductase.
NIRD Narcotic-induced respiratory depression; Non-immune renal disease.
NIRE National Institute for Rehabilitation Engineering.
NIRMP National Intern and Resident Matching Program.
NIRNS National Institute for Research in Nuclear Science.
NIRS National Institute of Radiological Sciences (Japan); Normal inactivated rabbit serum.
NIS Neuroimaging study; N-iodosuccinimide; No inflammatory signs; Normal intact skin; Nuclear-imaging system.
NISH National Institute of Safety and Health.
Nisi-67 Novicoff hepatoma cells.
NISP National Institute of Social Providence (= INPS).
NIT National Intelligence Test (psychology); Neuroimaging technology (see BIT); Non-invasive technique (see NIP)/ test/ therapy/ treatment; Nutrition Intervention Trial(s) (Study Group).
nit nitrous.
NITD Non-insulin treated disease.
Nitro; nitro Nitroglycerin(e); Nitroprusside

(sodium).
NITTS Noise-induced temporary threshold shift.
NIV Nodule-inducing virus; Non-invasive ventilation.
NJ Nasojejunal (feeding).
NJH National Jewish Hospital (Denver, Colorado).
NJHRC National Jewish Hospital and Research Center.
NJPC National Joint Practice Commission.
NK Natural killer (cells) - large granular lymphocytes, featuring about 1% of the peripheral blood lymphocytes, and producing Interferon, which destroys foreign cells such as tumors and viruses; Nomenclature Commission (ASG; Ger. Nomenklatur Kommission) - a committee on nomenclature of the German Anatomical Society; Not known (see n/k).
n/k not known (= NK).
NKA Natural Killer (cell) activity (see NK); Neurokinin A; No known allergies.
NKAD No known allergies to drugs.
nKat; nkat nanokatal (= 10^{-9} kat) (see kat).
NKC Natural Killer cell (granular lymphocyte) (see NK); Non-ketotic coma.
NKCA Natural Killer cell activity (see NK).
NKCF Natural Killer cytotoxic factor.
NKDA No known drug allergies.
NKEC Natural killer effector cell.
NKF National Kidney Foundation; Normal kidney function (see NRF).
NKFA No known food allergies.
NKH Non-ketogenic hyperglycemia; Non-ketotic hyperosmotic.
NKHA Non-ketotic hyperosmolar acidosis.
NKHS Non-ketotic hyperosmolar syndrome; Normal Krebs-Henseleit solution.
NKMA No known medicaton allergies.
NKPC National Kaiser Permanente Conference (see CHAIR; KPMG; SCPMG).
NL Nasolacrimal; Neural lobe; Neutral lipid; Nodular lymphoma; Normal (= nl); Normal libido/ limits (see n/l).
nL nanoliter (= nl).
nl nanoliter (= 10^{-9} l; 10^{-9} liter); normal (value) (see NL); normal limits (see n/l); not clear (L. non liquet); not permitted (L. non licet).
n/l normal limits (= NL; nl).
NLA National Leukemia Association; Neuroleptoanalgesia; Neuroleptoanesthesia; Normal lactase activity; Normal language ability (absent in autistic disorders).
NLADA National Legal Aid and Defender Association.
NLAP Neuroleptic antipsychotic (drug).
NLB Needle liver biopsy.
NLC National Laboratory Census (ASMT); National League of Cities; Nocturnal leg cramps (see BNLC; NLMC).
NLC&C Normal libido, coitus, and climax.
NLD Nasolacrimal duct; Necrobiosis lipoidica diabeticorum; Neuroleptic drug.
NLDL Normal low-density lipoprotein.
NLE Necrotizing leukencephalopathy; Neonatal lupus erythematosus; Nursing late entry.
Nle; Nleu Norleucine.
NLEC National Lipid Education Council (website, US).
NLF Nasolabial fold; Neonatal lung fibroblast; Non-lactose fermentation; Normal laparoscopic finding(s); Normal liver function (= NHF).
NLG National Lawyers Guild.
NLH Natural language habits.
NLHA Non-linear hearing aid.
NLI Non-linear increase.
NLK Neuroleukin.
NLM National Library of Medicine (PHS); Noise level monitor.
NLMC Nocturnal leg-muscle cramps (= NLC).
NLMIAF National League of Missing in Action Families.
NLMN National Library of Medicine News (journal).
NLN National League for Nursing, Inc; No longer needed.
NLNE National League for/of Nursing Education.
NLP Neurolinguistic Programming; No/ Normal light perception; Nodular liquefying panniculitis; Normal luteal phase.
NLPHPP National Legal Program on Health Problems of the Poor.

NLPK Non-linear pharmacokinetics.
NLR National legal requirement(s); Normal laboratory range.
NLRB National Labor Relations Board.
NLS Names Learning Test; Neighborhood legal services; Neonatal lupus syndrome; Non-linear least squares; Normal life span; Normal lymphocyte supernatant.
NLT Nephrolithotripsy (= PUL); No lactose tolerance; Normal lymphocyte transfer (test); Not later/ less than; Nucleus lateralis tuberis.
NLTAR Non-life-threatening adverse reaction.
NLV Norwalk-like virus (a small, 27-32 nm, round virus, of the family *Caliciviridae*, cause of 96% of the outbreaks of acute non-bacterial gastroenteritis in the United States).
NLX Naloxone.
NM Near-miss; Negro male; Neomycin (= NE); Neuromuscular; Nictitating membrane; Night and morning (see n et m); Nitrogen mustard; Nocturnal myoclonus; Nodular melanoma; Non-motile; Normetanephrine (see NMN); Non-/ Not malignant; Not measurable/red (see n/m); Not mentioned (see n/m); Not motile; Nuclear medicine (also technologist in); Nurse-midwife; Nursing Mirror (UK journal).
Nm Nutmeg (L. nux moschata) (= nm).
nM nanomolar/ nanomole (= 10^{-9} mol/mole) (see Symbols 5).
nm nanometer (= 10^{-9} meter; mμ; millimicron; 10 angstroms); night and morning (see n et m); non-metastatic (e.g. nm 23 - a non-metastatic gene, a protein with molecular weight 23); nutmeg (see Nm).
N/m newtons per meter.
n/m not measurable/red (= NM); not mentioned (= NM).
N-m newton-meter.
N&M; N et M Nerves and muscles; Night and morning (see n et m).
n et m night and morning (L. nocte et mane) (= NM; nm; N&M; N et M).
N x m newtons by meter.
N/m² newtons per square meter.
NMA National Malaria Association; National/ Newfoundland Medical Association; Neurogenic muscular atrophy; Neuromuscular activity/ agent (see NDNMA); N-nitroso-N-methylalanine.
NMAb Neutralizing monoclonal antibody (see IANA).
NMAC National Medical Audiovisual Center (NLM) (see NMAVC).
NMAF National Medical Association Foundation.
NMAJ National Medical Association Journal.
NMAM Non-menstrually associated migraine.
NM(ASCP) (Technologist in) Nuclear Medicine, certified by the American Society of Clinical Pathologists.
NMAVC National Medical Audiovisual Center (NLM) (= NMAC).
NMB Neuromuscular blockade.
NMBA Neuromuscular blocking agent.
NMC National Medical Center; Naval Medical Center; Neuromuscular control; No marked change(s); Non-motor condition; Normal motor control; Nuclear Medical Committee (AAPM); Nucleus reticularis magnocellularis; Nursing and Midwifery Council (UK).
NMCES National Medical Care Expenditure Survey.
NMCS National Medicinal Chemistry Symposium (DMC).
NMCUES National Medical Care Utilization and Expenditure Survey.
NMD Neuromotor disorder; Neuromuscular disease/ dysfunction; Neuro-myodysplasia; Nitroglycerin induced/-mediated (vaso) dilation (= NID); Non-malignant disease; Normal muscle/cular development.
NMDA N-methyl-D-aspartate.
NMDAA National Medical and Dental Association of America.
NMDAB National Medical and Dental Association Bulletin.
NMDEMS National Medical Device Experience Monitoring System (FDA).
NMDP National Marrow Donor Program.
NME National Medical Enterprises; Neuro-myelo-encephalopathy; Nursemaid's elbow (dislocation of small child's elbow, caused by excessive pulling on arm by an adult).
NMF National Medical Fellowships, Inc; National Migraine Foundation; Neuromuscular function; N-methylfor-

mamide; Non-migrating fraction (of spermatozoa) (see NMFS).

NMFI National Master Facility Inventory.

NMFS National Marine Fisheries Service (US - NOAA); Non-migrating fraction of spermatozoa (= NMF).

NMHA National Mental Health Association.

NMI No mental illness; No middle initial; Non-fatal myocardial infarction (see NFMI); Non-malignant illness (= NNI); Non-myelomatous monoclonal immunoglobulinemia; Normal male infant.

NMIS Nuclear Medicine Information System (FDA).

NMJ National Medical Journal (in NIMAJ); Neuromuscular junction.

NML National Medical Library; Nodular mixed lymphoma.

NMLI Neutrophil-mediated lung injury (= NDLI).

NMM Nodular malignant melanoma.

NMMJ Nursing Mirror and Midwives Journal (UK).

NMN Nicotinamide mononucleotide; No middle name; Normetanephrine (= NM).

NMNR Nicotinamide mononucleotide reduced.

NMNRU National Medical Neuropsychiatric Research Unit.

nmol nanomole (see nM).

nmol/L nanomoles per liter or millimicromolar (= nmol/l).

NMOR N-nitroso-morpholine (see NNM).

NMOS N-channel/ N-type metal-oxide semiconductor.

NMP Non-medical personnel; Normal menstrual period; Nucleoside monophosphate (= Nucleoside 5'-monophosphoric acids - generic designation for series of).

NMPC Non-metastatic prostate cancer/ carcinoma.

NMPCA Non-metric principal component analysis.

NMPTP N-methyl-4-phenyl-1,2,3,6-tetrahydropyridine.

NMR Neonatal mortality rate; Nictitating membrane response; Nuclear magnetic resonance (spectroscopy) (see MRI).

NMRDC Naval Medical Research and Development Command.

NMRF Non-modifiable risk factor.

NMRI Naval Medical Research Institute (NNMC); Nuclear magnetic resonance imaging (see MRI).

NMRI 448 A powerful insecticide and insect repellent developed by the NMR Institute.

NMRL Naval Medical Research Laboratory.

NMRS Nuclear magnetic resonance scanning.

NMRU Naval Medical Research/ Reserve Unit.

NMS National Medal of Science (awarded by the US President); National Merit Scholarship; Naval Medical School; Nerve myelin sheath; Neuroleptic malignant syndrome (associated sometimes with the administration of antipsychotic drugs and clinically manifested by altered mental status, evidence of autonomic instability [see AIS], hyperpyrexia, muscle rigidity, etc.); Neuromuscular spindle/ synapse; Normal mouse serum.

N-m/s newton meters per second.

NMSCIS National Model Spinal Cord Injury Systems (US).

NMSIDS Near-miss sudden infant death syndrome.

NMSQT National Merit Scholarship Qualification Test.

NMSR Normalized mean square root.

NMSS National Multiple Sclerosis Society.

NMT Nebulized mist treatment; Neuromodulation therapy; Neuromuscular tension/ transmission; N-methyltransferase; No more than; Nuclear Medicine Technician (ARRT); Nuclear medicine technologist/gy.

NMTB Neuromuscular transmission blockade.

NMTC National Medical Training Council (UK).

NMTCB Nuclear Medicine Technology Certification Board.

NMTD Non-metastatic trophoblastic disease.

NMTS National Milk Testing Service; Neuromuscular tension state.

NMU Neuromuscular unit; Nitrosomethylurea (= N-nitroso-n-methylurea).

NN Neonatal; Neuroelectric News (journal); Nevocellular nevus; Normal nursery/ nutrition; Normally nourished; Nurse's notes.

nn nerves (L. nervi); new name (L. nomen

novum).
N:N The azo group.
N/N Negative/negative.
NNA N-nitrosamine (see NAH; NAT; NNC); Non-narcotic analgesic (such as NSAIDs, paracetamol, salicylates).
NNAS Neonatal narcotic abstinence syndrome.
NNB Nature New Biology.
NNC National Nutrition Consortium; Navy Nurse Corps; N-nitroso compound (such as N-nitrosamine, produced by the conversion of dietary nitrate → nitrate → NNC, by microorganisms such as *Helicobacter* pylori in the stomach, and responsible for gastric cancer) (see Hp; NAH; NAT); Neonatal crisis; Non-neoplastic complication(s) (e.g. in immunosuppressed patients).
NNCD Nitro-naphthalene-chlorobenzene-diazonium sulfonate.
NND Neonatal death; New and Non-official Drugs - an annual publication of the American Medical Association (AMA) (formerly NNOR; NNR); Non-specific non-erosive duodenitis.
NNDC National Naval Dental Center.
NNE Neonatal necrotizing enterocolitis; No negative effect; Non-neuronal enolase.
NNEB National Nursery Examination Board.
NNG New nerve growth; Non-specific non-erosive gastritis.
NNH Neonatal hypocalcemia.
NNHS National Nursing Home Survey.
NNI Nature-nurture issue; Neonatal infection/ injury; Noise and number index; Non-neoplastic illness (see NMI).
NNIS National Nosocomial Infections Study.
NNJ Neonatal jaundice.
NNL Near-normal level(s); No new laboratory (test orders); Non-neoplastic lesion.
NNM Neonatal macrosomia (see PPRF)/ meningitis/ morbidity/ mortality; N-nitrosomorpholine (= NMOR); Nicolle-Novy-MacNeal (medium).
NNMC National Naval Medical Center.
NNN Novy-Nicolle-MacNeal (culture medium/ used in parasitology).
NNNMU N-nitroso-N-methylurethane.
NNO No new orders.
NNOR New and Non-official Remedies (now NND).
n nov new name (L. nomen novum) (= nov n).
NNP Neonatal nurse practitioner; Nerve net pulse.
NNR New and Non-official Remedies (now NND).
NNRTIs Non-nucleoside reverse transcriptase inhibitors ("non-nucs", which inhibit the reverse-transcriptase enzyme in AIDS therapy).
NNS Neonatal screen (hematocrit, total bilirubin, and total protein)/ sepsis/ survival; Non-neoplastic syndrome; Non-nutritive sweetener (e.g. acesulphame K, aspartame, cyclamate, saccharin, etc.) (see NS).
NNSA National Nurses Society on Alcoholism.
NNT Neonatal tetanus (see TNN); Nuclei nervi trigemini; Number needed to treat.
NNTC Neonatal thrombocytopenia.
NNU Net nitrogen utilization.
NNWI Neonatal Narcotic Withdrawal Index.
NO Narcotics officer; Nasal oxygen; Nitric oxide; None/ Not obtained (see n/o); Non-obese; Normally open (switch); Nurse's/ Nursing office; Nursing Outlook (journal).
No Nobelium (Z = 102) (see Elements - Nobelium); Number/ To the number of (L. numero) (= N; n; no).
no number (see No).
n/o none/ not obtained (= NO).
NO_2 Nitrous dioxide (see N_2O_4).
N_2O Nitrous oxide (an anesthetic - "laughing gas").
N_2O_3 Nitrogen trioxide.
N_2O_4 Nitrogen peroxide (= $2NO_2$).
N_2O_5 Nitrogen pentoxide.
NOA National Optometric Association; Non-opioid analgesic (see NNA); Nurse obstetric assistant.
NOAA National Oceanic and Atmospheric Administration.
NOAPP National Organization of Adolescent Pregnancy and Parenting.
nob to us (as a new species) (L. nobis).
NOBT Non-operative biopsy technique.
NOC Naturally-occurring chemical; Normo-ovulatory cycle; Not otherwise classified;

Nuffield Orthopaedic Center.
noc at night/ night/ nocturnal (see noct).
NOCAD Non-obstructive coronary artery disease.
noci- prefix meaning injury or deleterious agent (L. nocere).
noct at night (L. nocte)/ night or nocturnal (L. noctis) (= noc; Nox; nox).
noct maneq at night and in the morning/ night and morning (L. nocte maneque).
NOD Naturally occurring disease; Nodular (melanoma); Non-obese diabetic; Notify of death.
nod- combining form meaning knot (L. nodus).
NOED No effect dose (level) (in drug toxicity assessment = NEDL).
NOEL No observed effect level.
NOF National Osteopathic Foundation; Non-osteogenic fibroma (of bone); Normal oral flora.
NOFT Non-organic failure-to-thrive.
NOH Naturally occurring hormone.
NOHA Nutrition for Optional Health Association.
NOI Not otherwise indexed.
NOIBN Not otherwise indexed by name.
NOII Non-occlusive intestinal ischemia.
NOK Next of kin.
NOM Non-suppurative otitis media.
Nom Nomogram.
nom- combining form meaning custom or law (Gr. nomos).
nom dub a doubtful name (L. nomen dubium).
NOMI Non-occlusive mesenteric infarction.
nom nov new name (L. nomen novum).
nom nud a name without designation (L. nomen nudum).
non no; not (L.).
non- combining form meaning nine/ ninth (L. nonus).
non compos mentis Latin - not of sound mind.
Nonf G Non-flammable compressed gas.
NONMEM Non-linear mixed-effect modeling.
non pal not palpable.
non-REM Non-rapid eye movement (sleep).
non rep; non repetat do not refill/ repeat (prescription) (L. non repetatur) (see NR).
non segs non-segmented (neutrophils).
non seq it does not follow logically (L. non sequitur).
N_2O:O_2 Nitrous oxide/ Oxygen (ratio).
NOOB Not out of bed.
NOP Not otherwise provided for.
NOPHN National Organization for Public Health Nursing.
NOPW Non-obese pregnant woman/ women.
NOR Non-orthodox remedy (see AMP); Noradrenaline; Normal (see N. Normal); Nortriptyline; Nucleolar organizer region.
nor normal (see N. Normal).
NORC National Opinion Research Center.
NORD National Organization for Rare Disorders.
NORDA Naval Ocean Research and Development Activity (NRL).
Nord. P Nordic Pharmacopoeia (Pharmacopoea Nordica - official in Denmark, Finland, Iceland, Norway, and Sweden).
NOR-EPI Norepinephrine.
NORIF Natural (Cycle) Ovulation Retrieval in In-Vitro Fertilization.
NORIS Normal range information system.
Norleu Norleucine.
norm normal (see N. Normal).
NORML National Organization for the Reform of Marijuana Laws.
normo- prefix meaning usual (L. norma).
Norval Norvaline (= Dioctyl sodium sulfosuccinate) - a softening agent, lowering surface tension, used with laxatives in the treatment of constipation.
NOS Network operating system; No organisms seen; Non-organ-specific; Not on staff; Not otherwise specified.
Nos Nosology.
nos- combining form meaning disease (Gr. nosos) (= noso-).
NOSAC Non-steroidal anti-inflammatory compound.
NOSIE Nurses' Observation Scale for Inpatient Evaluation.
noso- prefix meaning disease (Gr. nosos) (see nos-).

NOSTA Naval Ophthalmic Support and Training Activity.
NOT Nocturnal oxygen therapy; Non-operative therapy/ treatment.
NOTA National Organ Transplant Act (US - 1984).
NOTB National Ophthalmic Treatment Board (UK).
noto- prefix meaning back (Gr. noton).
NOTT Nocturnal oxygen therapy trial.
Nov November.
nov new (L. novum).
nov n new name (L. novum nomen) (see n nov).
NOVS National Office of Vital Statistics.
nov sp new species (L. novum species).
NOW National Organization for Women (The); Negotiable orders for/of withdrawal.
NO_x Ozone, nitrous oxide and nitric oxide air pollutants (reported as parts per million of nitric oxide).
Nox; nox (L.) Night (see noct).
NP Nasal prongs; Nasopharyngeal/ynx; Naughton protocol (graded exercise tolerance test); Near point; Neer prosthesis (= PHP; SR; TSS) (Orthopedic Implants); Neonatal-perinatal; Neuritic plague; Neuropathology; Neurophysin (see Np); Neuropsychiatric/try; New patient; New Physician (The) (journal); New Psychiatry (UK journal); Newly presented; Niemann-Pick (disease); Nitrogen-phosphorus; Nitrophenide/phenol; No pain/ pressure/ protest; Non-palpable/ -paralytic/ -parasitic/ -pathogenic/ -perceptible/ -permeable/ -phagocytic/ -physical/ -physiological/ -poisonous/ -porous/ -practical/ -practicing/ -predictable/ -prevalent/ -progressive/ -protective/ -purulent; Nordic Pharmacopeia; Normal plasma/ pressure; Not perceptible/ performed/ practiced/ preferred/ pregnant/ present; Nuclear pharmacist/cy; Nucleocapsid protein; Nucleoplasmic (index) (see NPI); Nucleoprotein; Nucleoside phosphorylase; Nurse practitioner; Nursed poorly; Nursing procedure; Proper name (L. nomen proprium) (see n p).
Np Neper; Neptunium (Z = 93) (see Elements - Neptunium); Neurophysin (= NP).
np nucleotide pair.
n p proper name (label with) (L. nomen proprium) (= NP).
N-P Need-persistence.
NPA Nasal pharyngeal airway; National Parks/ Pharmaceutical/ Planning Association; National Pituitary Agency; Near point of accommodation (eye examination); Neuroprotective agent; Neuropsychiatric affect(ation)/(ivity); Nitrofural-dehyde p-arsonophenyl semicarbazone; Non-prescription analgesic.
NPAD Neuropsychiatric adverse event(s).
NPA-NIHHDP National Pituitary Agency - National Institutes of Health Hormone Distribution Program.
NPAP National Psychological Association for Psychoanalysis.
NPAT Non-paroxysmal atrial tachycardia.
NPB Nodal premature beat; Non-protein bound; Non-purulent blepharitis.
NPBC Node-positive breast cancer.
NPBD Non-protein bound drug.
NPBF Non-placental blood flow.
NPBI Non-protein bound insulin (see Insulin - NPBI); Non-puerperal breast infection.
NPC Nasopharyngeal cancer; National Petroleum/ Pharmaceutical Council; Near point of convergence (eye examination); Nitro-para-cresol; Nodal premature contractions; Non-parenchymal (liver) cell; Non-patient contact; Non-pregnant cycle (Obstetrics see NCC); Non-productive cough; Non-protein calorie; Non-purulent conjunctivitis; Nucleoprotein catabolism; Nucleus of posterior commissure.
NPCa Nasopharyngeal carcinoma.
NPCC National Program for Cancer Chemotherapy.
NPCCT Non-placebo controlled clinical trial (= NPCS).
NPCOA National Pest Control Operators Association.
NPCP National Prostatic Cancer Project; Non-Pneumocystis pneumonia.
NPCS National Prevention of Cancer Study; Non-placebo controlled study (see NPCCT).
NP cult Nasopharyngeal culture (procedure/ bacteriology).
NPD Narcissistic personality disorder;

National Program for Dermatology; Natriuretic plasma dialysate; Near (inter) pupillary distance; Negative pressure device; Neuropathologic/ psychiatric disorder; Neuropsychological development/ disorder/ disturbance; Niemann-Pick disease; Nitrogen-phosphorus detector (gas chromotography); Non-pathologic diagnosis; Non-prescription drug; Non-progressive disease; Normal protein diet.

NPDD Non-psychotic depressive disorder.

NPDES National Pollution Discharge Elimination System.

NPDI Non-psychotic depressive illness.

NPDL Nodular poorly differentiated lymphocyte/ lymphoma.

NPDR Non-proliferative diabetic retinopathy (characterized by cotton-wool spots, intraretinal hemorrhages, lipid exudates, macular edema and ischemia with visual loss, microaneurysms, venous beading and dilatation, etc.) (see PDR).

NPE Neurogenic pulmonary edema; Neuro(logic) psychiatric evaluation; Neuropathological examination; Neuroprotective effect; No previous exposure; Neuropsychologic examination; No palpable enlargement; Normal pelvic examination; Nutrition Program for the Elderly (AoA).

NPED Non-progressive exertional dyspnea.

NPF Nasopharyngeal fiberscope; National Paraplegic/ Parkinson/ Pharmaceutical/ Psoriasis Foundation; Negative prognostic factor (see MDRI); No predisposing factor; Not provided for.

NPFT Neurotic Personality Factor Test.

NPG No pregnancy; Non-pregnant.

NP-G Nurse practitioner - generalist.

NPH Nephrologist; Neutral protamine Hagedorn (globin insulin) (see Insulin - NPH) (= NPHi); No past/ present/ previous/ prior/ proper history; Normal pressure hydrocephalus.

NPHI National Public Health Institute (Finland).

NPHi Neutral protamine Hagedorn insulin (see Insulin - NPHi).

NPhx Nasopharynx.

NPI Narcissistic/ Netherlands Personality Inventory; Nasopharyngeal infection/ irritation; Neuropsychiatric institute/ution; No present illness; Nucleoplasmic index.

NPIC Neurogenic peripheral intermittent claudication.

NPII Neonatal Pulmonary Insufficiency Index.

NPJ Neuropathic joint (Charcot).

NPJT Non-paroxysmal (atrioventricular) junctional tachycardia.

NPK Neuropeptide K; Nitrogen/ phosphorus/ potassium (L. kalium) (fertilizer).

NPL National Physics Laboratory (UK); Neoproteolipid; Neuropathological lesion; Neurophysiology laboratory; Neutral protamine lispro (insulin) (fast acting human insulin analogue); Non-puerperal lactation; Nosocomial (hospital-transmitted) Pathogens Laboratory (CDC).

NPL suspension (intermediate acting h.i.a.) (see NPH).

NPM Non-pharmacological measure(s); Non-prescription medication; Nothing per mouth.

NPMC National Pediatric Myoclonus Center (US).

NPMRT Negative pi-meson radiation therapy.

NPMS Natural post-menopausal status.

NPN Negative-positive-negative (transistor); Non-protein nitrogen (test - supplanted by BUN) (see KFT - NPN).

nPNA Normalized protein nitrogen appearance (in 24-hr urine).

NPNG No pain, no gain (fact of/ philosophy in life).

NPNT Non-palpable, non-tender.

NPO Naphthyl-phenyl-oxazole (scintillator); Neurological-psychological outcome; Nothing by mouth (L. nulla per os); Nucleus preopticus.

NPOHS; NPO/HS Nothing by mouth at bedtime (L. nulla per os hora somni).

NPP Neural prosthesis program (NINCDS or NINDS - NIH); Nitrophenylphosphate; Non-progressive pregnancy; Normal pool plasma; Normal postpartum; Nucleus tegmenti pedunculopontinus.

NPPase Nucleotide pyrophosphatase.

NPPH Nucleotide pyrophosphohydrolase.

NPPNG Non-penicillinase-producing Neisseria gonorrhoeae.
NP polio Non-paralytic poliomyelitis.
NPR Narcotic pain reliever (see NBPK); National Public Radio; Net protein ratio; Neural-prostheses research; Normal pulse rate; Nothing per rectum; Nucleoside phosphoribosyl.
NPRL Navy Prosthetics Research Laboratory.
NPRQ Non-protein respiratory quotient (see PFT - NPRQ).
NPS Nail-patella syndrome; Nasopharyngeal speculum (Yankauer - Otolaryngology); National Park Service (DoI); Neuropsychiatric symptom(s); Nitrophenylsulfinyl; Non-pregnant state; Non-progressive sequence (in shock therapy for cardiac arrest); Non-pyrogenic solution.
NPSA National Patient Safety Agency (GMC, UK); Non-physician surgical assistant; Normal pilosebaceous apparatus.
NPSF National Patient Safety Foundation (AMA).
NPSH Non-protein sulfhydryl (group).
NPSP Net positive suction pressure.
NPT Negative pregnancy test; Neoprecipitin test; Neuropsychologic(al) test(s) (e.g. EMG; SFEMG; etc.); Nocturnal penile tumescence; Non-proliferation treaty (nuclear); Normal personality trait; Normal pressure and temperature; Nurse-physician team (see PNT).
NPT-10381 Synthesized inosine-alkyl-amino-alcohol compounds/ methisoprinol/isoprinosine.
NPTM Nocturnal penile tumescence monitor(ing).
NPTNAR National Peanut and Tree Nut Allergy Registry (US).
NPU National Pharmaceutical Union; Net protein utilization.
NPV Negative pressure value/ ventilation; Nuclear polyhidrosis virus; Nucleus paraventricularis.
NPW Non-pregnant woman/ women.
NPY Negative predictive value; Neuropeptide Y.
NQ Notes and queries.
N&Q Nostrums and Quackery (book).
NQA Nursing quality assurance.
NQMI Non-Q (wave) myocardial infection.
4NQO 4-nitroquinolone 1-oxide.
NQR Nuclear quadruple resonance.
NR Do not refill/ repeat prescription (L. non repetatur) (= non rep; non repetat); Nerve root; Neural retina; Neutral red (indicator); No radiation/ reaction/ record/ recurrence/ refill (prescriptions)/ rehearsal/ report/ respiration/ response/ result/ return; Noise reduction; Non-reactive/ -rebreathing (oxygen mask)/ -reimbursable/ -responder/ -retarded; Normal range/ reaction; Normotensive rat; Not reached/ readable/ ready/ recommended/ recorded/ remarkable (see N/R)/ reported/ resolved/ right; Nurse; Nursing Research (NLA and ANA journal); Nutrition/tive ratio; Nutrition Reviews (journal); Reynold's number (see NR).
nr near; normal; do not refill/ repeat (see NR).
N_R Reynold's number (= NR).
N/R Not remarkable (= NR).
NRA National Rehabilitation Association; National Research Act (1974); Nitrate reductase; Nucleus retroambigualis.
NRAF Non-rheumatic atrial fibrillation.
NRB Nerve root block (see SNRB); Non-rejoining break.
NRBC National Rare Blood Club; Normal/ Nucleated red blood cell (= NRbc; Nrbc).
NRbc; Nrbc Normal/ Nucleated red blood cell (see NRBC).
NRBS Non-rebreathing system.
NRC National Research Council (NAS - Canada, USA) (= NCR); Negative resistance characteristic; Non-renal clearance; Normal retinal correspondence (eye examination); Not routine care; Nuclear Regulatory Commission.
NRCA National Rehabilitation Counseling Association.
NRCC National Registry in Clinical Chemistry; National Research Council of Canada; National Resource for Computation in Chemistry (NRC).
NRCD National Register of Causes of Death.
NRCL Non-renal clearance.
NRC pad National Research Council pad (protective dressing).
NRCST National Referral Center for Science

and Technology.

NRD Nerve root damage (see PNR; PRG); Non-renal death.

NRDC National Research Development Corporation; National Respiratory Disease Conference; Natural Resources Defense Council.

NRDL Naval Radiological Defense Laboratory.

NRDS Neonate/ Newborn respiratory distress syndrome.

NREH Normal renin essential hypertension.

NREM Non-rapid eye movement (stage of sleep; "spindle" sleep).

NREM-REM Non-rapid eye movements - rapid eye movements (alternating cycles in sleep).

NREMS Non-rapid eye movement sleep.

NREMT National Registry of Emergency Medical Technicians.

NRF Neuro-rehabilitation facility; Neurosciences Research Foundation; Normal renal function.

NRFC Non-rosette-forming cell.

NRFD Not ready for data.

NRGC Nucleus reticularis gigantocellularis.

NRH National Rehabilitation Hospital (Washington, DC); Nitrate-related hypotension; Nodular regenerative hyperplasia.

NRI National Rehabilitation Institute; Neutral regular insulin (see Insulin - NRI); Nerve root involvement/ irritation; Non-respiratory infection; No real/ relevant increase; Noradrenaline reuptake inhibitor (5HT; Selective; Serotonin; Specific) (see SNRI); Nutrition Reports International (journal).

NRK Normal rat kidney.

NRL Naval Research Laboratory (US); Nerve root lesion (see SNRL); Nucleus reticularis lateralis.

NRM National Registry of Microbiologists; No return necessary; Normal range of motion; Nucleus reticularis magnocellularis.

NRMB News of Russian Medicine and Biochemistry (abstracts).

NRMC Naval Regional Medical Center.

NRMI National Registry of Myocardial Infarction.

NRMP National Resident Matching Program.

NRMR Non-reninmediated reduction (in systemic BP).

NRN No return necessary.

nRNA Nuclear ribonucleic acid.

nRNP Nuclear ribonucleoprotein.

NROM Normal range of motion.

NRNST Non-reactive non-stress test (of fetal status in diabetic pregnancies) (see BPS; NST).

NRP Notice of Research Project (SSIE); Nucleus reticularis parvocellularis.

NRPA National Recreation and Park Association.

NRPB National Radiological Protection Board (UK); Neurosciences Research Program Bulletin.

NRPC Nucleus reticularis pontis caudalis.

NRPG Nucleus reticularis paragigantocellularis.

NRR Nerve root retractor (Neurosurgery); Net reproduction rate; Normal reference range; Nursing Research Report (ANF journal).

NRRL Northern Regional Research Laboratory.

NRS National Research of Sciences; National Rosacea Society; National Runaway Switchboard (OYD); Neurobehavioral/ Numerical rating scale; Non-rising stem (gas valve); Normal rabbit/ reference serum.

NRSCC National Reference System in Clinical Chemistry.

NRSFPS National Reporting System for Family Planning Services.

NRT Neuromuscular reeducation techniques; Neutron radiation therapy.

NRTA National Retired Teachers Association.

NRTIs Nucleoside reverse transcriptase inhibitors ("nucs", as in AZT, ddC, ddl, d4T and 3TC, in AIDS therapy) (see NARTI; RTI; TDT).

NRV Nucleus reticularis ventralis.

NS Nasal septum/ sinus/ spray; National Spokesman (EFA journal); Natural science; Nelson's/ Nephrotic/ Noonan syndrome; Neosporin; Nerves (see Ns); Nervous system; Neuro(logical) signs/ surgery; Neuroelectric Society; Neuropathic symptom(s); Neurosecretion/tory; Neurosurgeon/gery; Neurosyphilis; Neurotic score; Nipple/ Non-stimulation; Nodular sclerosing/osis; Non-smoker; Non-specific (see ns); Non-structural; Non-stutterer; Non-symptomatic; Normal saline (see N/S)/ serum/ sodium (diet); No sample/ sequelae/ specimen (see ns); Norwegian scabies; Not seen/ significant (see ns)/ specified/ stated/ studied/ sufficient (on lab reports)/ symptomatic; Nuclear sclerosis; Nursing services; Nursing Sister; Nursing Standard (RCN journal); Nutrition Society (UK); Nutritive sweetener (fructose, sorbitol, etc.) (see NNS); Nylon suture (see ns).

Ns Nasospinale; Nerves (= NS).

ns nanosecond (= 10^{-9} sec; 10^{-9} second; nsec); non-specific (= NS); no sample/ sequelae/ specimen (= NS); not significant (= NS); nylon suture (= NS).

N/S Normal saline (solution) (= NS; NSS).

NSA National Stroke Association (US); Neurological Society of America; Neurosurgical anesthesiologist/gy; Non-selective antagonist; Non-surgical approach (to therapy) (see NST); No salt added; No serious/ significant abnormality/ anomaly; Normal serum albumin; No specific antidote; Nucleoside analogue (of cytidine) (= NA) - e.g. Lamivudine (used in the treatment of chronic hepatitis and AIDS).

NSAB National Scientific Advisory Board.

NSABBP National Surgical Adjuvant Breast and Bowel Project (NCI) (= NSABP).

NSABP National Surgical Adjuvant Breast Project (NCI).

NSAC National Society for Autistic Children.

NSAD No signs of acute disease.

NSAE Non-supported arm exercise.

NSAH Non-sedating antihistamine (see NSOAH).

NSAI Non-steroidal anti-inflammatory (drug); Non-steroidal aromatase inhibitor.

NSAIA Non-steroidal anti-inflammatory agent/ analgesic.

NSAID Non-steroidal anti-inflammatory drug.

NSAM Naval School of Aviation Medicine.

NSAP Non-steroidal anti-pruritic (see TNSAP).

NSAR Non-seasonal allergic rhinitis (see VMR).

NSB National Science Board (NSF); Nigrostriatal bundle; Normal sexual/ social behavior (see HSB).

NSBAB Non-selective beta-adrenergic blocker (see NCSBB).

NSBB Non-selective beta-blocker (see NCSBB).

NSBRI National Space Biomedical Research Institute (Houston, Texas).

NSC Bristol-Myers Co, Hoffman-La Roche, AD Little, National Cancer Institute code for experimental substances; National Safety Council; Neural stem cell (produces brain cells); Neurosecretory cell; No significant change (= nsc); Non-service connected (= nsc); Non-specific suppressor cell; Non-staining cream; Normal short child (i.e. Normal child with short stature).

nsc no significant change (see NSC); non-service connected (see NSC).

NSC 740 Methotrexate (= Amethopterin; α-Methopterin; MTX; 4-Amino-10-methylfolic acid) - a folic acid antagonist and cytotoxic agent, acting probably by interfering with purine synthesis. Used most effectively for the maintenance of remission in acute lymphoblastic leukemia.

NSC 8806 Melphalan (= CB 3025; PAM; Phenylalanine Nitrogen Mustard; Sarcolysin). A cytotoxic agent used in the treatment of multiple myelomatosis (see CB 3025).

NSC 12198 Drostanolone (= Dromostanolone; Methalone). An anabolic agent, which has been used in treating hypercholesterolemia, atherosclerosis, and advanced carcinoma of the breast.

NSC 14574 Lucanthone hydrochloride (= BW 57-233; Lucanth hydrochlor) - used in the treatment of schistosomiasis.

NSC 19893 Fluorouracil (= 5-Fluorouracil; FU; 5-FU; Ro 2-9757). An antimetabolite used in the palliative treatment of carcinoma, particularly of the breast, colon, and rectum.

NSC 23909 1-methyl-1-nitrosuria.

NSC 24559 Mithramycin (= A 2371; PA 144) (see A 2371).

NSC 25154 Pipobroman (see A 8103).

NSC 32065 Hydroxyurea (= SQ 1089). An antineoplastic agent used orally in chronic myeloid leukemia and other malignant diseases.

NSC 32074 Azauridine (= 6-Azauridine; 6-AzUR) (see 6-AzUR).

NSC 35770 Clomiphene citrate (see MRL 41).

NSC 37096 Benzodepa (see AB 103).

NSC 45383 Streptonigrin (= Flomycin). An antineoplastic agent produced by the growth of Streptomyces flocculus.

NSC 47547 1-(2-chlorethyl)-1-nitrosuria.

NSC 49842 Vinblastine sulfate (see LE 29060).

NSC 51325 Meturedepa (see AB 132).

NSC 64393 Spiramycin (see IC 5902).

NSC 64826 Azetepa. An antineoplastic agent used orally in various malignant conditions.

NSC 67574 Vincristine sulfate (= Leucocristine sulfate). An alkaloid obtained from Vinca rosea (of the Periwinkle family, Apocynaceae), and used as a cytotoxic agent principally in the treatment of leukemia in children, and in adults in Hodgkin's disease and reticulum-cell sarcoma.

NSC 77213 Procarbazine hydrochloride (= Ibenzmethyzin; Methylhydrazine; MIH; Ro 4-6467). A cytotoxic agent used in the treatment of malignant neoplasms.

NSC 409962 1,3,bis(2-chloroethyl)-1-nitrosurea/carmustine, BCNU (see BCNU).

NSC 521778 Hadacidin (= N-Formylhydroxyaminoacetic acid). An antimicrobial cytotoxic substance produced by the growth of Penicillium frequentans.

NSCAC National Society for Crippled Adults and Children (see NSCCA).

NSCC National Society for Crippled Children.

NSCCA National Society for Crippled Children and Adults, Inc (= NSCAC).

NSCCE National Study Commission on Cytotoxic Exposure (MCPAHS).

NSCD Non-service-connected disability; Non-specific cytotoxic drug.

NSCLC Non-small-cell lung cancer.

N Score Neuroticism score (Eysenck Personality Inventory).

NSCFPT No significant change from previous tracing.

NSD Nairobi sheep disease; Near-starvation diet; Neonatal staphylococcal disease; Nervous system disease/ disorder; Neurosecretory dysfunction; Neurostimulation device; Night sleep deprivation; No significant defect/ deficiency/ deviation/ difference/ disease; Nominal single/ standard dose; Non-significant decrease; Non-sudden death; Normal single/ singular/ standard dose; Normal spontaneous delivery.

NSDA Non-steroid dependent asthmatic.

NSDP National Society of Dental/ture Prosthetics/etists.

NSE Negative side effect(s); Neuron-specific enolase; Non-specific esterase; Normal saline enema.

N s E Nausea without (L. sine) emesis.

nsec nanosecond (see ns).

N-series X-radiation (transitions to n = 4).

NSF National Sanitation/ Science (formerly OST)/ Sleep Foundation; National Sex Forum; Nodular subepidermal fibrosis; Normal systolic function; Not sufficient funds.

NSFTD Normal spontaneous full-term delivery.

NSG Neurosecretory granule; Neutron Scattering Group (IOP); Nutrition Study Group (EASD).

Nsg; nsg Nursing.

NSGCT Non-seminomatous germ cell tumor.

NSG Hx Nursing history.

NSGI Non-specific genital infection.

NSH National Society for Histotechnology; No special hazard; Non-sedating histamine.

NSHA National Smoking and Health Association (Sweden); Non-sedating histamine antagonist.

NSHD Nodular sclerosing Hodgkin's disease; Non-selective heart defect(s).

NSHF Non-specific host factor.

NSI Nasal sinus irrigation; Needle-stick injury; Negative self-image; Nervous system impairment (includes anxiety, emotional instability, insomnia, introversion, irritability, loss of appetite, memory loss, tremors, etc. such as caused by inhaling high levels of mercury or other volatile chemicals); Nervous system involvement; Non-significant increase; Non-storage iron (in tissues other than the liver); Non-susceptible isolate; Non-

syncytium-inducing; No signs of infection/ inflammation.
NSIDS Near sudden infant death syndrome.
NSILA Non-suppressible insulin-like activity.
NSILP Non-suppressible insulin-like protein.
NSJ Nevus sebaceus of Jadassohn.
NSL Neoplastic skin lesion.
NSLSAA National Surf Life Saving Association of America.
NSM Nerve-sheath myxoma; Neurosecretory material/ motor (neuron); New smoking material; Non-antigenic specific mediator; Non-specific morphology; Nutrient sporulation medium.
NSM; NSMO Non-susceptible microorganism (see NSO).
N-s/m² newton seconds per square meter.
NSMHC National Society for Mentally Handicapped Children (UK).
NSMJ Nebraska State Medical Journal.
NSMOT Non-sexual mode(s) of transmission (of disease).
NSMR National Society for Medical Research.
NSMRB National Society for Medical Research Bulletin.
NSN Nephrotoxic serum nephritis; Nicotine-stimulated neurophysin; Number of similar negative (matches/ pairs).
NSNA National Student Nurses' Association.
NSND Non-symptomatic and non-disabling; No stroke, no dementia (see HAAS).
NSO Neosporin ointment; Non-susceptible organism (i.e. to antibiotics); Nucleus supraopticus; Nursing Service Office.
NSOAH Non-sedating oral antihistamine.
NSP Nasal septal/tum perforation; Neck and shoulder pain; Neurological Society of Paris; Neuron specific protein; Neurosensorial performance; Non-specific pruritus; Normal singleton pregnancy; No smoking please; Number of similar positive (matches/ pairs).
NSPB National Society for the Prevention of Blindness.
NSPE National Society of Professional Engineers.
NSPN Neurosurgery progress note.
NSPS Nanoshell-polymer system (see NST).
NSPVT Non-sustained polymorphic ventricular tachycardia.
NSQ Neuroticism Scale Questionnaire; Not a sufficient quantity (on lab reports).
NSQAN National Stream Quality Accounting Network (USGS).
NSR Nasal septal reconstruction; Nasoseptal repair; Neuroscientific research; Neurosurgery resident; Non-specific reaction; Normal sinus rhythm; No serious/ severe/ significant reaction/ response; Not seen regularly.
N-SRBC Neuraminidase(-treated) sheep red blood cells.
NSS Nerve-stimulation study; Neurosurgical service; Nigral striatal system (brain-stem); Non-specific symptom(s); Normal saline solution (see N/S); Normal size and shape; Not statistically significant; Nutrition support services.
1/2 NSS 1/2 Normal saline solution (sodium chloride 0.45%).
NSSD No statistically significant difference.
NSSL Normal size, shape, and location.
NSSP Normal size, shape, and position.
NSST Northwestern Syntax Screening Test.
NSSTT Non-specific ST and T (wave - on the electrocardiogram).
NSST-TWCS Non-specific ST and T wave changes.
NST Nanoshell technology (see NSPS); Negative self-talk; Neospinothalamic (tract); Nervous system toxicity; Neural shock therapy (for epilepsy); Nicotine substitution therapy; Non-shivering thermogenesis; Non-specific therapy/ treatment; Non-stress test; Non-surgical technique/ therapy (see NSA); No specific treatment; Not sooner than; Nutritional support team.
NSTA National Science Teachers Association (US).
NSTL National Space Technology Laboratories (NASA).
NSTP Neurosurgery-training program.
NSTT Non-seminomatous testicular tumor.
NSU Neurosurgical unit; Non-specific urethritis.
NSurg Neurosurgeon/gery.
NSV Non-specific vaginitis/nosis.
NSVD Normal spontaneous vaginal delivery.

NSVT Non-sustained ventricular tachycardia.
NSWJO New South Wales Journal of Optometry.
NSWMA National Solid Waste Management Association.
NSX Neurosurgical examination.
nsy nursery.
NSYF Natural Science for Youth Foundation.
NT Change in nuchal translucency (Obstetrics); Nasotracheal (tube); Neotetrazolium (histological stain); Neuroscience Translations (FASEB journal); Neurotensin; Neutralization technique/ test; Nicotine tartrate; Night terror; Nitrazine test (for pH of vaginal fluid); No test; Non-tender; Non-transplanting (see NTH); Non-tumoral; Non-typable; Normal temperature/ tissue; Normotensive; Nortriptyline; Nose and throat (see N&T); Not tender/ tested; Nourishment taken; N-terminal (fragment); Nuchal translucency (see NTA; NTM); Nuclear Technologist; Nuclear track (emulsion); Nucleotidase; Nucleotide (see nt); Nursing Times (UK journal); Nutrition Today (journal).
Nt Amino terminal; Niton, obsolete name for Radon (Rn, Z = 86) (see Elements - Radon).
nt nucleotide (= NT).
N&T Nose and throat (= NT).
5'NT 5'nucleotidase.
NTA Narcotic Treatment Administration (Washington, DC); National Tuberculosis Association; Natural thymocytotoxic autoantibody; Neurotoxic action (see NTE); Neutron monitoring film (Kodak); Nitrilotriacetic acid; Nuchal translucency assessment (Obstetrics); Nurse Training Act (see NT Act); Nursery Training Association.
NTAB Nephrotoxic antibody.
NT Act Nurse Training Act (= NTA).
NTB Neurotransmitter booster (see MAD; MAE; SED; SND).
NTBA National Tuberculosis Association.
NTBR Not to be resuscitated.
NTC Needs-treatment category; Neotetrazolium chloride; Neurotrauma center.
NTCC National Type Culture Collection.
NTD Nephrotoxic/ Non-toxic/ Neurotoxic drug; Neural tube defect; Nitroblue tetrazolium dye; No tissue damage; Noise tone difference; Normal therapeutic dose; 5'nucleotidase.
NTDAP Neural tube defect-affected pregnancy.
NTDT Neurotoxic drug therapy (such as Stavudine for AIDS, etc.).
NTE Neuropathy target esterase; Neurotoxic effect (see NTA)/ esterase; Non-test ear; Normal tidal expiration (see PFT); No toxic effect (of dose/ drug level); No treatment effect; Not to exceed.
NTF Neural tube fusion (see AAPP; NTD) (Obst.); Neurofibrillary tangle formation (in Alzheimer's disease) (see Ckk 5; NFT); Normal throat flora.
NTFEP Never-treated first-episode patient (e.g. schizophrenia).
NTFI National Tackle Football Injury (surveillance project).
NTG Nitroglycerin(e); Nitrosoguanidine; Non-toxic goiter; Non-target/ treatment group; Normal triglyceridemia; Normotriglyceridemia.
NTGE Non-teratogenic effect.
NTGO Nitroglycerin ointment.
NTH; NT Hospital Non-transplanting Hospital.
NTHH Non-tumorous hypergastrinemic hyperchlorhydria.
NTI Narrow therapeutic index; Non-thyroidal index; Non-thyroid illness.
NTIG Non-treated immunoglobulin.
NTIS National Technical Information Service (formerly CFSTI - US Dept. of Commerce).
NTL National Training Laboratories.
NTLI Neurotensin-like immunoreactivity.
NTM Neural tube malformation (see NTD) (Obstetrics); Nocturnal tumescence monitor; Non-tuberculous mycobacteria; Nuchal translucency measurement (see NTA).
NTMB Non-tuberculous mycobacteria (see NTM).
NTMI Non-transmural myocardial infarction.
NTN Nephrotoxic nephritis.
NTND Not tender, not distended.
NTO New Technology Opportunities; Normal target organ.
NTOS Neurogenic thoracic outlet syndrome.

NTP National Toxicology Program; Newly treated patient; Nitropaste (= Nitroglycerin ointment) (= NTGO); Nitroprusside; Non-target population; Normal temperature and pressure (see NT&P); Normal twin pregnancy; No-treatment period; Nucleoside triphosphate (generic designation for a series of nucleoside 5'-triphosphoric acids).
NT&P Normal temperature and pressure (of a gas) (= NTP).
NTPD Non-traumatic posterior dislocation (of the shoulder joint).
NTR Negative therapeutic reaction; Neurotoxic reaction; Neurotransmitter reception/tor; Non-therapeutic research; Normalized thyroxine ratio; Normotensive rat; Nutrition (see ntr).
Ntr; ntr Nutrition (= NTR).
NTRC National Toxins Research Center.
NTRDA National Tuberculosis and Respiratory Disease Association.
NTRS National Therapeutic Recreation Society.
NTS Nasotracheal suction; Nephrotoxic serum; Nicotine Transdermal System; Non-typhoid salmonellosis; Nucleus tractus solitarius.
NTSB National Transportation Safety Board.
NTSC National Television Standards Committee.
NTT Nasotracheal tube; Nearly total thyroidectomy; Neurotransmitter turnover; Nuclear transfer technology (see Neti); Nuchal translucency thickness (Obstetrics) (see FNTT).
NTTC Non-toilet trained child(ren).
Nt test Cross neutralization test.
NTTL National Tissue Typing Laboratory (see NTTRL).
NTTRL National Tissue Typing Reference Laboratory (UK) (= NTTL).
NTU Navy Toxicology Unit; Nephelometric turbidity unit.
NTV Nerve/vous tissue vaccine; Normotensive volunteer.
nt wt net weight.
NTX Naltrexone.
NTx (Urinary) N-telopeptides corrected (for creatinine).
NTZ Normal transformation zone.
NU Name unknown; Neuropathic ulcer.
Nu Nucleus (see Nuc).
nU nanounit (= 10^{-9} unit; one billionth of a standard unit).
nu nude (mouse).
NU 445 Sulfafurazole (= Sulfisoxazole). A sulfonamide especially useful in the treatment of urinary tract infections.
NU 1196 Alphaprodine hydrochloride (= Prisilidene HCl). A narcotic analgesic with an action similar to pethidine, but more rapid in onset and of shorter duration.
NU 1510 Piperidione (= 3,3-Diethyl-2,4-dioxopiperidine). A sedative, less powerful than phenobarbitone, used as a cough suppressant. It is not a narcotic and does not cause addiction.
NU 2121 Nicotinyl alcohol (= Nicotinic alcohol; 3-Hydroxymethylpyridine; 3-Pyridinemethanol; β-Pyridylcarbinol; 3-Pyridylmethanol; Pyrid-3-ylmethanol). A vasodilator used in the treatment of Meniere's disease and peripheral vascular disorders, including chilblains and frostbite.
NUB Non-ulcerative blepharitis.
NUC Nitrosourea compound; Non-specific ulcerative colitis; Normal umbilical cord; Sodium urate crystal.
Nuc Nucleated (= nuc); Nucleoside; Nucleus (= Nu; Nuc; nuc; Nucl; nucl).
nuc See Nuc.
Nucl; nucl Nucleus (see Nuc).
nucle- combining form meaning kernel (L. nucleus).
Nucleonics (journal).
NUD Nail unit disorder; Non-ulcer dyspepsia.
NUEA National University Extension Association.
NUG Necrotizing ulcerative gingivitis.
NUI National University of Ireland; Nocturnal urinary incontinence; Number user identification.
nullip nulliparous.
Number Marijuana cigarette (see Cannabis).
numc number concentration.
NUMS Northern University Medical School.
NUO Non-urgent operation.
NURB Neville upper reservoir buffer.

NURDD Northern Utilization Research and Development Division (US Dept. of Agriculture - formerly NRRL [Northern Regional Research Laboratory]).

Nurs Nursing (journal).

NUT Negative urine test; Norepinephrine-uptake transporter (see NEUP).

Nut Nutrients/ition.

nutri- combining form meaning nourish (L. nutrio).

NUV Near ultraviolet (light).

NV Naked/ Near vision (see Nv); Nausea and vomiting (see N&V); Negative variation; Neovascularization; Neurovascular; New vessels; Next visit; Non-vaccinated; Non-venereal; Non-verifiable; Non-veteran; Non-vital (tooth/ dead nerve); Non-volatile; Normal value (on laboratory reports); Norwalk virus; Not vaccinated/ venereal/ verified/ vital/ volatile.

Nv Naked/ Near vision (eye examination) (= NV).

N&V Nausea and vomiting (= NV).

NVA Near visual acuity (eye examination); Normal vascular anatomy.

NVAE Non-viral acute encephalopathy (e.g. Cryptococcal meningitis; Toxoplasma encephalitis, etc.).

NVAF Non-valvular atrial fibrillation.

NVB Neurovascular bundle.

nvCJD New variant Creutzfeldt-Jakob disease (see BSE; MCD; TSE).

NVD Nausea, vomiting, and diarrhea; Neck vein distension; No venereal disease; Non-valvular/ Non-venous disease; Non-vascularization of the disc; Newcastle virus disease; Normal vaginal delivery; Number of vessels diseased.

NVE Non-vascularization elsewhere; Non-vigorous exertion.

NVG Neovascular glaucome; Neoviridogrisein; Non-ventilated group.

NVIB Non-venomous insect bite.

NVL Neurovascular laboratory/ lesion; No visible lesion.

NVM Non-vascular membrane; Non-volatile matter.

NVMA National Veterans Medical Association.

NVMI Necropsy-verified myocardial infarction.

NVN Nature-versus-nurture.

NVP Nevirapine (a dipyridodiazepinone compound and non-nucleotide reverse transcriptase inhibitor [NNRTI] with activity against HIV-I virus. Its chemical name: 11-cyclopropyl-5,11-dihydro-4-methyl-6H-dipyrido[3,2-6:2',3'-][1,4]diazepin-6-one, and molecular formula is: $C_{15}H_{14}N_4O$) (see PIBCT); Non-viable pregnancy.

NVR Nausea, vomiting, regurgitation.

NVS Neurologic(al) vital signs; Neurovascular surgery.

NVSD National Vital Statistics Division (NCHS).

NVSS Normal variant short stature.

NVT Non-sustained ventricular tachycardia (see NSVT).

NW Naked/ Net weight; Nasal wash; Northwest; Not weighed.

NWB Non-weightbearing; Not weightbearing.

NWC Normal-weight child(ren); Number of words chosen.

NWD Neuroleptic withdrawal.

NWDA National Wholesale Druggists Association.

NWF National War Formulary; National Wildlife Federation.

NWHN National Women's Health Network.

NWL Net water loss (causing hypernatremia).

NWN National Warning Network (UK) (for nuclear attack; see CCP).

NWP Nitrogenous waste product(s).

NWR Normotensive Wistar rat.

NWRO National Welfare Rights Organization.

NWS Neonatal withdrawal symptoms/ syndrome; Nicotine withdrawal symptoms/ syndrome (e.g. agitation, insomnia, sweating, and tremors).

NWVB Non-withdrawal vaginal bleeding.

NX Naloxane.

Nx Nephrectomy.

NXG Necrobiotic xanthogranuloma.

ny nystagmus (see Nyst).

NYAM New York Academy of Medicine.

NYAS New York Academy of Sciences (The).

NYBC New York Blood Center.

NYC New York City (medium).
NYCDH New York City Department of Health.
NYD Not yet diagnosed/ discovered.
NYEEI New York Eye and Ear Institute.
NYHA New York Heart Association (classification of heart disease).
NYHA New York Heart Association (classification of heart disease): Class I - asymptomatic congestive heart failure (CHF), Class II - slightly symptomatic CHF, Class III - CHF symptoms, Class IV - severe CHF.
NYHAFC New York Heart Association Functional Class.
NYH-CMC New York Hospital - Cornell Medical Center.
NYHSC New York Health Science Center (Syracuse).
NYMC New York Medical College.
NYMC-MHC New York Medical College - Metropolitan Hospital Center.
NYMH New York Memorial Hospital.
NYNF New York Nephrology Foundation.
NYP Not yet published.
NYPI New York Psychiatric Institute.
NYPIRG New York Public Interest Research Group.
NYPUM National Youth Project Using Minibikes.
NYSHMAA New York State Hospitals Medical Alumni Association.
Nyst Nystagmus (= ny).
NYSVC New York State Veterinary College.
NYUHF New York's United Hospital Fund.
NYUSM New York University School of Medicine.
NZ Enzyme; New Zealand; Normal zone.
NZB New Zealand black (strain of inbred mice).
NZC New Zealand chocolate (mouse strain).
NZDA New Zealand Dental/ Dietitians Association.
NZDJ New Zealand Dental Journal (NZDA).
NZF New Zealand Formulary.
NZJMLT New Zealand Journal of Medical Laboratory Technology.
NZJP New Zealand Journal of Physiotherapy.
NZMJ New Zealand Medical Journal.
NZNA New Zealand Nurses Association.
NZNJ New Zealand Nursing Journal (NZNA).
NZO New Zealand obese (mouse strain).
NZR New Zealand red (strain of inbred rabbits).
NZSP New Zealand Society of Physiotherapists.
NZSPB New Zealand Society of Periodontology Bulletin.
NZSTA New Zealand Speech Therapists Association.
NZSTJ New Zealand Speech Therapists Journal.
NZT Nitrazine test (for pH of vaginal fluid in rupture of membranes).
NZVA New Zealand Veterinary Association.
NZVJ New Zealand Veterinary Journal (NZVA).
NZW New Zealand white (strain of inbred mice).

O

O Antigen (Somatic) (Ger. ohne Hauch = without breath or film) - the non-motile strain or somatic antigen, which occurs in the body of a microorganism (= Oa); Blood type in the ABO system; By mouth (orally); Eye (L. oculus); No special preparation necessary (for test); None (zero) (see ō); Objective findings (in problem-oriented medical records); Observed frequency (in a contingency table); Obstetrics; Obvious; Occipital (placement in electroencephalography); Occiput; Occlusal; Octarius (L. pint); Oculus (L.) eye; Office (doctor's); Often; Ohm (Symbol: Ω); Ohne Hauch (Ger.) without breath = Somatic antigen (above); Old; Omega (symbol Ω) - the 24th letter of the Greek alphabet) (see Symbols 4 - Greek alphabet); Open; Opening: i. An aperture or space, e.g. O. of bladder (= Urethral O; Ostium urethrae internum); ii. An opening of an electric circuit; Operator; Operon (geriatrics); Opium (see Papaver); Oral(ly); Orange (an indicator color); Orderly (respirations - anesthesia chart); Ortho- (see ortho-); Orthopedics; Osteocyte; Other; Output; Ovary; Ovine; Oxygen (Z = 8) (see Elements - Oxygen); Pint (L. octarius) (= o); Respirations (see O - Orderly); Size of suture; Tyrosine; Without film (bacteria) (Ger. ohne Hauch); Zero (none) (see ō).

o eye (L. oculus) (see O); octarius (L.) pint (see O); opening (see O); omicron (15th letter of the Greek alphabet); ortho (see o-); ovary (transplant) (= O); pint (L. octarius).

ō negative, none, without, or zero (= O).

o- ortho (in chemical formulas) (= o).

=o ketone group {see (O-)}.

(O-) keto-group (= =o).

Ω Ohm (see O - Ohm); Omega (24th Greek capital letter) (see O - Omega).

Ω^{-1} Ohm^{-1}, siemens.

ω Greek lower case letter "omega"; angular velocity.

O2; O_2 Both eyes (L. oculus); Opaque-2 (high-lysine corn); Oxygen (diatomic/ molecular) (= Ox; OXY; oxy).

O_2 Superoxide.

O_3 Ozone.

O_{12} Singlet oxygen.

^{15}O Radioactive oxygen.

OA Objective assembly (psychology); Obstructive apnea; Occipital artery; Occiput anterior (fetal position); Octanoic/ Oleic/ Orotic/ Oxalic acid; Ocular albinism; Old age; Opiate analgesia; Opsonic activity; Optic atrophy; Oral airway/ alimentation; Orthopedic assistant; Osteoarthritis; Osteopathic Annals (journal); Ovalbumin; Overall assessment; Overeaters Anonymous.

Oa Somatic antigen - see O - Antigen (Somatic).

O_2a Oxygen availability.

O&A Observation and assessment; Odontectomy and alveoplasty.

OAA Old Age Assistance; Older Americans Act (of 1965); Opioid agonist-antagonist (e.g. nalbuphine) (see OAAA); Opioid analgesic agent; Opticians Association of America; Orally active agent; Orientation association area (in the left parietal lobe of the brain); Oxaloacetic acid.

OAAA Opioid agonist-antagonist analgesic.

OAAD Ovarian ascorbic acid depletion (test).

OAB ABO blood group; Old age benefits; Overactive bladder (i.e. Urinary incontinence/ urgency) (= DHR; MUI).

OABG Osteoarticular bone graft.

OABP Organic anion binding protein.

OAC Oral anticoagulant drug; Oral anticoagulant(s); Osteoarticular candidiasis (see HCO); Ovarian adenocarcinoma; Overaction.

OACA Oral anticoagulant agent. OACD.

OACs Orphan Annie cells (seen in papillary carcinoma of the thyroid, looking like "Orphan Annie's eyes").

OACT Oral anticoagulant therapy/ treatment.

OAD Obstructive airway disease; Occlusive arterial disease; Once-a-day (dosage); Organic anionic dye; Osteoarthritis deformans.

OADA Oral antidiabetic agent (= OADD) - such as: 1) α-Glucoside inhibitors: Acarbose, 2) Biguanides: Metformin, Phenformin, 3) Non-sulphonylureas: Repaglinide, 4) Sulphonylureas: Acetohexamide,

Carbutamide (Glybutamide), Chlorpropamide, Glibenclamide, Glipizide, Glymidine, Netformide, Tolazamide, Tolbutamide, 5) Thiazolidinediones (PPARγ agonists): Rosiglitazone.

OADC Oleate (Oleic acid), albumin, dextrose, and catalase (culture medium).

OADD Oral antidiabetic drug (see OADA).

OAE Ocular adverse event (such as allergic conjunctivitis, asthenopia, blepharitis, cataract, eye pain, eyelid erythema, excessive tears, foreign body sensation, heterochromia or increase in pigmentation of conjunctivae, eyelashes, iris, or periocular skin, iritis, ocular burning, discharge, dryness, or irritation, photophobia, superficial punctate keratitis, and visual disturbance); Otoacoustic emissions.

OAEDC Ontario (Canada) Association for Emotionally Disturbed Children.

OAEP Overall adverse experience profile (of a drug).

OAET Otoacoustic emissions test (= OET).

OAF Open air factor; Oral airflow; Osteoclast activating/vity factor.

OAFP Oregon Academy of Family Physicians.

OAG Open angle glaucoma.

OAH Oral antihistamine; Ovarian androgenic hyperfunction.

OAI Oral active immunization; Osteoarticular involvement.

OAISO Overaction of the ipsilateral superior oblique.

OAJ Open apophyseal joint; Osteoarthritic joint.

OALF Organic acid-labile fluid/ fluoride.

OALL Ossification of the anterior longitudinal ligament.

OAM Office of Alternative Medicine; Office of Aviation Medicine (FAA); Outer acrosomal membrane.

OAMT Opioid-agonist maintenance therapy/ treatment (see OMT).

O antigen Somatic or body antigen (associated with the cytoplasm and cell wall of bacteria (see O - Antigen).

OAP Office of Adolescent Pregnancy; Old Age Pension(er); Omphaloangiopagus (twin fetuses of different sizes arising from one egg) (= AIAP or Allantoidoangiopagus); Ophthalmic artery pressure (procedure/ ophthalmology); Opioid antagonistic property; Organoacidopathy; Osteoarthropathy; Ovarian androgen production; Oxygen at atmospheric pressure.

OAPCC Ortho abnormal plasma coagulation control.

OAPP Office of Adolescent Pregnancy Programs.

OAQPS Office of Air Quality Planning and Standards (EPA).

OAR Other administrative reason.

OAS Old Age Security; Oral allergy syndrome; Organization of African/ American States; Osmotically active substance; Overall survival (e.g. in cancer patients).

2'5'-OAS 2'5'-oligoadenylate synthetase.

OASD Ocular albinism - sensorineural deafness (syndrome).

OASDHI Old-Age, Survivors, Disability, and Health Insurance (Program).

OASDI Old-Age, Survivors, and Disability Insurance (SSA).

OASDITF Old-Age, Survivors, and Disability Insurance Trust Fund (SSA).

OASI Old Age and Survivors Insurance.

OASO Overactive superior oblique.

OASP Organic acid soluble phosphorus.

OASR Overactive superior rectus.

OAT Optometrist Assistant Technician; Orbital adipose tissue; Ornithine aminotransferase.

OAV Oculo-auriculo-vertebral (dysplasia).

OAVD Obstructive aortic valvular disease; Oculo-auriculo-vertebral dysplasia.

OAW Oral airways.

OB Obese; Obesity; Objective benefit; Obliterative bronchiolitis; Obstetrician (see Obst); Obstetrics (= Ob; OBS; Obs; Obst); Occult bleeding/ blood; Olfactory bulb; Oligoclonal band; Orthodontic Bulletin (AAO journal).

Ob Obstetrics (see OB).

ob he/she died (L. obiit) (see obit); obese (mouse) (see ob/ob).

ob- prefix meaning i. death (L. obitus), or ii. in front of or towards (L. ob) (see oc-).

O&B Opium and belladonna (see Papaver).
OBA Oral bioavailability.
OBB Own bed bath.
OBD Obstructed bile duct; Organic brain damage (see ATP)/ disease/ disorder; Organic behavior disorder.
OBE Office of Biological Education; Order of the British Empire; Out-of-body experience.
OBE-CALP Placebo capsule or tablet.
OBEs Out-of-body experiences.
OBF Organ blood flow.
OBG; ObG; OB-GYN; Ob-Gyn; ob-gyn Obstetrician - Gynecologist; Obstetrics and Gynecology.
OBGS Obstetrical and gynecological surgery.
OB-GYN Obstetrician - Gynecologist (see OBG etc.).
Ob Gyn D OB/GYN Digest (journal).
Ob Gyn N OB GYN News (journal).
OB-GYN Ob OB-GYN Observer (journal).
obit he/she died or obituary (L. obiit) (= ob).
obj objective.
OBL Occult blood loss; Octave-band level.
obl oblique.
OBM Obesity and Bariatric Medicine (journal).
OBO Organic brain osmole(s).
ob/ob obese (mouse) (= ob).
OBP Obstetric brachial palsy (see SD - Shoulder dystocia); Ova, blood, parasites (in stool).
OBPC Optimal blood pressure control.
OBR Overall best response.
OBRA Omnibus Reconciliation Act.
OBRR Obstetric recovery room.
OBS Obstetrical service (see ObS); Obstetrics (see OB); Organic brain syndrome.
ObS Obstetrical service (= OBS).
Obs Observation/ved/ver (see obs); Obstetrician (see Obst); Obstetrics (see OB).
obs observation/ observed/ observer (= Obs); obsolete; obstructed/uction (see obstr).
Obst Obstetrician (= OB; Obs); Obstetrics (see OB).
obst; obstr obstructed/ obstruction (= obs).
OBT Obtained; Open-book type (pelvic fracture); Ortho brain thromboplastin.
OC Obstetrical conjugate; Occlusocervical; Office/ On call; On Call (journal); Onchauxis (overgrowth of nail); Only child; Onset and course (see O&C); Onychocryptosis (ingrown nail); Open/ Oral care; Operant conditioning (see OCA); Optic chiasma; Oral contraceptive (see OCA); Organ culture; Original claim; Outer canthal (distance); Outer canthus; Ovalocyte (an elliptical erythrocyte); Ovarian cancer/ carcinoma (see OCa); Oxygen capacity (see O_2 cap); Oxygen consumed/ consumption.
oc- prefix meaning in front of or towards (L. ob) (see ob-).
O&C Onset and course (of a disease) (= OC).
OC 43 Strain of corona virus.
OCA Occluded carotid/ cerebral/ coronary artery; Oculocutaneous albinism; Office of Consumer Affairs (HEW); Olivo-ponto-cerebellar atrophy; Open care area; Operant conditioning audiometry; Oral contraceptive agent; Osmotic cathartic agent (e.g. Lactulose); Osteochondral allograft (Orthopedics).
OCA; O_2CA Oxygen-carrying ability.
OCa Ovarian cancer/ carcinoma (= OC).
OCAD Occlusive carotid/ coronary artery disease.
O_2 cap Oxygen capacity (laboratory/ blood gas) (= OC).
OCAT Optometry College Admission Test.
OCAWU Oil, Chemical, and Atomic Workers Union.
OCB Obsessive-compulsive behavior (see OCD).
OCBF Outer cortical blood flow.
OCC Office of Cancer Communications (NCI); Oral contraception/ive (see OCA; PDA); Ovarian cancer cell; Oxygen-carrying capacity.
occ occasional(ly) (see occas); occipital/put (see occip); occlusal/sion/sive (see occl); occupation(al) (see occup); occurrence (see occur).
occas occasional(ly) (= occ).
OCCC Ontario Crippled Children's Center (Canada); Open chest cardiac compression.
OCCF Overt congestive cardiac failure.
occip occipital/put (= occ).
occl occlusal/sion/sive (= occ).
OCCM Open chest cardiac massage.

OCCPR Open chest cardiopulmonary resuscitation.
OCCT Oral contraceptive therapy (see OCT).
OccTh Occupational therapist (= OcTh)/ therapy (= occup Rx; OcTh).
occup occupation(al) (= occ).
occup Rx occupational therapy (see OccTh).
occur occurrence (= occ).
OCD Obsessive-compulsive disorder; Office of Child Development (HEW); Office of Civil Defense; Osmotic cell damage; Osteochondritis deformans/ dissecans; Ovarian cholesterol depletion (test).
OCE Office of Chief Executive; Osteocartilaginous exostosis; Osteoclastic erosion (Orthopedics).
OCF Occipito-cervical fusion (Orthopedics); Oral contraceptive failure; Orocutaneous fistula; Overt cardiac failure.
OCG Omnicardiogram/graph(y); Onychogryposis (Ingrowing toenail) (see ITN); Oral cholecystogram/graph(y); Ovarian cancer gene (= P 53).
OCH Oral contraceptive hormone (see Hormones - OCH); Ox cell hemolysin.
OCHA Office of Consumer Health Affairs.
OCHS Office of Cooperative Health Statistics.
OCHT Ox cell hemolysin test.
OCI Obsessive-compulsive illness (see OCD); Ontario Cancer Institute (Canada); Oxacillin.
OCIS Oncology Center Information System.
OCITA Office of the Chemical Industry Trade Adviser.
OCL Office of Clinical Laboratories (HEW); Oral colonic lavage; Osteochondral lesion (e.g. of the knee joint).
OCM Metamino-diazepoxide; Obstructive cardiomyopathy; Oral contraceptive medication.
OCMH Oklahoma Children's Memorial Hospital.
OCMM Oculo-cerebro-mucormycosis (fungal disease of the eyes and cerebrum).
OCN Oculomotor nucleus; Oncology-certified nurse.
OCNA Orthopedic/ Otolaryngologic Clinics of North America (journals).
OCO Optimal clinical outcome.
OCP Ochocerciasis Control Programme (West Africa); Octacalcium phosphate; Oral case presentation; Oral contraceptive pill; Osteoconductive properties/ty; Ova, cysts, and parasites; Ovarian cancer patient.
OCPG Ovarian cancer-predisposing gene.
OCR Ocular countertorsion reflex; Oculocardiac reflex; Oculo-cerebrorenal (syndrome) (see OCRS); Office for Civil Rights (HEW); Office of Coal Research (DI); Optical character reader/ recognition; Overall clinical response.
OCRC Onchocerciasis Chemotherapeutic Research Center (Ghana).
oCRF Ovine corticotropin-releasing factor.
OCRG Oxycardiorespirography.
oCRH Ovine corticotropin-releasing hormone.
OCRL Lowe's oculocerebrorenal (syndrome) (see OCRS).
OCRS Oculocerebrorenal syndrome (= OCR; OCRL).
OCS Occipital condyle syndrome; Ondine's curse syndrome; Open canalicular system; Open-chest surgery (= MS - Median sternotomy); Opiate cough suppression/ssor; Oral contraceptive steroid; Orderly cell self-destruction/ suicide (= Apoptosis) (see SCD); Outer continental shelf; Outpatient clinic substation; Ovarian Carcinoma Study.
Ocs Oral contraceptives.
11-OCS 11-Oxycorticosteroid.
OCSD Oculo-cranio-somatic disease.
OCSE Office of Child Support Enforcement (HEW).
OCSP Oxfordshire Community Stroke Project.
OCST Oral corticosteroid therapy (see OCT).
OCT Object classification test; Oculocutaneous telangiectasia (see AT); Optimal cutting temperature; Oral contraceptive therapy; Oral corticosteroid therapy (= OCST); Orbital connective tissue; Ornithine carbamyl/bomoyl/bomyl transferase; Orthotopic cardiac transplantation; Oxytocin challenge test.
Oct October.
oct- prefix meaning eight (L. octe).
OcTh Occupational Therapist/py (see OccTh).
OCTRF Ontario Cancer Treatment and

Research Foundation (Canada).

Octup Eight-fold (L. octuplus).

OCU Observation care unit; Oral-contraceptive use.

ocu ocular.

ocul- combining form meaning eye (L. oculus).

OCV Ordinary conversational voice.

OD Doctor of Optometry (see DO); Influence exerted upon the nervous system by magnetic agents; Obtained absorbance; Occipital dysplasia; Occupational dermatitis/ disease; Oculodynamic; Officer of the day; Ollier disease; On demand/ duty; Once a day (see od); Open drop (anesthesia); Ophthalmic Dispenser; Optic disc; Optical density (now called absorbance); Optimal dose; Organizational development; Originally derived; Orthopedics Digest (journal); Osmotic diuretic (e.g. Glucose, Mannitol, Urea, etc.); Out-of-date; Outdoor; Outside diameter/ dimension; Overdosage/ose (drugs) (= od); Oxygen demand; Right eye (L. oculus dexter) (= od).

od daily/ every day/ once a day/ once daily (L. omni die) (= OD); other significant disease (radiograph symbol); overdosage/ose (see OD); right eye (see OD).

O-D Obstacle-dominance.

od- combining form meaning road or path (Gr. odos).

ODA Occipito-dextra anterior (L.) - right occipitoanterior (position of fetus); Once-daily administration (see ODD); Ontario Dental Association; Osmotic driving agent; Overseas Doctors Association (GMC, UK).

ODAC On demand analgesia computer.

ODAJ Ontario Dental Association Journal.

ODAT One day at a time.

ODB Opiate-directed behavior.

ODC Once-daily challenge (medical therapy); Oritidine/ Ornithine decarboxylase; Orthodromic conduction (the transmission of a nerve signal along an axon in the normal direction); Outpatient diagnostic center; Oxygen dissociation curve.

ODCH Ordinary diseases of childhood.

ODD Oculodentodigital (dysplasia) (see ODDD); Once-daily dosage/ dose/ dosing/ drug (= ODA); Opioid drug dependence; Opium-derived drug (see MLD); Oppositional Defiant Disorder; Optical data digitizer.

OD'd Overdosed (drug).

ODDA Opioid-dependent drug addict.

ODDD Oculo-dento-digital dysplasia (= ODD).

ODDR Once-daily dosing regimen (= ODR).

ODE O-desmethylencalnide.

-ode- suffix meaning i. form (Gr. eidos), ii. path or road (Gr. odos).

ODEPA Oxapentamethylene-diethylene-phosphoramide.

ODF Orgasmic/astic dysfunction.

ODFR Oxygen-derived free radical.

ODG Oligodendroglia (a type of human 'support' brain cell); Oligodendroglioma.

ODJ Osteochondritis deformans juvenalis (= LPD - Legg-Perthes disease or OCD - Osteochondritis deformans).

ODM Occult distant metastases/stasis; Offspring of diabetic mother; Once-daily medication (see ODDR; ODMR; ODR); Ophthalmodynamometer/metry.

ODMC Office for Dependents Medical Care.

ODMDF Offspring of diabetic mothers and diabetic fathers.

ODMR Once-daily medication regimen (= ODDR; ODM; ODR).

ODN Optokinetic nystagmus.

ODOD Oculo-dento-osseous dysplasia.

Odont Odontogenic/tology.

odont- combining form meaning tooth (Gr. odontos).

odoram a perfume (L. odoramentum).

odorat fragrant, odoriferous, odorous, perfuming, scented, or smelling (L. odoratus).

ODP Obese diabetic patient; Occipito-dextra posterior (L.) - right occiputoposterior (position of fetus); Offspring of diabetic parents; Oocyte donation program; Opioid-dependent patient/ person.

ODPHP Office of Disease Prevention and Health Promotion.

ODR On-demand regimen; Once-daily regimen (see ODDR).

ODS Octadecyl silane; Office of Demographic Studies; Once-daily schedule; Open distal system; Osmotic demyelination syndrome; Oxygen delivery system (Trach-Mist).

ODSG Ophthalmic Doppler sonogram.

ODT Occipito-dextra transversa (L.) - right occipitotransverse (position of fetus); Oculodynamic tract; Omeprazole dual therapy (for *Helicobacter* pylori gastritis) - use of an acid pump inhibitor (API) such as omeprazole, with the antibiotic amoxycillin twice daily for two weeks (see BTT; OTT); On-demand therapy/ treatment; Orodispersible tablet.

ODTS Organic dust toxic syndrome.

ODU Optical density unit.

ODV O-desmethylvenlafaxine (the active metabolite of Venlafaxine, a drug used in the treatment of major depressive disorders or episodes).

ODW Oral drug withdrawal; Ovary-deprived woman/ women.

-odynia- suffix meaning pain (Gr. odyne).

OE On/ Orthopedic examination; Optical Engineering (journal of SPIE); Otitis externa; United States Office of Education (HEW).

Oe Oersted; Oesophagostomum (a genus of nematode worms).

O/E Observed/expected (ratio); On examination (= OE).

O&E Observation and examination.

OEA Obliquus externus abdominis (= Musculus OEA or External oblique muscle of abdomen); Obliterative endarteritis.

OEC Once-daily schedule; Oral epithelial cell (see BEC); Outer ear canal.

OEE Office of Environmental Education (HEW); Opaque enema examination (X-ray/CT, with Meglumine isoxitolamate, where Barium is contraindicated); Osmotic erythrocyte enrichment; Outer enamel epithelium; Oxygen-enriched environment (see MET-501).

OEF Oil immersion field; Oxygen extraction fraction.

OEIS Omphalocele, exstrophy, imperforate anus, spinal defects (complex).

OEL Occupational exposure limit.

OEM Open-end marriage; Opposite ear masked; Original equipment manufacturer; Overall excess morbidity/ mortality.

OEO Office of Economic Opportunity.

OEP Office of Emergency Preparedness (GSA).

OER Osmotic erythrocyte (enrichment); Oxygen enhancement ratio (see MET-501).

O_2ER Oxygen extraction ratio.

OERP Office of Education and Regional Programming.

OES Optical emission spectroscopy; Oral esophageal stethoscope.

Oes; oes; Oesoph; oesoph Oesophagus (= Esophagus).

OET Oral endotracheal/ esophageal tube; Oral estrogen therapy; Otoacoustic emissions test (see OAET).

OETT Oral endotracheal tube (= OET).

OF Occipitofrontal (diameter of head); Open field (test); Optical fiber/ fundus; Orbitofrontal; Osmotic fragility; Osteitis fibrosa; Outflow fraction (expressed as a percentage = V1/TVV x 100. Normal = 40-70%. APG - Air plethysmography: V1 = The amount of blood leaving the leg in the first second; TVV = Total venous volume); Outlet/ Ovum forceps (Obstetrics and Gynecology); Ovenstone factor; Oxidation-fermentation (see O/F).

Of Office/cial (see Off).

O/F Oxidation/fermentation ratio (medium) (= OF).

OFA Oncofetal antigen.

OFAGE Orthogonal field alternation gel electrophoresis.

OFBL Occult fecal blood loss (see FOBL).

OFBM Oxidation-fermentation basal medium.

OFC Occipital-frontal/ Occipitofrontal circumference (of head); Orbital frontal cortex; Orbitofacial cleft; Orofacial cleft; Osteitis fibrosa cystica.

OFCC Office of Federal Contract Compliance (Department of Labor).

OFCTAD Occipito-facio-cervico-thoraco-abdomino-digital (dysplasia).

OFD Object-film distance (= ofd); Occipital-frontal/ Occipito-frontal diameter; Oral-facial-digital (syndrome) (see OFD-I; OFD-II); Orofacial dyskinesia (see TOFD); Osteitis fibrosa disseminata (see AMSS).

ofd object-film distance (see OFD).

OFD-I Oral-facial-digital/ Oro-facial-digital (syndrome).
OFD-II Oral-facial-digital/ Oro-facial-digital (syndrome) (= Morh-Rimoin syndrome).
OFDA Office of Foreign Disaster Assistance (AID).
OFDS Oro-facial-digital syndrome Type I (cleft palate, lobed tongue, skeletal defects/ lethal in males/ a sex-linked derived, ectodermal dysplasia) (= PLS - Papillon-Leage and Psaume syndrome).
OFE Oral-facial episode.
Off Office/ Official (= Of).
OFHA Occipitofrontal headache.
OFHR Office of Federal Health Relations.
OFI Oral food intake; Overflow incontinence.
OFM Orofacial malformation.
OFR Office of the Federal Register; Oxygen-free radical.
O_2FR Oxygen-free radical (see OFR).
OFS Overall frequency shift.
OG Obstetrics and gynecology (see O&G); Obstetrics and Gynecology (ACOG journal); Occlusogingival; Oligodendrocyte; Oncogene (a cancer-activating gene/ proto-oncogene, being a mutant version of a normal gene e.g. the Ras gene, Mutated kinase gene, etc.); Onychogryphosis (ram's horn nail); Optic ganglion; Orange green (stain) (see OGS); Orogastric.
O-G Ortho-Gravindex (see OGT).
O&G Obstetrics and gynecology (= OG).
OGA Oculogyric attack (see OGC); Orogastric gonococcal aspirates.
OGB Ongoing basis; Optimal glucose balance.
OGC Oculogyric crisis (= OGA; OGS); Oral glucose challenge (see OGTT); Orogenital contact.
OGD Oculogyric dystonia; Oral gavage dose.
OGF Ovarian growth factor; Oxygen gain factor.
OGH Ovine growth hormone.
OGI Osteogenesis imperfecta.
OGIB Obscure gastrointestinal bleeding.
OGIM Osteogenesis imperfecta (see OGI).
OGIT Osteogenesis imperfecta tarda.
OGL Oral glucose load (test).
OGS Obstetrical and Gynecological Survey (journal); Oculogyric spasm (see OGC); Orange-green (stain) (= OG); Osteogenic sarcoma; Oxygenic/ Oxogenic steroid.
OGT Oral glucose tolerance (see OGTT); Orogastric tube; Ortho-Gravindex test (pregnancy test).
OGTT Oral glucose tolerance test.
OH Every hour (see oh); Hydroxide; Hydroxycorticosteroid (see 17-OH); Hydroxyl ion (in solution); Obstructive hydrocephalus/ hypopnea; Occipital horn; Occupational health/ history; Occupational Health (UK journal); On hand; Open heart (surgery); Oral Health (Canadian journal); Oral hygiene; Orthostatic hypotension; Osteopathic/ Out of/ Outpatient/ Outside hospital.
oh every hour (L. omni hora) (= OH).
=OH Hydroxyl group/ radical.
11-OH 11-beta-hydroxylase; 11-hydroxycorticosteroid (see 11-OHCS).
17-OH 17-alpha-hydroxylase; 17-hydroxycorticosteroid (see 17-OHCS).
18-OH 18-hydroxylase.
21-OH 21-hydroxylase.
OHA Ocular hypotensive activity (see SPA); Oral hypoglycemic agent.
OHAs Oral hypoglycemic agents.
4-OHA 4-hydroxyanisole.
17-OHA 17β-hydroxyandrogen.
OHAHA Ophthalmoplegia-hypotonia-ataxia-hypacusis-athetosis (syndrome).
OHB_{12} Hydroxy vitamin B_{12} (= Hydroxycobalamin; OH-Cbl).
18-OH-B 18-hydroxycorticosterone.
O_2Hb Oxyhemoglobin.
OHC Obstructive hypertrophic cardiomyopathy; Occupational health center; Outer hair cell.
25-OHC 25-hydroxycalciferol (= OHCC).
OH-Cbl Hydroxycobalamin (see OHB_{12}).
OHCBS Open-heart coronary bypass surgery (see CABG; OHS).
OHCC Hydroxycalciferol (see 25-OHC).
OHCS Hydroxycorticosteroid (= Oxyhydrocortisone).
11-OHCS 11-hydroxycorticosteroid(s) (= 11-hydroxycorticoids; 11-OH; 11-OH-CS).
11-OH-CS See 11-OHCS.

OHAs – Oral hypoglycemic agents

Class	Mechanisms of action	Brand names
Sulfonylureas	Increase insulin secretion	
Chlorpropamide		Diabenese
Glibenclamide		Daonil
Glimepiride		Amaryl
Glipizide		Glucotrol
Glyburide		DiaBeta, Glynase, Micronase
Tolbutamide		Orsinon
Non-sulphonylureas	Other insulin secratogogues	
Repaglinide		Novonorm, Prandin
Biguanides	Decrease hepatic gluconeogenesis and peripheral insulin resistance	
Netformin		Glucophage
Thiazolidinediones	Decrease peripheral insulin resistance and reduce fatty acids	
Proglitazone		Actos
Rosiglitazone		Avandia
Alpha-Glucosidase inhibitors	Slow absorption of carbohydrates	
Acarbose		Prandase, Precose
Miglitol		Glyset

17-OHCS 17-hydroxycorticosteroid(s) (= 17-hydroxycorticoids; 17-OH; 17-OH-CS; 17-OHS).

17-OH-CS See 17-OHCS.

OHD Hydroxyvitamin D; Office of Human Development (HEW); Oral hypoglycemic drug; Organic heart disease; Overt heart disease.

1.25-$(OH)_2D$ 1.25-dihydroxyvitamin D.

1.25-$(OH)_2D_3$ 1.25-dihydroxycholecalciferol.

1-α-OH-D_3 1-α-hydroxyvitamin D3 - an analogue of 1.25-$(OH_2)D_3$.

25-OHD; 25-OH-D 25-hydroxyvitamin D.

24,25-$(OH)_2D_3$ 24,25-dihydroxycholecalciferol.

OHDA Hydroxydopamine (see 6-OHDA).

6-OHDA 6-hydroxydopamine.

16-OH-DHAS 16-alpha-hydroxy-dehydroepiandrosterone sulfate.

18-OH-DOC 18-hydroxy-desoxycorticosterone.

8-OH-DPAT 8-hydroxy-2-(di-n-propylamino)tetralin.

OHDS Office of Human Development Services.

11-OH9-Δ THC 11-hydroxy-delta-9-tetrahydrocannabinol (see Cannabis).

OHE Obstetrical hemorrhagic emergency; Office of Health Economics (UK).

OHF Omsk hemorrhagic fever; Overhead frame; Overt heart failure.

OHFA Hydroxy fatty acid(s) (fecal).

OHFT Overhead frame trapeze.

OHG Oral hypoglycemic (agent/ drug).

OHI Occupational Health Institute; Ocular/ Operative hypertension indication/tor; Office for Handicapped Individuals (see OHD); Oral hygiene index; Oral Hygiene Instruction; Overall hormone intake.

OHIAA Hydroxy-indole-acetic acid.

OHI-S Oral Hygiene Instruction - Simplified.
OHL Oral hairy leukoplakia.
OHLys Hydroxylysine.
OHMO Office of Hazardous Materials Operations (MTB of DoT).
OHN Occupational health nurse; Occupational Health Nursing (AAIN journal).
OHP Hydroxyprogesterone (see 17-OHP); Hydroxyproline (see OHPro); Occupational health practice; Oncology health professional; Oxygen under high pressure (= Hyperbaric oxygenation; High-pressure O_2).
2-OHP 2-hydroxyphentidine.
17-OHP 17-hydroxyprogesterone.
OHPro Hydroxyproline (excretion) (= OHP).
OHR Office of Health Research.
OHRP Office for Human Research Protection (FDA).
OHRR Open heart recovery room.
OHS Obesity hypoventilation syndrome; Occupational Health Service; Ocular herpes simplex; Ocular histoplasmosis/ hypoperfusion syndrome; Open heart surgery; Ovarian hyperstimulation syndrome (see OHSS).
17-OHS 17-hydroxycorticosteroid (see 17-OHCS).
OHSC Oregon Health Sciences University.
OHSD Hydroxysteroid dehydrogenase.
OHSS Ovarian hyperstimulation syndrome (= OHS).
OHSU Oregon Health Sciences University (Portland).
OHT Occupational health technician; Ocular hypertension; Oral hypoglycemic therapy.
18-OH-THA 18-hydroxytetrahydro A.
18-OH-TH-DOC 18-hydroxy-tetrahydro-deoxycorticosterone.
OHTS Ocular Hypertension Treatment Study.
OHU Hydroxyurea (aka hydrea).
OHVS Open heart vascular surgery.
OI Obturator internus; Occasional insomnia; Opportunistic infection; Opsonic index (the name of the opsonic power of the serum of a person for a given organism as compared with normal; has been regarded as significant of the degree of resistance by the person to the particular infection); Optical Index (journal); Oral Implantology (AAID journal); Oral insulin (see Insulin - OI); Orgasmic impairment; Orientation inventory; Ortho-iodo-hippurate; Osteogenesis imperfecta; Otitis interna; Ouabain-insensitive/vity; Overuse injury (bursitis, capsulitis, capsulotendinitis; fibrositis myalgia, muscle strain, tendinitis, etc.) (= OUI); Oxygen income/ intake.
O-I Outer and inner.
OIA Obliquus internus abdominis (= AOM; IOM); Ocular anti-infective.
OIC Osteogenesis imperfecta congenita.
OID Opioid-induced depression (of the ventilatory response) (see OIRD); Optimal immunomodulating dose; Organism Identification Number; Ovulation-inducing drug.
-oid suffix meaning form, like, or resembling (Gr. eidos).
OIE Orthostatic idiopathic edema.
OIF Observed intrinsic frequency; Oil immersion field; Osteogenesis Imperfecta Foundation.
OIH Office of International Health; Ortho-iodo-hippurate; Ovulation-inducing hormone (see Hormones - OIH).
OIHA Orthoiodohippuric acid.
OII Optical intrinsic imaging.
Oil Hashish extract high in THC (see Cannabis).
OILD Occupational immunologic lung disease.
Oint; oint Ointment (see Ung).
OI/OP Orthopedic Implants/Orthopedic Prostheses: *ACS* Acetabular Cup System; *APR* Anatomic porous replacement; *CAP* Cup arthroplasty; *CHP* Cup hip prosthesis; *FSP* Femoral stem prosthesis; *GKR* Geometric knee replacement; *HJSR* Hip joint surface replacement; *ICK* Intracondylar knee; *KIS* Knee Instrumentation System; *PCKS* Porous Coated Knee System; *PHP* Proximal humerus prosthesis; *TCKR* Total condylar knee replacement; *THJR* Total hip joint replacement; *THP* Total hip prosthesis; *THR* Total hip replacement; *THS* Total Hip System; *TKP* Total knee prosthesis; *TKR* Total knee replacement; *TKRS* Total Knee Replacement System; *TKS* Total Knee System; *UHS* Universal Head System; *WJP* Wrist joint prosthesis.

OIP Organizing interstitial pneumonia.
OIR Office of International Research; Optimal/mum immune response.
OIRD Opioid-induced respiratory depression (= OID).
OIS Oral insulin secretagogue.
OIT Obstructive intestinal tumour; Oral iron therapy; Oregon Institute of Technology; Organic integrity test (psychiatry).
OJ Orange juice (diet order); Orthoplast jacket.
OJRO Optical Journal and Review of Optometry.
OJT On-the-job training.
OK Okay, i.e. All correct; All is correct; All right; Approved; Correct - The origins of this term are numerous, but none have been exclusively proved. Among them, are: i. "Ola Kola" (Gr.) - "all is fine". An expression said to have been used by early Greek sailors. ii. "Oll is Korrect". An expression used by the Pilgrim fathers in the early days. iii. "Old Kinderhook". First used in 1840 as an authorization or endorsement, after the O.K. Club, a name derived from the American Democratic organization supporting President Martin Van Buren for reelection, from the initials of his native village, his birthplace in New York State, Old Kinderhook. iv. "O Killed". An expression used by soldiers in World War I, each night, in reporting the number of deaths in their group.
OKAN Optokinetic after nystagmus.
OKN Optokinetic nystagmus.
OKT A group of monoclonal antibodies for typing lymphocytes (see OKT3).
OKT3 Orthoclone kilodalton glycoprotein T (molecule) - a murine monoclonal antibody for the (3) 20 kilodalton human T cell antigen receptor complex and an effective immunosuppressant in the treatment of allograft, transplant rejection.
OL Left eye (L. oculus laevus) (= ol); Off-label (prescription); Open label (study)/ lens (Lens implant); Origins of Life (journal); Osborne lesion (of the elbow)/ ligament (an arcuate ligament in the elbow); Other location (indicating place of service in insurance forms).
Ol Oil (L. oleum) (= ol).
ol left eye (see OL); oil (see Ol).
-ol suffix meaning oil (L. oleum).
OL 110 Thioxolone (= 4-hydroxy-2-oxo-1,3-benzoxathiole) - a dermatological agent, used externally in the treatment of acne vulgaris.
OLA Occipito-laeva (-laevo) anterior (L.) (Left occipitoanterior position of the fetal head during labor).
OLB Olfactory bulb; Open-liver/ lung biopsy.
OLC Output limiting compression (of hearing instruments).
OLD Obstructive liver/ lung disease; Orthochromatic leukodystrophy; Ototoxic labyrinthine damage.
OLDR Oral loading dose regimen.
ole- prefix meaning oil (L. oleum).
OLH Ovine lactogenic hormone (see Hormones - OLH).
oLH Ovine luteinizing hormone (see Hormones - oLH).
OLI Orbital lymphocytic infiltration.
OLIDS Open loop insulin delivery system.
oligo- prefix meaning few or small (Gr. oligos).
OLL Obstructive lymphatic lesion (as in, e.g. lymphatic filariasis).
-ologist suffix meaning specialist (Gr. logos).
-ologous suffix meaning relating to (Gr. logos).
-ology suffix meaning a branch of knowledge (Gr. logos).
Ol lini s i Cold-drawn linseed oil (L. oleum lini sine igne).
ol oliv olive oil (L. oleum olivae/vea).
OLP Occipito-laeva/laevo posterior (L.) (left occipitoposterior position of fetus); Open-label phase.
OLR Oak leaf roller; Otology, laryngology, and rhinology.
ol res oleoresin.
OLS Open-label study (of drugs); Ophthalmic laser surgery; Ouabaine-like substance.
OLT Occipito-laeva/laevo transversa (L.) (left occipitotransverse position of fetus); Open-label therapy; Orthotopic liver transplantation.
OLTC Office of Long-Term Care.
OLTx Orthotopic liver transplantation (=

OLT).

OM Obtuse marginal; Occipitomental (diameter of head); Occupational medicine; Occupational Medicine (journal); Ocular movement; Oculomotor; Optical/ Optometric Management (journals); Osborne Mendel (rat); Osteomalacia; Osteomyelitis; Osteopathic manipulation; Otitis media; Outer membrane; Ovulation method.

Om; om All or every (L. omnis); Every morning (L. omni mane).

OM 518 Mephenoxalone. An oxo-oxazolidine compound, and a mild tranquillizer with actions similar to those of meprobamate; used in the treatment of anxiety and tension.

OMA Ontario Medical Association (Canada); Optical multichannel analyzer; Oregon Medical Association.

-oma suffix meaning tumor (Gr. onkoma).

OMAC Otitis media, acute catarrhal.

OMALT Oral mucosal-associated lymphoid tissue (see MALT).

OMAR Office of Medical Applications of Research.

OMAS Occupational maladjustment syndrome; Otitis media, acute, suppurating.

OMB Office of Management and Budget (Executive Office of the President of the United States).

OMBE Office of Minority Business Enterprise (Department of Commerce).

om bid every two days (see omn bid).

om bih every two hours (see omn bih).

OMBR Osteoclast-mediated bone resorption.

OMC Open Mutual Commissurotomy; Optimal metabolic control.

OMCA Otitis media, catarrhalis, acute.

OMCC Otitis media, catarrhalis, chronic.

OMCS Oculomucocutaneous syndrome.

OMCT Orientation-Memory-Concentration Test.

OMD Occult metastatic disease; Ocular muscle/ muscular dystrophy; Oculo-mandibulo-dyscephaly; Omphalomesenteric duct (a vitteline duct connecting the mid-gut and yolk sac); On-line Medical Dictionary; Organic mental disorder; Oromandibular dystonia.

3-OMD 3-O-Methyldopa.

OMDP Office of Manpower Development Programs (DOL).

OME Object Memory Evaluation; Office of Medical Examiner; Otitis media with effusions.

Omega-3 Alpha-linolenic, polyunsaturated essential fatty acid found in flax and cold-water fish; said to reduce the risk of cancer and heart disease).

Omega-6 Linoleic, polyunsaturated essential fatty acid (found in corn, safflower and other vegetables; a possible tumor promoter).

7-OMEN Menogaril.

OMF Omsk hemorrhagic fever (a zoonotic disease); Organomercury fungicide.

OMFP Ovulation method of family planning (see NFPM).

OMFS Oral and Maxillofacial Surgeon/ery.

OMG Ocular myasthenia gravis.

OMH Office of Mental Health; Organic marine hydrocolloid.

OMI Office of the Medical Investigator; Ohio Medical Indemnity (Blue Shield); Old myocardial infarction.

OMM Outer mitrochondrial membrane.

OMN Oculomotor nerve.

omn bid every two days (L. omnibus bidendis) (= om bid).

omn bih every two hours (L. omni bihora) (= om bih; omn 2 hor; omn sec hor; om sec hor).

omn hor; om hor every hour (L. omni hora).

omn 2 hor every second hour (L. omni secunda hora) (see omn bih).

omn man; om man every morning (L. omni mane).

omn man vel noc; om man vel noc every morning or night (L. omni mane vel nocte).

omn noct; om noct; every night (L. omni nocte) (= ON; on).

omn quad hor; om quad hor; om quar hor every quarter of an hour (L. omni quadrante hora).

omn sec hor every second hour (L. omni secunda hora) (see omn bih).

OMP Olfactory marker protein; Oligo-n-methyl-morpholino-propylene oxide; Ornithine monophosphate; Outer membrane protein.

OMPA Octamethyl pyrophosphoramide (=

Octamethylphosphorodiamidic anhydride; Pestox III; Schradan) - an organophosphorus insecticide and anticholine esterase; Omega methyl pantothenic acid (a pantothenic acid antagonist); Otitis media, purulent, acute.

omphal- combining form meaning navel (Gr. omphalos).

OMPC; OMPCh Otitis media, purulent, chronic.

OMR Ontario Medical Review (Canada journal); Operative mortality rate.

OMRF Oklahoma Medical Research Foundation.

OMS Objectively measured sleep; Office of Medical Services (Department of State); Opsoclonus-myoclonus syndrome; Organic mental syndrome; Orthopaedic Medicine Surgery (UK journal); Otomandibular syndrome.

OM&S Osteopathic Medicine and Surgery.

OMSA Otitis media, secretory/ suppurative, acute.

OMSC; OMSCh Otitis media, secretory/ suppurative, chronic.

om sec hor every second hour (see omn bih; omn sec hor).

OMT O-methyltransferase; Opioid maintenance therapy/ treatment (see OAMT); Osteopathic manipulative therapy.

OMVC Open mitral valve commissurotomy (operation/ heart).

OMVI Operating motor vehicle (when/ while) intoxicated.

ON Every night (see omn noct); Obsessional neurosis; Occipitonuchal; Office/ Ophthalmic/ Orthopedic nurse; Onlay; Optic/ Otic nerve; Optic neuritis; Optic neuropathy; Oronasal; Ortho-Novum; Osteonecrosis; Overnight.

ONA Optic nerve atrophy.

ONAJ Orthopedic Nurse Association Journal.

ONB O-nitrobiphenyl.

ONC Oncogene; Oncology; Orthopaedic/ Orthopedic Nursing Certificate; Over-the-needle catheter.

Onc Oncology (journal).

onc- combining form meaning bulk (Gr. ogkos).

ONCLA Nursing Committee for Leprosy Control (Brazil).

onco- prefix meaning tumor (Gr. onkos).

OND Ophthalmic Nursing Diploma; Optic nerve damage/ demyelination; Orbitonasal dislocation; Other neurological disorders.

oneiro- prefix meaning dream (Gr. oneiros).

ONF O'nyong nyong fever (a viral arthritis of Central Africa, similar to that caused by the chikungunya virus in Africa and Asia).

ONHA Office of Nursing Home Affairs (HEW).

ONL Outer nuclear layer.

ONP Operating nursing procedure; Orthonitrophenyl.

ONPG O-nitrophenyl-beta-D-galactopyranoside.

ONR Office of Naval Research (USN); Optic-nerve regeneration.

ONS Office for National Statistics; Oncology Nursing Society.

ONTD Open neural tube defect (= NTD).

ONTG Oral nitroglycerin.

ONTR Orders not to resuscitate.

onych- combining form meaning claw or nail (Gr. onychos).

OO Oophorectomy; Ophthalmic Optician (BOA journal, UK); Oral order.

OÖ An egg.

oo- combining form meaning egg (Gr. oon).

o/o on account of.

O&O On and off.

OOA Oral opioid analgesic; Outer optic anlage.

OOB; OoB Out of bed.

OOBBRP Out of bed with bathroom priveleges.

OOC Onset of contractions; Oral-oral contact; Out of cast/ control.

OOD Optimal oral dose.

OOH Oliguric oligohydramnios (Obstetrics).

OOH; OoH; ooh Out-of-hospital (cardiac arrest; death; etc.).

OOHCA Out-of-hospital cardiac arrest.

OOH&NS Ophthalmology, otorhinolaryngology, and head and neck surgery.

OOL Onset of labor.

OOLR Ophthalmology, otology, laryngology, and rhinology.

OOM Oogonial metaphase.

OON Osteoid osteoma nidus (Orthopedics).
OOO One-on-one.
OOP Out of patience/ pelvis/ plaster; Out-of-pocket (expenses, etc.); Out on pass; Oxygen outlet pressure.
oophor- prefix meaning ovary (Gr. oophoros).
OOPR Oral opioid potency ratio (between dextromoramide, methadone, morphine, oxycodone, papaverine, pethidine, etc.).
OOR Oro-oral route (of infection); Out of room.
OORR Orbicularis oculi reflex response.
OOS Out of stock.
OOT Out of town; Outpatient oral therapy.
OOW Out of wedlock.
OOWS Objective opiate withdrawal scale.
OP Oblique presentation; Occipitoparietal; Occiput posterior; Octapeptide; Ocular prosthesis; Office Pathology (journal); Old patient (i.e. previously seen); Olfactory peduncle; Oncotic/ Opening/ Osmotic pressure; Open; Operating/ive procedure; Operation (see op); Operative; Ophthalmology (see Op); Opponens pollicis; Organophosphate/sphorus; Oropharynx; Orthomolecular Psychiatry (journal); Orthostatic proteinuria; Orthotics and Prosthetics (journal); Oscillatory potentials; Osteopathic Physician (British journal); Osteoporosis; Other than psychotic (= op); Outpatient (= OPT; Opt); Overproof; Ovine prolactin (see Hormones - OP; oPRL); Oviparous.
Op Operation (see op); Ophthalmology (= OP); Opisthocranion; Opium (see Papaver).
op operation (= OP; Op; oper); operator; ophthalmic; opposite; other than psychotic (see OP); work (L. opus).
op- combining form meaning see (Gr.).
O&P Ova and parasites (laboratory/ bacteriology).
OPA Obstetrical physician's assistant; Occupational physical activity; Opioid partial agonist/ antagonist; Oral pharyngeal airway; Outpatient anesthesia; Organ-procurement agency.
Op Amp Operational amplifier.
-opathy suffix meaning disease (Gr. pathos).
OPB Ophthalmic Pathology Branch (AFIP); Outpatient basis.
OPC Oculopalatocerebral (syndrome); Oral-penile contact; Organophosphorus compound (= OPI); Oropharyngeal candidiasis; Outpatient care; Outpatient clinic.
OPCA Olivopontocerebellar atrophy.
op cit in the work cited/ previously cited (L. opus citato/ citatum).
OPCOS Oligomenorrheic polycystic ovary syndrome.
OPCS Office of Population, Censuses and Surveys (UK).
OPD Obstetric prediabetic; Obstructive pulmonary disease (= OLD); Optical path difference; Orthophenylenediamine; Otopalatodigital (syndrome) (see OPDS); Outpatient Department/ Dispensary.
O'p-DDD Mitotane.
OpDent Operative dentistry.
OPDG Ocular plethysmodynamography.
OPDM Offspring of progestational diabetic mother.
OPDS Otopalatodigital syndrome.
OPE Outpatient evaluation.
OPEM Outpatient Electrolyte Mixture (of Queen Elizabeth Hospital for children, UK. - contains potassium and sodium chloride, potassium citrate, and sodium acid phosphate. Used with 5% sucrose solution orally for infants, for the treatment of acute dehydration).
Op Eng Optical Engineering (journal).
oper operation (see op).
OPF Osteoporotic fracture.
OPFRR ffice for Protection From Research Risks.
OPG Ocular/ Oculo pneumoplethysmograph(y) (= OPP; OPPG); Oculoplethysmograph(y); Oculoplethysmography (a non-invasive procedure for measuring carotid artery activity by the use of ultrasound) (= GEE-OPG; OPG-GEE); Osteoperiosteal graft; Osteoprotegerin (osteoclast inhibitor in the bone marrow stroma); Oxypolygelatin.
opg opening.
OPG-GEE Oculoplethysmography (test) (see GEE-OPG; OPG).
OPH Obliterative pulmonary hypertension; Ophthalmia; Ophthalmology (= Oph; Ophth);

Ophthalmoscope/copic/copy (= Oph; Ophth).
Oph Ophthalmologist; Ophthalmology (see OPH); Ophthalmoscope/copic/copy (see OPH).
OphD Doctor of Ophthalmology.
OPHE Office of Public Health Education (New York State).
Ophiophilia/lism Love of snakes (see -philia).
OPHS Office of Public Health and Science (USDA).
Ophth Ophthalmology (see OPH).
Ophthal Ophthalmologist (AAO journal).
ophthal- combining form meaning eye (Gr. ophthalmos).
OPI Oculoparalytic illusion; Omnibus Personality Inventory; Organophosphate/sphorus insecticide (see OPC).
OPIDN Organophosphorus-induced delayed neuropathy.
OPK; opk Optokinetic.
OPL Oropharyngeal lavage; Outer plexiform layer; Ovine placental lactogen.
OPLL Ossification of posterior longitudinal ligament.
OPM Occult primary malignancy; Ocular pseudomyasthenia (gravis); Ophthalmoplegic migraine; Out-patient Management.
OPMD Oculopharyngeal muscular dystrophy.
OPN Ophthalmic nurse.
OPP Obstetric prachial palsy (see SD - Shoulder dystocia); Ocular/ Oculo pneumoplethysmograph(y) (see OPG); Office of Pesticide Programs (EPA); Optimum prescribing practice; rganophosphate pesticide; Oropharyngeal preparation; Orthophenylphenol; Osmotic pressure of plasma; Outpatient practice/ procedure; Oxygen partial pressure.
opp opposed (to); opposite (of).
OPPG Ocular/ Oculo pneumoplethysmograph(y) (see OPG).
OPR Office of Population Research (AID); Overall potency ratio.
OPRR Office of Protection from Research Risks (NIH).
OPS Office of Product Safety (FDA); Oligo(hydramnios)-polyhydramnios sequence (Obstetrics); Operations; Oropharyngeal sample/ swab; Osteoporosis prevention study; Osteoporosis-pseudolipoma syndrome; Outpatient Service/ Surgery.
OPSA Ovarian papillary serous adenocarcinoma.
OPSC Osteopathic Physicians and Surgeons of California; Outpatient Surgery Center.
OpScan Optical scanning.
OPSI Overwhelming postsplenectomy infection.
OPSR Office of Professional Standards Review (HEW).
OPSR-BQA Office of Professional Standards Review - Bureau of Quality Assurance (HEW).
OPT Omphalopagus twins (see pagus); Opioid pharmacotherapy; Oropharyngeal thrush; Osteoporosis prevention trial; Outpatient (see OP); Outpatient treatment (see OpT)/ therapy.
OpT Outpatient treatment (= OPT).
Opt Optician (= opt); Option; Outpatient (see OP).
opt best (L. optimus); optic(s); optical; optician (see Opt); optimal/mum; optional.
OPT c CA Ohio pediatric test with compressed air.
OPT c O_2 Ohio pediatric test with oxygen.
OPTHD Optimal hemodialysis.
Optics (SAO journal).
opto- prefix meaning vision (Gr. optos).
OPU Oocyte pick-up (reproduction technique); Oropharyngeal ulcer(ation).
OPV Oral polio(myelitis)/ poliovirus vaccine; Outpatient visit.
OPVD Obstructive pulmonary valvular disease.
OPW Obese pregnant woman/ women.
OPWL Opiate withdrawel.
OQ Ostomy Quarterly.
OQD Oxyquinoline dressing.
OR A logical binary relation that is true, if any argument is true, and false otherwise; Oestrogen/ Olfactory receptor; Odds ratio; Oil retention (enema) (see ORE); Open reduction; Operating room; Operations research; Optic radiation/ recess; Oral; Oral rehydration; Orbital rhabdomyosarcoma; Orthopaedic/ Orthopedic; Orthopedic research; Orthopaedic Review (journal).

Or Orbitale.
O_R; O_r Rate of outflow.
O-R Oxidation-reduction (reaction).
or- combining form meaning mouth (L. oris).
ORA Opiate receptor agonist.
Orange Dexedrine tablet (see Amphet - Orange).
ORANS Oak Ridge Analytical System(s).
ORAU Oak Ridge Associated Universities.
ORB Odd repetitive behavior (as in Asperger syndrome, Autism, etc.) (see SMC).
orb- combining form meaning circle (L. orbis).
ORBC Ox red blood cell.
ORC Orthopedic Rehabilitation Center.
ORCH Orchiectomy.
orch orchitis.
orchi- prefix meaning testicle (Gr. orchis).
ORD Office of Research and Development (EPA); Off-set reverse dome (Podiatry) (see BE - Bunionectomy); Optical rotatory dispersion; Oral radiation death.
Ord Orderly.
ORDS Office of Research, Demonstration, and Statistics.
ORE Oil retention enema (= OR; OR enema); Operations readiness evaluation.
OREF Orthopedic Research and Education Foundation.
OR enema Oil retention enema (see ORE).
ORF Open reading frame (e.g. 73 - gene sequence) (= orf); Ortho Pharmaceutical Co (USA) code for experimental substances; Ortho Research Foundation; Osteoporosis-related fracture (of the spine, hip, rib, wrist, etc.).
ORF; orf Orthopox family (of [pox] viruses, such as cowpox, monkey-pox, smallpox, etc.).
OR&F Open reduction and fixation.
orf open reading frame (see ORF).
3'ORF gene A regulatory gene of the AIDS virus (HIV-1) genome, that exerts a regulatory effect reducing viral replication.
ORG Orexin-receptor gene (a key factor in narcolepsy and other sleep disorders, also known as the HRG - Hyocretin-receptor gene).
Org; org Organic; Organization(al) (= Organiz); Orgasm.
OR2G Orexin receptor 2 gene (see HR2G).
organ- prefix meaning implement (Gr. organon).
Organiz Organization(al) (see Org; org).
ORHL Otosclerosis-related hearing loss.
ORIF Open reduction with internal fixation (operation/ orthopedics).
orig origin(al)/ally/ated.
OrJ Orange juice.
ORL Otorhinolaryngology.
orl oral.
ORM Orosomucoid; Other regulated material.
ORMOSIL Organically modified silica.
ORN Operating Room Nurse; Orthopaedic/ Orthopedic Nurse.
Orn; Orni Ornithine.
Ornith Ornithology.
ORNL Oak Ridge National Laboratory (US).
ORO Oil red O (stain).
oro- prefix meaning mouth (Gr. oros).
OROS Oral osmotic; Ostomotic release oral system.
ORP Occiput right posterior (fetal position); Otolith Repositioning Procedure (see ESM - Epley/Semont maneuver); Oxidation-reduction potential.
ORPC Open-ring peptide compound.
ORPM Orthorhythmic pacemaker.
ORR Objective response rate; Overall response rate.
-orraphy suffix meaning repair or suture.
-orrhea suffix meaning discharge or flow (Gr. rhein).
orrho- prefix meaning serum (Gr. orrhos).
ORS Office of Research Safety (NCI); Office of Research and Statistics (SSA - HEW); Olfactory reference syndrome; Oncologic radiology service(s); Optimum revaccination schedule; Oral rehydration salt/ solution (see ORST); Oral replacement solution; Oral/ Orthopedic surgeon/ surgery (see OrS); Orthopaedic Research Society; Oxygen radical scavengers.
OrS Oral/ Orthopedic surgeon/ surgery (= ORS).
ORSA Operations Research Society of America.
ORSI Osteoarthritis Research Society

International.

ORST Oral rehydration salt Therapy (= ORT).

ORT Object relations technique; Occupational - Registered, Therapist; Operating room technician; Oral rehydration therapy (see ORST); Organization for Rehabilitation through Training (see AORTF - American ORT).

orth; ortho orthopaedic(s)/pedic(s) (= Ortho).

Ortho Ortho Diagnostics Inc; Orthopaedics/pedics (see orth; ortho); Orthopod (AOAO journal).

ortho- prefix meaning correct or normal (Gr. orthos).

ORU Ohio Resuscitation Unit (radiation warmer used in Newborn Nursery).

OR X1 Oriented to time.

OR X2 Oriented to time and place.

OR X3 Oriented to time, place, and person.

OS Left eye (L. oculus sinister) (see os); Occipitosacral; Occupational safety; Office surgery; Omenn's syndrome (a postnatal SCID disorder characterized by the development of generalized erythroderma, diarrhea, hepatosplenomegaly, hypereosinophilia, and marked elevation of serum IgE. This disease is fatal, unless it is corrected by bone transplantation) (see CSD; SCID); Oncostatin (naturally occurring protein that acts as a tumor inhibitor); Opening snap (heart valve/ sound); Operating system; Ophthalmic Surgery (journal); Oral surgery; Organ-specific; Orthopedic surgeon/ surgery; Ortolani's sign (clicking of the hip joint during abduction); Osgood-Schlatter('s disease); Osmotic (= os); Osteogenic sarcoma; Osteopathic Symposium (AOA journal); Osteosarcoma; Osteosclerosis; Ouabain-sensitive/vity; Outer segment (eye cone); Overall survival; Oxygen saturation (see O_2 sat).

Os Bone (L. os); Mouth or opening (L. oris); Osmium (Z = 76) (see Elements - Osmium).

os left eye (L. oculus sinister) (= OS); osmotic (see OS).

OS 2046 Mevinphos - an organophosphorus insecticide (see CMDP).

OSA Obstructive sleep apnea; Office of Services to the Aging; Optical Society of America; Ovarian sectional area.

OSAA Organ-specific autoantibody.

OSAHRC Occupational Safety And Health Review Commission (US).

OSAID Organ-specific autoimmune disease (e.g. Addison's disease, Alopecia areata, SLE, Vitiligo, etc.).

OSAS Obstructive sleep apnea syndrome.

O_2 sat Oxygen saturation (= OS) (laboratory/ blood gas).

OSC Orthopedics Spine Center (USC).

osc oscillation.

OSCD On the spot clinical diagnosis (= SD).

OSCE Objective Structered Clinical Exam.

OSCF Oligomycin-sensitivity-conferring factor (= F_0).

oscillo- prefix meaning oscillate (L. oscillare).

OSCOE Objective Structured Clinical and Oral Examination.

-oscopy suffix meaning view (Gr. skopein).

OSD Ocular-surface disorder (cornea); One-sided deafness; Orthostatic dysfunction; Orthotopic skull defect (Orthopedics); Osgood-Schlatter disease (Orthopedics) (= OS); Osteoporotic spinal degeneration; Overside drainage; Oxidative stress degree.

OSDW Obesity, Smoking, Drinking, and Worrying (effects on health).

OSE Office of Scientific Evaluation (FDA); Opioid side effect(s); Overall systemic exposure; Overall safety evaluation (of drugs); Ovine spongiform encephalopathy (i.e. in sheep - scrapie).

-ose suffix meaning carbohydrate.

OSES Office of Solar Energy Studies (ERDA).

OSETP Office of Science, Engineering and Technology Policy (White House, Washington, DC).

OSF Organ system failure; Organ system function (including hemapoietic, hepatic, and renal function); Outer spiral fiber; Overgrowth stimulating factor.

OSFA One-size-fits-all (therapy).

OSFET Oxide semiconductor field effect transistor.

OSFT Outstretched fingertip(s).

OSG Office of the Surgeon General (USAF).

OSH Orthostatic hypotension (see OH).

OSHA Occupational Safety and Health Act (see OSH Act)/ Administration (Dept of

Labor)/ Association.

OSH Act Occupational Safety and Health Act of 1970 (= OSHA).

OSI Oxidative stress index.

OSIS Office of Science Information Services (NSF).

-osis suffix meaning a condition or process, and especially an abnormal or morbid one (Gr.).

OSM Osmol(ality)/ar/arity/ Osmole/ Osmosis/ Osmotic (see Osm); Ovine submaxillary mucin; Oxygen saturation meter.

Osm; osm; Osmo (= OSM; osmol) Osmol; Osmolality (= mOsm/kg H_2O; milliOsmolalities per kilogram of water); Osmolar; Osmolarity; Osmole; Osmosis; Osmotic.

OSMA Ohio State Medical Association.

OsmC Osmotic concentration (= mOsm/l; milliOsmolalities per liter).

Osm/kg Osmoles per kilogram.

Osm/l Osmoles per liter.

osmo- prefix meaning impulse (Gr. osmos) or odor (Gr. osme).

osmol osmol(ality)/ar/arity/ osmole (see Osm).

OSM S Osmolarity serum.

OSM U Osmolarity urine.

OSN Off service note.

Os/O+ % Percentage pulmonary venous admixture.

OSOMOP Oral Surgery, Oral Medicine, and Oral Pathology (AAOP journal).

OSP Ovarian stimulation program; Overall safety profile (of a drug).

OSPAC Oral Surgery Political Action Committee.

OSR Overall safety/ survival rate.

OSRD Office of Scientific Research and Development (USA).

OSS Office of Special/ Strategic Services; Office of Strategic Studies (US); Ongoing Safety Surveillance; Over-the-shoulder strap.

oss osseous.

oss- prefix meaning bone (L. ossis) (see osteo-).

OST Object sorting test; Office of Science and Technology (US President - inactive since 1973; duties transferred to National Science Foundation) (see NSF); One-sided test; Oral steroid therapy; Ovarian screening test (e.g. CA-125, CEA, etc.); Oxytocin stress test (for monitoring fetal condition).

Ost Ostomy.

ost- combining form meaning bone (Gr. osteon).

OSTCMAD Organ-specific T-cell-mediated autoimmune disease (Thymus cell).

Osteo; osteo Osteoarthritis; Osteomyelitis; Osteopathy.

osteo- prefix meaning bone (Gr. osteon) (see oss-).

OStJ Office of the Order of St. John of Jerusalem.

-ostomy suffix meaning creation of an artificial opening.

OSTP Office of Science and Technology Policy.

Ost Quart Ostomy Quarterly.

OSTS Office of State Technical Services (Britain).

OSU Ohio State University.

OSUK Ophthalmological Society of the United Kingdom.

OSW Office of Saline Water (Department of the Interior).

OT Objective/ Orientation test (psychology); Oblique talus; Occiput transverse (fetal position); Occlusion/ Over time; Occupational/ Office therapist/py; Occupational Therapy (UK and US journals); Ocular tension (eye examination); Office of Telecommunications (Dept of Commerce); Old term (in anatomy) (vs. BNA term); Old tuberculin (see Tuberculin - OT; TO); Olfactory threshold; Opisthotonus (seen in tetanus); Optic tract; Oral therapy; Original tuberculin; Ornithine transcarbamylase (see OTC); Orotracheal (tube) (see OTT); Orthopedic treatment; Osteopathic Symposium (AOA journal); Otolaryngologist/ogy (see Ot); Otology; Oxytocin (see OXT); Oxytryptamine; Short for SGOT (see SGOT).

Ot Otolarngologist/ogy (= OT).

ot orotracheal (tube) (see OTT).

ot- combining form meaning ear (Gr. otos).

OTA Occupational therapy assistant; Office of Technology Assessment (US Congress); Open to air; Ornithine transaminase; Orthotoluidine arsenite (test for blood in the urine).

OTAF Office of Technology Assessment and Forecast (US Patent and Trademark Office).

OTC Ornithine transcarbamylase (= OT); Oval target cell; Over-the-counter (drug - with reference to drugs not requiring a prescription); Oxytetracycline (on culture and sensitivity reports).

OTC; O_2TC Oxygen-transporting component (e.g. of hemoglobin).

OTD Oil turbine dose (centrifuge); Onychotrichodysplasia (see CS - Cantu syndrome); Oral temperature device; Organ tolerance dose (that amount of radiation tolerated by the tissues of a normal organ); Ototome drill (Neurosurgery of the ear; pronounced "autotome") (= ATD); Ototoxic drug(s) (e.g. aminoglycoside antibiotics such as amikacin, dihydrostreptomycin, gentamycin, kanamycin, neomycin, streptomycin, tobramycin, and viomycin); Out (through) the door.

OTE Optically transparent electrode; Organ-toxic effect; Overall treatment evaluation.

OT&E Operational Test and Evaluation (program - USAF).

OTEC Ocean thermal energy conversion.

OTF Optical transfer function; Oral transfer factor.

Oth Other.

OTI Ovomucoid trypsin inhibitor.

OTM Orthotoluidine manganese sulfate; Ototoxic medication(s) (see OTD).

OTO Outflow tract obstruction.

OTO; Oto Otolaryngology (see Otolar); Otologist/gy (see Otol); Otorhinolaryngology.

oto- prefix meaning ear (Gr. otos).

Otol Otologist/ Otology (= OTO; Oto).

Otolar Otolaryngology (= OTO; Oto).

-otomy suffix meaning surgical incision or cut (Gr. tome).

OTP Office of Telecommunications Policy; Optimal test performance; Organ-transplant patient/ program; Overall tolerability profile (of a drug).

OTR Occupational Therapist, Registered (see OTReg); Organ-transplant recipient; Organ Transplant Registry (ACS - Am College of Surgeons); Ovarian Tumor Registry; Oxygen transfer rate.

OTRDA Ontario Tuberculosis and Respiratory Disease Association (Canada).

OTReg Occupational Therapist, Registered (= OTR).

OT/RT Occupational therapy/recreational therapy.

OTS Occipital temporal sulcus; Office of Toxic Substances (EPA); Officers' Training School (US armed forces); Oral tetratology study; Organ transplant service; Orotracheal suction.

OTT Omeprazole triple therapy (for *Helicobacter* pylori gastritis), using a combination of omeprazole with amoxycillin and clarithromycin (or metronidazole/tinidazole), or a combination of omeprazole with clarithromycin and metronidazole (or tinidazole) (see BTT; ODT); Oral tolerance test (for diabetes mellitus) (see GITT; GTT); Orotracheal tube; Osteoporosis treatment trial; Over-the-top (procedure) (Orthopedics).

OTU Olfactory tubercle; Operational taxonomic unit.

OU Both eyes together (see ou); Each eye (see ou); Observation unit; Oppenheimer-Urbach (syndrome).

ou both eyes together (L. oculi unitas) (= OU); each eye (L. oculus uterque) (= OU).

OUCH Organization of University of California House-staffs.

OUE Overall urinary excretion.

OUI Overuse injury (see OI).

OULQ Outer upper left quadrant (breast).

OURD Operated unilateral renovascular disease.

OURQ Outer upper right quadrant (breast).

OUS Obstructive urinary symptom(s); Overuse syndrome.

OV Objective vertigo; Oculovestibular; Office visit; Osteoid volume; Outflow volume (see O_v); Ovalbumin (see OVA); Ovary (see Ov); Overventilation → // v // → (see HV - Hyperventilation); Ovulation.

Ov Ovary (L. ovum = egg) (= OV).

ov ovarian; ovum.

O_v Outflow volume (= OV).

ov- prefix meaning egg (L. ovum).

O_{2v} Superoxide.

OVA Obstructive ventilatory alteration (see COVA; EOVA; POVA); Ovalbumin (= OV).
ova ovariectomy.
OVAL Ovalocytes.
OVC Ovarian cancer/ carcinoma.
OVD Obliterative/ Occlusive vascular disease; Obstructive valvular disease; Occlusal vertical dimension; Operative vaginal delivery (Obstetrics).
OvDF Ovarian dysfunction.
OVP Osteoporotic vertebral fracture.
OVR Office of Vocational Rehabilitation.
OVRFSA Office of Vocational Rehabilitation of the Federal Security Administration.
OVX Ovariectomized.
OW Once weekly; Open wedge; Optical World (UK journal); Optometric Weekly (journal); Optometric World (journal); Ordinary warfare; Outer wall; Out-of-wedlock; Oval window.
O/W Oil in water (emulsion - medication base); Oil/Water (ratio) (see o/w).
o/w oil/water (ratio) (= O/W).
OWCP Office of Workers' Compensation Programs (DoL).
OWD Once weekly dose/ dosing.
OWIG Office of the Welfare Inspector General (NYS).
OWL Older Women's League.
OWNK Out of wedlock not keeping/ knowing.
OWP Opiate/ Opioid withdrawal program (see OWR).
OWR Opiate/ Opioid withdrawal regimen (see OWP); Osler-Weber-Rendu (syndrome); Ovarian wedge resection.
OWRR Office of Water Resources Research (DoI).
OWRT Office of Water Research and Technology (DoI).
OWS Opiate/ Opioid withdrawal symptoms; Outerwear syndrome.
OWTP Oval window tympanoplasty.
OX Optic chiasma; Oxacillin; Oxalate; Oxide; Orthopedic examination; Oxytocin (see OXT).
Ox Oxygen (see O_2).
ox oxymel (honey, water, and vinegar).
OXA Oxaprotiline.
OXALAC Oxford Artificial Limb and Appliance Center.
Oxi Oximeter/try.
OXP Oxypressin.
OXT Oxytocin (= OT; OX).
OXY; oxy Oxygen (see O_2).
oxy- prefix meaning sharp (Gr. oxys).
OxyM Oxidizing material.
OXZ Oxazepam.
OYD Office of Youth Development (HEW).
OYE Old yellow enzyme.
OYS One-year survival.
OZ Oxazepam (see OXZ).
oz ounce (L. uncia).
oz ap apothecaries' ounce (US).
oz apoth apothecaries' ounce (UK).
oz t ounce troy (US).
oz tr ounce troy (UK).

P

P An electrographic wave corresponding to a wave of depolarization crossing the atria; By weight (L. pondere); Father (L. pater); Handful (L. pugilus); Near (L. proximum); Near point (L. punctum proximum); Pain; Para; Parent; Parietal (electrode placement in electroencephalography); Parity (obstetrics); Part; Partial pressure (blood gases); Pasteurella; Paternal; Patient; Pedicle/ Pediculus (a footlike or stemlike part, e.g. P. arcus vertebrae or Radix a v = Pedicle of the vertebral arch); Pelvis; Penicillin (on culture and sensitivity reports); Percent (= %) (see Symbols 2); Percentile; Percussion; Perforation; Peripheral; Permeability; Peta-; peta (10^{15}); Pharmacopeia; Phenacetin; Phenophthalein; Phenylalanine; Phosphate group; Phosphorus (Z = 15) (= phos) (see Elements - Phosphorus); Physiology; Pico- (= 10^{-12}) (see pico-); Pig; Pint (= O - from the L. octarius) (see Symbols 5); Placebo; Plan (on problem-oriented medical records); Plasma; Plasma concentration (e.g. P_{Na} - of sodium); Plasmodium; Pneumocystis; Point; Poise (the unit of viscosity of a liquid, being the number of grams per centimeter per second) - as in CP or centipoise (= one-hundredth of a poise); Poison(ing); Polarity/ization; Pole; Polymyxin; Pondere (L) - by weight (see above); Pons; Population; Porcelain; Porcine; Porphyrin; Position; Positive (= +; ⊥) (see Symbols 2); Posterior; Postpartum; Pott's shunt; Power; Precipitin; Precursor; Prednisone; Premolar; Presbyopia; Pressure; Primary; Primipara; Private (patient/ room); Probability; Product; Progesterone; Prolactin; Proline; Properdin; Propionate; Propranolol; Protein (on diet orders); Proteus; Proximal; Proximum (L.) - near (see above); Pseudomonas; Psychiatry/chology; Pulmonary; Pulse; Pupil; Radiant/ Sound power; Significance probability; Wave (ECG - see above); Weight (L. pondus).

p after (see p̄); atomic orbital with angular momentum quantum number 1; freeze preservation; frequency of the more common allele of a pair; momentum; papilla; phosphate; pico- (= 10^{-12}) (see pico-); pint (O) (see Symbols 5); pond (L. pondere = by weight); pressure; probability; proton; pupil; short arm of chromosome; sound pressure.

p̄ after/ following (L. post) (= p).

p- para- (chemical prefix).

~P energy-rich phosphate.

↓P Partial lower denture.

P↑ Partial upper denture.

π pi. the 16th lower case (small) letter of the Greek alphabet; the ratio of circumference to diameter: 3.1415926536 (see Symbols: 2).

Π Greek capital letter pi.

Φ Phi - the 21st (capital) letter of the Greek alphabet (small letter = φ); Magnetic flux; Osmotic coefficient.

Ψ Greek letter "psi"; Wave function.

^{32}P Radioactive phosphorus.

5p- Cri-du-chat syndrome.

3P (test) Plasma protamine paracoagulation (test).

$P_{0.1}$ Pressure/ at 100 milliseconds of inspiration (see PFT - $P_{0.1}$).

P_1; P-one First parental generation (symbol in genetics); Pulmonic first (heart) sound.

P_2 Second parental generation (genetics); Pulmonic second (ht) sound.

P_3 Proximal third.

P 12 Oxacillin sodium (see BRL 1400).

p 16 protein 16 (a tumor-suppressor gene, with molecular weight 16 - see MTS 1).

p24 Antigen in HIV infection.

P 25 Cloxacillin sodium (see BRL 1621).

P27; p27 Protein 27 (a cyclin-dependent kinase inhibitor).

P-32 Chromium phosphate.

P 35 Methicillin sodium (see BRL 1241).

P 50 Ampicillin (see BRL 1341).

P-50 Oxygen half-saturation pressure (= Oxygen pressure at 50% hemoglobin saturation).

P 53; p 53 Protein 53 (a tumor-suppressor gene, with molecular weight 53, located on the short arm of chromosome 17. Its malfunction or mutation leads to cancer).

P 55 Hydroxypregnanedione (a depressant).

P 152 Phenethicillin potassium (see BRL 152).

P 300 Polygraph 300 (a distinctive brain wave or spike occurring about 300 milliseconds after the stimulus, in the Lie detection test called Brain Fingerprinting).

P 301 Hydroxyphenamate (see Al 0361).

P 391 Pecazine hydrochloride (= Mecazine HCl). A phenothiazine tranquillizer, less potent than chlorpromazine, used for the control of nausea and vomiting, as a sedative in pre-anesthetic medication and obstetrics, and to control restlessness and agitation in the withdrawal stage of drug addiction and chronic alcoholism.

P450 Non-specific cytochrome inhibitor (e.g. Cimetidine; Hepatic cytochrome system, etc.).

P450 3A4 Cytochrome inducer (e.g. phenytoin, rifampicin, etc.); Non-specific cytochrome inhibitor (e.g. itraconazole, erythromycin, etc.).

P 607 Chlorpropamide (= Chlorglypropamide). A sulfonylurea; an orally active hypoglycemic agent used in the treatment of mild or moderately severe, uncomplicated diabetes mellitus.

P 638 Puromycin (see CL 13900).

P 725 Perazine (= Pemazine). A phenothiazine tranquillizer with a pronounced anti-emetic action.

P 1393 Benzthiaze. A thiazide diuretic, acting by reducing the resorption of electrolytes from the proximal renal tubules.

P 1742 Fluperolone acetate (= 9α-Fluoro-21-methylprednisolone acetate) - A synthetic corticosteroid used by topical application in the treatment of various skin disorders.

P 2105 Epithiazide. A thiazide diuretic and hypotensive agent.

P 2525 Polythiazide. A thiazide diuretic, acting within two hours after administration, reaching a maximum effect in about six hours, and lasting for 24 to 48 hours.

P 2647 Benzquinamide. A quinolizine derivative; a tranquillizer used in the treatment of anxiety and tension states.

P 4657B Thiothixene. A tranquillizer and antipsychotic agent of the phenothiazine group.

P 5048 Dimethisterone (= 6α,21-Dimethylethisterone). A synthetic sex hormone with actions and uses similar to those of progesterone.

PA Clinical pharmacology; Conduction times through the atrium; Panic attack; Pantothenic/ Periodic/ Phosphatidic/ Propionic/ Pyruvic acid; Paralysis agitans; Paranoia; Parents Anonymous; Passive aggressive; Pathologist/gy (see Pa); Periarteritis; Peridural artery; Periodontal abscess; Pernicious anemia; Personality accentuation (see PD - Personality difficulty); Phakic-aphakic; Phenylalanine; Phenylalcohol; Phenylalkylamine; Phosphoarginine; Photoablation (by light i.e. by laser); Photo-allergy; Phthalic anhydride; Physician('s) assistant(s); Pineapple; Pituitary-adrenal; Plasma adsorption/ aldosterone; Plasminogen activator (see rt-PA); Platelet adhesiveness; Platelet aggregating/ion; Platelet-/ Pregnancy-associated; Polyamine; Polyarteritis; Polyarthritis; Post-aural; Posterior-anterior (chest X-ray); Posteroanterior (see P-A); Pre-albumin; Predictive accuracy; Presents again; Pressure alopecia (see TA); Primary aldosteronism/ amenorrhea/ anemia; Prinzmetal's angina (Variant angina; Vasospastic angina) (= PMA; VA; VSA); Prior to admission; Proactivator; Proanthocyanidin; Procainamide; Professional associate/tion; Prolonged action (tablets); Prophylactic antibiotics; Prostate(tatic)/ Protective antigen; Proteolytic action; Prothrombin activity; Protrusio acetabuli; Pseudomonas aeruginosa (see Pa); Psychiatric aide; Psychoanalysis/yst; Psychogenic aspermia; Public address (system); Pulmonary artery/ atresia; Pulpoaxial; Puromycin aminonucleoside; Pyrrolizidine alkaloid; Yearly (L. per annum) (see pa).

Pa Pascal (unit of pressure, according to the International System of Units or SI) = $kg.m^2.s^{-2}$ (kg = kilogram; m = meter; s = second); Pathologist/gy (= PA); Protactinium (Z = 91) (see Elements - Proctactinium); Pseudomonas aeruginosa (= PA); Pulmonary arterial (pressure).

pA picoampere.

pa through the anus (L. per anum); yearly (L. per annum) (= PA).

P_A Alveolar pressure; Partial pressure of arterial fluid.
P-A Posteroanterior (= PA).
P&A Percussion and auscultation; Position and alignment.
$P_2 > A_2$ Pulmonic second heart sound greater than aortic second heart sound.
PA 105 Oleandomycin phosphate. The phosphate of an antimicrobial substance produced by the growth of Streptomyces antibioticus; active against a wide range of gram-positive bacteria.
PA 144 Mithramycin (see A 2371).
PA 248 Propicillin potassium (see BRL 284).
PAA Partial agonist/ antagonist activity; Passively acquired autoimmunity; Perianal area; Peripheral adrenergic activity; Phenylacetic/ Phosphonoacetic acid; Physical abilities analysis; Plasma angiotensinase activity; Plasminogen activator antigen; Platelet aggregation analysis; Polyacrylamide; Polyaminoacid; Potential/ Principal autoantigen; Pyridine acetic acid (see 3 PAA).
3 PAA 3-Pyridine acetic acid (= PAA).
PAA 701 Bialamicol hydrochloride (see CT 871).
$P(A\text{-}aDO_2)$ Alveolar-arterial oxygen tension difference (pulmonary function test) - see PFT - $P(A\text{-}aDO_2)$.
PAB Para-aminobenzoic acid (= Amben; Aminobenzoic acid; PABA; Pabacidum; Para-aminobenzoate; p-Aminobenzoic acid; Vitamin H'; $C_7H_7NO_2$). Is often included as a member of the vitamin-B group; was formerly used in the treatment of rickettsial infections (Tsutsugamushi disease), and topically as a sunburn cream (see Vitamins - Bx); Performance assessment battery; Peroneal artery bypass; Pes anserinus (Latin - "goose-foot") bursitis (Orthopedics); Pharmacologic autonomic block; Premature atrial beat(s); Pulmonary artery banding; Purple agar base.
PAb Specific antibody for Pemphigus.
PABA Para-aminobenzoic acid (see PAB).
PABD Peripheral adrenergic-blocking drug; Post-anoxic brain damage; Predeposit autologous blood donation.
PABE Post-antibiotic effect.
PABP Pulmonary artery balloon pump.
PAC Papular acrodermatitis of childhood/ children; Parent-adult-child; Phenacetin, aspirin, caffeine (medication orders/ prescriptions); Plasma albumin/ aldosterone concentration; Platelet-associated complement; Policy Advisory Committee; Political Action Committee; Portable air cleaner; Premature atrial/ auricular contraction; Primary auditory cortex; Pulmo-Aide compressor (De Vilbiss) - for nebulizer inhalation.
PACA Pancreatic acinar cell adenoma.
PACAB Port-Access coronary artery bypass.
PACC Pancreatic acinar cell carcinoma; Prospective Army Coronary Calcium (Study) (US).
pace pachytene.
PACE Pacing and Clinical Electrophysiology; Personal Assessment for Continuing Education; Personalized aerobics for cardiovascular enhancement; Pulmonary angiotensin I converting enzyme.
PACH Pipers to after coming head.
PA_{CO} Mean alveolar gas volume.
PA^{CO2}; PA_{CO2} Partial pressure/ tension of carbon dioxide in alveolar gas (see PFT - PA_{CO2}).
Pa^{CO2}; Pa_{CO2} Partial pressure/ tension of carbon dioxide in arterial blood (see PFT - Pa_{CO2}).
PACP Pulmonary alveolar-capillary permeability; Pulmonary artery counterpulsation.
PACS Picture archiving and communication system.
PACT Papillary carcinoma of thyroid; Periarticular connective tissue (Orthopedics); Precordial acceleration tracing.
PACU Post-anesthetic care unit; Post-operative anesthesia care unit.
PAC-V Platinum compd (cisplatin), Adriamycin (doxorubicin), and Cyclophosphamide (Vials).
PAD Parasite-associated diarrhea/ disease/ dysentery; Parenteral antineoplastic drug (see PAND); Percutaneous abscess drainage; Percutaneous automated discectomy; Peripheral arterial/ artery disease; Pharmacologically active dose/ drug; Phenacetin, aspirin, and desoxyephedrine;

Photon absorption densitometry; Physician-assisted death; Popliteal artery dilatation (Angioplasty); Portable assist device (artificial heart); Pre Aid to the Disabled; Primary affective disorder; Primary antibody deficiency; Prosthesis augmentation device (e.g. for prevention of recurrent hip dislocation); Psychoactive drug (e.g. lithium) (see CDT); Psychoaffective disorder; Public access defibrillation (see PADS); Pulmonary artery diastole; Pulsatile assist device.

PADP Pulmonary artery diastolic pressure.

PADR Pulmonary aerosol deposition rate.

PADS Public Access Defibrillation Study (NHLBI).

PADUA Progressive augmentation by dilating the urethra anterior.

PAE Peripheral arterial embolism; Persistent/ Potential/ Predominant/ Principal adverse effect(s)/ event(s) (= PAR); Post anoxic encephalopathy; Post-antibiotic era/ effect; Potentially additive effect; Pro-arrhythmic effect(s); Progressive assistive exercise; Psychiatric/ Pulmonary adverse event; Psychoactive effect.

P ae Equal/ In equal parts (L. partes aequales).

paed paediatric(s) (= pediatric/cs) (see Ped).

PAEDP Pulmonary artery end-diastolic pressure.

PAES Popliteal artery entrapment syndrome.

PAF Paroxysmal atrial (= PAFIB) / auricular fibrillation/ flutter; Paroxysmal atrial fibrillation Pathological auscultatory finding(s); Phosphodiesterase-activating factor; Pituitary-adrenal function; Platelet-activating/ -aggregating factor; Pollen adherence factor; Pre-adipocyte fibroblast; Premenstrual assessment form; Pulmonary arteriovenous fistula.

PA&F Percussion, auscultation, and fremitus.

PAF-A Platelet-activating factor of anaphylaxis.

PAFD Percutaneous abscess and fluid drainage; Pulmonary artery filling defect.

PAFI Platelet-aggregation factor inhibitor.

PAFIB Paroxysmal atrial fibrillation (see PAF).

PAFP Pre-Achilles fat pad.

PAG Periaqueductal gray (matter) (a pain control system, producing opioid peptides or endorphins, located in a tiny region of the center of the brain); Peripheral angiogram/graph(y); Phonoangiogram/graph(y); Polyacrylamide gel; Pregnancy-associated globulin/ $\alpha 2$-glycoprotein (an immunosuppressive protein); Protein Advisory Group (United Nations).

PA-G Physician's assistant - generalist.

pAg Protein A-gold (technique).

PAGA Prematurely appropriate for gestational age.

PAGE Polyacrylamide gel electrophoresis; Program for automatic gated evaluation (General Electric).

PAGIF Polyacrylamide gel isoelectric focusing.

PAGM Periaqueductal gray matter.

PAGMK Primary African green monkey kidney.

PAGP Pennsylvania Academy of General Practice.

pagus Greek suffix meaning "fastened" (as in Conjoined twins - CPT, IDT, OPT, PPT, TOPT, TPT, etc.) (Obstetrics).

PAH Para-aminohippurate/uric acid (see PAHA); Persistent asymptomatic hyponatremia (see AHH); Phenoxyacetate herbicide (weedkiller) (such as DCPA, MCPA, TCPA, Dichlorprop, Mecoprop, etc.); Phenylalanine hydroxylase; Polycyclic/ Polycystic aromatic hydrocarbon; Propylthiouracil-associated hepatotoxicity; Pulmonary artery hypertension/ hypotension.

pAH para-aminohippuric acid (see PAHA).

PAHA Para-aminohippuric acid (= Aminohippuric acid; N-p-Aminobenzoyl-aminoacetic acid; PAH; pAH; p-Aminobenzoylglycine; p-Aminohippuric acid; Para-aminohippurate). Used as a diagnostic agent to measure or test kidney function); Procainamide-hydroxylamine.

PAHD Penicillin-associated hepatic dysfunction.

PAHEF Pan American Health and Education Foundation.

PAHO Pan American Health Office/ Organization.

PAH sod Para-aminohippurate sodium.

PAHVC Pulmonary alveolar hypoxic vasoconstrictor.

PAI Passive-active immunization - with TIG(H) (see CAPI); Plasminogen activator inhibitor; Platelet accumulation index; Platelet aggregation inhibition (see IPA)/ impairment; Post-operative adynamic ileus.

PAIA Parents of Apneic Infants Association; Potential anti-inflammatory activity.

PAIA; Pα1A Peripheral α1 agonist (e.g. Midodrine).

PAIC Procedures, alternatives, indications, and complications.

PAIDS Paralyzed academic investigator's disease syndrome; Pediatric acquired immunodeficiency syndrome.

PAIgG Platelet-associated immunoglobulin G.

PAIRS Pain and Impairment Relationship Scale.

PAIS Partial androgen insensitivity syndrome; Phosphoribosylaminoimidazole synthetase.

PAI - type I Plasminogen-activator inhibitor type I (see TGF-β).

PAIVS Pulmonary atresia with intact ventricular septum.

PAJ Paralysis agitans juvenilis; Penicillin-associated jaundice.

PAL Paired-associate learning (how well new information is remembered); Papillary adenocystoma lymphomatosum (also called Adenolymphoma or Warthin's tumor); Pathology laboratory; Posterior axillary line; Procainamide level (toxicological test); Product of activated lymphocytes; Progressive bone loss; Pyogenic abscess of the liver.

pal palate.

PA level Procainamide level (toxicological test).

PaLine Pulmonary artery line.

PALN Para-aortic lymph node.

PALP Placental alkaline phosphatase.

palp palpable; palpate; palpation.

palpi; palpit palpitation(s).

PALS Parietolateral lymphocyte sheath; Patient Advocacy and Liaison Service (NHS, UK); Pediatric advanced life support; Physically active lifestyle; Prison-acquired lymphoproliferative syndrome.

PALSID Pernicious anemia-like syndrome and immunoglobulin deficiency.

PA-LS-ID See PALSID.

PALTA Plasma alanine aminotransferase activity.

PAL test Pathology laboratory test.

PAM Melphalan (see CB 3025); Pancreatic acinar mass; Parenteral antimicrobial (drug/ medicine/ therapy/ treatment etc.); Penicillin aluminium monostearate (= Procaine Penicillin G with 2% Aluminium Monostearate (suspension in oil) - used by I.M. injection as a long-acting penicillin; Perinatal Association of Michigan; Phagocyting alveolar macrophage; Phenylalanine mustard (= CB 3025; LPAM; L-PAM; Melphalan) - a nitrogen mustard derivative used in chemotherapy; P-methoxyamphetamine; Post-auricular myogenic; Posterior atlantoccipital membrane; Potential Acuity Meter; Practice/ Practitioner of alternative medicine (see AMP); Pralidoxime (Iodide) (= Pyridine-2-aldoxime methiodide; P-2-AM; 2-PAMI) - an antidote to poisoning with organic phosphate esters (insecticides) (see 2-FMPOI); Preconditioning adaption mechanism; Pregnancy-associated α-macroglobulin; Primary amebic meningoencephalitis (see PAME); Pro-asthmatic mediator(s) (= HMs - Humoral mediators or Spasmogens, released in the allergic and/or asthmatic reaction, from mast cells and eosinophils: 1. Bradykinin; 2. cAMP - Cyclic adenosine 3'-5'monophosphate; 3. cGMP - Cyclic guanosine monophosphate; 4. ECF-A - Eisinophil chemotactic factor of Anaphylaxis; 5. Histamine; 6. Kallikrein; 7. LTs - Leukotrienes (Cysteinyl leukotrienes [LTC4, LTD4, LTE4, etc.) - potent inflammatory eicosanoids; 8. NCF-A - Neutrophil chemotactic factor of Anaphylaxis; 9. PAF - Platelet activating factor; 10. PGs - Prostaglandins (F2α); 11. Serotonin; 12. SRS-A - Slow reacting substance of Anaphylaxis; 13. Tryptase); Pulmonary alveolar macrophage/ microlithiasis; Pulse amplitude modulation; Pyridine aldoxime methiodide (see above; 2-FMPOI).

2-PAM; P-2-AM Pralidoxime iodide (see 2-

FMPOI; 2-PAMI); 2-Pyridine aldoxime.

PAMA Pan American Medical Association.

PAMC Pterygo-arthro-myodysplasia congenita.

2-PAMCl Pralidoxime chloride (see 2-FMPOCl).

PAMD Primary adrenocortical micronodular dysplasia.

PAME Primary amebic meningoencephalitis (= PAM).

2-PAMI Pralidoxime iodide (see 2-FMPOI).

PAMIE Psychological and Medical Impairment of Function Evaluation.

2-PAMM Pralidoxime mesylate (see 2-FMPOMS).

PAMN Prampine methonitrate (= Propionyl atropine methyl nitrate; O-propionylatropine methonitrate). A parasympathetic and ganglion-blocking drug, reducing the volume and acidity of the gastric juice and decreasing the motility of the intestine. Used orally in the treatment of peptic ulcer, usually with the antacid magnesium trisilicate.

PAMP Pulmonary artery mean pressure.

PAMS Parents Advocating Morality Standards.

PAN Parenteral antineoplastic (see PAND); Periarteritis/ Polyarteritis nodosa; Periodic alternating nystagmus; Peroxyacetyl/ Peroxyacyl nitrate; Positional alcohol nystagmus; Puromycin aminonucleoside (= PANS).

pan pancreas/eatic/eatectomy.

Panama Red Marijuana (see Cannabis).

PAND Parenteral antineoplastic drug (= PAD; PAN); Primary adrenocortical nodular dysplasia.

PANE People Against Nuclear Energy.

Panendo Panendoscopy (procedure/ gastroenterology).

PANESS Physical and neurological examination for soft signs.

PANO Propofol/ Alfentanil/ Nitrous oxide (General anesthesia).

PANS Puromycin aminonucleoside (see PAN).

PANSS Positive and Negative Syndrome Scale.

Pansy Homosexual (see Homo).

PAO Peak acid output; Peripheral airway obstruction; Phenylarsine oxide; Plasma amine/ Polyamine oxidase; Psychiatric admitting office; Pustulotic arthro-osteitis.

PAo Airway opening pressure; Ascending aortic pressure; Pulmonary artery occlusion pressure.

PAO_2; PA_{O2}; P_{AO2} Partial alveolar oxygen (pressure/ tension) (= partial pressure of oxygen in alveolar gas (see PFT).

PaO_2; PaO_2; Pa_{O2} Partial arterial oxygen (pressure/ tension) (= partial pressure of oxygen in arterial blood (see PFT).

PAOD Peripheral arterial/teriosclerotic obstructive/ occlusive disease (see POAD); Pulmonary arterio-occlusive disease.

PAOO Pennsylvania Academy of Ophthalmology and Otolaryngology.

PAOP Pulmonary artery occlusion pressure.

PAP Meiklejohn-Eaton-Liu virus; Papanicolaou (smear/ test) (see Pap); Papaverine (see Papaver); Partial agonist/ antagonist profile (of a drug); Passive-aggressive personality; Patient assessment program; Peak/ Positive airway pressure; Perianal pain/ pruritis; Peroxidase antibody to peroxidase; Peroxidase-antiperoxidase (method); Phenolphthalein and paraffin (emulsion); Phosphoadenosine phosphate; Physician Augmentation Program; Physician's Assistant Program; Physiological ageing process; Placental acid/ alkaline phosphatase; Premenopausal anovulatory patient; Primary angioplasty procedure; Primary atypical pneumonia; Professional Assessment Program; Progressive ascending paralysis; Prostatic acid phophatase; Pseudoallergic reaction; Pulmonary alveolar proteinosis; Pulmonary arterial/ artery pressure (= Ppa); Purified alternate pathway.

PAR Persistent/ Predominant/ Principal adverse reaction(s) (see PAE); Plasma active renin; Procedures, alternatives and risks; Pseudo-allergic reaction.

Pap Papanicolaou (Dr. George N. Papanicolaou smear/ test for cancer - procedure/ gynecology) (= PAP).

pap papilla.

Papaver A genus of plants of the Poppy family, Papaveraceae. One of the species is the Opium poppy plant, P. somniferum, from the dried latex of which is obtained opium. This is a potent narcotic containing the alkaloids morphine, codeine, papaverine, narceine, noscapine, and theibane. Opium has other names, such as: Army disease; Black pill; Black stuff; Block; Brown stuff; Can (morphine); C&M (cocaine and morphine mixture); Dilaudid (dihydromorphinone hydrochloride); EX-10-029 (Dihydromorphine derivative); God's medicine (morphine); Gow; Gum (raw opium); HMC (heroin, morphine, and cocaine); Hop; Mary (morphine); Mash Allah (opium); M&C (morphine and cocaine); Metopon (methyldihydromorphinone); Mojo (morphine, heroine, or cocaine); Morph; MS (morphine sulfate); O; O&B (opium and belladonna); Op; Opium Crudum (crude opium/ opium crude); PAP (papaverine); Raw opium (= Gum); Tar (gum opium); Yerli (a fine quality of Turkish opium).

PAPF Platelet adhesiveness plasma factor.

papova papilloma-polyoma-vacuolating agent (virus).

PAPP Para-aminopropiophenone; Pregnancy-associated plasma protein.

PAPPC Pregnancy-associated plasma protein C.

PAPS 3'phosphoadenosine-5'-phosphosulfate.

Paps Papillomas.

PA/PS Pulmonary atresia/pulmonary stenosis.

Pap sm Papanicolaou smear (see Pap).

PAPUFA Physiologically active polyunsaturated fatty acid.

pa-pv pulmonary arterial (pressure) - pulmonary venous (pressure).

PAPVC Partial anomalous pulmonary venous connection.

PAPVR Partial anomalous pulmonary venous return.

PAPW Posterior aspect of the pharyngeal wall.

PAQ Personal Attitudes Questionnaire.

PAR Passive avoidance reaction; Perennial allergic rhinitis; Peripheral arterial resistance; Photosynthetically active radiation; Physiological aging rate; Platelet aggregate ratio; Post-anesthesia/thetic recovery/ room; Product Analytical Review; Program for Alcohol(ic) Recovery; Proximal absolute reabsorption (e.g. of water); Pulmonary arteriolar resistance.

par paraffin; parallel; paralysis.

PARA; Para; para To bring forth/ To bear (L. parere). The number of pregnancies producing viable offspring: *P*. number of pregnancies; *A*. number of abortions (or miscarriages); *RA*. number of living children. *para 0*. nullipara (having borne no children). *para I*. unipara/ primipara (having borne one child). *para II*. bipara/ secundipara (having borne two children). *para III*. tripara (having borne three children). *para IV*. quadripara/ quartipara (having borne four children). *para V*. quintipara (having borne five children). *para x*. the number designates the number of pregnancies that have resulted in the birth of viable offspring. It is not indicative of the number of children produced in the event of a multiple birth or births.

para paraplegic; parathyroid(ectomy).

Paranoia A psychotic personality disorder characterized by delusions of persecution and grandeur: Acute hallucinatory paranoia, in which hallucinations are added to delusions; alcoholic paranoia, developing in chronic alcoholism; Paranoia Hallucinatoria (L.) - acute hallucinatory paranoia; heboid paranoia, with prominent schizoid features: dementia paranoides, or the paranoid form of dementia praecox; litigous paranoia, with compulsion for litigation for any imagined cause; Paranoia Originaria (L.), found in children; querulous paranoia, associated with querulousness; Paranoia Simplex (L.), in which the delusions are related to the actual perceptions of the patient.

parasit parasite/tic/tology.

parasym parasympathetic.

PARC Perennial/ Prolonged allergic rhinoconjunctivitis.

PAR Cost Prescriptions at Reasonable Cost (Canada).

parent parenteral(ly).

PARF Post-anesthetic respiratory failure.

PARIS Persantin (Dipyridamole) - Aspirin Reinfarction Study (see RA8).

parkin gene The parkin gene - a gene in

which mutation, results in both sporadic and familial, autosomal, recessive Parkinson's disease (see ADPD; ARFPD; ARPD; EOPD; FPD; IPD; JOPD; LBs; PRD).

PAROM Passive assistance range of motion.

parox paroxysm(al).

PARR Post-anesthesia recovery room.

PARS Personal Adjustment and Roll Skills (Scale); Plastic and Reconstructive Surgery (= PRS).

pars aff the part affected (L. pars affecta).

part aeq equal parts (L. partes aequales).

part dolent painful parts (L. partes dolentes).

Partial agonist A ligand which has both agonist and antagonist properties (see Agonist; Antagonist; Ligand).

part vic in divided doses (L. partitis vicibus).

PARU Post-anesthetic recovery unit.

parv small (L. parvus).

PAS Para-aminosalicylic acid (= Aminosalicylic Acid; 4-Aminosalicylic acid; Aminosalylum; Para aminosalicylate; PASA; Pasalicylum; 4-Amino-2-hydroxybenzoic acid; $C_7H_7NO_3$). A salicylic acid derivative used as a bacteriostatic agent in the treatment of various forms of tuberculosis; Parent Attitude Scale; Patient absorbed serum; Patient appointments and scheduling; Patient's Aid Society; Pediatric Academic Societies (San Francisco, US); Pehr abduction splint (pronounced "Pier"); Periodic acid-Schiff (reaction/ stain/ technique) (see PAS technique); Peripheral anterior synechia; Peripheral appendicular skeleton (Orthopedics); Persistent atrial standstill; Personality Assessment Scale; Personality Assessment Schedule; Phobic anxiety state; Photo-acoustic spectroscopy; Phosphatase acid serum; Physician-assisted suicide; Physicians for Automobile Safety; Pneumatic antiembolic stocking; Polyethylene acetabular socket (see CAS); Post-anesthesia score; Posterior airway space; Precategorical acoustic storage; Precerebral artery stenosis; Pregnancy advisory service; Premature aging syndrome; Premature atrial stimulus/ systole; Problem Appraisal Scale; Professional Activity Study; Progressive accumulated stress; Pseudoachievement syndrome; Psychiatric Assessment Scale (see BPRS); Pulmonary arterial stenosis; Pulmonary artery systolic.

Pas Pascal-second.

PA-S Physician's assistant - specialist.

Pa x s Pascals per second.

PASA Para-aminosalicylic acid (see PAS); Primary acquired sideroblastic anemia; Proximal articular set angle.

PASAT Paced Auditory Serial Addition Task.

PAS-C Para-aminosalicylic acid (purified and crystallized with) vitamin C (ascorbic acid).

PASD After diastase digestion.

p'ase phosphatase (acid/ alkaline) (= p'tase).

PasEx Passive exercise.

PASG Pneumatic antishock garment.

PASH Periodic acid-Schiff hematoxylin (see PAS technique).

PASI Psoriasis area and severity index.

PASM Periodic acid-silver methenamine.

PASP Pulmonary artery systolic pressure.

pass passive.

PAS Sodique (Fr.) Sodium aminosalicylate (= Aminosalicylnatrium; Sodium PAS) - used, as in PAS, in the treatment of tuberculosis.

PAS stain Periodic acid-Schiff stain (see PAS technique).

PAST Periodic acid-Schiff technique (see PAS technique).

Past Pasteurella.

PAS technique Periodic acid-Schiff technique (a staining technique for histologic sections, e.g. for the detection of mucins in mucin-containing cancer cells).

PASVR Pulmonary anomalous superior venous return.

PAT Pain Apperception Test; Parents as Teachers (parent-education program, parenting and child development); Paroxysmal atrial tachycardia; Past/ Premature/ Previous/ Prolonged antibiotic therapy; Patient (see pt); Penetrating abdominal trauma (see PAW); Percent acceleration time; Periarteriolar transudate; Periarticular tissue; Peripheral arterial thrombosis (e.g. traumatic); Peripheral arteriolar tone; Phenylaminotetrazole; Physical abilities test; Picric acid turbidity; Platelet aggregation test; Polyamine acetyltransferase; Pre-admission assessment team/ test; Pre-admission testing; Predictive ability test; Pregnancy at term; Premature atrial tachycardia (see SVT); Psychoacoustic test; Pulmonary-artery tracing.

Pat; pat Patella; Patent; Paternal (origin); Patient (see pt).

PATCO Professional Air Traffic Controllers Organization.

PATE Psychodynamic and therapeutic education; Pulmonary artery thrombo-embolism.

PATH Pathological/gy (see Path); Pituitary adrenotropic hormone.

Path; path Pathogenesis/nic; Pathological/gy (= PATH; Pth).

PAT_m Maximal tubular excretory capacity for para-aminohippuric acid (PAH).

Pat med Patent medicine.

PAT-SED Pseudoachondroplastic dysplasia.

PA-T-SP Periodic acid - thiocarbohydrazide - silver proteinate.

PAU Post-approval use.

PAUSE Parents Against Unauthorized Sex Education.

PAV Pavulon; Percutaneous aortic valvuloplasty; Poikiloderma atrophicans vasculare; Posterior arch vein.

PAVC Partial atrioventricular canal.

pavex passive vascular exercise.

PAVF; PA-VF Pulmonary arteriovenous fistula.

PAVNRT Paroxysmal atrioventricular nodal reciprocal tachycardia.

PAW Penetrating abdominal wound (= PAT); Perianal wart (see EGW); Peripheral airways; Pulmonary arterial/ artery wedge.

Paw Mean airway pressure.

PAWP Pulmonary arterial/ artery wedge pressure (= Ppaw).

PAWS Primary withdrawal syndrome.

PB Blood pressure (see BP); Paradoxical bronchospasm; Paraffin bath; Paul-Bunnel (antibody/ test) (see P-B); Periodic/ Pressure breathing; Peripheral blood; Peroneus brevis (muscle); Pharmacopoeia Brittanica: British Pharmacopia (= Ph B); Phenobarbital (see Pb); Phenoxybenzamine; Phonetically/ Pressure balanced; Pinealoblastoma; Placental barrier; Polymyxin B (on culture and sensitivity reports); Powder board; Power building; Premature beat; Probiotic (a beneficial bacterium such as the *Lactobacillus*, found in the lower intestine and used in the treatment of diarrhea of adults and infants); 'Probiotic' (a species of friendly bacteria such as the *Lactobacillus*, found in the normal intestinal tract. Familiar sources include buttermilk, fermented cheese, cultured milk [kefir], fermented soybeans [miso], yoghurt, etc. The probiotics thrive on non-digested sugar foods known as prebiotics) (see BFB; FOS); Protein binding/-bound; Prussian Blue (see FHCF); Punch biopsy.

Pb Lead (L. plumbum) (Z = 82) (see Elements - Lead); Phenobarbital (= PB; pb); Presbyopia (eye examination).

pb phenobarbital (see Pb).

P-B Paul-Bunnel (test) - for infectious mononucleosis (= PB; PBT).

P&B Pain and burning; Phenobarbital and belladonna.

^{210}Pb Radioactive lead.

PBA Percutaneous bladder aspiration; Polyclonal B-cell activity; Polymer bonding agent (Dentistry); Pressure breathing assist(er); Problem-based approach (= POA); Prolactin-binding assay; Protein-binding affinity; Prune belly anomaly (= PBS); Pulpobuccoaxial.

PBB Peter Brent Brigham (Hospital) (see PBBH); Polybrominated biphenyl.

Pb-B Lead (level) in blood.

PBBB Parrot beak basket biter (arthroscopy).

PBBH Peter Brent Brigham Hospital (Boston, Massachusetts).

PBBs Polybrominated biphenyls.

PBC Peak blood concentration (see PDC); Peripheral blood cell/ count (see PBCC); Phalangeal bone cyst; Physio-biochemical challenge; Plasma bilirubin concentration; Platinum-based chemotherapy; Point of basal convergence; Prebed care; Primary biliary cirrhosis; Primary brain/ breast cancer; Progestin-binding complement; Protease-based combination (of drugs) (see PIBCT).

PBCA Priority-based clinical approach.

PBCC Peripheral blood cell count (= PBC).

$Pb(C_2H_3O_2)_2$ Lead acetate.

$PbCO_3$ Lead carbonate.

$PbCrO_4$ Lead chromate.

PBCS Population-based cohort study.

PBCs Packed blood cells (Blood transfusion); Pregnancy and birth complications.

PBD Paget's bone disease; Pancreatic and biliary disorder(s); Paucibacillary disease (as in leprosy); Percutaneous biliary drainage; Permanent brain damage; Photo(n) beam densitometer/metry (Estrogen receptor study); Pigeon breeder's disease (a breathing disorder or allergic alveolitis caused by allergic material in bird droppings. Also called BBL or Bird breeder's lung, HWL or Hen worker's lung, and PBL or Pigeon breeder's lung. Other kinds of allergic alveolitis include Anthracosis, Asbestosis, Bagassosis, Farmer's lung, Pneumoconiosis with the inhalation of various mineral dusts, Silicosis, etc.); Piggyback device (see PBH); Platinum-based drug; Postburn day; Primary bowel disease/ disorder; Protein-based debris (such as Amyloid); Protein-binding displacement; Protein bound drug.

PBE Partial breech extraction; Peripheral blood eosinophil(s); Perlsucht Bacillen-Emulsion (Ger) - tuberculin prepared from a culture of bovine tuberculosis bacilli (Mycobacterium tuberculosis bovis); Phage-borne epitope; Plant-based estrogen (as a natural-based remedy in HRT, found in black cohosh, soy products, wild yams and other vegetables); Previous bacterial endocarditis.

PBF Peripheral/ Placental/ Pulmonary blood flow.

PBF; +veBF Positive biopsy finding(s).

PBFe Protein-bound iron.

PBG Pedicle bone graft (Orthopedics); Plasmid-borne gene; Porphobilinogen (laboratory/ chemistry).

PBGC Post/Preprandial blood glucose concentration (see FPGC; PPGC).

PBG-D Porphobilinogen deaminase.

PBG-S Porphobilinogen synthase.

PBH Piggyback heart (= VAD or Ventricular assist device); Plant-based hormone (see PBE); Pulling both hands.

PBHb Polymerized bovine hemoglobin.

PBHB Poly-beta-hydroxybutyrate; Postbirth human being.

PBI Parental bonding instrument; Patient's/nts' best interest(s); Penile-brachial (pressure/ pulse) index (see PBPI); Phenformin (see DBI; PEDG); Protein-bound iodine (laboratory/ endocrinology) (= PBJ; SPBI); Puerperal breast infection.

$PB^{127}I$ Protein-bound radioactive iodine.

PbI Lead intoxication.

PbI_2 Lead iodide.

PBIgG Platelet surface bound immunoglobulin G.

PBJ Protein-bound iodine (see PBI).

PBK Phosphorylase B kinase; Pseudophakic bullous keratopathy.

PBL Paucibacillary leprosy (the milder form of Leprosy with fewer than six skin patches, and cured within six months with the same antibiotics as those employed in the multibacillary form of the malady see MBL); Peak blood level; Peripheral blood leukocyte/ lymphocyte; Pigeon breeder's lung (see PBD); Primary breast lymphoma; Problem-based learning (approach/ curriculum / seminar / student) (see PBLDC); Progressive bone loss.

PBLC Peripheral blood lymphocyte count.

PBLDC Problem-based-learning-dependent curriculum.

PBLN Peribronchial lymph node (Hilar, Interlobar, Lobar, and Segmental lymph nodes).

PBLT Peripheral blood lymphocyte count transformation.

PBM Peak bone mass; Periacinar/ Peripheral/ Placental basement membrane; Peripheral blood mononuclear (cell).

PBMC Peripheral blood mononuclear cell.

PBMD Particulate bone matrix derivative (Orthopedics); Psychosis, Bipolar, and Mood Disorder.

PBMNC Peripheral blood mononuclear cell (= PBMC).

PBMT Postbone-marrow transplant.

PBMV Pulmonary blood mixing volume.

PBN Paralytic brachial neuritis; Peripheral benign neoplasm; Pleural biopsy needle; Polymyxin (B sulfate), bacitracin, and neomycin.

PBNA Partial body neutron activation.

$Pb(NO_3)_2$ Lead nitrate.

PBO Partial biliary obstruction; Penicillin in beeswax and oil; Placebo (see pbo).
PbO Lead monoxide.
Pbo Placebo (= PBO; pbo).
pbo placebo (= PBO).
PbO_2 Lead dioxide.
PBP Penicillin-/ Prostate-binding protein; Porphyrin biosynthesis pathway; Postbulbar palsy (see BPM); Progressive bulbar palsy; Pseudobulbar palsy; Psychomotor behavior pattern/ performance; Pulsatile bypass pump.
PBPC Peripheral blood progenitor cell.
PBPI Penile-brachial pressure/ pulse index (= PBI).
PBR Periosteal bone repair (see EPBR); Population-based research; Progressive/ Prolonged/ Pronounced/ Protractive bone resorption; Prolonged bed rest.
PBS Paradoxical bronchospasm; Pennsylvania Blue Shield; Perfusion-pressure breakthrough syndrome; Periosteal/ Peripheral blood supply; Peripheral blood smear; Phenobarbital sodium; Phosphate-buffered saline; Physically/ Potentially/ Psychologically burdening situation; Planar bone scan; Population-based study; Preclinical bridging study (see PCBS); Predose blood sample; Premature beats; Primer binding site; Prune belly syndrome (see PBA); Public Broadcasting System; Pulmonary branch stenosis.
PBs Pick's bodies (see PD - Pick's disease).
PbS Lead sulfide.
PBSC Penicillin, bacitracin, streptomycin, caprylate (sodium) (a polyantibiotic paste/ Proprietary drug); Peripheral-blood stem-cell (see APBSCT).
PBSCR Peripheral-blood stem-cell rescue.
PBSCT Peripheral-blood stem-cell transplantation (see APBSCT; PBSC).
PBSN Penicillin, bacitracin, streptomycin, nystatin (polyantibiotic paste/ Proprietary drug).
$PbSO_4$ Lead sulfate.
PBSP Prognostically bad signs during pregnancy.
PBT Paul-Bunnel test (see P-B); Phenacetin breath test; Primary brain tumor; Profile-based therapy.
PBT_4 Protein-bound thyroxine.
PB (test); P-B (test) Paul-Bunnel (test) (see P-B).
PBU Primary bone union (Orthopedics).
PBV Percutaneous balloon valvuloplasty; Predicted/ Pulmonary blood volume; Patent Blue V (= Sulphan Blue; Sulphanum Caeruleum; Blue VRS; CI Food Blue 3; Color Index No: 42045) - a coloring agent for medicines and foodstuffs, little affected by variations in pH. Also used as a contrast coloring agent in lymphangiography, and to visualize the state of the circulation in normal and damaged tissues in assessing tissue viability in burns and soft tissue injuries; Plant/ Protein -based vaccine; Premature beat, ventricular (see PVB).
PBW Posterior bite wing; Predicted body weight.
PBZ Personal breathing zone; Phenoxybenzamine; Phenylbutazone; Pyribenzamine.
ΦBZ Phenylbutazone (= PBZ).
PC After food (L post cibum) (see pc); Avoirdupois weight (L. pondus civile); Pachyonychia congenita (an autosomal dominant, hereditary hypotrichosis with thickening of nail bed from birth, pronounced transverse curvature of the nails, palmoplantar keratoderma and leukoplakia); Packed cells; Palliative care; Paper chromatography; Para/ Piriform/ Posterior cortex; Parent/ Peritoneal/ Purkinje cell; Parent to child; Paroxysmal choreoathetosis (= PD - Paroxysmal dystonia); Particulate component; Partition coefficient; Patient compliance/ convenience (see PCC); Peak clipping (for limiting the output of hearing instruments); Pectoral; Penicillin (see Pen); Pentose/ Phosphate cycle; Personal computer; Pharmacology (see pharm); Pheochromocytoma (see PCC); Phosphatidylcholine; Phosphocreatine; Phosphorylcholine; Photocoagulation (by laser); Photoconduction; Physicians' corporation; Picture completion (psychology); Pill counter; Placebo-controlled (procedure/ study/ trial) (= P-C); Plasma concentration/ cortisol; Plasmacytoma; Plasmin complex; Platelet concentrate/ation/ count;

Pneumocystis carinii; Pneumotaxic center; Polar count (assay of urinary creatinine); Polycentric; Polyposis coli; Poor condition/ coordination; Popliteal cyst; Portacaval (anastomosis/ bypass/ shunt/ transposition); Portal cirrhosis; Postcoital; Posterior cervical/ chamber/ commissure; Postnatal/ Prenatal care; Precordial; Present complaint/ condition; Pressure-controlled; Primary closure; Printed circuit; Procollagen; Productive cough; Professional Corporation (physician); Prostatic carcinoma; Protein C; Provocation concentration (see PFT - PC); Proximal colon; Pseudocyesis; Pseudocyst; Pubococcygeus (muscle) (see PCG); Pulmonary capillary (wedge pressure) (see PCWP)/ circulation/ closure/ collapse/ congestion/ contusion; Pyloric canal; Pyruvate carboxylase.

P-C Placebo-controlled (see PC).

Pc Convergence near point (see PcB).

pC picocurie (see pc).

pc after food/ meals (L. post cibum) (= PC; post cib); parsec; percent (= pct; %); picocurie (= pC; 10^{-12} curie; ììc; micromicrocurie) - a unit of radioactivity, being the quantity of radioactive material in which the number of nuclear disintegrations is 3.7 x 10^{-2}, or 0.037, per second.

pc1 Platelet count (pretransfusion).

pc2 Platelet count (posttransfusion).

PC III Procollagen III (peptide) - a precursor of collagen synthesis.

PC4 Periscopic convex.

PCA Para-chloramphetamine; Parietal cell antibody; Passive cutaneous anaphylactic (reaction/ test)/ anaphylaxis; Patient care aide/ assistant/ audit; Patient-controlled analgesia; Perchloric acid; Percutaneous absorption/ application/ carotide/ coronary angioplasty; Peripheral conduit artery; Photocarcinogenicity assay; Photocontact allergic (reaction); Plasma catecholamine concentration; Polyclonal antibody; Porous coated anatomic (prosthesis); Portacaval anastomosis (operation/ liver) (= PCB; PCS; PCT); Postconceptional age; Posterior cerebral/ communicating artery; Posterior communicating aneurysm; Posterior cricoarytenoid; Potent chemotherapeutic agent (see PCD; PCT); Precoronary care area; President's Council on Aging; Primary cardiac arrest; Primary coronary angioplasty; Principal components analysis; Procainamide; Procoagulant activity; Progressive cerebellar ataxia (telangiectasia) (see AT); Prolonged central apnea; Prostatic cancer antigen (test); Prostatic carcinoma; Pyrrolidine carboxylic acid.

PCAA Porous-coated anatomic arthroplasty (see PCAI).

PCAC Per capita alcohol consumption.

PCAI Porous-coated anatomic implant (= PCAT).

PCB Pancuronium bromide; Paracervical block (procedure/ anesthesiology); Polychlorinated biphenyl (see PCBs); Poor cognitive behavior; Portacaval bypass (see PC; PCA); Pregnancy Category B; Prepared childbirth; Procarbazine (see PCZ); Protan color-blindness.

PcB Near point of convergence to the intercentral base line (L. punctum convergens basalis) (eye examination).

PCBA Plasma chain-breaking antioxidant.

PCBG Pig-cell brain graft (see PCT; POT).

PCBH Polychlorinated biphenyl hydrocarbon (see PCBs).

PC-BMP Phosphorylcholine - binding myeloma protein.

PCBS Preclinical bridging study (= PBS).

PCBs Polychlorinated biphenyls - petrochemicals; serious chemical contaminants of the environment in industry.

PCC Palliative care center (see PCS; PCU); Pasteur Culture Collection; Patient-care community; Patient convenience and compliance; Patient's current condition; Per capita consumption (see PCAC); Percutaneous cecostomy; Pericardiocentesis; Peterson cervical collar; Pheochromocytoma (= PC; Pheo); Phosphate carrier compound; Placental choriocarcinoma; Plasma catecholamine/ creatinine concentration; Platinum-containing compound (Chemotherapy); Platinum coordination complex(es) (chemotherapy); Pneumatosis cystoides coli; Poison Control Center (= PCIC); Postcentral cortex; Pre-conception/ Precoronary care; Pregnancy Category C; Premature chromosome condensation (= pcc); Primary Care Center/ Centre (UK); Primary care career/ clinic; Professional Conduct Committee; Prothrombin complex concentration; Physicochemical characteristic(s).

PCc Periscopic concave (eye examination).

pcc premature chromosome condensation (see PCC).

PCCC Pediatric critical care center.

PCCP Posterior-cruciate condylar prosthesis (Howmedica); Prostate Cancer Chemoprevention (trial).

PCCS Placebo-controlled clinical study (see PCCT; PCS; PCT).

PCCT Placebo-controlled clinical trial (= PCDRFS; PCS; PCT).

PCCU Postcoronary care unit.

PCD Papillary collecting duct; Paraneoplastic cerebellar degeneration; Paroxysmal cerebral dysrhythmia; Pediatric cardiology department; Phosphate-citrate-dextrose; Planned cesarian delivery (see ECD) (Obstetrics); Plasma cell dyscrasia; Polycystic disease; Poorly controlled diabetes; Posterior corneal deposits; Postmortem cesarean delivery; Potent chemotherapeutic dose/ drug (see PCA;PCT); Precancerous dermatitis (see IEC); Preclinical data; Prefrontal cortex damage (see PFCD); Premature centromere division; Premature cervical dilatation (Obstetrics); Primary-care doctor (= Family doctor; PCP); Primary ciliary dyskinesia; Programmed cell death (= Apoptosis); Progressive cartilage destruction; Prolonged contractile duration; Pulmonary clearance delay; Pyramidal cell discharge (neuron discharge - CNS).

PCDC Plasma clot diffusion chamber.

PCDF Polychlorinated dibenzofuran.

PCDK Polycystic disease of the kidney.

PCDRFS Placebo-controlled dose-range finding study (see PCCT).

PCDS Pediatric Care Delivery System (Kaiser-Permanente Medical Center).

PCE Erythromycin particles in tablets; Pericardiectomy; Physical capacity evaluation; Placebo-controlled evaluation; Plasma-cell endometritis; Positive cumulative effect; Primary care education; Protein-cutting enzyme (= Protease) - a family of such intracellular enzymes or proteases is called a Caspase, an enzyme responsible for cell destruction or apoptosis (see PCD; PCS); Pseudocholinesterase (= PCHE).

PCEC Purified chick embryo cell (vaccine) (a rabies v.).

PCET Pivotal clinical efficacy trial.

PCF Pancreatic cutaneous fistula; Pericentral fibrosis (see PVF); Peripheral circulatory failure; Pharyngoconjunctival fever; Plasma clotting/ converting factor (see Factor V); Platelet complement fixation; Posterior cranial fossa; Progressive cardiac failure (see PHF); Prothrombin conversion factor (see Factor V).

pcf pounds per cubic foot.

$PC_{20\text{-}FEV1}$ Provocation concentration producing a 20% reduction in forced expiratory volume (FEV1) (see PFT - $PC_{20\text{-}FEV1}$).

PCFO Pancreatic cutaneous fistula output.

PCFS Pacific Coast Fertility Society.

PCFT Platelet complement fixation test.

PCG Paracervical ganglion; Pharmacogenomics (a compound form of "omic" research in the Human Genome Project, beginning with Genomics and including CHOmics [for carbohydrates], Clinomics, Functional/compound genomics, Immunomics, Kinomics [for the kinases in aggregate], Metabolomics, Pharmacomethylomics, Proteomics, Structural/compound genomics, Toxicomics, etc.); Phono-/ Pneumocardiogram; Placebo/ Positive control group; Primate chorionic gonadotropin; Pubococcygeus (muscle) (= PC).

PCGG Percutaneous coagulation of gasserian ganglion.

PCH Paroxysmal cold hemoglobinuria; Polycyclic hydrocarbon; Primary Children's Hospital (Utah).

P-Ch Portico-cholecystostomy (hepatic).

PCHE Pseudocholinesterase (see PCE).

PCHGA Phenylcyclohexylglycolic acid (a pharmacologically inactive metabolic product of the antispasmodic, anticholinergic agent,

Oxybutinin) (see DOB).

PCHPE Pacific Center for Health Policy and Ethics (USC).

PCHR Porous-coated hip replacement.

PC&HS After meals (L. post cibum) and at bedtime (L. hora somnis).

PCI Peptide chain initiation; Percutaneous cardiovascular/ coronary intervention; Physician-computer interaction; Plasma-cell infiltration; Plastic corneal implant (= Intac); *Pneumocystis* carinii infection (a RMD - Resistance mechanism disorder, frequently affecting patients with AIDS); Porous-coated implant (Orthopedics); Pneumatosis cystoides intestinales; Preconception intervention (e.g. in pregestational diabetes) (= PPI); Prophylactic cranial irradiation; Prothrombin consumption index

pCi picocurie (10^{-12} curie) (see pc).

PCIC Poison Control Information Center (see PCC).

PCIOL Posterior chamber intraocular lens.

PCIOLI Posterior chamber intraocular lens implant (= PCLI).

PCIP Pneumocapillary infusion pump (EMS).

PC-IRV Pressure-controlled - inverted ratio ventilation.

PCIS Patient-Care Information System; Postcardiac injury syndrome.

PCK Polycystic kidney.

PCKD Polycystic kidney disease.

PCKS Porous Coated Knee System (Microloc - see OI/OP).

PCL Pacing cycle length; Persistent corpus luteum; Plasma cell leukemia; Posterior chamber lens; Posterior cruciate ligament; Pubococcygeal line.

PCLI Posterior chamber lens implant (see PCIOLI).

PCLN Posterior cervical lymph node.

PCM Paracetamol (Trade name for); Pelvicalyceal measurement(s see RPCM); Permanent Commission on Medicine (EEC - European Economic Council); Phase-contrast microscope; Plasma-cell myeloma; Primary cutaneous melanoma; Process control monitor; Prostate cancer mortality; Protein-calorie malnutrition; Protein carboxymethylase.

PCMC Chlorocresol (= Parachlorometacresol) - a chlorinated phenol; a potent bactericide with low toxicity, used in the process of sterilization of surgical instruments, and as a preservative in creams and other preparations for external use.

PCMCS Placebo-controlled multicenter study.

PCMO Principal Clinical/ Colonial (Britain) Medical Officer.

PCMT Pacemaker circus movement tachycardia.

PCMX Chloroxylenol (= Parachlorometaxylenol) - a chlorinated phenol; a potent non-irritant bactericide of low toxicity, used as an antiseptic for the skin in surgery and obstetrics.

PCN Palliative care need(s); Penicillin (see Pen); Percutaneous nephroscope/opy/ nephrostomy; Potts-Cournand needle (Angiography); Primary care nursing.

PCNA Pediatric Cardiology Nurse Associate; Proliferating cell nuclear antigen.

PCNB Pentachloronitrobenzene.

PCNL Percutaneous nephrolithotomy/tripsy (= PNL)/ nephrostolithotomy; Plantar calcaneonavicular ligament (= Spring ligament).

PCNS Penicillins.

PCNV Postchemotherapy nausea and vomiting; Provisional Committee on Nomenclature of Viruses.

PCO Patient complaints of; Polycystic ovary; Predicted cardiac output; Primary care orientation (see PCOS); Procytoxid.

P_{CO} Partial pressure of carbon monoxide (in alveolar gas/ arterial blood) (see PFT - P_{CO}).

P_{CO2}; pCO_2 Partial pressure of carbon dioxide (in alveolar gas/ arterial blood) (see PFT - pCO_2).

$\uparrow pCO_2$ Hypercapnia (respiratory acidosis) (see PFT - $\uparrow pCO_2$).

PCOB Permanent Central Opium Board (Geneva).

PCOD Polycystic ovarian disease.

PCO (disease/ syndrome) Polycystic ovarian (disease/ syndrome).

PCOS Placebo-controlled obesity study; Polycystic ovarian syndrome; Primary care-oriented system.

PCP Palpable carotid pulse; Pancytopenia; Para-chlorophenate; Para-chlorophenylalanine (see PCPA); Parvocellular/ (P) pathway (the slower light transmission awareness/ response to a moving object) (see MCP, LED); Patient care plan; Peace pill; Pediatric cerebral palsy; Pentachlorophenol (= Penta) - a chlorinated phenol, used industrially as a preservative for wood, jute sacks, glues and starch; 1-(1-Phenylcyclohexyl)piperidine; Periodic/ Persistent chest pain; Peripheral coronary pressure; Persistent cough and phlegm; Phencyclidine (hydrochloride) (see Hog); Physical-chemical properties/ty; Physiologic cardiac pacing (atrial/ dual - chamber); Pinky compression procedure (used in lens implant surgery); Plasma cell pneumonia, also called Pneumocystis carinii pneumonia (the disease caused by a protozoan organism of plasma cell pneumonia); Plasma concentration profile; Porous-coated prosthesis; Post-operative constrictive pericarditis; Precancerous polyp; Preclinical pharmacology/ phase; Primary care person/ physician/ practice; Primary chest pain; Prochlorperazine; Procollagen peptide; Progressive chronic polyarthritis; Psychotrophic (activity); Pulmonary capillary permeability/ pressure; Pulse cytophotometry.

PCPA Para-chlorophenylalanine (= PCP); Primary care physician's assistant.

PCPL Pulmonary capillary protein leakage.

pcpn perception; precipitation (see pcpt).

PCPP Posterior canal plugging procedure (in the surgical treatment of positional vertigo).

PCPT Prostate Cancer Prevention Trial (NCI).

pcpt perception; precipitation (see pcpn).

PCQ Polychloroquaterphenyl.

PCR Patient contact record; Percutaneous coronary revascularization; Percutaneous revascularization (heart); Phosphocreatine/tinine (see PCr); Photocoagulation of the retina (with the argon laser); Plasma clearance rate; Platinum-containing regimen (see PCT); Polymerase chain reaction - a gene amplification technology, used in gene identification or genetic "fingerprinting" (e.g. mother's blood analysis for sex of fetus, etc.); Poor cardiac reserve (= LCR); Postcoronary rehabilitation; Potential carcinogenic risk; Precocious/ Premature cervical ripening (in preterm labor, due to a congenital disorder of connective tissue, exposure to diethylstilbesterol in utero, local or intrauterine infection causing an increase of cytokines and prostaglandins, repeated bleeding or vascular lesions in the placenta in the second and third trimesters, traumatic damage to the structural integrity of the cervix and, finally, uterine overdistension); Prostate cancer risk; Protein catabolism rate; Protein-coupled receptor (G) (see GPCR).

PCr Phosphocreatine/tinine (= PCR).

PCR-ISH Polymerase chain reaction - in situ hybridization (see PCR).

PCRM Physicians Committee for Responsible Medicine.

PCRN Pittsburgh Clinical Research Network.

PCRT Placebo-controlled randomized trial.

PCS Palliative care service; Patient care standard(s); Patient Care System; Patterns of care study; Pelvic congestion syndrome; Peptide/ Polypeptide chain synthesis (RNA); Pericerebral space; Perichondrial sheath (of bone) (Orthopedics); Pharmacogenic confusional syndrome; Placebo-controlled study (see PCCT); Portable cervical spine; Portacaval shunt (see PC; PCA); Postcardiac surgery; Postcardiotomy/ Postcholecystectomy/ Postconcussion/ Prolonged crush syndrome; Postcontrast scan; Preclinical safety/ study; Preconscious (see pcs); Premature centromere separation; Primary cancer site; Primary care specialities/ty/ system (see PCOS); Programmed cell suicide (= Apoptosis) (see PCD); Prolonged chronic stress; Proportional counter spectrometry; Prospective cohort/ controlled study; Proximal coronary sinus; Pseudomotor/ Pseudotumor cerebri syndrome; Pyrophosphate crystal synovitis.

PCs Phytochemicals (plant chemical anti-carcinogens and/or coronary artery 'protectives', found in vegetables and fruits, which prevent the formation of various cancers by preventing carcinogens from binding to the DNA of the body's cells; such as:

1. Allylic sulfide - found in garlic and onions, which triggers a family of enzymes that detoxifies carcinogens, and protects against

stomach cancer;
2. Beta carotene and other antioxidants, such as Vitamin A, B, C, and so on - found in fruits and vegetables. These antioxidant vitamins have the power to subdue free radicals, the molecular vandals that harden the arteries and propogate various cancers;
3. Capsaicin - found in hot chili peppers. It keeps carcinogens like those of cigarette smoke from binding to DNA, thus reducing the risk of lung and other cancers;
4. p-Coumaric acid and chlorogenic acid - found in tomatoes, green peppers, strawberries, carrots and other vegetables, as well as in pineapples and other fruits. They neutralize nitric acid and nitrosamines produced by the body, and thus effectively detoxicate carcinogens;
5. Ellagic acid - found in strawberries, grapes, and raspberries. It neutralizes carcinogens before they can invade DNA;
6. Flavenoids - found in fruits and vegetables, from berries to yams, to citrus and cucumbers. These prevent cancer-causing hormones (including estrogen) from latching onto a cell;
7. Genistein - found in soybeans. It causes contraction of the tiny capillaries that carry oxygen and nutrients to the growing tumor, which without these supply lines cannot develop or metastasize, and thus dies; said to prevent cancer of the prostate;
8. Indole-3-carbinol - found in cauliflower and cabbage. It triggers enzymes that induce the precursor of estrogen, to break down into a harmless form, thus reducing the risk of breast cancer;
9. PEITC - Phenethyl isothiocyanate - found in cabbage and turnips. It protects DNA from a potent carcinogen in tobacco smoke, thus inhibiting lung cancer;
10. Sulforaphane - found in broccoli, cauliflower, Brussels sprouts, turnips, and kale. It boosts the activity of "phase 2" enzymes, which detoxify carcinogens in the body's cells. It is said to reduce the risk of breast cancer;
11. Anthocyanosides: red, blue and purple plants such as egg-plant, blood oranges, blueberries;
12. Catechins: tea;
13. Isoflavones: soybeans, other legumes, licorice;
14. Lignans: flaxseed, berries, whole grains, licorice;
15. Monoterpenes: oranges, lemons, grapefruit;
16. Phenolic acids: all plants;
17. Phytosterols: soybeans, other legumes, cucumbers, other fruits and vegetables;
18. Protease inhibitors: soybeans and all plants;
19. Saponins: garlic, onions, licorice, legumes;
20. Triterpenoids (such as glycyrrhizin): citrus fruit, mushrooms, licorice; Protein channels (or porins - found in the outer membrane of bacterial organisms).

pcs preconscious (= PCS).

P c/s Primary cesarean section.

PCSA Parent-compound-specific assay.

PCSD Preclinical safety data (= PSD)/ study (= PSS).

PCSM Percutaneous stone manipulation.

PCSS Potassium-containing salt substitute (see K+CSS).

PCT Palliative/ Potent/ Prolonged chemotherapy (see PCA; PCD); Palliative care team; Papillary carcinoma of the thyroid (see OAC); Paracoagulation test; Periarticular connective tissue; Peripheral carcinoid tumor; Pig-cell transplant (see POT); Pivotal clinical trial; Placebo-controlled trial (see PCCT); Plasma clotting time; Plasma cell tumor; Plasmacrit test (= Plasma Cri T; Plasma Cri test; Plasma Crit test; Plasma hematocrit test) - a reagin test for syphilis; Plasmacytoma; Platinum-containing therapy (cancer) (= PCR); Polychlorinated triphenyl; Porphyria cutanea tarda (a disorder of porphyrin metabolism with cutaneous manifestations); Portacaval transposition (see PC; PCA); Positron computed tomography; Postcoital test; Preclinical test(ing)/ trial; Primary Care Trusts (NHS, UK); Primary cerebral tumor; Progesterone challenge test; Prospective clinical/ cohort trial; Prothrombin consumption test/ time; Proximal convoluted tubule (of the kidney nephron).

pct percent (see pc).

PCTC Plasma concentration time curve (see AUC).

PCTF Percutaneous cerclage of tibial fracture(s) (Orthopedics).

PCTFE Polychlorotrifluoroethylene.

PCTMR Pecutaneous transmyocardial reperfusion (= PMR; PTMR).

PCTs Polychlorinated triphenyls.

PCU Pain control unit; Palliative/ Patient/ Primary/ Progressive/ Protective/ Pulmonary care unit; Periodic check-up; Postcoma unawareness; Proposed clinical usage.

PCV Packed cell volume (see Crit; Hct) (the volume of packed red cells in cubic centimeters per 100 cc of blood); Parietal cell vagotomy; Pathogenic chimeric virus (e.g. HIV-1/SIV); Placebo-corrected value(s); Pneumococcal/ Pneumoccoccal conjugate (= CPV; HCPV) vaccine; Polycythemia vera (= PV); Postcapillary venule; Posterior cervical vein; Prostate cancer vaccine (containing dendritic or specialized immune system cells, that activate disease-fighting T cells, obtained from the patient's blood).

PCVC Pes calcaneo-valgus congenitus (L.) (see CCV).

PCVI Percutaneous cardiovascular intervention (see PCI).

PCV-M Polycythemia vera with (myeloid) metaplasia.

PCvVC Paclitaxel plus Carboplatin versus Vinorelbine plus Cisplatin (study/ trial in the treatment of lung cancer).

PCW Pericanalicular web; Primary capillary wedge (pressure) (see PWCP); Pulmonary capillary wedge (see PCWP); Purified cell walls.

PCWP Pulmonary capillary wedge pressure (mean pressure - in mm Hg) (= PC; PCW; Ppw; PWP).

PCX Paracervical.

PCx Periscopic convex (wedge) (eye examination).

PCXR Portable chest radiogram/graph(y).

PCZ Procarbazine (= PCB); Prochlorperazine.

PD Doctor of Pharmacy (see Phar D); Dublin Pharmacopoeia; Interpupillary distance (see IPD); Paget/ Parkinson's disease; Pancreatic diabetes (see FCPD; PDPD)/ duct; Pancreaticoduodenectomy; Panic disorder; Papilla diameter (see Pd); Paralytic/ Paralyzing dose; Parkinsonian dementia; Paroxysmal discharge/ dystonia (see PC); Pars distalis (pituitary); Patent ductus; Pediatric(s) (see Pd); Per diem/ Pro die (see pd); Percentage difference; Percutaneous drain; Periodic disease (see FMF); Peritoneal dialysis; Personality difficulty (= PA - Personality accentuation); Personality disorder (Antisocial, Psychopathic, or Sociopathic/ Dependent, Histrionic, or Hysterical/ Inhibited, Anankastic, Compulsive, or Obsessional/ Withdrawn, Eccentric, Paranoid, Schizotypal, or Schizoid PD); Phenyldichlorarsine; Phosphate dehydrogenase (see G-6-PD)/ dextrose; Photosensitivity dermatitis; Pick's disease (asymmetrical lobar atrophy of the frontal or temporal lobes of the cerebrum - with neuronal loss, gliosis, and argyrophilic inclusion or Pick's bodies) (= ALA); Polydactyly; Postdose; Postural dizziness; Prescription drug; Progressive dementia; Plasma defect; Poorly differentiated (cells); Posterior division; Postnasal/ Postural drainage; Potential difference; Pregnanediol (see P-diol); Present/ Pulmonary disease; Pressor dose; Prism diopter (see p-d); Problem/ Protein degradation; Problem drinker; Progression of disease; Protein diet; Psychopathic deviate; Psychotic depression; Pulpodistal; Pulse duration; Pupillary distance (see IPD); Pyloric dilator; Pyruvate dehydrogenase (see PDH).

Pd Palladium (Z = 46) (see Elements - Palladium); Papilla diameter (= PD; pd); Pediatric(s) (= PD); Prism diopter (see p-d).

pd for the day (L. pro die)/ by the day (L. per diem) (= PD); interpupillary distance (see IPD); papilla diameter (see Pd); prism diopter (see p-d); pupillary distance (see IPD).

P-D Paranoid-destructive.

p-d prism diopter (= PD; Pd; pd).

p/d packs per day (cigarettes).

2-PD Two-point discrimination.

PDA Pacific Dermatological Association; Paraphenylamine diamine; Parenteral drug abuser; Patent/ Pulmonary ductus arteriosus;

Pediatric allergist/gy (see PdA); Persistent dilated airway(s) (as in bronchiectasis, emphysema, etc.); Personal Digital Assistant (www program); Pharmacodynamic activity; Posterior descending artery; PreDialysis Anemia; Previous dose adjustment; Prophylactic drug action (e.g. anticonvulsants, cardiac anti-arrhythmics, immunosuppressive agents, oral contraceptives, etc.); Pulmonary disease anemia; Pulmonary ductus arteriosus.

PdA Pediatric allergist/gy (= PDA).

PDAB Para-dimethylaminobenzaldehyde.

PD/AR Photosensitivity dermatitis and actinic reticuloid (syndrome).

PDAS Primary defective antibody synthesis (as in Agamma/ Hypogamma - globulinemia) (see PIDD).

PDAY Pathological Determinants of Atherosclerosis in Youth (Research group).

PDB Paget disease of bone; Paradichlorobenzene (= Dichlorobenzol; $C_6H_4Cl_2$) - an insecticide used against moths and furniture beetles; Phosphorus-dissolving bacteria; Postdengue "blah(s)" (see PDN or Postdengue neurasthenia); Presumptive diverticular bleeding (see CDH); Preventive dental (health) behavior.

PDC Parkinsonism dementia complex; Peak (see PBC)/ Plasma drug concentration; Pediatric cardiologist/gy (see PdC); Pentadecylcatechol; Peripheral dilatation catheter (used in artery angioplasty); Persistent dry cough; Physical dependence capacity; Plasma dioxin concentration; Poikiloderma congenitalis (sparse or absent scalp, axillary and pubic hair, erythema of face, ears and extensor limbs, followed by mottled pigmentation, possible cataracts and hypogonadism - an autosomal recessive, congenital hypotrichosis (= PAS; RTS); Poor diabetic control; Postdelivery care/ complication; Potential-dependent channel; Potts divisional clamp (Cardiovascular); Predose concentration (of drugs); Preliminary/ Primary diagnostic clinic; Pyridinol carbamate.

PdC Pediatric cardiologist/gy (= PDC).

PDCD Primary degenerative cerebral disease.

PD-CSE Pulsed Doppler cross-sectional echocardiography (= PDE).

PDD Pervasive development(al) disorder (or Asperger disorder, named after the pediatrician Hans Asperger of Vienna, Austria, who described mild variants of autism or the mindblindness syndrome, in the 1940s); Pharmacodynamic data; Platinum diamminodichloride (cisplatin); Pre-existing dysthymic disorder (see MDD); Premenstrual dysphoric disorder (see PMS); Primary degenerative dementia; Primary demyelinating disease (e.g. MS); Pyridoxine-deficient diet.

PDDD Polymeric drug delivery device.

PDE Paroxysmal dyspnea on exertion; Pharmacodynamic effect; Phosphodiesterase (= PDIE); Pigeon-dropping extract; Potassium-depleting effect(s) (of drugs such as furosemide, hydrochlorothiazide, etc.) (= K+DE); Progressive dialysis encephalopathy; Pulsed Doppler echocardiography (see PD-CSE).

PdE Pediatric endocrinology.

PDE 1-6 Phosphodiesterase - isoform types 1-6 (esp. 5).

PDEA Postdental extraction alveolitis.

PDE5I Phosphodiesterase type 5 inhibitor (e.g. Sildenafil [Viagra]).

PDES Phosphodiesterase (see PDE).

PDET-HBP Prevention, Detection, Evaluation and Treatment of High Blood Pressure (JNC).

PDF Parkinson's Disease Foundation; Peritoneal dialysis fluid; Predisposing factor; Psychological dysfunction.

PDFC Premature dead female child.

PDG Parkinsonism-dementia (complex) of Guam; Phosphogluconate/ Pyruvate dehydrogenase (see PDH); Pigment dispersion syndrome (intra-ocular).

PDGA Pteroyldiglutamic acid.

PDGF Platelet-derived growth factor (= PGF).

PDGS Partial form of DiGeorge's syndrome.

PDGXT Predischarge graded exercise test.

PDH Packaged Diaster Hospital; Past dental history; Phosphate dehydrogenase (see G-6-PD); Postdental history; Presumptive diverticular hemorrhage (see CDH); Progressive daytime hyperglycemia; Progressive disseminated histoplasmosis; Pyruvate dehydrogenase (= PD; PDG).

PDHa Pyruvate dehydrogenase in active form.

PDHC Pyruvate dehydrogenase complex.

PdHO Pediatric hematology-oncology.

PDI Periodontal disease index; Peripheral decarboxylase inhibitor; Pharmacodynamic interaction(s); Plan-do-integration; Power Doppler image (Ultrasound); Psychomotor development index.

PDI; PDIA Possible/ Predictable/(ted) drug interaction.

Pdi Transdiaphragmatic pressure.

PDIE Phosphodiesterase (see PDE).

P-diol Pregnanediol (= PD).

PDL Pancreatic duct ligation; Periodontal ligament; Poorly differentiated lymphocyte/ lymphoma (see PDLL).; Population doubling level; Progressive diffuse leukoencephalopathy.

pdl poundal; pudendal.

PDLC Poorly differentiated lung cancer.

PDLD Poorly differentiated lymphocytic-diffuse.

PDLL Poorly differentiated lymphocytic lymphoma.

PDLN Poorly differentiated lymphocytic-nodular.

PDM Primary dysmenorrhea; Progestational diabetes mellitus/ diabetic mother; Proper dietary management; Proxy decision maker (for the incapacitated patient in Scotland by the SEHD such as a welfare attorney, welfare guardian, or a person authorized under an intervention court order) (see AIA; SEHD); Pulmonary defense mechanism.

PDMC Premature dead male child.

PDMS Patient data management system; Pharmacokinetic drug monitoring service.

PDN Postdengue neurasthenia (= PDB); Prednisone; Private duty nurse.

pDNA Polymorphic/ Promoter deoxyribonucleic acid.

PdNEO Pediatric neonatology.

PdNEP Pediatric nephrology.

PDO Pyloroduodenal obstruction.

PDP Parallel distributing processor; Parenteral drug product(s) (i.e. injections); Pattern disruption point; Pediatric/ Peritoneal dialysis patient; Pharmacodynamic parameter/ profile (of a drug)/ property; Piperidinopyrimidine; Platelet-derived plasma; Pregestational diabetes pregnancy; Pregnant diabetic patient (= DPP); Primer-dependent deoxynucleic acid polymerase; Pro-drug phenomenon; Product Development Protocol; Protein-derived peptide.

PD&P Postural drainage and percussion.

PDPD Prolonged-dwell peritoneal dialysis; Protein deficient pancreatic diabetes (one of the two subtypes of MRDM - see FCPD; MRDM; PD).

PDPI Primer-dependent deoxynucleic acid polymerase index.

PDQ Personality Diagnostic Questionnaire; Physician's Data Query; Premenstrual Distress Questionnaire; Prescreening Developmental Questionnaire; Pretty darn quick; Protocol data query.

PDR Pediatric radiology (see PdR); Peripheral diabetic retinopathy; Proliferative diabetic retinopathy (characterized by fibrosis, neovascularization, retinal detachment, traction, vitreous hemorrhage, etc.) (see NPDR); Permanent dose reduction; Pharmacodynamic response; Physicians' Desk Reference (book); Postdelivery room; Primary drug resistance.

PdR Pediatric radiology (= PDR).

pdr powder (medical order/ prescription).

PDRB Permanent Disability Rating Board.

PDRcVH Proliferative diabetic retinopathy with vitreous hemorrhage.

PDRI Posteriorly directed rotary injury (knee).

PDRT Portland Digit Recognition.

PDS Pain-dysfunction syndrome; Parkinsonian Dementia Syndromes; Paroxysmal depolarizing shift; Passive dissemination strategy; Patient data system; Pediatric surgery (see PdS); Peritoneal dialysis solution/ system; Phosphorus depletion syndrome; Physiologic dead space; Plasma-derived serum; Polydimethylsiloxane; Polydioxanone sutures; Posterior drawer sign (posterior sag of the tibia) (see PDT); Predialyzed serum; Punch-drunk syndrome (occurring particularly in contact sports such as boxing); Purpose-designed software (CQ Analysis/ Doppler analysis).

PdS Pediatric surgery (= PDS).

PDSG Pigment dispersion syndrome glaucoma.

PDSP Postdental surgery pain.

PDSS Pharmacodynamic stimulation study.

PDT Pharmacodynamic test/ tolerability; Photodynamic therapy; Postdoctoral training; Posterior drawer test (for posterior sag[ging] [see PDS] of the tibia, with the knee in 90° flexion) (see DS - Drawer sign); Primary data source/ Problem drug taker; Prolactin-dependent tumor; Prolonged diuretic/ drug therapy.

PDU Perforated duodenal ulcer; Pulsed Doppler ultrasonography.

PDUF Pulsed Doppler ultrasonic flow-meter.

PDUR PreDischarge Utilization Review.

PDUS Pulsed Doppler ultrasound.

PDV Peak diastolic velocity; Pulsed Doppler velocimetry (Obstetrics).

PDVO Platelet-dependent vascular occlusion.

PDW Platelet distribution width.

PE Edinburgh Pharmacopoeia (see EP); Pancreatic/ Placental/ Powdered extract; Paper electrophoresis; Partial epilepsy; Pelvic examination; Penile erection; Percutaneous endoscopy; Peritoneal exudate; Pharyngoesophageal; Phenylephrine; Phenylethylamine (see PEA); Phosphatidyl ethanolamine; Photographic effect; Phycoerythrin; Physical education/ energy/ examination/ exercise; Physiological ecology; Pigmented epithelium; Pilocarpine-epinephrine; Placebo effect; Plasma exchange; Platinum compd (cisplatin) and etoposide; Pleural effusion; Point of entry/ exit; Polyethylene; Potential energy; Pre-eclampsia; Pre-excitation; Premature ejaculation; Present evaluation; Pressure equalization; Prior to exposure; Probable error; Professional engineer; Pseudoexfoliation; Pulmonary edema/ embolism; Pyrogenic exotoxin.

Pe; P_e Pressure on expiration (= Expiratory pressure) (respiratory therapy).

P_1E_1 Pilocarpine 1%, epinephrine 1% (ophthalmic solution).

PE_2 Prostaglandin E_2 (see PGE_2).

PEA Parenteral administration; Pelvic examination under anesthesia; Phasic electrical alternans (an abnormal finding on the ECG); Phenylethyl alcohol; Phenylethylamine (= PE); Polysaccharide egg antigen; Pre-existing arrhythmia/ asthma.

PEAP Positive end-airway pressure.

PEAR Princeton Engineering Anomalies Research (Laboratory) (see PEARL).

PEARL Princeton Engineering Anomalies Research Laboratory.

PEARLA Pupils equal and react to light and accommodation.

peau d'orange French - "orange skin" - pitted appearance of the skin, found in the late stages of carcinoma of the breast.

PEB Platinum compd (cisplatin), etoposide, and bleomycin.

PEBG Phenethylbiguanide (see DBI).

PEBT Pre-existing background therapy.

PEC Pelvic cramps; Peritoneal exudate cell; Phalangeal epidermal cyst (Orthopedics); Plain English Campaign (UK); Primary eosinophilopoietic cytokine; Prolactin-elevating compound; Pyrogenic exotoxin C.

PECA Pre-existing cardiac/ cerebral abnormality.

PECD Pre-existing cardiac/ cerebral disease/ disorder/ dysfunction.

PECHO Prostatic echogram.

$PECO_2$ Mixed expiratory carbon dioxide tension.

PECPD Polyendocrinopathic disease/ disorder.

PECS Picture Exchange Communication System.

PED Past/ Previous(ly) effective dose; Perforated ear drum; Performance-enhancing drug (see PES); Posterior elbow dislocation (see RPD); Pre-existing diabetes/ disease; Progressive exertional dyspnea.

PED; ped Pediatrics (see Ped).

PEd Physical education.

Ped Pediatrics (= paed; PED; ped).

PEDC Post/Pre-erythropoietin-dependent cell.

PEDG Phenformin hydrochloride (= Phenethyldiguanide HCl) - a diguanide oral anti-diabetic agent of value especially in elderly stable diabetes (see DBI; PBI).

PeDS Pediatric Drug Surveillance.

PEE Periodic eye examination (see PRE);

Polyethylenimine

PEEP Positive/ Peak end-expiratory pressure (respiratory therapy) (see PFT - PEEP); Primary efficacy end point.

PEEPi Intrinsic peak end-expiratory pressure.

PEF Peak expiratory flow (l/min) (see PFT - PEF); Peripheral endothelial function; Post-exercise facilitation; Psychiatric Evaluation Form; Pulmonary edema fluid.

PEFR Peak expiratory flow rate (pulmonary function test) (see PFT - PEFR).

$PEFR_n$ Peak expiratory flow rate through the nose (see PFT).

PEFT Peak expiratory flow time.

PEFV Partial expiratory flow volume.

PEG Patient Evaluation Grid; Percutaneous endoscopic gastrostomy; Pneumoencephalogram/raphy (procedure/ neurology); Polyethylene glycol (see PEGs).

PEG-ADA Polyethylene glycol-modified adenosine deaminase (replacement therapy for ADA deficiency).

PEG-ELS Polyethylene glycol and iso-osmolar electrolyte solution.

PEGG Parent Education and Guidance Group.

PEGIFA2a Peginterferon/ Pegylated interferon alfa-2a.

PEG 300/IMS Polyethylene glycol 300/ industrial methylated spirits (and other PEGs/IMS).

PEGs Polyethylene Glycols - macrogols or mixtures of condensation polymers of ethylene oxide and water. Used as stabilizers of emulsions and water-miscible bases for ointments, particularly where penetration of the skin is desired; also as solvents for drugs such as hydrocortisone, sulfonamides, etc., and as bases for pessaries and suppositories, e.g. PEG 300, 400, 1500, 1540, 4000 and 6000 - macrogols with various molecular weights and physical properties; those with an average molecular weight of 200-700 are liquids, and those with more than 1000 vary in consistency from soft unctions to hard wax-like solids.

PEHD Pre-existing hepatic disease (see PELD).

PEI Pancreatic exocrine insufficiency; Phosphate excretion index; Physical efficiency index; Polyethyleneimine; Potentially effective intervention; Progressive exercise intolerance.

PEITC Phenethyl isothiocyanate (a phytochemical found in vegetables such as cabbage and turnips, which inhibits lung cancer (see PCs).

PEJ Percutaneous endoscopic jejunostomy.

PEKD Pre-existing kidney disease/ disorder (= PERD).

PEL Peritoneal exudate lymphocyte; Permissible exposure limit; Plasma erythropoietin level; Primary effusion lymphoma (= β-cell or Bone marrow cell lymphoma, caused by the HHV-4 or Epstein-Barr virus) (see βCL; E-B; HHV-4).

PELD Pre-existing liver disease (= PEHD).

PELF Persistent elevated liver function.

pelidisi (L.) pondus decies linearis divisus sidentis (altitudo) = weight ten line divided sitting (height).

PEM Peritoneal exudate macrophage; Prescription event monitoring; Prespecified efficacy measure; Primary enrichment medium; Probable error of measurement; Protein energy malnutrition.

PEMA Phenylethylmalonamide.

PEMS Physical, emotional, mental, and safe(ty).

PEN Parenteral and enteral nutrition.

Pen Penicillin (= PC; PCN; PN; PNC).

Penic cam A camel's hair brush (L. penicillum camelinum).

Penicillin V Phenoxymethylpenicillin.

PEOT Pancreatic enzyme output test(s) (= LT; PSST).

PENS Percutaneous epidural nerve stimulation/ator.

Pent Pentothal (anesthetic agent).

Penta Pentachlorophenol (see PCP).

PEO Progressive external ophthalmoplegia.

PEP Past/ Previous ectopic pregnancy; Paths for Employee Progress; Patient education program; Performance Evaluation Procedure; Peptidase (see Pep); Physical exercise program; Phospho/Phosphoenol pyruvate; Pigmentation, edema, and plasma cell dyscrasia (syndrome); Polyestradiolphosphate; Positive expiratory pressure; Postencephalitic parkinsonism; Post/Pre-exposure prophylaxis (in infectious diseases); Pre-eclampic pregnancy; Pre-ejection period (heart); Primary efficacy parameter; Primary endpoint (e.g. coronary death, nonfatal myocardial infarction, etc.) (see SEP); Proficiency Evaluation Program (College of American Pathologists); Prolonged exposure period (to diseases, drugs, etc.); Protein electrophoresis; Public Education Program; Pupil Evaluation Project.

Pep Peptidase (= PEP).

PEPA Peptidase A; Protected environment units and prophylactic antibiotics.

PEPB Peptidase B.

PEPC Peptidase C.

PEP-C Patients' Evaluation of Performance in California (COH).

PEPc Pre-ejection period - corrected (for heart rate).

PEPCK Phosphoenolpyruvate carboxykinase.

PEPD Peptidase D; Post-encephalitic Parkinson's disease (see PEP); Pre-existing psoriatic disease.

PEPE Peptidase E.

PEPI Postmenopausal Estrogen-Projestin Interventions (Trial); Pre-ejection period index.

PEPP Positive expiratory pressure plateau (= PPEP).

Pep pill Amphetamines (see Amphet).

PEPR Precision encoder and pattern recognizer.

PEPS Peptidase S.

PER Peak ejection rate; Pediatric emergency room; Pronation, external rotation (fracture); Protein efficiency ratio.

per perineal; period(ic)/icity; peroneal (fibula/ outer side of leg).

PERB Public Employment Relations Board.

PERC Perchloroethylene (a solvent used in dry-cleaning).

Perc Perceptual; Percutaneous.

percus percussion.

PERD Pre-existing renal disease/ disorder (see PEKD).

perf perfect; perforated/tion; performed.

PERG Pattern electroretinogram.

perh perhaps.

PERI Pre-existing renal insufficiency; Psychiatric Epidemiology Research Interview.

peri perineum.

periap periapical.

PeriCare Perineum care.

Perio Periodontics.

PERK Prospective evaluation of radial keratotomy (protocol).

PERL Pupils equal, and react to light.

PERLA Pupils equal, react to light and accommodation.

perm permanent.

per op emet when the action of the emetic is over (L. peracta operatione emetici).

per os (L.). by mouth.

perp perpendicular.

PERR Pattern-evoked retinal response.

PERRLA Pupils equal, round, react to light and accommodation.

PERRRLA Pupils equal, round, regular, react to light and accommodation.

PERS Patient Evaluation Rating Scale.

PERs Planning estimating relationships.

pers personal.

Person-sievert/ Person-gray A unit of population exposure to nuclear radiation, obtained by summing dose-equivalent values for all exposed persons (see Gy; Gray; Sievert).

PERT Program Evaluation and Review Technique.

PERV Porcine endogenous retrovirus.

PES Paraffin-embodied section (Histology); Pediatric Endocrine Society; Performance-enhancing substance (such as ASI or Anticholinesterase inhibitor drugs, Donezepil and Rivastigmine, used in the treatment of Alzheimer's disease) (= PED); Pharmaco economic/ epidemiology study; Photoelectron spectroscopy; Physical, emotional, and spiritual (bond/ connection); Physicians' equity services; Polyethylene sulfonate; Post-exposure setting; Post-extrasystolic; Pre-epiglottic space; Pre-excitation syndrome; Pre-existing sepsis; Primary empty sella (syndrome); Pseudoexfoliative syndrome.

PESP Peak early systolic pressure; Post-extrasystolic potentiation.

peSPL Peak equivalent sound pressure level.

Pess Pessary. A device placed in the vagina to support a prolapsed uterus.
Bee-cell pessary - a soft rubber cube, on each face of which is a curved space, acting as a suction cup when the pessary is in the vagina.
Cup pessary - a pessary, the tip of which has a cup-like shape to fit over the os uteri.
Diaphragm pessary - a diaphragm inserted into the vagina as an occlusive contraceptive, and also used to hold up the uterus and vagina.
Doughnut pessary - a flexible rubber doughnut-shaped pessary supporting the uterus.
Emmert-Gellhorn pessary - a hollow-stemmed Gellhorn pessary (see).
Gariel's pessary - a hollow rubber inflatable pessary.
Gehrung pessary - a Hodge pessary bent on itself so as to form a double horseshoe; used in patients with Cystocele.
Gellhorn pessary - a single stem pessary for use in uterine prolapse.
Hodge's pessary - a pessary use in retrodeviation of the uterus.
Inflatable pessary - a rubber Doughnut that can be broken down and flexed to a flexible stem with a valve.
Lever pessary - a pessary acting on the principle of the lever.
Mange's pessary - a ring pessary with a fixed crossbar holding a detachable stem.
Ring pessary - a round or ring-shaped pessary.
Smith's pessary - used in retroversion of the uterus.
Stem pessary - it has a stem for introduction into the cervical canal.
Thomas pessary - a long narrow pessary for use in nulliparas.
Zwanck's pessary - a radium carrier pessary which can be fixed in the vault of the vagina.

Pestox 14 Dimefox (see BFPO).

PET Paraffin-embedded tissue; Parent effectiveness training; Peak ejection time; Peak/ Poor exercise tolerance; Performance-enhancement tool; Pocket Echo-Tone; Positron emission tomography (see SPECT); Pre-eclamptic toxemia; Pressure equalizing tubes; Progressive exercise test; Psychiatric emergency team; Psychic email transmitter.

PETA People for the Ethical Treatment of Animals.

peta- 10^{15} (= P).

PET$_{CO2}$ End-tidal pressure of carbon dioxide.

PETD Pre-existing thyroid disease.

PETH Pink-eyed, tan-hooded (rat).

petit pas French - shuffling short steps (see MAPP).

PETN Pentaerythrityl tetranitrate (= Erynite; Nitropentaerythrol; Nitropenthrite; Pentaerythrite/thritol/throl tetranitrate; Pentanitrol) - a slow-acting vasodilator nitrite, used prophylactically in the treatment of angina pectoris; its effect begins in about one hour and lasts about five hours. Also a powerful plastic explosive.

petr petroleum.

petrog petrography.

PETS Percutaneous energy transmission system (skin button); Perinatal Emergency Transport System.

PETT Pendular eye-tracking test; Positron emission transaxial/ transverse tomograph(y).

PEU Phacoemulsification unit (Ophthalmology); Plasma equivalent unit; Pre-existing ulcer(ation).

PEV Peak expiratory velocity; Pulmonary extravascular (fluid) volume (see PFT).

pev peak electron volts.

PEW Pulmonary extravascular water.

PEWV Pulmonary extravascular water volume (see PFT).

PEX Patient Resource Exchange (New York State).

PEx Physical examination (= PE).

PF Pair feeding; Palva flap (in tympanomastoidectomy); Peak flow (see PFT - PF; FEV); Perfusion/ Pericardial/ Peritoneal/ Pleural/ Prostatic fluid; Periodic fever; Peripheral field(s); Permeability/ Plasma/ Power/ Protection/ Pulmonary factor; Personality factor (questionnaire) (see PFQ); L-phenylalanine mustard and 5-fluorouracil - a cytotoxic chemical combination used in cancer therapy (see TPF); Picture-frustration (see P-F); Pilon fracture (comminuted intra-articular fracture of distal tibia and fibula): Type I - mild comminution, no displacement; Type II - comminution and slight displacement; Type III - extensive displacement and comminution (as in explosive fracture); Plantar flexion; Platelet factor (= CF - Coagulation factor) (see Factor VIII - PF-A or platelet cofactor 1; Factor IX - PF-B or platelet cofactor 2); Pontiac fever (non-pneumonia form of Legionnaire's disease caused by *Legionella* pneumophila; discovered in Pontiac, Michigan); Portal/ Pulmonary fibrosis; Pott's fracture; Preservative free; Primary fibrinolysin; Pulmonary function; Purkinje fiber; Purpura fulminans; Push fluids.

Pf Pfeifferella; Plasmodium falciparum.

pF picofarad.

P_f Final pressure.

P-F Picture-frustration (study/ test) (= PF).

PF_{1-4} Platelet (co)factors 1-4.

PF_3 Platelet cofactor 3 (antiplatelet antibody test) (= PF_c).

PF_4 Platelet cofactor 4 (= PF_d).

PFA Para-p-fluorophenylalanine; Phosphofructoaldolase; Phosphonoformalic acid; Phosphonoformate; Plaque-filled artery; Profunda femoris artery; Propylformic acid (also called Butanoic or Butyric acid).

PF-A; PF_a Platelet cofactor A (= PF_1).

PFAN Postfracture avascular necrosis (e.g. head of femur) (Orthopedics).

PFAS Performic acid-Schiff (reaction).

PFB Prefabricated functional brace (e.g. for treatment of fractures of the tibial diaphysis) (Orthopedics).

PF-B; PF_b Platelet cofactor B (= PF_2).

PFBD Placental-fetal blood distribution (Obstetrics).

PFC Pair-fed control (mice); Pelvic flexion contracture; Perfluorocarbon; Pericardial fluid culture; Persistent fetal circulation; Plaque-forming cell; Prefrontal cortex; Pregnancy Food Chart; Preventative/ Preventive foot care; Pulmonary function criteria.

PF-C; PF_c Platelet cofactor C (= PF_3).

pFc Noncovalently bonded dimer of the C-terminal immunoglobulin of the Fc fragment.

PFCD Prefrontal cortex damage (= PCD).

PFCs Perfluorocarbons (a group of chemicals that act like red blood cells by carrying oxygen through the blood vessels; also called Artificial blood).

PFD Patellofemoral disorder (Orthopedics); Pelvic fracture-diastasis; Peripheral field defect (see PVD); Polyostotic fibrous dysplasia; Primary flash distillate; Purine-free diet (used in gout).

PF-D; PF_d Platelet cofactor D (= PF_4).

PFDA Perfluoro-n-decanoic acid.

PFE Pelvic floor exercise(s).

PFF Prophylactic forearm fasciotomy; Proximal femoral fracture.

PFFD Proximal focal femoral deficiency.

PFFFP Pall filtered fresh frozen plasma.

PFG Peak flow guage.

PFGE Pulsed field gel electrophoresis.

PFH Positive family history (see +veFH).

PFI Potential fungal infection; Press-fit implant (of a trial prosthesis); Pulmonary function impairment.

PFIB Perfluoroisobutylene.

PFJS Patellofemoral joint syndrome.

PFK Phosphofructokinase.

PFKL Phosphofructokinase, liver type.

PFKM Phosphofructokinase, muscle type.

PFKP Phosphofructokinase, platelet type.

PFL Prefrontal lobotomy; Profibrinolysin; Protect(ed)/(ion) from light.

PFM Peak flow meter/ monitor(ing) (expiratory flow); Porcelain fused to metal.

PFN Parafascicular nucleus (thalamotomy - Neurosurgery); Partially functional neutrophil; Perifascicular necrosis.

PFO Patent foramen ovale; Postfusion orthosis (orthopedic brace).

PFP Partial/ Peripheral facial paralysis; Perfluoropropane (gas used in scleral buckling); Pill-free period (see PFW); Platelet-free plasma; Prevailing Fee Plan (Blue Shield).

PFPC Pall filtered packed cells.

Pf/Phag Phlogistic phagocytosis.

PFPS Patellofemoral pain syndrome.

PFQ Personality factor questionnaire.

PFR Parietofrontal region; Parotid/ Peak flow rate (see PFT); Plain film radiogram/graph(y); Popular folk remedies/dy (see TYRs); Preputial flap repair (for severe hypospadias); Proximal fractional reabsorption.

PFRC Plasma-free red cells; Predicted functional residual capacity (see PFT).

PFS Panview fiberscope; Penile flow study; Prefilled syringe; Preservatory-free solution; Primary fibromyalgia syndrome; Progression-free status/ survival; Protein-free supernatant; Pulmonary function score/ studies/dy (see PFT).

PFS-B Panviewfiberendoscope with biopsy (equipment).

PFT Pancreatic function test; Parafascicular thalamotomy; Pituitary function test(s): 1. Metapyrone, 2. Cortrosyn stimulation, 3. GnRH (Factrel), LHRH, TRH, etc., and 4. Insulin hypoglycemia; Platelet-fibrin thrombi/bus; Posterior fossa tumor; Prednisone, fluorouracil and tamoxifen; Pulmonary function test(s) (= RFT - Respiratory function test):
A-a: Difference of gas pressure between alveolus (A) and pulmonary artery (a); see PFT - P(A-adO_2).
A-aDO_2: Alveolar-arterial oxygen difference; see PFT - P(A-aDO_2).
AaPO_2: Alveolar-arterial oxygen tension difference; see PFT - P(A-aDO_2).
AFM: Air-flow meter (unit).
ATPD: Ambient temperature and pressure, dry.
ATPS: Ambient temperature and pressure, saturated with water vapor BTPD. Body temperature and ambient pressure, dry.
BTPS: Body temperature and ambient pressure, saturated with water vapor.
C_L: Lung compliance/ stiffness.
CO_2 comb: Carbon dioxide combining power (blood gas).
CO_2 cont: Carbon dioxide content (blood gas).
CVS_{O2}: Central venous oxygen saturation.
D_{CO}: Diffusing capacity for carbon monoxide.
DC/P: (Oxygen) diffusing capacity/perfusion (ratio).
D_L: Diffusing capacity of the lung.
DLCO; D_LCO; DL_{CO}: Diffusing capacity of the lungs for carbon monoxide.
DLCO-SB; $DL_{CO\text{-}SB}$: Single-breath diffusing capacity of the lungs for carbon monoxide.
DLCO-SS; $DL_{CO\text{-}SS}$: Steady-state diffusing capacity of the lungs for carbon monoxide.
D_O: Diffusing capacity of oxygen.
dP_{O2}: Rate of pressure change.
DS: Dead-air space.
E: Expiration/red (gas).
EFR_{max}: Maximum expiratory flow rate.
EFVC: Expiratory flow-volume curve.
E/I: Expiration/inspiration (ratio).
ERV: Expiratory reserve volume.
ET_{CO2}: End tidal carbon dioxide.
f: respiratory rate.
FEF: Forced expiratory flow (l/sec) (= FEFR; FEFV; MEF; MEFR).
$FEF_{25\text{-}75\%}$: Forced midexpiratory flow (rate) - between 25 to 75 per cent of the forced vital capacity (FVC) (= MMEF; MMEFR; MMF; MMFR; MMFV).
FEFR: Forced expiratory flow rate (l/sec) (see PFT - FEF).
FEFV: Forced expiratory flow volume (see PFT - FEF).
FER: Forced expiratory ratio (= FEV1/VC or the ratio of the Forced expiratory volume in 1 second to the Vital capacity).
FES: Forced expiratory spirogram.
FET: Forced expiratory time.
FETS: Forced expiratory time, in seconds.
FEV: Forced expiratory volume (= FVE; PF) - a test of the Forced vital capacity (FVC).
$FEV_{1/2}$: Forced expiratory volume in half a second.
$FEV_{0.75}$: Forced expiratory volume in 3/4 of a second.
FEV_1: Forced expiratory volume (ml) in one second.
FEV 1%; %FEV_1: Percent vital capacity in one second.
%>FEV_1: Mean percentage decrease in one second forced expiratory volume.
$FEV_{25\text{-}75\%}$: Maximal midexpiratory flow (between 25 to 75% of the VC or Vital capacity).
FEV1/VC: Forced expiratory volume as a proportion of the vital capacity (see PFT - FER).
IF: Forced inspiratory flow (l/sec) (= FIFR; MIF; MIFR).
FIFR: Forced inspiratory flow rate (see PFT - FIF).

FRC: Functionalreserve/ residual capacity (= RLC or Resting lung capacity).
FSVC: First-second vital capacity.
FVC: Forced ventilatory/ vital capacity - vital capacity during forced full expiration (see PFT - FEV).
FVC_1: Mean forced vital capacity (expiratory volume).
FVE: Forced volume, expiratory (see PFT - FEV).
IC: Inspiratory capacity.
I/E: Inspiratory-expiratory ratio.
IFR: Inspiratory flow rate.
IMBC: Indirect maximum breathing capacity.
IRV: Inspiratory reserve volume.
I_v: Volume inflow.
IVC: Inspiratory/ Inspired vital capacity.
K_{co}: Pulmonary diffusion coefficient.
MAC: Minimum alveolar concentration.
MBC: Maximum breathing capacity (l/min) (see PFT - MVVF).
MEF: Maximal/imum expiratory flow (l/sec) (now FEF; see PFT - FEF).
MEF_{50}: Mean maximum expiratory flow.
MEFR: Maximum expiratory flow rate (l/sec) (now FEF; see PFT -FEF).
MEFV: Maximum expiratory flow volume (see PFT - FEF).
MEP: Maximal/imum expiratory pressure.
MET: Midexpiratory time (oxygen expenditure at rest, equivalent to 3.5 ml of oxygen per kilogram of body weight per minute.
MIF: Maximal/imum inspiratory flow (l/sec) (now FIF; see PFT - FIF).
MIFR: Maximal/imum inspiratory flow rate (now FIFR; see PFT - FIFR).
MIP: Maximum inspiratory pressure.
MMEF: Maximal/imum midexpiratory flow (see PFT - $FEF_{25-75\%}$).
MMEFR: Maximal/imum midexpiratory flow rate (see PFT - $FEF_{25-75\%}$).
MMF: Maximal/imum midexpiratory flow (see PFT - $FEF_{25-75\%}$).
MMFR: Maximal/imum midexpiratory flow rate (see PFT - $FEF_{25-75\%}$).
MMFV: Maximal/imum midexpiratory flow volume (see PFT - $FEF_{25-75\%}$).
MOI: Maximum oxygen intake.
MRE: Maximum respiratory excursion.
MV: Minute ventilation/ volume.
MVV: Maximum voluntary ventilation.
MVVF: Maximum voluntary ventilation, free (formerly, MBC).
NEEP: Negative end expiratory pressure.
NPRQ: Non-protein respiratory quotient.
ODC: Oxygen dissociation curve.
$P_{0.1}$: Pressure at mouth at 100 milliseconds of inspiration.
$P(A\text{-}aDO_2)$: Alveolar (A) - pulmonary arterial (a) oxygen pressure difference (= A-a; A-aDO_2; $AaPO_2$).
$PACO_2$; PA_{CO2}; P_{ACO2}: Partial pressure of carbon dioxide in alveolar gas).
$PaCO_2$; Pa_{CO2}; P_{aCO2}: Partial pressure of carbon dioxide in arterial blood.
PAO_2; PA_{O2}; P_{AO2}: Partial pressure of oxygen in alveolar gas.
PaO_2; Pa_{O2}; P_{aO2}: Partial pressure of oxygen in arterial blood (i.e. arterial oxygen pressure tension; partial arterial oxygen-blood gas).
PC: Provocation concentration.
$PC_{20\text{-}FEV1}$: Provocation concentration producing a 20% reduction in FEV1.
PCO: Partial pressure of carbon monoxide in alveolar gas/ arterial blood.
pCO_2; PCO_2; P_{CO2}: Partial pressure of carbon dioxide in alveolar gas/ arterial blood (= $PACO_2$; PA_{CO2}; P_{ACO2}; $PaCO_2$; Pa_{CO2}; P_{aCO2}).
$\uparrow pCO_2$: Hypercapnia (respiratory acidosis).
PEEP: Positive end expiratory pressure.
PEF: Peak expiratory flow (l/min).
PEFR: Peak expiratory flow rate (l/min).
$PEFR_n$: Peak expiratory flow rate through the nose.
PEP: Positive expiratory pressure.
PEV: Pulmonary extravascular (fluid) volume.
PEWV: Pulmonary extravascular water volume.
PF: Peak flow (see PFT - FEV).
PFR: Peak flow rate.
PFRC: Predicted functional residual capacity.
PFT: Pulmonary function test(s).
P_I: Inspiratory pressure.
PI_{CO2}; P_{ICO2}: Partial pressure of carbon dioxide in inspired air.
PIF: Peak inspiratory flow.

PIFR: Peak inspiratory flow rate.
PIO_2: Intra-alveolar oxygen tension.
P_{IO2}: Partial pressure inspired oxygen.
PIP Peak inflation/ inspiratory pressure.
PL_{CO}; PL_{co}: Single breath diffusing capacity for carbon monoxide.
pO_2; PO_2; P_{O2}: Partial pressure of oxygen in alveolar gas/ arterial blood (= PAO_2; PA_{O2}; P_{AO2}; PaO_2; Pa_{O2}; P_{aO2}).
$\downarrow pO_2$: Hypoxemia.
P_{Tr}: Inspiratory triggering pressure.
PV: Pressure-volume.
P_vO_2: Partial pressure of venous oxygen (blood gas).
PVT: Pulmonary ventilation test.
$\dot{Q}$: Alveolar perfusion.
Qo: Cubic millimeters of oxygen used per milligram of tissue per hour.
QO_2: Oxygen consumption.
$\dot{Q}s/\dot{Q}t$: Shunt blood flow (directly to the left heart, without perfusing ventilated alveoli) (= Oxygen quotient).
RAW; Raw; R_{aw}: Resistance of the airways to gas flow (= Airway Resistance).
RFT: Respiratory Function Test(s).
RLC: Residual/ Resting lung capacity (see PFT - FRC).
RMV: Respiratory minute volume.
Rp: Pulmonary resistance (vascular).
RQ: Respiratory quotient.
RV: Residual volume.
RV/TLC: Residual volume per total lung capacity/ compliance.
SG_{aw}: Specific airways conductance.
SO_2: Percentage saturation of hemoglobin with oxygen (oxygen saturation in the blood).
S_{VO2}: Oxygen saturation in the pulmonary artery.
TC: Total capacity (of the lungs).
T_{CO}: Transfer factor for carbon monoxide.
T_E: Expiratory phase time.
T_I: Inspiratory phase time.
T_I/T_E: Inspiratory-expiratory phase time ratio.
TLC: Total lung capacity/ compliance.
TLV: Total lung volume.
T^{Pe}: Expiratory pause time.
T^{Pi}: Inspiratory pause time.
TV: Tidal/ Total volume.
TVC: Timed vital capacity; Total volume capacity.
V: Ventilation (alveolar); Volume of gas (respiration) (see PFT - V).
$\dot{V}$ Rate of gas flow (vol/min), i.e. Volume of gas per unit of time (= V).
VA: Alveolar aspiration; Volume of alveolar gas (see PFT - V_A).
V_A: Volume of alveolar gas (= VA).
V_A: Alveolar ventilation.
VA/f: Volume of gas entering the alveolar space.
$\dot{V}A/\dot{Q}$; $\dot{V}a/\dot{Q}$; $\dot{V}a/\dot{Q}c$; VAQT: Ventilation/perfusion ratio.
VC: Ventilatory capacity (in milliliters); Vital capacity (in milliliters) - the maximum amount of gas that can be expelled from the lungs by forceful effort (slow full expiration), after maximal inspiration (= Vit Cap).
V_C: Pulmonary capillary blood flow/ volume.
VC/kwt: Vital capacity in milliliters per kilogram of body weight.
V_{CO}: Endogenous production of carbon monoxide.
$\dot{V}_{CO2}$: Amount of carbon dioxide eliminated per minute.
V_D:. Volume of dead air space/ dead space gas/ physiologic dead space (= Vd; VDA; Volume of air/ gas in the conducting airways).
V_d: See PFT - V_D.
VDA: Anatomic dead space (see PFT - V_D).
V_{Dp}: Physiologic dead space volume.
VDp/Vt: Physiologic dead space/tidal volume ratio (see PFT - VD/VT).
VD/VT: Ratio of dead space ventilation to total ventilation, i.e. proportion of tidal volume which is dead space ventilation - not delivered to perfused alveoli (= VDp/Vt).
V_E: Volume of expired gas (Ventilation).
$\dot{V}_E$: Minute volume (= expired volume of ventilation per minute).
V_{EO2}; V_{eO2}: Ventilatory equivalent for oxygen.
V_E period: Volume ejection period.
V equiv: Ventilatory equivalent for oxygen in liters.
V_e/V_{O2} 100 ml: Vcntilatory equivalent.
Vit cap: Vital capacity (see PFT - VC).
$\dot{V}$ max: Maximal rate of airflow during

forced expiration.

VO_2; $\dot{V}_{O2}$: Oxygen consumption/ uptake per minute (at rest).

$\dot{V}_{O2\ max}$: Maximum oxygen consumption per minute (i.e. maximal rate of oxygen uptake per minute).

$\dot{V}/\dot{Q}$; $\dot{V}$-$\dot{Q}$: Ventilation-perfusion ration.

VT; V_T; V_t: Tidal ventilation/ volume.

VTG; V_{TG}; V_{tg}: Respiratory trapped gas/ Thoracic gas volume/ Total gas volume.

PFT$_4$ Proportion free thyroxine.

PFTBE Progressive form of tick-borne encephalitis.

PFU Plaque-/ Pock-forming unit; Preventive follow up.

PFUO Prolonged fever of unknown origin.

PFV Physiologic full value.

PFW Pill-free week (oral contraception); pHisoHex face wash.

PFWB Pall filtered whole blood.

PG Glycerate/rol-3-phosphate (see G3P; G-3-P); Paged (in hospital); Paregoric; Parotid gland; Pectin-(poly)galacturonase (= Pectinase; Pectolase) - an enzyme produced by most thallophytes, including algae, fungi and lichens. It hydrolyses pectin and pectic (polygalacturonic) acids, and is used in wine making and in the manufacture of fruit juices, to reduce their viscosity; Pentagastrin; Pepsinogen; Peptidoglycan; Pharmacogenomics (tailoring drugs to fit genes); Pharmacopoeia Germanica (= German Pharmacopeia; PhG); Phosphate glutamate; Phosphatidyl glycerol/ glycine (test on amniotic fluid to determine maturity of fetus); Phosphogluconate (see 6PG); Pigment granule; Pigmentary glaucome; Pituitary gonadotropin; Pineal germinoma; Plasma gastrin/ glucose/ (tri)glyceride; Polygalacturonate; Postgraduate; Pregnancy/nant (see Pg); Pregnanediol glucuronide; Progesterone; Prolyl hydrolase; Propylene glycol; Prostaglandin (= PGl); Proteoglycan; Pseudogout; Pyoderma gangrenosum.

Pg Nasopharyngeal electrode placement in electroencephalography; Gastric pressure; Pogonion; Pregnancy/nant (= PG; pg).

pg picogram (= 10^{-12} g; μμg; γγ ; micromicrogram); pregancy/nant (see Pg).

P/G Pediatric/Geriatric.

PG Plasma glucose (arterial) (= PG).

6PG 6 Phosphogluconate (= PG).

PGA Patient(s')/ Physician(s') general/ global assessment; Pepsinogen A; Phosphoglyceric/ Polyglycolic acid; Phylogenetic analysis; Polyglandular autoimmune (syndrome); Post/Prenatal genital ambiguity; Prostaglandin A; Prostaglandin analogue (e.g. Misoprostol); Pteroylglutamic acid (a folic acid) (see 3HPGA).

PGA$_{1,\ 2\ and\ 3}$ Prostaglandin A_1, A_2, and A_3.

PG-AC Phenylglycine-acid chloride.

PGAM Phophoglycerate mutase.

PGAS Persisting galactorrhea-amenorrhea syndrome; Polyglandular autoimmune syndrome.

PGB Porcelain gallbladder (opaque or porcelain appearance on X-ray); Prostaglandin B.

PGC Percentage of goblet cells; Placental growth restriction (Obstetrics); Plasma/ Preprandial glucose concentration; Poor glycemic control; Postgraduate course; Presystemic glucuronide conjugation; Primordial germ cell; Prophylactic glucocorticoid.

PGD Phosphogluconate dehydrogenase (see 6- PGD); Phosphoglyceraldehyde dehydrogenase; Pre-implantation genetic diagnosis (a procedure combining in-vitro fertilization with genetic testing of fertilized cells) (= PIGD); Prostaglandin D; Prostaglandin dehydrogenase (see PGDH).

PGD$_2$ Prostaglandin D_2 (an inflammatory mediator).

6-PGD 6-Phosphogluconate dehydrogenase (see G6PD).

PGDF Pilot Guide Dog Foundation.

PGDH 15-Hydroxyprostaglandin/ Phosphogluconate dehydrogenase (see G6PD).

PGDM; Pre-GDM Pregestational diabetes mellitus (Obstetrics).

PGDR Plasma glucose disappearance rate.

PGE Parotid gland enlargement; Platelet granule extract; Posterior gastroenterostomy; Prostaglandin E.

PGE$_1$ Prostaglandin E_1.

PGE_2 Prostaglandin E_2 (= PE_2).
PGEA Postgraduate Education Appraisal (GMC, UK).
PGEm Prostaglandin E metabolite.
PGES Postgastroenteritic syndrome.
PGF Paternal grandfather; Peptide/ Protein growth factor; Platelet (derived) growth factor (see PDGF); Prostaglandin F.
PGF_1 Prostaglandin F_1.
PGF_{1a}; $PGF_{1\alpha}$; PGF_1^a Prostaglandin F_1 alpha.
PGF_2 Prostaglandin F_2.
PGF_{2a}; $PGF_{2\alpha}$; PGF_2^a Prostaglandin F_2 alpha.
PGFT Phosphoribosylglycinamide formyltransferase.
PGG Polyclonal gamma globulin; Prostaglandin G.
PGG_2 A cyclic endoperoxide - a derivative of arachidonic acid and a precursor of prostacyclin (PGI_2); Prostaglandin G_2.
PGGE Polyacrylamide gradient gel electrophoresis.
PGH Past/ Poo/ Present/ Previous general health; Philadelphia General Hospital; Pituitary/ Porcine growth hormone (see Hormones - GH); Pineal gland hormone (Melatonin) (see AAH); Prostaglandin H.
PGH_2 A cyclic endoperoxide (see PGG_2); Prostaglandin H_2.
PGI Phosphoglucose isomerase; Potassium, glucose, and insulin; Postaglandin I.
PGI_2 Epoprostenol; Prostacyclin - a derivative of arachnoid acid, a precursor of the cyclic endoperoxides PGG_2 and PGH_2, and a vasodilator, preventing platelet aggregation (= PGX); Prostaglandin I_2.
PGK Phosphoglycerate kinase.
PGL Persistent generalized lymphadenopathy; Phosphoglycolipid; Plasma glucose level.
PGl Prostaglandin (see PG).
PGL_2 Prostaglandin$_2$.
PGlyM Phosphoglyceromutase.
PGM Paternal grandmother; Phosphoglucomutase.
PGM_1 Phosphoglucomutase$_1$.
PGMA Polyglyceryl methacrylate.
PGMD Polyethylene glycol-modified ("pegylated") derivative (of interferon alfa-2B) (see PIFN-2B).
PGME Monomethyl ester of propylene glycol; Postgraduate medical education.
PGMT p-Glycoprotein-mediated transport (see GMT).
PGN Postinfectious glomerulonephritis; Proliferative glomerulonephritis.
PGO Ponto-geniculo-occipital (spike).
PGP Paternal grandparent; Patient's/ Personal genetic profile; Phosphoglyceroyl phosphatase; Postgamma proteinuria; Prepaid group practice; Progressive general paralysis.
PGR Platelet glycoprotein-receptor; Prandial glucose regulation; Principles governing research; Progesterone receptor (see PgR); Psychogalvanic resistance/ response (audiometry) (see PGSR).
PgR Progesterone receptor (= PGR).
PGRA Platelet glycoprotein-receptor antagonist (see GRA).
PGS Pantagastrin-stimulated (peak acid output, in the stomach); Parallel group study (= PGT); Persistent gross splenomegaly; Pharmacogenomic study; Plant Genetic Systems; Plant growth substance; Postsurgical gastroparesis syndrome; Prostaglandin synthetase; Protected genital sex.
PGs Pharmacogenetics (gene receptors, enzymes, and vulnerability to drugs); Prostaglandins; Pyoderma gangrenosum.
PGSI Prostaglandin synthetase inhibitor.
P_2G Solution Two percent phenol w/v with 30% glycerine v/v in water for injection. Used as a local sclerosing agent for varicose veins.
PGSR Psychogalvanic skin resistance/ response (audiometry) (= PGR).
PGSW Penetrating gun-shot wound.
PGT Parallel group trial (see PGS); Pharmacological gene therapy; Polygraph test (see LDT); Postgraduate training.
PGTR Plasma glucose tolerance rate.
PGTT Prednisolone glucose tolerance test.
PGU Peripheral glucose uptake; Postgonococcal urethritis.
PGUT Phophogalactose uridyl transferase.
PGV Proximal gastric vagotomy.
PGW Psychogeriatric ward.

PGWB Psychological General Well-Being (Index).
PGX Prostacyclin (see PGI_2).
PGY Postgraduate year.
PGYE Peptone, glucose yeast extract.
PH Parathyroid/otropic hormone (see PTH); Partial hepatectomy/ hysterectomy; Passive hemagglutination; Past/ Patient's/ Personal/ Physical/ Previous history; Peliosis hepatis (blood-filled cysts in the liver, following androgenic steroid therapy); Persistent hepatitis; Pharmacopeia/poeia (see Ph); Pinhole; Poor/ Public health; Porphyria hepatica; Posterior hypothalamus; Postural hypotension; Primary hyperparathyroidism; Prospect Hill (virus); Prostatic hypertrophy; Pseudohermaphroditism; Pubic hair; Pulmonary hypertension/ hypoplasia.
Ph Pharmacopeia/poeia (= PH); Phenyl (chemical symbol); Philadelphia (chromosome) (see Ph'); Phosphate.
pH Hydrogen ion concentration (= negative logarithm of the hydrogen ion concentration of a solution, i.e. measurement of acidity or alkalinity.
ph phial; phot.
Ph' Philadelphia chromosome (laboratory/ hematology) (= Ph; Ph^1c).
pH_1 Isoelectric point.
PH 203 Hypacom (a proprietary drug containing a mixture of methanesulfonates).
PHA Passive hemagglutination (technique); Passive hemagglutination-inhibition assay; Pelger-Hüet anomaly (see PNA - Pelger's nuclear anomaly); Peripheral hyperalimentation; Phenylalanine (= PA; Phe); Phytohemagglutinin (= Phytohemagglutin) - a complex mucoprotein extract from the seeds of the bean Phaseolus vulgaris, causing hemagglutination, serum-protein precipitation, and the stimulation of mitosis in leukocytes. Has been tried in the treatment of aplastic anemia, with equivocal results; Phytohemagglutinin activation/ antigen; Post-hoc (L. after this) analysis; Primary hyperaldosteronism; Pseudohypoaldosteronism; Public Health Administrator/ Authority; Public health approach; Pulse-height analyzer.
pHa acid pH; Arterial blood pH.
pH_A Arterial blood hydrogen tension.
PHAL Phytohemagglutinin-stimulated lymphocyte.
phal phalangeal/anx.
PHA-LCM Phytohemagglutinin-stimulated leukocyte conditioned medium.
PHAM; PHA-m Phytohemagglutinin-mucopolysaccharide (fraction).
PHAP; PHA-P Phytohemagglutinin-protein (fraction).
phar pharmaceutical/acist/acology/acopeia/acopoeia/acy (see Pharm); pharynx (= phx).
Phar B Bachelor of Pharmacy (L. Pharmaciae Baccalaureus).
Phar C Pharmaceutical Chemist (= PhC).
Phar D Doctor of Pharmacy (L. Pharmaciae Doctor) (= PD; PhD).
Phar G Graduate in Pharmacy (= PhG; PhmG).
PHARM Pharmacy (see Pharm; pharm).
Pharm; pharm Pharmaceutical/acist/acology/acopeia/acopoeia/acy (= PC; phar; PHARM).
Phar M Master of Pharmacy (L. Pharmaciae Magister) (= PhM).
PharmD Doctor of Pharmacy (see Phar D).
Pharm Soc Lab Rep Pharmaceutical Society's Laboratory Report (British).
Ph-ase Phosphorylase.
PHB Polyhydroxybutyrate; Potential health benefit; Preventive health behavior.
PhB Bachelor of Philosophy.
PhB; Phb Pharmacopoeia Brittanica (see BP).
PHBB Propylhydroxybenzyl benzimidazole.
PHC People's Health Center; Personal health costs; Physically handicapped child; Post-hospital care; Premolar hypodontia, hyperhidrosis, (premature) canities (syndrome); Preventive/ Primary/ Professional health care; Primary Health Center (India); Primary hepatic/ tocellular carcinoma; Primary hypercholesterolemia (types IIa and IIb); Proliferative helper cell; Prostate Health Council (AFUD); Public Health Committee (BMA).
PhC Pharmaceutical chemist.
Ph^1c Philadelphia chromosome (see Ph^1).

PHCC Primary hepatocellular carcinoma.
PHCP Physically Handicapped Children's Program; Primary health care professional.
PHCR Productivity and Health Care Resources.
PHCT Primary health care team.
PHD Pathological habit disorder; Post-heparin (plasma) diamine oxidase; Potentially harmful drug; Pre-existing/ Premature/ Pulmonary heart disease; Primary/ Progressive hepatic disease/ disorder (see PLD); Progressive hereditary disease (e.g. Cystic fibrosis); Pseudohypertrophic dystrophy (see DPHD).
PhD Doctor of Pharmacy (L. Pharmaciae Doctor) (see Phar D); Doctor of Philosophy (L. Philosophiae Doctor).
PHE Periodic health exam(ination); Post-operative hyponatremic encephalopathy.
Phe Phenylalanine (see PHA).
PhEEM Photoemission electron microscope/py.
PHEMA Poly-2-hydroxyethylmethacrylate.
Phe-Mer-Nite Phenyl mercuric nitrate (a germicide) (= Phe-Ni-Mer).
Phen Phenformin (see DBI).
Phe-Ni-Mer Phenyl mercuric nitrate (see Phe-Mer-Nite).
Pheno Phenotype.
Pheo Pheochromocytoma (see PCC).
pheresis (Gr.) apheresis = to remove, separate, or take away.
PhEur European Pharmacopia.
PHEW-O Patient Health Education and Welfare Office.
PHF Paired helical filament; Personal hygiene facility; Phagocytosis frequency; Progressive heart failure (= PCF).
PHFG Primary (cultures of) human fetal glia.
PhG Graduate in Pharmacy (see Phar G); Pharmacopoeia Germanica (see PG).
PHGHG Post-hypoglycemic hyperglycemia (= SP - Somogyi phenomenon).
Phgly Phenylglycine.
PHH Post-hemorrhagic hydrocephalus.
PHI Passive hemagglutination inhibition; Past history of illness; Phagocytosis/ Prehospital index; Phosphohexose isomerase; Physiological hyaluronidase inhibitor; Programmable hearing instrument; Public health intervention; Public Home Infirmary.
PhI Pharmacopoeia Internationalis (see PI).
-philia Greek: philein - to regard with affection/ to love - Word termination, designating notable or abnormal attachment, attraction, combination, fondness, fixation, interaction, and/or interest for the particular subject, indicated by the stem to which it is attached.
I. Emotional/ Psychological/ Sympathetic attachment to or love for, as in:
algophilia (= algophily) - Sexual perversion marked by a desire for experiencing pain;
ailurophilia (= galeophilia; gatophilia) - a morbid or inordinate fondness for cats;
alcoholophilia - a morbid appetite for alcoholic drinks;
autophilia - Pathological self-esteem;
claustrophilia - a morbid desire to be shut in, to close all doors, windows, etc.);
coprophilia - a psychopathologic interest in filth, especially in feces and in defecation (= mysophilia);
dendrophilia - Erotic love for trees;
epistemophilia - an abnormal or marked interest in learning;
galeophilia - inordinate fondness for cats (see ailurophilia);
gatophilia - inordinate fondness for cats (see ailurophilia);
gerontophilia - special fondness for old people;
hyphephilia - Sexual gratification by contact, friction or rubbing, with fabrics such as silk, velvet, etc.;
lipophilia - (i) Affinity for fat, (ii) A tendency of the obese for fat fixation;
lygophilia - abnormal longing for dark places;
mysophilia - a form of paraphilia in which there is a lustful attitude toward excretions (see coprophilia; paraphilia);
necrophilia (= necrophilism) - a morbid attraction to corpses, sexual intercourse with a dead body;
nosophilia - a morbid desire to be sick;
nyctophilia - Abnormal preference for night over day;
ophidiophilia/ ophiophilia - Morbid fondness for snakes;
osphresiophilia - Abnormal interest in odors;

paraphilia - Aberrant sexual activity; expression of the sexual instinct in practices which are socially prohibited, unacceptable, or biologically undesirable;
pathophilia - The condition in which a patient adapts himself and his mode of life to some chronic affection;
pedophilia - A morbid interest in children;
pedophilia erotica - Sexual perversion toward children;
pharmacophilia - Morbid fondness for drugs;
photophilia - Fondness of light; scatophilia - a perverted fondness for dung;
scophophilia (= soptophilia) (i) active scophophilia - The derivation of sexual pleasure from looking at genital organs, (ii) passive scophophilia - A morbid desire to be seen (naked);
scoptophilia (see scophophilia);
scotophilia - Love of darkness;
taphophilia - Morbid interest in graves and cemetries;
traumatophilia - a subconscious delight in one's own injuries or surgical operations.
II. Chemical/ Physiological/ Synergistic combination or interaction as in:
achromatophilia - The property of resisting the coloring action of stains;
aneosinophilia (= eosinopenia) - Decrease in the number of eosinophils (see hypoeosinophilia);
angiohemophilia (= pseudohemophilia; vascular hemophilia; von Willebrand's disease) - A congenital hemorrhagic diathesis, characterized by integumentary and mucosal surface bleeding, with or without associated platelet defects or deficiencies of blood coagulation factor VIII or IX;
azurophilia - a condition in which the blood contains cells having azurophil (staining well with blue aniline dyes) granulations;
barophilia - preferentially best growth, such as bacterial, under high atmospheric pressure;
basophilia - (i) An abnormal increase in basophilic erythrocytes in the blood, as in Punctate/ Stippling basophilia or Diffuse basophilia/ polychromasia, (ii) basocytosis - An abnormal increase in basophilic leukocytes in the blood;
calciphilia - A tendency to absorb lime salts from the blood and thus become calcified;
carbophilia - Tendency to grow best in the presence of carbon dioxide;
carcinophilia - Special affinity for cancerous tissue;
chromatophilia (= chromophilia) - the condition of staining easily;
hromophilia (see chromatophilia); crymophilia (see cryophilia);
cryophilia (= crymophilia) - the condition of growing best at low temtemperatures (e.g. bacteria);
deuterohemophilia - a condition resembling classical hemophilia, a hemophilioid state (see hemophilia);
eosinophilia -(i) A large increase in blood eosinophils, (ii) The condition of being readily stained with eosin;
euchsinophilia - the property of staining readily with fuchsin dyes;
glycerophilia - having a special affinity for glycerine;
glycophilia - an illness in which a small amount of dextrose causes hyperglycemia;
hematophilia (see hemophilia);
hemoglobinophilia - Fondness for hemoglobin (bacteriology);
hemophilia (= hematophilia; hemorrhaphilia) - A hereditary hemorrhagic diathesis characterized by internal bleeding, and due to deficient generation of thromboplastin;
hemorrhaphilia (see hemophilia);
hydrophilia - the property of absorbing water;
hypereosinophilia - excessive eosinophilia;
hypoeosinophilia (= eosinopenia) - abnormal deficiency of eosinophilic leukocytes in the blood (see aneosinophilia);
iodophilia - Staining of leukocytes with iodine (intra/extracellular staining);
mesophilia - Fondness for moderate temperature (bacterial growth);
neutrophilia (= neutrophilic leukocytosis) - Increase in the number of neutrophil leukocytes in the blood;
opsonophilia - Affinity for opsonins (antibacterial antibodies);
parahemophilia (= Owren's disease) - a hemophilia-like condition caused by the con-

genital absence of blood coagulation factor V;
polychromatophilia (= polychromophilia) (i) The quality of affinity for all sorts of stains, (ii) A condition in which the erythrocytes on staining, show various shades of blue combined with tinges of pink;
polychromophilia (see polychromatophilia);
pseudohemophilia (see angiohemophilia);
spasmophilia - A condition in which the motor nerves show abnormal sensitiveness to mechanical or electric stimulation and the patient, a tendency to spasm, tetany, and convulsions;
sudanophilia - (i) Affinity for Sudan stain, (ii) A condition in which the leukocytes contain particles that stain readily with Sudan red (indicative of suppuration);
thermophilia - Growing best or having a fondness for high temperatures (microorganisms);
thrombophilia - A tendency to the occurrence of thrombosis.

philos philosophy.

PHIM Post-hypoxic intention myoclonus.

PHIS Post-head injury syndrome.

p^{HisoHex} Trade mark for an emulsion containing hexachlorophene.

PHK Platelet hexokinase (phospho); Postmortem human kidney (cells).

PHL Permanent/ Persistant/ Persisting/ Profound hearing loss; Philadelphia (chromosome); Progressive hair loss; Public Health Laboratory.

PHLA Post-heparin lipolytic activity.

PHLS Public Health Laboratory Service (Britain).

PHLSHC Public Health Laboratory Service Hydatid Centre (Liverpool, UK).

PHM Peptide histidine methionine; Posterior hyaloid membrane; Predominant human metabolite; Promoter hypermethylation; Public health measure/ medicine (= Community medicine) (UK); Pulmonary hyaline membrane.

PhM Master of Pharmacy (L. Pharmaciae Magister) (see Phar M); Pharyngeal muscle.

pHm Muscle surface pH.

PHMG Post-heparin monoglyceridase.

PhmG Graduate in Pharmacy (see Phar G).

PHN Paroxysmal nocturnal hemoglobinuria; Passive Heymann nephritis; Post-herpetic neuralgia; Primary human neoplasia; Public Health Nurse; Public health nursing.

PHO Periarticular heterotopic ossification; Public health official.

PH_2O Partial pressure of water vapor.

phob- Greek: phobos - combining form meaning morbid dread or fear, e.g.:
Acarophobia - morbid dread of mites (*Acarus*), or of small objects;
Acousticophobia - morbid fear of sounds;
Acrophobia (= Aerophobia; Hypsiphobia; Hypsophobia) - morbid fear of high altitudes;
Aelurophobia (see Ailurophobia);
Aerophobia - i) Morbid dread of air, air drafts, air-borne influences, or bad air (e.g. body odor), ii) Morbid fear of being up in the air (= Acrophobia);
Agoraphobia (= Kenophobia) - morbid fear of open spaces;
Aichmophobia - abnormal fear of sharp-pointed objects;
Ailurophobia (= Aeurulophobia; Elurophobia; Galeophobia; Gatophobia) - morbid fear of cats;
Algophobia (= Odynophobia) - morbid dread of experiencing or of witnessing pain;
Amathophobia - morbid fear of dust;
Amaxophobia - insane dread of vehicles;
Amychophobia - morbid fear of being scratched, as by the claws of a cat;
Androphobia - morbid fear or dislike of the male sex;
Anemophobia - morbid fear of wind or of drafts;
Anginophobia - morbid dread of angina pectoris;
Ankylophobia - morbid fear of ankylosis in cases of fracture or joint disease;
Anthophobia - morbid dislike or dread of flowers;
Anthropophobia - morbid fear of crowds, human gatherings, or society;
Aphephobia - morbid dread of touching or being touched;
Apiphobia - morbid fear of bees and their sting;

Arachnophobia - morbid fear of spiders;
Asthenophobia - morbid fear of being weak or losing weight;
Astraphobia - i) (= Astrophobia) morbid fear of the stars, ii) (= Astrapophobia) morbid fear of lightning;
Astrophobia (= Astraphobia) - morbid fear of the stars and celestial space;
Astrapophobia (= Astraphobia) - morbid fear of lightning;
Ataxiophobia (see Ataxophobia);
Ataxophobia (= Ataxiophobia) - morbid or insane dread of disorder;
Automysophobia - abnormally exaggerated dread of personal uncleanliness;
Autophobia (= Eremophobia) - abnormal dread of being alone;
Bacillophobia, Bacteriophobia - morbid fear of disease-producing microorganisms;
Ballistophobia - a morbid dread of missiles;
Basiphobia (see Basophobia);
Basophobia (= Basiphobia) - morbid fear if walking, or fear of being unable to walk;
Bathmophobia - morbid fear of stairways or steep slopes;
Bathophobia - morbid fear of depths, or looking down from a high place with fear of falling;
Batophobia - morbid fear of passing near or among high objects (e.g. buildings, mountains, etc.);
Belonephobia - dread of pins and needles;
Bromidrosiphobia - morbid dread of bodily odors, with delusions as to their perception;
Cainotophobia (see Cenophobia; Cenotophobia; Neophobia) - morbid fear of novelty or new things;
Cancerophobia, Cancerphobia, Carcinomatophobia (see Carcinophobia);
Carcinophobia (= Cancerophobia; Cancerphobia; Carcinomatophobia) - morbid fear of/ Delusion of being affected with cancer;
Cardiophobia - morbid dread/ fear of heart disease;
Carnophobia - abnormal aversion to meat/ meat foods;
Cathisophobia (= Acathisia; Akathesia) - a condition of motor restlessness with inability to sit or lie down quietly, or to sleep;
Catoptrophobia. (= Eisoptrophobia) - morbid fear of mirrors;
Cenophobia (see Cainotophobia; Cenotophobia; Neophobia) - i) morbid dread of large open spaces, ii) morbid fear of new things;
Cenotophobia (= Neophobia) - morbid fear of novelty or new things;
Cheimaphobia - morbid fear of cold;
Cherophobia - morbid dislike or fear of gaiety;
Cholerophobia - an abnormal dread of cholera;
Chrematophobia - morbid dread of money;
Chromatophobia (= Chromophobia) - morbid aversion to certain colors;
Chromophobia - i) a morbid aversion to colors (see Chromatophobia), ii) The quality of staining poorly to dyes;
Chronophobia - a morbid fear of time; a psychoneurosis found commonly in prison inmates;
Cibophobia - abnormal loathing of food;
Claustrophobia (= Cleisiophobia; Cleithrophobia; Clithrophobia) - morbid fear of closed spaces or of being shut up in a confined space;
Cleisiophobia, Cleithrophobia - (see Claustrophobia);
Cleptophobia - insane dread of becoming a thief or of being stolen (see Kleptophobia);
Clithrophobia (see Claustrophobia);
Coitophobia - morbid fear of coitus;
Cometophobia - morbid fear of comets;
Coprophobia - abnormal repugnance to defecation and to feces;
Crystallophobia (= Hyalophobia) - morbid fear of glass or objects made of glass;
Cynophobia - i) Morbid fear of dogs, rabies, etc., ii) Pseudorabies - a disease resembling rabies (see Lyssophobia);
Delanophobia - abnormal dread of fear itself;
Demonophobia - morbid fear of demons;
Dermatopathophobia - morbid anxiety with regard to the skin, its diseases, etc. (see Dermatophobia);
Dermatophobia (= Dermatopathophobia; Dermatosiophobia; Dermophobia) - morbid

fear of having some cutaneous lesion;
Dermatosiophobia, Dermophobia (see Dermatophobia);
Dextrophobia - morbid dread of objects on the right side of the body;
Diabetophobia - an abnormal fear of diabetes;
Dikephobia - morbid fear of justice;
Dinophobia - morbid fear of becoming dizzy;
Diplopiaphobia (= Horror fusionis - L - Horror of fusion) - antipathy to single binocular fusion, and manifested in the tendency of one eye to move away from the fixation state in which the retinal image falls on the macula in each eye;
Domatophobia - abnormal or morbid dread of being in a house;
Doraphobia - a morbid dread of the skin or fur of animals;
Dromophobia - morbid fear of roaming;
Dysmorphophobia - morbid fear of bodily deformity or of becoming deformed;
Ecophobia (= Oikophobia) - morbid aversion to home surroundings;
Eisoptrophobia - morbid fear of mirrors (see Catoptrophobia);
Elurophobia (see Ailurophobia);
Emetophobia - abnormal fear of vomiting;
Enissophobia - fear of reproach for sin, fear of unpardonable sin;
Entomophobia - morbid dread of insects (cockroaches, mites, ticks, etc.);
Eosophobia - morbid fear or dread of daybreak/ dawn;
Equinophobia - morbid fear of horses;
Eremophobia - morbid fear of being alone (see Autophobia);
Ergasiophobia (see Ergophobia);
Ergophobia (= Ergasiophobia) - i) Morbid fear of work, ii) Undue fear of performing surgical operations;
Erotophobia - morbid dislike for sex, sexual love, or the sexual act (see Genophobia);
Erythrophobia - i) A neurotic manifestation marked by blushing at the slighest provocation, ii) Morbid fear of blushing, iii) Morbid aversion to red;
Febriphobia - anxiety produced by a rise of body temperature;
Galeophobia - morbid fear of cats (see Ailurophobia);
Gamophobia - morbid fear of marriage;
Gatophobia - morbid fear of cats (see Ailurophobia);
Genophobia (= Erotophobia) - morbid dread of sex and sexuality;
Geumaphobia - morbid fear of tastes;
Glossophobia (see Lalophobia);
Graphophobia - abnormal dread of writing;
Gymnophobia - morbid aversion to the sight of the naked body; Gynephobia, Gynophobia - morbid aversion to or dread of the society of women;
Hadephobia - morbid fear of hell;
Haemophobia (= Hemophobia) - morbid dread of blood;
Haphephobia, Haptephobia - morbid fear of being touched;
Heliophobia - morbid avoidance or dread of sunlight;
Helminthophobia (= Vermiphobia) - morbid fear of being infected with worms;
Hemaphobia, Hematophobia (see Hemophobia);
Hemophobia (= Haemophobia; Hemaphobia; Hematophobia) - morbid dread of blood;
Hierophobia - fear of sacred or religious objects/ things (see Theophobia);
Homilophobia - dread of sermons;
Hyalophobia - morbid fear of glass (see Crystallophobia);
Hydrophobia - 'fear of water' - Rabies;
Hydrophobophobia - morbid dread of rabies (see Lyssophobia);
Hygrophobia - morbid fear of dampness or water;
Hylephobia - morbid fear of materialism;
Hypengyophobia - morbid fear of responsibility;
Hypophobia - lack of fear;
Hypsiphobia (see Acrophobia; Hypsophobia), Hypsophobia (= Hypsiphobia) - morbid fear of great heights (see Acrophobia);
Ichthyophobia - abnormal aversion to fish;
Iophobia - a morbid fear of poisons;
Kainophobia - morbid fear of new things;
Kathisophobia (= Acathisia; Akathisia) - a condition of motor restlessness, ranging from a feeling of inner disquiet to inability to sit or

lie quietly, or to sleep;
Kenophobia - morbid dread of large open spaces (see Agoraphobia);
Kinesophobia - dread of movement;
Kleptophobia (= Cleptophobia) - insane dread of becoming a thief or of being stolen;
Koinoniphobia - morbid fear of a room filled with people;
Kopophobia - morbid fear of fatigue;
Kynophobia - morbid fear of dogs or of hydrophobia;
Laliophobia - morbid fear of talking, stammering, and stuttering (see Lalophobia);
Lalophobia (= Glossophobia; Laliophobia) - morbid or extreme dislike of speaking, often associated with stuttering;
Lepraphobia - morbid dread of leprosy;
Levophobia - morbid dread of objects on the left side of the body (see Sinistrophobia);
Lyssophobia (= Cynophobia; Hydrophobophobia) - morbid dread of rabies, with symptoms simulating those of that disease;
Maieusiophobia - morbid dread of childbirth;
Maniaphobia - fear of insanity;
Melissophobia - abnormal dread of bees and other stinging insects;
Meningitophobia - morbid fear of meningitis, or with any condition simulating the disease;
Metallophobia - morbid fear of metals and metal objects;
Meteorophobia - morbid fear of meteors;
Microbiophobia - morbid dread of microbes (see Microphobia);
Microphobia - i) morbid fear of small objects, ii) insane dread of germs or microbes;
Molysmophobia (= Mysophobia) - morbid dread of filth and contamination.
Monophobia - morbid dread of being left alone;
Musophobia - morbid fear of mice;
Mysophobia (= Molysmophobia) - morbid dread of filth and contamination;
Mythophobia - morbid fear of myths or stating an untruth;
Necrophobia - i) Morbid fear of death, ii) Morbid dread of dead bodies;
Neophobia (= Cenotophobia) - morbid fear of novelty or new things;
Noctiphobia - morbid dread of night, darkness, and silence;
Nosophobia - abnormal fear of disease;
Nucleomitophobia - morbid fear of an atomic explosion;
Nudophobia - an abnormal aversion to being unclothed;
Nyctophobia - morbid fear of darkness or night;
Ochlophobia - morbid fear of crowds;
Odontophobia - an abnormal dread associated with or aroused by the sight of teeth; immense fear of dental operations;
Odynophobia - a morbid dread of pain (see Ponophobia);
Oikophobia (= Ecophobia) - morbid aversion to home surroundings;
Olfactophobia - morbid aversion to odors (see Osmophobia);
Ombrophobia - fear of rain;
Onomatophobia - morbid dread of hearing a certain name or word;
Ophidiophobia - morbid dread of snakes;
Osmophobia (= Olfactophobia; Osphresiophobia) - abnormal dread of odors;
Osphresiophobia - morbid dislike of odors (see Osmophobia);
Panophobia, Panphobia (see Pantophobia);
Pantaphobia - absence of fear;
Pantophobia (= Panophobia; Panphobia) - i) Fear of everything, ii) A vague morbid dread of some unknown evil;
Paralipophobia - morbid apprehension of neglecting something;
Parasitophobia - i) Morbid dread of parasites, ii) Morbid delusion that one is infested with parasites;
Parthenophobia - morbid dread of girls;
Pathophobia - morbid dread of disease;
Peccatiphobia - morbid fear of sinning;
Pediophobia - morbid dread of infants or of small dolls;
Pedophobia - fear or dread of children;
Peladophobia - morbid fear of baldness;
Peniaphobia - morbid fear of poverty;
Phagophobia (= Sitophobia) - morbid fear of eating;
Pharmacophobia - morbid dread of drugs or medicines;

Phasmophobia - fear of ghosts;
Phengophobia (= Photophobia) - abnormal intolerance to light;
Phobophobia - a condition in psychoasthenia, marked by fear of one's own fears;
Phonophobia - morbid dread of sounds or of speaking aloud;
Photaugiaphobia - abnormal intolerance to a glare of light;
Photophobia (= Phengophobia) - abnormal intolerance to light;
Phthisiophobia (= Tuberculophobia) - morbid dread of phthisis (tuberculosis);
Pnigophobia - abnormal dread of choking;
Polyphobia - morbid dread or fear of many things;
Ponophobia - i) abnormal dread of pain, ii) dread of work; morbid laziness;
Potamophobia - morbid dread of rivers, streams, lakes, etc.; Proctophobia - the mental state of apprehension in rectal disease;
Proteinphobia - morbid aversion to protein foods;
Pseudohydrophobia (= Aujeszky's disease; Pseudorabies) - an infectious viral disease causing bulbar paralysis of cattle, horses, and other domestic animals, first observed in Hungary and Brazil, where it is called the "scratching pest" (peste de cocar);
Psychrophobia - abnormal dread of cold;
Pyrexiophobia - morbid fear of fever;
Pyrophobia - abnormal dread of fire;
Radiophobia - morbid anxiety concerning the damaging effects of X-rays and radium;
Rectophobia - morbid foreboding peculiar to patients with rectal disease;
Rhabdophobia - morbid dread of a stick or of a beating;
Rhypophobia (= Rupophobia) - morbid dread of filth;
Rupophobia (see Ryphophobia);
Scabiophobia - morbid fear of scabies;
Scopophobia (= Scoptophobia) - morbid dread of being seen;
Scoptophobia (see Scopophobia);
Scotophobia - morbid fear of darkness;
Siderodromophobia, Siderophobia - morbid fear of railway travel;
Sinistrophobia (= Levophobia) - morbid dread of objects on the left side of the body;
Sitophobia (= Phagophobia) - morbid fear of eating;
Spectrophobia - morbid dread of mirrors or of seeing one's face in a mirror;
Spermatophobia - morbid fear of being affected with spermatorrhea (involuntary, frequent and excessive ejaculation or discharge of semen, without copulation);
Stasibasiphobia (= Stasobasiphobia - morbid distrust of one's ability to stand or walk (see Stasiphobia);
Stasiphobia (= Stasophobia) - morbid dread of standing erect;
Stasobasiphobia (see Stasibasiphobia);
Stasophobia (see Stasiphobia);
Symbolophobia - a morbid fear that one's acts may contain some symbolic meaning;
Syphiliphobia (see Syphilophobia);
Syphilophobia (= Syphilomania; Syphiphobia) - i) Morbid fear of syphilis (= Syphiliphobia), ii) The delusion of being infected with syphilis (= Syphilomania; Syphiphobia);
Syphiphobia. (see Syphilophobia);
Tabophobia - a morbid fear of tabes (dorsalis);
Taphophobia - Obsessive fear of being buried alive;
Telephonophobia - pathologic fear of telephones;
Teratophobia - i) Morbid fear or aversion to monsters, ii) Morbid dread of giving birth to a teratism (malformed fetus of fetal monster;
Thalassophobia - morbid dread of the sea;
Thanatophobia - morbid fear of death or the unwarrented apprehension of imminent death;
Thassophobia - morbid dread of sitting idle;
Theophobia - morbid fear of the Wrath of God;
Thermophobia - morbid dread of high temperatures;
Tocophobia - abnormal dread of childbirth;
Tonitrophobia, Tonitruphobia - morbid fear of thunder;
Topophobia - morbid dread of particular places;
Toxicophobia (= Toxiphobia) - morbid dread of poisons;

Toxiphobia (see Toxicophobia);
Tremophobia - morbid fear of trembling;
Trichinophobia - morbid dread of trichinosis;
Trichopathophobia - morbid anxiety with regard to the hair, its growth, disease, etc. (see Trichophobia);
Trichophobia - morbid dread of hair (see Trichopathophobia);
Tuberculophobia (= Phthisiophobia) - morbid dread of tuberculosis (phthisis);
Uranophobia - morbid dread of heaven;
Urophobia - fear of passing urine;
Vaccinophobia - morbid and perverse dread of vaccination;
Venerophobia - morbid dread of venereal infection;
Vermiphobia (= Helminthophobia) - morbid fear of being infected with worms;
Xenophobia - morbid dislike or fear of foreigners and strangers;
Xerophobia - Inhibition of saliva flow with dryness of the tongue, caused by fear, anger, or excitement;
Zoophobia - abnormal dread of animals.

Phobias Fear of: Air - Aerophobia; Almighty Wrath - Theophobia; Angina pectoris - Anginophobia; Animal fur - Doraphobia; Animals - Zoophobia; Ankylosis - Ankylophobia; Atomic explosion - Nucleomitophobia; Baldness - Peladophobia; Bees - Apiphobia, Melissophobia; Being seen - Scopophobia, Scoptophobia; Blood - Haemophobia, Hemaphobia, Hematophobia, Hemophobia; Blushing - Erythrophobia; Cancer - Cancerophobia, Cancerphobia, Carcinomatophobia, Carcinophobia; Cats - Aeurolophobia, Ailurophobia, Elurophobia, Galeophobia, Gatophobia; Childbirth - Maieusiophobia, Tocophobia; Children - Pedophobia; Choking - Pnigophobia; Cholera - Choleraphobia; Closed space - Claustrophobia, Cleisiophobia, Cleithrophobia; Clithrophobia; Cold - Cheimaphobia, Psychrophobia; Colors - Chromatophobia, Chromophobia; Comets - Cometophobia; Corporeal punishment - Rhabdophobia; Crowds - Anthropophobia, Koinoniphobia, Ochlophobia; Darkness - Scotophobia; Dawn - Eosophobia; Death - Necrophobia, Thanatophobia; Deformity (bodily) - Dysmorphophobia; Depths - Bathophobia; Diabetes - Diabetophobia; Dirt/ Filth - Automysophobia, Mysophobia, Molysmophobia, Rhypophobia; Disease - Nosophobia, Pathophobia, Rupophobia; Disorder - Ataxiophobia, Ataxophobia; Dolls - Pediophobia; Dust - Amathophobia; Dyes - Chromophobia; Eating - Phagophobia, Sitophobia; Fatigue - Kopophobia; Fear - Delanophobia, Phobophobia; Fear of everything - Panophobia, Panphobia, Pantophobia, Polyphobia; Fear, absence of - Pantaphobia; Fearlessness - Hyphophobia; Feces - Coprophobia; Fever - Febriphobia, Pyrexiophobia; Fire - Pyrophobia; Fish - Ichthyophobia; Flowers - Anthophobia; Food - Cibophobia; Gaiety - Cherophobia; Ghosts - Phasmophobia; Girls - Parthenophobia; Glass - Crystallophobia, Hyalophobia; Hair - Trichopathophobia, Trichophobia; Heart disease - Cardiophobia; Heaven - Uranophobia; Heights - Acrophobia, Hypsiphobia, Hypsophobia; Hell - Hadephobia; High temperatures - Thermophobia; Horses - Equinophobia; House/ Home surroundings - Domatophobia, Ecophobia, Oikophobia; Idleness - Thassophobia; Insanity - Maniaphobia; Insects - Entomophobia, Melissophobia; Justice - Dikephobia; Lakes - Potamophobia; Left side of body - Levophobia, Sinistrophobia; Leprosy - Lepraphobia; Light - Phengophobia, Photaugiaphobia, Photophobia; Lightning - Astrapophobia, Astraphobia; Loneliness - Autophobia, Eremophobia; Marriage - Gamophobia; Materialism - Hylephobia; Meat - Carnophobia; Medicines/ Drugs - Pharmacophobia; Meningitis - Meningitophobia; Metals - Metallophobia; Meteors - Meteorophobia; Microorganisms - Bacillophobia, Bacteriophobia, Microbiophobia, Microphobia; Mirrors - Catoptrophobia, Eisoptrophobia; Missiles - Ballistophobia; Mites - Acarophobia, Entomophobia; Money - Chrematophobia; Monsters (fetal and other) - Teratophobia; Mountains/ High buildings - Batophobia; Movement - Kinesophobia; Myths -

Mythophobia; Names - Onomatophobia; Neglect - Paralipophobia; Night - Noctiphobia, Nyctophobia; Novelty - Cainotophobia, Cenophobia, Cenotophobia, Kainophobia, Neophobia; Nudity - Gymnophobia, Nudophobia; Odors - Aerophobia, Bromidrophobia, Olfactophobia, Osmophobia, Osphresiophobia; Open spaces - Agoraphobia, Cenophobia, Kenophobia; Pain - Algophobia, Odynophobia, Ponophobia; Parasites - Parasitophobia; Particular places - Topophobia; Pins & Needles - Belonephobia; Poisons - Iophobia, Toxicophobia, Toxiphobia; Poverty - Peniaphobia; Protein foods - Proteinphobia; Pseudorabies - Pseudohydrophobia; Rabies/ Dogs - Cyophobia, Hydrophobia, Hydrophobophobia, Kynophobia, Lyssophobia; Railway travel - Siderodromophobia, Siderophobia; Rain - Ombrophobia; Rectal disease - Proctophobia, Rectophobia; Red (color) - Erythrophobia; Religious objects - Hierophobia; Responsibility - Hypengyophobia; Restlessness - Cathisophobia, Kathisophobia; Right side of body - Dextrophobia; Rivers; - Potamophobia; Robbery - Cleptophobia, Kleptophobia; Scabies - Scabiophobia; Scratches - Amychophobia; Sea - Thalassophobia; Seeing one's image in the mirror - Spectrophobia; Self-internment (burial) - Taphophobia; Sermons - Homilophobia; Sex, Coitus - Coitophobia, Erotophobia, Genophobia; Female society - Gynephobia,Gynophobia; Dislike of sex in males - Androphobia; Sharp objects - Aichmophobia; Sin - Enissophobia; Sinning - Peccatiphobia; Skin disease - Dermatphobia, Dermatopathophobia, Dermatosiophobia; Dermophobia; Small objects - Microphobia; Snakes - Ophidiophobia; Sounds - Acousticophobia, Phonophobia; Speaking/ Stammering - Glossophobia, Lalophobia, Laliophobia; Spermatorrhea (seminal discharge) - Spermatophobia; Spiders - Arachnophobia; Stairways/ Steep slopes - Bathmophobia; Standing erect - Stasibasiphobia, Stasiphobia, Stasobasiphobia, Stasophobia; Stars - Astrophobia, Astrophobia; Strangers/ Foreigners - Xenophobia; Sunlight - Heliophobia; Symbols - Symbolophobia; Syphilis - Syphiliphobia, Syphilophobia, Syphiphobia; Tabes - Tabophobia; Taste - Geumaphobia; Teeth - Odontophobia; Telephones - Telephonophobia; Thunder - Tonitrophobia, Tonitruphobia Time - Chronophobia; Tongue (dryness of) - Xerophobia; Touch - Aphephobia, Haphephobia, Haptephobia; Trembling - Tremophobia; Trichinosis - Trichinophobia; Tuberculosis - Phthisiophobia, Tuberculophobia; Urination - Urophobia; Vaccination - Vaccinophobia; Vehicles - Amaxophobia; Venereal disease - Venerophobia; Vertigo - Dinophobia; Vision (single binocular fusion) - Diplopiaphobia; Vomiting - Emetophobia; Walking - Basiphobia, Basophobia; Wandering - Dromophobia; Weakness - Asthenophobia; Wind - Anemophobia; Work - Ergasiophobia, Ergophobia, Ponophobia; Writing - Graphophobia; Worms - Helminthophobia, Vermiphobia; X-rays - Radiophobia.

phon phonology.

Phos Phosphorus (= P) (see Elements - Phosphorus).

phos phosphate.

photog photography.

PHP Persistent hyperphenylalaninemia; Post-heparin phospholipase; Post-hypophysectomy polydipsia/ polyuria; Prehospital program; Prepaid health plan; Primary hyperparathyroidism (see pHPT); Proximal humerus prosthesis (Neer II - see OI/OP); Pseudohypoparathyroidism (see PHPT); Public health physician/ perspective/ problem.

p-HPPO p-Hydroxyphenyl pyruvate oxidase.

PHPT Primary hyperparathyroidism (see pHPT); Pseudohypoparathyroidism (= PHP).

pHPT Primary hyperparathyroidism (= PHP; PHPT).

PHPV Persistent hyperplastic primary vitreous.

PHQ Patient Health Questionnaire (Primary Care Study Group).

PHR Peak heart rate; Photoreactivity;

Proximal humerus reconstruction; 'Pseudohypoglycemic' reaction (to anxiety and hyperventilation); Public-health risk.

PHRI Public Health Research Institute.

PhRMA Pharmaceutical Research and Manufacturers of America (Foundation).

PHS Partial hospitilization program; Patient-heated serum; Physicians' Health Services/ Study; Pooled human serum; Post-hypnotic suggestion; Post-hysterectomy syndrome; Program for Human Sexuality; Public Health Service; Pudenz-Heyer-Schulte (valves used in neurosurgery in shunt operation).

PHSACIP Public Health Service Advisory Committee on Immunization Practices.

PHSC Pleuripotent homopoietic stem cell.

PHSL Public Health Service Laboratory (UK).

PHSRG Physicians' Health Study Research Group (US).

PHSS Pathological human social behavior.

pH-stat Apparatus for maintaining the pH of a solution.

PHT Passive hyperimmune therapy (= PIT); Permanent hypothyroidism; Peroxide hemolysis test; Phenytoin (= PT); Pinhole test (to eliminate refractive error - eye examination); Portal/ Pulmonary hypertension; Post-hepatic transplant(ation); Postural hypotension; Primary hyperthyroidism.

PHT Act Public Health Training Act.

PhTD Doctor of Physical Therapy.

PHTN Paradoxical/ Portal/ Primary (= EHTN)/ Pulmonary hypertension.

PHTS Psychiatric Home Treatment Service.

PHV Peak height velocity; Peak hypercapnic ventilation (see VFR); *Pediculus* humanus varcorporis (Body louse); *Pediculus* pubis (Crab or Pubic louse); *Pediculus* varcapitus (Head louse); Periodic home visit(s); Pivot/ Porcine/ Prosthetic heart valve (Lillehei-Cruz-Kaster prosthesis); Prospect Hill virus.

PHVT Prosthetic heart valve thrombosis.

PHX Pulmonary histiocytosis X.

PHx; Phx Past history (see PH).

Phx; phx Pharynx (see phar).

PHY Pharyngitis; Physical (see Phys); Physics (see Phys); Physiology (see Physio); Phytohemagglutination.

PHYS Physiology (see Physio).

PhyS Physiologic(al) saline (solution) (= PSS; pss).

Phys; phys Physical (= PHY); Physician; Physics (= PHY); Physiology (see Physio).

phys dis physical disability.

Phys Ed Physical education.

Physio; physio; Physiol; physiol Physiology (= PHY; PHYS; Phys; phys); Physiotherapist/py (see PT).

Phys Med Physical medicine (see PM).

Phys Ther Physical therapist/py (see PT).

PI First meiotic prophase; Isoelectric point (see pI); Pacing impulse; Package insert; Pancreatic insufficiency; Parainfluenza; Paranoid ideation (see MDP); Pars intermedia; Past/ Present illness; Patient's interest; Pearl index (number of pregnancies/ 100 women years) of oral contraceptive steroids; Performance intensity; Perinatal injury; Periodontal/ Permeability/ Phagocytic/ Plaque/ Ponderal (height/ weight)/ Prematurity/ Pulsatility index; Peripheral iridectomy (operation/ ophthalmology)/ ischemia; Permanent incidence; Peroral insulin (see Insulin - PI i); Personal injury; Personality inventory; Pharmacopoeia Internationalis (= PhI); Phosphatidylinositol; Phosphoinositide; Physically impaired; Pineal body; Plant insulin (see Insulin - PI ii); Plasmin inhibitor; Pneumatosis intestinalis; Poison ivy; Porcine insulin (see Insulin - PI iii); Post-ictal immobility; Post-infection; Post-influenza; Post-injury; Post-inoculation; Pre-induction (examination); Premature infant; Preparatory interval; Pressure index (= ASP/BSP = Ankle/Brachial systolic pressure); Pressure in/of inspiration (see Pi); Primary infarction/ infection; Principal investigation/ator; Proactive interference; Product information; Programmed instruction; Proinsulin; Prolactin inhibitor (= Pi); Protease inhibitor(s) (= Pi) (see AIDS) including indinavir, nelfinavir, ritonavir and saquinavir: Indinavir - Crixivan (Merck), Sequinavir - Invirase (Hoffmann La Roche), Ritonavir - Norvir (Abbot Labs); ABT-378 (Abbot Labs), Nelfinavir (Agouron Pharmaceuticals) - formulated for children as well as adults; Protamine insulin (see Insulin - PI iv); Protocol Internationale (International Protocol); Proximal intestine; Pulmonary incompetence/ infarction/ infection/ insufficiency; Pulsatility index (in fetal blood vessels); Pulsed immunization (of communities, in successive 'pulses').

pi platelet (count) increment.

p.i. post ingestion/ inhalation/ intake (of a drug).

Pi Inorganic phosphate/ phosphorus (serum); Parental generation; Pressure in/of inspiration (respiratory therapy) (= PI); Prolactin/ Protease inhibitor (see PI).

pI Isoelectric point (= PI).

P_I Inspiratory pressure (see PFT - P_I).

P_i Inorganic phosphate (see Pi).

PIA Peripheral interface adapter; Photoelectric intravenous angiography; Plasma insulin activity (laboratory/ endocrinology); Post-infarction angina; Post-infectious arthritis; Pre-infarct(ion) angina; Primary insurance amount; Prolactin-induced amenorrhea; Psychiatric Institute of America.

PIAT Peabody Individual Achievement Test.

PIAVA Polydactyly-imperforate anus-vertebral anomalies (syndrome).

PIB Poisons Information Bureau (UK); Positive iron balance.

PIBC Percutaneous intraaortic balloon counterpulsation (catheter).

PIBCT Protease inhibitor-based combination therapy (for AIDS) (Protease inhibitors such as Amprenavir, Indinavir, Nelfinavir, Ritonavir, Saquinavir, etc., with Nucleoside reverse transcriptase inhibitor analogues [NRTIs or "Nucs"] such as Azidothymidine or Zidovudine [AZT; ZDV], ddC, d4T, 3TC, Didanosine or Dideoxyinosine [ddI; DDI], Lamivudine, Stavudine, Zalcitabine, Abacavir, etc., and Non-nucleoside reverse transcriptase inhibitors [NNRTIs or "Non-nucs"] such as Delavirdine, DMP - 266 or Efavirenz, NVP or Nevirapine, MXC-442, etc.) (see RTI).

PIBS Post-infectious bronchospasm; Post-intestinal bypass syndrome.

PIC Pandemic influenza control (see IPP); Pediatric intensive care; Peripherally inserted catheter; Personality Inventory for Children; Physician-in-chief; Polymorphism information content; Population investigation committee; Potentially inoperable cancer/ carcinoma/ case; Proinflammatory cytokine (e.g. tumor necrosis factor-α, interleukin-1, rheumatoid factor, etc.).

PIC; PICa Preinvasive carcinoma (= CIS; IEC which see).

PIC; PICs Poisons Information Center(s).

PI:C Polyinosinic: polycitidylic.

P-IC Post-intercourse.

PICA Percutaneous transluminal coronary angioplasty; Porch Index of Communicative Abilities/ty; Posterior inferior cerebellar/ communicting artery.

Pica An abnormal appetite/ craving for unnatural foods such as chalk, clay, earth, etc.

PICC Peripherally inserted central catheter.

PICD Primary irritant contact dermatitis.

PICFS Post-infective chronic fatigue syndrome.

PICH Pancreatic islet cell hyperplasia; Primary intracerebral hemorrhage.

pico- 10^{-12} (= P), e.g. pg (= picogram; ìig; micromicrogram; 10^{-12} gram).

P_{ICO2} Partial pressure of carbon dioxide in inspired air (see PFT - PI_{CO2}).

PICSI Picture Identification for Children - Standardized Index.

PICSO Pressure-controlled intermittent coronary sinus occlusion.

PICT Primary intracranial tumor.

PICU Pediatric/ Pulmonary intensive care unit.

PID Pain intensity difference (score); Pelvic inflammatory disease; Photoionization detector; Plasma iron disappearance; Post-inertia dyskinesia; Primary immunodeficiency (see PIDD); Progessively increased dosage/ dose; Progressive intellectual deterioration; Potentially interacting drug; Prolapsed/ Protruded/ding intervertebral disk.

PIDA Public Interest Disclosure Act (of 1998 - UK).

PIDD Primary immunodeficiency disease/ disorder (e.g. ARA - Autosomal recessive agammaglobuninemia; Autosomal recessive SCID [severe combined immunodeficiency], etc.)

(see IIDD).

PIDJ Pediatric Infectious Disease Journal.

PIDM Phenothiazine-induced dyskinetic movement(s).

PIDRA Portable insulin dosage-regulating apparatus.

PIDS Pediatric infectious disease specialist; Primary immunodeficiency syndrome.

PIDT Plasma iron disappearance time.

PIE Paradoxical inhibitory effect (of the LHRH agonist) (see Hormones - LHRH); Para-infectious encephalopathy; Pill-induced esophagitis; Post-infectious encephalomyelitis; Potent inflammatory eicosanoid(s) (released from various cells, including mast cells and eosinophils) (see CLT; PAM); Pre-implantation embryo; Prosthetic infectious endocarditis; Pulmonary infiltration with eosinophilia (= Tropical eosinophilia; Weingarten syndrome); Pulmonary interstitial emphysema.

PIF Paratoid isoelectric focusing (variant protein); Peak inspiratory flow (see PFT - PIF); Plague-infected flea; Potentially important factor; Proinsulin-free; Prolactin-inhibiting factor (released by the hypothalamus) (see Hormones - PIH); Proliferation-inhibiting factor; Prostatic interstitial fluid.

PIFG Poor intrauterine fetal growth.

PIFL Post-implantation fetal loss (teratology study in laboratory animals).

PIFN Peginterferon (see PIFNα-2B).

PIFNα-2B Peginterferon alfa-2b (a covalent conjugate/ation of recombinant interferon alfa-2b with monomethoxy polyethylene glycol, used in the treatment of adult patients with histologically proven chronic hepatitis C) (see IFN).

PIFR Peak inspiratory flow rate (respiratory therapy) (see PFT - PIFR).

PIFT Platelet immunofluorescence test.

PIG Pertussis immune globulin.

PIGD Pre-implantation genetic diagnosis (see PGD).

PIGI Pregnancy-induced glucose intolerance.

pigm pigment(ation)/ed.

PIGP Pyruvate inosine glucose phosphate.

PIGPA Pyruvate inosine glucose phosphate adenine.

PIGT Pre-implantation genetic testing (see PGD; PIGD).

PIH Periventricular-intraventricular hemorrhage; Phenyl isopropylhydrazine; Pregnancy-induced hypertension; Prolactin-inhibiting hormone (see Hormones - PIH).

PIHH Post-influenza-like hyposmia and hypogeusia.

PIHTN Pregnancy-induced hypertension.

PII Parainguinal incision (see inc.); Plasma inorganic iodine; Primary irritation index.

PIIP Portable insulin infusion pump.

PIIS Posterior inferior iliac spine.

PIK Posterior instability of the knee (see KJI).

PIL Patient Information Library; Platelet information leaflet; Progressive intestinal lesion.

pil pill (L. pilula).

PILBD Paucity of interlobular bile ducts.

PIM Penicillamine-induced myasthenia; Porcine intestinal mucosa; Post-infectious myocarditis.

PIMC Phoenix Indian Medical Center (Arizona).

PIMI Post(erior) inferior myocardial infarction.

PIMM Antitrypsin phenotype (normal).

PIMS Programmable implantable medication system.

PIMS; PIMZ Antitrypsin phenotype.

PIN Posterior interosseous nerve (see PINP; PIP); Post-infective neuropathy (= GBS or Guaillain-Barré syndrome); Product identification number.

PINL Posterior interosseous nerve lesion (see PIN; PINP; PIP; TTE).

PINN Proposed international nonproprietary name.

PINP Posterior interosseous nerve palsy (= PIP).

PINS Person(s) in need of supervision.

PINV Post-imperative negative variation.

PIO Pemoline (see LA 956); Phenyl-imino-oxo-oxazolidine (= Yh 1); Progesterone in oil.

PIO_2; P_IO_2 Partial pressure of inspired oxygen (= Intra-alveolar oxygen tension (see PFT - PI_{O2}).

PIOL Phakic intraocular lens.

PION Posterior ischemic optic neuropathy.

PIP Paralytic infantile paralysis; Patients' Insurance Package/ Policy; Peak inflation/ inspiratory pressure (see PFT - PIP); Piperacillin; Posterior interosseous palsy (see PINP); Post-immunization pyrexia; Post-inflammatory pigmentation (skin); Post-infusion phlebitis; Post-injection pain; Post-insertion period (IDD) (Gynecology); Pressure inversion point; Primary inflammatory process; Proximal interphalangeal (joint); Psychotic Inpatient Profile; Psychosis, intermittent hyponatremia, polydipsia (syndrome); Posterior interphalangeal; Probable intrauterine pregnancy.

PIP2 Phosphoinositide.

PI-PB Performance intensity - phonemically balanced.

PIPE Persistent interstitial pulmonary emphysema.

PIPIDA N-para-isopropyl-acetilinide-iminodiacetic acid (hepatobiliary scanning agent/ radioisotope scan).

PIPJ Proximal interphalangeal joint.

PIPSRO Private initiative in professional standards review organizations.

PIPT Posterior iliopsoas transfer (Orthopedics).

PIQ Performance Intelligence Quotient.

PIR Parent-infant relationship (as in "Binding"); Peripheral insulin receptor/ resistance; Post-inhibition rebound; Post-introduction report; Post-ischemic reperfusion; Protective immune response.

Pir Pirenzepine (see LS 519).

PI-R Pacing impulse to ventricular activation time.

PIRG Public Interest Research Group.

PIRGIM Public Interest Research Group in Michigan.

PIRI Plasma immunoreactive insulin.

PIROL Prevention of recurrent infections of the upper and lower respiratory tract (study/ trial).

PIRS Plasma immunoreactive secretion.

PIS Pharmacological immune suppression; Poisons information service(s) (UK); Post-infarction syndrome (see BIP; DS); Pre-infarction syndrome; Primary immunodeficiency syndrome; Proteasome-inhibiting substance (such as LDP 341) (used in the treatment of multiple myeloma & chronic lymphocytic leukemia); Provisional International Standard.

pIs Isoelectric point.

$\bar{p}$Is Isoproterenol inhalation.

PISA Phase invariant signature algorithm.

PISCES Percutaneously inserted spinal cord electrical stimulation.

P_{ISH} Interstitial hydrostatic pressure.

PIST Protease inhibitor-sparing therapy (in AIDS) - with use of NNRTIs and NRTIs (see PIBCT; RTI).

PIT Pacing-induced tachycardia; Parenteral iron therapy; Passive immunotherapy (see PHT); Patella inhibition test; Picture identification test; Pitocin; Pitressin; Plasma iron turnover; Poor injection technique; Proliferative intestinal tuberculosis; Protease inhibitor therapy (for AIDS).

pit pituitary.

PITC Phenylisothiocyanate.

PITP Pseudo-idiopathic thrombocytopenic purpura.

PITR Plasma iron turnover rate; Primary intrathoracic rhabdomyosarcoma (see ITRMS).

Pi type Phenotype.

Pi type (analysis) Antitrypsin phenotype (analysis).

PIU Polymerase-inducing unit.

PIV Parainfluenza virus; Peripheral intravenous; Polydactyly - imperforate anus - vertebral anomalies (syndrome).

PIVD Post-ischemic vasodilatation; Prolapsed/ Protruded intervertebral disk.

PIVH Peripheral intravenous hyperalimentation; Periventricular-intraventricular hemorrhage.

PIVKA Protein induced by vitamin K absence or antagonism.

PIVR Pulseless idioventricular rhythm (with cardiac arrest).

PIWI Puppit in the Window Illuminated (test).

PIWT Partially impacted wisdom teeth/ tooth.

PIXE Particle-induced/ Proton-induced x-ray emission.

pixel picture element (in CT scanning).
PJ Pancreatic juice; Peutz-Jeghers (syndrome).
P3J Jijoye strain of Burkitt lymphoma cells.
PJB Premature junctional beat (ECG).
PJC Permanent joint contracture; Premature junctional contractions.
PJD Progressive joint destruction.
PJM Passive joint motion/ movement.
PJP Pancreatic juice protein.
PJS Peritoneo-jugular shunt; Peutz-Jeghers syndrome.
PJT Paroxysmal junctional (A-V) tachycardia.
PK Passive transfer; Penetrating keratoplasty; Pericardial knock; Pharmacokinetics; Phosphokinase; Pig kidney; Prausnitz-Küstner (reaction/ test) (see PKT); Protein kinase (see PKase); Psychokinesis; Pyruvate kinase (assay) (laboratory/ chemistry).
pK Negative logarithm of the dissociation or ionization constant.
pk peck.
pK' Apparent value of a pK; Negative logarithm of the dissociation or ionization constant of an acid.
P-K Prausnitz-Küstner (reaction/ test) (see PKT).
PKA Pharmacokinetic assessment; Prokinetic agent (see GIPKA); Protein kinase A (an enzyme that modulates the function of other proteins).
PkA Prekallikrein activator.
pK_a Negative logarithm of the acid ionization content.
PKAR Protein kinase activation ratio.
PKase Protein kinase (= PK).
PKB Pharmacokinetic behavior (of drugs); Prone knee bend; Protein kinase B (a key element enzyme in growth factor, signalling cell protection and survival from apoptosis, and transformation to a cancerous phenotype).
PKC Pharmacokinetic characteristic; Protein kinase C.
PKD Pain-killing drug; Persistent kidney dysfunction (see PRD); Polycystic kidney disease (i. ADPKD or Autosomal dominant polycystic kidney disease, ii. APD or Adult polycystic disease, iii. CPD or Childhood polycystic disease, and iv. Congenital polycystic disease) (see ADPKD; ARPKD); Proliferative kidney disease; Pyruvate kinase deficiency (a blood disorder).
PKDL Post-kala-azar dermal leishmaniasis (with multiple nodules, butterfly erythema and hypopigmented or depigmentation macules).
PKE Pharmacokinetic evaluation.
PKF Phagocytosis and killing function; Progressive kidney failure (see PRF).
PKI Potato kallikrein inhibitor; Pharmacokinetic interaction(s) (between two or more medications).
PKK Plasma prekallikrein.
PKN Parkinsonism.
PKP Penetrating keratoplasty; Pharmacokinetic parameter/ pathway/ profile/ property.
PKR Phased knee rehabilitation; Prausnitz-Küstner reaction (see PKT).
PKS Parker-Kerr suture (see Sut.); Pharmacokinetic(s) study.
PKT Prausnitz-Küstner test (= PR; P-R; PKR; PK test).
PK test Prausnitz-Küstner test (see PKT).
PKU Phenylketonuria (an autosomal recessive, hypotrichosis with atopic dermatitis and mental retardation).
PKV Killed poliomyelitis vaccine; Pharmacokinetic value/ variability.
pkV Peak kilovolt(age)/(s).
PL Palmaris longus (tendon); Pancreatic lipase; Perception of light (see LP); Peroneus longus; Phospholipase; Phospholipid(s) (= PLP); Photoluminescence; Placebo (= Pla; PLBO); Placental/ Platelet lactogen; Plantar; Plasma lemma; Plastic surgery; Polarized light; Preleukemia; Prolymphocytic leukemia; Pulpolingual; Purkinje's layer.
Pl Poiseuille.
pl picoliter; place; placenta; plasma (on laboratory reports); plate; platelet (see plat); plural.
P_L Transpulmonary pressure.
PL/1 Programming language 1 (one).
PL 3/5003 Pseudoephedrine hydrochloride.
PLA Percutaneous laser ablation (see PNPN; PVPD); Peripheral laser angioplasty; Phenyl lactate; Phospholipase A; Phospholipid anti-

body; Placebo therapy; Plasminogen activator; Platelet antigen; Polylactic acid; Potentially lethal arrhythmia; Procaine/ lactic acid; Pulpolinguoaxial.

PLa Pulpolabial.

Pla Left atrial pressure (see LAP); Placebo (see PL).

P_{LA} Left atrial pressure (see LAP).

PLA2 Phospholipase A2.

PLAB Professional and Linguistic Assessments Board (test).

PLAC-II Pravastatin, Lipids, and Atherosclerosis in the Carotid Arteries - II (AJC, 1995).

PLANASA National Sanitation Plan (Brazil).

PLAP Placental alkaline phosphatase.

plasia Growth (Gr. Plasma = Formation/ Growth) - Anaplasia or backward/ poorly differentiated growth, Dysplasia or deranged growth, Hyperplasia or increased rate of growth, Hypoplasia or arrested/ decreased/ diminised growth, and Neoplasia or new growth.

plat platelet (laboratory/ hematology) (= pl; PLT).

PLB Parietal lobe battery; Phospholipase B; Porous layer bead.

PLBO Placebo (see PL).

PLC Phospholipase C; Pituitary lactotrophic cell; Primary liver/ lung cancer; Proinsulin-like component; Pro-Life Caucus (House of Representatives); Protein-lipid complex; Pseudolymphocytic choriomeningitis.

PLCC Primary liver cell cancer.

PLCO Post-operative low cardiac output.

PL_{CO} Single-breath diffusing capacity for carbon monoxide (see PFT - PL_{CO}).

PLCOCST Prostate, Lung, Colon and Ovarian Cancer Screening Trial (NCI).

PLD Percutaneous laser decompression (see PLDD); Perilunate dislocation; Peripheral light detection; Phospholipase D; Phospholipidosis (see IPA); Pigment-like discoloration (of the skin); Platelet defect; Polycystic/ Primary/ Progressive liver disease; Posterior latissimus dorsi (muscle); Potentially lethal damage; Progressive lenticular degeneration (Wilson's disease) (see HLD).

PLDD Percutaneous laser disc decompression (of herniated intervertebral disc) (Orthopedics).

PLDH Plasma lactic dehydrogenase.

PLDR Potentially lethal damage repair.

PLE Paraneoplastic limbic encephalopathy; Protein-losing enteropathy; Pseudolupus erythematosus.

PLED Periodic lateral epileptiform discharge.

PLEDS Periodic lateral(ized) epileptiform discharges (EEG).

PLES Parallel-line equal space.

PLET Polymyxin, lysozyme, EDTA, and thallous acetate (in heart infusion agar).

PLEVA Pityriasis lichenoides et varioliformis acuta.

PLF Perilymphatic fistula; Phospholipid fraction; Posterior lung fiber.

PLFC Premature living female child.

PLFS Perilymphatic fistula syndrome.

PLG Plasminogen; L-propyl-L-leucylglucinamide.

P-LGV Psittacosis-lymphogranuloma venereum.

PLH Palaemontes lightening hormone; Paroxysmal localized hyperhidrosis; Placental lactogenic hormone; Pulmonary lymphoid hyperplasia.

$PLHCO_3$ Plasma bicarbonate.

PLI Partial luteal insufficiency (with dysovulation, menstrual irregularities, etc.); Paternal leukocyte immunization; Posterior lens implant; Professional Liability Insurance; Proinsulin-like immunoreactivity.

PLIF Posterior lumbar interbody fusion (same as Cloward fusion).

PLL Peripheral light loss; Perturbation level lethality (Psychiatry); Poly-L-lysine; Posterior longitudinal ligament; Preferred listening level (hearing aid); Pressure length loop; Prolymphocytic leukemia.

PLM Percent labeled mitoses; Periodic leg movement; Persistent low mood; Plasma level monitoring; Polarized light microscopy.

PLMC Premature living male child; Professional Liability Management Council.

PLME Polymorphous light eruption(s).

PLMV Posterior-leaf mitral valve.

PLN Palpable lymph node; Pelvic/ Peripheral/

Popliteal lymph node; Percutaneous laser nucleolysis (see PNPN; PVPD); Proliferative lupus nephritis (see DPLN).

PLND Pelvic lymph node dissection.

PLO Polycystic lipomembranous osteodysplasia.

PLP Papillon-Leage and Psaume (syndrome) (see OFDS); Phantom limb pain (Causalgia); Phospholipid (see PL); Plasma leukapheresis; Plasma lipid profile (total cholesterol, high and low density lipoproteins, and triglycerides); Polypeptide (see PP); Polystyrene latex particles; Pressure-like pain (e.g. chest pain); Pyridoxal-5'-phosphate; Pyroxidal-5'-phosphate.

PLPD Pseudoperiodic lateralized paroxysmal discharge(s).

PLPT Potentially life-prolonging treatment.

PLR Painful local reaction; Pupillary light reflex.

PLS Papillon-Lefèvre/ Polydactylyluxation/ Preleukemic syndrome; Parkinsonism-like syndrome (rigidity and tremor); Parsons Language Sample; Pediatric Life Support (CPR) (AHA); Perfusion lung scan (= XVS); Plastic surgery (= PLSURG); Preschool Language Scale; Primary/ Progressive lateral sclerosis (see ALS); Prostaglandin-like substance; Pseudo-lupus syndrome; Pulmonary leukostasis syndrome.

PLSDs Platyspondylic lethal skeletal dysplasias (Obstetrics).

PLSD-SD PLSD -San Diego type, -Torrance type and -Luton type, TD variants, with straighter femora, metaphyseal flaring, better preservation of growth plate and large rER inclusion bodies (see PLSDs, rER, TD1 and TD2 Obstetrics).

PLSO Posterior leafspring orthosis.

PLSURG Plastic surgery (see PLS).

PLT Pancreatic lymphocytic infiltration; Peptide leukotriene (C4, D4, and E4) (see PAM); Platelet (see plat); Primed lymphocyte test; Primed lymphocyte-defined typing (LD typing) (in transplants); Prolonged laxative therapy/ treatment; Psittacosis - lymphogranuloma venereum - trachoma (group).

Plt Platelet (see plat).

PLTC Post-liver transplant care.

PLT EST Platelet estimate.

PLTS Platelets.

Plumb Lead (L. plumbum) (see Elements - Lead).

PLUT Plutchnik (geriatric rating scale).

PLV Panleukopenia virus; Partial/ Permanent loss of vision (= PVL); Phenylalanine, lysine, and vasopressin; Poliomyelitis live vaccine; Posterior left ventricle; Preload volume (heart).

PLV2 Felypressin (= Phelypressine; 2-[Phenylalanine]-8-lysine vasopressin). A vasopressor agent with anti-diuretic and coronary vasoconstrictive effects less than those of vasopressin. Has been used intravenously in the treatment of hemorrhage from esophageal varices.

PLW Proximal limb weakness.

PLWS Prader-Labhart-Willi syndrome.

plx plexus.

PLZ Phenelzine.

PM After death (L. post mortem); After noon (L. post meridiem); Evening; Mean pressure; Night; Pacemaker(s) (Cardiology): Activitrax pacemaker, Arcolithium pacemaker, Biotronik pacemaker, Classix pacemaker, Cordis Atricor pacemaker, Cordis Etrocor pacemaker, Cordis Multicor II pacemaker, Cordis Omni Stanicor Theta transvenous pacemaker with endocardial lead, CPI Microthin D I lithium powered programmable pacemaker, CPI Microthin D II pacemaker, CyberTach 60 bipolar pacemaker, Daig ESI-II or Daig DSI-III atrial screw-in lead, Diplos 04 pacemaker, Ectocor pacemaker, Elecath pacemaker, Electrodyne pacemaker/ cardiac monitor, Eligoloy lead tip pacemaker, Fast-Pass endocardial lead, Ferrule (on pacemaker wires), Finned pacemaker lead, Genisis dual chamber pacemaker, Hermetically sealed standby pacemaker, Intermedics Cyberlith X multiprogrammable pacemaker, Intermedics lithium powered pacemaker, Intermedics Quantum programmable pulse generator, Lambda pacemaker, Lithium pacemaker, Medtronic Byrel-SX pacemaker, Medtronic pacemaker, Medtronic Symbios pacemaker, Multicor Gamma pacemaker, Neos pacemaker, Omni-Theta pacemaker, Omni Stanicor

Gamma pacemaker with pervenous lead, Omni Stanicor Theta pacemaker, Optima-MP programmable pulse generator, Optima 274 bipolar pulse generator, Pacesetter programmable pulse generator, Permathane Pacesetter lead, PolyFlex implantable pacing lead, Programalith A-V pacemaker, Programalith pacemaker (bipolar & unipolar), Programalith II VVI/AAI bipolar programmable pacemaker, Prolith pacemaker, Quantum pacemaker, Screw-in lead, Sensor Kelvin 500 system pacemaker, Sequicor II pacemaker, Siemens-Elema multiprogrammable pacemaker, Spectrax bipolar pacemaker battery, Standby pacemaker, Stanicor Gamma pacemaker, Stanicor pacemaker, Starr-Edwards hermetically sealed pacemaker, Symbios 7005C dual chamber pacemaker, Telectronic pacemaker, Tined lead, Tined 1 mm lead, Ventricor pacemaker, Versatrax pacemaker, VVI bipolar Programalith pacemaker, VVI/AAI bipolar programmable pacemaker, Xytron pacemaker; Papillary muscle; Papular mucinosis; Partial meniscectomy; Perinatal mortality; Peritoneal macrophage; Petit mal (Fr.) (epileptic seizures); Photo multiplier; Physical medicine (= Phys Med); Plasma membrane; Platelet membrane/ microsome; Pneumomediastinum; Poliomyelitis; Polymorph(s) (WBCs); Polymorphonuclear (leukocytes) (see PMNL); Polymyositis; Poor metabolizer(s); Porokeratosis of Mibelli; Posterior mitral; Postmenstrual; Postmortem (see above); Premarketing (approval); Premenstrual; Premolar; Prescription medication/cine; Presents mainly; Presystolic murmur; Pretibial myxedema; Preventive mastectomy/ medicine; Primary motivation; Prostatic massage; Protein methylesterase; Protocol management; Pterygoid muscle; Pubertal macromastia; Pulmonary macrophage; Pulmonary melioidosis (an infection caused by the microorganism *Pseudomonas* pseudomallei, also known variously as *Actinobaccilus* pseudomallei, *Bacillus* whitmori, *Lofflerella* whitmori, *Malleomyces* pseudomallei, *Pfeifferella* pseudomallei and *Pfeifferella* whitmori); Pulpomesial.

Pm Paratid middle (band protein); Promethium (Z = 61) (see Elements - Promethium).

pM picomolar.

pm picometer.

πm pi meson.

PM 396 Methsuximide - an anticonvusant, used in the treatment of petit mal and psychomotor attacks of epilepsy.

PM 671 Ethosuximide (see H 940).

PMA Expression or index of the prevalence and severity of Gingivitis in large groups of persons, where P represents the papillary gingiva, M the marginal gingiva, and A the attached gingiva; Papillary, marginal, attached (gingiva); Paralysis of muscles of accommodation (causing blurred vision); Para-methoxyamphetamine (= P-methoxyamphetamine); Peroneal muscular atrophy; Pharmaceutical Manufacturers Association; Phenylmercuric acetate (= Phenylhydrargyri acetas) - an antibacterial and antifungal agent, used as a preservative in the storage of antigens; also as a spermicide in chemical contraceptives; Phorbol myristate acetate; Phosphomolybdic acid; Photomutagenicity assay; Plant-made antibody; Platelet membrane antigen; Point Mutation Assay (*Saccharomyces* cerevisiae, etc.); Postmenarchal/chial adolescent; Premarket approval; Premature abortion; Premenstrual asthma; Primary Mental Abilities (test); Prinzmetal's angina; Progressive muscular atrophy; Prompt medical attention; Psychomotor activity; Pyridylmercuric acetate.

PMAB Plasmin Modulate Amyloid Beta (in Alzheimer's disease).

PMAU Postmenopausal atrophic urethritis.

PMAV Postmenopausal atrophic vaginitis.

PMB Papillomacular bundle; Para-hydroxymercuribenzoate; Partial myelographic block (of cervical or other spinal nerves); Polychrome methylene blue; Polymorphonuclear basophil (leukocyte); Polymyxin B (sulfate); Postmenopausal bleeding.

PMBC Post/Premenopausal breast cancer.

PMBL Postmenopausal bone loss.

PMBT Primary malignant bone tumor.

PMC Pain Management Center (UCSF); Paramagnetic complex; Patient medical compliance; Phenylmercuric chloride; Physical medicine clinic; Pleural mesothelial click; Precautionary Measure(s) and Contraindication(s); Premature mitral closure; Private/ Professional medical care; Professional misconduct; Pseudomembranous colitis.

PMCBS Postmenopausal Craggy Breast Syndrome.

PMCF Private Medical Care Foundation.

PMCP Para-monochlorophenol.

PMCS Post/Premenopausal climacteric syndrome.

PMCT Premarketing clinical trial.

PMD Doctor of Primary Medicine; Pain-modulating drug; Pelizaeus-Merzbacher disease; Perceptual motor development; Periodic mood disorder (see MRPMD); Polymorphic microsatellite dinucleotide; Posterior mandibular depth; Postmarketing data; Premature delivery; Premenstrual disorder; Primary mitochondrial/ myocardial disease; Private medical doctor; Programmed multiple development; Progressive muscle/ muscular degeneration; Progressive muscular dystrophy; Pseudohypertrophic muscular dystrophy (Duchenne's - see DMD); Psychomotoric disorder; Psychotic manifestation(s) of dementia; Psychotic mental disease/ disorder.

PM/DM Polymyositis/dermatomyositis.

PMDS Persistent müllerian duct syndrome; Primary myelodysplastic syndrome.

PME Periodic medical examination; Polymorphonuclear eosinophil (leukocyte); Postmarketing experience; Postmenopausal estrogen; Postmortem examination; Premarketing evaluation/ experience; Primary medical education; Progressive myoclonic/nus epilepsy; Pseudomembranous enterocolotis (see PMEC).

PMEA 9-(2-Phosphomethoxyethyl) adenine.

PMEC Pseudomembranous enterocolitis.

PMED Postmenopausal estrogen deficiency.

PMF Pathological mammographic finding; Post/Premenarchal/(chial)/ menopausal female; Progressive massive fibrosis; Proton motive force (= pmf); Psychomotor function; Pterygomaxillary fossa.

pmf proton motive force (see PMF).

PMFC Premotor frontal cortex.

PMG Postmenopausal gonadotrophin (see HMG; HPMG; LHPMG)/ grandmother; Professional medical group.

PMGCT Primary mediastinal germ-cell tumor.

PM gene Polymerase gene, found in the AIDS virus (HIV-1) genome. It codes proteins, including reverse transcriptase which first transcribes viral RNA to single stranded DNA and then transcribes single stranded DNA to double stranded DNA.

PMH Past/ Patient's/ Personal/ Previous/ Programmed medical history; Pharmacologically-mediated hypocalcemia; Posteromedial hypothalamus; Postmenopausal Health; Prolonged maintenance hemodialysis; Public Mental Hospital.

PMHR Predicted maximum heart rate.

PMI Pacemaker implant; Past/ Present/ Previous medical illness; Patient medical instruction; Pennsylvania Muscle Institute; Perioperative/ Posterior myocardial infarction; Plea of mental incompetence; Point of maximal impulse/ intensity; Postmyocardial infarction; Potent mediator of inflammation (see HMs; PMsI); Premedicated induction (of anesthetic); Premixed insulin (see Insulin); Preventive Medicine Institute; Psychomotor(ic) inhibition.

PMIS Postmyocardial infarction syndrome; Professional (Standards Review Organization or PSRO) Management Information System.

PMK Primary (rhesus) monkey kidney.

PML Pacemaker lead (see FPL); Polymorphonuclear leukocyte; Posterior/ Prolapsing mitral leaflet; Progressive multifocal leukodystrophy/ leukoencephalitis(alopathy); Pulmonary microlithiasis; Pulsed-mode laser.

PMLE Polymorphous light eruption.

P_{50}(mm Hg) Partial pressure of oxygen at which hemoglobin is 50% saturated.

PMM Passive motion machine; Pentamethylmelamine; Postmenopausal mother; Protoplast maintenance medium.

PMMA Polymethylmethacrylate.
PMMC Polymethylmethacrylate.
PMMF Pectoralis major myocutaneous flat.
PMN Peripheral/ Proximal motor neuropathy; Phenylmercuric nitrate (= Phenylhydrargyri nitras) - properties and uses as in Phenylmercuric acetate (PMA); Polymorphonuclear neutrophil (leukocyte) (see PMNL); Polymorphonucleotide; Primary mediastinal neoplasm; Prostatic malignant neoplasm.
PMNC Percentage of multinucleated cells; Peripheral (blood) mononuclear cell.
PMNG Polymorphonuclear granulocyte.
PMNL Peripheral (blood) monocytes and (polymorpho)nuclear leukocytes; Polymorphonuclear leukocyte(s) (= PM; PMN; Poly; polys); Polymorphonuclear neutrophil leukocyte(s) (= PMN; PMNN; PNL).
PMNN Polymorphonuclear neutrophil (see PMNL).
PMNR Periadenitis mucosa necrotica recurrens.
PMNs Polymorphonucleosites.
PMO Postmenopausal osteoporosis; Principal Medical Officer; Progressive myositis ossificans (see MOP).
pmol picomole (= 10^{-12} mole; μμmol; micromicromole).
PMOT Pseudomalignant osseous tumor (Orthopedics).
PMOW Postmenopausal osteoporotic woman/ women.
PMP Pain/ Patient management program; Parenteral medicinal product; Past/ Previous menstrual period; Patient medication profile; Perras mammary prosthesis; Persistent mentoposterior (fetal position); Personal memory program (for stimulating memory, especially in old age)/ BCESTV- B. Breathing (deep, slow), C. Concentration (on the subject in question), E. Exercise (time off for), S. Speaking (reading aloud the specific items or words), T. Triggers (creating a personal mnemonic device, like a thread tied around the finger, etc.), V. Visualization (mentally rehearsing thc facts); Phenoxymethyl penicillin; Placental membrane protein (= Fibronectin); Postmarketing period; Private medical practitioner; Psychomotor performance; Psychotropic medication plan.
PMPO Postmenopausal palpable ovary.
PMPS Postmastectomy pain syndrome.
PMQ Phytylmenaquinone.
PMR Percutaneous myocardial reperfusion (see PCTMR); Perinatal mortality rate; Periodic medical review; Peri/Post-operative mortality rate (see POMR); Peripherally mediated reflex; Physical medicine and rehabilitation (see PM&R); Plasma-membrane receptor; Polymorphic reticulosis; Polymyalgia rheumatica; Post-marketing report; Prior medical record; Proportionate morbidity/ mortality rate; Proton magnetic resonance.
PMR&MI Periodic medical repair and medical inspection.
PM&R Physical medicine and rehabilitation (= PMR).
PMRAFNS Princess Mary's Royal Air Force Nursing Service.
PMRS Physical Medicine and Rehabilitation Service; Proton magnetic resonance spectroscopy.
PMS Pacemaker syndrome (see RVC); Partial monosomy (chromosomes); Patient management system; Pennsylvania Medical Society; Perimenstrual/ Postmenopausal syndrome; Periodic minimal surface; Periodic movements (during) sleep; Petit mal seizure (= AS - Absence seizure); Phenazine methosulfate; Pituitary microsurgery (for Cushing' s disease); Postmarket(ing) surveillance; Postmeasles state; Postmenopausal status (see NPMS; PMS); Postmenstrual stress; Postmitochondrial supernatant (= PSM); Postmortem study; Potential myelosuppressant/ession; Pregnant mare(s') serum (gonadotropin) (see PMSG); Premenopausal status/ syndrome; Premenstrual symptoms/ syndrome (see PMTS); Progressive multiple sclerosis; Psoas minor syndrome (Orthopedics); Psychomotor seizure/ status; Psychotic motor syndrome.
PMSC Pluripotent myeloid stem cell.
PMSF Phenylmethylsulfonyl fluoride.
PMSG Pregnant mare/ mares' serum gonadotropin (see Hormones - PMSG).

PMsI Potent mediators of inflammation (such as histamine, leukotrienes, etc.) (see HMs - Humoral mediators).
PMST Psychological mental and social trauma (resulting from IHC or In-hospital care, etc.).
PMT Parametric test (in statistical analysis) (such as CST or Chi-square[d] test, STT or Student's t test, and Welch's test); Peripheral meniscal tear (Knee joint) (Orthopedics); Phenol O-methyltransferase; Photomultiplier tube; Porteus maze test; Premenstrual tension (see PMTS); P Premolar tooth (or Bicuspid); rimary malignant tumor; Prolonged maintenance therapy; Properly monitored treatment; Pyridoxyl-methyltrytophan; Pyrrolidino-methyltetracycline (= Rolitetracycline) - a derivative of tetracycline with similar actions and uses as this antibiotic.
PMTS Premenstrual tension symptoms/ syndrome (= PMS; PMT).
PMTT Pulmonary mean transit time.
PMU Preventive Medicine Update (journal).
PMV Paramyxovirus; Peak minute ventilation (see VFR); Percutaneous mitral (balloon) valvotomy; Plus-minus value(s); Postmenopausal vaginitis (see PMAV); Prolapse of mitral valve.
PMVL; pMVL Posterior mitral valve leaflet.
PMW Pacemaker wires; Pre/Postmenopausal woman/ men.
PN Nightmares (L. pavor nocturnus); Pancreatic; Papillary necrosis; Parenteral nutrition; Penicillin (see Pen); Perceived noise; Percussion note; Percutaneous nephrostogram; Periarteritis nodosa; Perinatal; Peripheral/ Phrenic nerve; Peripheral/ Poly neuropathy (see PNP); Phobic neurosis (includes simple phobia, agoraphobia, social phobia and panic disorder); Plaque neutralization; Pneumonia (see Pn); Polyarteritis nodosa; Polymorphonuclear; Polynephritis; Polyneuritis; Polynucllear; Polynucleotide; Poorly nourished; Positional nystagmus; Posterior nares; Postnasal/ natal; Practical/ Primary nurse; Predicted normal; Premie nipple; Progress note; Protease nexin; Psychchiatry and neurology (see P&N); Psychoneurosis/rotic; Pyelonephritis; Pyridine nucleotide.
Pn Pneumatic; Pneumonia (= PN; pneu).
pn pain.
P/N Positive/negative.
P&N Psychiatry and neurology (= PN).
PN2. Protease nexin 2 (= APP or Amyloid precursor protein).
P_{N2} Partial pressure of nitrogen.
PNA Paris Nomina Anatomica; Peanut agglutinin; Pediatric nurse associate; Pelger's nuclear anomaly (a hereditary anomaly in the form of the nuclei of leukocytes) (= PHA or Pelger-Hüet anomaly); Pentose nucleic acid; Potent narcotic analgesic (e.g. cannabis, cocaine, etc.); Protein nitrogen appearance (see nPNA); Purine nucleoside analogue (such as the synthetic analogue ddI or didenosine, abacavir, etc., of the naturally occurring nucleoside Deoxyadenosine, used in the treatment of AIDS) (see SNA).
P_{Na} Plasma sodium.
PNAB Percutaneous needle aspiration biopsy.
PNAG Primary narrow angle glaucoma.
PNAS Proceedings of the National Academy of Sciences; Prudent no added salt (i.e. Prudently not to add salt).
PNAvQ Positive-negative ambivalent quotient.
PNB Percutaneous/ Perineal needle biopsy; p-Nitrobiphenyl; Premature newborn/ nodal beat; Proximal nail bed.
PNBF Periosteal new-bone formation.
PNBT Para- or p-nitroblue tetrazolium.
PNC Penicillin (see Pen); Peripheral nerve conduction; Peri/Prenatal cardiology; Perinatal complication(s); Peripheral nucleated cell; Pneumotaxic center; Postnecrotic cirrhosis; Premature nodal contraction/acture; Prenatal care/ course; Psychiatric Nurse Clinician.
PND Paroxysmal nocturnal dyspnea; Partial neck dissection; Pelvic node dissection; Peri/Postnatal development/ dilemma; Peripheral nerve damage/ disease/ distribution; Permanent neurologic(al) damage; Postnasal drain(age)/ drip; Postnatal death; Postnatal depression; Post/Prenatal diagnosis/ disease/ disorder; Pregnancy, not delivered; Principal neutralizing determinant/ domain

(antibody) - a specific protein contained in GP 120, one of the four molecules identified in the outer coating of the AIDS virus; Pronephric duct (the duct of the pronephros or primordial kidney of the developing embryo) (see ANC; AND); Progressive neurologic disease; Purulent nasal drainage.

PNdB; PNdb Perceived noise (level) decibel.

PNDS Peri/ Postnatal developmental study.

PNDT Prenatal diagnostic testing.

PNE Peripheral nerve ending; Peroneal nerve exploration (Orthopedics); Plasma norepinephrine; Pneumoencephalography; Prolonged nucleoside exposure (see PNA; SNA); Pseudomembranous necrotizing enterocolitis.

PNed Nederlandsche Pharmacopee (Dutch Pharmacopeia).

PNER Plasma norepinephrine response (to exercise, exertion, etc.).

PNET Peripheral neuroepithelioma; Primitive neuroectodermal tumor.

PNET-MB Primitive neuroectodermal tumor - medulloblastoma.

pneu pneumonia (see Pn).

pneumo pneumothorax (see Pnx).

Pneumoconiosis A lung dust disease caused by chronic fibrous reaction in the lungs to long-term inhalation of dust, with resulting fibroid induration and pigmentation (see JRLD; LDD). Examples are:
Aluminosis - a form of pneumoconiosis caused by aluminium-bearing dust, especially alum, bauxite, or clay in the lungs. Also called Aluminosis pulmonum.
Anthracosis - a form of pneumoconiosis caused by the inhalation of coal dust. Also called Anthracosis linguae or Black tongue.
Asbestosis - a form of pneumoconiosis caused by inhaling particles of asbestos.
Byssinosis - a form of pneumoconiosis caused by inhaling cotton dust, as in factories.
Cadmiosis - a form of pneumoconiosis caused by breathing in cadmium dust.
Chalicosis - a form of pneumoconiosis caused by inhalation of fine stone particles as occurs among stone-cutters.
Ptilosis - a form of pneumoconiosis caused by inhaling the dust from ostrich feathers.
Siderosis - a form of pneumoconiosis caused by the inhalation of iron or other metallic particles.
Silicosis - a form of pneumoconiosis caused by the inhalation of the dust of sand, stone, or flint containing silicone dioxide (= Grinders' disease).
Tabacosis - a form of pneumoconiosis caused by the inhalation of tobacco dust. Also called Tabacosis pulmonum.

PNF Proprioceptive neuromuscular facilitation.

PNG Penicillin G; Peroneal nerve graft(ing) (Orthopedics).

PNH Paroxysmal nocturnal hemoglobinuria; Polynuclear hydrocarbon; Prolonged neonatal hypoglycemia.

PNHA Physicians National Housestaff Association.

PNI Peripheral nerve injury; Postnasal infection; Prognostic nutrition index; Psychoneuroimmunology.

PNID Peer Nomination Inventory for Depression.

PNK Polynucleotide kinase.

PNL Percutaneous nephrolithotomy/tripsy (see PCNL); Peripheral nerve lesion; Polymorphonuclear neutrophil(ic) leukocyte (see PMNL).

PNLA Percutaneous needle lung aspiration.

PNLI Postnatal lung immaturity (Obstetrics).

PNM Paraneoplastic manifestation(s) (e.g. of thymoma, such as myasthenia gravis, hypogammaglobulinemia, and red-cell aplasia); Peri/Post/Prenatal management/ mortality; Peripheral dysostosis, nasal hypoplasia, and mental retardation (syndrome); Peripheral nerve myelin.

PNMG Persistent neonatal myasthenia gravis.

PNMR Peri/Post/Prenatal mortality rate; Postnatal mortality risk.

PNMT Phenyl-ethanolamine-N-methyl transferase.

PNN Peripheral nerve neuroma; Prenatal nutrition.

PNO Peri/Postnatal outcome; Principal Nursing Officer.

PNP Pancreatic polypeptide; Para-nitrophenol

(see P-NP); Peak negative pressure; Pediatric nurse practitioner; Perinatal outcome; Peripheral neuropathy (= PN); Peripheral/ Peroneal nerve palsy; Pneumoperitoneum; Polyneuropathy (= PN); Polynucleotide phosphorylase (see PNPase); Poorly nourished patient; Postnatal period/ prognosis; Progressive nuclear palsy; Prominent neurological problem; Psychogenic nocturnal polydipsia; Pure Natural Process (in cholesterol food control); Purine nucleoside phosphorylase.

P-NP Para-nitriphenol (= PNP).

PNPase Polynucleotide phosphorylase (= PNP).

PNPB Positive-negative pressure breathing.

PNPD Purine nucleoside phosphorylase deficiency.

PNPN Percutaneous nucleus pulposus denaturization (Orthopedics) (see PVPD).

PNPP Para-nitrophenylphosphate.

PNPR Positive-negative pressure respiration.

P-NPS Para- or p-Nitrophenylsulfate.

PNR Peroneal nerve reconstruction/ repair (Orthopedics); Posterior nerve root (see NRD; PRG); Postnatal repair.

PNRP Pulmonary Neoplasm Research Project.

PNS Paraneoplastic syndrome; Parasympathetic/ Peripheral nervous system; Partial nonprogressive stroke; Peri/Postnatal study; Peripheral nerve stimulation/ supply/ surgery; Persistent night sweats; Poor nutritional status; Posterior nasal spine; Postnasal/natal surgery (Obstetrics); Practical nursing student; Premature nodal systole; Prenatal screening; Pseudoneurotic schizophrenia (see BLS).

PNSD Peripheral nervous system disease/ disorder/ dysfunction.

PNSP Prenatal screening program.

PNT Paroxysmal nodal tachycardia; Partial nodular transformation; Patient (see pt); Percutaneous nephrostomy tube; Peripheral nerve trunk; Physician-nurse team (= NPT); Prenatal therapy/ treatment.

Pnt; pnt Patient (see pt).

pnthx pneumothorax (see Pnx).

PNU Postnatal uropathy (Obstetrics); Protein nitrogen unit.

PNV Penicillin phenoxymethyl; Post/Prenatal virility/lization; Prenatal vitamins.

Pnx Pneumonectomy; Pneumothorax (= pneumo; pnx; PT; PTX; PTx; Px).

pnx pneumothorax (see Pnx).

PNZ Posterior necrotic zone.

PO By mouth/ orally (see po); Parietal operculum; Parieto-occipital; Period of onset; Peri/Post/Pre-operative (see POp); Phone order; Posterior (see post); Predominant organism.

Po Polonium (Z = 84) (see Elements - Polonium); Porion.

po by mouth/ orally (L. per os) (= PO).

P/O Phone order; Protein/osmolar (ratio).

PO# Post-operative fracture (see POF).

P_o Opening pressure.

PO_2; P_{O2}; pO_2 Partial pressure/ tension of oxygen (i.e. in alveolar gas or arterial blood) (see PFT - pO_2).

$\bar{p}O_2$ Hypoxemia (see PFT).

PO_4 phosphate.

^{210}Po Radioactive polonium.

POA Pancreatic oncofetal antigen; Parenteral opioid analgesic; Partial opioid agonist; Patient's own assessment; Peripheral opioid action; Phalangeal osteoarthritis; Poor oral absorption; Post/Pre-operative administration/ alignment (Orthopedics); Potent opioid analgesic (such as dextromoramide, dipipanone, heroin, methadone, morphine, pentazocine and pethidine); Pre-operative arthrogram/graph(y)/ assessment (see RNN); Pre-optic area; Primary optic atrophy; Primary osteoarthritis; Problem-oriented approach (see PBA); Professional older adult.

POAD Peripheral obstructive/ occlusive arterial/ iosclerotic disease (= PAOD; Fontaine Stage III - daily rest pain; Fontaine Stage IV - focal tissue necrosis).

POAG Primary open-angle glaucoma.

POA-HA Pre-optic anterior hypothalamic area.

POAT Post-operative adjuvant therapy.

POB Penicillin, oil, beeswax; Periosteal osteoblastoma (Orthopedics); Phenoxybenzamine; Pituitary ovarian blockade; Place of birth.

POC Particulate organic carbon; Performance-obsessed culture; Perioperative complication(s); Post-operative care/ chemotherapy/ complication(s); Primary-oriented care (see SOC); Probability of chance; Product of conception; Progesterone/tin -only contraceptive.

Po/C Ocular pressure ratio ("C" represents tonographic value).

POCC Procarbazine, Oncovin, Cyclophosphamide and CCNU (Lomustine) (Chemotherapy).

pocill a small cup (L. pocillum).

POCR Patient-oriented clinical research.

POCT Peri/Post/Pre-operative chemotherapy.

pocul a cup (L. poculum).

POD Pacing on demand; Periodontal disease (pyorrhea); Perioral dermatitis; Peroxidase (see PX); Place of death; Podiatry; Polycystic ovarian/ry disease; Post-obstructive diuresis; Post Office Department; Post-operative day/ death; Potential organ donor; Pre-operative deformity (Orthopedics, Plastic surgery, etc.).

POD I Post-operative day one.

PODP Post-operative dental pain.

PODs Points of delivery.

PODT Post/Pre-operative drug therapy/ treatment.

PODx Post-operative diagnosis.

POE Pediatric orthopedic examination; Peri/Post/Pre-operative episode/ evaluation/ exacerbation/ examination; Periorbital edema; Point/ Portal of entry (= PofE); Polyoxyethylene; Position of ease; Post-operative endophthalmitis/ epilepsy; Primary outcome event; Proof of eligibility.

POEMS (Plasma cell dyscasia with) polyneuropathy, organomegaly, endocrinopathy, monoclonal (M-) protein, and skin changes (syndrome); Post-operative Expert Medical System.

POF Position of function; Post-operative fracture (= PO#) (Orthopedics); Premature/ Primary ovarian failure; Pyruvate oxidation factor.

PofE Point/ Portal of entry (see POE).

PofI Proof of illness.

POG Pediatric Oncology Group; Penthrane - oxygen gas (nitrous oxide); Polymyositis ossificans generalisata; Products of gestation.

Pog Pogonion.

POH Post-occlusive hyperemia.

pOH The hydroxide/xyl ion concentration (alkalinity = OH) of/in a solution.

POHA Pre-operative holding area.

POHI Physically or otherwise health-impaired.

POHS Presumed ocular histoplasmosis syndrome.

POHT Post/Pre-operative hyper/hypothyroidism.

POI Personal Orientation Inventory; Post-operative ileus/ immobilization (Orthopedics); Pre-op(eration/tive) injection/ interview; Pre-operative image/ging (MRI - brain surgery).

POIW Physician-Oriented Information Website (Internet).

POIC Post-operative indwelling catheter.

POIK Poikilocytosis.

poik poikilocyte/tosis (blood cells).

POIS Parkland On-Line Information Systems.

pois poison(ed)/(ing).

Poker spine Ankylosing spondylitis (see MSD).

POL Polymerized flagellin; Premature onset of labor.

Pol Poland; Polish.

pol polish(ed)/(ing).

POLI Post-operative local irradiation.

polio poliomyelitis.

Pol P Polish Pharmacopoeia (Farmakopea Polska).

Pol/Vac (Inactivated) Poliomyelitis Vaccine (Inactivated) - grown in cultures of monkey kidney tissue and inactivated; developed from the Salk vaccine.

Pol/Vac (Oral) Poliomyelitis Vaccine (Oral) - an aqueous suspension of live attenuated strains of poliomyelitis virus (developed from the original work of Albert Sabin); grown in cultures of monkey kidney tissue, and used for active immunization against poliomyelitis.

POLY Polychromic (erythrocyte).

Poly Polymorphonuclear (see PMNL).

poly-A; poly(A) Polyadenylic acid.

poly A:U Polynucleotide.

poly-C; poly(C) Polycytidylic acid.

POLYCHR Polychromatophilia.

poly(CM)-oligo(dG) Poly(2'-O-methycytidylate)-oligoxyguanylate.
poly-G; poly(G) Polyguanylic acid.
poly-I; poly(I) Polyinosinic acid.
poly-IC; poly-I:C Copolymer of polyinosinic and polycytidylic acids; Synthetic RNA polymer.
polys polymorphonuclear leukocytes (see PMNL).
poly-T; poly(T) Polythymidylic acid.
poly-U; poly(U) Polyuridylic acid.
POM Pain on motion/ movement; Polyoximethylene; Peri/Post/Pre-operative management/ measure/ medication/mobility; Prescription-only medication/cine; Primary outcome measure.
POMC Propiomelanocortin (a protein which plays a role in hair color, energy storage and adrenal gland function; a gene mutation on chromosome 2 coding for this protein, results in red hair, early-onset obesity and hormonal disturbances.
POMP Prednisolone, oncovin, methotrexate, and 6-mercaptopurine (cancer chemotherapy); Principal outer material protein.
POMR Peri/Post-operative mortality rate (= PMR); Problem-oriented medical record.
POMS Profile of Mood States.
PON Paraoxonase; Particulate organic nitrogen.
pond by weight (L. pondere); heavy (L. ponderosus).
PONI Post-operative narcotic infusion.
POOC Progestin-only oral contraceptive (see POC).
POP Diphosphate group; Painful ophthalmoplegia (see THS - Tolosa-Hunt syndrome); Pain on palpation; Paroxypropione; Pelvic organ prolapse (Gynecology/ Obstetrics); Peri/Post/Pre-operative patient/ period; Peri/Post/Pre-ovulatory period (Obs/Gyn); Persistent occipitoposterior (fetal position); Personal ozone protection (clothing/ headwear); Pituitary opioid peptide; Plasma oncotic/ osmotic pressure; Plaster of Paris; Polymyositis ossificans progressiva; Post-obstructive pneumonia; Post-operative pain/ physiotherapy/ problem/ prognosis; Posterior occipital proturburance (Orthopedics); Progestogen-only (contraceptive) pill (the 'mini-pill') (= POOC).
POp Peri/Post/Pre-operative (= PO).
Pop; pop Popliteal (= Poplit); Popular; Population.
POPE Parents for Orthodox Parochial Education.
Poplit Popliteal (see Pop).
POPM Post-operative pain management.
POPOP 1,4-bis-(5-phenoxazol-2-yl) benzene.
Poppers Amyl nitrite (see).
poppet part of an aortic valve prosthesis.
POR Patient-oriented research (see POCR); Physician of record; Post-occlusive oscillatory response; Post-operative recovery/ recurrence/ remobilization (Orthopedics); Prevalence odds ratio; Problem-oriented record (see POMR).
PORD Post-operative respiratory depression.
PORH Post-operative reactive hyperemia.
PORK Porkilocytosis.
PORP Partial ossicular reconstructive/ replacement prosthesis.
PORT Patient Outcome Research Team; Peri/Post-operative respiratory therapy; Post-operative radiation therapy.
Port P Portuguese Pharmacopoeia (Farmacopeia Portuguesa).
Portagen Medium chain triglyceride diet.
POS Partial onset seizure (epilepsy); Peri/Post/Pre-operative sedation/ state; Periosteal osteosarcoma; Point-of-service Plan; Polycystic ovarian/ ovary syndrome; Portable oxygen system (Traveler); Pre-operative sterilization (of bowel, etc.); Prolongation of survival (see PoS); Protected oral sex; Psycho-organic syndrome; Purchase of service(s).
PoS Prolongation of survival (= POS).
pos position; positive.
POSC Problem-oriented system of charting.
POSCH Prognostic Outcome for the Surgical Control of the Hyperlipidemias.
POSE Parents Opposed to Sex Education.
POSM Patient-operated selector/ sensing mechanism.
POSP Post-orthopedic surgery/gical pain.
pos press positive pressure.
POSS Percutaneous on-surface stimulation;

Proximal over-shoulder strap.
poss possible.
POSSUM Pictures of Standard Syndromes and Undiagnosed Malformations.
Post Posterior (see post); Postmortem (autopsy) (see PM).
post posterior (= PO; Post).
post cib after meals (L. post cibum) (see pc).
postgangl postganglionic.
Post ãS Serum immunoglobulin concentration after dialysis.
postinoc post-inoculation.
postop; post-op Post-operative.
Post Sag D Posterior sagittal diameter.
post sing sed liq after very loose stool (L. post singulas sedes liquidas).
post tib posterior tibial.
POSW Post-operative sutured wound.
POT Peri/Post/Pre-operative therapy/ transfusion/ treatment; Periostitis ossificans toxica; Porcine organ transplant (see PCT); Post-operative tachycardia.
Pot Marijuana (see Cannabis); Potash (L. potassa); Potassium (= K; Kalium; pot; potass) (Z = 19) (see Elements - Potassium); Potential (see pot); Potion.
pot potassium (see Pot); potential (see Pot).
potass potassium (see Pot).
POTO Pulmonary outflow tract obstruction (as in Fallow's Tetralogy).
POTP Post-operative time period.
POU Pediatric oncology unit; Placenta, ovary, and uterus; Post-operative ulcer (gastric/ duodenal).
pouce flottant French - floating thumb.
POV Post-operative vomiting.
PoV Portal vein.
pov pants-over-vest (overlapping sutures in hernia repair).
POVA Permanent/ Persistent obstructive ventilatory alteration.
POVT Puerperal ovarian vein thrombophlebitis.
POW Period off-work (Working inability); Powassan (encephalitis); Prisoner of war (= PW).
powd powder (see pulv).
POX Point of exit.
PP Diphosphate group; Emphysema (pink puffers); Near point of accommodation (L. punctum proximum) (eye examination - see pp); Pace-setter potential; Palatal palsy/ paralysis; Palatoplasty (Plastic and Reconstructive Surgery); Palmoplantar; Pancreatic polypeptide (= PPY); Paradoxical/ Parietal/ Pedal/ Peripheral pulse; Partial/ Perfusion/ Pulmonary/ Pulse pressure; Partial (upper) and partial (lower) (dentures); Pellagra-preventing (substance) (see PPS); Periodic paralysis; Peritoneal pseudomyxoma; Per-protocol (analysis); Persisting proteinuria; Peyer patches; Photopheresis (immunosuppressive therapy in transplant medicine); Pinprick; Placenta previa; Placental protein (in maternal blood during pregnancy); Planned parenthood; Plasma pepsinogen/ protein; Plasmapheresis; Plaster of Paris; Polypeptide (= PLP); Polypharmacy; Polypropylene; Polystyrene agglutination plate; Poor person; Population planning; Posterior papillary/ pituitary; Postpartum (see pp); Postprandial (after meals) (see pp); Pott's paraplegia; Precocious puberty; Poulard procedure (scar revision); Preferred provider; Presenting part; Primipara (see primip); Private patient/ practice; Proactivator plasminogen; Prothrombin-proconvertin (see Factors II & VII) (see P&P); Protoporphyria/yrin (= PROTO); Proximal phalanx; Pseudomyxoma peritonei; Pseudoparkinsonism (caused by drugs such as reserpine, tetrabenazine, phenothiazines, butyrophenones, etc.); Pseudophake/kia/kos (a lens implant); Pterygoid process; Puerperal psychosis; Pulsus paradoxus; Purulent pericarditis; Push pills; Pyrophosphate (see P-P).
Pp Pressure.
pp near point of accommodation (L. punctum proximum) (eye examination) (= PP); pages; postpartum (= PP); postprandial (after meals) (= PP); privately printed.
P-P Prothrombin - proconvertin (see P&P).
P&P Pins and plaster; Policy and procedure; Prothrombin and proconvertin (= PP; P-P) (see Factors II and VII).
P-5'-P Pyridoxal-5'-phosphate.
PP_1 Free/ Labeled pyrophosphate; Polynoxylin - a condensation product of formaldehyde and urea. An antibacterial and

antifungal agent, used in the treatment of skin infections.

PPA First shake well (see Ppa); Palpation, percussion, & auscultation (see PP&A); Pepsin A; Phenylpropanolamine (a CNS stimulant); Phenylpyruvic/ Polyphosphoric acid; Pittsburgh pneumonia agent; Population pharmacokinetic analysis; Postpartum/ Postpill amenorrhea; Pure pulmonary atresia.

Ppa First shake well/ The bottle first having been shaken/ The bottle to be first shaken (L. phiala prius agitata) (= PPA); Pulmonary arterial/ artery pressure (see PAP).

PP&A; pp&a Palpation, percussion, and auscultation (= PPA).

PPAD Practical Procedures and Aesthetic Dentistry (IDJ).

PPARγ Peroxisomal proliferator activated gamma (nuclear) receptor (see OADA - Thiazolidinediones).

PPAS Peripheral pulmonary artery stenosis; Postpolio atrophy syndrome.

Ppaw Pulmonary artery wedge pressure (see PAWP).

PPB Partial placental barrier (Obstetrics); Percutaneuous pleural biopsy; Plasma protein binding; Platelet-poor blood; Pneumococcal pneumonia and bacteremia; Polymeric phosphate binder/ binding (restoring serum Ca and P balance by lowering serum phosphorus in dialysis patients with ESRD - e.g. treatment with Sevelamer HCl); Positive pressure breathing; Postpartum bleeding (see PPH).

PPb Postparotid basic (protein).

ppb parts per billion.

PPBD Plasma protein-bound drug.

PPBE Postpartum breast engorgement/ enlargement.

PPBS Postprandial blood sugar.

PPC Patient-physician cooperation; Patient's past/ poor/ present/ previous condition (see PPMC); Peak plasma concentration; Pentose phosphate cycle; Peri/ Post/ Prepartal/tum care; Peripheral posterior curve; Persistent peripheral cytopenia; Phosphatidylcholine; Plasma paracetamol concentration; Plasma/ Proserum prothrombin conversion; Pluripotential cell; Pneumopericardium; Poor patient compliance; Postpartum complication (s); Prepregnancy counselling; Preliminary Proceedings Committee; Primary peritoneal cancer (an Ovarian cancer); Progressive patient care; Pronounced pharmacodynamic change(s); Proximal palmar crease; Psychiatric pain clinic; Psychotherapy-pharmacotherapy combination; Pyopericardium.

PpC Pregnancy per cycle.

PPCA Plasma/ Proserum prothrombin conversion accelerator (see Factor - VII).

PPCD Polymorphous posterior corneal dystrophy.

PPCE Postproline cleaving enzyme.

PPCF Peripartum cardiac failure; Plasma/ Proserum prothrombin conversion factor (see Factor - VII).

PPCH Piperazinylmethyl cyclohexanone.

PPCM Postpartum cardiomyopathy.

PPCP Personal primary care physician.

PPD Packs per day; Parallel plate dialyzer (Hemodialysis); Paraphenylenediamine; Percussion and postural drainage; Permanent partial disability; Phenyldiphenyloxadiazole; Posterior polymorphous dystrophy; Postpartum day/ deterioration; Postprandial distress; Primary physical dependence; Primary polydipsia; Progressive perceptive deafness; Purified protein derivative (procedure/ tuberculin skin test) (see Tuberculin); (Siebert) purified protein derivative (of tuberculin).

P&PD Percussion and postural drainage (= PPD).

PPD-B Purified protein derivative - Battey (strain) (tuberculin).

PPD-S Purified protein derivative - standard (tuberculin).

PPE Palmar-plantar erythrodysesthesia; Patient-protection ethic(s); Permeability/ Prepulmonary edema; Personal protective equipment; Physician/patient encounter (seeDPE); Polyphosphoric ester; Porcine pancreatic elastase; Postpartum endometritis; Pre-pregnancy evaluation; Primary pharmacological effect; Programmed physical examination; Pulmonary permeability edema.

PPEM Postpartum endomyometritis.

PPEP Positive expiratory pressure plateau (see PEPP).

PPES Palmar-plantar erythrodysesthesia syndrome.

PPF Pellagra preventive factor; Perfusion pressure flow (of urine); Phagocytosis promoting factor; Phosphonoformate; Phototoxic protection factor; Plasma protein fraction (see HPPF); Polypropylenefumarate; Poor prognostic factor; Posterior pituitary function; Prepubertal female; Progressive pulmonary failure/ fibrosis; Protein-producing factory (= Cytoplasmic ribosome, in cell replication).

PPFA Planned Parenthood Federation of America (formerly BCFA).

PPG Photo(electric) plethysmogram/aph(y); Physiologic-pacing group (heart see VPG); Posterior pituitary gland; Postprandial glucose; Powered/ Programmable pulse generator (pacemaker).

ppg picopicogram (= 10^{-24} g; 10^{-12} picogram).

PPGA Postpill galactorrhea-amenorrhea.

PPGC Post/Preprandial plasma glucose concentration (see FBGC; PBGC); Postprandial glucose control.

PPGF Polypeptide growth factor.

PPGI Psychophysiologic gastrointestinal (reaction).

PPGL Postprandial glucose level.

PPGP Prepaid group practice.

ppGpp 3'-Pyrophosphoryl-guanosine-5'-diphosphate.

PPG-RT Photoplethysmography recovery time.

PPH Past pertinent history; Permanent physical handicap; Persistent/ Postpartum/ Primary pulmonary hypertension; Postpartum hemorrhage; Postprandial hyperglycemia/ hypotension; Primary palmar hyperhidrosis; Protocollagen proline hydroxylase.

pphm parts per hundred million.

PPHN Persistent pulmonary hypertension of the newborn.

PPHP Pseudo-pseudohypoparathyroidism.

ppht parts per hundred thousand.

PPI Benzylpenicilloylpolysine; Partial permanent impairment; Patient package insert; Peripartum infection; Physician Performance Index; Poor prognostic indicator; Pre-pregnancy intervention (see PCI); Present pain intensity; Proton (or acid) pump inhibitor (i.e. omeprazole, lansoprazole, and pantoprazole); Purified porcine insulin.

PPi; PP_i Inorganic pyrophosphate.

PPIC Peak plasma insulin concentration.

PPID Peak pain intensity difference (score).

PPIE Prolonged post-ictal encephalopathy.

PPK Palmoplantar keratosis.

PPKA Population pharmacokinetic analysis (see PPKS).

PPKS Population pharmacokinetic study (see PPKA).

PPL Pars plana lensectomy; Peak/ Prolactin plasma level; Penicilloyl-polylysine; Permathane Pacesetter lead; Planned Parenthood League.

Ppl Intrapleural pressure.

PPLF Postperfusion low flow.

PPLO Pleuropneumonia-like organism (such as Mycoplasma, a genus of highly pleomorphic, gram-negative, wall-defective microorganisms, e.g. M. pneumoniae or Eaton agent, a species causing viral pneumonia) = PPO.

PPM Pasta Picis Mitis (= Mild Tar Paste of St. John's Hospital, UK) - contains coal tar solution, zinc oxide, boric acid, starch, emulsifying wax, light liquid paraffin or yellow soft paraffin; Permanent pacemaker; Phosphpentomutase; Pigmented pupillary membrane; Posterior papillary muscle; Postpartum mastitis; Postprandial mood; Prepubertal male; Professor of Preventive Medicine; Protected passive mobilization (Orthopedics).

ppm parts per million; pulses per minute.

PPMA Postpoliomyelitis/ Progressive postmyelitis muscular atrophy; Pre-pregnancy medical asssessment.

PPMC Patient's past/ poor/ present/ previous medical condition (= PPC).

PPMM Postpolycythemic myeloid metaplasia (a disease characterized by anemia, dacryocytosis, extensive bone marrow fibrosis, leukoerythroblastic polycythemia vera, myelofibrosis, and increasing splenomegaly).

PPMS Primary progressive multiple sclerosis; Psychophysiologic musculoskeletal (reaction).

PPN Partial/ Peripheral/ Prolonged parenteral nutrition; Pedunculopontine nucleus;

Postprandial nausea; Pulmonary parenchymal nodule.

PPNA Peak phrenic nerve activity.

PPNAD Primary pigmented nodular adrenocortical disease.

PPNG Penicillinase-producing Neisseria gonorrhoeae.

PPNRP Philadelphia Pulmonary Neoplasm Research Project.

PPO Platelet peroxidase; Pleuropneumonia-like organism (see PPLO); Postprandial output (of gastric acid) (see APG; BAO); Preferred physician/ provider organization.

PPP Palatopharyngoplasty; Palmoplantar pustulosis; Particularly poor prognosis; Pedal pulse present; Pentose phosphate pathway; Peripheral pulses palpable; Personal primary physician (see PPCP); Pickford projective pictures; Pin-point pupil(s); Plasma protamine paracoagulation (see PPPC)/ precipitation; Platelet-poor plasma; Poison prevention packaging; Poker players' pneumonia (an outbreak of Q fever following exposure to a parturient cat); Polyphloretin/phoretic phosphate; Porcine pancreatic polypeptide; Portal perfusion pressure; Postpartum period/ psychosis; Post/Preprostatectomy patient; Powered programmable pacemaker; Prepatent period (the time between infection e.g. by *Giardia* lamblia and the appearance of parasites in the stools); Primary prevention project; Prospective Pravastatin Pooling (Project) (see PPPP); Protamine paracoagulation phenomenon; Protopathic prescription; Psychopathic personality (= Antisocial/ Sociopathic personality) (see ASPD or Antisocial personality disorder); Purified placental protein.

PPPA Poison Prevention Packaging Act.

PPPBL Peripheral pulses palpable in both legs.

PPPC Plasma protamine paracoagulation (test).

PPPD Pylorus-preserving pancreaticoduodenectomy.

PPPG Postprandial plasma glucose.

PPP(H) Purified placental protein (human).

PPPI Primary private practice insurance.

PPPP Prospective Pravastatin Pooling (PPP) Project.

PPPS Pistonless pulsometer pumping system (e.g. of the Umbilical cord)

PPP (test) Plasma protamine paracoagulation/ precipitating/ation test (= 3P [test]).

PPR Palliative/ Prompt pain relief; Patient progress record/ report; Physician-patient relation(ship); Posterior primary ramus; Postpartum relapse; Preterm premature rupture (of the membranes); Price's precipitation reaction.

PPr Paraprosthetic.

PPRC Physician Payment Review Commission.

PPRF Paramedial (zone of the)/ Paramedian pontine reticular formation; Postpartum renal failure; Pre-pregnancy risk factor(s) (such as Age, Diabetes mellitus, Genes, Multiparity, Obesity, etc., leading to birth of macrosomic offspring or Fetal Macrosomia, among other developmental problems).

PP-Ribose-P; PPRP 5-Phosphoribosyl-1-pyrophosphate.

PPRM Preterm premature rupture of the membranes.

PPROM Prolonged premature rupture of membranes.

PPRWP Poor precordial R-wave progression.

PPS Pain producing substance; Pellagra-preventing substance; Peripheral pulmonary stenosis; Personal Preference Scale; Phosphoribosyl-1-pyrophosphate synthetase; Physicians Placement Service (AMA); Pollution prevention strategy; Polyp Prevention Study (see CPPS; PPT); Polyvalent pneumococcal polysaccharide; Poor performance status; Poor prognostic sign; Popliteal pterygium syndrome; Postpartum sterilization; Postperfusion/ Postpericardiotomy/ Postpolio/ Postpump syndrome; Postprandial sleep(iness); Premature placental separation; Prepsychotic state; Primary (acquired) preleukemic syndrome; Primary-prevention strategy; Prospective payment system; Protein plasma substitute; Pseudopsychopathic schizophrenia (see BLS); Pulse per second; Purified protein solution.

PPs Peyer's patches.

PPSC Pluripotent stem cell.

PPSH Pseudovaginal perineoscrotal hypospadias.
PPSL Postprandial sugar level.
PPT Parietal pleural tissue; Partial prothrombin time; Peak-to-peak threshold; Person-to-person transmission (of disease/ infection); Plant protease test; Podophyllotoxin (e.g. Etoposide); Polyp Prevention Trial (US Study Group) (with high dietary fiber, fruit and vegetables, and low fat); Polypurine tract; Positive pregnancy test; Postpartum thyroiditis; Postprandial thermogenesis; Postprimary tuberculosis; Prolonged physiotherapy; Pulmonary platelet trapping; Pyopagus twins (see pagus).
ppt parts per trillion; precipitate; precipitated (see pptd); precipitation (see pptn); preparation (see prep); prepared (= prep).
pptd precipitated (= ppt).
PPTL Postpartum tubal ligation.
pptn precipitation (= ppt).
PPU Perforated peptic ulcer.
PPV Papillomavirus; Paroxysmal positional vertigo; Pneumococcal polysaccharide vaccine; Porcine parvovirus; Positive predictive value; Positive pressure ventilation (respiratory therapy); Postpayment verification; Progressive pneumonia virus; Pulmonary plasma volume.
P_{pvO2} Oxygenating ability.
PPVr Regional pulmonary plasma volume.
PPVT Peabody Picture Vocabulary Test.
PPVT-R Peabody Picture Vocabulary Test, Revised.
PPvVP Physiologic pacing versus Ventricular pacing.
PPW Postpartum woman/ women; Prepregnancy weight.
Ppw Pulmonary wedge pressure (see PCWP).
PPY Pancreatic polypeptide (see PP).
PQ Paraquat; Permeability quotient; Physician's questionnaire; Plastoquinone; Pronator quadratus (muscle); Pyrimethamine-quinine; Wave, in the ECG.
PQRST Probucol Quantitative Regression Swedish Trial (LDL oxidation in atherosclerosis).
PQTI Prolonged QT interval (ECG - in SIDS).
PR Far point (of accommodation) (L. punctum remotum) (see pr); Interval (ECG) (see P-R); Palindromic rheumatism; Panama red (variation of marijuana) (see Cannabis); Parallax and refraction; Paralytic rabies (= rabies with flaccid paralysis) (see FR - Furious rabies); Partial reinforcement/ remission/ response; Patient relations; Peer review; Perfusion/ Pregnancy/ Production (see Pr)/ Pulse rate; Peripheral neuritis; Peripheral/ Progressive resistance; Per rectum (L.) by way of the rectum (rectal examination) (see pr); Phenol red; Photoreaction; Physical/ Pulmonary rehabilitation; Pityriasis rosea; Pneumatic retinopathy; Posterior root; Postmyalgia rheumatica; Postural/ Preyer's reflex; Potency ratio; Potential relation(ship); Preference record; Pregnancy/ant (see pregn); Premature; Preretinal; Pressoreceptor; Pressure (see press); Prevention/ive (see prev); Previous (see prev); Procedure/ceedings/cess (see proc); Proctologist/ogy (see Proct); Proctoscope/opy (see procto); Production rate (see Pr); Profile; Progesterone receptor; Progress report; Progressive relaxation; Prolactin (see Pr); Proliferative retinopathy; Prolonged remission; Propranolol (see PROP); Prosthion; Protein (see prot); Public relations; Puerto Rican; Pulse repetition; Punctum remotum (L.) (see pr); Pyramidal response.
PR# Pelvic ring fracture (see PRF).
PR; P.R. Prolonged release (dose/ injection/ tablet etc.).
PR; P/R; P-R Poor-risk (patient).
Pr Praseodymium (Z = 59) (see Elements - Praseodymium); Prednisolone (see PSL); Prednisone (see PRED); Presbyopia (eye examination); Primary; Prism (see pr); Proctologist/ogy (see Proct); Production rate (of steroid hormones) (= PR); Prolactin (serum) (= PR); Propyl.
pr far point (of accommodation) (L. punctum remotum) (= PR); pair; per rectum (L.) by way of the rectum (rectal examination) (= PR); prism (= Pr).
P-R Interval (ECG) - the interval or time between the P wave and the beginning of the QRS complex in electrocardiography (= PR).

P&R Pelvic and rectal (examination); Pulse and respiration.

PRA Phosphoribosylamine; Physician's Recognition Award (AMA); Plasma renin activity (laboratory/ endocrinology); Platelet reducing agent (e.g. Anagrelide); Posterior rim of acetabulum; Progesterone receptor assay; Prospective randomized assessment (of medical treatment) (see PRS).

PRAC Pharmaceutical Reimbursement Advisory Committee (HEW).

prac; pract practical; practice; practitioner.

PRACTIS Practitioner's Award Computer Tabulated Information Service.

PrA-HPA Protein A hemolytic plaque assay.

PRAISE Prospective randomized amiodipine individual survival evaluation.

PRAP Pregnancy risk assessment program (CDC).

PRAS Prereduced, anaerobically sterilized (culture medium); Pseudorenal artery syndrome.

PRAT Platelet radioactive antiglobulin test.

p rat aetat in proportion to age (L. pro ratione aetatis).

PRAVD Prednisolone, cytarabine (= cytosine Arabinoside), vincristine sulfate, daunorubicin.

PRB Pharmaceutical Reimbursement Board (HEW); Prosthetics Research Board; Psychopharmacology Research Branch (NIMH).

PRBC Packed red blood cells (blood transfusion) (= PRC); Placental residual blood capacity (see PRBV).

PRBV Placental residual blood volume (= PRBC).

PRC Packed red cells (see PRBC); Peer review committee; Perennial rhinoconjunctivitis; Phase response curve; Photoreceptor cell(s) (light-sensing cells in the retina); Physicians' Review Committee (UMS); Plasma renin concentration; Potentially risky condition; Primate Research Center (University of California); Professional review commission/ committee; Prolonged release capsule (see PR; P.R.).

PRCA Pure red cell aplasia.

PRCSG Pediatric Rheumatology Collaborative Study Group.

PRCT Preresectional chemotherapy.

PRD Panic-related disorder (= PD); Parkin-related disease (see parkin gene); Partial reaction of degeneration; Pediatric rheumatic disease; Perceptions of Racial Discrimination; Persistent renal dysfunction (= PKD); Polycystic/ Progressive renal disease; Postradiation dysplasia; Pregnancy and the rheumatic diseases; Pregnancy-related death (= PRM).

PRDS Prolonged release delivery system.

PRDU Poorly responsive duodenal ulcer.

PRE Painful red eye; Passive/ Progressive resistance/tive exercise(s) (physiotherapy); Periodic retinal examination (see PEE); Photoreacting enzyme; Pigmented retinal epithelium; Preclinical research experience; Prospective randomized evaluation.

pre before or preliminary.

pre-AIDS Pre-acquired immune deficiency syndrome.

precip precipitate(d)/ating/ation.

PRED Prednisone (= Pr).

pred predicate (affirm/ declare).

Preemy Premature infant (see Premie).

pref preference.

prefd preferred.

Preg Pregestimil.

preg pregnancy/ant (see pregn).

Pregang Preganglionic.

pregn pregnancy/ant (= PR; preg).

Pre γS Serum immunoglobulin concentration before dialysis.

preinoc pre-inoculation.

prelim preliminary.

prem premature/urity.

PreMACE Prednisone, methotrexate, (calcium folinate or leucovorin), Adriamycin (doxorubicin), cyclophosphamide, and etoposide.

Premie Premature infant (= Preemy).

Prenat Prenatal.

preop; pre-op pre-operative.

prep preparation (= ppt); prepare; prepared (see prepd); preposition.

PREPARE Preventing Postmenopausal Memory Loss and Alzheimer's with Replacement Estrogens (study).

prepd prepared (= ppt; prep).

PRERLA Pupils round, equal, react to light and accommodation.
Pre-Rx Before treatment.
pres present(ed)/(ing).
preserv preservation/ve(d).
PRESS Preschool Readiness Experimental Screening Scale.
press pressure (= PR).
prev prevent(ed)/(ion)/(ive) (= PR); previous (= PR).
PREVMEDU Preventive medical/cine unit.
PRF Partial reinforcement; Patient report form; Pelvic ring fracture (= PR#); Perceivable/ Permanent/ Personal/ Persumable/ Plausible/ Possible/ Potential/ Predictable/ Predisposing/ Presumptive/ Prevailing/ Previous/ Primary/ Probable/ Profound/ Progressive/ Prominent/ Pronounced/ Proven/ Psychological risk factor ([in heart disease - Age, Cigarette smoking, Family history, High blood cholesterol (LDL/ TGL), Hypertension, Physical inactivity, etc.] and other diseases); Plasma recognition factor; Pontine reticular formation; Progressive renal/ respiratory failure; Prolactin-releasing factor (see Hormones - PRH); Prolonged release formulation (of a drug).
pRF Polyclonal rheumatoid factor.
PRFA Plasma recognition factor activity.
PRFCC Prompt, rapid, forceful chest compression (in CPR) (see MtM).
PRFM Premature rupture of fetal membranes.
PRFN Percutaneous radio frequency.
PRFR (valve) Pressure-retaining flow-relieving (valve).
PRFS Postrheumatic fever syndrome (= Jaccoud arthritis).
PRG Phleborrheogram/graph(y); Posterior root ganglia/ion; Purge.
PRGS Phosphoribosylglycineamide synthetase.
PRGU Poorly responsive gastric ulcer.
PRH Past relevant history; Preretinal hemorrhage; Prolactin-releasing hormone (see Hormones - PRH).
PRHBF Peak reactive hyperemia blood flow.
PRHO Preregistration house officer.
PRI Pain Rating Index; Pararectus incision (see inc.); Passive rabies immunization; Phosphate reabsorption index; Phosphoribose isomerase; Practice-related issue(s); Pronounced renal impairment/ insufficiency (see SRI).
PRIAS Packard's radioimmunoassay system.
PRICES Protection, rest, ice, compression, elevation, and support (first aid).
PRIH Prolactin release - inhibiting hormone.
prim primary.
PRIME Pediatric research, informed (consent), and medical ethics; Prematriculation Program in Medical Education.
PRIME-MD Primary Care Evaluation of Mental Disorders.
PRIMEX Primary (care) extender (i.e. Nurse practitioners for extension of primary care).
Primip Primipara (woman bearing first child) (= PP).
primip primipara (a woman who has had one pregnancy which resulted in a viable child) (see Para I).
prim luc first thing in the morning (L. prima luc).
prim m first thing in the morning (L. primo mane).
PRIMS Pediatric Risk of Mortality Score.
PRIN Professional Rescue Instructors of Nevada.
Princ Principal; Principle.
PRIND Prolonged reversible ischemic neurologic defect.
P-R int P-R interval - time from beginning of atrial contraction to beginning of ventricular contraction (in the ECG) (see P-R).
Prion. Proteinaceous infectious particle (causing TSE) (see BSE; MCD).
PRISM Policy Research in Science and Medicine.
PRIST Paper radioimmunosorbent test.
Pristine gloves No powder on gloves (Surgery).
Priv Private; Privilege.
PRK Photorefractive keratectomy/atonomy/atotomy; Primary rabbit kidney.
PRL Plasma renin level.
PRL; Prl Prolactin (see Hormones - LH i).
PRLA Pupils react to light and accommoda-

tion.

PRM Pain relief/ relieving medication; Passive range of movement (of a joint); Peri/Post/Prenatal morbidity/ mortality; Peripheral rhabdomyosarcoma; Phosphoribomutase; Photoreceptor membrane; Pitanguey reduction mammoplasty; Postreceptor mechanism; Pregnancy-related mortality (see PRD Premature rupture of the membranes; Primary Reference Material.

PrM Preventive medicine.

PRMJ Peer-reviewed medical journal.

PRMR Public Responsibility in Medicine and Research (US trade group).

PRM-SDX Pyrimethamine sulfadioxine.

PRN as required (see prn); Phenyltoloxamine (citrate) (see C 5581); Physician's Radio Network; Physicians' Research Network; Polyradiculoneuropathy.

prn according to circumstances/ as circumstances may require/ as needed/ as required/ when required, occasionally/ whenever necessary/ whenever required (L. pro re nata).

PRNT Plaque reduction neutralization test.

PRO Professional Review Organization; Pronated/tion/tor (see pron).

Pro Proline; Prophylactic/laxis (see proph); Prothrombin (see Prothr).

pro protein (see prot).

prob probable/ly.

PROBE Prospective, Randomized, Open with Blinded Endpoint (evaluation program).

proc procedure/ceedings/cess (= PR; Proc).

PROCAM Prospective Cardiovascular Munster (Study).

Pro-Con Prophylactic contraceptive.

Procs Proceedings (see proc).

Proct Proctologist/gy (= PR; Pr).

procto proctology; proctoscope/opy (procedure/ rectal) (= PR).

prod product(ion).

Prof Profession/ Professor.

prog prognathism; prognosis (see progn); program; progress(ive).

progn prognosis (= prog; Prx).

Proj Project.

prolong prolongation/ged.

PROM Passive range of motion; Premature/ Prolonged rupture of (fetal) membranes; Preterm rupture of membranes (Obstetrics); Programmable read only memory.

ProMACE Prednisone, Methotrexate, Adriamycin, Cyclophosphamide and Etoposide (Epipodopophyllotoxin) (Chemotherapy for the treatment of aggressive lymphomas).

PROMIS Problem-Oriented Medical Information System.

Promotoras de Salud Promotors of Health (program - SFMS; TSRI).

Promy Promyelocyte(s) (= PROMYELO).

PROMYELO Promyelocyte(s) (see Promy).

pron pronated/tion/tor (= PRO).

PROP Prop. Propionate; Propranolol (= PR).

ProPac Prospective Payment Assessment Commission.

Prop graft see H graft.

proph prophylactic/laxis (= Pro).

pro rect rectal (L. pro recto).

pros; prost prostate/ prostatic.

prosth prosthesis/thetic.

Prot Protestant.

prot protein (= PR; pro).

Prothr Prothrombin (= Pro).

Prothr cont Prothrombin content (laboratory/ coagulation).

Pro time Prothrombin time (laboratory/ coagulation) (see Pro-X).

PROTO Protoporphyria/yrin (see PP).

prov provisional(ly).

PROVIMI Proteins, vitamins, and minerals.

prox proximal(ly).

Pro-X Prothrombin time (laboratory/ coagulation) (= Pro-X).

prox luc the day before (L. proxima luce).

PRP Pain relief program; Pan retinal photocoagulation (laser therapy); Penicillinase-resistant penicillin; Physiologic rest position; Pityriasis rubra pilaris; Plasma-replacement preparation; Platelet-rich plasma (transfusion); Polyradiculopathy; Poly ribo/ribosyl phosphate; Polyribosyl-ribitol-phosphate (capsular polysaccharide); Poor-risk patient; Poorly-responsive patient; Postural rest position; Pregnancy-related problem(s); Pressure rate product; Primary Raynaud's phenomenon; Progressive rubella panencephalitis; Proliferative retinopathy; Proliferative retinopathy photocoagulation; Psychotic Reaction Profile.

PrP Prion protein (a gene/ protein that encodes the protein's normal version of the prion (see Prion).

PRPP Phosphoribosyl pyrophosphate.

PRPU Poorly responsive peptic ulcer.

PRR Proton relaxation rate; Pulse repetition rate.

PrR Progesterone receptor.

PRRE Pupils round, regular, and equal.

PRR&E Periodic Resident Review and Evaluation.

PR-RSV Prague Rous sarcoma virus.

PRS Pain resting splint (used in rehabilitation therapy); Penicillin resistant strain (of bacteria); Personality Rating Scale; Pierre Robin syndrome; Plasma renin substrate; Plastic and Reconstructive Surgery (see PARS); Polyester Retrieval System; Prospective randomized study (see PRA); Psychiatric Rating Scale (see BPRS).

PRSA Plasma renin substrate activity; Public Relations Society of America.

PRSIS Prospective Rate Setting Information System.

PRSM Peripheral smear.

PRS$_r$ Plasma renin substrate reactivity.

PRSs Positive rolandic spikes.

PRT Penicillium roqueforti toxin; Pharmaceutical research and testing; Phosphoribosyl transferase (see PRTase); Pill-rolling tremor (seen in parkinsonism); Post-operative respiratory therapy; Prerequisite training; Prospective randomized trial.

PRTase Phosphoribosyl transferase (= PRT).

PRTH-C Prothrombin time control.

PRU Peripheral resistance unit (i.e. unit of peripheral resistance).

PRUJ Proximal radio-ulnar joint (Orthopedics).

PRV Polycythemia rubra vera; Pseudo-rabies virus.

PRVA Peripheral vein renin activity.

PRVEP Pattern reversal visual evoked potential.

PRW Polymerized ragweed.

PRX Pseudoexfoliation.

Prx Prognosis (see progn).

PRZ Pirenzepine - a pyrido-benzodiazepine compound used in the treatment of gastric and duodenal ulcer (see LS 519); Prazepam.

PRZF Pyrazofurin.

PS Chloropicrin; Pacemaker/ Paired stimulation (electric); Pacemaker syndrome (fatigue, palpitations, & presyncope): The "Pointing sign" - typical of functional dyspepsia or duodenal ulcer, as demonstrated in the sculpture of the Dying Slave by Michelangelo, exhibited in the Louvre, Paris; Prefilled syringe (see PFS); Presenilin (1 & 2) - abnormal proteins, mutant versions of which purportedly cause Alzheimer's disease: they are found on the inner surface of the nuclear membrane; Paper speed; Paradoxical sleep; Paranoid schizophrenia; Paranoid state; Paraspinal; Parasympathetic; Parotid sialography; Partial seizure; Pathological stage/ging; Patient('s)/ Pigeon/ Pregnant serum; Pediatric/ Plastic surgeon/ery; Performance status; Performing scale (IQ); Periodic (see FMF)/ Proteus syndrome; Peripheral smear; Pferdestarke; Phosphate saline (buffer); Phosphatidyl serine; Photosensitivity/tization; Photosynthesis; Phrenic stimulation; Physical status; Physiologic(al) saline; Platelet survival; Point of symmetry; Polysaccharide; Polystyrene; Population sample; Porter-Silber (chromogen) (see P-S); Postscript; Prescription (see Ps); Presenting symptom; Pressure support; Pronator syndrome; Prostatic secretion; Protamine sulfate; Protective services; Protein S/ synthesis; Psychiatric/ry (see PSY; Psy); Psychiatric surgery/ Psychosurgery; Pulmonary/ Pyloric stenosis.

Ps Prescription (= PS); Pseudo; Pseudocyst; Pseudomonas; Psoriasis.

ps per second; picosecond.

P/S Polisher-stimulator; Polyunsaturated/saturated (fatty acid ratio).

P-S Pancreozymin-secretion; Porter-Silber (chromogen) (= PS); Pyramid-surface (kidney dialysis machine).

P&S Pain and suffering; Paracentesis and suction (procedure/ gastrointestinal); Physicians and Surgeons (College of) (Columbia University).

PS1 Presenilin 1 (the Alzheimer's gene, found

on chromosome 14) (see PS2).

PS2 Presenilin 2 (the Alzheimer's gene, found on chromosome 1, and identified by Gerard Schellenberg and Thomas Bird in 1995 at the University of Washington's Alzheimer Disease Center in Seattle).

P2S Pralidoxime mesylate (see 2-FMPOMS).

PS I Healthy patient with localized pathological process.

PS II A patient with mild to moderate systemic disease.

PS III A patient with severe systemic disease limiting activity, but not incapacitating.

PS IV A patient with incapacitating systemic disease.

PS V Moribund patient not expected to live.

PSA Paroxystic symptoms of anxiety; Patient self-assessment (see IA - Investigator assessment); Polyethylene sulfonic acid; Posterior spinal artery; Presystolic accentuation (late diastolic murmur - mitral stenosis); Product selection allowed; Progressive spinal ataxia; Prolonged self-administration; Prolonged sleep apnea; Prostate-specific antigen (a glycoprotein) (test for cancer of the prostate); Psoriatic arthritis; Psycho-social aspect (e.g. of self); Public service announcement.

Psa Psoriatric arthritis (= PSA); Systemic arterial (blood) pressure.

PSAC President's Science Advisory Committee.

PSAD Psychoactive substance abuse and dependence (see PSDA); Psychostimulant antidepressant/essive (drug).

PSAGN Poststreptococcal acute glomerulonephritis.

PSAL Peak serum antibody level.

PSAn; PsAn Psychoanalysis.

PSAP Pulmonary surfactant apoprotein.

PSAR Postsynaptic acetylcholine receptor.

PSα1R Postsynaptic alpha-1 receptor.

PSB Pathological sexual/ social behavior (see HSB); Proctosigmoid biopsy; Protected specimen brush.

PSbetaG Pregnany-specific beta-1-glycoprotein.

PSC Partial subligamentous calcification; Patient services coordination; Pediatric Symptom Checklist; Porter-Silber chromogen; Posterior semicircular canal (in the labyrinth of the inner/ internal ear); Posterior subcapsular cataract; Primary sclerosing cholangitis; Psychosocial counseling; Psychosomatic complaint; Public Service Commission; Pulse synchronized contractions.

PSCA Prostate stem cell antigen (gene).

PSCC Portosystemic collateral circulation.

PSCD Postsurgical cognitive difficulty/ disturbance.

PSCEE Presystemic Clearance, Elimination and Excretion (of a drug).

PsChE Pseudocholinesterase.

PSCI Primary Self Concept Inventory.

Psci Pressure at slow component intercept.

PSCs Polar stratospheric clouds.

PSCT Peripheral stem cell transplant.

PSD Particle size distribution; Peptone, starch and dextrose; Periodic synchronous discharge; Photosensitive drug; Platelet serotonin depletion; Pooled standardized difference (see SD; SMD); Positive significant difference (see HSD); Poststenosis dilation; Postsynaptic density; Presenile dementia; Potassium-sparing diuretic/ drug (e.g. amiloride, spironolactone, triamterine, etc.); Preclinical safety data; Pre-existing seizure disorder; Presynaptic disorder; Psycho sexual/ social/ somatic development/ disorder/ distress/ disturbance/ dysfunction.

PSDA Psychoactive substance dependence and abuse (see PSAD).

PSDES Primary symptomatic diffuse esophageal spasm.

PSE Paradoxical systolic expansion; Penicillin-sensitive enzyme; Point of subjective equality (psychology); Portal system episode; Portal systemic encephalopathy; Potassium-sparing effect (see K+SD; K+SE); Potential sedative/ side effect(s); Present State Examination; Prolonged sedative effect; Proven superior efficacy; Purified spleen extract; Protein sparing effect (of growth hormones, etc.).

PSEC Poststress ethanol consumption.

psec picosecond.

PSES Parental socioeconomic status.

PSF Peak scatter factor; Peak systolic flow;

Polysaccharide fraction; Posterior spinal fusion; Potential seizure frequency (epilepsy); Pseudosarcomatous fasciitis; Psychosocial function.

PSG Peak systolic gradient; Phosphate, saline, and glucose; Polysomnogram/graph(er)/graphy; Presenilin gene (in Alzheimer's disease); Presystolic gallop.

PSGBI Pathological Society of Great Britain and Ireland.

PSGI Post surgical gynecologic infection.

PSGN Poststreptococcal glomerulonephritis.

PSH Past surgical history; Postspinal headache; Puncture-site hemorrhage.

PsHD Pseudoheart disease.

PSI Parascapular incision (see inc.); Periodic somatic inactivity; Physiologic Stability Index; Policy Studies Institute (UK); Posterior sagittal index; Problem solving information; Professional Services Index; Prostaglandin synthetase/etic inhibition/tor; Psychosomatic inventory; Pyrimidine synthesis inhibitor (see TFMA).

psi pounds per square inch (pressure measurement).

psia pounds per square inch absolute.

PSIa Problem Solving Information apparatus.

pSIDS Partially unexplained sudden infant death syndrome.

PSIFT Platelet suspension immunofluorescence test.

PSIG Pounds per square inch guage.

PSIL Preferred (frequency) speech interference level.

PSIS Posterior sacro/ superior iliac spine.

PSL Parasternal line; Partial skin loss (superficial, 2nd degree burn with no loss of dermis); Percent stroke length (cardiology); Potassium, sodium chloride, and sodium lactate (solution); Prednisolone (= Pr); Progressive sensory loss.

PSM Paraspinous musculature (parallel to spinal cord); Patient self-management; Postmitochondrial supernatant (see PMS); Poststenotic myocardium; Post/Presynaptic membrane; Practical surrogate marker; Presystolic murmur.

PSMA Progressive/ Proximal spinal muscular atrophy.

PSMD Portable Spacelab (90207) monitoring device (for monitoring ambulatory blood pressure).

PSMed Psychosomatic medicine.

PSMF Protein-sparing modified fast.

PSMT Psychiatric services management team.

PSN Peripheral sensorimotor/sory neuropathy; Post/Presynaptic neuron.

PSO Proximal subungual onychomycosis.

PSOF Public Safety Officers Foundation.

Psol Partly soluble.

P/sore Pressure sore.

PSP Pancreatic spasmolytic peptide; Paralytic shellfish poisoning; Parathyroid secretory protein; Patient safety program; Peak systolic pressure; Penicillinase-stable penicillin; Periodic short pulse; Peripheral sensory potential(s) (see SNAP); Phenolsulfonphthalein (Phenosulphthalein test) (see KFT - PSP); Phosphoserine; Phosphatase; Photosensitivity potential; Positive spike pattern (EEG); Posterior spinal process; Postsurgical pain/ patient; Postsympathectomy patient; Postsynaptic potential (= psp); Prednisone sodium phosphate; Preseizure period (in epilepsy); Progressive supranuclear palsy/ paralysis; Proximal spacer prosthesis; Pseudopregnancy (= Pseudocyesis or False pregnancy); Psychosomatic phenomena/menon.

PSPA Prolactin-secreting pituitary adenoma.

PSPE Purine-salvage-pathway enzyme (adenosine deaminase) (see ADD).

PSPT Postsurgical physical therapy.

PSQ Parent Symptom Questionnaire; Patient Satisfaction Questionnaire.

PSR Pain sensitivity range; Pap(anicolaou) screening routine; Patient survival rate; Phosphatidylcholine/Sphingomyelin ratio (in amniotic fluid); Photosensitivity reaction; Photosensitivity skin reaction (see PSSR); Physicians for Social Responsibility (Boston, USA); Poor subjective result; Portal systemic resistance; Postsurgical recovery; Premature spontaneous rupture (see PSRBOW); Proliferative sickle retinopathy; Pruritic skin reaction; Psychosomatic reaction; Pulmonary stretch receptor.

PSRBOW Premature spontaneous rupture of

bag of waters (= PSR).

PSRC Plastic Surgery Research Council.

PSRM Precise surgical road map (prior to brain surgery, etc.).

PSRO Professional Standards Review Organization (see CLAPSRO).

PSS Painful shoulder syndrome; Phase specific substance; Physiologic(al) saline solution (see PhyS); Porcine stress syndrome; Potts-Smith scissors (Vascular surgery); Preclinical safety study (see PCSS); Primary Sjögren syndrome (see pSS); Problem-solving skill (psychotherapy); Proctosigmoidoscopy; Progressive systemic scleroderma/ sclerosis; Pseudo-Cushing's syndrome; Psoriasis severity scale; Psychiatric Status Schedule; Psychological and social sciences; Psychosomatic syndrome; Pulmonary surfactant system; Pure sensory stroke; Pursestring suture (see Sut).

pSS Primary Sjögren syndrome (= PSS).

pss physiologic(al) saline solution (see PhyS).

PSSR Photosensitivity skin reaction (= PSR).

PSST Pancreozymin/ secretin stimulation test (see PEOT).

PSSU Potential stroke screening unit (= PSU).

PST Pancreatic suppression test; Paroxysmal supraventricular tachycardia (see PSVT); Patient-specific therapy/ treatment; Penicillin, streptomycin and tetracycline; Pentagastrin stimulation test (a pentapeptide given IV for gastric secretion/ stimulation test); Peristimulus time; Phenolsulfotransferase; Platelet survival time; Poststenotic; Poststimulus time; Postsurgical therapy/ treatment; Prefrontal sonic therapy/ treatment; Presumptive self-treatment; Protamine sulfate test (see PS test); Protein-sparing therapy; Proximal straight tubule; Psychosuggestion/ive therapy; Pulmonary surface tension.

PSTA Predictive Screening Test of Articulation.

P_{stat} Static recoil pressure (measure of lung elasticity) increased in pulmonary fibrosis, and reduced in emphysema.

PS test Protamine sulfate test (see PST).

P-S test Patient Self test.

PSTH Poststimulus time histogram (= PTSH).

PSTI Pancreatic secretory trypsin inhibitor.

PSU Pennsylvania State University; Photosynthetic unit; Potential stroke (screening) unit (see PSSU); Primary sampling unit.

P-substance Protein substance (antigen).

PSurg Plastic surgery.

PSV Pressure supported ventilation; Proximal selective vagotomy.

PSVC Postsurgical venous congestion.

PSVER Pattern shift visual evoked response.

PSVS Portal systemic venous shunting.

PSVT Paroxysmal supraventricular tachycardia (= PST).

PSW Primary surgical ward; Protective service worker; Psychiatric social worker.

PSWD Postsurgical wound dressing.

PSWL Placebo-subtracted weight loss.

PSWOP Public Service Work Opportunity Program.

PSWT Psychiatric social work training.

PSX Pseudoexfoliation.

PSY; Psy Psychiatric/ry (= PS; psych; psychiat); Psychological/gy (see psych).

psych psychiatric/ry (see PSY); psychological/gy (= PSY; psychol).

psychiat psychiatric/ry (see PSY; Psy).

psychoan; psychoanal psychoanalysis/lytical.

psychol psychological/gy (see psych).

psychopath psychopathological/gy.

psychosom psychosomatic.

psychother psychotherapist/apy (see PT).

psy-path psychopathic.

Ps-ZES Pseudo-Zollinger-Ellison syndrome.

PT Cisplatin (Platinum compd); Pancoast's tumor (see ALC); Parathormone; Parathyroid; Parkinsonian/ Physiological/ Postural tremor; Paroxysmal tachycardia; Part time; Patient (see pt); Pericardial tamponade; Permanent and total (see P&T); Pertussis toxoid; Pharmacy and therapeutics (see P&T); Phenylthiocarbamide/moyl (see PTC); Phenytoin (see PHT); Photophobia; Phototoxicity; Physical therapist/py (= Phys Ther)/ training; Physiotherapist/apy (= Physio; physio); Pine tar; Plasma thromboplastin; Pneumothorax (see Pnx); Polyvalent tolerance; Positional testing (for nystagmus); Posterior tibial (artery/ pulse); Postgraduate trainee(ship); Posttetanic; Posttransfusion;

Posttransplant(ation); Posttraumatic; Premature termination (of pregnacy); Preterm; Proficiency test(ing); Pronator teres (muscle); Propylthiouracil (see PTU); Prothrombin time (laboratory/ coagulation) (see LFT iv); Proverbs Test (psychology); Psychotherapist/apy (= psychother); Psychotherapy (such as behavioral, cognitive, emotional, hypnotic, and interpersonal therapy); Pulmonary thrombosis; Pulmonary tuberculosis (see PTb); Pyramidal tract; Pyloric tumor; Temporal plane (see TP).

Pt Patient (see pt); Platinum (Z = 78) (see Elements - Platinum); Psychoasthenia.

pt let it be continued (L. perstetur); part; patient (= PAT; Pat; pat; PNT; Pnt; pnt; PT; Pt); pint; point.

P&T Paracentesis and tubing (of ears); Peak and trough; Permanent and total (disability) (= PT); Pharmacy and therapeutics (= PT).

PT 9 Betahistine hydrochloride (= 2-[2-Methylaminoethyl]pyridine dihydrochloride) - a diamine oxidase inhibitor with histamine-like activity. Used in the treatment of histamine headache and Meniere's syndrome.

PT-14 Palatin Technologies - 14 (a peptide molecule derivative of a melanocyte-stimulating hormone causing penile vasodilation and now used in the treatment of ED - Erectile dysfunction).

PT 150 Cuprophane.

PTA Pain, tears, and agony; Parallel tubular arrays; Parathyroid adenoma; Percutaneous transluminal angioplasty; Peritonsillar abscess; Peroxidase-labeled antibody; Persistent truncus arteriosus; Pharmacotherapeutic agent; Phosphotungstic acid; Physical therapy assistant; Plasma thromboplastin antecedent (see Factor XI); Platelet thromboplastin antecedent; Phototoxic activity; Posterior tibial artery; Posttherapeutic amenorrhea; Posttraumatic amnesia/ amputation (Orthopedics); Posttraumatic arachnoiditis; Pretreatment anxiety; Prior to admission/ arrival; Prothrombin activity; Pure-tone acuity/ average(s) (see PTAT)/ audiometry (see Audiometry).

P-TAG Target-attaching globin precursor.

PTAH Phosphotungstic acid hematoxylin; Plasma thromboplastin factor I (= blood coagulation factor I) (see factor I).

PTAN Post-traumatic anoxic necrosis (of muscle).

PTAP Purified (diphtheria) toxoid (precipitated by) aluminium phosphate.

p'tase phosphatase (laboratory/ chemistry) (see p'ase).

PTAT Pure tone average threshold.

PTB Patellar tendon bearing (prosthesis); Post/Preterm baby/ birth (see PTD; PTL; PTP); Prior to birth.

PTb Pulmonary tuberculosis (= PT).

PTBA Percutaneous transluminal balloon angioplasty.

PTBD Percutaneous transhepatic biliary drainage (= PTD; PTH); Percutaneous transluminal balloon dilatation.

PTBD-EF Percutaneous transhepatic biliary drainage - enteric feeding.

PTBE Pyretic tick-borne encephalitis.

PTBI Post total body irradiation.

PTBNA Protected transbronchial needle aspirate.

PTBP; ptBP Paratertiary/ Peritertiary butylphenol.

PTBPD Posttraumatic borderline personality disorder.

PTBS Posttraumatic brain syndrome.

PTBSC-SP Patellar tendon bearing - supracondylar-suprapatellar (prosthesis).

PTC Papillary transitional carcinoma (urinary bladder see FCIS); Patient to call; Percutaneous transhepatic cholangiography; Pharmacy and therapeutic committee; Phase transfer catalyst; Phenothiocarbazine; Phenylthiocarbamide/moyl (= PT); Phosphatidylcholine (a phospholipid); Plasma thromboplastin component (= Christmas factor - see factor IX); Poisoning Treatment Center; Premature tricuspid closure; Prior to conception; Prothrombin complex; Pseudotumor cerebri.

PT-C Prothrombin time control.

PTCA Percutaneous transluminal coronary angioplasty; Peripheral thrombosis of the coronary artery.

PTCC Posttraumatic chest condition (see

PTCD).

PTCD Posttraumatic chest disease/ disorder (= PTCC).

PTCE Percutaneous transcatheter embolization (for massive bleeding in pelvic fractures).

$PtcCO_2$ Transcutaneous partial pressure of carbon dioxide.

PTCER Pulmonary transcapillary escape rate.

PTCL Peripheral T-cell lymphoma.

$PtcO_2$ Transcutaneous oxygen tension.

PTCR Percutaneous transluminal coronary recanalization/ revascularization.

PTD Percutaneous transhepatic drainage (see PTBD); Percutaneous transluminal dilatation; Period to discharge; Permanent total disability; Persistent tardive dyskinesia; Personality trait disorder; Post/Preterm delivery (see PTB; PTL; PTP); Posttraumatic disorder (see PTSS); Prior to delivery; Psychotropic drug(s) (Antidepressants, Antipsychotics and Anxiolytics); Pyramidal tract degeneration.

PTDC Posttraumatic degenerative change(s) (Orthopedics).

PTDI Posttraumatic diabetes insipidus.

PTDP Permanent transvenous demand pacemaker.

PTE Parathyroid extract; Partial/ Potential toxic effect(s); Positive treatment effect; Post/Pretransplant(ation) evaluation; Posttreatment exacerbation (of an illness); Posttraumatic epilepsy; Pretibial edema; Proximal tibial epiphysis; Psychotomimetic effect; Pulmonary thromboembolism.

PTED Pulmonary thromboembolic disease.

PteGlu Pteroylglutamic acid.

PTEI Picture Test of English Inflections.

PTEN Pentaerythritol tetranitrate; Primary thymic epithelial neoplasm.

PTEP Past/ Present/ Previous thromboembolic process.

pter end of short arm of chromosome.

PTF Patient treatment file; Peritubular fibroblast (kidney); Pittsburgh triangular frame (for ext. fixation of pelvic fracture); Plasma thromboplastin factor (X) (see factor X); Posttuberculous fibrosis; Primary treatment failure.

PTFA Prothrombin time fixing agent.

PTFE Polytetrafluoroethylene (Teflon).

PTFS Posttraumatic fibromyalgia syndrome.

PTG Parathyroid gland; Teniposide; Pharmaco-therapeutic group; Phosphatidylglycerol (associated with FLM - Fetal lung maturity); Placebo-treatment group (see PTS); Plasma triglyceride.

PTH Parathormone; Parathyroid; Parathyroid/ Parathyrotropic hormone (see Hormones - PTH); Percutaneous transhepatic (drainage) (see PTBD); Phenylthiohydantoin; Plasma thromboplastin (component); Posttransfusion hepatitis; Posttraumatic headache; Prior to hospitalization.

Pth Pathology (see Path).

PTHC Percutaneous transhepatic cholangiography.

PTHL Plasma total homocysteine level (see tHCY).

PTHLP Parathyroid-hormone-like protein.

PTHrP Parathyroid-hormone-related protein.

PTHS Parathyroid hormone secretion (rate).

PTI Pancreatic trypsin inhibitor; Parenterally transmitted infection; Persistent tolerant infection; Pictorial Test of Intelligence; Preterm infant (i.e. premature baby); Primary topical (i.e. skin) infection; Pulsatility transmission index.

PTJS Posttraumatic joint stiffness.

PTJV Percutaneous transtracheal jet ventilation.

PTL Peritoneal telencephalic leukoencephalomyopathy; Pharyngotracheal lumen; Plasma thyroxine level; Posttransplant lymphoma; Posterior tricuspid leaflet; Preterm labor; Pretreatment level; Sodium Pentothal.

PTLC Precipitation thin-layer chromatography.

PTLD Posttransplantation lymphoproliferative disorder; Prescribed tumor lethal dose.

PTLH Pseudotumoral lymphocytic hypophysitis.

PTLS Posttraumatic limb swelling; Preterm labor syndrome (Obstetrics).

PTM Perforated tympanic membrane (see PED); Posterior trabecular meshwork; Posttransfusion mononucleosis; Posttraumatic meningitis; Pressure time per minute; Proximal tibial metaphysis (Orthopedics);

Psychotropic medication; Pulse time modulation.

Ptm Pterygomaxillary (fissure).

PTMA Phenyltrimethylammonium.

PTMD Pharmacotoxic myocardial disease.

PTMDF Pupils, tension, media, disc, and fundus.

PTMF Post-term macrosomic fetus (Obstetrics).

PTMR Percutaneous transmyocardial reperfusion (see PCTMR).

PTN Pain transmission neuron; Posterior tibial nerve; Preterm newborn.

pTNM Primary Tumor, (regional) Nodes, and Metastasis (TNM) (staging of tumors as determined by correlation of clinical, pathological, and residual findings.

PTO Patent and Trademark Office; Perlsucht Tuberculin Original (Ger.) - Klemperer's tuberculin (= Spengler's t) (see Tuberculin); Please turn over.

PTOI Posttraumatic osseous infection.

PTP Pain transmission pathway; Pancreas transplant(ation) program; Pancreatic thread protein; Pediatric transplant patient; Peptide-transporter protein; Percutaneous transhepatic portography; Phototoxic potential; Placebo-treated patient/ population; Planned therapeutic program; Posterior tibial pulse; Post/Preterm parturition (see PTB; PTD; PTL); Postterm pregnancy; Posttetanic potential; Posttransplant patient/ period; Posttransfusion purpura; Posttraumatic pain/ problem(s); Previously-treated patient; Prothrombin-Proconvertin; Proximal tubular pressure.

PtP Person-to-person; Transpulmonary pressure.

PTPH Posttraumatic pelvic hemorrhage.

PTPI Posttraumatic pulmonary insufficiency.

PTPM Posttraumatic progressive myelopathy.

PTPN Peripheral (vein) total parenteral nutrition.

PTPP Posttransplantation plasmacytic proliferation (related to Kaposi's sarcoma-associated herpesvirus) (see KSARV; MIP).

PTPS Postthrombophlebitis syndrome.

PTR Patellar tendon reflex; Patient termination record; Patient to return; Peripheral total resistance; Perlsucht Tuberculin Rest (Ger.) - a tuberculin prepared from the bovine bacillus, Mycobacterium tuberculosis bovis, similar to Koch's new tuberculin; Phototoxic reaction; Plasma transfusion reaction; Prothrobin time ratio (see PT-R)/ response; Proximal tibial resection (Orthopedics); Psychotic trigger reaction.

PTr Porcine trypsin.

PT-R Prothrombin time ratio (= PTR).

P_{Tr} Inspiratory triggering pressure (respiratory therapy) (see PFT).

PTRA Percutaneous transluminal renal angioplasty.

PTRIA Polystyrene-tube radioimmunoassay.

Ptrx Pelvic traction (see PTx).

PTS Painful tonic seizure; Para-toluenesulfonic (acid); Past/ Post/ Previous thrombotic stroke; Past/ Previous tubal surgery; Patellar tendon suspension; Patients (see pt; Pts); Permanent threshold shift; Phosphoenolpyruvate-phosphotransferase system; Placebo-treated subject (see PTG); Pneumatic tube system; Postthrombotic syndrome; Posttraumatic syndrome (see PTSS); Potent topical steroid; Preclinical toxicity study; Premenstrual tension syndrome; Prior to surgery; Pseudothalidomide syndrome (see HHFH).

PTSD Posttraumatic shock disorder (see PTSS).

Pts; pts Patients (= PTS) (see pt).

PTSD Posttraumatic stress disorder.

PTSH Poststimulus time histogram (see PSTH).

PTSS Posttraumatic shock (= PTSD)/ syndrome (= PTD; PTS).

PTT Partial thromboplastin time (see ptt); Particle transport time; Patellar tendon transfer (Orthopedics); Patient's tolerance threshold; Platelet transfusion therapy; Positive tourniquet test (petechial hemorrhages/ bleeding below the tourniquet site, seen in hemorrhagic illnesses e.g. Dengue HF); Posterior tibial tendon/ transfer; Pulmonary transit time; Pulse transmission time.

PtT Peak-to-trough (drug fluctuation).

ptt partial thromboplastin time (test) (= PTT).

PTT-C Partial thromboplastin time control.

PTTI Posttraumatic tissue infection.
PTTS Pre-Trial Treatment Status.
PTU Pain treatment unit; Propylthiouracil (= PT).
PTV Paralysis, tracheostomy, and ventilation (treatment for tetanus) (see MRTV); Posterior tibial vein; Posttransplantation variable(s) (such as presence or absence of acute rejection, delayed graft function, immunosuppressant therapy, etc.); Pretreatment value.
PTVT Placental terminal villous tree (Obstetrics).
PTW Partial-thickness wound; Placebo-treated woman/ women; Pork tapeworm (= *Taenia* solium).
PTWTKG Patient's weight in kilograms.
PTX Parathyroidectomy (see PTx); Pelvic traction (see PTx); Pentoxifylline; Phototoxic (reaction); Picrotoxinin; Pneumothorax (see Pnx).
PTx Parathyroidectomy (= PTX); Pelvic traction (= Ptrx; PTX).
PTZ Pentylenetetrazole; Phenothiazine.
PU Palindromic/ Pepsin unit; Pass(ed)/ Pregnancy urine; Pelvic, ureteric; Peptic ulcer; Per urethra (L.) - by way of the urethra; Potential uncitedness; Pregnancy urine hormone (see Hormones - HCG); 6-Propyluracil; Prostatic urethra.
Pu Plutonium (Z = 94) (see Elements - Plutonium); Purine; Purple.
PUAT Phosphotungstate uric acid test (for serum uric acid).
PUB Perforation, ulcer(ation), or bleed(ing) - upper gastrointestinal.
pub pubic; public.
PUBS Percutaneous umbilical blood sampling; Purple urine bag syndrome.
PUC Painful/ Prolonged uterine contraction(s) (see RPC); Pediatric urgent care; Pediatric urine collector.
PUCL Percutaneous umbilical cord ligation (Obstetrics).
PUD Papulo-urticarial dermatitis; Peptic ulcer disease (= AGU; APD; APUD; DUD; GUD); Pudendal (see pud); Pulmonary disease (see PuD).
PuD Pulmonary disease (= PUD).
pud pudendal (= PUD).
PUE Persistent undesirable effect(s); Potential undesirable effect (of drugs); Pyrexia of uncertain/ undetermined/ unknown etiology (see PUO).
PUF Peak urinary flow; Poly-unsaturated fat (found especially in oily fish); Poor urinary/ne flow; Pure ultrafiltration.
PUFA Polyunsaturated fatty acid (cicosapentaenoic and docosahexanoic acids).
PUFR Peak urinary flow rate (mL/sec) (= PFR).
PUH Peptic ulcer hemorrhage; Pregnancy urine hormone (see Hormones - HCG).
PUI Platelet uptake index; Primary uterine inertia.
PUJ Pelvi-ureteric junction.
PUK Prourokinase (a new clot-dissolving, thrombolytic drug used in cerebral thrombosis).
PUL Percutaneous ultrasonic lithotripsy (see NLT); Plasma urate level.
PUL; Pul; pul Pulmonary (see Pulm).
pulleys A, C pulleys A (angular shaped), C (cruciform shaped) - i.e. slings for tendons of the hands and phalanges.
Pulm; pulm Gruel (L. pulmentum); Pulmonary (= PUL; Pul; pul).
pulv powder (L. pulvis) (= powd).
pulv gros a coarse powder (L. pulvis grossus).
pulv subtil a smooth powder (L. pulvis subtilis).
pulv tenu a very fine powder (L. pulvis tenuis).
PUM Peanut(-reactive) urinary mucin.
PUMC Peking Union Medical College.
PUMS Permanently unfit for military service.
PUN Plasma urea nitrogen.
PUO Pyrexia of uncertain/ uncertified/ unclassified/ unconfirmed/ undefined/ undetermined/ undisclosed/ undiscovered/ undivulged/ unfathomed/ uninterpreted/ unknown/ unrevealed/ unsubstantiated/ untraced/ unverified origin (= FUE; FUO; PUE).
PUP Percutaneous ultrasonic pyelolithotomy; Peri-umbilical pain.
PU-PC Polyunsaturated phosphatidylcholine.
PUPP Pruritic urticarial papules and plaques (of pregnancy) (see PUPPP).
PUPPP Pruritic urticarial papules and plaques

of pregnancy (= PUPP).

PUR Polyurethrane.

Pur Purple.

pur purulent.

purg purgative.

PUS Paraurethral suspension (Endoscopic suspension of the bladder neck = Stamey procedure).

PUT Preparation, Understanding, and Treatment (Physical training program); Provocative use test; Putamen.

PUU Puumala (virus).

PUVA Prednisone, Ultraviolet therapy, Vincristine and Adriamycin (Combined chemotherapy); Psoralens and Ultraviolet Application/ A-range (therapy) - in the treatment of depigmentation; Pulsed ultraviolet actinotherapy.

PUVD Pulsed ultrasonic velocity detector (blood).

PV Pancreatic/ Popliteal/ Portal/ Pulmonary vein; Papilloma/ Polyoma virus; Papovavirus; Paraventricular; Paravertebral; Parvovirus; Pemphigus vulgaris; Per vaginam (L.) - by the way of the vagina; Peripheral vascular/ vein/ vessel; Phonation/ Plasma/ Pressure volume (see P-V; PFT); Pinocytotic vesicle; Pityriasis versicolor; Plasma viscosity; Polio vaccine; Polycythemia vera (see PCV); Polyvinyl; Postvasectomy; Postvoiding; Pressure velocity; Process variable; Projectile vomiting; Pulmonary ventricle.

Pv Proteus vulgaris; Venous pressure.

P-V Pressure-volume (curve) (= PV) (see PFT).

P&V Peak and valley; Pyloroplasty and vagotomy (operation/ stomach).

PVA Paralyzed Veterans of America; Paravertebral abscess; Parovirus arthritis; Placental vascular anastomoses/osis; Polyvinyl acetal (a thermoplastic resin used chiefly in moulded products and adhesives); Polyvinyl acetate (a polymer of vinyl acetate used in adhesives and textile processes) (= PVAc); Polyvinyl alcohol (a polymer of vinyl alcohol, a thermoplastic resin used in moulded products, emulsifiers, etc.); Prinzmetal's variant angina.

PVAc Polyvinyl acetate (see PVA).

PVB Cis-platinum, vinblastine, and bleomycin; Paravertebral block; Premature ventricular beat (= PBV; VBP; VEB; VPB; VPC); Prolonged vaginal bleeding.

PVC Partial Vision Center; Pelvic/ Peripheral venous circulation; Peripheral vascular constriction; Permanent vegetative condition (see PVS); Persistent vaginal cornification; Pityriasis versicolor (= TVC); Polyvinyl catheter; Polyvinyl chloride (a polymer of vinyl chloride, used for pipes, floors, electrical installations, etc.); Postvoiding cystogram; Predicted vital capacity; Premature ventricular contraction; Primary visual cortex; Pulmonary venous confluence (= CPC)/ congestion.

PVCM Paradoxical vocal cord motion.

PV_{CO2} Partial pressure of carbon dioxide in mixed venous blood.

PVD Past/ Placental/ Present/ Previous vascular disease; Patient very disturbed; Peripheral/ placental vascular disease/ disorder; Peripheral vasodilatation/lation; Peripheral visual defect (= PFD); Plasma volume depletion; Postvagotomy diarrhea; Portal venous dilation; Posterior vitreous detachment (eye); Postural vertical dimension; Premature ventricular depolarization; Progressive valgus deformity (of the heel); Pulmonary vascular/ valvular disease (see OPVD).

PVdC Polyvinylidene chloride.

PVE Perivenous encephalomyelitis; Periventricular edema (of the brain, in hydrocephalus); Postvaccinal encephalitis/lomyelitis; Premature ventricular extrasystole; Prosthetic valve endocarditis.

P-VEP Pattern visual evoked potential.

PVF Paravenous extravasation; Pericentral venous fibrosis (in chronic liver disease) (= CPF; PCF); Peripheral ventilatory failure; Peripheral visual field; Portal venous flow; Posterior vaginal fornix; Primary ventricular failure/ fibrillation.

PVFS Postviral fatigue syndrome (= Akureyri disease; Atypical poliomyelitis; Benign myalgic encephalomyelitis; Chronic mononucleosis syndrome; Iceland disease; Neuromyasthenia; Royal Free disease - the Royal Free Hospital in London in 1955, probably caused by the human herpesvirus 6 - HAV6).

PVG Pulmonary valve gradient.

PVGM Periventricular gray matter.

PVH Periventricular hemorrhage; Primary vasoactive hormone; Pulmonary valve hypoplasia; Pulmonary vascular hypertension.

PVI Paravenous injection; Parovirus infection; Peripheral vascular insufficiency; Perivascular infiltration; Pulmonary valve insufficiency.

PV/IF Plasma volume/interstitial fluid volume ratio.

PVK Penicillin V Potassium (Kalium) (= PVP).

PVL Partial/ Permanent vision loss (see PLV); Perivalvular leakage; Periventricular leukomalacia; Permanent vision loss; Plasma viral level/ load; Progressive vision/ visual loss.

PVM Pneumonia virus of mice; Proteins, vitamins, and minerals; Pyloric vein of Mayo (= Prepyloric vein - a tributary of the right gastric vein).

PVMA-119 See PVM/MA.

PVMed Preventive medicine.

PVM/MA A water-soluble linear copolymer consisting of alternating methyl vinyl ether and maleic anhydride units. Used as a suspending agent (= PVMA-119).

PVN Paraventricular nucleus; Predictive value negative.

PVNO Polyvinylpyridine-N-oxide.

PVNPS Post-Vietnam psychiatric syndrome.

PVNS Pigmented villonodular synovitis.

PVO Peripheral vascular occlusion; Pulmonary venous obstruction.

PV_{O2}; PvO_2 Partial oxygen pressure in mixed venous blood (laboratory/ blood gas) (see PFT).

PVOD Pulmonary vascular obstructive disease; Pulmonary veno-occlusive disease.

PVOS Peripheral vascular obstructive/ occlusive syndrome.

PVP Penicillin V Potassium (see PVK); Percutaneous venous puncture (Whitaker test); Peripheral vein plasma; Peripheral/ Portal/ Pulmonary venous pressure; Platinum compd (cisplatin) and (etoposide-)VP; Povidone (= Polyvidone; Polyvinylpyrrolidone; Poly[vinylpyrrolidone]) (a polymerized form of vinylpyrrolidone; has been used as a plasma expander in the emergency treatment of shock due to trauma, hemorrhage, and burns; also as a vehicle for drugs such as iodine, insulin, cortisone, penicillin and procaine to delay their absorption and thus prolong their action).

P-VP-B Platinum compd (cisplatin), VP (etoposide), and bleomycin.

PVPD Percutaneous vaporization of (intervertebral) protruded disc (Orthopedics) (see PNPN).

PVP-I Povidone iodine (= Polyvinylpyrrolidone-iodine-complex) (see PVP).

PVR Peripheral vascular resistance (mmHg/l/min/kg); Postvoiding residual; Proliferative vitreoretinopathy; Prosthetic valve replacement; Pulmonary vascular resistance = 80 (PAP-PCWP)/CO = 80 (Pulmonary arterial pressure - pulmonary capillary wedge pressure)/cardiac output ($dynes/s/cm^{-5}$); Pulse volume recorder/ding; Renin (activity) in peripheral vein(s).

PVRI Pulmonary vascular resistance index.

PVRV Postvoid residual volume (urine); Purified verocell rabies vaccine.

PVS Percussion, vibration, and suction; Peripheral vascular system; Permanent Vegetative State; Peroneovenous shunt; Persistent vegetative state (= PVC); Persistent viral/ Plummer-Vinson/ Postviral syndrome; Pigmented villonodular synovitis (Orthopedics); Poliovirus susceptibility; Polyvinyl sponge; Portal venous shunting (see PSVS); Premature ventricular systole; Programmed ventricular stimulation; Pulmonary valve/ valvular/ vein/ venous stenosis.

PVSG Polycythemia Vera Study Group.

PVT Paroxysmal ventricular tachycardia; Peripheral vascular tone; Portal vein thrombosis; Pressure, volume, and temperature (gas); Private (patient) (see pvt); Pulmonary ventilation test (see PFT).

pvt private (patient) (= PVT).

PVV Polyvalent vaccine; Primary varicose veins.

PVW Posterior vaginal wall.
PVY Potato virus Y.
pvz pulverization/ze(d).
PW Pacing waves; Patient walking; Peristaltic/ Pressure/ Pulsed wave; Physician's World (journal); Plantar wart; Posterior wall (of the heart); Prisoner of war (see POW); Psychological warfare; Pulmonary wedge (pressure); Puncture wound.
Pw Progesterone withdrawel.
P&W Pressures and waves.
PWA Person(s) with AIDS.
PWB Partial weight-bearing; Psychological well-being.
PWBC Peripheral white blood cell.
PWBRT Prophylactic whole brain radiation therapy.
PWC Peak/ Physical work(ing) capacity.
PWCA Pure white cell aplasia.
PWC max Maximum physical work(ing) capacity.
PWCR Prader-Willi chromosome region.
PWD Psychogenic water drinker; Public Welfare Department; Pure water depletion (see PWL).
Pwd; pwd Powder (= Pwdr).
Pwdr Powder (see Pwd).
PWDS Postweaning diarrhea syndrome.
PWE Pinwheel exam(ination); Posterior wall excursion.
PWH Pinwheel hypesthesia (hypoesthesia) (see PWE).
PWI Pediatric walk-in (clinic); Posterior wall infarct.
PWL Pure water loss (= PWD).
PWLV Posterior wall of left ventricle.
PWM Pokeweed/ Pokewood mitogen.
PWP Pulmonary wedge pressure (see PCWP).
PWR Pressurized-water reactor.
PWS Palmar wrist support; Physical withdrawal syndrome (from narcotics, etc.); Popliteal web syndrome (brittle and sparse hair, hypodontia with enamel defects and toe nail dysplasia) (see PPS - Popliteal PS); Port wine stain; Prader-Willi syndrome.
pwt pennyweight.
PWV Polistes wasp venom; Posterior wall velocity; Pulse wave velocity.
PX Pancreatectomized; Past history (see PH); Peroxidase (= POD; Px); Physical examination (see Px).
Px Past history (see PH); Peroxidase (see PX); Physical examination (= PX); Pneumothorax (see Pnx); Prognosis.
PXE Pseudoxanthoma elasticum.
PXG Porcine xenograft (aortic valve replacement).
PXI Puboxyphoid incision (see inc.).
PXM Protection x-ray microscopy; Pseudoexfoliation material.
PXS Pseudoexfoliation syndrome.
PY Pack/ Peak years.
Py Phosphopyridoxal; Polyoma (virus); Pyridine (see Pyr); Pyridoxal (see Pyr).
PYA Psychoanalysis.
PYC Protease-yeast, castione (culture medium).
PyC Pyogenic culture.
PYE Peptone yeast extract.
PYG Peptone yeast (extract) - glucose (agar broth).
PYGM Peptone-yeast-glucose-maltose (broth).
PYLL Potential years of life lost.
PYM Psychosomatic; Psychosomatic medicine.
PYP Pyrophosphate.
PYP-TC^{99m}; ^{99m}TC-PYP Stannous pyrophosphate labeled with radioactive technetium.
Pyr Pyridine (= Py); Pyridoxal (= Py); Pyruvate.
PyrP Pyridoxal phosphate.
PZ Pancreozymin (= Pz); Peripheral/ Pregnancy/ Proliferative zone.
Pz Pancreozymin (see PZ); Parietal midline electrode placement in electroencephalography; 4-Phenylazobenzylcarbonyl.
pz pièze.
PZA Pyrazinamide (an antitubercular drug).
PzB Parenzymes buccal.
PZ-CKK Pancreozymin - cholecystokinin (see CKK-PZ).
PZD Partial zona drilling - a drilling procedure into the zona pellcida, the egg or ovum's outer membrane, in order to enhance entry of sperm, and attachment of the embryo to the

womb.

PZE Piezoelectric.

PZI Protamine zinc insulin (see Insulin - PZI).

PZP Polyzygotic pregnancy; Pregnancy zone protein; Prozone phenomenon (caused by antibodies binding to antigen but not agglutinating it, thus producing false-negative results).

PZQ Praziquantel.

PZT Lead zirconate titanate (L. plumbum = lead); Piezoelectric ceramic.

Q

Q Cardiac output; Coulomb (unit of electrical energy); Electric charge/ quantity (see q); Fever (Queensland/ Query fever) (see Q fever); 1-4-Glucan branching enzyme; Glutamine; Heat; Perfusion; Qualitative; Quantity; Quart; Quartile; Queensland/ Query fever (see Q fever); Question; Quinacrine; Quinidine; Quinone; Quotient; Radiant/ Reaction energy; Reactive power; Temperative coefficient (see Q10); Volume of blood flow (cardiac output); Wave (Q) on the electrocardiogram (see QRS).

q each/ every (L. quaque); electric charge/ quantity (= A); long arm of chromosome; quart (see quart); quintal.

$\dot{Q}$ Alveolar perfusion; Rate of blood flow.

Q10 Temperature coefficient (increase in rate of any process caused by raising the temperature 10 degrees); Coenzyme Q10 (a powerful antioxidant used in the treatment of cardio/ cerebrovascular and neoplastic disease).

QA Quality assurance.

QAC Quaternary ammonium compound.

QAF Quality adjustment factor.

QAIP Quality assessment and Improvement Program (Health Program, US).

QALE Quality-adjusted life expectancy.

QALY Quality-adjusted life years.

QAM Quality assurance monitor(ing).

qam every morning (L. quaque ante meridiem).

QAP Quality Assurance Program (American Hospital Association); Quinine, atabrine/ atebrin, and pamaquin/ plasmoquine.

QAR Quantitative autoradiography.

QARANC Queen Alexandra's Royal Army Nursing Corps (UK).

QARNNC Queen Alexandra's Royal Naval Nursing Service (UK).

QAS Quality assurance standard.

Q&As Questions and Answers (GMC, UK).

QAT Quality assurance testing.

QAUR Quality assurance and utilization review.

QB Queen's Bench (UK); Whole blood.

Q_B Blood flow (milliliters per minute); Total body clearance.

QBCA Quantitative buffy coat analysis.

QBD Quantitative bone density (Orthopedics).

QBS Quaduple bypass surgery (see CABG).

QBV Whole blood volume.

QC Quality control; Queen's Counsel (UK); Quick catheter; Quinine chloroquine/ colchicine.

Qc Pulmonary capillary blood flow.

QCA Quantitative coronary angiography.

QCABG Quadruple coronary artery by-pass graft.

q-CARin Onset q-wave to the carotid incisura.

QCC Quality control criteria.

QCD Quinolone-class drug.

QCI Quantitative computer imaging.

QCIM Quarterly Cumulative Index Medicus.

Q_{CO2} Carbon dioxide evolution by a tissue (manometer) (microliters of carbon dioxide discharged per milligram of dry weight of tissue per hour).

QCR Quality control range (for susceptibility to microorganisms).

QCT Quantitative computed/ computerized tomography.

Q-CU Carotid upstroke.

QD Qi deficiency; Every day (see qd); Once daily (see qd).

qd every day (L. quaque die).

q2d every second day (L. quaque secunda die).

QDR Quantitative digital radiography.

qds four times a day (to be taken) (L. quater die sumendum).

QE Quantum of energy - the smallest quantity of energy associated with a given phenomenon. The quantum of electromagnetic radiation of a particular frequency equals the product of this frequency and Planck's constant, h (= 6.624×10^{-27} erg-second).

qe which is (L. quod est).

QED Quantum electrodynamics; Quite easily done; Which was to be proved/ demonstrated (L. quod erat demonstrandum).

QEE Quadriceps extension exercise.

QEEG Quantitative electroencephalogram/graphy.

QEF Quail embryo fibroblasts; Which was to be done (L. quod erat faciendum).

QENF Quantifying examination of neurological function.

QEONS Queen Elizabeth's Overseas Nursery Service (UK).

QEW Quick early warning.

QF Q fever (see Q fever); Quadriceps femoris (muscle); Quality factor; Queensland/ Query fever (see fever); Quick freeze; Relative biological effectiveness.

Qf see Q fever.

Q fever Queensland or Query fever - a febrile rickettsial infection, usually respiratory, caused by Coxiella burnettii (= Rickettsia diaporica), described in Australia but of world-wide distribution, including the Balkan "flu" in the Mediterranean region (= A; QF; Qf).

Q fract Quick fraction.

qh each/ every hour (L. quaque hora) (= qq hor).

q2h every second hour/ two hours (L. quaque secunda hora) (= qsh).

q3h every three hours (L. quaque tertia hora) (= qth).

q4h every four hours (L. quaque quarta hora) (= qqh).

Q-HA Interval between onset of QRS on the electrocardiogram and the aortic second heart sound.

QHCP Qualified health care professional.

QHDS Queen's Honorary Dental Surgeon (UK).

QHM Qualitative/ Quantitative histomorphometry (biopsy) (see HME).

QHNS Queen's Honorary Nursing Sister (UK) (= QNS).

QHP Queen's Honorary Physician (UK).

Q-HP Interval between onset of QRS on the electrocardiogram and the pulmonic second heart sound.

qhr every hour (L. quaque hora) (= qh).

QHS Qualitative/ Quantitative histologic study; Queen's Honorary Surgeon (UK).

qhs every hour of sleep (L. quaque hora somni).

Qi ("chee") Acupuncture energy point (TCM or Traditional Chinese medicine).

qid four times a day/ daily (L. quater in die).

QIDD Quintessense International Dental Digest.

QIDN Queen's Institute of District Nursing (UK).

QIG Quantitative immunoglobulins.

QIS Quality-improvement strategy.

QJ Quadriceps jerk.

ql as much as desired (L. quantum libet).

QLS Quality of Life Scale.

QLT Quadra Logic Technologies.

QM Quinacrine mustard.

qm every morning (L. quaque mane).

QMI Q-wave myocardial infarction.

QMP Qualified medical personnel.

QMRP Qualified mental retardation professional.

QMT Quantitative muscle test.

QMWS Quasi-morphine withdrawal syndrome.

qn every night (L. quaque nocte) (= qPM).

QNB Quinuclidinyl benzilate.

QNS Quantity not sufficient (see qns); Queen's Nursing Sister (UK) (see QHNS).

qns quantity not sufficient (on laboratory reports) (= QNS).

Qo Cubic millimeters of oxygen used per milligram of tissue per hour (see PFT - Qo).

QO_2 Oxygen consumption (see PFT - QO_2); Oxygen quotient/ utilization.

QoC Quality of Care.

qod every other day (L. quaque altera die).

qoh every other hour (L. quaque altera hora).

QoL Quality of Life.

qon every other night (L. quaque altera nocte).

QOS Quality of sleep.

Q-oTc Corrected Q-oT interval, on the electrocardiogram.

QP quanti-Pirquet (reaction) - expresses the activity or level of the tuberculous infection; Quantum pacemaker.

Qp Pulmonary blood flow.

qp as much as desired/ as much as you please/ at will (L. quantum placeat) (= qpl).

QPC Quality of patient care.

Qpc Pulmonary capillary blood flow.

QPEEG Quantitative pharmaco-electroencephalography.

QPL Quadrupedal locomotion (Orthopedics).

qpl as much as desired (see qp).
qPM every night (see qn).
qpq quid pro quo (L.) something for something i.e. option; substitute.
Qp/Qs Pulmonary (right)/Systemic (left) shunt ratio.
QPVT Quick Picture Vocabulary Test.
qq each/ every (L. quaque; quoque).
qqd every day (L. quoque die).
qqh every four hours (L. quaque quarta hora) (see q4h).
qq hor each/ every hour (L. quaque hora) (see qh).
qqv which see (see qv).
QR Quality review; Quantity is correct (see qr); Quellung reaction (response of pneumococci to immune serum); Quiet room; Quieting response; Quinaldine red.
qr quadriradial; quantity is correct (L. quantum rectum) (= QR); quarter (see qto).
QRB Quality Review Bulletin.
QRS Ventricular complex/ wave on the electrocardiogram, consisting of Q, R, and S waves; the interval/ loop traced by QRS vectors, representing ventricular depolarization.
QRS-ST The junction between the QRS complex and the ST segment in the electrocardiogram.
QRST; QRS-T The angle or M complex between the QRS and T vectors in vectorcardiography.
QRS STAT Sensing device for rapid determination of heart activity.
QRZ Wheal reaction time (Ger. Quaddel Reaktion Zeit).
QS Every shift; Quiet sleep.
Qs; $\dot{Q}$s Systemic blood flow.
qs as much as suffices/ as will suffice (L. quantum sufficit) (= q suff); a/ to a sufficient quantity/ enough (L. quantum satis) (= q sat).
Q-S1 First heart sound.
QS_2 Electromechanic systole.
qs ad (make) up to a sufficient quantity (L. quantum sufficit ad).
QSAR Quantitative structure-activity relationship.
q sat to a sufficient quantity (L. quantum satis) (see qs).
QSEs Quad-setting exercises (Rehabilitation therapy).
qsh every second hour/ two hours (L. quaque secunda hora) (see q2h).
QS_2I Shortened electrochemical systole.
QSP Physiological shunt fraction.
QSPV Quasistatic pressure volume.
Qs/Qp Systemic (left)/Pulmonary (right) shunt ratio.
Qs/Qt; $\dot{Q}$s/$\dot{Q}$t Intrapulmonary shunt fraction, shunt blood flow, or venous admixture ratio (see PFT).
QSS Quantitative sacroiliac scintigraphy.
QST Quantitative sensory test.
q suff as much as suffices (L. quantum sufficit) (see qs).
QS_z Time of systole (electromagnetic).
QT Cardiac output (see $\dot{Q}$t); Quick test; Quiet/ In secret/ "On the QT" (slang); Quinine tetracycline; Quinton tube (used for small bowel biopsy).
$\dot{Q}$t Total cardiac output (= QT).
qt quantity; quart (see quart); quiet.
Q-T The interval between/ time from the beginning of the QRS complex and/ to the end of the T wave (on the electrocardiogram).
QTC Quantitative tip cultures.
QTc Q-T interval corrected for heart rate.
Q-Tc Corrected Q-T (interval).
qter end of long arm of chromosome.
qth every three hours (L. quaque tertia hora) (see q3h).
QTI QT interval (see Q-T).
qto a fourth/ a quarter (L. quarto) (= qr).
QU Quiet.
qu quart (see quart); quarterly; query; question.
quad quadrant; quadriceps; quadriplegic.
quadrupl four times as much (L. quadruplicato).
qual qualitative; quality.
QUALY Quality adjusted life year (medication).
quan quantitative; quantity.
quar quarantine.
QUART Quadrantectomy, axillary (dissection), and radiotherapy.
quart the fourth part of a gallon (= 946 cc or ml; q; qt; qu) (L. quartus = fourth).
Quat; quat Four (L. quattuor).

Queer Homosexual (see Homo).
QUEST Quality, Utilization, Effectiveness, and Statistically Tabulated.
QUI Queen's University of Ireland.
QUICHA Quantitative inhalation challenge apparatus.
Quinolones An expanding class of antibiotics, acting by selectively inhibiting bacterial DNA gyrase enzymes crucial to DNA replication. They include nalidixic acid, oxolinic acid, acrosoxacin, etc. (see Fluoroquinolones).
quinq five (L. quinque).
quint fifth or quintan (L. quintus).
quot quotient.
quotid daily or quotidian (L. quotidie).
quot op sit as often as necessary (L. quoties opus sit).
qv as much as you desire/ see fit/ will (L. quam volvens)/ wish (L. quantum vis); which see (L. quae vide; quod vide) (= qqv).
qwk every week/ once a week (L. quaque = every).
QYD Qi and Yin deficiency.
QZ 2 Methaqualone hydrochloride (= TR 495; WB = Wall-banger) - a hypnotic, acting within 30 minutes; its hypnotic effect lasts 6-10 hours. It has no analgesic action.

R

R A conjugative plasmid responsible for resistance to various elements; Any chemical (alfyl/ alkyl) group of an alkane (paraffin hydrocarbon); Arginine; Behnken's unit - a unit of roentgen-ray dosage or exposure which, when applied in 1 cc of air at 18 °C and 760 mm Hg of pressure, produces electric conductivity equal to one electrostatic unit, as measured by the saturation current; Broadbent registration point; Electrical resistance; Exchange ratio; Far point (L. remotum); Gas constant (8.315 joules); In electrocardiography, the first positive deflection during the QRS complex (wave); Organic radical (in chemical formulas); Race; Racemic; Radioactive; Radiologist/gy; Radius; Ramus; Rankine (temperature scale) - an absolute scale on which each unit corresponds with that of the Fahrenheit scale, and the ice point is at 459.67 °R; Rate; Ratio; Reaction; Reading; Reaumur (temperature scale) - the ice point is at 0 and the normal boiling point of water at 80 °R; Receptor; Recessive (gene) - a gene producing an effect in the organism only when it is transmitted by both parents; Rectal/tum; Rectified; Red (an indicator color); Registered trademark; Regression coefficient (Galton's law of regression) - the coefficient or ratio of certain factors, plus or minus, present in parents and their offspring, whereby the offspring inherit these parental peculiarities in a less marked or regressive degree than are manifested in the parents themselves; Regular; Regular insulin; Regulator (gene); Reiz (Ger.) - stimulus; Rejection factor; Relapse; Relaxation; Release (factor); Remission; Remote; Remotum (L.) - far/ far point; Repressor (a compound that represses the formation of a specific enzyme); Repressor (gene) - a gene that controls the formation of a repressor, which in turn controls the function of a structural gene (a gene that governs the formation of an enzyme); Resazurin; Residue; Resistance (e. g. bacterial, pulmonary vascular, etc.); Resistant (bacteriology); Respiration; Respiratory coefficient/ exchange rate or ratio/ quotient - the ratio between the volume of carbon dioxide expired and the volume of oxygen inspired in a given time; Responder; Response; Rest (in cell cycle); Restricted; Reticulocyte; Reverse (banding/ Giemsa method); Review; Rhythm; Rib; Ribose (= Rib); Rickettsia; Right (= Rt; rt); Right eye; Rinne (test); Roentgen (= Rontgen) - the international unit of X- or ã (gamma) radiation, i.e. it is the quantity of exposure or administered radiation, such that the associated corpuscular emission per 0.001293 g of air produces ions carrying 1 electrostatic unit of electrical charge of either sign; Roentgenologist/logy; Rough (colony) - irregular and opaque variant type of bacterial colony (on bacterial cultures); Rub; Symbol (used in formulas of aminoacids, denoting characteristic side chain); Take (L. recipe); Wave (in the electrocardiogram).

r former symbol for roentgen, now officially replaced by the capital letter R (see R); radius (see R); ratio (see R); recombinant; regional; ribose (see R); ribosomal; ring chromosome; roentgen; sample correlation coefficient.

R' In electrocardiography, the second positive deflection during the QRS complex.

® Registration/ Trade Mark (see R); Right (see R).

(R) Rectal (on temperature records) (= R).

R_x Take/ Take treatment (see Rx; Rx).

°R Degree on the Rankine/ R,aumur scale (see R - Rankine; Réaumur).

+R Rinne's test positive (test for hearing).

-R Rinne's test negative (test for hearing).

ρ; p; P; rho the 17th letter of the Greek alphabet; correlation coefficient; electric charge density; electrical resistivity; mass density; reactivity.

r1/2 half life.

R1; R2; R3 etc. Years of resident study.

r^2 coefficient of determination.

R 79 Isopropamide iodide (= SKF 4740) - a peripherally acting anticholinergic drug, used in the treatment of peptic ulcer and other functional disorders of the gastrointestinal tract.

R 100 Ambutonium bromide (see BL 700 B).
R 381 Phenbutrazate hydrochloride - an anorecting agent, used with phenmetrazine theoclate in the treatment of obesity.
R 382 Phenmetrazine theoclat - a potent anorecting agent used in the treatment of obesity.
R 516 Cinnarizine (see 516 MD).
R 875 Dextromoramide (see MCP 875).
R 1132 Diphenoxylate hydrochloride - used in the treatment of acute and chronic diarrhea.
R 1303 Carbophenothion (= Trithion) - an organophosphorus insecticide.
R 1406 Phenoperidine hydrochloride - a narcotic analgesic with similar actions to morphine, particularly useful for children, the elderly, and the severely ill.
R 1575 Cinnarizine (see 516 MD).
R 1625 Haloperidol (= Haloperidole) - a tranquillizer chemically related to gamma-aminobutyric acid, a naturally occurring brain aminoacid. By competing with this acid it may influence brain metabolism and thereby affect motor activity.
R 3345 Dipiperon (see McN-JR 3345).
R 4263 Fentamyl citrate (= Fentanyl citrate) - a potent narcotic analgesic with actions similar to those of morphine. Given with droperidol (a neuroleptic drug) to produce anesthesia (see R 4749).
R 4749 Droperidol (= Dehydrobenzperidol) - a tranquillizer pharmacologically similar to chlorpromazine. Used with analgesics to produce a state of calm in laboratory and radiodiagnostic procedures.
R 8299 Tetramisole hydrochloride (see ICI 50,627).
R 13423 Dicloxacillin sodium (see BRL 1702).
R 33812 Domperidone (= "Motilium" - Janssen Pharmaceutica) - a peripheral dopamine antagonist, used as a gastrokinetic and anti-emetic in the treatment of digestive disorders, such as nausea, vomiting and hiccups, gastric pain and heart-burn, etc.
RA Radioactive; Radionuclide angiography; Ragocyte; Ragweed antigen; Rales; Rapidly adapting (receptors); Reciprocal asymmetrical; Refractory anemia/ ascites; Relative allocation; Renal anemia/ artery; Renin-angiotensin; Repeat action; Research Associate (VA); Residual/ Room air; Respiratory acidemia/dosis / alkalemia/kalosis; Retinoic acid; Retrospective analysis (= RSA); Rheumatoid agglutinins (laboratory/ serology); Rheumatoid arthritis; Right angle/gulation (orthopedics); Right arm/ atrial/ atrium/ auricle.
Ra Airflow/ Airway resistance (see RA); Radial/ius; Radiation (see Rad); Radium (Z = 88) (= Rad) (see Elements - Radium).
rA riboadenylate.
R_A Afferent vascular resistance (kidneys); Airflow/ Airway resistance (pulmonary function test) (= Ra).
Ra 5 Ragweed pollen antigen.
RA 8 Dipyridamole (= Persantin) - a synthetic coronary vasodilator used in the treatment of myocardial ischemia (see PARIS).
RA 27/3 Rubella virus strain, effective by intranasal route.
RAA Renin-angiotensin-aldosterone (system); Rotational ablation angioplasty.
RAAMC Royal Australian Army Medical Corps.
RAAS Renin-angiotensin-aldosterone system.
RAB Remote afterloading brachytherapy; Renin-aldosterone bond (angiotensin II - mediated) (see RAAS).
RABA Rabbit antibladder antibody (test).
Rab Rabbit; Rabies.
RABBI Rapid Access Blood Bank Inputer.
RABD Respiratory acid-base dosorder/ disturbance.
RABG Room air blood gas.
$RaBr_2$ Radium bromide.
Rab/Ser Rabies antiserum - used for the prevention of rabies in cases of bites on the head and neck, and other areas of special danger. It is given in conjunction with Rabies Vaccine (Rab/Vac).
Rab/Vac Rabies vaccine (= Antirabic vaccine) - used for the prevention of rabies. Rabies antiserum (Rab/Ser) may be given before commencing treatment with Rabies vaccine.
RAC Recombinant DNA Advisory Committee (NIH); Regenerated articular cartilage; Rest activity cycle (video documentation in preg-

nancy, including twin activities) (Obstetrics); Right atrial catheter/ chamber; Royal Agricultural College.

rac racemate; racemic.

RACB Robotic-assisted coronary bypass.

RACCO Right anterior caudocranial oblique.

RACGP Royal Australian College of General Practitioners.

RACP Royal Australasian College of Physicians.

RACS Recurrent acute chest syndrome.

RACT Recalcified (whole blood) activated clotting time.

RAD Radial artery catheter; Radiation absorbed dose (see rad); Radical (see rad); Reactive airways disease (in bronchial asthma); Recommended adult dose; Reversible airways disease; Right atrium diameter; Right axis deviation (on the electrocardiogram); Roentgen administered dose.

RAD; Rad; rad Radiation-absorbed dose (= 100 ergs/g; 0.01 Gy).

Rad Ionizing radiation unit; Radiation (= Ra); Radiology; Radiotherapy (see RADIO); Radium (see Ra).

rad radial; radian; radiation absorbed dose (= RAD) - a unit of measurement of the absorbed dose of ionizing radiation equal to 100 ergs per gram of any absorbing material (including tissues). The roentgen (R) and the rad in soft tissue are approximately equivalent in magnitude; radical (= RAD); radius; root (L. radix).

RADA Right acromiodorsoanterior (position of fetus); Rosin amine-D-acetate.

RADAR Radio detection and ranging - discovered by Sir Robert Wattson-Watt, the Scottish physicist (1892-1973) in 1935.

RADC Royal Army Dental Corps.

RADIO Radiotherapy (= Rad).

Radiol; radiol Radiologist/gy.

Radionuclide(s) Radioactive materials released through ionizing atomic radiation: Barium - 140, Half-life 12.8 days, Activity, PBq 4,800; Cerium - 141, Half-life 33 days, Activity, PBq 5,600; Cerium - 144, Half-life 285 days, Activity, PBq 3,300; Cesium - 134, Half-life 2 years, Activity, PBq 180; Cesium - 137, Half-life 30 years, Activity, PBq 280; Curium - 242, Half-life 163 days, Activity, PBq 26; Iodine - 131, Half-life 8 days, Activity, PBq 3,200; Molybdenum - 99, Half-life 67 hours, Activity, PBq 4,800; Neptunium - 239, Half-life 2.4 days, Activity, PBq 27,000; Plutonium - 238, Half-life 86 years, Activity, PBq 1; Plutonium - 239, Half-life 24,400 years, Activity, PBq 0.85; Plutonium - 240, Half-life 6,580 years, Activity, PBq 1.2; Plutonium - 241, Half-life 13.2 years, Activity, PBq 170; Rubidium - 103, Half-life 39.6 days, Activity, PBq 4,800; Rubidium - 106, Half-life 1 year, Activity, PBq 2,100; Strontium - 89, Half-life 52 days, Activity, PBq 2,300; Strontium - 90, Half-life 28 years, Activity, PBq 200; Tellurium - 132, Half-life 78 hours, Activity, PBq 2,700; Xenon - 133, Half-life 5.3 days, Activity, PBq 6,500; Zirconium - 95, Half-life 1.4 hours, Activity, PBq 5,600.

RadLV Radiation leukemia virus.

RADP Right acromiodorsoposterior (position of fetus).

RADR Royal Association for Disability and Rehabilitation (UK).

RADS Reactive airways dysfunction syndrome; Retrospective assessment of drug safety.

rad/s rad/ radian per second.

rad ther radiation therapy.

RADTS Rabbit antidog thymus serum.

RAE Rare/ Relevant adverse event(s); Regular active/ aerobic exercise(s); Right atrial enlargement.

RAEB Refractory anemia, erythroblastic/ with excess blasts.

RAEBiT; RAEB-T Refractory anemia with excess blasts in transformation.

RAEM Refractory anemia with excess myeloblasts.

RAF Repetitive atrial firing; Rheumatoid arthritis factor (see RA factor); Right-angle forceps.

RA factor Rheumatoid arthritis factor (laboratory/ serology) (= RAF).

RAFMS Royal Air Force Medical Services.

RAG Ragweed; Room air gas.

RAG 1, 2 Recombinase-activating gene 1, 2.

Ragg Rheumatoid agglutinin.

RAH Regressing atypical histiocytosis; Right atrial hypertrophy.
RAHD Recommended adult human dose.
RAHM Resume-at-home medication.
RAHO Rabbit antibody to human ovary; Robotically-assisted heart operation (see CARS).
RAHTG Rabbit antihuman thymocyte globulin.
RAI Radioactive iodine (nuclear medicine); Rapid-acting insulin (see Insulin); Receptive anal intercourse; Residual adrenal impairment; Resting ankle index; Right atrial involvement/ isomerism (Asplenia).
RAIA Rapid-acting insulin analogue (see FAHIA).
RAID Radioimmunodetection.
RAim Radioimmunoassay.
RAIS Reflection-absorption infrared spectroscopy.
RAIU Radioactive iodine uptake (test).
RAL Refractory acute leukemia.
RALPH Renal-anal-lung-polydactyly-hamartoblastoma (syndrome).
RALT Routine admission laboratory tests.
RAM Radioactive material; Random-access memory; Rapid alternating movements; Rectus abdominis muscle/ myocutaneous (flap); Redox-active metal(s) (used in the treatment of neurological disorders); Research aviation medicine; Right anterior measurement; Risk-associated mutation (of genes, leading to cancer).
RAMC Royal Army Medical Corps (British).
RAMP Radioactive antigen microprecipitin; Right atrial mean pressure.
RAMS Random access memories.
RAMT Rabbit antimouse thymocyte.
RAN Resident's admission notes.
$R_{1,2,3,...}$AN First, second, third,.. year resident's admission notes.
RANA Rheumatoid arthritis nuclear antigen.
RANN Research Aimed at National Needs.
rANP Rat atrial natriuretic peptide.
RAO Renal/ Retinal artery obstruction/ occlusion; Reversible airways obstruction; Right anterior oblique (projection/ radiology).
RaONC Radiation oncology.
RAOR Robot-assisted operating room (see CARS).
RAP Recurrent abdominal pain; Regression-associated protein; Renal allograft patient; Renal arterial/ artery pressure; Residency Assistance Program; Rheumatoid arthritis precipitin (RA precipitin); Right atrial pressure; Risk-assessment program.
RAPD Random amplified polymorphic DNA; Relative afferent pupillary defect.
RAPD-PCR Random amplified polymorphic DNA - polymerase chain reaction.
RAPE Right atrial pressure elevation.
RAPID Register for the Ascertainment and Prevention of Inherited Diseases.
RAPK Reticulate acropigmentation of Kitamura.
RAPM Refractory anemia with partial myeloblastosis.
RAPO Rabbit antibody to pig ovary.
RAPORT Computer Assisted Radiographic Reporting System Utilizing Mark-Sense Format.
RAQ Right anterior quadrant.
RAR Rat insulin receptor; Renal allograft recipient/ rejection; Right arm reclining/ recumbent.
RARE Rehabilitation of Addicts by Relatives and Employers.
RARLS Rabbit anti-rat lymphocyte serum.
RARS Refractory anemia with ring(ed) sideroblasts (= RA-S).
RARTS Rabbit anti-rat thymocyte serum.
RAS Rapid atrial stimulation; Recurrent aphthous stomatitis; Reflex activating stimulus; Renal artery stenosis; Renin activity serum (see RA Serum); Renin-angiotensin system; Reticular activating/ activation system; Retinal artery stenosis; Rheumatoid arthritis serum; Robot(ically)-assisted surgery (see CARS).
RAS; ras Rat sarcoma (gene/ oncogene/ protein) (assoc. with cancer).
ras retrovirus-associated DNA sequence; filings or scrapings (L. rasurae).
RA-S Refractory anemia with (ring/ ringed) sideroblasts (see RARS).
RA Serum Renin activity serum (= RAS).
RASI Renin-angiotensin system inhibitor (e.g. losartan).

RASS Rheumatoid arthritis and Sjögren syndrome.
RASSF1A A new candidate TSG - Tumor suppressor gene (found on the human chromosome 3) (see TSG).
RAST Radioallergosorbent technique/ test (for the measurement of IgE in the serum).
RAT Radioactive tracer; Recurrent arterial thrombis; Repeat action tablet; Resting arterial tone; Rheumatoid arthritis test; Right anterior thigh (injection site).
RATA Radioimmunological assay antithyroid antibody.
RATG; R-ATG Rabbit-antithymocyte globulin.
RATHAS Rat thymus antiserum.
RATN Repeated avulsion of the toenail.
rAT-P Recombinant antitrypsin Pittsburgh.
RATx Radiation therapy/ Radiotherapy (= RT).
RAU Radioactive uptake.
RAV Radioautographic visualization; Rous-/ Roux-associated virus.
RAVC Retrograde atrioventricular conduction; Royal Army Veterinary Corps.
RAVLT Rey Auditory Verbal Learning Test.
RAW; R(AW); R_{aw} Airway resistance (Resistance of the airways to gas flow) (see PFT - RAW).
RAYNET Radio Amateurs Emergency Network.
RAZ Razoxane.
RB Radiation burn; Rating board; Rebreathing; Receptor-binding; Rectal biopsy; Reticulate body; Retinoblastoma (see Rb); Retrobulbar; Right bundle; Right buttock (injection site); Round bodies (intracellular); Rubriblast (immature erythrocyte with a relatively large nucleus).
Rb Rabbit; Retinoblastoma (= RB); Rubidium (Z = 37) (see Elements - Rubidium).
R&B Right and below.
Rb 86 Rubidium chloride.
R (bacterial colony) Rough (bacterial colony) (see R. Rough).
RBA Radioligand binding assay (see RLBA); Relative binding affinity; Rescue breathing apparatus; Right basilar/ brachial artery; Rose bengal antigen; Ruptured brain aneurysm.
RBAF Rheumatoid biologically active factor.
RBAP Repetitive bursts of action potential; Risk-based audit programme (GMC, UK).
RBAS Rostral basilar artery syndrome.
RBB Repeated breakthrough bleeding; Right breast biopsy; Right bundle branch; Risk-benefit balance.
RBBB Right bundle-branch block.
RBBsB Right bundle-branch system block.
RBBx Right breast biopsy.
RBC Rapid brain cooling (in cardiac resuscitation); Recurrent Bartholin cyst; Recurrent breast cancer; Red blood cell/ cell count/ corpuscle/ count (= rbc); Regular biological control (see SRBCC).
rbc red blood cell (see RBC).
^{84}RbCBF Radioactive rubidium measured coronary blood flow.
RBCD Right border cardiac dullness.
RBCH Rainbow Babies and Childrens Hospital.
RBCM Red blood cell mass.
RBC:P Red blood cell/ plasma ratio.
RBC s/f Red blood cells spin filtration.
RBCV Red blood cell volume (laboratory/ hematology).
RBD Recurrent brief depression; Relative biological dose; Renal and bladder disease/ disorder/ dysfunction; Renal bone disease; Right border of dullness (of heart to percussion).
RBE Receptor blocker effect; Reduced bilirubin excretion (jaundice-associated); Relative biological effectiveness (the inverse ratio of the absorbed doses of two different ionizing radiations required to produce a given biological effect).
RBF Regional/ Renal/ Retinal blood flow; Regional bone mass; Research-based facility; Resting blood flow (ml/min).
RBG Random blood glucose.
RBI Respiratory bacterial infection; Retrobulbar inflammation.
Rb Imp Rubber base impression (dentistry).
RBK Robert Brigham Knee (Orthopedics Implants).
RBL Rat basophilic leukemia; Reid's baseline.
RBM Repetitive body movement(s) (such as rocking, head banging, self-stimulation, and complex twirling movements of the hands

and arms) - seen in psychiatric illness patterns.

RBMMA Rat Bone Marrow Metaphase Analysis.

RBN Retrobulbar neuritis; Reverse barrier nursing.

RBNA Royal British Nurses Association.

RBO Relative betting odds.

RBOW Rupture of the bag of waters (i.e. of the amniotic sac in labor).

RBP Receptor-binding profile; Retinol-/ Riboflavin-binding protein; Retrobulbar pain/ pressure.

RBR Radiation bowel reaction; Records-based research; Reduced blinking reflex; Risk- balance/ benefit ratio.

RBRF Reproductive Biology Research Foundation.

RBRVS Resource-based relative value scale.

RBS Radical breast surgery; Radionuclide bone scan(ning); Random blood sugar; Resistant bacterial strain; Reversible bronchospasm; Rich blood supply; Rutherford backscattering.

RbSA Rabbit serum albumin.

RBSPD Recurrent bacterial sinopulmonary disease (see AT).

RBT Repeated blood transfusions; Retrobulbar tissue/ tumor; Rifabutin (an antibody used with CLA [Clarithromycin], in the treatment of MAC [*Mycobacterium* avium Complex] disease).

RBV Rectilinear biphasic waveform (defibrillation) (see BWD); Right brachial vein.

RB-V Right bundle-ventricular (conduction time).

RBW Recommended/ Reduced/ Relative body weight.

RBZ Rubidazone.

RC An electronic circuit containing a resistor and capacitor in series; Radiocarpal; Reaction/ Respiratory center; Recrystallization; Red cell/ cell casts/ corpuscle/ Cross; Referred/ Respiratory care; Regenerated cellulose; Respiration ceases; Rest cure; Retention catheter; Retrograde cystogram; Rheumatic chorea; Rib cage; Roman Catholic; Root canal; Rotator cuff; Routine cholecystogram/graphy; Rubricyte (immature erythrocyte with a relatively small nucleus); Rutner catheter (has a basket on the end to remove ureteral calculi) (= RSB).

Rc Conditioned response; Receptor.

R/C Reclining/ Rocking chair.

R&C Resistance and capacitance.

RCA Radionuclide cerebral angiogram; Recurrent cardiac arrest; Red cell agglutination/ antibody (see AKA)/ aplasia (see PNM); Relative chemotactic activity; Renal cell anemia; Retrograde conduction to the atria; Right carotid/ coronary artery; Ruptured cerebral aneurysm.

RCAF Royal Canadian Air Force.

RCAMC Royal Canadian Army Medical Corps.

RCB Regular cyclic bleeding.

RCBF; rCBF Regional cerebral blood flow.

RCBV; rCBV Regional cerebral blood volume.

RCC Radio-Chemical Center; Radiological control center; Radiotherapy-combination/ned chemotherapy (see ARC); Rape crisis center; Ratio of costs to charges; Receptor-chemoeffector complex; Red cell cast/ count; Reduced cycle control (menstruation); Regular clinical control (see SRBCC); Renal cell carcinoma; Response-concentration curve (see CRC); Right common carotid (artery); Roman Catholic Church.

RCCA Right common carotid artery.

RCCM Regional Committee for Community Medicine.

RCCT Random(ized) controlled clinical trial (= RCT).

RCD Radiocarbon dating; Radiocarpal dislocation; Recommended clinical dose (see HCD; RHCD); Reduced-calorie diet; Relative cardiac dullness; Remote-control device; Ruptured cervical disc (Orthopedics).

RCDA Recurrent chronic dissecting aneurysm.

RCDP Rhizomelic chondrodysplasia punctata.

RCDR Relative corrected death rate.

RCDS Royal College of Dental Surgeons.

RCE Reasonable compensation equivalent; Routine cervical examination (Gynecology/ Obstetrics).

RCEC Retinal capillary endothelial cell.

RCF Red cell ferritin/ folate; Reiter complement fixation; Relative centrifugal field/ force; Relevant clinical finding(s); Ristocetin cofactor.
RCG Radioelectrocardiogram/graph(y).
RCGP Royal College of General Practitioners (UK).
RCH Rectocolic hemorrhage; Reversible clinical hepatoxicity; Royal Children's Hospital (Melbourne, Australia).
RCHF Right congestive heart failure.
RCHMS Regional Committee for Hospital Medical Services.
RCI Recurrent chest infection; Respiratory control index; Reversible cholinesterase inhibitor.
RCIA Red cell immune adherence.
RCIRF Radiologic contrast-induced renal failure.
RCIT Red cell iron turnover.
RCITR Red cell iron turnover rate.
RCJ Radiocarpal joint.
RCL Renal clearance; Repair of cleft lip; Retro-cochlear lesion; Rib-cage level (spine).
RCM Radiographic contrast media/ium; Red cell mass; Regular clinical monitor(ing); Reinforced clostridial medium; Replacement culture medium; Restrictive cardiomyopathy; Retinal capillary microaneurysm; Right costal margin; Royal College of Midwives.
RCMA Red cell membrane acetyl-cholinesterase.
RCMAC Red Cross Mid America Chapter.
RCME Royal Commission on Medical Education (Brit).
RCMI Red cell morphology index.
rCMRGlc Regional cerebral metabolic rate for glucose.
$rCMRO_2$ Regional cerebral metabolic rate for oxygen.
RCN Right caudate nucleus; Royal College of Nursing (Brit).
RCNA Radiologic Clinics of North America (journal).
RCO Aliphatic acyl radical.
RCoF Ristocetin cofactor.
RCOG Royal College of Obstetricians and Gynaecologists (Brit).
RCP Rate-controlling polymer; Recombinant capsid protein; Red cell protoporphyrin; Retrocorneal pigmentation; Riboflavin carrier protein; Rotator cuff pathology (see RCT); Routine clinical practice; Royal College of Pathologists (London, UK)/ Physicians (London, UK)/ Psychiatrists.
rCP Regional cerebral perfusion.
rcp reciprocal (translocation).
RCPA Royal College of Pathologists of Australia.
RCPath Royal College of Pathologists (Brit).
RCPCH Royal College of Paediatrics and Child Health (UK).
RCPE Royal College of Physicians, Edinburgh.
RCPH Red cell peroxide hemolysis.
RCPL Royal College of Physicians of London (UK) (see RCP).
RCPM Raven colored progressive matrices.
RC-Prep Root canal preparation.
RCP&S Royal College of Physicians and Surgeons (Scotland).
RCPSGlas Royal College of Physicians and Surgeons, Glasgow.
RCPT Registered Cardiopulmonary Technician.
RCR Recommended combination regimen; Relative consumption rate; Respiratory control ratio; Response-concentration relationship (see CRC); Rotator cuff repair (shoulder joint).
RCRA Resource Conservation and Recovery Act.
RCS Rabbit (aorta-)contracting substance; Randomized controlled study (= RCT); Red cell suspension; Repeat cesarean section; Replication-competent source (of infection); Reticulum cell sarcoma; Retrospective cohort study; Right coronary sinus; Royal College of Science/ Surgeons (England); Rural communal settlement (Israeli kibbutz).
RCSE Royal College of Surgeons, Edinburgh.
RCSI Royal College of Surgeons, Ireland.
RCT Random(ized) clinical/ controlled trial (see RCCT); Recapitulation theory (= BGL; Haeckel's law); Red cell transfusion; Registered Care Technologist; Retrograde conduction time; Root canal therapy (dentistry); Rorschach Content Test; Rotator cuff

tear (shoulder ligaments/ tendons).

rct a marker showing the ability of virulent strains to replicate at 40 °C, while vaccine strain shows no replication.

RCU Respiratory care unit.

RCV Red cell/ corpuscular volume.

RCVS Royal College of Veterinary Surgeons.

RD Radial deviation; Rapid dissolution; Rate difference; Raynaud's/ Reiter's/ Renal/ Respiratory/ Reye's/ Rheumatoid disease; Reaction of degeneration (= DeR; DR; EaR); Reactive depression (= ED or Exogenous d); Reflex decay; Refsum's disease (a heredodegenerative disorder characterized by progressive nerve deafness, cerebellar ataxia, peripheral neuropathy, and often pigmentary changes in the retina); Registered dietician/titian; Renal dysfunction (see RDF); Respiratory depression; Respiratory distress; Retinal detachment; Right deltoid (injection site); Riley-Day/ Rolland-Desbuquois (syndrome); Rubber dam; Ruminal drinking; Ruptured disk.

5α-RD 5-alpha-reductase deficiency (causing female-to-male sex change at puberty).

Rd Rate of disappearance; Reading.

rd rutherford (a unit of radioactivity) (see Rf).

R&D Research and development.

RD 1572 Homidium bromide (= 3,8-Diamino-5-ethyl-6-phenylphenanthridinium bromide) - a trypanocide used in veterinary medicine.

RD 3803 Diloxanide (see DHM).

RD 13962 Quinacillin sodium - a semi-synthetic penicillin, reported to be resistant to staphylococcal penicillinase.

RDA Recommended daily allowance (= MDAR; MDR); Recommended dietary allowance (= MDR); Registered Dental Assistant; Right dorsoanterior (position of fetus).

RdA Reading age.

RDAD Recommended daily adult dose.

RDB Random double-blind (trial); Recurrent diverticular bleeding (see CDH).

RDC Research diagnostic criteria.

RDCT Repeat-dose charcoal therapy (for drug poisoning).

RDD Reactive depressive disorder (see RDP); Recommended daily/ diagnostic dose.

RDDA Recommended daily dietary allowance.

RDDP Ribonucleic acid (RNA) - dependent/ directed deoxyribonucleic acid (DNA) polymerase.

RDE Receptor-destroying enzyme; Recurrent dislocation of the elbow; Repeated daily exposure.

RDES Remote data entry system.

RDF Renal dysfunction (= RD).

RDFC Recurring digital fibroma of childhood.

RDG Right dorsogluteal.

RDH Recurrent diverticular hemorrhage (colon); Registered Dental Hygienist.

RDHBF Regional distribution of hepatic blood flow.

RDI Recommended daily/ dietary intake; Respiratory disturbance index; Rupture-delivery interval.

RDIH Right direct inguinal hernia.

RDLBBB Rate-dependent left bundle-branch block.

RDLP Research-and-development limited partnership.

RDM Re-admission; Recommended dilution method; Registration Development Manager (GMC, UK); Renal dialysis machine; Rhabdomyolysis.

RDMA Royal Dutch Medical Association.

rDNA Recombinant deoxyribonucleic acid (see DNA); Ribosomal deoxyribonucleic acid.

RDOD Retinal detachment, right eye (L. oculus dexter).

RDOS Retinal detachment, left eye (L. oculus sinister).

RDP Rapid dissolution powder; Reactive depressive psychosis (= RDD); Right dorsoposterior (fetal position).

RDPE Reticular degeneration of the pigment epithelium.

RDQ Respiratory disease questionnaire.

RdQ Reading quotient.

RDR Recommended/ Reduced dosage/ dose/ dose range/ dosing regimen; Reduced death.

RDS Recurrent dislocation of the shoulder; Reduced drug susceptibility; Renal Data System; Repeat-dose study (e.g. in rats and other laboratory animals); Research diagnostic criteria; Respiratory distress syndrome (of the neonate or newborn; it develops immediately after delivery due to low concentration of the pulmonary surfactant or surfactant factor in the amniotic fluid, causing the formation of alveolar hyaline membranes in the lungs - also known as HDS or Hyaline membrane disease); Reticuloendothelial depressing substance; Revolving-door surgery (see OPS; SDS); Reward-deficiency syndrome; Rhodanese; Rural Development Service (USDA).

R-DS Riley-Day syndrome.

RDSG Rheumatic Diseases Study Group.

RDT Radical dietary therapy; Regular/ Routine dialysis therapy/ treatment (hemodialysis); Repeated dose toxicity; Retinal damage threshold.

RDTD Referral, diagnosis, treatment, and discharge.

RDTS Repeated dose toxicity study.

RDU Rational drug use.

RDV Rice dwarf virus.

RDVT Recurrent deep vein thrombosis.

RDW Red (blood cell) distribution width (index).

RDX Hexogen (= Cyclotrimethylene trinitramine) - a plastic explosive.

RE Concerning; Radium emanation; Re-admission (see readm); Rectal examination; Re-examine/nation (see reex); Reflux esophagitis; Refractory; Regional enteritis; Renal and electrolyte; Resistive exercise; Resting energy; Restriction endonuclease/ enzyme; Reticuloendothelial/lium; Retinol equivalent; Retrograde ejaculation; Right ear/ eye.

Re Rhenium (Z = 75) - formerly known as Bohemium (Bo) (see Elements - Rhenium).

R_E Efferent vascular resistance (kidneys); Respiratory exchange ratio.

R_e Reynold's number.

R&E Research and education (program); Rest and exercise; Round and equal.

R^E Right upper extremity.

R_E Right lower extremity.

RE√ Recheck.

REA Radiation emergency area; Radio-enzymatic assay; Renal anastomosis; Right ear advantage; Rural Electrification Administration (USDA).

REAB Refractory anemia with (excess of) blasts.

REACT Roche European American Cataract Trial (to investigate the efficacy of an oral antioxidant micronutrient mixture to low progression of age-related cataract).

readm re-admission (= RE).

REAG Real-ear aided gain (hearing measurement procedure - see RECD; RESR).

REAP Rural Environmental Assistance Program (USDA).

REAR Real-ear aided response.

REAS Reasonably expected as safe; Retained, excluded antrum syndrome.

REAT Radiological emergency assistance team.

REB Roentgen-equivalent biological.

REC Receptor; Research Ethics Committee (NHS, UK); Reticuloendothelial cell.

rec fresh (L. recens) (= recen); recessive; recombinant (chromosome); recombination; recommend; record(ing); recovery; recreation; recur(red)/(rence/(rent).

Rec 7-0267 Dimefline hydrochloride (see DW 62).

RECA Right external carotid artery.

RECD Real-ear-to-coupler difference (hearing measurement procedure).

RE cells Reticuloendothelial cells.

recen fresh (see rec).

RECG Radioelectrocardiography; Radioelectrocardiology (telemetry).

recip recipient; reciprocal.

recip titer reciprocal titer.

recomm recommendation.

Recommend Recommendation/ded (= recomm).

recon The smallest unit of DNA capable of recombination (recombination or "rec" + quantum or "on" - Gr.).

recond recondition(ed)/(ing).

reconstr reconstruction.

RECP Rural Environmental Conservation Program (USDA).

recryst recrystallization.

rect rectal/tum; rectification/fied (L. rectifica-

tus); rectus (muscle).
recumb recumbent.
recur recurrence/ent.
RED Radiation experience data; Rapid erythrocyte/cytic degeneration; Rapidly eliminated drug; Relevant epidemiological data; Reticulo-endothelial disease/ disorder.
red reduction.
REDC Race, Equality, and Diversity Committee (formerly REG) (GMC, UK).
REDD Real-ear-to-dial difference (hearing measurement procedure).
REG Racial Equality Group (now REDC) (GMC, UK).
REH Recombinant erythropoietin hyporesponsiveness.
ReHuEPO Recombinant human erythropoietin (see rHuEPO; r-HuEPO).
red in pulv reduced to powder (L. reductus in pulverem).
redig in pulv let it be reduced to powder (L. redigatur in pulverem).
redox "reduction-oxidation", i.e. oxidation-reduction.
RED SUBS Reducing substances.
redupl reduplication.
REE Rapid extinction effect; Rare earth element; Resting energy expenditure.
REEDS Retention (of tears), ectrodactyly, ectodermal dysplasia, and strange (hair, skin, and teeth) (syndrome).
REEG Radioelectroencephalogram/graphy.
R-EEG Resting electroencephalogram/graphy.
ReEND Reproductive endocrinology.
REEP Right end-expiratory pressure.
reev re-evaluate.
reex re-examine/nation (= RE).
REF Ejection fraction at rest; Refer(ence)/(red)/(ring) (see ref); Refused (see ref); Renal erythropoietic factor.
ref refer/ reference/ referred/ referring (= REF); reflective/ reflex/ reflux (see refl); refractive; refused (= REF).
ref → refer to.
Ref Doc Referring doctor.
REFI Regional ejection fraction image.
ref ind refractive index.
refl reflective/ reflex/ reflux (= ref).
REFMS Recreation and Education for Multiple Sclerosis (Victims).
Ref Phys Referring physician.
REFRAD Released from active duty.
REG Radiation exposure guide; Radioencephalogram/graph(y); Random Event Generator; Rheoencephalogram/graph(y).
Reg Registered.
reg regarding; region; regular.
Reg block Regional block (anesthesia).
regen regenerate(d)/ting/tion.
reg rhy regular rhythm.
reg umb region of the navel or umbilical region (L. regio umbilici).
regurg regurgitation.
REH Renin essential hypertension.
rehab; rehabil rehabilitated/ation.
REL Rate of energy loss; Recommended exposure limit; Resting expiratory level (pulmonary).
rel related/tion/tive; religion/ous.
RELE Resistive exercise of lower extremities.
reliq remainder (L. reliquus).
REM Rapid eye movement (paradoxical sleep) (= D sleep); Recent-event memory; Reticular erythematous mucinosis; Return electrode monitor; Roentgen-equivalent-man - a unit of ionizing radiation equal to the absorbed dose in rads (radiation absorbed dose), multiplied by the RBE (Relative biological effectiveness) of the radiation used (1 rem = 1 rad x RBE) (= rem).
rem removal/ve; roentgen-equivalent-man (a biologic unit) (see REM).
REMA Repetitive excess mixed anhydride.
REMAB Radiation-equivalent-manikin absorption.
REMCAL Radiation-equivalent-manikin calibration.
remit remittent.
REMP Roentgen-equivalent-man period.
REMS Rapid eye movement sleep (see REM).
REN Renal.
ren renew (L. renovetur).
ren sem renew/ shall be renewed only once (L. renovetum semel).
reNVA Recombinant Norwalk virus antigen.
REO Respiratory enteric orphan (virus) (see

Reovirus).

Reovirus Respiratory and enteric origin/ Respiratory and entero/ Respiratory enteric orphan virus - one of a subgroup of the ECHO viruses, with ECHO 10 as the prototype strain. There are three serotypes of this virus (see ECHO).

REP Regular/ Residual/ Ruptured ectopic pregnancy; Regular/ Rest exercise program; Retrograde pyelogram; Roentgen/ Röntgen equivalent-physical - a unit of the amount of ionizing radiation, which when delivered to a given mass of tissue, produces the same real energy conversion as one roentgen of hard X- or gamma (γ) radiation delivered to the same mass of air (i.e. about 84 ergs per gram) (= rep).

rep repair; repeat or let it be repeated (see rept); replicate/tion; report (= rept); roentgen-equivalent-physical (see REP).

repet repeat/ to be repeated (L. repetatur) (= rept).

repol repolarization.

REPS Reactive extensor postural synergy; Repetitions.

rept repeat or let it be repeated (L. repetatur) (= rep); report (see rep).

Reqd Required.

RER Regular exercise regimen; Renal excretion rate; Respiratory exchange ratio; Rough endoplasmic reticulum (see rER).

rER Rough endoplasmic reticulum (= RER).

RERF Radiation Effects Research Foundation.

RES Radiological evaluation score; Radionuclide esophageal scintigraphy; Refractive eye surgery; Reticuloendothelial system.

res research; resection; reserve; residence/nt; residue; resistance/nt (see resist).

RESC Resuscitation (see resus).

resist resistance/ resistant (= res).

RESNA Rehabilitation Engineering Society of North America.

resp respective(ly); respiration/tory; response/onsible.

RESPL Real ear sound pressure level/ loss.

RESR Real-ear saturation response (hearing measurement procedure - see REAG; RECD).

REST Raynaud's phenomenon, esophageal motor dysfunction, sclerodactyly and telangiectasia (syndrome); Regressive electroshock therapy; Restoration/red.

resus; resusc resuscitation.

RET Rational-emotive therapy (cognitive behavior psychotherapy of Albert Ellis - USA); Retained; Retention (see ret); Reticular; Reticulocyte; Retina; Reverse electron transport; Right esotropia.

ret rad equivalent therapeutic; retention (= RET); retired; return.

retard retardation/ded.

ret cath retention catheter.

retic reticulocyte.

retic ct reticulocyte count (laboratory/ hematology).

retics reticulocytes.

REV Reticuloendotheliosis virus.

ReV Regulator of virion.

rev reverse; review; revise(d)/sion; revolution.

Rev of Sym Review of symptoms.

Rex Regulator x.

re-x reexamination.

RF Radial fiber; Radiofrequency (see rf); Receptive field; Recognition/ Release/ Releasing/ Resistance/ Rheumatoid/ Risk factor; Reitland-Franklin (unit); Relative flow (rate)/ fluorescence; Renal/ Respiratory failure; Replicative form; Respiratory frequency (see Rf); Reticular/ Rosette formation; Retroperitoneal fibromatosis; Rheumatic fever; Riboflavin (= Rib); Root (canal) filling.

Rf Respiratory frequency (= RF); Rutherfordium - a unit representing one million disintegrations of radioactive matter per second (= rd).

rf radiofrequency (= RF).

R^F Rate of flow (chromatography).

R_f The distance that a spot of a substance has moved from the point of application (in paper or thin-layer chromatography.

R&F Radiographic and fluoroscopic.

RFA Radiofrequency ablation (electrode blockage applied in cardiac arrhythmia); Right femoral artery; Right frontoanterior (position of fetus).

RFB Retained foreign body.

RFC Retrograde femoral catheter; Right frontal craniotomy; Rosette-forming cell.
RFD Renal functional disorder; Residual functional deficit (Orthopedics); Respiratory function data (see PFT); Retarded fetal development.
RFDS Royal Flying Doctor Service (Australia).
RFE Relative fluorescence efficiency.
RFF Right fifth finger.
RFFIT Rapid fluorescent focus inhibition test.
RFH Right femoral hernia; Royal Free Hospital (London, UK).
RFI Recurrence-free interval; Recurrent/ Refractory fungal infection; Renal failure index.
RFIT Risk factor intervention trial.
RFL Right frontolateral (fetal position).
RFLA Rheumatoid-factor-like activity.
RFLP Restriction fragment length polymorphism.
RFLS Rheumatoid factor-like substance.
RFM Renal function monitoring.
Rfm Rifampin (= RIF; Rif; RMP).
RFN Registered Fever Nurse (Brit).
RFNNSP Relapsing febrile nodular non-suppurative panniculitis (= WCD - Weber-Christian disease).
RFP Radio-frequency probe; Recurrent facial palsy/ paralysis; Request for proposal; Right facial palsy; Right femoral pulse; Right frontoposterior (fetal position).
RFPS (Glasgow) Royal Faculty of Physicians and Surgeons of Glasgow.
RFR Refraction; Ring field of radiation (Waldeyer - radiation therapy).
RFS Radical flexor synovectomy; Rapid frozen section (see RFR); Relapse-free survival (e.g. in cancer patients); Renal function studies/dy.
RFT Radio-frequency technology; Renal function test(s) (see KFT); Respiratory function test(s) (see PFT); Right frontotransverse (fetal position); Rod-and-frame test; Routine fever therapy.
R-F unit Reitman-Frankel unit.
RFV Right femoral vein.
RFW Rapid filling wave.
RFX Multiprotein transcription factor complex (regulator).
RG Reagent grade (= GR); Replicator gene (a cancer-related gene); Right gluteal/eus (injection site).
rG Regular gene.
RGA Regurgitated gastric acid; Retrograde amnesia.
RGB Renal graft biopsy.
RGBMT Renal glomerular basement membrane thickness.
RGC Radio-gas chromatography; Rapidly growing children; Regional genetic clinic; Remnant gastric cancer; Retinal ganglion cell; Retrograde cystogram/graph(y); Right giant cell.
RGD An artificial peptide, containing the tripeptide arginine-glycine-aspartic acid and binding to metastatic cells' receptors for fibronectin, blocking their attachment to the matrix and ultimately suppressing metastasis; Radio Gas Dispenser; Range-gated Doppler; Recessive gene disorder.
RGE Relative gas expansion; Respiratory gas exchange.
R-Gene Arginine hydrochloride - an essential aminoacid used in the treatment of hepatic coma.
RGF Renal growth factor (see RHGF).
RGH Rat growth hormone; Recurrent genital herpes.
RGK Retrograde knife.
RGM Recurrent glioblastoma multiforme; Right gluteus medius.
rGM-CSF Recombinant granulocyte-macrophage colony-stimulating factor.
RGMT Reciprocal geometric mean titer.
RGN Registered General Nurse (Brit).
RGO Reciprocating gait orthosis.
RGP Retrograde pyelography; Rural general practitioner.
RGR Recurrent gastric reflux; Relative growth rate; Renal graft rejection.
RGT Regional gene therapy (for cancer); Retroviral gene transfer; Reversed gastric tube.
RGU Regional glucose utilization.
RH Radiant heat; Radiological health; Reactive hyperemia; Recurrent herpes; Reduced haloperidol; Regulatory/ Releasing

hormone; Relative hazard/ humidity; Renal hemolysis; Rest home; Retinal hemorrhage; Right hand/ heart/ hemisphere/ hyperphoria; Room humidifier.

Rh Rhesus (antigen) (blood group); Rhesus (factor) (Rh system of red cell agglutinogens); Rheumatoid (= rheu; rheum); Rhinion; Rhipicephalus (a genus of cattle ticks, species of which transmit Babesia, Borrelia, Rickettsia, Theileria and other diseases in animals and man), e.g. Rh sanguineus - the Common Dog Tick transmitting Rickettsia connori, the causal agent of Spotted Fever); Rhodium (Z = 45) (see Elements - Rhodium); Rhonchi (or rales) (see rh).

rh rales (L. rhonchi) (= Rh); rheumatic.

r/h roentgens per hour.

Rh+ Rhesus positive (laboratory/ blood bank).

Rh- Rhesus negative (laboratory/ blood bank).

^{106}Rh Radioactive rhodium.

RHA Rat hepatocyte assay; Regional Health Authority; Right hepatic artery; Rural Health Association.

RhA Rheumatoid arthritis.

Rh agglut Rheumatoid agglutinins (laboratory/ serology).

Rham Rhamnus - a genus of trees and shrubs of the family Rhamnaceae, e.g. Rham purshiana (= R. purshiana) - The Cascara Sagrada or Sacred Bark, used as a mild purgative in the treatment of constipation due to colonic stasis.

Rham cat Rhamnus cathartica - the buckthorn plant.

rhAPC Recombinant human activated protein C (e.g. Drotrecogin alfa - lifesaving antithrombolytic used in acute organ dysfunction).

RHB Raise head of bed; Reactive hypertrophy of bone (Orthopedics); Regional Hospital Board; Right heart border/ bypass.

RHBF Reactive hyperemia blood flow.

RHBs Regional Hospital Boards.

RHBV Right-heart blood volume.

RHC Reproductive healthcare; Resin hemoperfusion column; Respiration(s) has/ have ceased; Right heart catheterization; Right hypochondrium; Rural Health Clinic.

RHCD Recommended human clinical dose (see HCD; RCD); Rural Health Care Delivery.

RHCSA Regional Hospitals Consultants' and Specialists' Association.

RHD Radial head dislocation; Radiological health data; Recommended human dose (see HRDD; RHDD); Recurrent hip dislocation (esp. with prostheses); Relative hepatic dullness; Relevant human data; Renal hypertensive disease; Resting hemodynamics; Rhesus hemolytic disease (see Rh-HD); Rheumatic heart disease (= Rheu ht dis).

RhD Rhesus (hemolytic) disease (see Rh-HD).

RHDD Recommended human daily dose (= HRDD).

rhDNA Recombinant human deoxyribonuclease (= Dornase alfa - see rDNA).

RH(DNA)RA Rat Hepatocyte Deoxyribonucleic Acid Repair Assay.

RHE Recombinant human erythropoietin; Retinohepatoendocrinologic (syndrome).

rhe (Gr. rheos = current). The unit of fluidity, being the reciprocal of the unit of velocity or centipoise.

RHEED Reflection high-energy electron diffraction.

RHEHPPD Regional Health Education, Health Promotion and Prevention Department (SCPMG).

rheo rheology.

rheu rheumatic/ism (= rheum); rheumatoid (see Rh).

Rheu fev Rheumatic fever.

Rheu ht dis Rheumatic heart disease (see RHD).

rheum rheumatic/ism (see rheu); rheumatoid (see Rh).

RHF Refractory/ Right heart failure.

Rh factor Rhesus factor (laboratory/ blood bank).

RHG Right hand grip.

rhG-CSF Recombinant human granulocyte colony-stimulating factor.

RHGF Renal hepatocyte growth factor (= RGF).

rhGM-CSF Recombinant human granulocyte macrophage colony-stimulating factor.

RHH Right homonymous hemianopsia.

Rh-HD Rhesus hemolytic disease (= RHD; RhD).
RHHED app-Hodgkin hypohidrotic ectodermal dysplasia.
RHI Rural Health Initiative.
RHIG; RHIg Rho(D) immune globulin.
Rhin Rhinologist/gy.
rhino rhinoplasty.
Rhiz Rhizobium - a genus of microorganisms of the family Rhizobiaceae; rod-shaped, gram-negative, symbiotic, nitrogen-fixing bacteria, producing nodules on the roots of leguminous plants and fixing free nitrogen in this symbiosis, e.g. Rhiz japonicum (= R. japonicum).
RHJSC Regional Hospital Junior Staff Committee.
RHL Radioactive half-life (see EHL; Half-life); Recurrent herpes labialis; Right hemisphere lesions; Right hepatic lobe.
RHLN Right hilar lymph node.
rhm roentgen-hour-meter - roentgens per hour at one meter radiation (therapy).
rHmEPO Recombinant human erythropoietin.
RhMK Rhesus monkey kidney (cells) (= RhMkK; RMK).
RhMk Rhesus monkey.
RhMkK Rhesus monkey kidney (see RhMK).
RHMV Right heart mixing volume.
RHN Rochester Health Network (New York); Rockwell hardness number.
RHO Right heeloff.
Rho(D) Red cell antigen.
RhoGAM Rh immune globulin.
RHP Rare health/ hereditary problem.
rhPDGF Recombinant human platelet-derived growth factor.
RHR Rapid/ Regular/ Renal hypertensive rate; Rapid (tachycardia)/ Regular/ Resting heart rate.
r/hr roentgens per hour.
RHRA Rat Hepatocyte (DNA) Repair Assay {see RH(DNA)RA}.
RHRD Recurrent hip replacement dislocation.
RHS Ramsay-Hunt syndrome (geniculate herpes zoster, associated with lower motor neurone paralysis of the facial nerve); Reciprocal hindlimb-scratching (syndrome); Right hand side; Right heelstrike.
rHS Recombinant human somatotropin.
RHSA Regional health-system administrator.
RHSC Research in Health and Social Care (UK).
RHT Recurrent hyperthyroidism; Renal homotransplantation; Right hypertropia.
rH-TNF Recombinant human tumor necrosis factor.
RHU Registered health underwriter; Rheumatology (see Rhu).
Rhu Rheumatology (= RHU).
rHuEpo; r-HuEPO Recombinant human erythropoietin.
rHuGM-CSF Recombinant human granulocyte-macrophage colony stimulating factor (e.g. Molgramostim - used in cancer therapy).
rHuIL-2 Recombinant human interleukin-2 (e.g. Aldesleukin - used in cancer therapy).
rHuKGF Recombinant human keratinocyte growth factor.
rHuLH Recombinant human luteinizing hormone.
rHuPDGF Recombinant human platelet-derived growth factor.
rHuTNF Recombinant human tumor-necrosing factor.
RHW Radiant heat warmer.
rhy rhythm.
RI Radiation/ Relative intensity; Radioactive isotope; Radioimmunology; Rapid-acting/ Regular Insulin (see Insulin - RI); Recession/ Reflux/ Refractive/ Regenerative/ Respiratory/ Reticulocyte/ Rosette index; Recombinant inbred (strain); Recovery Incorporated; Regional ileitis; Release-inhibiting; Release/ Rosette inhibition; Remission induction; Renal insufficiency; Replicative intermediate; Resistance index (in fetal blood vessels); Respiratory illness; Retroactive inhibition (psychology)/ interference; Ribosome; Rooming in; Roseola infantum (= ES - Exanthema subitum) - a multivirus infection); Rubeosis iridis.
R/I Rheumatic fever recurrence rate per streptococcal infection.
r_i Interclass correlation.
RIA Radioimmunoassay (laboratory method); Rare Isotope Accelerator (Nuclear physcics); Reduced iron availability; Remission-induc-

ing agent (see RID); Research Institute on Alcoholism.

RIA-DA Radioimmunoassay-double antibody (procedure/ test).

RIAS Roter International Analysis Scheme.

RIAT Radioimmune antiglobulin tes; Radioimmunoassay test.

RIB Reduced insulin breakdown; Rest in bed; Retirement Insurance Benefit.

Rib Riboflavin (see RF); Ribose (see R).

RIBA Radioimmunoblotting assay.

RIBS Rutherford ion backscattering.

RIC Radiation-induced cancer (see RIT); Renomedullary interstitial cell(s); Right iliac crest; Right internal carotid (artery); Royal Institute of Chemistry.

RICA Right internal carotid artery.

RICE Rest, Ice, Compression, and Elevation (in treatment of sports and similar injuries).

RICH Right intracerebral hemisphere.

RICM Right intercostal margin.

RiCoF Ristocetin cofactor.

RICS Right intercostal space.

RICU Respiratory intensive care unit.

RID Radial/io immunodiffusion; Recommended initial dosage/ dose; Remission-inducing drug; Remove Intoxicated Drivers (Inc); Reversible intravas device; Ruptured intervertebral disc.

RIE Rocket immunoelectrophoresis.

RIF Release-/ Rosette-inhibiting factor; Rifampin (see Rfm); Right iliac fossa (injection site); Right index finger; Rigid internal fixation.

Rif Rifampin (see Rfm).

RIFA Radioiodinated fatty acid.

RIFC Rat intrinsic factor concentrate.

rIFN Recombinant interferon.

RIG Rabies immune globulin.

RIGH Rabies immune globulin, human.

RIGHA Rhode Island Group Health Association.

RigiScan Rigidity Scan (a take-home exam that monitors penile rigidity and tumescence).

RIH Right inguinal hernia.

RIHSA Radioactive iodinated human serum albumin.

RIITD Radioiodine-induced thyroid damage.

Riker 594 Sulthiame (= Sultiame) - a sulfamoylphenyl-thiazine compound. An anticonvulsant used in the treatment of all forms of epilepsy, with the exception of petit mal.

Riker 595 Butaperazine (see Bayer 1362).

rIL Recombinant interleukin.

RILT Rabbit ileal loop test.

RIM Radiation-induced mucositis; Radioisotope medicine; Recurrent induced malaria; Relative-intensity measure.

RIMA Right internal mammary anastomosis/ artery.

RIMN Research Institute of Metabolism and Nutrition.

RIMR Rockefeller Institute for Medical Research.

RIMS Resonance ionization mass spectrometry.

RIN Radiocontrast-induced nephropathy; Rat insulinoma; Reversible interstitial nephritis.

RINB Reitan-Indiana Neuropsychological Battery.

RIND Resolving/ Reversible ischemic neurologic(al) deficit; Reversible ischemic neurological defect/ disorder.

RINN Recommended international non-proprietary name.

RIO Right inferior oblique.

RIP Radiation-induced pneumonitis; Radioimmunoprecipitation; Rapid infusion pump; Reduced lipid peroxidation; Reflex inhibiting pattern; Renally impaired patient; Respiratory inductance plethysmogram-graph(y) (rib cage & abdominal excursion monitor, used in assessment of SDB or Sleep disordered breathing); Rest In Peace; Run-in period.

RIPA Radioimmunoprecipitation assay.

RIPH Royal Institute of Public Health.

RIPHH Royal Institute of Public Health and Hygiene.

RIPP Resistive-intermittent positive pressure.

RIR Rapid initial response; Relative incidence rates; Right interior rectus (muscle).

RIRB Radioiodinated rose bengal.

RIS Rapid immunofluorescence staining; Reduced inspiratory stretch (in the treatment of lung injury); Residual insulin secretion; Resonance ionization spectroscopy.

RISA Radioactive iodinated/nized serum albumin (= $RISA^{131}$) (nuclear medicine); Radioimmunosorbent assay.

$RISA^{131}$ See RISA.

RIST Radioimmunosorbent test (for measurement of the total IgE concentration in the serum); Radioisotope scanning test.

RIT Radiation-induced tumor (= RIC); Radioimmune trypsin; Radioimmunotherapy; Radioiodinated triolein; Radioiodine treatment; Recherche et Industrie Thérapeutiques (Fr.) (Research and Therapeutical Industry); Rosette inhibition titer.

RITA Random Intervention Treatment of Angina.

RITC Rhodamine isothiocyanate.

RITD Recommended initial target dose.

RITDR Recommended initial target dose range.

RIU Radioactive iodine uptake (nuclear medicine).

RIV Resistant influenza variant.

RIVC Right inferior vena cava.

RIVD Ruptured intervertebral disc.

RIVS Ruptured interventricular septum.

RIX Radiation-induced xerostomia.

RJS Residual joint stiffness.

RK Rabbit kidney (tissue culture); Radial keratotomy; Refractive keratoplasty; Right kidney.

RK 13 Cell line.

RKD Resistant kidney disease.

RKF Reduced/ Retarded kidney function.

RKG Radiocardiogram.

RKH Rokitansky-Küster-Hauser (syndrome).

RKI Robert Koch Institute (Germany).

RKJ Rheumatoid knee joint.

RKL Right-to-Know legislation.

RKM Rokitamycin.

RKV Rabbit kidney vacuolating (virus).

RKY Roentgen kymography.

RL Coarse rales (on chest auscultation); Radiation laboratory; Reduction level (reciprocal of respiratory quotient); Reiz lumen (stimulus); Resistive load; Reticular lamina; Right lateral/ leg/ lower/ lung; Ringer lactate (solution).

Rl Medium rales.

rl fine rales.

R_L Pulmonary resistance.

R → L Right to left.

R&L Right and left.

rl_1 few fine rales.

Rl_2 Moderate number of medium rales.

Rl_3 Many coarse rales.

RLA Reduced language abilities/ty (see SMI); Regional lymphadenopathy.

RLBA Radioligand binding assay (= RBA).

RLBCD Right lower border of cardiac dullness.

RLBD Right-left battery discrimination.

RLC Residual/ Resting lung capacity (see PFT - RLC); Retinoid-like compound.

RLCAA Rat Lymphocyte Chromosomal Aberration assay.

RLD Radiolabelled dose/ drug; Related living donor; Right later decubitus; Ruptured lumbar disc.

RLE Right lower extremity.

RLF Retrolental fibroplasia; Right lateral femoral (injection site).

RLI Routine laboratory investigation (see RLT).

RLL Radiolucent line; Right lower limb/ lobe (of lung).

RLM Radiolabelled metabolite; Regional Library of Medicine; Right lower medial.

RLMD Rat liver mitochondria digitonin (i.e. rat liver mitochondria and submitochondrial particles derived by digitonin treatment).

RLN Recurrent laryngeal nerve; Regional lymph node.

RLNC Regional lymph node cell.

RLND Recurrent laryngeal nerve damage; Regional lymph node dissection.

RLO Residual lymphatic output; Residual lymphocyte count.

RLP Radiation leukemia protection; Ribosome-like particle.

RLQ Right lower quadrant (of the abdomen).

RLR Right lateral rectus (muscle of the eyeball).

RLS Radiolabelled study; Reproductive life span; Restless leg syndrome; Ringer's lactate solution; RLS person (who stammers, mispronounces, or has difficulty in enunciating the letters "R", "L", and "S"); Roussy-Lévy syndrome.

RLSB Right lower scapular border.

R-L sh Right-left shunt.
RLSMD Royal London School of Medicine and Dentistry.
RLT Right lateral thigh (injection site); Right lower thorax; Routine laboratory test(s).
RLTSC Repeat lower transverse cesarean section.
RLV Rauscher leukemia virus; Recurrent labyrinthine vertigo (caused by vestibular hydrops, a clinical variant of Meniere's disease).
RLW Right lateral wall (of chest, etc.).
RLWD Routine laboratory work done.
RM Radical mastectomy (operation/ breast); Random migration; Range of motion/ movement (see ROM); Red marrow; Reference material; Reflectance meter (dextrostix); Rehabilitation Medicine; Reinforced maneuver; Relative mobility (see Rm); Repetitions maximum; Rescue medication; Resistive/ Respiratory movement; Riehl's melanosis; Rhinitis medicamentosa; Right median; Routine management; Ruptured membranes (obstetrics).
Rm Relative mobility (= RM); Remission (= rm).
rm remission (see Rm); room.
R&M Routine and microscopic.
RMA Raised/ Relevant/ Rough maternal age (Obstetrics); Registered Medical Assistant; Relative medullary area; Reverse mutation assay (Ames); Right mentoanterior (position of fetus).
RMB Regular menstrual bleeding; Right mainstem bronchus.
RMBF Regional myocardial blood flow.
RMC Registered medical center; Regular menstrual cycle; Reproductive medical center; Reticular magnocellular (nucleus); Reversible mental confusion; Right middle cerebral (artery); Rush Medical College.
RMCA Right main coronary artery; Right middle cerebral artery.
RMCL Right midclavicular line.
RMCT Rat mast cell technique.
RMD Doctor of Research Medicine; Rapid movement disorder; Recommended maximum dose; Recurrent major depression; Recurrent metastatic disease; Repetitive motion disorder (see RSI); Resistance mechanism disorder; Retromanubrial dullness.
RME Rapid maxillary expansion; Receptor-mediated endocytosis; Resting metabolic expenditure; Right mediolateral episiotomy; Routine medical examination.
RMEC Recurrent metastatic endometrial carcinoma; Regional medical education center.
RMEE Right middle ear exploration.
R meter Radiation meter.
RMF Right middle finger.
RMFP Rhythm method of family planning (see CMFP; NFPM).
RMG Recurrent malignant glioma; Routine morning grumpiness.
RMI Reading Miscue Inventory; Recent/ Recurrent myocardial infarction.
RMK Rhesus monkey kidney (see RhMK).
RMK #1 Remark number 1.
RML Radiation myeloid leukemia; Regional medical library; Rhabdomyolysis; Right mediolateral (episisotomy) (operation/ obstetrics); Right middle lobe (of lungs).
RMLB Right middle lobe bronchus.
RMLE Right mediolateral episiotomy.
RMLS Right middle lobe syndrome.
RMLV Rauscher murine leukemia virus (see RMuLV).
RMM Rapid micromedia method; Read mostly (from) memory; Receptor-mediated mechanism.
RMMD Radiomorphometric data.
RMN Registered Mental Nurse (England and Wales).
RMO Regional/ Registered Medical Officer (Brit).
RMP Rapidly miscible pool; Regional Medical Program(s) (NIH); Registered Medical Practitioner; Resting membrane potential; Ribulose monophosphate pathway; Rifampin (see Rfm); Right mentoposterior (position of fetus).
RMPA Royal Medico-Psychological Association.
RMPS Regional Medical Programs Service.
RMR Relative maximum response; Renin-mediated reduction (in systemic BP); Resting metabolic rate; Right medial rectus (muscle of the eyeball).

RMS Recovered/ Restored memory syndrome; Rectal morphine sulfate (suppository); Red/ Rigid man syndrome; Repetitive motion syndrome; Respiratory muscle strength; Rhabdomyolysis syndrome (caused by "statin" drugs such as simvostatin, etc., in the treatment of hyperlipidemia); Rhabdomyosarcoma; Rheumatic mitral stenosis; Rhodomyosarcoma; Rigorous medical supervision; Root-mean-square (see rms).

rms root-mean-square (= RMS) (i.e. square root of mean square).

RMSD Root-mean-square deviation.

RMSE Root mean square error.

RMSF Rocky Mountain spotted fever (caused by *Rickettsia* rickettsii and transmitted by ticks) (see SF - Spotted fever).

RMT Registered Music Therapist; Regular maintenance therapy; Relative medullary thickness; Retromolar trigone; Right mento-transverse (position of fetus); Routine medical treatment (= RTM).

RMUI Relief medication unit index.

RMuLV Rauscher murine leukemia virus (= RMLV).

RMV Raised/ Reduced minute ventilation (see VFR); Respiratory minute volume (see PFT).

RN Radionuclide; Red/ Reticular nucleus; Registered Nurse; Residual nitrogen; Royal Navy.

Rn Radon (Z = 86) (see Elements - Radon).

RNA Radionuclide angiography; Refractory nocturnal asthma; Registered Nurse Anesthetist; Rough, noncapsulated, avirulent (bacteria); Ribonucleic acid (see also DNA) (= Plant nucleic acid; Ribose nucleic acid; Yeast nucleic acid) - a nucleic acid found in all living cells, and originally isolated from yeast; a nucleotide polymer, it contains a complex mixture of phosphorus-containing organic acids, one of two distinct varieties of nucleic acid (the other is DNA - Deoxyribonucleic acid):
RNA hydrolyses, yielding adenine, guanine, cysteine, uracil, ribose, and phosphoric acid. These acids are composed of chains of nucleotides (phosphate esters of purine or pyrimidine bases and pentose-sugars), and act as "building blocks" of the chromosomes in all cell nuclei;
messenger RNA - an RNA fraction of intermediate molecular weight, which transfers information from DNA to the protein-forming system of the cell;
soluble RNA - see transfer RNA;
transfer RNA - an RNA fraction of low molecular weight, found in 20 species, each of which combines with one aminoacid species, transferring it from activating enzyme to ribosome.

RNAA Radiochemical neutron activation analysis.

RNAse; RNase Ribonuclease.

RNAse A; RNase A Ribonuclease A.

RNB Reflex neurogenic bladder.

RNBS Radionuclide bone scanning (= RBS).

RNC Respiratory nerve center.

RND Radical neck dissection (operation/ neck); Radionuclide dacryography; Reactive/ Refractory neurodermatitis; Reactive neurotic depression; Recurrent neurological dysfunction.

RNEF Radionuclide/ Resting nuclide ejection fraction.

RNF (Von) Recklinghausen's neurofibromatosis (see VRNF).

RNFP Registered Nurse Fellowship Program.

rNGF Recombinant nerve-growth factor.

RNH Recurrent nocturnal hypoglycemia.

RNHRD Royal National Hospital for Rheumatic Diseases (Bath, UK).

RNI Recommended nutrient intake.

RNIB Royal National Institute for the Blind.

RNICU Regional neonatal intensive care unit.

RNID Royal National Institute for the Deaf.

RNL Radial nerve lesion.

RNMD Registered Nurse for Mental Defectives (Brit).

RNMS Registered Nurse for the Mentally Sub-Normal (Brit).

RNN Retinopathy, neuropathy and nephropathy (preoperative assessment).

RNP Radial nerve palsy; Radical neck procedure (= CP - Commando procedure); Ribonucleoprotein.

RNR Ribonucleotide reductase.

RNS Radionuclide scan (seleniomethionine)/ study; Reference normal serum; Repetitive nerve stimulation.

RNSC Radionuclide superior cavography.

RNSS Repetitive nerve-stimulation study (see RNS).

RNST Repetitive nerve-stimulation test (for myasthenia gravis, etc.).

Rnt Roentgenologist/logy.

rNTP Ribonuclease-5'-triphosphate.

RNV Radionuclide venography; Resting nuclear ventriculography (see SNV); Ritonavir (HIV protease inhibitor).

RNVG Radionuclide ventriculography.

RO Radiation output; Ratio of; Relative odds; Realignment osteotomy; Reverse osmosis; Ritter-Oleson (technique); Routine order; Rule out (see R/O).

Ro Roche (Hoffmann-La Roche AG) (British subsidiary - Roche Products).

R/O Rule out (= RO).

R_0 Resting radium.

RO8 RO8 - 0074/003 sodium salt.

Ro 1-6463 Methyprylone (= Methypryl; 3,3-Diethyl-5-methyl-2,4-dioxopiperidine) - a depressant of the central nervous system, with a sedative and hypnotic action, taking effect within half an hour, and lasting about 6 hours. Used in the treatment of anxiety, tension, and moderate insomnia.

Ro 1-7683 Tropicamide (= Bistropamide; N-ethyl-N-pyrid-4-ylmethyltropamide; $C_{17}H_2ON_2O_2$) - a rapidly acting mydriatic and cycloplegic agent; used as eyedrops it acts within 10-15 minutes, the dilated pupils returning to normal in 8-9 hours. Does not elevate intraocular pressure in preglaucoma.

Ro 1-9569 Tetrabenazine (= TBZ) - has central effects similar to those of reserpine, causing depletion of serotonin and noradrenaline in brain tissues. Has been used in the treatment of acute and chronic mental disorders.

Ro 1-9934 Dehydroemetine hydrochloride (see DHE).

Ro 2-2453 Diamthazole hydrochloride (= Amycazol HCl; Diamthazol Dihydrochloride) - an antifungal agent effective against species of Trichophyton and Microsporum, and against Candida albicans. Used externally as an ointment, dusting-powder, and tincture.

Ro 2-3248 Azapetine phosphate (= Azepine phosphate) - a mild adrenolytic and sympatholytic drug, used in the treatment of peripheral vascular disorders due to arterial spasm.

Ro 2-3773 Clinidium bromide (= 3-Benziloyloxy-1-methylquinualidinium bromide) - a peripheral parasympatholytic agent, reducing secretion of gastric juice and having an antispasmodic action on the gastrointestinal tract. Used in the symptomatic treatment of peptic ulcer and other gastrointestinal disorders, in conjunction with a tranquillizer such as chlorodiazepoxide.

Ro 2-9757 Fluorouracil (see NSC 19893).

Ro 4-0403 Chlorprothixene (see N 714).

Ro 4-1544/6 Stibocaptate (= Antimony sodium dimercaptosuccinate; Sb-58; TWSb/6) - an organic antimony compound used in the treatment of schistosomiasis, the dimercaptosuccinate salt most commonly used in this disease (see TWSb; TWSb/1).

Ro 4-1778 Metofoline hydrochloride (= Methofoline HCl; Methopholine HCl) - an analgesic used for pre-anesthetic medication and for the relief of acute and chronic pain.

Ro 4-3076 Dehydroemetine and Bismuth Iodide - a combination product used successfully in the treatment of intestinal amebiasis.

Ro 4-3816 Alcuronium chloride (= Allnortoxiferin chloride; Diallylnortoxiferine dichloride; Diallyltoxiferine chloride; Diallyldinortoxiferin dichloride pentahydrate) - a nondepolarizing muscle relaxant with a speed of onset and duration of action similar to those of tubocurarine chloride.

Ro 4-4393 Sulphormethoxine (= Sulphorthodimethoxine) - a long-acting sulfonamide, its period of half-elimation being 100 to 200 hours.

Ro 4-5360 Nitrazepam - a benzodiazepine hypnotic agent used for insomnia associated with anxiety or organic disease.

Ro 4-6467 Procarbazine hydrochloride (see NSC 77213).

Ro 5-0690 Chlordiazepoxide hydrochloride (see CMPB).

Ro 5-0831 Isocarboxazid (= 3-N'-Benzylhydrazinocarbonyl-5-methylisoxazole) - a monoamine oxidase inhibitor drug used in the treatment of exogenous and reactive

depression.
Ro 5-2807 Diazepam (see LA 111).
Ro 5-3307/1 Debrisoquine sulfate (= Isocaramidine sulfate; 2-Amidino-1,2,3,4-tetrahydroisoquinoline sulfate) - a hypotensive agent acting by selectively blocking transmission in post-ganglionic adrenergic nerves. Used in the treatment of hypertension.
ROA Rat ovarian augmentation; Repeated oral administration; Right occipitoanterior (fetal position).
ROAC Repeated oral (doses of/ treatment with) activated charcoal.
ROAD Reversible obstructive airways disease (see COLD).
ROAT Repeat open application test.
ROATS Rabbit ovarian antitumor serum.
rob robertsonian (translocation).
ROC Receiver/ Relative operating characteristic; Receptor-operated channels; Remote obstetrical care; Resident on call; Residual organic carbon; Retained Organs Commission (UK); Royal Observer Corps (UK).
ROC; RO_2C Reduced oxygen consumption (see LOC; LO_2C).
ROCF Rey-Osterrieth Complex Figure.
Rock Cocaine (see Erythroxylum).
ROD Radiation Oncology Department; Renal osteodystrophy.
RODAC Replicate organism detection and counting.
rOEF Regional oxygen extraction fraction.
Roent; roent Roentgonologist/logy.
ROER Rapid-onset extended release (capsule/ drug/ medication/ tablet).
R of N Review of need (of health facilities).
ROH Rat ovarian hyperemia (test).
ROI Reactive oxygen intermediate; Region of interest.
ROIDS Hemorrhoids.
ROIH Right oblique inguinal hernia.
ROL Right occipitolateral (position of fetus).
ROM Range of motion/ movement (= RM); Read only memory (EDP - Electronic data processing); Right otitis media; Rupture of membranes (obstetrics).
Rom Roman; Romberg (sign).
rom reciprocal ohm meter.
Romb Romberg (see Rom).
ROM CP Range of motion complete and painfree.
ROMSA Right otitis media, suppurative, acute.
ROMSC Right otitis media, suppurative, chronic.
ROP Retinopathy of prematurity; Right occipitoposterior (position of fetus).
ROPS Rollover protective structure.
ROR Radiological objective response; Refractory organ rejection (see RRAR; RRE; RRR).
Ror Rorschach (intelligence test).
RoRx Roentgen radiation (therapy).
ROS Reactive oxygen species; Reconstituted oral suspension; Review of symptoms/ systems; Rod outer segment.
RoS Rostral sulcus.
ROSC Restoration of spontaneous circulation.
ROSS Review of subjective symptoms.
ROT Real oxygen transport; Remedial occupational therapy; Right occipitotransverse (position of fetus); 'Rule of thirds' (e.g. one in three patients).
rot rotate(d)/ating/ation/ator.
ROTC Reserve Officer Training Corps.
ROU Recurrent oral ulcer.
ROUL Rouleaux.
Roum. P Roumanian Pharmacopoeia (Farmacopeea Romana).
rout routine.
ROW Rat ovarian weight; Rendu-Osler-Weber (syndrome).
Roy. Child. Hosp Royal Children's Hospital (Melbourne, Australia).
Roy. Free Hosp Royal Free Hospital (London, UK).
ro-zha see Maladie-de-Roger.
RP Radial pulse; Radical prostatectomy; Radiopharmaceutical; Rapid processing (of film); Raynaud's phenomenon; Reactive/ Regulatory protein; Readiness/ Resting potential; Rectal prolapse; Refractory period; Relapsing polychondritis; Repair; Respiratory rate : pulse rate (index) (see R/P); Resection of prostate; Rest pain; Resting pressure; Retinitis pigmentosa; Retinitis proliferans (see RPr); Retrograde pyelogram/aphy; Retroperitoneal; Reverse phase; Rheumatic

pain; Rheumatoid polyarthritis; Ribose phosphate (see R-5-P); Rickettsialpox (an urban-associated spotted fever, caused by *Rickettsia* akari and transmitted to man by the rodent [mouse] mite) (see SF - Spotted fever); Ripstein procedure (proctopexy); Roche Products code for experimental substances; Russe procedure (see IBG).

Rp Take (L. recipe) (see Rx).

R_p Pulmonary resistance (vascular) (see PFT); Take (see Rx).

R/P Respiratory rate : pulse rate (index) (= RP; RPI; RP index).

R-5-P Ribose-5-phosphate (= RP).

RP 2168 Meglumine antimoniate (= Antimony meglumine; N-methylglucamine antimoniate; Protostib) - an organic antimony compound used in the treatment of cutaneous leishmaniasis and Kala-azar.

RP 2512 Pentamidine mesylate (= Pentamidine methanesulfonate; Pentamidine dimethylsulfonate) - a trypanocidal drug used in the treatment of early cases of African trypanosomiasis.

RP 2987 Diethazine hydrochloride (= Eazamine HCl) - used in the palliative treatment of Parkinson's disease; the drug mainly reduces rigidity, and to a lesser extent tremor and akinesia; it has no effect on excessive salivation.

RP 3359 Proguanil hydrochloride (= Bigumal; Chlorguanide HCl; Chloriguane HCl; Proguan HCl; Proguanide HCl; Proguanili hydrochloridum; SN 12,837) - a synthetic diguanide antimalarial drug used for the prevention and treatment of malaria. It kills the parasites undergoing schizogony in the red blood cells.

RP 3377 Chloroquine sulfate - a synthetic 4-aminoquinoline antimalarial drug used for the suppression and treatment of malaria. It kills the erythrocytic forms of malarial parasites at all stages of development. Chloroquine has also been used in the treatment of amebic hepatitis and liver abscess, and for the remission of symptoms in rheumatoid arthritis; it has also been found useful in the treatment of lupus erythematosus and giardiasis. Prolonged therapy may give rise to toxic effects, such as irreversible retinal damage and corneal opacities.

RP 3554 Thiazinamium methyl sulfate - an antihistamine and anticholinergic drug.

RP 3854 Melarsoprol (see Mel B).

RP 4516 Pamaquin (= Aminoquin; Gametocidum; Pamachin; Pamaquine Naphthoate; Plasmoquine; Plasmoquinum; SN 971) - a synthetic 8-aminoquinoline antimalarial drug, formerly used extensively in the treatment of malaria, but has been almost entirely replaced by the use of primaquine and other drugs (see SN 13,272).

RP 4632 Methoxypromazine maleate (= Methopromazine maleate) - a phenothiazine tranquillizer.

RP 4753 Pyrimethamine (see BW 50-63).

RP 4763 Diphetarsone - an organic arsenical compound used in the treatment of intestinal amebiasis, usually in conjunction with a broad-spectrum antibiotic.

RP 4909 Chlorproethazine - a phenothiazine derivative similar in its chemical composition, action, and uses as chlorpromazine. Used as a tranquillizing agent.

RP 6171 Amphotalide (see M&B 2948A).

RP 6753 Diphetarsone - Spiramycin - the spiramycin salt of diphetarsone. Has been used in the treatment of intestinal amebiasis and in threadworm infestation in children (see RP 4763).

RP 7044 Methotrimeprazine (= Levomepromazine; SKF 5116) - a tranquillizing agent used in the treatment of moderate depression and psychosis.

RP 7162 Trimipramine (see IL 6001).

RP 7293 Pristinamycin - a mixture of two antibiotics, produced by the growth of Streptomyces pristina spiralis. A bacteriostatic agent especially useful in the treatment of infections due to gram-positive bacteria (particularly Staphylococcus aureus) and penicillin-resistant Neisseria gonorrhoeae.

RP 7522 Sulfamethoxypyridazine (see CT 879).

RP 7676 Pralidoxime mesylate (see 2-FMPOMS).

RP 7843 Thioproperazine mesylate (= Thioproperazine methanesulfonate;

Thioproperazine dimethanesulfonate) - a phenothiazine tranquillizer having sedative, hypotensive, and hypothermic properties less than those of chlorpromazine. Used in the treatment of schizophrenia, mania, and delirious states to control excitement, and disturbed or aggressive behavior.

RP 8599 Dimethothiazine (= Dimethitazine) - an antihistamine used in the treatment of migraine.

RP 8823 Metromidazole (see Bayer 5360).

RP 8909 Pericyazine (= Propericiazine; SKF 20716) - a phenothiazine derivative with sedative, anti-emetic, and adrenolytic properties. Used in the treatment of severe anxiety and tension states, and in acute and chronic schizophrenia.

RP 9955 Melarsonyl potassium (see Mel W).

RPA Radial photon absorptiometry; Recognized pharmacological action; Registered Physician's Assistant; Regular physical activity; Resultant physiologic acceleration; Reverse passive anaphylaxis; Right pulmonary artery.

RPase Ribonucleic acid polymerase.

RPAW Right pulmonary artery withdrawel.

RPB Research to Prevent Blindness; Retroperitoneal/ Retroplacental bleeding (see RPH).

(rpb)[7] Point-biserial correlation.

RPBI Resting penile-brachial index.

RPBS Randomized placebo-blind study.

RPC Radiographic pulmonary congestion; Radiographically-pronounced cardiomegaly; Recurring productive cough; Regional Physician Coordinator; Regular painful contraction(s) (of the uterus during labor); Relapsing polychondritis; Relative proliferative capacity; Renal-pelvis cancer/ carcinoma/ cavitation; Renin producing cell (kidney); Retroplacental clot (Obstetrics); Routine post/prenatal care.

RPCC Regional Poison Control Center.

RPCF Reiter protein complement fixation (test) (see RPCFT).

RPCFT Reiter protein complement fixation test (for treponemal antibody-serological test for syphilis) (= RPCF; RPF) (see STS-RPCFT).

RPCGN Rapidly progressive crescenting glomerulonephritis.

RPCM Renal pelvi-calyceal measurement (e.g. antenatal Obstetrics).

RPCT Randomized placebo controlled trial.

RPD Rapidly progressive dementia/ disease/ disorder; Recurrent posterior dislocation (of the elbow); Recurrent prosthesis/etic dislocation (of the hip joint); Removable partial denture; Renal pelvic diameter/ dilation (see APRPD).

RPDE; RPDES; RPDIE Retinal phosphodiesterase.

RPE Radioprotective effect; Rapid plasma exclusion (see STS-RPE); Rate of perceived exertion; Recurrent pulmonary embolism; Regular physical exercise; Retinal pigment epithelium; Retrograde push enteroscopy; Routine physical/ psychological examination.

RPF Recurrent pyrexial fit(s) (in children); Reiter protein fixation (test) (see RPCFT); Relaxed pelvic floor; Renal perfusate/ plasma flow; Retroperitoneal fibromatosis/ fibrosis.

RPG Radiation protection guide; Retrograde pyelogram/aphy (X-ray/ kidneys); Rheoplethysmography.

RPGMEC Regional Postgraduate Medical Education Committee.

RPGN Rapidly progressive glomerulonephritis.

RPGS Renal prostaglandin synthesis.

RPH Retroperitoneal/ placental hemorrhage (= RPB).

RPh Registered Pharmacist.

RPHA Reversed passive hemagglutination.

RPHAMFCA Reversed passive hemagglutination by miniature fast centrifugal analysis.

RP-HPLC Reverse phase - high performance liquid chromatography.

RPI Racial Perceptions Inventory; Recurrent psychiatric illness; Recurrent pyogenic infection(s); Relative percentage index; Resolved pulmonary infiltrate(s); Respiratory rate : pulse rate index (see R/P); Reticulocyte production index; Ribose 5-phosphate isomerase.

RPICCE Round pupil intracapsular cataract extraction.

RPID Recurrent pelvic inflammatory disease.

RP index Respiratory rate : pulse rate index

(see R/P).

RPIPP Reverse phase ion-pair partition.

RPL Recurrent pregnancy loss; Retroperitoneal lymphadenectomy (see RPLAD).

RPL-12 Infectious lymphoid neoplasm (of chickens).

RPLAD Retroperitoneal lymphadenectomy.

RPLC Reverse phase liquid chromatography.

RPLD Repair of potentially lethal damage.

RPLs Random peptide libraries.

RPM Rapid processing mode.

rpm revolutions per minute.

RPMD Rheumatic pain modulation disorder.

RPMI Roswell Park Memorial Institute (Buffalo, New York) (medium).

RPMS Relapsing progressive multiple sclerosis (see RRMS; SPMS); Royal Postgraduate Medical School (London).

RPN Registered Practical Nurse; Renal papillary necrosis; Resident's progress notes.

R_2PN Second year resident's progress notes.

RPNV Regular prenatal visit(s).

RPO Right posterior oblique.

RPP Rate pressure product (= HR {heart rate} x SBP {systolic blood pressure}); Rapidly progressing pancytopenia; Regional placental perfusion (Obstetrics); Retropubic prostatectomy (operation/ urology); Reversible phosphorylation pathway (of metabolism) (see DDP).

RPPC Regional Pediatric Pulmonary Center.

RPPI Role perception picture inventory.

RPPR Red cell precursor production rate.

RPR Rapid plasma/ plasmin reagin (card/ Portnoy's/ serological test for syphilis) (= RPRCF; RPRCT); Reiter protein reagin.

RPRCF Rapid plasma/min reagin complement fixation (test) (see RPR).

RPRCT Rapid plasma/min reagin card test (see RPR).

"r" product moment coefficient of correlation.

RPS Rapid symptom resolution; Reconstructive plastic surgery; Regional pain syndrome (back); Renal pressor substance; Renal Protection Study; Reproductive performance study; Revolutions per second (see rps); Royal Pharmaceutical Society (UK).

rps revolutions per second (= RPS).

RPT Randomized prevention trial; Rapid pull-through; Refractory period of transmission; Registered Physical Therapist; Renal proximal tubule; Retroperitoneal tissue; Rifapentine (a drug used in the treatment of tuberculosis); Routine pregnancy test.

Rpt Report.

RPTA Registered Physical Therapist Assistant; Renal percutaneous transluminal angioplasty.

RPTC Regional Poisoning Treatment Center.

Rptd Ruptured.

RPU Recurrent peptic ulcer.

rPUK Recombinant prourokinase (an anticoagulant used in CVA therapy).

RPV Right portal/ pulmonary vein.

rPV Recombinant protein vaccine.

RPVP Right posterior ventricular pre-excitation.

RPW Repatriated prisoners of war.

RQ Recovery quotient; Reportable quantity; Respiratory quotient (see PFT - RQ).

RQT Ruptured quadriceps tendon.

RR Radiation reaction/ response; Radiation-related; Random/ Relaxation response; Rapid recompression; Rate/ Risk ratio; Recovery room; Reflex relaxation; Regular rate/ respiration(s)/ rhythm; Relative response/ risk; Renin release; Respiratory rate/ reserve/ resistance; Responder rate; Response rate/ ratio; Retinal reflex; Rhematoid rosette(s); Richards-Rundle (syndrome); Riva-Rocci (sphygmomanometer).

R/R Rales-rhonchi.

R&R Rate and rhythm (heart & pulse); Recent and remote; Recession and resection; Rest and recuperation.

R-R Relapsing-remitting (disease).

RRA Race Relations Act (UK); Radioreceptor assay; Refractory recurrent angina; Registered Record(s) Administration/rator; Right renal artery.

RR(A)A Race Relations (Amendment) Act 2000 (UK).

RRAM Rapid rhythmic alternating movements.

RRAR Refractory renal allograft rejection (see ROR; RRE; RRR).

RRC Residency review committee; Risk reduction component; Routine respiratory care; Royal Red Cross (Brit).
R/Rc Renal vein ratio.
RRCA Recurrent renal cell anemia.
RRCC Recurrent renal cell carcinoma (see MRCC).
RR cells Radiation reaction cells.
RRCT Randomized reference controlled trial.
RRCT, no(m) Regular rate, clear tones, no murmurs.
RRD Rhegmatogenous retinal detachment; Roughage-rich diet (see FRD; HBD).
RRE Radiation-related eosinophilia; Rapid renal elimination (= FRE); Refractory/ Renal rejection episode (see ROR; RRAR; RRR); Relative risk estimate; Round, regular, and equal (see RR&E).
RR&E Round, regular, and equal (pupils) (= RRE).
RREF Resting radionuclide ejection fraction.
RRF Reduced/ Residual renal fraction; Right ring finger; Ross River fever (Epidemic polyarthritis) - a viral infection of Eastern Australia, the arthritis component of which appears to be associated with HLA-DR7).
RRHF Rate-related heart failure.
RR-HPO Rapid recompression - high pressure oxygen.
RRI Recurrent respiratory infection; Reflex relaxation index; Relative response index.
RRIS Recurrent respiratory infection syndrome.
RRL Rabies Research Laboratory; Registered Record(s) Librarian.
RRM Riordan repair of muscles (Orthopedics).
RRMS Recurrent rhabdomyosarcoma; Relapsing-remitting multiple sclerosis.
rRNA Ribosomal ribonucleic acid.
RRND Right radical neck dissection.
rRNP Ribosomal ribonucleoprotein.
RROM Resistive range of motion.
RRP Relative refractory period (heart).
RRpm Respiratory rate per minute.
RRQ Rage relief quotient.
RRR Refractory renal rejection (see ROR; RRAR; RRE); Regular rate and rhythm (see RR&R); Relative risk reduction; Renal renin release; Renin release rate/ ratio; Risk rescue rating.
RR&R Regular rate and rhythm (heart/ pulse) (= RRR).
RRRN Round, regular, and react normally (pupils).
RRS Retrorectal space; Richards-Rundle syndrome.
RR (sphyg) Riva-Rocci (sphygmomanometer).
RRT Radio-resistant tumor (Orthopedics); Random response technique; Registered Respiratory Therapist; Relative retention time; Resazurin reduction time.
RRU Respiratory resistance unit.
RS Rabbit serum; Random sample; Rat spleen/ stomach; Rating schedule; Rauwolfia serpentina (see Rs); Raynaud/ Reiter/ Rett/ Roberts/ Russell-Silver syndrome; Recipient's serum; Rectal sinus/ suppository; Rectosigmoid; Reed-Sternberg (cell); Reinforcing/ Relative stimulus; Renal specialist; Resorcinol-sulfur; Respiratory syncytial (virus) (see RSV); Response to stimulus (ratio); Resting subject; Reticulated siderocyte; Review of symptoms; Reye's syndrome (a combination of acute brain disease such as life-threatening encephalitis and fatty invasion of the internal organs in infants and young children; linked to Influenza B, Varicella, the Enteroviruses, Epstein-Barr virus, etc.); Rhythm strip (ECG); Rienke's space (a potential subepithelial space at the margin of the true vocal cord); Right sacrum/ septum/ side/ stellate (ganglion); Ringer's solution; Risus sardonicus (the "sardonic smile" seen in tetanus); Ritchie sedimentation; Robosurgeon/ery; Rocher's sign (see DS - Drawer sign); Romana's sign (palpebral edema, conjunctivitis and satellite lymphadenopathy) - seen in Chagas's disease, when the portal of entry of the parasite, *Trypanosoma* cruzi is the eye (see IC - Inoculation chagoma); Rous sarcoma (virus) (see RSV); Rovsing's sign (for appendicitis).
Rs Rauwolfia serpentina (used in the treatment of hypertension and psychosis); Systemic resistance (total).
rS; r_s Rank correlation coefficient

(Spearman's).
R/S Rest stress; Rupture, spontaneous.
R/s Roentgens per second.
RS 1401 AT Fluocinolone acetonide - a synthetic glucocorticoid used by topical application in the treatment of various allergic and allied skin diseases, such as contact dermatitis, seborrhoeic dermatitis, infantile eczema, neurodermatitis, psoriasis and intertrigo.
RS 2177 Flumethasone pivalate (= Flumethasone trimethylacetate). A synthetic corticosteroid with anti-inflammatory properties, and used by topical application in the treatment of various skin diseases.
RS 3540 Naproxen - a propionic acid derivative and an anti-prostaglandin, used in the treatment of rheumatoid and osteo-arthritis.
RSA Rabbit serum albumin; Regular spiking activity; Rehabilitation Services Administration (HEW); Relative specific activity; Relative standard accuracy; Reticulum (cell) sarcoma; Retrospective analysis (see RA); Right sacroanterior (fetal position); Right subclavian artery.
Rsa Systemic arterial resistance (total).
RSAS Royal Swedish Academy of Sciences.
RSB Regimental Stretcher Bearer; Reticulocyte standard buffer; Right sternal border; Rutner stone basket (see RC - Rutner catheter).
RSC Rat spleen cell; Reed-Steinberg cell; Regional Steering Committee; Reliable statistical comparison; Rested state contraction; Reversible sickle-cell; Rubber shod catheter/ clamp.
RScA Right scapuloanterior (position of fetus).
Rsch Research.
RSCI Right-sided cardiac insufficiency.
RSCN Registered Sick Children's Nurse (Brit).
RScP Right scapuloposterior (postion of fetus).
rscu-PA Recombinant, single-chain, urokinase-type plasminogen activator.
RSD Recommended starting dose; Recurrent shoulder dislocation; Reflex sympathetic dystrophy; Relative standard deviation; Respiratory stress disease (= RSS); Respiratory system disorder; Robotic surgery device (see CARS); Rochester School for the Deaf; Ruptured spinal disc.
RSDS Reflex sympathetic dystrophy syndrome.
RSE Robotic surgery equipment (see CARS).
RSEP Right somatosensory evoked potential.
RSES Rosenberg Self-Esteem Scale.
RSF Renal stone formation (= Nephrolithiasis); Rheumatoid synovial fluid; Right-sided failure (congestive/ cardiac).
RSH Royal Society of Health.
RSI Radiation 'seed' implant; Repetition/itive strain/ stress injury.
RSIC Radiation Shielding Information Center.
R-SICU Respiratory-surgical intensive care unit.
R-SIRS Revised, Seriousness of Illness Rating Scale.
RSIVP Rapid-sequence intravenous pyelogram/raphy (X-ray/ kidneys).
RSL Right sacrolateral (position of fetus).
RSLD Repair of sublethal damage.
RSM Reversible systemic metabolism; Risk screening model; Royal Society of Medicine.
RSMR Relative standard mortality rate.
RSN Right substantia nigra.
RSNA Radiological Society of North America.
RSO Resident Surgical Officer; Right salpingo-oophorectomy (operation/ gynecology); Right superior oblique (muscle).
RSP Raster scanning process (heavy ion beam therapy for cancer tumors); Removable silicone plug; Repeated self-poisoning; Resting size of pupil (Neurology); Retrosternal pain; Right sacroposterior (position of fetus); Rucksack palsy (caused by traction on the upper trunk of the brachial plexus).
RSPA Royal Society for the Prevention of Accidents.
RSPCA Royal Society for the Prevention of Cruelty to Animals.
RSP dialyzer Recirculating single pass dialyzer.
RSPH Royal Society for the Promotion of Health (Brit).
RSPK Recurrent spontaneous psychokinesis.
RSR Regular sinus rhythm (heart); Relative

survival rate; Renal sodium retention; Right superior rectus (muscle).
rSr An electrocardiographic complex.
RS(RA) Latex fixation test for rheumatoid arthritis.
R/S ratio Response/stimulus ratio.
RSS Rat stomach strip; Rectosigmoidoscopy; Resectoscope (Wolf); Respiratory stress syndrome (see RSD); Right-sided stomach; Robotic Surgery/ Surgical System (see CARS); Russell-Silver syndrome; Russian spring-summer (encephalitis) (see RSSE).
RSSE Russian spring-summer encephalitis.
RSSR Relatively slow sinus rate.
RST Radiosensitivity test(ing); Rank-sum test (Wilcoxon) (see WRST); Raster scan(ning) technique (see RSP); Reagin screen test; Renal support treatment (i.e. dialysis); Reticulospinal/ Rubrospinal tract; Right sacrotransverse (position of fetus); Right-sided thoracotomy.
R_{st} The distance that a spot of a substance has moved, relative to a reference standard spot (in paper or thin layer chromatography).
RSTI Radiological Service Training Institute.
RSTL Relaxed skin tension lines.
RSTMH; RSTM&H Royal Society of Tropical Medicine and Hygiene (Brit).
RSTS Retropharyngeal soft tissue space.
RSTs Rodney Smith tubes.
RSV Recombinant subunit vaccine; Resistant strain of virus (see RVS); Respiratory syncytial virus (= CCA or Chimpanzee coryza agent); Right subclavian vein; Rous sarcoma virus).
RSVC Right superior vena cava.
RSVP Please reply (Fr. Repondez s'il vous plaît); Retired senior volunteer program.
RSW Right-sided weakness.
RT Radiation therapy (see RATx); Radiologic/ Respiratory Technologist/gy; Radiotelemetry; Radiotherapy (see RATx); Radium/ Recreational/ Respiratory therapy; Rapid tranquilization; Reaction/ Recovery/ Reduction/ Repetition/ Response/ Retention time (= TR); Reading task/ test; Reciprocating tachycardia; Rectal/ Room temperature; Registered Technician (American Registry of X-Ray Technicians); Renal transplant(ation); Resistance transfer; Respiratory Therapist/ tract; Rest tremor; Retransformation; Reverse transcriptase; Ribose titer; Right (see R); Right thigh; Rubinstein-Taybi (syndrome); Rubin tube (for insufflation of fallopian tubes); Running total.
Rt Right (see R); Total resistance.
rT Ribothymidine.
rt right (see R).
R/t Related to.
RT3; rT_3 Resin/ Reverse triiodothyronine.
RT4; rT_4 Resin/ Reverse thyroxin(e) (serum).
RTA Renal tubular/le acidosis/ atrophy; Reverse transcriptase assay; Road traffic accident.
RTAD Renal tubular acidification defect.
RT(ARRT) Radiologic Technologist (certified by the American Registry of Radiologic Technologists).
RTC Random Trial Control (see RCT); Rape/ Residential treatment center; Renal transplant clinic; Renal tubular cell; Research and training center; Return to clinic; Ribofuranosyl-triasole-carboxamide; Round the clock.
RTD Reaginic tissue damage; Recent trophoblastic disease; Recommended therapeutic/ total dose; Renal tract dilation (pathological/ physiological); Renal-transplant donor; Renal tubular damage; Reproductive/ Respiratory tract disease/ disorder (see RTI); Routine test(ing) dilution(s).
Rtd Retarded.
RTDS Right-to-Die Society (Canada).
RTE Restricted tendon excursion; Reverse-transcriptase enzyme (see NNRTIs; NRTIs; RTI).
RTECS Registry of Toxic Effects of Chemical Substances.
RTER Return to emergency room.
R test Reductase test.
rt^{ext} right upper extremity.
rt_{ext} right lower extremity.
RTF Resistance transfer factor; Respiratory tract fluid; Return to flow.
RTG Radiotherapy group (of patients); Revalidation Technical Group (GMC, UK); Reverse transcriptase gene.
RTG-2 Rainbow trout gonadal tissue cells.
RTI Research Triangle Institute (US);

Respiratory tract illness/ infection; Reverse transcriptase inhibition/tors (see AIDS): AZT - Zidovidine or Retrovir (Glaxo-Wellcome) (Azidothymidine, 3'-azido-3'deoxythymidine; BW A509U; Compound S; ZVD) (see AZT); ddl - Didanosine or Dideoxyinosine = Videx (Bristol-Myers Squibb) (see ddl); ddC - Dideoxycytidine or HIVID (Hoffmann La Roche) (see ddC); d4T - Zerit (Bristol- Myers Squibb); 3TC - Epivir (Glaxo-Wellcome); Nevirapine - Viramine (Boehringer Ingelheim); "1592" (Glaxo-Wellcome), reputedly ten times as powerful as AZT; Delaviridine (Pharmacia & Upjohn); Reversible thrombin inhibitor (see SRDTI).

RTL Reaction/ive to light.

RtL Right-to-left; Ropinirole-to-levodopa (ratio, in the treatment of Parkinson's disease).

rtl rectal.

rt lat right lateral.

RTM Radioisotope test meal; Registered trademark; Routine treatment, medical (see RMT).

RTN Renal tubular necrosis; Retrograde transvenous neuroperfusion.

RT(N)(ARRT) Radiologic Technologist (Nuclear Medicine) (certified by the American Registry of Radiologic Technologists).

rTNF Recombinant tumor necrosis factor.

RTNM Retreatment staging of cancer.

RTO Return to office; Right toe-off.

RTOG Radiation therapy oncology group.

RTP Regional Transplant Program; Renal transplant(ation) patient; Retro-transposon (see CMD-FT); Reverse transcriptase-producing (agent).

rt-PA Recombinant human tissue-type plasminogen activator.

RTPCR; RT-PCR Reverse-transcriptase-polymerase-chain-reaction (assay).

RTR Recreational Therapist, Registered; Red blood cell turnover rate; Renal transplant recipient (see KTR); Renal tubular reabsorption; Retention time ratio.

RT(R)(ARRT) Radiologic Technologist (Radiography) (certified by the American Registry of Radiologic Technologists).

RTRD Registry of Tissue Reactions to Drugs (AFIP).

RTRR Return to recovery room.

RTS Real time scan; Regional tracking system; Renal tubular secretion/ system; Reproductive toxicity study; Return to sender; Right toe-strike; Rothmund-Thomson syndrome (see PDC); Rubinstein-Taybi syndrome.

RTT Radiation Therapy Technician; Refractory testicular tumor.

RT(T)(ARRT) Radilogic Technologist (Radiation Therapy) (certified by the American Registry of Radiologic Technologists).

RTU Relative time unit.

RtU Ready-to-use.

RT3U; rT_3U Resin/ Reverse triiodothyronine uptake (laboratory test/ endocrinology).

RTUS Realtime ultrasound.

RTV Room temperature vulcanization (= Room-temperature-vulcanizing).

RTW Return to work (see R/W).

RTWD Return to work determination.

RTx Radiation therapy.

RU Radioulnar; Rat/ Reading/ Resistance/ Roentgen (Röntgen) unit; Reading of unknown; Residual urine; Resin uptake; Retrograde urogram; Right upper; Routine urinalysis (see RUA).

Ru Ruthenium (Z = 44) (see Elements - Ruthenium).

ru radiation unit.

RU-1 Human embryonic lung fibroblasts.

RU 486 Mifepristone (an abortifacient, contraceptive drug).

RUA Refractory unstable angina; Right upper arm; Routine urine analysis (= RU).

RUAF Recurrent uric acid formation.

rub red (L. ruber).

RUCM Rutgers University College of Medicine.

RU_{creat} Urine concentration of creatine, right kidney.

RUD Recreational use of drugs (see CDUD; CUD; EUD); Recurrent ulcer of the duodenum (duodenal bulb).

RUE Rare undesirable effect; Right upper extremity.

RU-EF-Tb Isoniazid.
RUG Retrograde urethrogram.
RUI Royal University of (Northern) Ireland.
RUL Right upper lid (eyelid)/ lateral/ limb/ lobe (of lung).
RuMP Ribulose monophosphate pathway.
RU_{Na} Urine concentration of sodium, right kidney.
RUO Right ureteral orifice.
RUOQ Right upper outer quadrant (site of injection).
RUP Right upper pole (of kidney).
Ru5-P Ribulose-5-phosphate.
rupt rupture(d).
RUQ Right upper quadrant.
RUR Resin-uptake ratio (nuclear medicine).
RURTI Recurrent upper respiratory tract infection.
RUS Radioulnar synostosis; Renal ultrasound.
RUSB Right upper sternal border.
Rus P Russian Pharmacopeia.
Russ Russian.
RUT Rapid urease test (see HUT).
RUV Residual urine volume.
RUX Right upper extremity.
RV Random variable; Rat/ Rauscher/ Rhino/ Rubella virus; Rectovaginal; Reinforcement value; Renal vein; Reserve volume; Residual/ Respiratory volume - the volume of air left in the lungs after full forced expiration (see PFT); Resveratrol (a natural antifungal antioxidant found in grapes, thus making wine, particularly red wine, an effective cardiovascular protective, since it is said to raise HDL cholesterol in the liver, reducing 'stickiness' of thrombocytes or blood platelets and deterring formation of artery-blocking clots); Retroversion; Retrovirus; Return visit; Rheumatoid vasculitis; Rhinovirus (cause of the common cold); Ribavirin (a guanosine analogue used in treating Lassa fever and other viral diseases); Right ventricle/cular; Rotavirus; Rubella vaccine; Russell viper.
R_v Radius of view.
RVA Re-entrant ventricular arrhythmia; Resistant ventricular arrhythmia (see torsade de pointes); Retinal visual acuity; Right ventricle/cular activation; Right vertebral artery.
RVAD Right ventricular assist device.
RVAW Right ventricle anterior wall.
RVB Red venous blood.
RVC Rectovaginal constriction; Retrograde ventriculoatrial conduction (a harbinger of symptoms of the pacemaker syndrome); Rinse-vomit cycle - associated with binge eating or the "bingeing syndrome" in bulimia nervosa.
RVD Regurgitant/ Renal/ Reno valvular disease; Relative/ Right vertebral density; Retinal vein/ venous dilatation; Right ventricular dilatation/ dimension/ dysfunction/ dysplasia.
RVDO Right ventricular diastolic overload.
RVDV Right ventricular diastolic volume.
RVE Right ventricular enlargement.
RVECP Right ventricular endocardial potential.
RVEDD Right ventricular end-diastolic diameter.
RVEDP Right ventricular end-diastolic pressure.
RVEDV Right ventricular end-diastolic volume.
RVEDVI Right ventricular end-diastolic volume index.
RVEF Right ventricular ejection fraction; Right ventricular end-flow.
RVET Right ventricular ejection time.
RVF Renal vascular failure; Residual volume fraction (of the calf muscle pump) - RVF = RV/VV x 100 (RV = Residual volume; VV = Functional venous volume) - after ten tiptoe movements at the rate of one per second; Rift Valley fever (caused by a flavivirus of the *Phlebotomus* group of the *Bunyaviridae* and transmitted by the *Culex* mosquito); Right ventricular failure/ function; Right visual field.
RVFP Right ventricular filling pressure.
RVG Radionuclide ventriculography; Relative Value Guide; Right ventral gluteus (muscle); Right visceral ganglion.
RVH Recurrent vascular headache; Renal/ Reno vascular hypertension; Right ventricular hypertrophy.
RVHD Rheumatic valvular heart disease.
RVI Relative value index; Right ventricle infarction.

RVIDd Right ventricle internal dimension diastole.
RVIT Right ventricular inflow tract.
RVL Radical vein ligation; Right vastus lateralis (muscle).
RVLG Right ventrolateral gluteal (site of injection).
RVM Right ventricular mean.
RVO Regional Veterinary Officer; Relaxed vaginal outlet; Retinal vascular/ vein occlusion; Right ventriclar outflow/ overactivity.
RVOT Right ventricular outflow tract.
RVP Red veterinary petrolatum; Resting venous pressure; Revascularization procedure; Right ventricular pressure.
RVPEP Right ventricular pre-ejection period.
RVPFR Right ventricular peak filling rate.
RVPRA Renal vein plasma renin activity (= RVR).
RVPW Rat ventral prostate weight.
RVR Rapid/ Repetitive ventricular response; Reduced vascular response; Renal vascular resistance; Renal vein renin (activity) (see RVPRA); Resisitance to venous return; Rhinovirus receptor (= ICAM-1) (see ICAM-1).
RVRA Renal vein/ venous renin activity/ assay.
RVRC Renal vein renin concentration.
RVS Rabies vaccine, adsorbed; Recto/ Retro vaginal space; Relative value scale/ schedule/ studies/ study; Reported visual sensation; Resistant viral strain (= RSV).
RVSF Right ventricular systolic function.
RVSO Right ventricle/cular stroke output.
RVSW Right ventricle/cular stroke work.
RVSWI Right ventricle/cular stroke work index.
RVT Recurrent venous thrombosis; Recurrent ventricular tachycardia; Renal/ Retinal vein thrombosis.
RVTE Recurrent/urring venous thromboembolism.
RV-TLC; RV/TLC Residual volume/total lung capacity (= Ratio of residual volume to total lung capacity or compliance) (see PFT).
RVU Relative value unit.
RVV Reassortant/ Rota virus vaccine; Reserve venous volume; Rubella vaccine-like virus; Russell viper venom (time).
RVVT Russell's viper venom time (= RVV).
RW Radiological warfare; Ragweed; Respiratory work; Round window.
R/W Return to work (= RTW).
R-W Rideal-Walker (phenol coefficient test); Romano-Ward (syndrome); Rose-Waaler (test) (see SCAT; DAT).
RWAGE Ragweed antigen E.
RWE Renal water excretion (see WED).
RWG Recommend weight gain (Obstetrics).
RWIS Restraint and water immersion stress.
RWL Rapid weight loss.
RWM Regional wall motion.
RWP Ragweed pollen; R-wave progression.
RWS Ragweed sensitivity.
Rx Radiotherapy (see RXT).
Rx; R_X (= Rp; R_p) Drug(s); Medication; Pharmacy; Prescribe; Prescription; Prescription drug; Take (thou) (L. recipe); Therapy; Treatment.
r(X) Right X chromosome.
RXLI Recessive X-linked ichthyosis.
RXN Reaction.
RXT Radiation therapy (= Rx); Right exotropia.
RxTFC "Rx. Twenty First Century" (a computer software program, used among other things, to document pharmaceutical services).
R-Y Roux-en-Y (anastomosis).

S

S Antigen - found in human sera (challenged by sarcoma); Code (Wyeth Laboratories USA), for experimental substances; Desoxycortisol; Electrocardiography (S wave), a negative deflection following an R wave; Entropy; Exposure time; Half (L. semis) (see s); Left (L. sinister) (see s); Mean dose per unit cumulated activity; Midpoint of the sella turcica (point); Relative storage capacity; Sacral (in vertebral formulas); Saline; Salmonella; Saturated/ration; Schistosoma; Schizophrenia; Second (see sec); Secretion, e.g. S_{cr} = Secretion of creatinine; Section (see s); Sedimentation coefficient (see S - Svedberg unit) (= s); Sella (turcica); Semilente (insulin) (see Insulin - SI i); Semis L. = half; Sen - coin representing one hundredth of a riel (Cambodia), rupiah (Indonesia), or yen (Japan); Senate (US); Senile/lity; Sensation/ Sensorium/ Sensory (see sens); Sensitive/vity (see sen); Sepsis (see s); Septum; Sequential analysis (drug study); Serine; Serum; Shigella (= Sh; Shig); Siderocyte; Siemens; Signa (L.) - label, let it be labeled, marked or written, mark, write (= Signetur; s); Signature (prescription); Signetur (L.) (see S - Signa); Silicate; Simulium; Sine (L.) = without; Single (marital status/ unmarried) (= s); Singular (see sing); Sister; Slope; Smooth (colony) (= see S - bacterial colonies); Soft (diet) (see S diet); Solid; Soluble, e.g. S antigen, S insulin (see Insulin - SI ii), etc.; Solute; Son (= s); Sone (unit); South (= So); Space; Spatial; Special (precautions necessary for test) (see sp); Spherical; Spherical lens; Spirillum; Spleen; Standard (normal deviation); Staphylococcus; Stem (cell); Stimulus; Streptococcus; Streptomyces; Streptomycin (on culture/ sensitivity reports); Subject (of an experiment/ psychlology/ etc.); Subjective findings; Substrate; Suction; Sulfur (Z = 16) (see Elements - Sulfur); Sum (of an arithmetic series) (= s); Supervision; Supramamillary (nucleus); Supravergence; Surface; Surgeon/ery; Susceptible (to antibiotics - see MS; R); Suture; Svedberg (unit of sedimentation coefficient) (= 10^{-13} second); Swine; Swiss (mouse); Symbol (see Symbols); Synthesis (of DNA in cell cycle); Systole; Wave (on the electrocardiogram); Without (L. sine) (see s; Write/ Let it be written (prescription notation) (see S - Signa).

s atomic orbital with angular momentum quantum number 0; distance; half (L. semis) (= S); left (L. sinister) (= S); length of path; sample standard deviation; satellite (chromosome); scruple (apothecaries); second (unit of time) (see sec); section (see S); sedimentation coefficient (see S - Swedberg); see; sensation/ sensorium/ sensory (see sens); sensitive/vity (see sen); sepsis (= S); series; sign(ed); single (see S); singular (see sing); smooth (see S); soluble (see S); son (see S); suckling; sum (see S); without (L. sine) (= S; Σ; s̄); write/ label (see S - Signa).

s̄ without (L. sine) (see s; Symbols - 5, Medicine and Pharmacy).

Σ Sigma - the 18th (Capital) letter of the Greek alphabet; See Symbols 5, Medicine and Pharmacy: Sum/ Summation of series (= S); Syphilis (euphemistic abbreviation); Without (L. sine) (see s).

σ conductivity; cross section; millisecond or one-thousandth part of a second; molecular bond/ type; sigma - the 18th (lower case/ small) letter of the Greek alphabet; standard deviation (population); stress; surface tension; wave number (see Symbols - 5).

s- symmetric isomer.

ΔS Entropic variation (see Symbols - 2, Calculation).

S1-S5 First to fifth sacral nerves.

S_1 First heart sound.

s^{-1} cycles per second.

S_2 Second heart sound.

$-S_2-$ Dithio (Chemical group).

s^2 sample variance.

S_3 Third heart sound (ventricular gallop).

4 S Scandinavian Simvastatin Survival Study.

S_4 Fourth heart sound (atrial gallop); A protein fraction in normal serum with a sedimentation coefficient of four S-units (= Sedimentation or Svedberg units).

S_7 A protein fraction in normal human serum.

S_{19} Normal ultracentrifugal macroglobulin, a protein fraction in normal human serum.

Sλ Symptoms or signs (see Symbols - 6, Numeration - λ/ lambda/ 30).

S 46 Pheneturide (= Ethylphenacemide). An anticonvulsant drug, used chiefly in the treatment of major and temporal lobe epilepsy.

S 62 Chlorphentermine hydrochloride. An anorectic agent used in the treatment of obesity.

S 768 Fenfluramine hydrochloride. An anorectic agent used in obesity and claimed to have no stimulating effect on the central nervous system.

S 1942 Bromophos. An organophosphorus insecticide.

SA According to the art (L. secundum artem) (see sa); Saddle area (i.e. pelvis); Salaam activity (i.e. seizures); Salicylic acid; Saline (solution) (see Sa); Salt added; Salvation Army; Sarcoidosis; Sarcoma (see Sa); Scalenus anticus; Science Abstracts (IEE, UK/ journal); Science American (journal); Secondary amenorrhea/ anemia/ arrest; Self/ Semen/ Spectrum analysis; Self assessment (see S-A); Sensitizing antibody; Serum albumin/ aldolase; Sex appeal; Sexual addict; Short-acting (drug); Simian adenovirus; Sinoatrial/ Sinoauricular (node) (see S-A); Sinus arrest/ arrhythmia; Skin-adipose (unit); Sleep apnea; Slightly active; Slowly adapting (receptors); Social acquiescence; Society of Actuaries; Soluble in alkaline (medium/ solution); South Africa/ America; Soybean agglutinin; Spanish American; Specific/ Spiking/ Sympathetic activity; Spinal anesthesia; Standard accuracy; State of anxiety; Statistical analysis; Stimulus artifact; Stokes/ Adams (attacks/ syndrome); Subarachnoid; Subject to approval; Succinylacetone; Suicide alert/ attempt; Surface antigen/ area; Surgical assistant; Sustained action (see S-A); Systemic aspergillosis.

Sa Saline (solution) (= SA); Samarium (now, symbol: Sm; Z = 62) (see Elements - Samarium/Sm); Sarcoma (= SA); Staphylococcus aureus; The most anterior point of the anterior contour of the sella turcica.

sA Statampere.

sa according to the art/ by skill (L. secundum artem) (= SA); sufficient water (L. sufficiente aqua).

S-A Self-assessment (= SA); Sinoatrial/ Sinoauricular (node) (= SA); Sustained action (= SA).

S/A Same as.

S/A; S&A Sickness and accident (insurance); Sugar and acetone (laboratory/ urinanalysis).

S_2A Second heart sound, aortic component.

SA 446 2R,4R-2-(hydroxyphenyl)-3-(3-mercaptopropionyl)-4-thizolidine-carboxylic acid - Santen, Osaka, Japan. An angiotensin-converting enzyme inhibitor (see SQ 14225).

SAA Same as above (S = Same, A = As, A = Above); Serum A related protein; Serum amyloid A; Serum aspartate aminotransferase; Severe aplastic anemia; Short-/Slow-acting agent/ analgesic (see SAD); Sidero-achrestic anemia; Single article announcement (ACS custom information service); Small-airway abnormalities/ty; Specific anesthetic agent; Speech Association of America; Spondylarthritis ankylopoetica (Ankylosing spondylitis); Stokes-Adams attack (see SA; SAS); Sympathoadrenal axis.

SAADD Society for the Advancement of Anaesthesia in Dentistry Digest (UK journal).

SAAM 26 A computer program for the analysis of data in terms of models.

SAAOT South African Association of Occupational Therapists.

SAAP Span-aid abduction pillow (Orthopedics).

SAARD Slow-acting antirheumatic drug.

SAAST Self-administered alcohol screening test.

SAAT Serum alanine aminotransferase; Serum aspartate aminotransferase (= SAST).

SAB Science Advisory Board (EPA); Serum albumin; Short-acting barbiturate (e.g. Thiopental); Significant asymptomatic bacteriuria; Sinoatrial/ Subarachnoid block; Society of American Bacteriologists; Spontaneous abortion; Stomach acid barrier; Subacromial bursa; Subarachnoid bleed.

Sα1AB Selective alpha 1A - blocker (e.g.

Tamsulosin) (used in the treatment of BPH).

SAb Spontaneous abortion (= SAB).

SABE Subacute bacterial endocarditis (see SBE).

SABENA Such a bloody experience never again! (after the terrorist PLO attack on the Sabena aircraft at Ben Gurion Airport, Lod, Israel, on May 8, 1972).

SABP Spontaneous acute bacterial peritonitis.

SABS Span-aid bed support (for patients with back injury or after laminectomy).

SABT Systemic antibacterial therapy (= SAT).

SAC Saccharin (see sacch); Sacrum; Screening and acute care; Seasonal allergic conjunctivitis; Self-Assessment of Communication (scale); Serum albumin concentration; Shock-absorbing cartilage; Short-arm cast; Single-agent chemotherapy; South Australian Clinics (journal); Sub-area advisory council; Subarticular cyst; Substance abuse counselor.

Sac LSD-25 (sacrament) (see LSD; LSD 25).

SACA Synergistic anticonvulsant activity.

SACB Selective adrenoceptor blocker (see SACBA); South African Cancer Bulletin (NCASF journal); Stereotactic automated core biopsy (= SALCB).

SACBA Selective adrenoreceptor blocking agent (α1-; β1-).

SACC Short arm cylinder cast.

sacc cogwheel (respiration).

sacch saccharin (= SAC).

SACD Subacute combined degeneration (of the spinal cord).

SACE Serum angiotensin-converting enzyme.

SACED Self-Assessment and Continuing Education Program.

SACG Secondary angle closure glaucoma.

SACH Save A Child's Heart (a volunteer Israeli, worldwide cardiac surgery, organization program since 1995); Small Animal Care Hospital; Solid ankle, cushioned heel (prosthesis or prosthetic foot).

SACHT Serum antichromotrypsin.

SACS Secondary anticoagulation system; Systemically administered corticosteroid.

SACSF Subarachnoid cerebrospinal fluid.

SACT Single-agent chemotherapy (see SAT); Sinoatrial conduction time.

SAD Scale of Anxiety and Depression; Schizo-affective disorder (mania, depression, and psychosis); Seasonal affective disorder; Selective antibiotic decontamination (with oral systemic antibiotics); Self-Assessment Depression (scale); Serious/ Severe/ Significant allergic disease/ disorder; Sexual aversion disorder; Short-/Slow-acting drug (= SAA); Short -axis diameter; Skin appendages disease/ disorder; Small airway disease; Small-artery disease (= SAL); Social-anxiety disorder/ distress; Source-to-axis distance; Subacute dialysis; Substance-abuse disorder (such as alcohol, cocaine and other drugs, on the brain); Sugar, acetone, and diacetic acid; Sugar and acetone determination; Suppressor-activating determinant; Symptomatic atherosclerotic disease/ disorder; Systemic autoimmune disease.

SaD Supply-and-demand (see S/D).

SADD Short-Alcohol Dependence Data (questionnaire); Standardized assessment of depressive disorders; Students Against Drunk Driving.

SADH Succinic acid dimethyl hydrazide.

SADL Satisfaction with amplification in daily life (hearing aid); Simulated activities of daily living.

SADQ Severity of Alcohol Dependence Questionnaire.

SADR Suspected adverse drug reaction.

SADS Schedule for Affective Disorders and Schizophrenia; Self-assessment depression scale.

SADS-C Schedule for Affective Disorders and Schizophrenia - Change.

SADS-L Schedule for Affective Disorders and Schizophrenia - Lifetime.

SADT Stetson Auditory Discrimination Test.

SAE Self-addressed envelope (see sae); Serious/ Severe/ Sexual/ Significant/ Solicited/ Systemic adverse effect (see SAR)/ event/ experience(s); Short above-elbow (cast); Specific action exercise; Subcortical arteriosclerotic encephalopathy; Supported arm exercise.

sae self-addressed envelope (= SAE).

SAEB Sinoatrial entrance block.

SAEM Society for Academic Emergency

Medicine.

SAEP Salmonella abortus equi pyrogen; Supra-aural earphone (hearing aid).

SAF Polysilicic acid gel impregnated with a fluorescent indicator; Saturated animal fat; Scrapie-associated fibrils; Self-articulating femoral; Serum accelerator factor; Simultaneous auditory feedback; *Staphylococcus* aureus folliculitis; Systolic antigrade flow (heart).

SAFA Soluble antigen fluorescent antibody (test).

SAFE Self Abuse Finally Ends (Psychiatric Program); Simulated aircraft fire and emergency.

SAFSASC Society for the Advancement of Free-Standing Ambulatory Surgical Care.

SAFT Systemic antifungal therapy (= SAT).

SAG Salicyl acyl glucuronide; Swiss agammaglobulinemia.

Sag D Sagittal diameter.

SAGE Senior Action in a Gay Environment.

SAGM Sodium chloride, adenine, glucose, and mannitol.

SAH S-adenosyl-L-homocysteine; Small animal hospital; Subarachnoid hemorrhage; Systemic arterial hypertension.

SaH Sandoz Pharmaceutical (USA) code for experimental substances.

SAHA Seborrhea-hypertrichosis/ -hirsutism-alopecia (syndrome).

SAH-Gr Subarachnoid hemorrhage grade (I to V).

SAHH S-adenosylhomocysteine hydrolase.

SAHIGES Staphylococcus aureus hyperimmunoglobulinemia E syndrome.

SAHMEE Simulator of Assorted Hazardous Malfunctions in Electrical Equipment.

SAHS Sleep apnea-hypersomnolence (syndrome).

SAI Self-Analysis Inventory; Severe aortic insufficiency; Sexual Arousability Inventory; Short-acting insulin (see Insulin); Social Adequacy Index (hearing); Sodium Amytal interview; Steroidal aromatase inactivator/ inhibitor (see ISAI); Systemic active immunotherapy; Without other qualification (L. sine altera indicatione).

SAIA Short-acting insulin analogue.

SAICAR Succino-amino-imidazole-carboxamide ribotide (= Aminoimidazole-N-succinocarboxamine).

SAID Sexually acquired immunodeficiency (syndrome) (see SAIDS); Specific adaptation to imposed demand (principle); Systemic autoimmune disease (e.g. Lupus erythematosus, Polymyositis, Scleroderma, etc.).

SAIDS Sexually acquired immunodeficiency syndrome; Simian acquired immune deficiency syndrome.

SAIMR South African Institute for Medical Research.

SAIT Systemic anti-inflammatory therapy.

SAJ Synarthrodial joint (or Junctura fibrosa) - a form of articulation in which the bony elements are united by continuous intervening fibrous connective tissue or synarthrosis (BNA).

SAJHM South African Journal of Hospital Medicine.

SAJLCM South African Journal of Laboratory and Clinical Medicine (supplement to SAMJ).

SAJMLT South African Journal of Medical Laboratory Technology.

SAJMS South African Journal of Medical Sciences.

SAJOG South African Journal of Obstetrics and Gynecology.

SAJOT South African Journal of Occupational Therapy.

SAJS South African Journal of Surgery (ASSA).

SAKH Surgical assist knee holder (Lanny-Johnson - Orthopedics).

SAL Secondary acute leukemia; Sensorineural activity/ acuity level; Sexual arousal level (esp. in the female); Small-artery lesion (see SAD); Suction-assisted lipectomy.

Sal Salicylate/ylic (see Salicyl); Saline (= sal); Salmonella (see S; Salm); Salt (L. sal) (= sal).

sal according to the rules of art/ the art (L. secundum artis leges/ legis); salicylate/ylic (see Salicyl); saline (see Sal); saliva; salt (see Sal).

sAl Serum aluminium (level).

SAL 12 Sequential analysis of 12 chemistry constituents.

s alc soluble in alkalis.
SALCB Stereotactic automated large-core biopsy (see SACB).
SALH Surgical assist leg holder (knee).
Salicyl Salicylate/ylic (= Sal; sal).
Salm Salmonella (= Sal) (see S).
SALP Serum (total) alkaline phosphatase (see LFTiv; SAP).
salping- prefix meaning tube (Gr. salpigx).
SAM S-adenosyl-L-methionine (= SAME; SAMe); Scanning acoustic microscope; Scanning Auger microphobe; School of Aerospace Medicine (USAF); Scientific American Medicine (publication); Self-administered medication; Severe allergic manifestation(s); Sex arousal mechanism; Society for Adolescent Medicine; Sore aching muscle(s); Sound-activated monkey; Staphylococcal absorption method; Sulfated acid mucopolysaccharide; Surface active material; Surface-to-Air missile; Sympathetic-adreno-medullary (axis) responsible for the flight-or-fight response; Systolic anterior motion/ movement (e.g. of the mitral valve apparatus).
SAM; sAM Soluble adhesion molecule (see sCAM; sICAM; sVCAM).
SAMA Scientific Apparatus Makers Association; South Africa Medical Association; Student American Medical Association.
SAMD S-adenosyl-L-methionine decarboxylase (see SAM-DC); Schizoaffective manic disorder (= SMD).
SAMDC South African Medical and Dental Council.
SAM-DC S-adenosyl-L-methionine decarboxylase (= SAMD).
SAME; SAMe S-adenosyl-L-methionine (see SAM).
SAMEN South African Medical Equipment News (journal).
SAMF Single antibody millipore filtration.
SAMHSA Substance Abuse and Mental Health Services Administration.
SAMI Socially acceptable monitoring instrument (hearing).
SAMJ South African Medical Journal.
"Sammy" 5-adenosyl-L-methionine (= "Happy pill"; SAME; SAMe; SAM-E) - an anti-depressant and anti-rheumatic drug.
SAMO Senior Administrative Medical Officer.
SAMP Simulation analysis and modeling program (PHS).
SAMPE Society for the Advancement of Material and Process Engineering.
SAMS Society for Advanced Medical Systems.
SAMs Surface-to-Air missiles.
SAMT Systemic antimicrobial therapy (= SAT).
S-AMY Serum amylase.
SAN Short-acting nitrate; Side-arm nebulizer; Sinoatrial/ Sinoauricular node (see S-A node); Skin and Allergy News (journal); Slept all night; Solitary autonomous nodule(s) (thyroid); Spinal accessory nerve (= Accessory nerve; 11th Cranial nerve; Nervus accessorius).
S-AN Sinoatrial/ Sinoauricular node (see S-A node).
SANA Sinoatrial-node arrest; South African Nursing Association.
Sanat Sanatorium.
SANC Short-arm navicular cast.
SAND Sinoatrial/ Sinoauricular nodal disease (see SSS).
SANDR Sinoatrial nodal reentry.
sang sanguinous.
sangui- prefix meaning blood (L. sanguis).
sani; sanit sanitarium/tary/tation.
SANJ South African Nursing Journal (SANA).
SA node See S-A node.
S-A node Sinoatrial/ Sinoauricular node (= SA; S-A; SAN; S-AN; SA [node]).
SANS Scale for the assessment of negative symptoms.
SANTA South African National Tuberculosis Association (journal).
S antigen Soluble antigen.
SANWS Sinoatrial node weakness syndrome.
SAO Scottish Association of Opticians; Small airway obstruction; Splanchnic artery occlusion; Systemically administered opioid.
SA_{O2} Oxygen saturation in alveolar gas.
S_{aO2} Oxygen saturation in arterial blood.

SAOB Sulfide antioxidant buffer.

SAODAP Special Action Office for Drug Abuse Prevention.

SAP Schizo-affective psychosis; School-age population; Sensory action potential; Serum acid phosphatase; Serum alkaline phosphatase (see LFT iv); Serum amyloid P; Severe abdominal pain; Shock-absorbing property; Situs ambiguus with polysplenia; SLAM-associated adaptor protein (see SH2D1A; SLAM); Society of Analytical Psychology (UK); Stable angina pectoris; Standardized Assessment of Personality; Staphylococcus aureus protease; Strong Approach Group; Surfactant-associated protein; Systemic arterial pressure.

s ap Apothecary's scruple.

SAPA Science-A Process Approach (AAAS).

SAPD Self-administration of psycho active/tropic drugs.

saph saphenous.

SAPHO Synovitis-acne-pustulosis-hyperostosis-osteomyelitis (syndrome).

SAPK Stress-activated protein kinase.

SAPM Society for the Aid of Psychological Minorities.

Sapon Saponification.

SAPP Self-Assessment Program for Pediatricians; Sodium acid pyrophosphate; Sulfosalicylic acid precipitation procedure (for urine protein) (see KFT).

sapro- prefix meaning putrid (Gr. sapros).

SAPS Short arm plaster splint; Simplified Acute Physiology Score.

SAPX Salivary peroxidase.

SAQ Self-administered questionnaire; Short arc quadriceps (muscle).

SAQC Statistical analysis of quality control.

SAQS Short-arc quadriceps setting (exercise).

SAR Seasonal allergic rhinitis; Seminars in Arthritis and Rheumatism (journal); Serious/ Severe/ Specific/ Systemic adverse/ allergic/ antigenic reaction(s); Serious/ Severe/ Sudden/ System anaphylactic/toid reaction (see FAR; FHR); Sexual Attitude Reassessment (Seminar); Sexual attitude reconstruction; South African Refractionist (Society of Opticians journal); Specific airway resistance; Structure-activity relationship (dentistry); Suspected adverse reaction(s); Sympathoadrenal regulation (of ACS - Adrenocortical steroidogenesis); Systemic arterial resistance.

SAr; Sar Sulfarsphenamine/ Sulpharsphenamine.

SARA Sexually acquired reactive arthritis; Skeletal antiresorptive agent; Superfund Amendments and Reauthorization; System for anesthetic and respiratory administration.

SARAA Serum acetylcholine-receptor-antibody assay (for binding, blocking, and modulating antibody, and used in the diagnosis of myasthenia gravis) (see BAA; MAA).

SARB Selective angiotensin receptor blocker (= AIIA; ARB) (such as Candesartan, Irbesartan, Losartan, Valsartan), used in the treatment of hypertension.

SARC Seasonal allergic rhinoconjunctivitis.

Sarc Sarcoma; Sarcosine.

sarc- prefix meaning flesh (Gr. sarx).

SARD Severe active renal disease.

SARI Selective 5-alpha reductase inhibitor (e.g. Finasteride).

SARS Severe acute respiratory syndrome (the potentially lethal viral infection first appearing in the city of Hong Kong in China, in early spring of the year 2003).

SART Society for Assisted Reproductive Technology.

SART O_2; $S_{ART\ O2}$; $S_{Art\ O2}$ Oxygen saturation in systemic artery.

SAS Saline, agent, and saline; Scalenus anticus syndrome (entrapment of scalene nerve under first rib); Self-rating anxiety scale; Short-acting sedative/ steroid; Short arm spint; Sickle-anemia syndrome; Simpson-Angus Scale (for extrapyramidal disorders); Single agent/ application study; Sinoatrial standstill; Sklar Aphasia Scale; Sleep apnea study (see SAT; SDS)/ syndrome (= SDS); Small animal surgery; Small aorta syndrome; Society for Applied Spectroscopy; Sodium acetate solution; Sodium aluminium sulfate; Sodium amylosulfate; Somatostatin; Space/ Stress adaptation syndrome; Spinal artery stenosis; Standard Arthroscope System (Arthroscopy); Statistical Analysis System; Sterile aqueous solution/ suspension; Stokes-

Adams syndrome; Strategic Armed Services (USA); Students Advocate System (AMA); Subacromial sclerosis/ space; Subaortic stenosis; Subarachnoid space; Subaxial subluxation; Subvalvular aortic stenosis (see ISAS); Sulfasalazine; Supravalvular aortic stenosis; Surface-active substance(s); Synchronous atrial stimulation; Synthetic absorbable suture.

Sas Skeletal anomalies (such as Clubfoot, Hypoplastic limbs, Pes equinovarus, Polydactyly, and Sacral hypoplasia and agenesis (see DRMs).

SASA Sulfapyridine and 5-aminosalicylic acid.

SASE Self-addressed stamped envelope.

Saser Sound amplification by stimulated emission of radiation (of sound quanta or phonons) ("Sound laser").

SASH Saline, agent, saline, and heparin.

SASHEP Study of Accreditation of Selected Health Education Programs.

SASMAS Skin-adipose superficial musculo-aponeurotic system.

SASP Salicylazosulfapyridine.

SASPP Syndrome of absence of the septum pellucidum with preencephaly.

SAST Self-administered Alcoholism Screening Test; Selective arterial secretin injection test; Serum aspartate transferase (see SAAT).

SAT Oxygen saturation (blood); Satellite (see Sat); Scholastic Aptitude Test (psychology); School Ability Test (psychology); Senior Apperception Test (assesses personality conflicts); Serum antitrypsin; Short-acting tablet; Single-agent chemotherapy/ therapy (see SACT)/ trial; Sleep apnea test (see SAS; SDS); Slide agglutination test; Sodium ammonium thiosulfate; Speech awareness threshold; Spermatogenic/ Spontaneous activity test; Standard achievement test; Subacute thyroiditis; Suitable alternative therapy/ treatment; Supraventricular atrial tachycardia (see SVAT); Symptomless autoimmune thyroiditis; Systematic assertive therapy; Systemic antibacterial (see SABT)/ biotic/ fungal (see SAFT)/ microbial (see SAMT) therapy/ treatment; Without thymonucleic acid (L. sine acido thymonucleinico).

Sat Satellite (= SAT); Saturate(d)/turation (see sat); Saturday.

sat saturate (= Sat); saturated (= Sat; satd; sat'd); saturation (= Sat; satn; sat'n).

SATA Spatial average, temporal average.

SATB Special aptitude test battery.

satd; sat'd saturated (see sat).

SATL Surgical Achilles tendon lengthening.

satn; sat'n saturation (see sat).

SATP Spatial average temporal peak; Substance-abuse treatment problem/ program.

sat sol saturated solution.

SAU Statistical analysis unit.

SAUS Statistical Abstract of the United States.

SAV Sequential atrioventricular (pacing); Severe acne vulgaris; Strong Avoidance (group).

SAVAJ South African Veterinary Association Journal.

SAVD Spontaneous assisted vaginal delivery.

SAVE Survival and Ventricular Enlargement (Trial).

SAVMA South African Veterinary Medical Association.

SAW Sexually active woman/ women; Surface acoustic wave.

SaW Sit-and-wait (pathogens) - infectious agents such as viruses.

SAX Strong anion exchanger (chromatography).

SB Bachelor of Science (see BSc); Safety belt; Sandbag; SANTA Bantu (journal); Schwartz-Barter (syndrome); Sengstaken-Blakemore (tube); Serum bilirubin (see LFT iv); Shortness of breath; Sick bay; Sideroblast; Single blind (study)/ breath; Sinus bradycardia; Skin button (see PETS); Small bowel/ business; Sodium balance; Social Biology (journal); Soybean; Spastic bronchitis; Sperm bank; Spina bifida; Spontaneous blastogenesis/ breathing; Standby; Stanford-Binet (Intelligence Scale/ Test) (see SBIS); Stereotyped behavior; Sternal border; Still birth/ born; Sucrida Berna (butylmetanilylurea); Surface binding; Surgical Business (journal); Syringobulbia.

Sb Antimony (L. stibium) (Z = 51) (see Elements - Antimony); Strabismus (eye examination).

sb stilb.

S-B Stanford-Binet (Intelligence Scale) (see SBIS).

S/B Side bending.

S/ß Sickle cell beta-thalassemia.

Sα1B Selective alpha 1 - blocker (e.g. Doxazosin) (used in the treatment of BPH, HTN, etc.).

S-B II Schoemaker-Billroth II (type of intestinal anastomosis).

SBA Septic brucellar arthritis; Serum bactericidal activity; Serum bile acid; Severe bronchial asthma; Sick bay attendant (Navy); Sideroblastic anemia; Small Business Administration; Soybean agglutinin; Spina bifida aperta; Spina Bifida Association (see SBAA); Stand-by assistance/nt; Sympathetic-blocking agent (see SBD); Systemic bioavailability.

SB2A Selective β2 agonist (see SB2-AS).

SBAA Spina Bifida Association of America (= SBA).

S bacterial colonies Smooth bacterial colonies (= S).

SB2-AS Selective beta 2 - adrenoceptor stimulant (e.g. Formoterol, Sal -butamol, Salmeterol, Terbutaline, etc.) - causes less cardiac excitation as the non-selective B2-AS (= SB2A).

SBB Small bowel biopsy; Specialist in Blood Bank (technology); Stimulation-bound behavior.

SBC Serum bactericidal concentration; Small bladder capacity; Society of Biological Chemists; Special back care; Spina bifida cystica (= MMC); Standard bicarbonate (blood); Sterile blood culture; Strict bed confinement; Strict biological control (see SRBCC); Superficial (urinary) bladder carcinoma; Suspected breast cancer/ carcinoma.

$SbCl_3$ Antimony trichloride.

SBCS Standard breast cancer surgery.

SBD Senile brain disease; Severe bone destruction (caused by osteoclasts - as in Multiple myeloma); Small bowel disease/ diverticulitis (e.g. Meckel's diverticulitis); Specific birth defect; Spine/ Spinal bone density; Sputum bacterial density; Structural brain damage/ disease/ disorder; Sympathetic-blocking drug (= SBA); Systemic bleeding disorder.

S-BD Seizure-brain damage (see CVA).

SbDH Sorbitol dehydrogenase.

SBE Breast self-examination; Short below-elbow (cast); Shortness of breath on exertion; Small bowel enema/ enteritis; Standard base excess; Subacute bacterial endocarditis (SABE).

SBECD Sulphobutyl ether beta-cyclodextrin sodium (an excipient).

SBET Society of Biomedical Equipment Technicians.

SB experiment/ study Single blind experiment/ study.

SBF Serologic/ Serum/ Specific blocking factor(s); Skin Bank Fluid - containing a balanced salt solution with sodium, potassium, calcium and magnesium chloride, potassium acid and sodium phosphate, phenol red solution, and plasma, sterilized by filtration, with addition of the antibiotic neomycin sulfate; Skin blister fluid; Soy-based formula (see FFI; IMF); Splanchnic/ Subendocardial/ Subcutaneous blood flow; Stillborn fetus; Synovium biopsy forceps (Arthroscopy).

SB&F AAAS Science Books and Films (journal).

SBFT Small bowel follow-through.

SBG Selenite brilliant green; Stand-by guard; Steroid-binding globulin (see HBG); Strut bone graft; Synthetic bone graft (= SBS).

SBGM Self blood glucose monitoring.

SBH Sea-blue histiocyte; State Board of Health.

SBI Secondary bacterial infection; Severe baseline infection; Small bowel intussuception; Soybean (trypsin) inhibitor (see STI); Spectrum Bioelectrical Impedance (see BIA); Systemic bacterial infection.

SBIC Small Business Investment Company (SBA).

SBIS Stanford-Binet Intelligence Scale (= SB; S-B).

SbKT Antimony potassium tartrate (a drug used to treat infection caused by the parasite *Schistosoma* japonicum) (also called Tartar emetic).

SBL Secobarbital level; Serious/ Severe bone loss; Serious/ Severe/ Significant blood loss; Serum bactericidal level/ lysin; Soybean lecithin; Specific bacteriolysin; Systolic baseline.

sBL Sporadic Burkitt's lymphoma.

SBLA Sarcoma, breast and brain tumors, leukemia, laryngeal and lung cancer, and adrenal cortical carcinoma.

SB-LM Stanford-Binet (Intelligence Test) - Form LM.

SBM Science-based medicine; Spinal bone mass (see SBD).

SBMJ Selections from the British Medical Journal.

SBMS-UC School of Basic Medical Sciences at Urbana Champaign (Illinois).

SBN Skin benign neoplasia (see BSN); Standard book number (now ISBN).

SBN_2 Single-breath nitrogen (test) (see SBNT).

SBNS Society of British Neurological Surgeons.

SBNT Single-breath nitrogen test.

SBNW Single-breath nitrogen washout.

SBO Small bowel obstruction; Spina bifida occulta.

Sb_2O_3 Antimony trioxide.

Sb_2O_5 Antimony oxide (pentoxide).

Sb_4O_6 Antimonious oxide.

SBOD Scleral buckle, right eye (L. oculus dexter).

SBOM Soybean oil meal.

SBOS Scleral buckle, left eye (L. oculus sinister).

SBOT Single-breath oxygen test; Speech, Behavior, and Occupational therapy (see DBEMOS therapy).

SBP Schizobipolar; School breakfast program; Scleral buckling procedure; Seated blood pressure; Semi-barber position (see SSP); Serotonin-binding protein; Severe back pain; Sitting/ Standing blood pressure; Small bowel phytobezoars; Society of Biological Psychiatry; Spontaneous bacterial peritonitis; Standby pacemaker; Steroid-binding plasma (protein); Streptavidin-biotin-peroxidase (linked method or analysis of bound antibodies); Sulfobromophthalein (see BSP); Supine/ Systemic/ Systolic blood pressure.

SBPD Severe borderline personality disorder.

SBPR Society for Back Pain Research (UK).

SBQ Smoking Behavior Questionnaire.

SBQC Small based quad cane.

SBR Scleral and blepharostat ring (keratoplasty - Ophthalmology); Small bowel resection; Spleen-to-body (weight) ratio; Strict bed rest; Styrene-butadiene rubber.

SBRB Small bowel resection bypass.

SBRN Sensory branch of radial nerve.

SBS Sealed/ Sick/ Stuffy building syndrome (see TBS); Serial blood sample(s); Shaken baby syndrome; Short bowel syndrome; Single/ Standard-bypass surgery (see CABG); Sinobronchial syndrome; Skin-biopsy specimen; Small bowel series; Social breakdown syndrome; Split-brain syndrome (an association of symptoms produced by disruption of, or interface with, the connection between the hemispheres of the brain); Standard buffer solution; Straight back syndrome; Synthetic blood (see ABS)/ bone (= SBG) substitute.

SbS Step-by-step (approach to diagnosis; medical/ operative procedure).

SBSS Seligmann's buffered salt solution.

SBStJ Serving Brother Order of St. John (of Jerusalem).

SBT Serum bactericidal titer; Single-blind therapy/ treatment/ trial; Single-breath test; Skull base tumor; Standard behavioral therapy/ treatment; Sulbactam.

SBTI Soybean trypsin inhibitor (see STI).

SBTPE State Boards Test Pool Examination.

SBTT Small bowel transit time.

SBV Singular binocular vision; Symptomatic bacterial vaginosis.

Sbv Pentavalent antimony.

SC Closure of the semilunar valves; Conditioned stimulus; Namely (L. scilicet); Sacrococcygeal; Safety code; Sanitary Corps; Satellite/ Schwann/ Sezary/ Sick/ Sickle (see S-C) cell; Scalenus (muscle); Scapula (see Sc); Schizophrenia (= Schiz); Sciatica; Science/ntific (see Sc); Scintillation counter; Scruple (L. scrupulus) (see sc); Searle, GD & Co. (USA) code for experimental substances; Secondary cleavage; Secretory component; Self/ Supportive care; Semicircular;

Semiclosed; Semilunar (valve) closure; Serum cholinesterase (see LFT iv); Serum calcium (ionized)/ complement/ creatinine; Service-connected; Sex chromatin; Short circuit; Sierra Club (The); Sigmoid colon; Silicone-coated; Single chemical; Skin condition/ conduction; Slow component; Snellen's chart (test type/ eye); Society of Chiropodists (UK); Society for/of Cryosurgery; Sodium citrate; Soluble complex; Spastic colon (see IBS); Special/ Stepped care; Specific conductance; Spinal canal/ cord; Sqamous carcinoma; Statistical control; Statistics Canada; Sternoclavicular (joint); Stratum corneum; Subcellular; Subclavian; Subcommittee; Subcorneal; Subcortical; Subcutaneous(ly) (= sc; scu; SQ; sq; subcut; subq); Succinylcholine (see SCh); Sugar-coated; Sulfur-carbon/ colloid; Superior colliculus; Supracolliculus (brain); Surface colony; Sydenham's chorea (= RC - Rheumatic chorea); Systemic candidiasis; Systolic click.

Sc Scandium (Z = 21) (see Elements - Scandium); Scapula (= SC; SCAP); Science/ Scientific (= SC); Screening.

sC statcoulomb.

sc scruple (L. scrupulus) - measure of weight (= SC); staff constant (cconstant watch over a patient by psychiatric staff); subcutaneous(ly) (see SC); without correction (L. sine correctio) - in eye examination.

S-C Sickle-cell (hemoglobin C anemia/ disease) (= SC).

S&C Sclerae and conjunctivae.

SC# Spinal column/ Supracondylar fracture (see SCF).

5-SC 5-Scysteinyl dopa.

SC 3497 Aminometradine (= Aminometrad; Aminometramide). A relatively weak diuretic whose precise mode of action is unknown; used to control edema in mild cases of congestive heart failure.

SC 9387 Pipamazine. A phenothiazine tranquillizing agent, used chiefly in controlling vomiting associated with anesthesia, radiation therapy, cytotoxic drug therapy, etc. In antiemetic doses it has little sedative action.

SC 9420 Spironolactone (= Spirolactone). A synthetic steroid with a structure resembling that of the natural adrenocortical hormone aldosterone. It acts as a competitive inhibitor of aldosterone, which promotes the retention of sodium and the excretion of potassium by the distal renal tubules. It thus increases sodium and reduces potassium excretion, and so differs from chlorthiazide and similar diuretics which act on the proximal tubules increasing sodium excretion, but do not prevent the excretion of potassium by the distal tubules. Used as a diuretic in the management of edema associated with congestive heart failure, hepatic cirrhosis and ascites, and the nephrotic syndrome, and also in idiopathic edema.

SC 10363 Megestrol acetate (see BDH 1298).

SC 11585 Oxandrolone. A synthetic sex hormone with anabolic and androgenic actions; contraindicated in patients with liver disturbances.

SC 11800 Ethynodiol diacetate. A synthetic sex hormone with progestational actions and a potent inhibitor of ovulation. Used in the treatment of primary and secondary amenorrhea and of functional uterine bleeding, and as a contraceptive, usually in combination with an estrogen such as mestranol.

SCA Self-care agency; Severe congenital anomaly; Sickle-cell anemia (see S-C); Significant clinical activity; Single-channel analyzer; Single-contrast arthrogram/graph(y); Sperm-coating antigen; Spinocerebellar ataxia; Steroidal-cell antibody; Subclavian artery; Subcutaneous abdominal (block)/ administration; Sudden cardiac arrest; Superficial cystic acne; Superior cerebellar artery; Suppressor cell activity; Supracervical amputation (of uterus).

S_{Ca} Serum calcium (see SC).

SCAA Skin Care Association of America; Sporadic cerebral amyloid angiopathy.

SCAB Streptozoticin, CCNU (Lomustine), Adriamycin and Bleomycin (Chemotherapy).

SCAb Autoantibodies/dy to stratum corneum.

SCABG Single coronary artery bypass graft (operation/ heart).

SCACM South Central Association for Clinical Microbiology.

SCAG Sandoz Clinical Assessment - Geriatric

(rating/ scale).
SCAH Self-contained artificial heart.
Scalp The Scalpel (journal).
sCAM Soluble cell adhesion molecule (= SAM; sAM).
SCAMC Symposium on Computer Applications in Medical Care.
SCAMIN Self-Concept and Motivation Inventory.
SCAN Suspected child abuse and/or neglect; Systolic coronary artery narrowing.
Scand Scandinavia(n).
SCAP Scapula (see Sc); Single-chamber atrial pacing.
scapho- prefix meaning boat-shaped (Gr. skaphe).
SCARF Skeletal abnormalities, cutis laxa, craniostenosis, psychomotor retardation, facial abnormalities (syndrome).
SCAT School and College Ability Test; Sheep cell agglutination test (= Rose Waaler test) - immunological assay for Rheumatoid factor; Sickle cell anemia test; Sports Competition Anxiety Test; Stanford Crash Analysis Team.
S-CAT Spaceflight Cognitive Assessment Tool (Psychology test on aeronauts).
Scat Box or package (L. scatula); Scatological.
Scat orig Original/ Manufacturer's package (and label) (L. scatula originalis).
SCB Sentence construction board; Stem cell biology; Strictly confined to bed.
SCBA Self-contained breathing apparatus.
SCBC Small cell bronchogenic carcinoma.
SCBF Spinal cord blood flow.
SCBG Symmetric calcification of the basal cerebral ganglia.
SCBH Systemic cutaneous basophil hypersensitivity.
SCBP Stratum corneum basic protein.
SCBS Serial core-biopsy specimen.
SCBU Special care baby unit.
SCC Science Council of Canada; Sentinel community clinic; Sequential combination chemotherapy; Serum creatinine concentration; Service(s) for Crippled Children; Short-circuit current; Short-course chemotherapy; Sickle Cell Center(s) (NHLI); Sickle cell crisis; Small/ Squamous cell carcinoma (see SCCa); Small cleaved cell; Society of Cosmetic Chemists (New York); Spinal cord compression; Standard cubic centimeter (of a gas); State Curriculum Commission; Strict clinical control (see SRBCC); Subcortical cytoplasm.
SCCA Semi-closed circle absorber; Single-cell cytotoxicity assay.
SCCa Small/ Squamous cell carcinoma (= SCC).
SCCB Small-cell carcinoma of the bronchus.
SCCC Squamous cell cervical carcinoma.
SCCH Sternocostoclavicular hyperostosis.
SCCL Small cell carcinoma of the lung.
SCCM Sertoli cell culture medium; Society for Critical Care Medicine.
SCCT Severe cerebrocranial trauma; Subcapsular cell tumor (e.g. Benign adrenal tumor).
SCD Selective cell death (see OCS); Sequential compression device; Service-connected disability; Severe cardiac decompensation; Sickle-cell disease; Spinal canal/ cord damage/ disease; Spinocerebellar degeneration; Stable cardiac disease; Stem-cell donor; Subacute combined degeneration (of the spinal cord); Subacute coronary disease; Subcortical dementia; Sudden cardiac death; Systemic carnitine deficiency.
ScD Doctor of Science (see DSc).
ScDA Scapulodextra anterior (L.) (right scapuloanterior) - position of the fetus.
SCDB Self-contained dropping bottle.
SCDIC Sickle-Cell Detection and Information Center.
S-C disease Sickle-cell hemoglobin C disease.
ScDP Scapulodextra posterior (L.) (right scapuloposterior) - position of the fetus.
SCDS Sprengel's congenital deformity syndrome (see SIT).
SCE Secretory carcinoma of the endometrium; Single contrast enema; Sister chromatid exchange; Split hand - cleft lip/ palate ectodermal (dysplasia); Subcutaneous edema/ emphysema; Sudden coronary event; Supraciliary effusion.
SCe Somatic cell.
SCEH Society for Clinical and Experimental Hypnosis.

SCEMIA Self-contained enzymic membrane immunoassay.
SCEP Sandwich counterelectrophoresis; Spinal and cortical evoked potential (see SSEP).
SCER Sister chromatid exchange rate.
SCF Save the Children Federation/ Fund; Severe cardiac failure; Sigmoidocutaneous fistula; Skin Cancer Foundation; Spinal column fracture (Orthopedics) (= SC#); Standard cubic feet (gas); Supracondylar fracture (e.g. of the femur) (= SC#).
SCFA Short-chain fatty acid (serum).
SCFE Slipped capital femoral epiphysis.
SCFH Standard cubic feet per hour (gas flow).
SCFM Standard cubic feet per minute (gas flow) (= SCF/min; Scf/min).
SCF/min; Scf/min See SCFM.
SCFN Subcutaneous fat necrosis (seen sometimes in pancreatic disease).
SCG Serum chemistry graph; Serum chemogram; Serum chorionic gonadotropin (mIU/ml) (= CGL; SCGL); Sodium cromoglycate; Superior cervical ganglion; Supportive care guideline(s).
SCGL Serum chorionic gonadotropin level (see SCG).
SCGMB La Société Canadienne de Génie Médical et Biologique (= CMBES).
SCGT Somatic-cell gene therapy/ transfer.
SCh Succinylchloride; Succinylcholine (= SC; SUX).
Sch Schering Corporation (USA) code for experimental substances.
SChE Serum cholinesterase.
Sched Schedule.
SCHF Southern California Housestaff Federation.
SCHIN Sowerby Centre for Health Informatics at Newcastle (DoH, UK).
SCHIP State Children's Health Insurance Program (US, since 1997).
SCHISTO Schistocytes.
schisto- prefix meaning split (Gr. schizo).
SCHIZ Schizocytes.
Schiz; schiz Schizophrenia.
Schizo Schizophrenia (journal, now Orthomolec Psychiat).
schizo- prefix meaning divided (Gr. schizein).
SCHL Subcapsular hematoma of the liver.
SCHLP Supracricoid hemilaryngopharyngectomy.
Schoolboy Codeine (see Cod; cod).
SCHT Subclinical hypothyroidism.
SCI Science Citation Index; Science of Creative Intelligence (TM Transcendental Meditation); Seroconversion illness (associated with AIDS); Single component insulin (see Insulin - SCI); Specific cellular immunity; Spinal cord injury; Spontaneous clinical improvement; Structured clinical interview.
Sci Science/ntific.
SC-ICR Southern California Islet Cell Resource (center at COH).
SCID Severe combined immune/ immuno deficiency (disease, disorder or syndrome) (see CSD).
SCIDS Severe combined immunodeficiency syndrome (= SIDS).
SCIDS; SCIDs Severe combined immune/ immuno deficiency syndrome (see CSD).
Science (journal).
SCII Strong-Campbell Interest Inventory.
SCIM Scripps Center for Integrative Medicine (La Jolla, CA).
SC-insulin Single component insulin (see Insulin - SCI).
scint scintigram.
SCIPP Sacrococcygeal to inferior pubic point.
SCIR Society of Cardiovascular and Interventional Radiology (Baltimore, Md, USA).
Sci Res Scientific Research (journal).
SCIS Science Curriculum Improvement Study (NSF funded); Spinal cord injury service.
SCIT Subcutaneous injection technique.
SCITEC Scientific, Engineering and Technological Community of Canada Association.
SCIU Spinal cord injury unit.
SCIV Subclavian/ Subcutaneous intravenous.
SCIWORA Spinal cord injury without radiographic abnormality.
SCJ Sacrococcygeal joint (= Junctura sacrococcygea; SCS; SSC); Scapuloclavicular joint (= ACJ; Articulatio acromioclavicularis); Sclerocorneal junction (between the sclera

and the cornea, marked on the outer surface of the eyeball by a slight furrow); Squamocolumnar junction; Sternoclavicular/ Sternocostal joint.

SCK Serum creatine kinase (laboratory/ chemistry); Straight cutting knife (Arthroscopy).

SCL Scleroderma (= Scl; Scld; Scler; Sclero); Serum copper level; Sinus cycle length; Skin conductance level; Soft contact lens; Sonographic cervical length (Obstetrics); Spinal cord lesion (cervical/ lumbar); Symptom/ Syndrome checklist.

Scl Scleroderma (see SCL); Sclerosed/osis/otic (see scl).

scl sclerosed/osis/otic (= Scl; Scler; Sclero).

ScLA Scapulolaeva anterior (L.) (left scapuloanterior) - position of the fetus.

SCLC Small cell lung carcinoma.

SCLD Sickle-cell chronic lung disease; Suction cup-like device (used in VAD - Vacuum-assisted delivery).

Scld Scleroderma (see SCL).

SCLE Sub/ Subacute cutaneous lupus erythematosus.

Scler Scleroderma (see SCL); Sclerosed/osis/otic (see scl).

Sclero Scleroderma (see SCL); Sclerosed/osis/otic (see scl).

sclero- prefix meaning hard (Gr. skleros).

SCLN Supraclavicular lymph node.

ScLP Scapulolaeva posterior (L.) - left scapuloposterior (position of the fetus).

SCLS Systemic capillary leak syndrome.

SCLs Soft contact lenses.

SCLW Stout continuous loop wire (intradental fixation procedure).

SCM Schwann/ Streptococcal cell membrane; Sensation, circulation, and motion; Society for Computers in Medicine; Society of Community/ Computer Medicine; Sodium colistimethate; Soluble cytotoxic medium; Sonor cephalometry (used in twin pregnancy, etc.) (Obstetrics); Spleen cell-conditioned medium; Spondylitic caudal myelopathy; Standard cubic meter (of gas at STP - Standard temperature and pressure); State Certified Midwife (UK); Sternocleidomastoid; Structure of the cytoplasmic matrix; Superconductive magnet; Surface-connecting membrane.

SCMBP Saratoga Conference on Molecular Biology and Pathology.

SCMC S-carboxymethyl-L-cysteine (a mucoregulatory agent); Select Committee on Medical Ethics (UK); Sodium carboxymethylcellulose (= Sodium cellulose glycollate) - used as a suspending agent for insoluble powders in aqueous preparations; Spontaneous cell-mediated cytotoxicity.

SCMD Senile choroidal macular degeneration.

SCME Select Committee on Medical Ethics (UK).

SCMO Senior Clerical Medical Officer.

SCN Potassium thiocyanate; Severe chronic nephritis/ neurosis/ neutropenia; Special care nursery/sing; Spindle cell nevus (see BJM); Suprachiasmatic nucleus.

SCNA Surgical Clinics of North America (journal).

SCNB Stereotactic core needle biopsy.

SCNM . Sulfur colloid nuclear membrane (a radiopharmaceutical used in nuclear scanning of bone marrow, lymph nodes and spleen).

SCNRL Soft → Casual → Normal → Raised → Loud (vocal recording with an overall span of about 20 dB - see IL-TASS).

SCNS Subcutaneous nerve stimulation.

SCO Sclerocystic ovary; Sex-change operation; Society for Contemporary Ophthalmology; Society for Cryo-Ophthalmology; Somatic crossing-over; Southern Council of Optometrists; Stem cell operation; Subcapital/ Supracondular osteotomy (Orthopedics); Subcapsular opacity (crystalline lens); Subcommissural organ.

SCOI Southern California Orthopaedic Institute.

SCOLRCS Single-center, open-label, randomized, crossover study.

SCOP; Scop Scopolamine.

SCOPE Scientific Committee on Problems of the Environment; Study on Cognition and Prognosis in the Elderly (Clinical Hypertension Research, Uppsala, Sweden) (see SCOPE).

-scope suffix meaning view (Gr. skopeo).

SCOR Specialized Centers of Research (NHLI).
SCORAD Clinical score of atopic dermatitis.
SCORE Service Corps of Retired Executives (see ACTION).
Scot Scotland/ Scottish.
SCP Self-Care Program; Senior Companion Program (see ACTION); Severe chest pain; Single cell(ed) protein; Single-chamber pacing (= Ventricular pacing); Skin care programme; Sodium cellulose phosphate; Soluble cytoplasmic protein; Somatosensory cortical potential (see SSCP); Spastic cerebral palsy; Spherical candle power (see scp); Squamous cell papilloma; Submucous cleft palate; Sugar-coated pill; Superior cerebral peduncle; Supracondyloid process (of the humerus).
scp spherical candle power (= SCP).
SCPC Serum ceruloplasmin concentration (see CT - Copper toxicosis).
SCPK Serum creatine phosphokinase.
SCPMG Southern California Permanente Medical Group (KPMG or Kaiser Permanente Medical Group).
SCPNT Southern California Postrotary Nystagmus Test.
SCPV Special Virus Cancer Program (see SVCP).
SCR Same/ Similar clinical response; Schick conversion rate; Scruple (see scr); Seclusion/ Special care room; Serious/ Severe cutaneous reaction(s); Severe caloric restriction; Silicon-controlled rectifier; Skin conductance response; Slow-cycling rhodopsin; Solar cosmic rays; Spondylitic caudal radiculopathy; Stem-cell recipient/ replacement/ rescue/ research; Subcutaneous route; Swedish Cancer Registry.
SCr Serum creatinine.
Scr; scr Scruple (= SCR) - a measure of weight = 20 gr (grains or 1.296 g (grams).
SCRAD Standing Committee on Radiation Dosimetry (AAPM).
SCRAM Speech-controlled respirometer for ambulation measurement.
SCRAP Simple complex reaction-time apparatus.
SCRDP Stanford Center for Research in Disease Prevention.
SCRF Scripps Clinic and Research Foundation.
scRNA Small cytoplasmic ribonucleic acid.
SCS Sacrococcygeal symphysis (see SCJ); Saethre-Chotzen syndrome; Schilder's cerebral sclerosis; Severe cerebellar/ cerebral syndrome; Shared computer system; Silicon-controlled switch; Society of Clinical Surgery; Soil Conservation Service (USDA); Spinal cord stimulation/ syndrome (= CSCS; NCSCS); Stable clinical status; Stem-cell science; Still-Chauffard syndrome (see JCA - Juvenile chronic arthritis; Juvenile form of FS or Felty's syndrome; SD - Still's disease); Subchondral spongiosa; Subcutaneous stripping (removal of a varicosed saphenous or other vein, as in Babcock's operation); Supracondular spur (of the humerus) (see SCP); Surgical Classification System (see SGO TLR): (1) easy to use, (2) universally applicable, (3) consistent with oncological principles of treatment, (4) based on staging studies and surgical and functional anatomy, (5) correspondent to the magnitude of surgery, and (6) reproductible. Malawer and Meller developed an SCS for limb-sparing shoulder-girdle resections, divided into six types: Type I. Intraarticular proximal humeral resection, Type II. Partial scapular resection, Type III. Intraarticular total scapulectomy, Type IV. Extraarticular total scapulectomy and humeral head resection, Type V. Extraarticular humeral glenoid resection, and Type VI. Extraarticular humeral and total scapular resection; Systemic corticosteroid; Systolic click syndrome.
SCSA Soil Conservation Society of America.
SCSB Static charge sensitive bed.
SCSIT Southern California Sensory Integration Test.
SCSP Senior Community Service Project (NCA).
SCT Salinity, conductivity, and temperature (meter); Salmon calcitonin (see sCt); Secondary cerebral tumor; Sentence completion test; Sex chromatin test; Sexual compatibility test; Sickle-cell trait; Specific cognitive task; Sperm cytotoxicity; Spinal computed

tomography; Spinocerebellar tract; Spinocervicothalamic; Standard chemotherapy; Standard cytogenetic technique; Staphylococcal clumping test; Stem cell technology/ therapy/ transplant(ation) (bone marrow, for cancer) (see BMT); Sugar-coated tablet; Systemic chelation/ corticosteroid therapy.

sCt Salmon calcitonin (= SCT).

SCTAT Sex cord tumor with annular tubules.

SCTx Spinal cervical traction.

SCTZ Chloromethiazole edisylate (= Chlormethiazole ethanedisulfonate; Chloroethyl-methyl-thiazole; Wy 1485) - a hypnotic drug, with muscle-relaxant and anti-convulsant properties, used in the treatment of delirium tremens and other acute alcoholic states, acute mania, and some types of insomnia.

SCU Self-care/ Special care unit; Sulfur-coated urea (fertilizer).

scu subcutaneous(ly) (see SC).

SCUBA Self-contained underwater breathing apparatus.

SCUD Septicemic cutaneous ulcerative disease.

SCUF Slow continuous ultrafiltration therapy.

SCUFT Slow continuous ultrafiltration therapy (see SCUF).

SCUM Secondary carcinoma of the upper mediastinum.

SCU-PA Single-chain urokinase plasminogen activator.

SCUT Schizophrenic chronic undifferentiated type.

SCV Sacrocaudal vertebrae; Sensory nerve conduction velocity; Smooth, capsulated, virulent (bacteria); Squamous-cell carcinoma of the vulva; Subclavian vein; Subcutaneous vaginal (block).

SCV-CPR Simultaneous compression ventilation - cardiopulmonary resuscitation.

SCVD Supracristal ventricular defect (Cardiovascular).

SCVE Significant cardiovascular event(s).

SCVP Single chamber ventricular pacing.

SCWS Society of Civil War Surgeons (Reynoldsburg, OH).

SCX Strong cation exchanger.

SD Sandhoff/ Stable/ Still's disease; Science Development (program - NSF); Science Digest (journal); Scleroderma; Seborrheic dermatitis; Segmental demyelination; Senile degeneration/ dementia; Septal/ Serum defect; Serodiagnosis; Serologically defined/ detectable/ detected/ determined (antigen); Severely disabled; Sexual dysfunction (see ED - Erectile dysfunction; FSD; MSD); Shell Development Corporation; Shine-Dalgarno (sequence); Short dialysis; Shoulder disarticulation/ dislocation; Shoulder dystocia (occurring by impaction of the anterior shoulder of the newborn against the maternal symphysis pubis, after the delivery of the head, resulting in fractures of the collarbone and humerus, and damage to the brachial plexus with OBP or Obstetric brachial palsy); Shy-Draper (syndrome); Sickle-cell hemoglobin D (see S-D); Single-dose (study/ therapy/ treatment/ trial) (= S/D); Skeletal dysplasia; Skin destruction/ dose; 'Slim disease' (or Enteropathic AIDS, common in Africa and associated with chronic diarrhea); Somatization disorder; Spectrodensitometer; Sperm diaphorase; Sphincter dilatation; Spontaneous delivery; Sporadic/ Spreading depression; Spot diagnosis (see OSCD); Sprague-Dawley (rat); Standard deviation/ diet/ dose (= S/D); Standardized difference (see PSD; SMD); Star dust (cocaine) (see Erythroxylum); Statistical documentation; Steinert's disease (see DM - Dystrophia myotonica); Stensen duct; Stent/ Sterile dressing; Steroid-dependent (see S-D); Stimulus, discriminative (see Sd); Stimulus drive (see Sd); Stone disintegration; Straight drainage; Strength duration (see S-D); Streptodornase; Streptozocin and doxorubicin; Study-disease (drug cost); Sudden death; Superintendent of Documents (GPO); Superoxide dismutase; Surgical drain; Swank diet (a low-saturated fat diet recommended for patients with multiple sclerosis); Systolic discharge.

Sd Stimulus drive (psychology) (= SD).

S-D Sickle-cell hemoglobin D (disease) (= SD); Steroid-dependent (= SD); Strength-duration (curve) (= I-D; SD); Suicide-depression.

S/D Sharp/ dull; Single/ Standard dose (see SD); Supply/ demand; Systolic/ diastolic (blood pressure).

S^d Discriminative stimulus (= SD - Stimulus, discriminative).

S&D Stomach and duodenum.

SDA Sabouraud dextrose agar; Sacrodextra anterior (L.) - right sacroanterior (position of fetus); Same day admission; Serologically defined/ detectable/ detected/ determined antigen(s); Seventh-Day Adventist; Sialodacryoadenitis; Single-dose administration (see SD; S/D); Specific dynamic action/ activity; State Dental Association; Steroid-dependent asthma; Study-drug administration; Succinic dehydrogenase activity; Synthetic decapeptide analogue (e.g. Triptorelin - an analogue of natural GnRH).

SD antigens Serologically defined/ detectable/ detected/ determined antigen(s).

SDAS Same day admission for surgery.

SDAT Senile dementia of Alzheimer's type.

SDB Second degree burn (see PSL); Self-destructive behavior; Sleep-disordered breathing; Society for Developmental Biology; Standards Development Branch (EPA).

SDBP Seated/ Standing/ Supine diastolic blood pressure.

SDC Serum digoxin (= SDL)/ drug concentration; Sleep Disorders Center; Sleep-disorders clinic; Sodium deoxycholate; Specialist drug clinic (for alcohol and drug addicts, UK); Subacute combined degeneration (see SCD); Subclavian (hemo) dialysis catheter; Succinyldicholine.

SD&C Suction, dilation, and curettage.

SDCI Subdermal collagen implant (Zyplast implant - Plastic and Reconstructive Surgery).

SDCL Symptom distress check list.

SDD Selective digestive (tract) decontamination; Severe/ Sporadic depression/ive disorder; Severely debilitating disease (= SDI; SDM); Single/ Standard daily dosage/ dose/ dosing/ drug (see ODA; ODD); Spondylodiscitis; Sporadic distress disease/ disorder; Sterile dry dressing; Sulfonamide-derived drug.

Sd/d Standard deviation of the absolute differences.

SDDS 2-Sulfamoyl-4,4'diaminodiphenylsulfone.

SDE Skin depot effect; Specific dynamic effect; Standard diagnostic evaluation; Subdural empyema.

SDEEG Stereotactic depth electroencephalography.

SDES Symptomatic diffuse esophageal spasm.

SDF Slow death factor; Speech dysfunction (= Dysphonia); Stress distribution factor.

SDFP Single donor frozen plasma.

SDG Self-destruct gene; Sucrose density gradient.

SDH Serine dehydrase; Severe diverticular hemorrhage (colon); Sorbitol/ Succinate/nic dehydrogenase; Spinal dorsal horn; Subdural hematoma.

SDHD Sudden death heart disease.

SDI Selective Dissemination of Information (SSIE) (see SDILINE); Severe depressive illness; Severely debilitating infection/ illness (see SDD); Short duration infusion; Spine Deformity Index; Standard deviation interval; State disability insurance (plan); Survey diagnostic instrument.

S diet Soft diet (= S - Soft).

SDIHD Sudden death ischemic heart disease.

SDILINE Selective Dissemination of Information On-Line (NLM - National Library of Medicine/ data bank) (= SDI).

SDJ Skeletal deformity of jaw.

SDL Serum digoxin (see SDC)/ drug level; Speech discrimination level/ loss.

sdl sideline; subline.

SDM Sensory detection method; Severely debilitating malady (see SDD); Standard deviation of the mean; Streptomycin dependent mutant (Shigella); Superficial dermatomycosis.

SDMC Severe debilitating medical condition.

SDMT Symbol Digit Modalities Test (psychology).

SDN Sexually dimorphic nucleus.

SDNA Single-strand deoxyribonucleic acid.

SDO Sudden dosage/ dose onset.

SDP Sacrodextra posterior (L.) - right sacroposterior (fetal position); Single-dose protocol;

Stomach, duodenum, and pancreas; Systems development project.

SDPD Self-defeating personality disorder.

SDPH Sodium diphenylhydantoin (= Phenytoin).

SDR Signal-to-distortion ratio; Slow dissociation rate (of a drug); Specific dosage regimen; Spontaneously diabetic rat; Standard density reference; Standardized death rate; Surgical dressing room.

SDR; S/DR Systolic/ Diastolic ratio.

S/D ratio Supply/demand ratio.

SDRT Standard Diagnostic Reading Test.

SDS Same day surgery; School Dental Service(s); Self-rating depression scale; Sensory deprivation syndrome; Severe decompression sickness (= Caisson disease) - with aseptic/ avascular necrosis of bone (see CAD); Sexual differentiation scale; Shy-Drager syndrome; Single-dose study/ suppression/ syringe; Sleep disorder syndrome (see SAS); Sodium dodecylsulfate; Specific Diagnosis/ Diagnostic Service; Speech discrimination score; Standard deviation score; Stooped dorsal spine; Sudden death syndrome (see SAS); Sulfadiazine silver; Sulfonamide-derived substance (e.g. HCTZ or Hydrochlorthiazide); Surgical drainage system; Sustained depolarizing shift.

S/DS Sharp/dull sensation.

Sds Sounds.

SD-SK Streptodornase-streptokinase (enzymes).

SDSP Safe dietary-supplement products (see SDSS).

SDS/PAGE; SDS-PGE Sodium dodecylsulfate - polyacrylamide gel electrophoresis.

SDSS Safe dietary-supplement substances (= SDSP).

SDT Sacrodextra transversa (L.) - right sacrotransverse (position of the fetus); Self-/Sero-/Specific diagnostic test; Severe drug toxicity; Signal detection theory; Single donor transfusion; Single-dose trial; Single-drug therapy; Specific drug therapy; Speech detection threshold; Standardized dilution technique (laboratory procedure); Substance-dependence therapy/ treatment.

SD_t Standard deviation of total scores.

SDU Selective drug use; Standard deviation unit; Step-down unit.

SDUB Short double upright brace.

SDV Subdiaphragmatic vagotomy.

SDVB Styrene divinylbenzene.

SDW Separated, divorced, or widowed; Sterile distilled water.

SDWA Safe Drinking Water Act (1974).

SE Saline enema; Sanitary engineer(ing); Seeing Eye (dog for the blind); Self-explanatory; Series elasticity; Side effect(s) (see S/E); Skin electrode; Smoke/ Systemic exposure; Society for Endocrinology (UK); Soft exudates; Solid extract; Southeast; Spatial-emotional (stimulus); Sphenoethmoidal (suture); Spherical/ Starch equivalent; Spin-echo; Spongiform encephalopathy; Spurway-Eddowes (syndrome) (see S-E); Standard error; Staphylococcal endotoxin/ enterotoxin; Starr-Edwards (prosthesis) (see S-E); Status epilepticus; Sterol ester; Subendothelial.

SE# Supination-eversion fracture (see SEF).

Se Secretion; Selenium (Z = 34) (see Elements - Selenium).

S-E Side-effect (see S/E); Spurway-Eddowes (syndrome) (= SE); Starr-Edwards (prosthesis) (= SE; S-E prosthesis; S-E valve).

S/E Side effect(s) (= SE).

S&E Safety and efficiency.

^{75}Se Radioactive selenomethionine (75) (nuclear medicine).

SEA Serotonergic agent; Sheep erythrocyte agglutination (test) (see SEAT); Shock-elicited aggression; Soluble egg antigen; Spontaneous electrical activity (physiology); Staphylococcal enterotoxin A; Subepidermal abscess; Surgical Educational Authorities/ity.

SEAE Severe esophageal adverse experience.

SEAMHO Southeast Asia Medical and Health Organization (WHO - UN).

SEAT; SEA test Sheep erythrocyte agglutination test (= SEA).

SEB Seborrhea; Society for Experimental Biology (US); Staphylococcal enterotoxin B.

SEBA Staphylococcal enterotoxin B antiserum.

Se-bis Cibis ski needle (Ophthalmology).

SEBL Self-emptying blind loop.

SEBM Society for/of Experimental Biology

and Medicine.

SEC Secretin; Securities and Exchange Commission; Singapore epidemic conjunctivitis; Soft elastic capsule; Subendometrial contractility (Obs/Gyn); Subepidermal cyst.

Sec Seconal (see Seccy); Second(ary) (see sec); Secretary; Section (see Sect).

sec second (unit of time) (= S; s; Sec); secondary (= Sec); section (see Sect).

sec-Bu sec-butyl or butyl seconal.

Seccy Seconal capsule (= Sec; Seggy).

SECD Science of Early Childhood Development (NAS).

SECG Stress electrocardiography.

SECPR Standard external cardiopulmonary resuscitation.

SECSY Spin-echo coorelated spectroscopy.

Sect; sect Section (= Sec; sec).

sect- combining form meaning cut (L. sectus).

SED Sedimentation (rate); Serotonin-enhancing drug (e.g. 5-Hydroxytryptamine [= 5HT, Enteramine, or Serotonin] reuptake inhibitors such as Citalopram, Fluoxetine, Fluvoxamine, Imipramine, Nefazodone, Paroxetine, Sertraline, etc.) (= SSRI) (see MAD; MAE; NTB; SND); Skin erythema dose; Socioeconomic data; Solar Energy Division ERDA); Spondyloepiphyseal dysplasia (congenita); Standard error of deviation/ difference; Staphylococcal enterotoxin D; Sub-erythemal dose.

Sed; sed Sediment(ation); Stool (L. sedes).

SEDA Susquehanna Economic Development Association.

SeDBP Seated diastolic blood pressure.

Sed rate; sed rt Sedimentation rate.

Sed time Sedimentation time (= Sed rate; sed rt).

SEE Standard error of estimate.

SEEG Stereotactic electroencephalography.

See lit See literature.

SEER Surveillance Epidemiology and End Results (Program).

SEF Sodium excreting factor; Somatically-evoked field; Staphylococcal enterotoxin F; Supination-eversion fracture (ankle joint) (= SE#) (Orthopedics); Suppressed ejaculation/tory function.

SEG Segment(ed) (see segm); Soft elastic gelatin; Sonoencephalogram.

seg segment(ed) (see segm).

Seggy Seconal capsule (see Seccy).

segm segment(ed) (= SEG; seg) (see Segs).

SEGNE Secretory granules of neural and endocrine (cells).

Segs Segmented neutrophils (polymorphonuclear leukocytes).

SEH St. Elizabeth's Hospital (HEW); Subependymal hemorrhage.

SEHD Scottish Executive Health Department.

SEI Self-Esteem Inventory; Severe ethanol intoxication (see AEI); Severe exercise intolerance; Spin-echo image (MRI); Subepithelial (corneal) infiltrate.

SEIU Service Employees International Union.

SEKF Sister Elizabeth Kenny Foundation, Inc.

SEL Systemic exposure level (to drugs).

SELECT Selenium and Vitamin E Prostate Cancer Prevention Trial.

SELF Self-Evaluation of Life Function (scale).

SELFVD Sterile elective low forceps vaginal delivery.

SEM Sample evaluation method; Scanning electron micrograph(y); Scanning/ Shadow electron microscope/py; Secondary enrichment medium; Serummethylguanidine; Specified efficacy measure; Standard error of the mean; Systolic ejection murmur.

Sem Semitic.

sem one-half (L. semis); semen (L.)/ seminal - seed.

SEMDJL Spondyloepimetaphyseal dysplasia with joint laxity.

SEMI Subendocardial myocardial infarction.

semi- prefix meaning half or part (L.).

semid; semidr half a drachm/ dram (L. semidrachma).

semih half an hour (L. semihora).

SEMPRO Southeastern Massachusetts Professional Review Organization.

Sem ves Seminal vesicle.

SEN Scalp-ear-nipple (syndrome); State Enrolled Nurse (UK).

sen sensitive/vity (= S; s).

SENIC Study on the efficacy of nosocomial infection control (Gr. nosokomeion, from

"nosos" disease + "komeion" to take care of, i.e. a hospital or an infirmary). CDC project.
Sens Sensitivity (test/ culture report).
sens sensation; sensorium/ry (= S; s).
sens- combining form meaning feel (L. sensus).
SENSOR Sentinel Event Notification System for Occupational Risks.
SENTAC Society for Ear, Nose and Throat Advances in Children.
SEOO State Economic Opportunity Office.
SEP Secondary/ Specific/ Study (= PEP)/ Surrogate endpoint; Self-empowering personality; Sensory/ Somatosensory/ Spinal evoked potential; Septum (see sept); Serum electrophoresis; Sperm entry point; Standard Employer Plan; Surface epithelium; Systolic ejection period.
Sep September (see Sept).
sep separate(d)/(ly)/tion (see separ); septum (see sept).
sep- combining form meaning decay (Gr. sepo).
separ separate(d)/(ly)/tion (L. separatum) (= sep).
SEPI Specific enzyme polymorphic isoform (e.g. CYP 2 C meph).
S-E prosthesis Starr-Edwards prosthesis (see S-E).
Sept September (= Sep).
sept septum (= SEP; sep); seven (L. septem).
sept- combining form meaning fence off (L. saepio) or seven (L. septem).
SEQ Side effects questionnaire; Sleep evaluation questionnaire.
seq sequel(a)/(ae); sequence/ntial; sequester/trum; that which follows or the following (L. sequela).
seq luc; seq luce the following day (L. sequenti luce).
SER Scanning equalization radiography; Sebum excretion rate; Sensory/ Somatosensory evoked response; Service; Smooth/ Smooth-surface endoplasmic reticulum (see sER); Spontaneous epileptic rat; Stomach emptying rate; Subendocardial region (heart); Supination, external rotation (fracture); Systolic ejection rate.
Ser Serine; Serology; Serous; Serum; Service.
sER Smooth/ Smooth-surface endoplasmic reticulum (= SER).
ser serial; series.
ser- combining form meaning watery material (L. serum).
SERA Serological Evaluation and Research Assembly (Study) (PHS).
SerCl Serum chloride.
SERHOLD National Biomedical Serials Holding Database.
SERI Spondee Error Index.
SER-IV Supination, external rotation - type IV (fracture).
SERLINE On-Line Biomedical Serial Titles (Serials on Line - NLM).
SERM Selective estrogen receptor modulator (anti/ 'designer'- estrogen).
sero; serol serological/gy.
SERS Stimulus Evaluation/ Response Selection (test).
SERT Sustained ethanol release tube.
serv keep or preserve (L. serva); service(s).
SERVE Standardization, expense reduction, and value enhancement.
SERVHEL Service and Health Records.
SES Sero-epidemiological survey; Serotoninergic syndrome (due to drug overdosage or combination of psychotropic medicines with MAO inhibitors, and characterized by any of the following symptoms: Motor {hyper activity/ reflexia, myoclonus, rigidity, tremor}, Psychiatric {agitation, confusion, hypomania, possibly coma}, and Vegetative {chills, hyper/hypothermia, sweating, tachycardia}); Sesone (= sodium dichlorophenoxyethyl sulfate); Sick euthyroid syndrome; Society of Eye Surgeons; Socioeconomic status; Spatial emotional stimulus; State Employment Service (New York); Subendothelial space; Synchroton energy source (radiation/ detection of breast cancer).
SESA Social and Economic Statistics Administration (Department of Commerce).
SESAP Surgical Education and Self-Assessment Program (American College of Surgeons).
SeSBP Seated systolic blood pressure.
sesqui- prefix meaning one-and-a-half (L.).
sesquih an hour and a half (L. sesquihora).

SEST Standardized exercise-stress test.
sesunc an ounce and a half (L. sesuncia).
SET Sex-enhancement therapy/ treatment; Systolic ejection time.
SETD Sulfaethidole (= Aethazolum; Ethazol; Sulfaethylthiadazole) - a sulfonamide compound and a chemotherapeutic agent, readily absorbed from the gastrointestinal tract, with duration of action longer than that of sulfamethizole. In sustained release form it is administered once every 12 hours.
SETI Search for extraterrestrial intelligence (NASA project).
SEU Smallpox Eradication Unit.
sev several; severe; severed.
S-E valve Starr-Edwards (heart) valve (see S-E).
SEWHO Shoulder-elbow-wrist-hand orthosis.
SEX Supination-external (rotation fracture) (see SER).
sex sexual.
sex- prefix meaning six (L.).
SeXO Serum xanthine oxidase.
s expr without expressing/pressing (L. sine expressio/ expressione).
SF Sabin-Feldman (test) (see S-F test); Safety/ Scale/ Serum/ Stable (see Factor VII)/ Sulfation/ Suppressor factor; Salt/ Sugar/ Symptom free; Saturated fat (mostly of animal origin); Scarlet/ Swine fever; Scintillation fluor; Seizure frequency; Seminal/ Serosal/ Spinal/ Synovial fluid; Serum ferritin (Iron status) (see IS); Serum fibrinogen; Sham feeding; Shell/ Shrapnel fragment; Short Form; Shunt flow (arteriovenous); Sickle-cell hemoglobin F (disease); Simian foam (virus); Skin fibroblast; Slow function (initial, transplantation); Sodium azide, fecal (culture medium); Soft feces; Spectroflow; Spectrofluorometer; Spontaneous fibrillation; Spotted fever (RMSF - Rocky Mountain spotted fever, TT - Tick typhus and RP - Rickettsial pox) (see RMSF; TT; RP); Squibb, E.R & Sons (USA) code for experimental substances; Sterile female; Streptococcus fecalis (= Sf; Str F) - on bacteriology reports; Stress formula; Strykerframe; Sulfonamide; Superior facet; Suprasternal fossa; Svedberg flotation (unit) (see SFU).
Sf Streptoccocus fecalis (see SF); Svedberg flotation (unit) (see SFU).
S&F Soft and fat.
SFA Saturated fatty acid; Seminal fluid assay; Serum folic acid; Severely fractured ankle; Stimulated fibrinolytic activity; Structure-function analysis (mode of action of antibiotics, etc.); Stuttering Foundation of America; Superficial femoral artery; Synovial fluid analysis.
SFAP Single-fiber action potential (in SFEMG).
SFB *Salmonella* food poisoning; Sanfilippo syndrome type B; Saphenofemoral bypass; Sarmiento functional brace (with plastic heel cup) (Orthopedics); Subglottic/ Surgical foreign body.
SFBL Self-filling blind loop.
SFC Sexual-function complaint (female/ male) (see FSD; MSD); Soluble fibrin/ fibrin-fibrinogen complex; Spinal fluid count.
SFCE Sudden fatal coronary event.
SFD Sacral fracture-diastasis; Sheep factor delta; Silo filler's disease; Single fixed dose; Skin-film distance; Small for date; Spectral frequency distribution; Sudden fetal death/ demise.
SFDs Somatiform disorders (see CFS, FMS, GWI, GWS, PTSD, PTSS & CMI).
SFE Slipped femoral epiphysis (Orthopedics); Smoke-free environment; Systemic fibrinolytic effect.
SFEMG Single fiber electromyography.
SFF Speaking fundamental frequency.
SFFA Serum free fatty acid.
SFFF Sedimentation field flow fractionation.
SFFV Spleen focus-forming virus.
SFG Segmental fibular graft(ing) (e.g. for tumors) (Orthopedics).
SFGA Small-for-gestational-age (infant).
SFGH San Francisco General Hospital.
SFH Schizophrenia family history; Serum/ Stroma-free hemoglobin.
SFHD Single fixed high dose (see BRR).
SFI Severe febrile illness; Sexual/ Social Function Index; Solid fat index; Systemic fungal infection (esp. blastomycosis, coccidioidomycosis, cryptococcosis, histoplasmosis

and paracoccidioidomycosis).

SFICH Spontaneous fetal intracranial hemorrhage (Obstetrics).

SFJ Sapheno-femoral junction.

SFK Single functioning kidney.

SFL Sexual Freedom League; Synovial fluid lymphocyte.

SFLT Standard first-line therapy.

SFM Serum-free medium.

SFMC Soluble fibrin monomer complex.

SFMS Scripps Foundation for Medicine and Science (La Jolla, CA).

SFN Sore fissured nipple; Subcutaneous fat necrosis (see ASN).

SFO Subfornical organ.

SFODF French Orthodontic Society.

SFP Screen filtration pressure; Simultaneous foveal perception; Single-fiber potential(s) (see SFAP; SFEMG); Spinal fluid pressure; Stop(ped) flow pressure (kidneys); Symptom-free period.

SFPC Safety and Fire Protection Committee (MCA).

SFPS Skin-flap plastic surgery.

SFPT Standard fixation preference test.

SFR Screen filtration resistance; Stroke with full recovery.

SFS Serial focal/ foveal seizures; Serofast syphilis (positive serology test for syphilis) (see STS); Skin and fascia stapler; Split function study.

SFT Sabin-Feldman test; Sensory feedback therapy; Serum-free thyroxine; Skinfold thickness.

S-F test Sabin-Feldman test (= SF; SFT).

SFTR Sagittal, frontal, transverse, and rotation; Society for Family Therapy and Research.

SFU Surgical follow-up; Svedberg flotation unit (= SF; Sf; Sf).

S_f unit Svedberg flotation unit (see SFU).

SFV Semliki Forest virus; Shipping fever virus; Shope/ Squirrel fibroma virus; Superficial femoral vein.

SFW Sexual function of women; Shell/ Shrapnel fragment wound; Slow-filling wave.

SG Sachs-Georgi (test) (see S-G); Salivary gland; Scintillogram/graph(y); Serum globulin/ glucose; Signs; Silica gel; Skin graft; Soluble gelatin (with reference to capsules); Sonogram/graph(y); Specific gravity; Subgluteal; Substantia gelatinosa; Surgeon General; Swan-Ganz (catheter); Synthetic gonadotropin (see Hormones - LH-RH).

sg specific gravity (see sp gr).

S-G Sachs-Georgi (test for syphilis) (= SG; SGR; S-Gt) (see STS - SG).

s-g subgenus (L.).

SGA Second generation agent/ assay; Single-gene aberration; Small for gestational age; Subgroup analyses/sis; Subjective Global Assessment.

SGa; SG_a Specific conductance.

SGA DC Small-for-gestational age dichorionic (twin).

SGA MC Small-for-gestational age monochorionic (twin).

SG_{aw} Specific airway(s) conductance (see PFT).

SGB Seagull bruit (in aortic stenosis); Sparsely granulated basophil.

SGC Slate grey cyanosis (methemoglobinemia, caused by inhalation of volatile nitrates) (see VSA); Soft/ Soluble gelatin capsule (see SG capsule); Spermicide-germicide compound; Strain-guage controller; Subgingival curettage; Swan-Ganz catheter; Systemic glucocorticoid.

SG capsule Soft/ Soluble gelatin capsule (= SGC).

SGD Salivary gland disease/ disorder; Second-generation drug; Single gene defect/ disease/ disorder (such as Cystic fibrosis, Fragile X syndrome [a common form of mental retardation], Huntington's disease, Muscular dystrophy, Severe combined immune deficiency [syndrome - SCID], Sickle-cell anemia, Tay-Sachs disease [with loss of brain cells], etc.); Specific granule deficiency; Straight gravity drainage.

SGE Secondary generalized epilepsy; Significant glandular enlargement; Significantly greater extent; Sporadic gastroenteritis; Starch gel electrophoresis; Superficial gastric erosion.

SGF Sarcoma/ Skeletal growth factor.

s-gg subgenera (L.).

SGGT Serum gamma-glutamyl transferase

(see GGT).
SGH Serum/ Synthetic (= Somatropin) growth hormone; Subgluteal hematoma.
SGHWR Steam-generating heavy-water reactor.
SGI Schizophrenia Genetics Initiative (NIMH).
SGL Salivary gland lymphocyte.
s gl without glasses/ (correction of) glasses.
SGM Single-gene malady (see SGD); Society for General Microbiology; Strain guage manometer (Cardiac catheterization).
SGO Shoulder-girdle operation(s) - include 1. Classical interscapulo- thoracic resection (TLP - Tikhoff-Linberg procedure), 2. Total scapulectomy (forequarter amputation), 3. Nearly total scapulectomy, 4. Radical subtotal scapulectomy, and 5. Subtotal or partial scapulectomy (see SCS; TLR); Society of Gynecologic Oncologists; Surgeon General's Office; Surgery, Gynecology, and Obstetrics (journal).
SGOC Second-generation oral contraceptive (containing a progestogen such as levonorgestrel, lynestrol, norethisterone, etc.).
SGOT Serum glutamic oxaloacetate/acetic transaminase (enzyme) (= Serum aspartate aminotransferase; Serum glutamic oxalacetate/acetic transaminase) (see AST; LFT iv).
SGP Serine glycerophosphatide; Sialoglycoprotein; Skin-graft patient; Society of General Physiologists; Soluble glycoprotein; Strain guage plethysmography.
SGPT Serum glutamate/mic pyruvate/vic transaminase (= Serum alanine/ pyruvic aminotransferase) (see ALT; LFT iv); Strain guage pressure transducer.
SGR Sachs-Georgi reaction (see STS - SG); Satisfactory global response; Schwartzman generalized reaction; Science and Government Report (journal); Shoulder-girdle resection (including the upper end of the humerus, the scapula, the clavicle, and the surrounding soft tissues and axillary contents) (see SGO); Skin galvanic reflex; Submandibular gland renin; Substantia gelatinosa Rolandi.
SGRH Synthetic gonadotropin releasing hormone (see Hormones - LH-RH).
SGRQ Saint George's Respiratory Questionnaire.
SGS Second generation sulfonylurea; Senile gait syndrome (see MAPP - Marche à petit pas); Subglottic stenosis.
SGS 1 *Saccharomyces* cerevisiae (brewer's yeast) gene (a gene similar to the human gene responsible for Werner's syndrome, a condition associated with aging in the young, with early grey hair, osteoporosis, cataracts and hardening of the arteries).
SGSR Society for General Systems Research.
SGT Salivary gland tumor; Slow-growing tumor; Somatic-gene therapy; Suicide gene therapy (in which a gene inserted into a cancer cell, renders it supersensitive or "suicidal to some drug that ordinarily has no anticancer effect") (see HGT).
S-Gt Sachs-Georgi test (for syphilis) (see S-G; STS - SG).
SGTT Standard glucose tolerance test.
SGV Salivary gland virus; Selective gastric vagotomy.
SGVHD Syngenic graft-versus-host disease.
SH Pseudohypoparathyroidism; Salter-Harris (fracture); Schönlein-Henoch (purpura); Self-help; Self-hypnosis; Seminars in Hematology (journal); Serum hepatitis (antigen; antiserum; virus B; or long-incubation SH virus); Sex hormone(s) (see Hormones - SH); Sexual harassment; Shell Development Corp (USA) code for experimental substances; Sherman (rat); Shigella flexeri hybrid; Sick in hospital; Sinus histiocytosis; Social/ Surgical history; Somatic-gene therapy; Somatotropic hormone (see Hormones - GH); Southern Hospitals (journal); Spontaneously hypertensive (rat); State Hospital; Steric hindrance; Student health; Sulfhydryl; Symptomatic hypoglycemia; Syndrome of (hyporeninemic) hypoaldosteronism (see SHH); Systemic hyperthermia.
Sh Sheep; Sherwood (number); Shigella (see Shig); Shoulder (see sh).
sh short; shoulder (= Sh; SHLD); shower; shunt; slender.
S/H Sample and hold; Suicidal/ homicidal.
S&H Speech and hearing.
-SH Sulfhydryl group.

S-H Sims-Huhner (fertility test).
SH# Spontaneous hip fracture (see SHF).
SH 714 Cyproterone acetate.
SH 717 Glymidine (= Glycodiazine; Sodium glymidine) - an hypoglycemic agent, not related to the diguanides or the sulfonylureas. Active only in diabetic patients who produce some endogenous insulin, and is used in the treatment of maturity-onset diabetes.
SH 742 Fluocortolone (= Fluoromethyl dehydrocortisone) - a synthetic glucocorticoid, used topically in the treatment of various skin disorders.
SH 770 Fluocortolone caproate - has a more powerful but less rapid action than fluocortolone (see SH 742).
SHA Self-health assessment; Staphylococcal hemagglutinating antibody; Superheated aerosol.
sHa Suckling hamster.
SHAA Serum hepatitis-associated antigen; Society of Hearing Aid Audiologists.
SHAA-Ab Serum hepatitis-associated antigen - antibody.
SHAb Specific humoral antibody.
SHAFT Sad, hostile, anxious, frustrating, tenacious (patient) (syndrome).
shagreen Lesions of the lens of the eye.
SHAME Society to Humiliate, Aggravate, Mortify and Embarrass (Smokers).
SHARP School health additional referral program.
SHB Sequential hemibody (irradiation); Smoking and Health Bulletin (USPHS); Sulfhemoglobin (see S-Hb).
SHb Sickle hemoglobin (screen).
S-Hb Sulfhemoglobin (= SHB).
SHBD Serum hydroxybutyrate/butyric dehydrogenase.
SHBG Sex hormone-binding globulin.
SHC Severe hepatic cholestasis/ cirrhosis; Sexual Health Clinic; State Health Commissioner.
SHCC State Health Coordinating Council.
SHCO Sulfated hydrogenated castor oil.
SHCOGP Special Health Career Opportunity Grants Program (HRA).
SHCs State Health Corporations.
SHD Senior hospital doctor; Severe hepatic disease/ disorder/ dysfunction (= SLD); Sex hormone deprivation; Single high dose; State health department (US); Structural/ Syphilitic heart disease.
SH2D1A The adapator protein also referred to as DSHP and SAP (see DD; DSHP; SAP).
SHDC Severe hemodynamic compromise.
SHDI Supraoptical hypophysial diabetes insipidus.
SHDPP Stanford Heart Disease Prevention Program.
SHE Severe hemorrhagic enteritis; Subject headings for engineering (EI); Syrian hamster embryo.
SHEC Syrian hamster embryo cell.
SHECTA Syrian Hamster Embryo Cell Transformation Assay.
shee-ba Chiba eye needle (Ophthalmology).
SHEENT Skin, head, eyes, ears, nose, and throat.
SHEP Systolic Hypertension in the Elderly Program.
SHF Scalp hair follicle; Severe/ Symptomatic heart failure; Simian hemorrhagic fever; Spontaneous hip fracture (Orthopedics) (= SH#).
shf super-high frequency.
SHG Self-help group; Society for Human Genetics (ASHG; ESHG); Synthetic human gastrin.
SHG; SHGd; SHG diet Sauerbruch-Herrmannsdorfer-Gerson diet.
SHH Syndrome of hyporeninemic hypoaldosteronism (= SH).
SHHD Scottish Home and Health Department.
SHHH Self Help for Hard of Hearing (People Inc.) (Bethesda, MD).
SHHS Scottish Heart Health Study; Sleep Heart Health Study.
SHHV Society for Health and Human Values.
SHI *Schistosoma* hematobium infection (= Urinary schistosomiasis caused by S. hematobium and transmitted through the intermediate snail host of the genus *Bulinus*) (see WCP); Semisynthetic human insulin (see Insulin); Sequence hypersecretion-infection (as in bronchiectasis); Severe hepatic impairment/ insufficiency; Severe hepatocellular

insufficiency; Severe hospital infection; Soluble human insulin (see Insulin).

Shig Shigella (= Sh).

Shin Shinto (religion).

SHIV Simian-human immunodeficiency virus (mucosal virus - infection).

SHK Syrian hamster kidney.

SHL Scalp hair loss; Sensorineural/ Serious/ Severe/ Slight/ Sudden hearing loss; Short half-life; Supraglottic horizontal laryngectomy.

SHLA Soluble human lymphocyte antigen.

SHLD Shoulder (see sh).

SHM Self-help manual; Single heterozygous mutation (gene).

SHML Sinus histiocytosis with massive lymphadenopathy.

SHMO Senior Hospital Medical Officer (UK).

SHMT Serine-hydroxymethyl transferase.

SHN Spontaneous hemorrhagic necrosis; Subacute hepatic necrosis.

SHO Secondary hypertrophic osteoarthropathy; Senior House Officer (UK); Student Health Organization; Symptomatic heterotopic ossification.

SHORT; S-H-O-R-T Short stature, hyperextensibility of joints or hernia or both, ocular depression, Rieger anomaly, and teething delayed.

SHOT Society for the History of Technology.

SHOTS Statewide House Officer Training System (Michigan).

SHP Schönlein-Henoch purpura; Secondary hyperparathyroidism; State Health Plan; Strongin-Hinsie-Peck (test).

SHPDA State Health Planning and Development Agency.

SHR Serious health risk; Severe hypersensitivity reaction/ respone (to drugs etc.); Slow heart rate (bradycardia); Spontaneously hypertensive rat (genetic).

ShR Shading response (Rorschach).

SHRT Sequential hormone replacement therapy (estrogen → progestin).

SHS Sayre head sling; Schönlein-Henoch syndrome (= Anaphylactoid purpura) (see HSP; HSS; SHP); Second-hand smoke/ smoking (breathing someone else's smoke or passive smoking); Senate Health Subcommittee; Severe hepatic steatosis; Sex hormone synthesis; Sheep hemolysate supernatant; Student health service.

SHSP Spontaneously hypertensive stroke-prone (rat).

SHSS Stanford Hypnotic Susceptibility Scale.

SHT Self-hypnosis technique(s); Serious/ Severe hepatic toxicity; Severe/ Spontaneous hyper/ hypothyroidism; Simple hypocalcemic tetany; Speech and hearing therapy; Standard hematologic test; Standard histologic technique; Subcutaneous histamine test; Suspected hyperthyroidism (CMHT) (see GHT) (see Scheme); Symptomatic hypotension; Systemic hematologic toxicity.

S-HT Serotonin.

SHTN; Sys Htn Systolic hypertension.

SHuC Synthetic human calcitonin.

SHUR System for Hospital Uniform Reporting.

SHV Simian herpes virus.

SHZ Simian herpes zoster (laboratory-acquired encephalomyelitis).

SI International System of Units (= Le Système International d'Unités; rationalized metric system); Sacro-iliac; Saline infusion/ injection; Salk Institute; Saturation/ Severity/ Singh/ Stimulation/ Stroke/ Suppression Index; Self-inflicted; Semilente insulin (see Insulin - SI i); Sensory integration; Septic inflammation; Serious illness; Seriously ill; Serum insulin/ iron; Sex inventory; Shober's index (test for spondylitis); Single injection; Small intestine; Smithsonian Institute (= Smith I); Social introversion; Soluble Insulin (= Insulin; Insulin Injection; Ordinary Insulin; Regular Insulin; Unmodified Insulin) (see Insulin - II i; SI ii); Spirochetosis icterohaemorrhagica; Stress incontinence; Strict isolation; Substantia innominata (of the brain); Swimmer's itch (a form of schistosomiasis that is endemic in avian schistosomes, such as *Trichobilharzia* sp).

Si Silicon (Z = 14) (see Elements - Silicon); Sinus (venous); The most anterior point on the lower contour of the sella turcica (point).

S&I Suction and irrigation.

SIA International Society of Audiology (Fr. Société Internationale d'Audiologie) (= ISA);

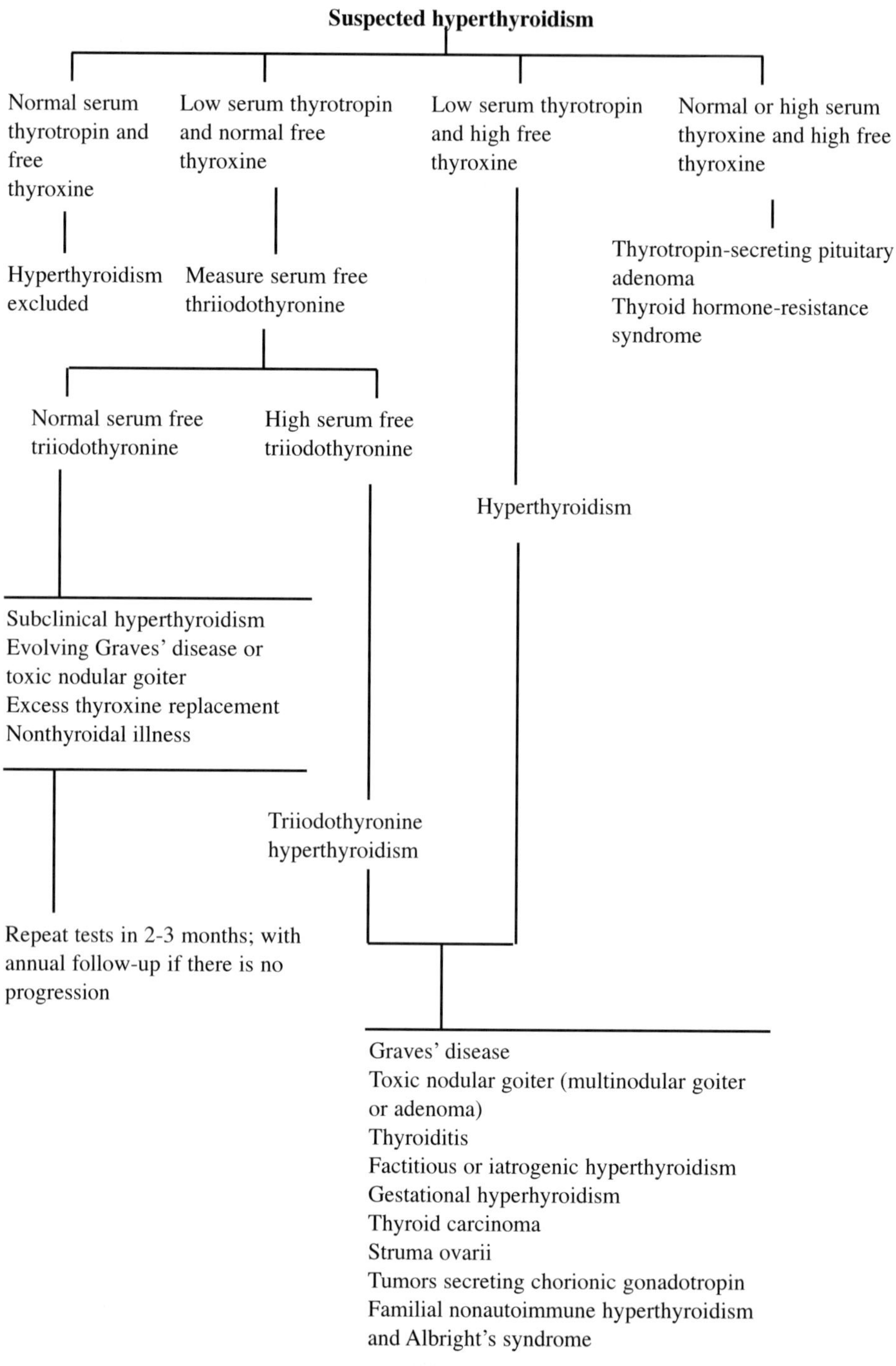

Suspected hyperthyroidism
Normal serum thyrotropin and free thyroxine
Low serum thyrotropin and normal free thyroxine
Low serum thyrotropin and high free thyroxine
Normal or high serum thyroxine and high free thyroxine
Hyperthyroidism excluded
Measure serum free thriiodothyronine
Thyrotropin-secreting pituitary adenoma
Thyroid hormone-resistance syndrome
Normal serum free triiodothyronine
High serum free triiodothyronine
Hyperthyroidism
Subclinical hyperthyroidism
Evolving Graves' disease or toxic nodular goiter
Excess thyroxine replacement
Nonthyroidal illness
Triiodothyronine hyperthyroidism
Repeat tests in 2-3 months; with annual follow-up if there is no progression
Graves' disease
Toxic nodular goiter (multinodular goiter or adenoma)
Thyroiditis
Factitious or iatrogenic hyperthyroidism
Gestational hyperhyroidism
Thyroid carcinoma
Struma ovarii
Tumors secreting chorionic gonadotropin
Familial nonautoimmune hyperthyroidism and Albright's syndrome

Serum inhibitory activity; Severe intrinsic asthma; Stress-induced analgesia/ anesthesia; Subacute infectious arthritis; Sympathetic-induced arrhythmia; Synalbumin-insulin antagonism.

SIAD; SIADH Syndrome of inappropriate antidiuretic hormone (secretion).

sial- prefix meaning saliva (Gr. sialon).

SIAM Society for Industrial and Applied Mathematics.

SIAS Specific interaction study.

SIB Self-injurious behavior.

SIBS Salk Institute for Biological Studies (La Jolla, Calif.).

sib(s) sibling(s) (Anglo Saxon: sib-kin) - a blood relative/ one of a group of persons all of whom are descendants of a common ancestor.

SIC Serum insulin concentration; Sidewall infusion cannula (Ophthalmology); Standard Industrial Classification (System); Standardized inoculum concentration (of antibiotics); Structurally inadequate cervix.

sic (L.) as follows/ as one is/ as stated/ as things are/ so/ this way/ thus/ thus so; dry (L. siccus).

SICCE Syndrome of intermittent claudication of the cauda equina.

SICCU Satellite Industrial Coronary Care Unit.

SICD Sequenced Inventory of Communication Development; Serum isocitrate/ric dehydrogenase.

SICH Symptomatic intra cerebral/ cranial hemorrhage.

SICSVA Sequential impaction cascade sieve volumetric air (sampler).

SICT Selective intracoronary thrombolysis.

SICU Spinal/ Surgical intensive care unit.

SID Selective immunoglobulin deficiency; Severe immunodeficiency; Severe iron deficiency; Single intradermal (test); Society for Investigative Dermatology; Source-image distance (receptor, X-rays); Streptozotocin-induced diabetes (Obstetrics); Sucrase isomaltase deficiency; Sudden inexplicable death; Sudden infant death (= crab death) (see SIDS); Suggested indication of diagnosis; Surgically implanted device (artificial heart); Systemic inflammatory disease.

SIDA Steroid-induced dermal atrophy; Sudden Infant Death Association.

sidero- prefix meaning iron (Gr. sideros).

SIDI Superficial intradermal implant (Plastic and Reconstructive Surgery).

SIDS Severe immunodeficiency syndrome (see SCIDS); Sudden infant death syndrome (= Crib death; SID).

SIE Severe ischemic enteritis; Static isometric exercise(s); Stroke in evolution.

SIECOP Sex Information and Educational Council of Physicians.

SIECUS Sex Information and Educational Council of the United States.

Sievert A unit of ionizing radiation equal to 100 rems (see REM).

SIF Serum-inhibition factor.

SIFT Selector ion flow tube.

SIg; sIg Surface immunoglobulin.

Sig; sig Label/ Let it be labeled or written/ mark thou/ write/ write on label (L. signa; signetur) - in prescriptions (= S); Sigmoidoscope/py (= Sigmo); Signal; Significant.

SIgA; S-IgA; s-IgA Secretory immunoglobulin A (dimeric IgA); Surface immunoglobulin A.

sig col sigmoid colon.

sig n pro label with the proper name (L. signa nomine proprio).

Sigmo Sigmoidoscope/py (see Sig).

SIH Seminars in Hearing (US); Stimulation-induced hypalgesia; Stress-induced hyperthermia.

SIHE Spontaneous intramural hematoma of the esophagus.

SII Self-inflicted injury; Sucrase-isomaltase insufficiency.

SIJ Sacroiliac joint.

SIJD Sacroiliac joint diastasis (see DSH).

SIL Screw-in lead (Pacemaker); Soluble interleukin; Speech interference level.

SILD Sequenced Inventory of Language Development.

SILFVD Sterile indicated low forceps vaginal delivery.

SILI Stretch-induced lung injury (see EIS).

SIM Selected ion monitoring; Similac; Small

intestinal metaplasia; Society of Industrial Medicine/ Microbiology; Spontaneous involuntary movement; Sulfide, indole, motility (culture medium); Surgically-induced menopause.

sim simple (see simp).

SIMA Single internal mammary artery.

Sim c Fe Similac with iron.

simp simple (L. simplex) (= sim).

SIMS Scripps Institutions of Medicine and Science; Secondary ion mass spectroscopy; Students' International Meditation Society.

simul simultaneous(ly).

SIMV Synchronized intermittent mandatory ventilation.

sin six times a night (L. sex in nocte).

sin- combining form meaning hollow (L. sinus).

SINB Succinylcholine-induced neuromuscular blockade.

sing of each (L. singulorum); singular (one) (= S; s).

sinist- prefix meaning left (L. sinister).

si non val if it is not enough (= if of no value; if it does not answer) (L. si non valeat) (= si n val).

Sinsemilla Marijuana (Spanish American) (see Cannabis).

sinu sinusoidal.

si n val if it is not enough (see si non val).

SIO Sacroiliac orthosis.

SiO_2 Silicon dioxide.

si op sit if (it is) necessary (L. si opus sit) (see SOS).

SIP Self-injection procedure (see SIT); Seriously ill/ Severely injured patient/ person; Severe intractable pain; Sickness Impact Profile; Slow inhibitory potential; State Implementation Plan (NAAQS); Surface inductive plethysmography; Systemic inflammatory process (such as Sarcoidosis, SLE, etc.).

SIPI Scientists' Institute for Public Information.

sIPTH Serum immunoreactive parathyroid hormone.

SIQ Symptom Interpretation Questionnaire.

SIR Severe immune reaction (to a vaccine, virus, etc.); Significant intrinsic repair (Orthopedics); Single isomorphous replacement; Specific immune release; Standardized incidence ratio; Syndrome of immediate reactivities; Systemic inflammatory response.

SIRA Scientific/ Standard Instrument Research Association (British).

SIREF Specific immune response enhancing factor.

SIRF Severely impaired renal function.

siRNA Small interfering RNA (small pieces of RNA used in inhibiting viral growth, such as HIV, in infected cells).

SIRS Soluble immune response suppressor; Structured Interview of Reported Symptoms.

SIS Sacro-iliac scintogram/aph(y); Science Information Services (FIRL); Selective/Systemic immunosuppressant (see IST; SIST); Serotonin irritation syndrome; Shoulder impingement syndrome (= CIS); Simian sarcoma; Simulator-induced syndrome; Social information system; Spontaneous interictal spike; Sterile injectable solution/ suspension; Sterilized injection syringe; Subintensional suicide (= Benign suicide); Surgically implanted system (see SID); Symptom improvement score; Synthetic Immune System (computer program).

Sis; sis Sister.

-sis suffix meaning condition or state (Gr) (also Gr. -asis; - iasis; -osis).

SISA Selective immunosuppressive agent (e.g. Etanercept).

SISD Scottish Information Services for the Disabled.

SISI Short increment sensitivity index.

SISO Sisomycin.

SISS Serum inhibitor of streprolysin S; Small inducible secreted substances.

SIST Selective/ Systemic immunosuppressive therapy (see IST).

SISV; SiSV Simian sarcoma virus.

SIT Sedative-induced torpor; Self-injection technique (= SIP); Serum inhibiting titer; Silicon intensified target; Situs inversus totalis (= SCDS or Sprengel's congenital deformity syndrome) (Orthopedics); Slosson Intelligence Test; Sperm/ Suggested immobilization test; Structured interrupted therapy (antiviral therapy in AIDS); Supraspinatus, infraspinatus, teres minor (group of muscles).

sit- prefix meaning food (Gr. sitos).

SitBal Sitting balance.

SITH Stereoisomeric tetrahydrosteroid.

SitTol Sitting tolerance.

Si Tr Silent treatment (= SlTr).

SIV Self-induced vomiting (see GR - Gag reflex); Simian immunodeficiency virus; Sprague-Dawley-Ivanovas (rat).

SIVagm Simian immunodeficiency virus from African green monkeys.

S_{ivcO2} Oxygen saturation inferior vena cava.

si vir perm if strength permits/ if the strength will permit (L. si vires permittant).

SIVMAC Simian immunodeficiency virus of macaques.

SIW Self-inflicted wound.

SIWIP Self-induced water intoxication and psychosis.

SIWIS Self-induced water intoxication and schizophrenic disorders.

Six-o-six (606) Arsphenamine.

S_j Jaccard coefficient.

SJ 1977 Methixene hydrochloride. A parasympatholytic antispasmodic drug used in the treatment of paralysis agitans and other types of parkinsonism.

SJCLI Scandinavian Journal of Clinical and Laboratory Investigation.

SJID Scandinavian Journal of Infectious Diseases.

SJN Spontaneous jerk nystagmus.

SJO Southern Journal of Optometry (SCO).

SJOT Southern Journal of Occupational Therapy.

SJR Shinowara-Jones-Reinhart (unit) (= S-JU; S-J unit); St John Review (UK journal).

SJS Stevens-Johnson/ Swyer-James syndrome (= S-J syndrome); Stiff joint syndrome; Subtalar joint stiffness (Orthopedics).

SjS Sjögren syndrome.

S-J syndrome Steven-Johnson/ Swyer-James syndrome (see SJS).

SJT Simple/ Single joint trauma.

S-JU; S-J unit Shinowara-Jones unit (see SJR).

SK A strain of Poliovirus; Seborrheic/ Senile keratosis; Sloan-Kettering (Cytosine arabinoside, 6-Thioguanine, Doxorubicin, L-asparaginase - Chemotherapy); Sloan-Kettering code for experimental substances used in the treatment of cancer at the SKICR (New York City); SmithKline; Solar keratosis; Spontaneous killer (cell); Streptokinase (= STK); Swine kidney.

Sk; sk Skeletal/ton (= Skel; skel); Skin (= Skn; skn).

SK 65 Propoxyphene HCl 65 mg.

SKA Supracondylar knee-ankle (orthosis, plate, or prosthesis).

SK 331 A Xanthinol niacinate/ nicotinate - a peripheral vasodilator used in the treatment of peripheral vascular disease, cerebral vascular accidents, and hypercholesterolemia.

Skag Cheap, low-grade heroin (see Diamorph HCl).

SKAO Supracondylar knee-ankle orthosis.

SKAT Sex Knowledge and Aptitude/ Attitude Test.

SKD Serious/ Severe kidney damage/ disease/ dysfunction (see SRD); Severe keratinisaturation disorder; Structural kidney damage.

Skel; skel Skeletal/ton (see Sk; sk).

SKF Severe/ Sudden kidney failure (see ESRD; SKD; SRF); Smith, Klein and French (pharmaceutical firm code for experimental substances).

SKF 385 Tranylcypromine sulfate (= Tranylcypromine Sulf; Transamine sulfate) - a non-hydrazine monoamine oxidase inhibitor used in the treatment of severe mental depression, where the patient does not respond satisfactorily to other antidepressant drugs, or for whom electroconvulsive therapy is considered unsuitable.

SKF 525 A Proadifen - a calcium antagonistic agent.

SKF 688 A Phenoxybenzamine hydrochloride (= Phenoxybenz HCl) - an adrenergic receptor blocking drug, used to control the hypertension caused by phaeochromocytoma; also employed in the treatment of peripheral disorders characterized by excessive vasospasm, including Raynaud's disease, acrocyanosis, chilblains, and causalgia.

SKF 4740 Isopropamide iodide (see R 79).

SKF 5019 Trifluoperazine hydrochloride (=

Trifluoper HCl) - a phenothiazine derivative and a tranquillizing agent, used in the treatment of acute mania, delirium tremens, and schizophrenia. Also used in cases of psychoneurosis, and in nausea and vomiting due to various causes, such as pregnancy vomiting and post-radiation sickness.

SKF 5116 Methotrimeprazine (see RP 7044).

SKF 5137 Dextromoramide (see MCP 875).

SKF 6539 Flurothyl (= Hexafluorodiethyl Ether) - a volatile non-inflammable liquid, which has been used as an alternative to electroconvulsive therapy in the treatment of severe depression.

SKF 8542 Triamterene (= 2,4,7-Triamino-6-phenylpteridine) - a diuretic acting mainly on the distal tubules, and increasing the excretion of sodium and chloride, and reducing the excretion of potassium. Used as an adjuvant to mercurial or thiazide diuretics in the treatment of refractory edema associated with hepatic cirrhosis, congestive heart failure, and the nephrotic syndrome.

SKF 12141 Diphenicillin sodium (see BLP 413).

SKF 14287 Idoxuridine (see IDU).

SKF 20716 Pericyazine (see RP 8909).

SKF-D 2623 Detrothyronine (see DT3; Hormones - TH, Thyroid hormones B).

SKG Sperm-killing gene (injected into insects such as the mosquito, in order to cut down infectivity).

SKI Sloan-Kettering Institute (see SKICR).

skia- prefix meaning shadow (Gr. skia).

SKICR Sloan-Kettering Institute for Cancer Research (New York City) (see SK).

SKIP Scholarships for Kids of International Physicians (AMA).

SKL Serum killing level.

Skn; skn Skin (see Sk; sk).

SKS Symptomatic kidney stone.

SKSAP Surgical Knowledge Self-Assessment Program.

SKSD; SK-SD Streptokinase-streptodornase.

sk trx skeletal traction.

SL According to rule/ to the rules (L. secundum legem) (= sl); Sarcolemma; Satellite-like; Sclerosing leukoencephalopathy; Secondary leukemia; Sensation level (of hearing); Sensory latency; Short-leg (brace); Sibley-Lehninger (unit); Sidney line; Signal/ Sound level; Sinding Larsen/ Sjögren-Larsson/ Stein-Leventhal syndrome; Slit lamp (eye examination); Small lymphocyte; Sodium lactate; Solidified liquid; Streptolysin; Subliminal; Sublingual(ly) (= sl); Sutton's law (directing attention to the most obvious medical problem).

S-L Scapholunate (dissociation, with rupture of the interosseous membrane i.e. between the scaphoid and lunate carpal bones) (see L-T; SLAC).

Sl Steel (mouse).

sl according to the rules (see SL); broadly speaking/ in a broad sense (L. sensu lato); slight(ly); slow(ly); stemline; sublingual(ly) (see SL).

S/L Slit lamp (examination).

SL 501 Chlophedianol hydrochloride (see Bayer B 186).

SLA Sacrolaeva anterior (L.) - left sacroanterior (position of fetus); Second-line antibiotic; Single-cell liquid (cytotoxic) assay; Slide latex agglutination (test); Soluble liver antigen; Surfactant-like activity.

SLAA Sex and Love Addicts Anonymous.

SLAC Scapholunate advanced collapse (wrist); Stanford Linear Accelerator Center.

SLAM Scanning laser acoustic microscope; Signaling lymphocyte activation molecule (a mutant protein).

slan without place, year, or name (L. sine loco, anno, vel nomine).

SLAP Serum leucine aminopeptidase.

s lat in a broad sense (L. sensu lato).

SLB Short-leg brace.

SLC Secondary lymphoid cancer; Self-limiting condition (see SLI); Semilunar cartilage (Orthopedics); Severe liver cirrhosis; Short-leg cast; Suction lipectomy cannula (for facial area) (= Gram's cannula).

SLCC Short-leg cylinder cast.

SLCG Sulfolithoe-cholecystogram/aph(y).

SLCT Sertoli-Leydig cell tumor (of the ovary whose cells release male sex hormones; also called Andreioma, Andreoblastoma, Androma, Arrhenoblastoma, Arrhenoma).

SLD Second-line data/ drug (see SLDT); Self-limiting disease (see SLI); Serum lactate dehydrogenase; Severe learning disability; Severe liver damage/ disorder/ dysfunction (see SHD); Specific learning deficit/ disorder (see CBD).

SLDH Serum lactate dehydrogenase.

SLDS Slit lamp delivery system (for the Argon laser).

SLD/SLDH activity Serum lactate dehydrogenase activity.

SLDT Second-line drug therapy (in RA) - such as Gold salts, Penicillamine, Sulfasalazine and Antimalarial drugs.

SLE Saint/St. Louis encephalitis (virus); Selectin ligand expression (in activated T cells in cancer); Self-limiting episode; Slit lamp examination; Subacute lupus erythematosus; Systemic lupus erythematosus (= LED; LES).

SLEA Sheep erythrocyte antibody.

SLEE St. Louis equine encephalitis (Serology test) (= SLE).

SLEF Systemic Lupus Erythematosus Foundation.

SLEP Short latent evoked potential.

SLEV St. Louis encephalitis virus.

SLFVD Sterile low forceps vaginal delivery.

SLGS 'Start low, go slow' (drug prescribing policy/ strategy).

SLGXT Symptom limited graded exercise test.

SLH Standard liter per hour (gas) (= SLPH).

SLHR Sex-linked hypophosphatemic rickets (vitamin D - resistant).

SLI Selective lymphoid irradiation; Self-limiting illness/ infection (= SLC; SLD); Serious/ Severe liver impairment/ Severe liver insufficiency; Somatostatin-like immunoreactivity (see SLIR); Specific language impairment; Splenic localization index; Stepladder incision (see inc).

SLIR Somatostatin-like immunoreactivity (= SLI).

SLJ Sclerolimbal junction (of the sclera and limbus in the eye).

SLK; SLKC Superior limbic keratoconjunctivitis.

SLL Serum lipid level.

SLM Secondary lymphoid malignancy; Sound level meter; Sphingolipid metabolism; Standard liter per minute (gas) (= SLPM).

SLMC Spontaneous lymphocyte-mediated cytotoxicity.

SLMFVD Sterile low mid-forceps vaginal delivery.

SLMP Since last menstrual period.

SLN Secondary lymphoblastic/ lymphoid neoplasm; Sublentiform nucleus; Superior laryngeal nerve.

SLNB Sentinel lymph node biopsy.

SLNE Sentinel lymph node evaluation.

SLNM Sentinel lymph node mapping (in breast cancer, for detection of metastases).

SLNs Sentinel lymph nodes (see CAD; SLNM; SNR); Shotty lymph nodes.

SLNTG Sublingual nitroglycerin.

SLNWBC Short-leg non-weightbearing cast.

SLNWC Short-leg non-walking cast.

SLO Scanning laser ophthalmoscope; Smith-Lemli-Opitz (syndrome); Streptolysin O.

Sloan Alfred P. Sloan Foundation.

SLOS Smith-Lemli-Opitz syndrome.

SLP Sacrolaeva posterior (L.) - left sacroposterior (fetal position); Second-line pharmacotherapy (= SLT); Segmental limb (systolic) pressure; Senior-level people; Sex-limited protein; Shelf-life/ Short latency period; Short luteal phase; Standard laboratory protocol; Subligamentous protrusion (roof disk - Neurosurgery); Subluxation of the patella.

SLPC Six lumen perfused catheter (EMS - Esophageal Motility Studies).

SLPH Standard liter per hour (gas) (see SLH).

SLPM Standard liter per minute (gas) (see SLM).

SLPP Serum lipophosphoprotein.

SLR Shwartzman local reaction; Single lens reflex; Straight leg raising; Streptococcus lactis R (rhizopterin) (factor).

SLRD Sex-linked recessive disease (as in FD; AKCD).

SLRT Straight leg raising test.

SLS Second-line study; Sedentary lifestyle; Segment long-spacing (collagen fibers); Short-leg splint; Single limb support; Sinding Larsen/ Sjögren-Larsson/ Stagnant loop/ Stein-Leventhal syndrome; Soft laser stimulation (or QI Gong acupuncture electrotherapy used in pregnancy); Sublingual spray.

SLSP Sarcolemmal sodium pump.

SLT Sacrolaeva transversa (L.) - left sacro-transverse (fetal position); Second-line therapy (see SLDT; SLP); Sick-leave time; Solid logic technology; Standard laboratory test; Sublingual tablet; Swing light test.

SlTr Silent treatment (see SiTr).

sl tr slight trace (on laboratory reports).

SLTSA Society of Laboratory Technologists of South Africa.

SLU Superficial leg ulcer.

S-LU Sibley-Lehninger unit.

SLUD Salivation, lacrimation, urination, and defecation.

SLVD Systolic left ventricular dysfunction.

SLWC Short-leg walking cast.

SM Master of Science (see MSc); Sadomasochism (see S/M); Scientific Monthly (journal); Self-monitoring; Seminars in Medicine (journal); Sexual Myths (scale); Shigella mutant; Simple mastectomy; Skim milk; Smooth/ Stapedius muscle; Society for Microbiology; Somatomedin; Southern Medicine (journal, formerly Southern Medical Bulletin); Southwest Medicine (journal); Space/ Sports medicine; Sphingomyelin; Splenic macrophage; Splenomegaly; Spurling maneuver (diagnostic test in patients suffering from low back pain with lumbosacral radiation); Streptomycin (= STM; Strep); Stria medullaris; Strumpell-Marie (syndrome); Submandibular; Submaxillary; Submucous; Suckling mouse (see sM); Sucrose medium; Suction method; Superior mesenteric; Sustained medication; Symptom (see Sym); Synaptic/ Synovial membrane; Syringomyelia; Systolic mean/ motion/ murmur.

Sm Samarium (Z = 62) (formerly Sa, see Elements - Samarium); Serratia marcescens (formerly Erythrobacillus m) - gram-negative, saprophytic microorganisms of the family Enterobacteriaceae.

sM Suckling mouse (= SM).

sm small; smear.

S/M Sadism/masochism (= Sadomasochism) (= SM).

SMA Selective monoaminergic antagonist; "Self-matched" analysis; Self-Mutilators Anonymous; Sequential/ Serial multiple analysis/yzer; Sequential/ Simultaneous multichannel autoanalyzer; Serum muramidase activity; Severe metabolic acidosis/ alkalosis; Smooth muscle antibody; Society for Medical Anthropology; Somatomedin A (see SM-A); Sound medical advice; Southern Medical Association; Spinal muscular atrophy; Spontaneous motor activity; Standard method agar; Superior mesenteric artery; Supplementary motor area; Surface modulating assembly; Surgical muscle analysis (in DMD or Duchenne muscular dystrophy in children).

SM-A Somatomedin A (= SMA).

SMA-6 Sequential Multiple Analysis/yzer - 6 different serum tests, viz.: for sodium, potassium, carbon dioxide, chloride, glucose, and blood urea nitrogen (BUN) (laboratory/ chemistry).

SMA-6/60 Sequential Multiple Analysis - 6 tests in 60 minutes.

SMA-7 Sequential multipler analyzer for sodium, potassium, carbon dioxide, chloride, glucose, blood urea nitrogen (BUN), and creatine.

SMA-12 Sequential Multiple Analysis/yzer - 12 different serum tests, viz: for glucose, blood urea nitrogen (BUN), uric acid, calcium, phosphorus, total protein, albumin, cholesterol, total bilirubin, alkaline phosphatase, SGOT, and LDH.

SMA-23 Sequential multiplier analyzer, which includes the entire SMA-12, plus sodium, potassium, carbon dioxide, chloride, direct bilirubin, triglyceride, SGPT, indirect bilirubin, R fraction, and BUN/creatinine ratio.

SMABF Superior mesenteric artery blood flow.

SMABV Superior mesenteric artery blood velocity.

SMAC Sequential Multiple Analyzer and Computer (for blood chemistry profile); Supramolecular activation cluster (the point of contact between a T cell and an APC or Antigen-presenting cell as in CD4 and CD8 T cells).

Smack Heroin (see Diamorph).

SMAE Superior mesenteric artery embolism.
SMAF Smooth muscle activating factor; Specific macrophage arming factor.
SMAG Special Medical Advisory Group.
SMAL Serum methyl alcohol level.
sm amts small amounts.
sm an small animal.
SMAO Superior mesenteric artery occlusion.
SMART Simultaneous multiple angle reconstruction technique.
SMAS Sub/ Superficial muscular/lo aponeurotic system; Superior mesenteric artery syndrome.
SMAs Spinal muscular atrophies.
SMAST Short Michigan Alcoholism Screening Test.
SMB Selected mucosal biopsy; Southern Medical Bulletin (journal, now Southern Medicine - see SM); Standard medical base (medium) (= Smb); Suppressed mating behavior.
Smb Standard medical base (see SMB).
sMB Suckling mouse brain.
SMBFT Small bowel follow-through (X-ray/ intestines).
SMBG Self-monitoring blood glucose.
SMC Scientific Manpower Commission; Scottish Medical Council; Sensitized mast cell; Skeletal/ Smooth muscle cell; Socially maladroit child(ren) as in Autism [first discovered in 1943 by Johns Hopkins psychiatrist Leo Kanner]; in Asperger syndrome [after the work of Austrian pediatrician Hans Asperger in 1944]; and in other PPDs or Pervasive developmental disorders see ORB); Somatomedin C (see SM-C); Special mouth care; Standard medical care; State Medical Society; Subendometrial-myometrial contractility/ contractions (Obs/Gyn); Succinylmonocholine.
SM-C; Sm-C Somatomedin C (= SMC).
SMCA Smooth muscle contracting agent; Suckling mouse cataract agent.
SMCD Senile macular chorioretinal/horoidal degeneration; Systemic mast cell/ meningococcal disease.
SM-C/IGF Somatomedin C / insulin-like growth factor.
SMD Schizoaffective manic disorder (see SAMD); Senile macular degeneration; Single morning dose; Slow mental development; Spatial memory deficit; Standardized mean difference (see PSD; SD); Submanubrial dullness; Sympathomimetic drug (see âAA); Systemic mycobacterial disease.
SMDA Safe Medical Devices Act (of 1990); Starch methylenedianiline.
SMDC Sodium-N-methyl dithiocarbamate (dihydrate) - a soil sterilizant.
SMDS Secondary myelodysplastic syndrome.
SME Severe myoclonic epilepsy; Skeletal muscle effect(s) (see RML - Rhabdomyolysis); Sound medical evidence; Structure-modifying effect.
SMEAT Skylab medical experiment altitude test (NASA).
SMEDI Stillbirth-mummification, embryonic death, and infertility (syndrome).
SMEI Severe myoclonic epilepsy of infancy.
SMEM Supplemented (Eagle's) minimum essential medium.
S-Mez Sulfamezathine - a sulfonamide chemotherapeutic agent.
SMF Severe (bone) marrow failure; Sociedad Mexicana de Física (Mexican Physical Society); Streptozocin, mitomycin C, and 5-fluorouracil; Stylomastoid foramen.
smf sodium motive force.
SMFP State medical facilities plan.
SMFVD Sterile mid-forceps vaginal delivery.
SMG Submandibular gland.
SMGO Something more going on.
SMGT Streptococcus MG titer.
SMH Scripps Memorial Hospital; Scripps Mercy Hospital (see MOST); Soviet Ministry of Health (late USSR, now Russian M. of H.); State mental hospital; Strongyloidiasis with massive hyperinfection.
SMI Secondary mechanical imbalance; Self-Motivation Inventory; Senior Medical Investigator (VA); Sensory motor integration (group); Serious/ Severe/ Shadow mental illness; Serious/ Severe motor impairment (such as CP or Cerebral Palsy, RLA or Reduced language ability, UI or Urinary incontinence, etc.); Severe mental impairment; Silent myocardial infarction/ ischemia; Small (volume) infusion (see SVI); Stress myocardial

image; Style of Mind Inventory; Supplementary medical insurance; Sustained maximal/imum inspiration; Systemic mycoplasmal/ mycotic infection.

SmIg Surface membrane immunoglobulin.

SMILE Safety, monitoring, intervention, length of stay, and evaluation; Sustained maximal inspiratory lung exercises.

SMITF Supplementary Medical Insurance Trust Fund (SSA).

Smith Smithsonian (Institute) (see SI) (journal).

SMJ Society of Medical Jurisprudence; Southern Medical Journal (SMA); Squamomucosal junction; Sternomanubrial joint.

SMJAB State medical journal advertising bureau.

SMJ node Sister Mary Joseph node (in the superior pole of the umbilicus; diagnostic of metastatic carcinoma of the pancreas).

SML Severe memory loss; Sixth molar lactate (for electrolyte replacement therapy); Skylab Mobile Laboratory (NASA); Smouldering leukemia; Spleno medullary/ myelogenous leukemia.

$SMLD_{50}$ Suckling (mouse) mean lethal dose.

SMLs SM Laboratories (see SML).

SMM Science, Medicine, and Man (journal); Spinal myelomeningocele; Sternomastoid muscle (see SCM).

SMMD Specimen mass-measurement device.

SMN Second malignant neoplasm.

SMNB Submaximal neuromuscular block.

SMO Medical Officer of Schools; School Medical Officer; Senior Medical Officer (Navy); Serum monoamine oxidase (levels); Site-management organization; Slip made out.

SMOH Senior Medical Officer of Health; Society of Medical Officers of Health (UK).

SMOI Selective monoamine oxidase inhibitor (e.g. selegilene).

SMON Subacute myelo-optical neuropathy/ myelo-opticoneuropathy.

SMOT Sole mode of transmission (of disease).

SMN Sensorimotor neuropathy.

SMP Selfmanagement program; Sensory-motor paralysis; Skeletally mature patient/ person; Slow(est) moving protease; Smooth muscle proliferation; Special monthly pension; Spondylotic myelopathy; Standard medical practice/ procedure; Steroid metabolic pathway; Submitochondrial particle; Sulfamethoxypyrazine/ridazine - a long-acting sulfonamide compound (see CT 879).

SMR Senior medical resident; Sensorimotor rhythm; Severe mental retardation; Severe mitral regurgitation; Skeletal muscle regeneration/ relaxant (drug); Smooth muscle relaxant; Somnolent metabolic rate; Specific membrane receptor; Sphygmomanometer reading; Standard(ized) mortality rate; Stroke with minimum residuum; Submucosal/ Submucous resection (operation/ nose); Supportive medical resource(s).

SMRR Submucosal resection and rhinoplasty.

SMRV Squirrel monkey retrovirus.

SMS Senior medical student; Serial motor seizures; Severe myelosuppression; Shared Medical Systems; Smooth muscle spasm; Social Maturity Scale (psychological test assessing capacity for independent functioning); Sodium 2-mercaptoethane sulfonate; Somatostatin - a tetradecapeptide or octapeptide (see Hormones - SMS); Southern Medicine and Surgery (journal); Standard (damped sine wave) monophasic shock (used in TVD - Transthoracic ventricular defibrillation in cardiac arrest (see SWMV; TBS); Stiff-man syndrome; Strict medical supervision; Supplemental minimum sodium.

SMSA Standard metropolitan statistical area.

SMSG Submandibular salivary gland.

SMSV San Miguel sea-lion virus.

SMSW State Medical Society of Wisconsin.

SMT *Salmonella* Microsome Test; Significant maternal toxicity; Smooth muscle tone; Snider Match Test; Spontaneous mammary tumor; Stereotactic mesencephalic tractomy; Sternomastoid tumor (see SCM; SMM).

SMuLV Scripps murine leukemia virus.

SMV Slow-moving vehicle; Stenotic mitral valve; Submentovertical (fetal position); Superior mesenteric vein.

SMVB Sign mechanism for ventilator breathing.

SMVT Sustained monomorphic ventricular tachycardia.

SMW Severe muscular weakness (e.g. due to hypokalemia).

SMWDSep Single, married, widowed, divorced, or separated.

SMX; SMZ Sulfamethoxazole.

SN Parke, Davis & Co (USA) and Wintrop Sterling Research Laboratories (USA) code for antimalarial experimental drugs; School Nurse (NEA journal); Sciatic/ Suprasternal notch; Sclerema neonatorum; Scrub/ Staff/ Student/ Surgical Nurse; Sensorineural; Sensory neuron; Serendipitous neologism; Serum neutralization; Single nephron; Sinus node; Society for Neuroscience (Canada); Spastic News (SS journal, UK); Spontaneous nystagmus; Standard nomenclature (records); Subnormal; Substantia nigra (of the brain); Supernatant; Supernormal; Supervisor Nurse (journal); Surgical Neurology (CNS journal).

Sn Subnasale; Tin (L. stannum) (Z = 50) (see Elements - Tin).

sn according to nature (L. secundum naturam); swaged needle (with no eye and permantly swaged to or stamped on the suture material).

S/N Signal/noise (ratio) (see SNR).

SN 44 Dalanated Insulin - an insulin derivative prepared by removal of the C-terminal alanine from the B-chain of insulin (see Insulin - DI)

SN 46 Dinex (see DNOCHP).

SN_{50} Serum neutralizing antibody.

SN 971 Pamaquin (see RP 4516).

SN 3115 Plasmocide (see F 710).

SN 6771 Bialamicol hydrochloride (see CT 871).

SN 7618 Chloroquine Phosphate (= Chlorochinum diphosphoricum; Chloroquin diphosphate; Chloroquini diphosphas; Chloroquinium phosphate) - a 4-aminoquinoline synthetic drug used for the suppression and treatment of malaria, killing the erythrocytic forms of the parasites at all stages of development. Also found useful in the treatment of amebic hepatitis and liver abscess, but has no effect in intestinal amebiasis. Remission in rheumatoid arthritis has been achieved after 2 to 3 months, but prolonged therapy may give rise to toxic effects such as corneal opacity or irreversible retinal damage ("chloroquine retinopathy"). Chloroquine has also been found of value in the treatment of giardiasis and lupus erythematosus.

SN 10751 Amodiaquine hydrochloride (= Amodiachin HCl; Amodiaquini hydrochoridum) - a 4-aminoquinoline synthetic antimalarial drug with actions similar to those of choroquine (SN 7618).

SN 12837 Proguanil hydrochloride (see RP 3359).

SN 13272 Primaquine phosphate (= Primachin phosphate; Primaquini diphosphas; Primaquinium phosphate) - an 8-aminoquinoline synthetic antimalarial drug which kills the exoerythrocytic forms of the malarial parasites but has little action on other erythrocytic stages, and therefore it should not be used alone in the treatment of a malarial attack. It is chiefly used for the radical cure of Plasmodium vivax infections.

SN 13276 Pentaquin phosphate (= 8-[5-Isopropylaminopentylamino]- 6-methoxyquinoline phophate) - an 8-aminoquinoline synthetic antimalarial drug with actions similar to those of pamaquin (see RP 4516; SN 13272).

SN 16168 Hydroxychloroquine sulfate (= Win 1258-2) - a 4-aminoquinoline synthetic antimalarial drug with action similar to that of chloroquine (see SN 7618).

SNA Seronegative arthritis; Serum neutralizing antibody; Specimen not available; Student Nurses Association; Synthetic nucleoside analogue (see NA; NSA).

SNa Serum sodium concentration.

SNagg Serum normal agglutinator.

SNAI Standard nomenclature of athletic injuries.

snake graft sequential graft (CABG).

SNAP RCN journal, UK; Sensory nerve action potential.

Snapper Amyl nitrite capsule/vial (see Amyl nitrite).

SNAT Serotonin n-acetyltransferase.

SNB Scalene node biopsy (operation/ chest); Sentinel node biopsy (in malignant

melanoma) (see SLNB); Spastic neurogenic bladder; Spinal nerve block.
SNBF Single nephron blood flow (see SNGBF).
SNC Sensory/ Slowed nerve conduction; Serious/ Stabilized neurologic(al) condition; Single needle catheter (Coke, Cook, or Shiley needle catheters - attached to the dialysis machine as a double blood pump {Hemodialysis}); Skilled nursing care; Skinny needle cholangiography; Spontaneous neonatal chylothorax.
SNCL Sinus node cycle length.
SNCS Sensory nerve conduction studies.
SNCV Sensory nerve conduction velocity.
SND Sensorineural deafness; Serotonergic drug - i.e. Serotonin enhancer or serotonin releaser (see MAE; SED); Single needle device; Sinus node disease/ disorder/ disturbance/ dysfunction; Striatonigral degeneration; Stroke, no dementia (see HAAS); Suspected notifiable disease (see KND); Systemic nasal decongestant; Swan-neck deformity (of the interphalangeal joint) (see FAC).
SNDA Student National Dental Association.
SNDO Standard Nomenclature of Diseases and Operations.
SNE Severe necrotizing enteritis; Sinus node electrogram; Spatial-nonemotional (stimulus); Subacute necrotizing encephalomyelopathy.
SNES Suprascapular nerve entrapment syndrome.
SNF Sinus node formation; Skilled nursing facility; Sympathetic nerve fiber.
SNG Solidified nitroglycerol.
SNGA Sodium (salt of) n-glycoloyl-arsanilic acid.
SNGBF Single nephron glomerular blood flow (= SNBF).
SNGFR Single nephron glomerular filtration rate.
SNHL Sensorineural hearing loss.
SNI Severe neurological impairment.
Sniff Cocaine (see Erythroxylum).
Snip(s) Pronunciation of SNP or Single nucleotide polymorphism(s) (see SNP; SNPS).
SNIT Single needle insertion technique (Obstetrics).
SNL Sciatic nerve lesion.
SNM Society of Nuclear Medicine; Sulfanilamide.
SNMA Student National Medical Association.
SNMN Society of Nuclear Medicine Newsletter.
SNMT Society of Nuclear Medicine Technologists.
SNO S-nitrosothiol.
SNOBOL String-Oriented Symbolic Language.
SNODO Standard Nomenclature of Diseases and Operations.
SNOMED Standardized/ Symmetrical Nomenclature of Medicine.
SNOOP Systemic Nursing Observation of Psychopathology.
SNOP Standard/ Standardized/ Systematized Nomenclature of Pathology (College of American Pathologists).
Snop Marijuana (see Cannabis).
Snort Cocaine (see Erythroxylum); Small alcoholic drink.
Snow Cocaine (see Erythroxylum).
SNP Parathion (see DNTP); Saturday night palsy (compression lesion of the radial nerve against the humerus occurring in inebriated individuals, especially on Saturday or weekend nights); School nurse practitioner; Sensory neuropathy; Severe neutropenia; Single-nucleotide polymorphism (database) (see SNPS); Sinus node potential; Sodium nitroprusside; Soviet Neurology and Psychiatry (now Russian, translation journal).
SNPS Single-nucleotide polymorphisms (one-letter genetic differences in the human genome).
SNR Sentinel node resection (in breast cancer see CAD; SLNM; SLNs); Signal-to-noise ratio (= S/N); Spinal nerve regeneration/ root; Substantia nigra (zona) reticulata (see SNZR); Supernumerary rib.
SNRA; sNRA Soluble ribonucleic acid (see sRNA).
SNRB Selective nerve root block.
SNRI Selective/ Serotonin/ Specific noradrenaline/ norepinephrine reuptake inhibitor.
SNRL Spinal nerve root lesion (= NRL).

snRNA Small nuclear ribonucleic acid.
snRNP Small nuclear ribonucleoprotein.
SNRT Sinus node recovery time.
SNRTd Sinus node recovery time, direct measuring.
SNRTi Sinus node recovery time, indirect measuring.
SNS Senior Nursing Sister; Society of Neurological Surgeons; Statistically non-significant; Sterile normal saline (0.9% sodium chloride); Sympathetic nervous system.
SNSA Seronegative spondyloarthritis/ spondyloarthropathy.
SNSP Seronegative sex(ual) partner (see S-SP; S-ve SP).
SNST Sciatic nerve stretch test.
SNT Serious/ Severe neurological toxicity (e.g. irreversible paraparesis/ quadriparesis); Sinuses, nose, and throat; Suppan nail technique.
SNV Spleen necrosis virus; Stress nuclear ventriculography (see RNV).
SNW Slow negative wave.
SNZR Substantia nigra zona reticulata (= SNR).
SO Sale only; Salpingo-oophorectomy (see S&O); Schlatter-Osgood (disease/ test); Second opinion; Seminars in Oncology (journal); Sex offender; Shoulder orthosis; Significant offer/ other; Society of Opticians (South Africa); Spheno-occipital (synchondrosis); Sphincter of Oddi; Standing orders; Suboccipital; Superior oblique (muscle) (see SOM); Supraoptic (nucleus) (see SON); Supraorbital; Sutures out.
So South (see S. South).
S-O Salpingo-oophorectomy (see S&O).
S&O Salpingo-oophorectomy (= SO).
SO_2 Oxygen saturation (of hemoglobulin) (see PFT); Sulfur dioxide.
$^{35}SO_2$ Radioactive-labeled sulfur dioxide.
SO_3 Sulfite (radical).
SO_4 Sulfate (radical).
SOA Secondary osteoarthritis; Serum opsonic activity; Sex Offenders Act 1997 (UK); Single oral administration (see SOD); Spinal opioid analgesia; Supraorbital artery; Swelling of ankles.
SoA Signs of anxiety: *Appearance*: Muscle tension (rigidity) - Skin blanches, pales - Perspiration, clammy skin - Fatigue - Small motor activity (e.g. restlessness, tremor); *Behavior*: Attention span - Ability to follow directions - Acting out - Somatizing - Immobility; *Conversation*: - Number of questions - Constant seeking of reassurance - Frequent shifting of topics of conversation - Describes fears with sense of helplessness - Avoids focusing on feelings - Focuses on equipment or procedures; *Physiological signs mediated through autonomic nervous system*: - Heart rate - Rate or depth of respirations - Rapid extreme shifts in body temperature, blood pressure, menstrual flow - Diarrhea Urinary urgency - Dryness of mouth - Appetite - Perspiration - Dilation of pupils - Signs of anxiety are dependent on their degree. Mild anxiety heightens the use of capacities, whereas severe and panic states severly paralyze or overwork capacities; Symptoms of asthma.
SOAA Signed out against advice (see SOAMA).
SOAM Sutures out in the morning.
SOAMA Signed out against medical advice (= SOAA; SOMA).
SOA-MCA Superficial occipital artery to middle cerebral artery.
SOAP Subjective, objective, assessment, and plan (in problem-oriented records).
Soaper Methaqualone.
SOAPIE Subjective, objective, assessment, plan, implementation/ intervention, and evaluation (in problem-oriented records).
SOB See order blank/ book; Short(ness) of breath; Side of bed; Son of a bitch!; Suboccipitobregmatic.
SOC Second Opinion Clinic (Breast Center, COH, Ca, USA); Sequential oral contraceptive; Socialization; Specialty-oriented care (see POC); Spontaneous ovulatory cycle; Standard Occupational Classification; Standards of care; Synthetic oxygen carrier (Perfluorocarbons used in preparation of oxygen-absorbing, synthetic blood); Syphilitic osteochondritis; System organ class.
SoC State of consciousness.
S&OC Signed and on chart.

Soc econ Socioeconomic.
SOCMA Synthetic Organic Chemical Manufacturers Association.
SocSec Social Security.
SocServ Social Services.
S-OCT Serum ornithine carbamyl transferase.
SOD Septo-optic dysplasia; Severity of diseaase; Single oral dose (= SOA); Sinovenous occlusive disease; Specific organ damage; Spray-on dressing (Reziplast); Superoxide dismutase (a drug erroneously touted as a retardant of the aging process); Surgical officer of the day.
Sod; sod Sodium (see Na).
Soda Sodium carbonate or Washing soda (see Na_2CO_3).
SODAS Spheroidal Oral Delivery Absorption System (Elan, Dublin, Ireland); Spheroidal oral drug absorption system.
Sod/Soda bicarb Sodium bicarbonate or Baking soda (see $NaHCO_3$).
SODH Sorbitol dehydrogenase.
SODQ Severity of Opiate Dependence Questionnaire.
SOEH Society for Occupational and Environmental Health.
SOF Secondary ovarian failure; Superior orbital fissure.
SOG Suggestive of good.
SOH Sub-optimal health; Sympathetic orthostatic hypotension.
SOHN Supraoptic hypothalamic nuclei/eus.
SOI Severe ocular infection/ inflammation/ irritation; Severe opportunistic infection (occurring in AIDS, and caused by parasites such as: *Coccidiodes* immitis, *Cryptococcus* neoformans, the Cryptosporidium protozoan parasite, the Cytomegalovirus [CMV], the Hepatitis-B virus, *Histoplasma* capsulatum, the Human papilloma virus [HPV], *Mycobacterium* avium [MAC] and M. tuberculosis [TB], *Pneumocystis* carinii, and *Toxoplasma* gondii) (see LTOI); Severity of disease.
SOL Solution (see sol); Space-occupying lesion; Spontaneous onset of labor.
SoL Sanctity-of-life (principle, in medicine).
Sol See sol.
sol solidification (= solidif); soluble (= Sol); solution (L. solutio) (= SOL; Sol; Soln; soln).
SOLAS Safety of Life at Sea (ship company rules).
SOLEC Stand on (one) leg eyes closed.
soleno- prefix meaning pipe or tube (Gr. solen).
solidif solidification (see sol).
Soln; soln Solution (see sol).
solut- combining form meaning dissolve or free (L. solutus) (see solv-).
Solv; solv Dissolve (L. solve); Solvent.
solv- combining form meaning dissolve or free (L. solvo) (see solut-).
SOLVD Survival of Left Ventricular Dysfunction (Study).
SOM Scanning optical microscope; Secondary outcome measures; Secretory/ Serous/ Suppurative otitis media; Sensitivity of method; Society of Occupational Medicine (UK); Somatic/ Somatostatin/ Somatotropin (see Somat); Superior oblique muscle (eye) (= SO); Suppurative otitis media.
Som Somatic/ Somatostatin/ Somatotropin (see Somat).
SOMA Signed out against medical advice (see SOAMA); Student Osteopathic Medical Association.
soma- prefix meaning body (Gr.).
Somat; somat Somatic/ Somatostatin/ Somatotropin (= SOM; Som).
-some suffix meaning body (Gr. soma).
SOMI Sternal occipital mandibular immobilization.
SOMJ Society of Occupational Medicine Journal.
SOMOS Society of Military Orthopedic Surgeons.
SON Spontaneous osteonecrosis (e.g. of the medial femoral condyle) (= ION); Superior olivary nucleus; Supraoptic nucleus (= SO).
SONAR Sound navigation and ranging.
Sonix (journal).
Sono Sonogram.
SONP Solid organs not palpable.
SO nucleus Superior olivary nucleus (see SON); Supraoptic nucleus (see SON).
SOP Stabilized oncotic pressure; Standard operation(al) procedure; Standing operating procedure.

SoP Standard of performance.
SOPA Syndrome of primary aldosteronism.
SOPCA Sporadic olivopontocerebellar ataxia.
SOPM Stitches out in the afternoon.
Sopor Methaqualone; Soporific.
SOPP Society for Oncology Pharmacy Practitioners (UK) (see ISOPP).
s op s if (it is) necessary (L. si opus sit) (see sos).
SOQ Suicide Opinion Questionnaire.
SOR Sign out release; Stimulus-organism-response (see S-O-R); Sorbitol (see Sorb); Superoxide release.
SOr Supraorbitale.
Sor; sor Sorbitol (see Sorb).
S-O-R Stimulus-organism-response (theory of behavior) (= SOR).
Sorb; sorb Sorbitol (= SOR; Sor; sor).
SorbD; SORD Sorbitol dehydrogenase.
SOS If (it is)/ Only if necessary (see sos); International distress signal ("Save our souls"); Scandinavian Orthodontic Society; Self-obtained smear; Self- organizing system; Silicon-on-sapphire (computer memory); Supplemental oxygen system.
sos if/ if it is/ only if necessary (L. si opus sit) (= s op s; SOS).
SoSAI Springfield Outpatient Symptom and Adjustment Index.
SOSF Single organ system failure.
SOSH Sub-optimal subjective health.
SOSSUS Study on Surgical Services for the United States.
SOT Sensory organization test; Solid-organ transplant(ation); Something other than; Stream of thought; Sub-optimal treatment; Systemic oxygen transport.
SOTA State-of-the-Art (care/ treatment).
SOTT Synthetic medium old tuberculin trichloracetic acid (precipitated).
SOWS Subjective opiate withdrawal scale.
SP Sacroposterior; Sacrum to pubis; Salivary progesterone; Schizotypal personality; Schwangerschafts-protein (pregnancy-associated plasma protein); Scientia Pharmaceutica (journal); Secretary piece; Semi-private (room) (see S/P); Senile plaque; Septum pellucidum; Sequential pulse; Seropositive; Serum/ Surfactant protein; Settleable particulates (air pollution); Shunt/ Systolic pressure; Shunt procedure (group/ arteriovenous); Sigura/ Sugiura procedure (devascularization of esophagus and stomach) (= SS - Segura surgery); Silent period; Sippy's point (on the epigastrium); Skin/ Steady/ Summation potential (= Sp); Sleep deprivation; Soft palate; Solid phase; Somogyi phenomenon (see PHGHG); Spastic paraparesis/ paraplegia (see SPP); Special precautions (see S/P); Speech pathologist/gy; Spleen; Spontaneous proliferation; Squinting patella (skin crease over the patella of a knee affected with chondromalacia); Stamey procedure (see PUS); Stand pivot; Standard practice/ procedure; Staphylococcal protease; Status post (see s/p); Step-parent; Stool preservative (Hajna); Subliminal perception; Substance P (polypeptide); Suicide precautions (see S/P); Sulfopropyl (sulfonic acid); Suprapatellar; Suprapubic (S. puncture); Symphysis pubis.
Sp Skin/ Study/ Summation potential (see SP); Space/ Special/ Species/ Specific/ Speech/ Spinal(ne)/ Spouse (see sp); Spanish (see Span); Sphenoid(al); Spirillum; Spirit (L. spiritus) (see Spt); The most posterior point on the posterior contour of the sella turcica.
sP Senile parkinsonism.
sp space/ special/ species/ specific/ speech/ spinal(ne)/ spouse (= Sp); spirit (alcohol) (see Spt); without issue (L. sine prole).
S/P Scientific Products (Div of AHSC); Semi-private (room) (= SP); Serum protein (= SP); Special precautions (= SP); Spinal/ne (= Sp; sp); Stand and pivot; Status post (see s/p); Suicide precautions (= SP); Suprapubic (= SP); Systolic pressure.
s/p status post (as before/ condition after/ no change) (= SP; S/P).
S_P Serum phosphorus.
S2P Second heart sound (pulmonic component).
S7P Sedoheptulose 7-phosphate.
SP-6 Acupuncture point (Sanyinjiao) - as in Hegu (Anatomical location, 3 'cun' or three times the breadth of the patient's thumb, proximal to the peak of the ankle behind the tibia, and used to evaluate the influence of acupuncture, in the blood flow in the umbili-

cal artery, fetal aorta, and uterine artery - see LI-4).

SP 732 Prolintane hydrochloride (= 1-Phenyl-2-pyrrolidinopentane HCl) - a central nervous stimulant with a potency intermediate between that of amphetamine and caffeine. Used as a tonic for convalescence in cases of stress, strain, or overwork, and in the elderly.

SPA Salt-poor (human) albumin (IV therapy); Scapuloperoneal atrophy; Schizophrenia with premorbid asociality; Screening panel arbitration; Serum prothrombin activity; Severe persistent asthma; Sheep pulmonary adenomatosis; Simultaneous peroxidase activity (for occult blood); Single-photon absorptiometry; Smith-Petersen arthrodesis (of the wrist); Southern Perinatal Association; Speech-processing area (of the brain; i.e. Brocha's area in the left temporal lobe of the cerebrum); Sperm penetration assay; Spinal progressive amyotrophy; Spondyloarthropathy; Spontaneous platelet aggregation; Staphylococcal protein A; Stimulation-produced analgesia; Suprapubic aspiration (bladder); Synthetic prostamide analog (of prostaglandin, with ocular hypotensive activity).

SP-A Surfactant protein A.

SPACE Secondary prevention with antioxidants of cardiovascular disease in endstage renal disease.

sp act specific activity.

SPAD Stenosing peripheral arterial disease; Subcutaneous peritoneal access device (used in the treatment of refractory diabetes mellitus).

SPAG Small particle aerosol generator.

SPAI Steroid protein activity index.

SPAM Scanning photoacoustic microscope/py.

SPAMM Spatial modulation of magnetization.

SP amputation Suprapatellar amputation.

Span Spanish (= Sp).

sp an spinal anesthesia.

SPAN-80 Sorbitan mono-oleate.

Span-K Potassium chloride.

Span P Spanish Pharmacopeia (= Sp P).

span(s) spansule(s) (prescription).

SPAR Sensitivity prediction by acoustic reflex.

spas- prefix meaning pull (Gr.).

SPAT Slow paroxysmal atrial tachycardia.

SPB Serum protein binding; "Slash, poison, and burn" (traditional cancer therapy); Spontaneous preterm birth.

SP-B Surfactant protein B.

SPBI Serum protein-bound iodine (see PBI).

SPBT Suprapubic bladder tap.

SPC Salicylamide, phenacetin, and caffeine; Self-perpetuating condition; Serious/ Severe/ Similar/ Suicidal psychiatric condition; Seropositive carrier; Serum phenylalanine concentration; Severe persistent cough; Sickle-shaped particle cell; Single palmar crease; Single photoelectron count; Spleen cell; Standard plate count; Statistical process control; Subgenual prefrontal cortex (degenerates in hereditary and other forms of severe depression); Subperiosteal chondroma (Orthopedics); Suicide Prevention Center; Summary of Product Characteristics; Sun-protective clothing (see SPF; SPP); Synthetizing protein complex.

SPCA Serum prothrombin conversion accelerator (= Proconvertin) (see Factor VII); Society for Prevention of Cruelty to Animals.

SPCC Society for Prevention of Cruelty to Children; Spill Prevention, Control, and Countermeasure (plan).

SPCD Severe peripheral circulatory disturbance (as in Buerger's disease, Raynaud's disease, etc.); Syndrome of primary ciliary dyskinesia.

SpCd; sp cd Spinal cord.

SPCDC Stress, Pain and Chronic Disease Clinic (Toronto General Hospital, Canada).

SPCF Serine-protease coagulation factor.

SPD Salmon poisoning disease; Schizoid/ Schizotypal/ Severe/ Sociopathic personality disorder; Serum protein binding/ bound; Severe periodic/ psychic disturbance; Severe peripheral dysesthesia; Severe psychiatric disorder; Shadow panic disorder; Single-photon densitometer/metry (of bones, etc.); Sociopathic disorder (see ASP; ASPD); Specific paroxysmal discharge; Speech-processing device (i.e. artificial cochlear implant); Spontaneous preterm delivery; Standard peak dilution; Storage pool deficiency; Stupor-producing dose/ drug; Subcorneal pustular dermatosis; Symptomatic Parkinson's disease.

SPDC Strio-pallido-dentate calcinosis.

SPE Septic pulmonary edema; Serum protein electrolytes/ electrophoresis; Splash-proof equipment (MET-501) (see also, APE); Spontaneous perforation of the esophagus; Streptococcal pyrogenic exotoxin; Sucrose polyester (a synthetic food fat substitute); Sustained physical exercise; Symptomatic pleural effusion.

SPEAR Selective parenteral and enteral antisepsis regimen; Stanford Positron Electron Accelerating Ring (synchotron radiation).

Spec Specialist; Speciality; Specification (see specif).

spec special; specific (see specif); specimen.

SPE-C Streptococcal pyrogenic exotoxin - type C.

SpecEd Special education.

spec gr specific gravity (see sp gr).

specif specific(ation) (= Spec).

SPECT Single photon emission computed/erized tomography (see PET).

spectr- combining form meaning appearance (L. spectrum).

Spectrum (journal - IEEE).

Speed Methamphetamine (see Amphet).

Speedball A mixture of cocaine and heroin (see Erythroxylum; Diamorph).

SPEG Serum protein electrophoretogram.

SPEM Smooth pursuit eye movement.

SPEP Serum protein electrophoresis (laboratory/ chemistry).

SPEPB Society of Pharmacological and Environmental Pathologists Bulletin.

sperm- combining form meaning seed (Gr. sperma).

spers- combining form meaning scatter (L. -spersus).

SPET Single-photon emission tomography.

SPF Shared professional facility; Skin protection factor; Specific-pathogen free; Spectrophotofluorometer; S-phase fraction; Split products of fibrin; Standard perfusion fluid; Stuart-Prower factor (see SP-F); Sun protection/ive factor (see SPC; SPP); Symptomatic pleural fibrosis; Systemic pulmonary fistula.

SP-F Stuart-Prower factor (= SPF) (see Factor X).

sp fl spinal fluid.

SPG Separate/ Small/ Special parent group; Serine phosphoglyceride; Sliding pulse generator; Sphenopalatine ganglion; Strain guage plethysmograph(y); Sucrose, phosphate, and glutamate; Symmetrical peripheral gangrene.

SpG Specific gravity.

spg sponge.

SPGA Bovarnik's solution; Sucrose.

sp gr specific gravity (= sg; spec gr; SpG).

SP group Shunt procedure group (see SP).

SPH School of Public Health; Secondary pulmonary hemosiderosis/ hypertension; Severely and profoundly handicapped; Severe pregnancy hypertension; Society of Public Health (UK); Spherocyte/tosis; Sphyngomyelin (see Sph).

Sph Sphenoidale; Sphyngomyelin (= SPH).

sph spherical; spherical lens; spheroid.

SPHE Society for Public Health Education.

sphen- combining form meaning wedge (Gr.).

spher- combining form meaning round (Gr. sphaira).

SPHERO Spherocytes (see SPH).

sp ht specific heat.

sphygm- prefix meaning pulse (Gr. sphygmos).

SPI Selective/ Serum protein index; Self-Perception Inventory; Serum precipitable iodine; Severe pelvic/ pulmonary infection; Severe pulmonary insufficiency; Shipley Personal Inventory; Silicone penile implant; Single peak insulin (see Insulin - SPI); Smith-Petersen incision (Total hip replacement) (see inc.); Speech processor interface.

SP-I Podophyllinic acid ethylhydrazide.

SPIA Solid-phase immunoabsorption/ immunoassay.

SPIF Spontaneous peak inspiratory force.

SPICU Surgical pulmonary intensive care unit.

SPID Summed pain intensity difference.

SPIE Society of Photo-Optical Instrumentation Engineers.

SPIF Solid-phase immunoassay fluorescence.

SPIH Signal Processing and Information

Handling (Committee) (GEMB).
SPIN Searchable physics information notices (computer-readable) (NERAC).
spin spinal/ne/nous.
spin- combining form meaning spine (L. spina).
sp indet indeterminate species (L. species indeterminata).
sp inquir species of doubtful status/ uncertain species (L. species inquirendae).
SPIP Scrotal-perineal incontinence prosthesis (placed either around the urethra or the bladder neck to control incontinence due to neurogenic bladder).
Spir Alcohol/ spirit (see Spt); Spirometry.
spir alcohol/ spirit (see Spt); spiral; spiritual.
spirat- combining form meaning breathe (L. spiratus).
spis; spiss dried (L. spissus); inspissated/ thickened by evaporation (L. spissatus).
SPIT Society for the Prevention of Involunatary Tranquilization.
S-PITC Sulfo-phenylisothiocyanate.
SPK Serum pyruvate kinase; Spinnbarkeit (with reference to cervical mucus); Superficial punctate keratitis.
SPL Serum progesterone level (ng/ml; nmol/L); Skin potential level; Sound pressure level; Speech perception level; Splanchnic; Split; Spontaneous lesion; Staphylococcal phage lysate; Superior parietal lobule.
splanchn- combining form meaning entrails (Gr. splagchna).
Splash Amphetamines (see Amphet).
SPLATT Split anterior tibial tendon.
splen- combining form meaning spleen (Gr.).
sPLM Sleep-related periodic leg movement.
SPLV Serum parvovirus-like virus.
SPM School of Postgraduate Medicine; Serious professional misconduct (GMC, UK); Shocks/ Syllables per minute; Slow-paced management; Spectinomycin; Spinal poliomyelitis (see APM); Subhuman primate model; Superparamagnetic (properties of iron oxide nanoparticles, etc.); Suspended particulate matter; Synaptic plasma membrane.
SpM Spiriformis medialis (nucleus).
SPMA Spinal progressive muscular atrophy.
SPMR Standard proportionate mortality rate/ ratio.
SPMS Secondary progressive multiple sclerosis (see RPMS; RRMS).
SPMSQ Short Portable Mental Status Questionnaire.
SPN Serotonin-producing neuron; Severe/ Symmetrical peripheral neuropathy; Smith-Petersen nail (Orthopedics); Solitary pulmonary nodule; Student practical nurse; Supplemental parenteral nutrition; Sympathetic paraganglionic neuron.
sp n; sp nov new species (L. species novum).
SPO Sodium benzyl penicilloate.
SPO; SPO_2; SpO_2 Single pulse oximetry.
SpO_2 Oxyhemoglobin saturation measured by pulse oximetry; Pulse oximetry.
SPOD Spouse's perception of disease.
spon spontaneous (see spont).
spongio- combining form meaning sponge (L. spongia).
spont spontaneous (= spon).
SPOOL Simultaneous peripheral operation on-line.
spor- combining form meaning seed (Gr. sporos).
Spork Combining spoon and fork.
SPP Schizophreniform psychosis; Scrabicphtiriasis pediculosis (inguinal skin, louse infestation); Secondary pharmacological properties/ty; Sexuality Preference Profile; Skin perfusion pressure; Small porous particle; Sociopathic personality (see ASP; ASPD; PPP); Spastic paraparesis/ paraplegia (= SP); Species (pl.) (see spp); Sun-protection program (see SPC; SPF); Suprapubic pain/ prostatectomy; Synthetic polypeptide.
spp species (plural of) (= SPP).
Sp. P Spanish Pharmacopoeia (Farmacopea Oficial Española) (see Span P).
SPPD Sociopathic personality disorder; Standard parallel-dose design.
SPPP; sppp subspecies (plural of).
SPPS Solid phase peptide synthesis; Stable plasma protein solution.
SPPSR School of Public Policy and Social Research (UCLA).
SPPT Superprecipitation (response).
SPR Serial probe recognition; Significant pressor release; Skin potential response;

Society for Pediatric Radiology/ Research; Society for Physical/ Psychical/ Psychoanalytical/ Psychophysiological Research; Solid phase radioimmunoassay (see SPRIA); Stimulated prolactin release; Surface protein marker.

SPR; S/PR; S/PR Staff-patient ratio.

Spr Scan projection radiography.

spr sprain.

SPRIA Solid phase radioimmunoassay (= SPR).

SPROM Spontaneous premature rupture of membrane(s).

SPS Scapuloperoneal syndrome; Serial-parallel-serial (shift register); Shoulder pain and stiffness; Simple partial seizure(s); Slow(ly) progressive schizophrenia; Society of Pelvic Surgeons; Sodium polyethanol sulfonate; Sound Production Sample (test); Special Pap(anicolaou) smear (see Pap); Stable Parkinsonian syndrome; Sterile physiological saline; Stimulated protein synthesis; Storage photoconductor scan (converter); Suicide Probability Scale; Sulfite polymyxin sulfadiazine (agar); Systemic progressive sclerosis.

SpS Sphenoid sinus.

sps without surviving issue (L. sine prole supersite).

SPSE Society of Photographic Scientists and Engineers.

spSHR Stroke-prone spontaneously hypertensive rat.

SPSP Seropositive sex(ual) partner (see S+ SP; S+ve SP).

SPSS Statistical Package for the Social Sciences.

SPST Symonds Picture-Story Test.

SPS test Sound Production Sample test.

S/P surgery Status post surgery.

SPT Secretin-pancreazymin test; Serum pyruvic transaminase; Signal-processing technology; Simple patch technique; Skin-prick test; Sleep period time; Sound production task(s); Speech Pathology and Therapy (journal, now in BJDC); Spondee Picture Test; Static pelvic traction (see SPTx); Station pull-through (technique); Strenuous physical training; Systolic pressure time.

SpT Spinal tap (= Sp tap).

Spt; spt Alcohol/ Spirit(s) (L. spiritus) (= Sp; sp; Spir; spir).

Sp tap Spinal tap (see SpT).

SPTB Spontaneous preterm birth (see SPTD).

SPTD Spontaneous preterm delivery (see SPTB).

SpTh Spino-thalamic (tract).

SPTI Systolic pressure time index.

SPTS Subjective posttraumatic syndrome.

SPTx Static pelvic traction (= SPT).

SPU Sample processing unit; Short procedure unit; Society of Pediatric Urology; Special precautions for use; Stenosing peptic ulcer.

SPUC Society for the Protection of Unborn Children.

SPV Selective proximal vagotomy; Selective pulmonary vasodilator; Severe peripheral vasospasm; Shope papilloma virus; Smallpox virus; Sulfophosphovanillin.

SpVol Specific volume.

SPVR Systemic peripheral vascular resistance.

SPW factor Single present worth factor.

SPZ Sulfinpyrazone.

SQ E.R. Sqibb & Sons (USA) code for experimental substances; Social quotient; Status quo; Subcutaneous(ly) (see SC); Survey question; Symptom questionnaire.

Sq Subcutaneous(ly) (see SC).

sq following (L. sequentia); squamous (cell); square; subcutaneous(ly) (see SC).

SQ 1089 Hydroxyurea (see NSC 32065).

SQ 9453 Dimethyl sulfoxide (see DMSO).

SQ 9538 Testolactone - an antineoplastic agent.

SQ 9993 Estradiol undecylate (= Oestradiol undecenoate) - an estrogenic hormone with properties similar to those of estradiol; administered by intramuscular injection in oily solution, to provide a depot from which the drug is slowly released.

SQ 14225 Captopril (= D-3-mercapto-2-methylpropanoyl-L-proline) - a dipeptidyl carboxypeptidase and hypotensive drug acting by the active inhibition of angiotensin I-converting enzyme and inactivation of bradykinin.

SQ 15761 Sodium Ipodate (= Sodium iopodate) - an organic iodine compound used as a contrast medium for examination of the biliary tract.

SQ 16150 Estradiol ethanate (= Oestradiol ethanate; Oestradiol 17-heptanoate) - an estrogen with properties similar to those of estradiol undecylate (see SQ 9993).

SQ 16374 Methenolone enathate (= Methenolone oenanthate) - an anabolic sex hormone, with anabolic properties more pronounced than its androgenic effects. It increases retention of nitrogen, calcium, sodium, potassium, chloride and phosphate, leading to an increase in skeletal weight, water retention, and increased growth of bone.

SQ 16401 Halquinol (= Chlorhydroxyquinoline) - an antibacterial, antifungal, and anti-amebic agent used topically in the treatment of infected skin conditions, and given internally as tablets in bacterial, non-specific and amebic diarrheas.

SQ 20881 Teprotide - a snake venom peptide, prepared from the species Bothrops jararaca, a specific inhibitor of the angiotensin-converting enzyme, and highly effective as an antihypertensive agent.

SQA Systematic quality assurance.

SQC Semi-quantitative criteria; Statistical quality control.

SqCCa Squamous cell carcinoma (see sq cell ca).

sq cel ca See sq cell ca.

sq cell ca squamous cell carcinoma (= SqCCa; sq cel ca; squamous cancer cell).

sq cm square centimeter(s).

SQE Semi-quantitative estimation (e.g. urinary sugar, etc.).

sq epith squamous epithelium.

sq ft square foot/ feet.

SQID Superconducting quantum interference device (see SQUID).

sq in square inch(es).

Sql Squirrel.

sq m square meter(s) (= M^2; m^2).

sq mm square millimeter (= mm^2).

SQP Spastic quadriparesis.

sqq and following (L. sequentia).

SQ3R Survey, question, read, review and recite (study method in psychology) (= SQRRR).

SQRRR See SQ3R.

SQS Semiquantitative score.

squam- combining form meaning scale (L. squama).

SQUID Superconducting quantum (mechanical) impedance/ interference device (= SQID; SQuID).

SQuID See SQUID.

sq yd square yard(s) (= yd^2).

SR Sarcoplasmic reticulum; Scanning radiometer; Screen; Secretion/ Sedimentation rate; Seizure resistant; Selective reduction (of fetuses in multiple pregnancies); Self-relaxation; Seminars in Radiology (journal); Senior (see Sr); Senior Registrar; Sensitivity/ Sensitization/ Sexual/ Specific/ Stimulus response (see S-R); Service record; Sex ratio; Shorthair (guinea pig); Short range; Shoulder replacement (see PHP); Sick role (in hysteria and psychosomatic syndromes); Side rails; Sigma reaction; Silent rehearsal; Sinus rhythm; Skin/ Steroid/ Systemic resistance; Slow release (see SRO); Smooth-rough (see S-R); Sneeze/ Stretch reflex; Society of Radiographers (UK); Soluble repository (with reference to penicillin); Specific/ Sustained release (see S-R); Spontaneous respiration; Stage of resistance (stress, in general adaptation syndrome); Stomach rumble; Stress related; Sulfonamide-resistant; Sulforaphane (an anticancer agent found in the sprouts of broccoli, which acts by turning on detoxifying phase-2 enzymes); Superior rectus; Sustained release; Systems research; Systems review (patient's history).

Sr Senior (= SR; sr); Sister; Strontium (Z = 38) (see Elements - Strontium).

sr senior (see Sr); steradian.

S-R Self-reported (medication, use of drugs, etc.); Smooth-rough (= SR); Sensitivity/ Sensitization/ Sexual/ Specific/ Stimulus - response (= SR); Specific/ Sustained-release (see SRT).

S&R Search and rescue; Seclusion and restraint.

^{85}Sr Radioactive strontium (nuclear medicine).

Sr^{90} Strontium 90.

SRA Science Research Associates; Segmental

renal artery (branch); Serum renin activity; Spinal reflex arc (see H response); Spleen repopulating activity.
SRAM Static random access memory.
S_{RAO2} Oxygen saturation right atrium.
SR_{AW}; SR_{aw}; SRaw Specific airway resistance.
SRB Serotonin-receptor blocker.
SRBC Sheep/ Sickle red blood cell(s).
SRBCC Strict and regular biological and clinical control(s) (= RBC; RCC; SBC; SCC).
SRBD Sleep-related breathing disorder.
SRBOW Spontaneous rupture of bag of waters.
SRBT Surgery-related brain trauma.
SRBV Silicon rubber ball valve (aortic/ mitral).
SRC Scandinavian Radiological Society; Science Research Council (UK); Scientific Review Committee; Sedimented/ Sheep red cell(s); Self-retaining catheter (Urology); Semi-rigid condom; Sleep Research Center; Spondylotic root compression; Steroid responsible condition (= CRD; CSRC); Survey Research Center (University of Michigan); Swiss Red Cross.
src Rous sarcoma oncogene.
SRCA Specific red cell adherence.
SRCBC Serum reserve cholesterol binding capacity.
SRCD Society for Research in Child Development.
SR cells Sensitization response cells (in vaginal smears).
SR/CP Schizophrenic reaction, chronic paranoid.
SRD Seizure-related death; Serious/ Severe/ Structural renal damage/ defect/ deficit/ disease/ dysfunction (= SKD); Serious/ Severe respiratory depression; Serious/ Severe retinal detachment; Service-related disability; Smoking-related disease; Society for the Relief of Distress; Society for the Right to Die; Sodium-restricted diet; Soluble, repository, plus dihydrostreptomycin (with reference to penicillin); Specific reading disability; Standard recommended dose; Stress-related disease/ disorder (= SRP).
SRD5A2 Steroid 5alpha-reductase (enzyme/ gene found in the prostate, which controls the metabolic 'activation' of testosterone into dihydrotestosterone).
SRDS Severe respiratory distress syndrome.
SRDT Single radial diffusion test.
SRDTI Specific reversible direct thrombin inhibitor (e.g. Bivalirudin) (= DTI; RTI; STI).
SRE Schedule of Recent Experiences; Society for Radiologic Engineering; Scoring based on a regression-derived weighing system; Severe reflux esophagitis; Skeletal-related event.
sREM Stage rapid eye movement.
SRF Secondary/ Serious/ Severe/ Significant/ Social/ Strong(est) risk factor (in heart and other diseases): Gender, Obesity, Status, etc.; Self-reported frequency (concerning drug use, medication, etc.); Severe renal/ respiratory (see COLD; COPD) failure; Skin reactive factor; Somatotropin-releasing factor (see Hormones - GH-RH); Split renal function; Sporadic relapsing fever (caused by spirochetes of the *Borrelia* family, which thrive in cave-dwelling, argasid or soft-bodied ticks); Subretinal fluid.
SRF-A Slow-reacting/ -releasing factor of anaphylaxis.
SRFD Severe renal functional disorder.
SRFS Split renal function study.
SRG Schering Corp (USA) code for experimental substances; Society of Remedial Gymnasts (UK); Suprarenal gland (also called Accessory renal or Adrenal gland = [L.] glandula suprarenalis).
SRG 95213 Diazoxide - an antihypertensive agent, chemically related to chlorothiazide, but without any diuretic activity. It acts directly on the arterioles, reducing peripheral resistance and increasing cardiac output.
SRH Signs/ Stigmata of recent hemorrhage; Single radial hemolysis; Somatotropin-releasing hormone (see Hormones - GH-RH); Spontaneously responding hyperthyroidism.
SRHS Self-reported health status.
SRI Scripps/ Stanford Research Institute (both California); Severe renal impairment/ insufficiency; Severe respiratory insufficiency (see SRF; COLD; COPD); Short-range implication; Significant renal impairment/ insufficiency; Stress response involvement;

Subretinal implant.
SRID Single radial immunodiffusion.
SRIF Somatotropin-release inhibiting/ inhibition/ inhibitory factor (= Somatostatin; SS; SST) (see Hormones - GH-IH).
SRL Safety Research Laboratory; Specific risk level; Suppurative regional lymphadenitis.
SRLC Severe recurrent leg cramp(s).
SRM Spontaneous rupture of membrane(s) (see SROM); Standard Reference Material (NBS); Superior rectus muscle (eye); Sustained-release mechanism.
SRMD Stress-related mucosal damage.
SRN Serotonin-releasing neuron; State/ Student Registered Nurse (England and Wales).
SRNA See sRNA.
sRNA Soluble ribonucleic acid (= SNRA; sNRA; SRNA).
SR/NE Sinus rhythm, no ectopy.
SRNG Sustained release nitroglycerin.
SRNS Steroid-responsive nephrotic syndrome.
SRNVM Senile retinal/ Subretinal neovascular membrane.
SRO Sex-ratio organism; Single room occupancy (halfway house); Slow-release oral (form of drug); Smallest region of overlap; Steele-Richardson-Olszewski (syndrome).
SROM Spontaneous rupture of membrane(s) (= SRM).
S romanum The sigmoid colon.
SROS Steele-Richardson-Olszewsky syndrome (progressive supranuclear palsy).
SRP Salt-replacement preparation; Short rib-polydactyly (syndrome); Signal recognition particle; Slow/ Sustained -release preparation; Society for Radiological Protection (UK); Stapes replacement prosthesis; State Registered Physiotherapist; Stress-related problem (see SRD); Surgery-related pain; Synchronized retroperfusion.
SRPS Short rib-polydactyly syndrome.
SRQ Self-Reporting Questionnaire.
SRR Self-retaining retractor (Oral and General Surgery); Serotonin receptor research; Skin resistance response; Standardized rate ratio; Surgery recovery room; Sustained response rate (to medication); Systemic reaginic reaction.
SRRS Social Readjustment Rating Scale.
SR-RSV Schmidt-Ruppin (strain) - Rous sarcoma virus.
SRS Scandinavian Radiological Society; Schizophrenic residual state; Sex reassignment surgery; Silver-Russell syndrome; Slow-reacting substance (see SRS-A); Social and Rehabilitation Service (HEW); Splenorenal shunt; Square root sign (in cardiac catheterization); Steroid reference substance (USP); Subretinal space (see ARI); Symptom Rating Scale.
SRSA Slow-reacting substance of anaphylaxis (see SRS-A); Social and Rehabilitation Services Administration (HEW).
SRS-A Slow-reacting substance of anaphylaxis (= SRS; SRSA).
SRT Schild Regression Technique (for assessment of the pharmacological potency of a drug); Sedimentation rate test (see ESR); Simple reaction time; Sinus (node) recovery time; Slow reaction time (e.g. in alcohol intoxication) (see AEI); Slow/ Sustained release tablet; Speech reception test/ threshold (hearing); Spontaneously resolving thyrotoxicosis; Stress-reduction technique(s) - such as relaxation, meditation, music therapy, visualization and guided imagery tapes, and prayer (see MBA); Stroke rehabilitation technician; Surfactant replacement therapy; Sustained-release theophylline/ therapy (see S-R)/ tablet; Symptom Rating Test.
SRTP Science Research Training Program (NYAS).
SRU Sample ratio units; Side rails up; Solitary rectal ulcer; Structural repeating unit.
SRUS Solitary rectal ulcer syndrome.
SRV Schmidt-Ruppin virus; Simian retrovirus; Substantial residual variability; Superior radicular vein.
S_{RVO2} Oxygen saturation right ventricle.
SRVT Sustained re-entrant ventricular tachyarrhythmia.
SRW Short ragweed (test).
SS Disulfide; Immediately to be taken (L. statim sumendum); In a/ the strict sense (L. sensu stricto) (see s str); Sacrosciatic; Safe(r) sex (practice[s]); Saline soak; Saline/

Saturated/ Sterile solution (ss); Saliva sample; Salmonella-Shigella (agar); Salt substitute (see S/S); Schizophrenia Subscale; Schopf syndrome (see MEHS); Science Service (News); Scintillating scotoma (= Flittering s; Fortification spectrum; Scotoma scintilans; Teichopsia - Gr. teichos wall + opsis vision + ia); Seckel's syndrome (see BHD; PAS); Segura surgery (for esophageal varices) (see SP - Sigura/ Sugiura procedure); Seizure-sensitive; Selective shunt; Serotonin syndrome (associated with the use of SSRIs; it includes one or more of the following symptoms: agitation, anxiety, ataxia, confusion, diaphoresis, disorientation, dysarthria, emesis, excitement, hemiballismus, hyperreflexia, hyperthermia, hypomania, incoordination, loss of conciousness, motor weakness, myoclonus, pupillary dilation, restlessness, shivering, tachycardia and tremor); Serum sickness; Sezary/ Sjögren/ Staccato/ Stickler/ Sweet syndrome; Shedding syndrome (Obstetrics and Gynecology); Shirodkar suture (for the short cervix) (see under Sut.); Short single (cone - eye); Short sleep; Siblings; 'Sicca syndrome'; Sickle cell (anemia); Side-to-side; Signs and symptoms (see S&S); Single-strand(ed) - DNA (= ss); Skull series (radiographs); Sleeping sickness (Gambian trypanosomiasis - a protozoan disease caused by *Trypanosoma* brucei gambiense and transmitted to humans by various species of *Glossina* or tsetse fly); Sliding scale; Slip sent; Soap solution/ suds (= ss); Social Security/ Services; Somatostatin (see SRIF); Sparingly soluble; Spastics Society (UK); Staccato speech; Stainless steel; Standard score (psychology); Statistically significant; Steady state; Steroid sensitivity/ sulfurylation; Subaortic stenosis; Subscapular; Substernal; Suction socket; Sudan stain (Iodine compound used as a test for stool fat); Sum of squares; Sun spot (excess pigment forming in the skin from years of exposure to the sun's UV rays) (= ARSC - Age-related skin changes [with greater vulnerability to cosmetic and medical problems]; AS - Age spot; LF - Lipofuscin); Supersaturated; Support and stimulation; Suppressor sensitive (see SuS); Susceptible; Symmetrical strength; Systemic sclerosis.

Ss One half (see ss); Shigella sonnei; Subjects.

ss in a/ the strict sense (see s str); namely (L. scilicet); one-half (= semis) (= Ss; ss; ss); saline solution (= SS); single-strand(ed) (see SS); soap solution/ suds (= SS); subspinale.

Ss; ss one-half (see ss).

S/S Salt substitute (= SS).

-S-S- Interchain disulfide bridge.

S&S Shower and shampoo; Signs and symptoms (= SS); Support and stimulation.

SSA Sagittal split advancement; Salicylsalicylic/ Sulfosalicylic acid; Semi-synthetic antibiotic; Severe seasonal asthma; Sickle cell anemia; Sjögren's syndrome antigen; Skin-sensitizing antibody; Skin surface area; Skin sympathetic activity; Smooth surface antigen; Social Security Administration (HEW); Somatostatin analogue (e.g. Octreotide); Southern Surgical Association; Sperm-specific antiserum; Statistically significant advantage/ association; Subjective Symptoms Assessment; Sufficient systemic absorption; Systems safety analyst.

SS-A Sjögren's syndrome A (antibody) (= SSA).

SSA/BW Skin surface area/Body weight ratio.

SS agar Salmonella-Shigella agar.

SSAl Smallest Space Analysis.

SSAP Subjective Symptoms Assessment Profile.

SSAT Society for Surgery of the Alimentary Tract.

SSA test Sulfosalicylic acid test (for albumin) (= SSA).

SSAV Simian sarcoma-associated virus.

SSB Segura stone basket (Urology); Short spike burst; Single-stranded binding (protein); Specific sexual behavior; Stereospecific binding.

SS-B Sjögren syndrome B.

SSBG Sex steroid-binding globulin.

SSBL Steady-state blood level.

SSBP Seated/ Standing/ Supine systolic blood pressure.

SSBS Significant symptomatic bronchospasm.

SSC Sensitive solar cell (photoreceptor); Shear stress component (Orthopedics); Shoulder spica cast; Sister strand crossover;

Somatosensory cortex; Southern Surgical Congress; Spectroscopy Society of Canada; Sperm stem cell (of spermatogonium); Stainless steel crown (see SSCr); Standard saline/ sodium citrate; Statistically significant change(s); Steady state condition/ concentration (of drugs, time-profile, etc.) (see CTP); Subsequent symptom control; Symphysis sacrococcygea (BNA) (see SCJ); Syngenetic spleen cell; Synthetic salmon calcitonin.

SSc Systemic scleroderma/ sclerosis.

SSCA Single shoulder contrast arthrography; Spontaneous suppressor cell activity.

SSCC Superficial squamous cell carcinoma.

SSCCS Slow spinal cord compression syndrome.

ss(c)DNA Single-stranded circular deoxyribonucleic acid.

SSCF Sleep stage change frequency.

SSCP Somatosensory cortical potential (see SCP); Substernal chest pain.

SSCr Stainless steel crown (on tooth) (dentistry) (= SSC).

SSCVD Sterile spontaneous controlled vaginal delivery.

SSD Salem sump drain (used in cholecystectomy); Scalp seborrheic dermatitis; Severe skin disease/ disorder; Severe structural defect; Severe systemic disease; Sickle cell disease; Silver sulfadiazine; Single saturating dose; Social Security disability; Social Services Department; Source skin/ surface distance (radiology); Spastic spinal disease; Special Science Development (program, NSF); Special senses disorder (e.g. parosmia, taste perversion, etc.); Speech-sound discrimination; Statistically significant decrease/ difference; Strong sex desire/ drive; Subsequent sudden death; Subsyndromal depression; Succinate semi-aldehyde dehydrogenase; Sudden sniffing death (syndrome); Sum of square deviations; Syndrome of sudden death.

SSDBS Symptom schedule for the diagnosis of borderline schizophrenia.

SSDI Social Security disability income.

ssDNA Single-stranded deoxyribonucleic acid.

SSDS Subsyndromal depressive symptoms.

SSDST Standard single-disk susceptibility test (of bacteria, to antimicrobial compounds).

SSE Saline solution enema (see SS enema); Serious/ Severe/ Significant/ Systemic side effect(s); Serotonin syndrome effect (e.g. blushing, cognitive dysfunction, confusion, delirium, diaphoresis, hyperpyrexia, restlessness, and tremor); Severe subcutaneous emphysema; Sheep spongiform encephalopathy (= Scrapie) (see BSE; TSE); Significant systemic exposure; Skin self-examination; Soapsuds enema (see SS enema); Statistically significant effect/ extent; Steady state exercise; Stratified squamous epithelium; Subacute spongiform encephalopathy; Sustained stretching exercise(s); Systemic side effects.

SSEA Sensitized sheep erythrocyte agglutination; Stage-specific embryonic antigen.

SS enema Saline solution/ Soapsuds enema (= SS; ss; SSE).

SSEP Somatosensory evoked potential (cortical and spinal).

S seq Without sequel (L. sine sequela).

SSER Somatosensory evoked response.

SSES Sexual Self-Efficacy Scale.

SSF Soluble suppressor factor; Subscapular skinfold (thickness); Supplemental sensory feedback.

SSFI Social stress and functionability inventory.

SSG Sublabial salivary gland; Submarine Survivors Group.

SSGA Southern Surgical and Gynecological Association.

SSH Salt-sensitive hypertensive; Severe symptomatic hyponatremia; Severe systemic/ systolic hypertension.

SSHb Fetal hemoglobin (see Hb); Homozygous for sickle hemoglobin.

SSHD Severe sensorineural hearing defect (see SSNHD).

SSI *Sarcoptes* scabies infection; Segmental sensory innervation; Segmental sequential/ sequestral irradiation; Severe/ Superficial/ Surface skin infection/ inflammation/ irritation; Shoulder subluxation inhibition; Skin structure infection; Slit/ Split-size incision; Small-scale integration (circuits); Somatic Symptom Inventory; Sound scientific inquiry; Staphylococcal skin infection; Statistically significant improvement/ increase; Steroid synthesis inhibitor (e.g. Aminogluthemid); Subshock insulin; Substandard intelligence; Supplemental Security Income (program) (SSA); Swanson Silastic implant (wrist); System Sign Inventory.

SSIDS Sibling of sudden infant death syndrome (victim).

SSIE Smithsonian Science Information Exchange, Inc. (formerly, MSIE).

SSIPFM Single-signed integral pulse frequency modulation.

SSIS Smithsonian Science Information Service.

SSKI Saturated/ Supersaturated solution of potassium iodide.

SSL Skin surface lipid; Steady-state level; Sufficient sleep; Synthetic sentence list(s).

SSLI Serum sickness-like illness.

SSM Serosanguinous material (Orthopedics); Standard supportive measure(s); Subsynaptic membrane; Sulphamate-substituted monosaccharide; Superficial spreading melanoma; Supraspinatus muscle; Synthetic suture material.

SSME Society for the Study of Medical Ethics.

SSN Severely subnormal; Sliding scale normogram (anti-coagulation therapy); Social security number; Stainless steel needle; Subacute sensory neuropathy; Suprasternal notch; Symmetrical sensory neuropathy.

SSNCV Sural sensory nerve conduction velocity.

SSNHD Severe sensorineural hearing defect (= SSHD).

SSNS Steroid-sensitive nephrotic syndrome.

SSO Society of Surgical Oncology; Spanish speaking only; Special sense organ.

SSOP Second Surgical Opinion Program.

SSP Safe sex practice(s) (see USS); Sanarelli-Schwartzman phenomenon; Second (see ASP)/ Superficial surgical procedure; Semi-sitting position (= SBP); Semi-synthetic penicillin; Sequence-specific primer (DNA); Sex-specific prevalence (e.g. of autoimmune diseases); Soapsuds and peppermint enema; Standard susceptibility pattern (see SSTP); Standard system of psychiatry; Stereoscopic parallax (see BOP); Subacute sclerosing panencephalitis (see SSPE); Subspecies (see ssp); Sudden severe pain; Supersensitivity perception.

ssp subspecies (= SSP).

S+ SP Seropositive sex(ual) partner (= SPSP; S+ve SP).

S- SP Seronegative sex(ual) partner (= SNSP; S-ve SP).

SSPC Steady-state plasma concentration (= SSPL).

SSPE Subacute sclerosing panencephalitis (= SSP).

SSPG Steady state plasma glucose.

SSPI Steady state plasma insulin.

SSPL Saturation sound pressure level; Steady-state plasma level (see SSPC).

SSPP Subsynaptic plate perforation.

SSPS Side-to-side portacaval shunt.

SSPs Safer sex practices.

SS-PSE Schizophrenic Subscale of the Present State Examination.

SSPU Surgical short procedure unit.

SSQ Significant scientific question(s); Social Support Questionnaire.

SSR Severe skin reaction (= Hypersensitivity reaction); Sight Saving Review (NSPB journal); Site-specific recombination; Somatosensory response; Statistically significant reaction/ reduction/ relation/ result; Surgical supply room.

SSRG Scottish Schizophrenia Research Group.

SSRI Selective serotonin reuptake inhibitor; Serotonin syndrome receptor inhibitor.

SSRL Stanford Synchotron Radiation Laboratory.

ssRNA Single-stranded ribonucleic acid.

SSRP Stanford Synchotron Radiation Project.

SSS Saliva, serum, sputum (drug concentration); Scalded skin syndrome; Secondary Sjögren syndrome; Sick sinus syndrome (= SAND; SA nodal disease); Simvastatin Survival Study; Slit-skin smear; Specific soluble substance (polysaccharide hapten); Stanford Sleepiness Scale; Statistically significantly superior; Sterile saline soak/ solution; Symbolic shorthand system; Systemic sicca syndrome.

SSs Stroke symptoms - These include sudden 1. confusion; 2. dizziness or severe headache with no known cause; 3. numbness or weakness of face, arm, or leg; 4. trouble speaking or understanding; and 5. trouble seeing or walking.

sss layer upon layer (L. stratum super stratum).

SSSA Soil Science Society of America.

SSSB Sagittal split setback.

SSSE Steady-state systemic exposure.

SSSS Scandinavian Simvastatin Survival Study (= 4S); Society for the Scientific Study of Sex; Staphylococcal scalded skin syndrome (Phase II Staphylococcus) - found especially in young children.

SSST Superior sagittal sinus thrombosis.

SSStJ Serving Sister, Order of St. John of Jerusalem.

SSSV Superior sagittal sinus (blood) velocity.

SST Sagittal sinus thrombosis; Same-sex twin (Obstetrics); Serum sensitivity test(s); Soapsuds and turpentine (enema); Social-skills therapy (for autism, etc.); Sodium sulfite titration; Somatostatin (see SRIF); Specific shock therapy/ treatment; Sum of ST segment elevations (see ΣST); Supersonic transport; Systemic steroid therapy.

ΣST Sum of ST segment elevations on the electrocardiogram in millivolts (mV), i.e. from multiple epicardial sites (= SST).

SSTA Statistically significant therapeutic activity.

SSTF Social Security Trust Funds (SSA).

SSTP Standardized susceptibility test procedure.

SSTPC Steady-state trough plasma concentration.

s str in a/ the strict sense (L. sensu stricto) (= SS; ss).

SSU Self-service unit; Sterile supply unit.

SSV Schulman-Schwartz virus; Simian sarcoma virus; Steady state volume (see MSSV); Synthesized scorpion venom (used in the treatment of brain cancer, especially glioma); Under/ With a poison label (L. sub signo veneni) (= ssv).

ssv under/ with a poison label (see SSV).

S_{SVCO2} Oxygen saturation superior vena cava.

SSVHP Serpentine supravenous hyperpigmentation.

SSW Small superficial wound.

SSX Sulfisoxazole (= Sulphafurazole).

S/SX Signs/ symptoms.

ST Esotropia; Sacrotransverse (fetal position); Scala tympani; Sclerotherapy; Sedimentation/ Starting/ Survival/ Systolic time; Segment/ Wave on the electrocardiogram (the portion of the segment between the end of the S wave and the beginning of the T wave) (= S-T); Semitendinosus; Sensitivity/ Skin/ Standard(ized)/ Stress test; Shock/ Speech therapy; Sickle-cell thalassemia (see S-T); Sinus tachyarrhythmia/ tachycardia/ tympani; Skin/ Split thickness; Slight trace; Slow twitch; Society for Toxicology; Somatotherapy; Spasmodic/ Spastic torticollis; Speech therapist; Sphincter tone; Stable toxin (i.e. heat-stable bacterial enterotoxin); Standard taper (joint); Station (see Sta); Sternothyroid; Stimulus (see St); Store; Stretcher; Stria terminalis; Striation; Subtalar (see st); Subtotal; Subtype (see St); Surface tension; Surgical treatment; Syndrome of the trephined.

St Ciba Pharmaceutical Products, Inc. (USA) code for experimental substances; Let it/ them stand (see st); Saint; Stab form(s) - of leukocytes (see Stab); Standing; Status (see st); Sterile; Stimulate/lus (= ST; stim); Stimulation (= stimn); Stokes; Stomach; Stroke; Subtype (= ST).

st do not change/ let it stand/ make no change (L. stet) (= St; stet); do not make changes/ let them stand/ make no changes (L. stent) (= St; stent); stage (of disease); status (= St); stere; stone (unit); straight; stomion; subtalar (= ST).

S-T (segment) or wave on the ECG (see ST); Sickle-cell thalassemia (= ST; STh; S-Thal).

ST 37 Hexylresorcinol (= Caprokol) - a proprietary disinfectant.

STA Second trimester abortion/ amniocentesis (Obstetrics); Serum thrombotic accelerator; Serum thymic activity (= TA); Sexually transmitted agent; Short term absence/ adjustment/ administration; Soft tissue affliction(s); Specialist Training Authority; Superficial temporal artery; Syme's terminal amputation (Orthopedics).

Sta Staphylion; Station (= ST).

S-Ta Atrial S-T segment change(s) on the electrocardiogram.

sta- combining form meaning stop (Gr.).

Stab; stab Stabilization/ze(d); Stabnuclear neutrophil (= Band cell; Non-segmented polymorphonuclear leukocyte; St).

STAD Short-term arterial damage.

STAG; S-TAG Slow-binding target-attaching globulin (= Slow-target attaching globulin); Split-thickness autogenous graft.

STAI State Trait Anxiety Inventory.

stal- combining form meaning send (Gr.).

STA-MCA Superficial temporal artery to middle cerebral artery.

Stan Standard(ization)/(ize)/(ized) (= std).

StanPsych Standard psychiatric (nomenclature).

Staph; staph Staphylococcus; Staphylococcal.

staphyl- combining form meaning grapes (Gr. staphyle).

STAR Study of Tamoxifen and Raloxifene (trial, in breast cancer).

Star (journal on Hansen's disease).

Star dust Cocaine (see Erythroxylum).

STARPAHC Space Technology Applied to Rural Papago Advanced Health Care.

START Special treatment and rehabilitation training.

STASH Student Association for the Study of Hallucinogens, Inc.

-stasis suffix meaning hold in check/ stop (Gr.).

STAT Short term adjunctive therapy.

Stat Statistics.

stat at once/ immediately (L. statim); Radiation emanation unit (Ger.) - unit for measuring the amount of radiation emanation, equivalent to 0.364 μc (microcurie).

STAT-I State-Trait-Anxiety Index - I.

STB Short-term/ Synergistic therapeutic benefit(s); Short-term blindness (= Amaurosis fugax) (see APF; STPB).

Stb Stillborn (= stillb).

StBal Standing balance.

St. Bart's Hosp St. Bartholomew's Hospital (London, UK).

StBy Stand by.

STC Saw-toothed/ Serrated curet (Neurosurgery); Secondary thrombocytosis (see BTC); Serum trough/ theophylline concentration; Short-term cost/ culture; Society for Technical Communications; Soft tissue calcification/ cancer/ carcinoma/ component/ correction; Stimulate to cry; Stroke treatment center; Subtotal colectomy; Sugar tongue cast.

STD Science and Technology Division (LC); Sexually transmitted disease; Short-term decongestant (nasal); Skin/ Standard test dose; Skin-tumor distance; Sodium tetradecyl (sulfate); Sotradecol.

std saturated; standard(ized) (see Stan).

STDH Skin test for delayed hypersensitivity.

STDT Standard tone-decay test.

StdTF Standard tube feeding (see STF).

STE Serology test for encephalitis (see CEE); Short-term efficacy/ exposure; Systemic therapeutic exposure (level, to drugs).

STEAM Stimulated-echo acquisition mode; Streptonigrin, Thioguanine, Endoxan (= cyclophosphamide), Actinomycin D and Mitomycin C (= Zymosan) - combination treatment in neoplastic disease.

stear-; steat combining forms meaning fat (Gr.).

STEL Short-term exposure limit.

STEM Scanning transmission electron microscope.

sten stenosed/osis.

sten- prefix meaning constricted or narrowed (Gr. stenos).

-stenosis suffix meaning constriction of a passage (Gr. stenos).

stent do not make changes/ let them stand/ make no changes (L.) (see st).

STEP Sequential Tests of Educational Progress; Society for Total Emergency Programs.

ster- prefix meaning solid (Gr. stereos).

sterc- combining form meaning dung (L. stercus).

Stereo; stereo Stereogram.

stern- combining form meaning sternum.

Steroids (journal).

STESS Subject's treatment emergent symptom scale.

STET Submaximal treadmill exercise test.

stet do not change/ let it stand/ make no change (L.) (see st).

STETH Stethoscope.

steth- combining form meaning chest (Gr. stethos).

STEV Short-term exposure value.

STF Salter type fracture (fractures that involve the cartilaginous growth plate of a bone): Type I - epiphysis separates without a fracture, Type II - metaphysis fractures and a spike of it remains attached to the displaced epiphyseal fragment, Type III - epiphysis fractures and the fracture is usually parallel to the long axis of the bone, Type IV - both the epiphysis and metaphysis fracture and the fracture crosses the epiphyseal plate, Type V - the epiphyseal plate is crushed and compressed; Scar-tissue formation; Serum thymus factor; Slow-twitch fiber; Special/ Standard (= StdTF) tube feeding; Specialized treatment center; Sudden transient freezing.

STFM Society of Teachers of Family Medicine.

STG Second trimester of gestation; Serotonin transporter gene; Serum triglyceride; Severe tophaceous gout; Short-term goal(s)/ growth; Soft tissue hemorrhage; Split-thickness graft (operation/ plastic surgery); Subtotal gastrectomy.

STH Seminars in Thrombosis and Hemostasis (journal); Soft tissue healing/ hemorrhage/ hemostasis; Somatotropic hormone (Growth hormone of the anterior pituitary) (see Hormones - GH; STH); Subtotal hysterectomy (operation/ gynecology); Supplemental thyroid hormone (see Hormones - STH ii).

STh; S-Thal Sickle-cell thalassemia (see S-T).

STHC Serum thyroid hormone concentration (raised in Graves' disease).

sthen- combining form meaning strength (Gr. sthenos).

STHRF Somatotropic hormone releasing factor.

STHV Science, Technology, and Human Values (NEH program).

STI Scientific and Technical Information; Secondary topical (i.e. skin) infection; Serum/ Soybean (= SBI; SBTI) trypsin inhibitor; Sexually transmitted illness/ infection (see STD; STP) (includes AIDS, Chlamydia, Gonorrhea, Herpes, Lymphogranuloma venereum; Syphilis, Trichomoniasis, etc.); Short-term immobilization (Orthopedics)/ improvement/ insomnia; Signal transduction inhibitor (anti-cancer drug such as STI-571 or Gleevec); Soft-tissue infection/ inflammation/ injury; Soil-transmitted infection; Specific thrombin inhibitor (see SRDTI); Structured treatment interruption(s) (antiviral treatment in AIDS); Systolic time interval.

STIA Science, Technology, and International Affairs.

STIC Serum trypsin inhibition capacity; Solid-state transducer intracompartment.

Stick Marijuana twig (see Cannabis).

stil; stillat by drops/ drop by drop/ in small amounts or quantities (L. stillatim).

stillb stillborn (see Stb).

stim stimulate(d)/ stimulation/ stimulus (see St).

stimn stimulation (see St).

STIQ Surface technique for immunoquantitation.

STI/SIT Structured treatment interruptions/Structured interrupted therapy (cycles) (as in AIDS medication).

STIMS Swedish Ticlopidine Multicenter Study.

stirred heme blood within the eye.

STJ Subtalar joint.

STK Serine-threonine kinase (an enzyme associated in the kidney with two genes, hWNKI and hWNK4 found on chromosome I7, and associated with the more common forms of hypertension); Streptokinase (see SK).

STL Second-trimester loss; Serum theophylline level; Soft tissue lesion (bursitis, capsulitis, enthesopathy, muscle injury, tendinitis, tendon rupture, etc.); Status thymicolymphaticus; Swelling, tenderness, and limitation (of movement)/ limited (motion) (= STLOM).

STLA Surface tension-lowering activity.

STLE; StLE St. Louis encephalitis.

STLL Severly traumatized lower limb (Orthopedics).
STLOM Swelling, tenderness, and limitation of motion/ movement (= STL).
STLS Subacute thyroiditis-like syndrome.
STLV; STLV-3 Simian T-lymphotropic virus - infecting the "spider" or "green" monkey.
STM Scanning tunneling microscope; Short-term management/ memory; Soft-tissue mass; Streptomycin (see SM).
STMFP Symptothermal method of family planning (see NFPM).
STML Short-term memory loss (see STMP).
STMP Short-term memory problem(s) (see STMS); Sodium thymolphthalein monophosphate.
STN Subthalamic/ Supratrochlear nucleus.
sTNM TNM (primary tumor, regional nodes, metastasis) staging of tumors as determined by surgical procedures.
STNR Symmetric tonic neck reflex.
STNV Satellite tobacco necrosis virus.
STO Short-term outcome; Store; Subtrochanteric osteotomy (e.g. for Perthes' disease) (Orthopedics).
stol- combining form meaning send (Gr.).
stom stomach.
stom- prefix meaning mouth (Gr. stoma).
Stomahesive Adhesive material used with stomal bags to secure the bag.
-stomy suffix meaning a surgical opening (Gr. stomoun).
STOP-HTN Swedish Trial in Old Patients with Hypertension.
STORCH Syphilis, toxoplasmosis, rubella, cytomegalovirus, and herpesvirus.
STP Methyl-dimethoxy-methylphenethylamine (= 2,5-dimethoxy-4-methylamphetamine; BZ; DOM) (see Amphet); Schizotypal personality (see SMI; SPD - Shadow panic disorder); Scientifically-treated petroleum (a motor oil additive); Second trimester of pregnancy; Serenity, tranquility and peace (Timothy Leary); Severe toxemia of pregnancy; Sexually transmitted pathogen (see STI); Short-term pain/ phase/ plan(ning)/ potentiation/ preceptorship/ prescribing/ problem/ procedure/ prophylaxis/ prospect/ prospective/ protection; Sibling Training Program; Sodium thiopental; Soft tissue pain; Spastic tetraparesis/ tetraplegia; Spontaneous twin pregnancy; Standard temperature and pressure/ pulse (i.e. normal t & p/p); Standard treatment program; 'Stuck twin' phenomenon (Obstetrics); Successfully treated patient; Superficial thrombophlebitis.
STPAb Serum thyroid peroxidase antibody (concentration, etc.).
STPB Short-term partial blindness (= APF).
STPD Standard temperature and pressure, dry, i.e. a volume of gas at standard conditions of temperature and pressure, "dry" or containing no water vapor.
STPP Sodium tripolyphosphate.
STPS Specific thalamic projection system.
STPT Short-term prospective trial.
STQ Superior temporal quadrant.
STR Selective therapeutic regimen; Short-term relief/ response/ result (see STRs)/ risk; Society of Therapeutic Radiologists; Soft tissue reconstruction/ relaxation/ repair/ resection; Stirred tank reactor.
Str Streptococcal; Streptococcus (see S - Streptococcus).
str straight; stretcher.
Strab; strab strabismus (eye examination).
Strep Streptococcus (see S - Streptococcus); Streptomycin (see SM).
strep- prefix meaning to twist (Gr. strepho).
strict- combining form meaning close or tight (L. strictus).
-stringent suffix meaning to draw tight or cause pain (L. stringo).
Stroke (AHA journal).
stroph- combining form meaning twist (Gr.).
STRs Short tandem repeats (tiny snips/ stretches of DNA coding, two to seven base-pairs long); Short-term results.
STRT Skin temperature recovery time.
struc; struct structural/ure.
struct- combining form meaning pile up (L. structus).
STS Serological test(s) for syphilis:
BST: Blood serological test;
BW: Blood Wassermann (see STS - WR);
CMT: Cardiolipin microflocculation test;
CSF-WR: Cerebrospinal fluid - Wassermann reaction;

CSL: Cardiolipin synthetic lecithin (test);
FTA: Fluorescent treponemal antibody (see STS - FTA-ABS);
FTA-ABS: Fluorescent treponemal antibody - absorption (test);
FTA-Abs: See STS - FTA-ABS (= FTA; FTA-Abs; TPFA);
HATTS: Hemagglutination treponemal test for syphilis;
Hint: Hinton (flocculation test for syphilis);
KCCF: Kolmer cardiolipin complement fixation (test);
KT: Kahn test;
LT: Lues test(s) (= STS);
MHATP: See STS - MHA-TP;
MHA-TP: Microhemagglutin assay for Treponema pallidum antibodies (= MHATP);
MTR: Meinicke turbidity reaction;
PCT: Plasma Cri Test";
RPCF: Reiter protein complement-fixation (test) (see STS - RPCFT);
RPCFT: Reiter protein complement-fixation test (= RPCF; RPF);
RPE: Rapid plasma exclusion (test);
RPF: Reiter protein fixation (test) (see STS - RPCFT);
RPR: Rapid plasma reagin (test) (= Portnoy's card test; RPRCF);
RPRCF: Rapid plasma reagin complement fixation (see RPR) (= RPRCT);
RPRCT: Rapid plasma reagin card test (see STS - RPR);
SG; S-G: Sachs-Georgi reaction/ test (= SGR; S-Gt);
SGR: Sachs-Georgi reaction (see STS - SG);
S-Gt: Sachs-Georgi test (see STS - SG);
STS: Standard test for syphilis;
SWR: Serum Wassermann reaction (see STS - WR);
TIT: Treponema immobilization test;
TPC: Treponema pallidum complement (fixation test) (see TPCF);
TPCF: Treponema pallidum complement fixation (test) (= TPC);
TPFA: Treponema pallidum fluorescent antibody (test) (see FTA-ABS);
TPHA: Treponema pallidum haemagglutination (test);
TPI: Treponema pallidum immobilization (test);
TPIA: Treponema pallidum immune adherence (test);
USR: Unheated serum reagin (test);
VDRL: Venereal Disease Research Laboratory (test);
VDRT: Venereal disease reference test (Harris);
WR: Wassermann reaction (= BW; SWR; Was; Wass);
Was; Wass: Wassermann test (see STS - WR)

STS Short-term sequelae/ strategy/ study/ supplementation; Society of Thoracic Surgeons; Sodium tetradecyl sulfate; Sodium thiosulfate; Soft tissue sarcoma/ swelling; Space Transportation System (NASA); Standard test for syphilis (see STS - STS); Stereotactic surgery; Steroid sulfatase; Stuck twin syndrome (see STP); Subacute toxicity study; Sugartong splint (for splinting of fracture, usually of wrist); Superior temporal sulcus.

ST(s) Serology Test(s): Histoplasma myecelial, Histoplasma yeast, Toxoplasmosis tests, ELISA-Ig, IFA-IgM, RA latex slide test and California/ St. Louis/ and Western equine encephalitis.

StS Side-to-side (anastomosis).

STSA Southern Thoracic Surgical Association.

ST Schick test (skin test for diphtheria); Schlicter test (serum inhibition); Scrub typhus (= Tsutsugamushi disease caused by *Rickettsia* tsutsugamushi and transmitted by the larvae of trombiculid [chigger] mites); Self-treatment; Sonotrode (ultrasonic device used to pulverize kidney stones); Streptozyme test/ titer (replaces ASO in measuring antibodies in rheumatic fever, etc.) (= SZT); String test (for peptic ulcer).

STSE Split-thickness skin excision.

STSG Split-thickness skin graft.

STSS Staphylococcal toxic shock syndrome.

STT Salt tolerance test; Scaphotrapeziotrapezoid (joint); Sensitization test; Serial thrombin time; Short-term therapy; Skin temperature test; Soft-tissue trauma (see STI)/ tumor; Snapped/pping triceps tendon; Spinothalamic tract; Student's t test (a parametric test in statistical analysis) (see

PMT); Subtotal thyroidectomy; Supratentorial tumor (brain); Systemic thrombolytic therapy.

sTt Titmus stereotest (Ophthalmology) (see DPT; TST).

StTol Standing tolerance.

STU Shock trauma unit; Short-term use; Sigma Tietz unit; Skin test unit.

STV Short term variability; Stenosing tendovaginitis (see TFP); Superior temporal vein.

STVA Subtotal villose atrophy.

STVS Short-term visual storage/ store (eye).

STX Saxitoxin.

stylo- prefix meaning pole (Gr. stylos).

STZ Streptozocin; Streptozyme.

SU Salicyluric (acid); Secretory/ Sensation/ Shinowara/ Siegbahn (approx. 10^{-13} meter)/ Somogyi/ Sorbent/ Spectrophotometric/ Strontium/ Sub unit; Sensory urgency; Solar urticaria; Status uncertain; Sulfonamide (see sulfa); Sulfonylurea; Supine (see sup).

Su Sulfonamide (see sulfa).

su let him take/ take (L. sumat).

S&U Supine and upright.

SU 1906 Diphenylthiourea (see DPT).

SU 3088 Chlorisondamine chloride - a ganglion-blocking agent used in the treatment of severe hypertension.

SU 3118 Syrosingopine (= Methyl carbethoxysyringoyl reserpate) - a drug chemically related to reserpine, and having a mainly peripheral action. Used in the treatment of mild or moderate hypertension, usually in combination with other hypotensive agents.

SU 4885 Metyrapone - a drug which inhibits the synthesis of the glucocorticoids, cortisone and hydrocortisone, and to a lesser extent, aldosterone. It has been used to investigate the ability of the anterior pituitary to synthesize and release corticotropin in puitary function tests; also used in the treatment of resistant edema of unkown origin.

SU 5864 Guanethidine sulfate (= Guaneth sulf) - a hypotensive agent acting by selectively blocking transmission in post-ganglionic adrenergic nerves, thus preventing the release of adrenaline and noradrenaline from the nerve endings. Guanethidine is used in the treatment of severe hypertension, or in mild hypertension when other drugs have proved ineffective.

SU 6518 Dimethindene maleate (= Dimethpyrindene maleate) - an antihistaminic agent with an effect more potent than that of promethazine.

SU 8341 Cyclopenthiazide - a diuretic with similar actions and uses to chlorthiazide, but effective in much smaller doses. It reduces the resorption of electrolytes from the proximal renal tubules, thereby increasing the excretion of sodium, potassium, and chloride ions, and consequently of water.

SUA Serum uric acid; Single umbilical artery; Single unit activity; Special unemployment assistance (USDL).

SUB Skene's urethra and Bartholin's (glands).

sub frequently (L. subinde); prefix meaning less or under (L.).

subac subacute.

subclav subclavian; subclavicular.

subcrep subcrepitant (rales).

subcut subcutaneous(ly) (see SC).

sub fin coct toward the end of boiling (L. sub finem coctionis).

subgenus subgenus (L.) (see s-gg).

subl subliminal (see sublim); sublingual (see subling).

sublim subliminal (= subl).

subling sublingual (= subl).

subman; submand submandibular.

SubN Subthalamic nucleus.

subq subcutaneous(ly) (see SC).

subsp subspecies (L.) (see sppp).

substan; substd substandard.

SUC Serious underlying condition(s) (see SUD).

suc juice (L. succus).

Succ Succinate/nic.

SUD Senile uncomplicated dementia; Serious underlying disease (= SUC); Skin unit dose; Sudden unexpected/ unexplained death; Sulphonylurea derivative/ drug (such as Chlorpropamide, Glibenclamide, Glipizide, Netformide, and Tolbutamide).

SuDBP Supine diastolic blood pressure.

SUDH Succinyldehydrogenase.

SUDS Subjective Unit of Distress Scale.

SUE Serious/ Severe undesirable effect(s).
suf; suff sufficient.
suf- prefix meaning less or under (L.).
SUG Sustained upward gaze.
Sug Sugar - a sweet carbohydrate of various kinds, of both animal and vegetable origin. These are the monosaccharides (with the formula $C_6H_{12}O_6$), including glucose, fructose, and galactose; the disaccharides (with the formula $C_{12}H_{22}O_{11}$), including sucrose or cane sugar, hydrolyzed by enzymes into glucose (dextrose) and fructose (levulose), lactose or milk sugar, hydrolyzed into glucose and galactose, and maltose or malt sugar, hydrolyzed into glucose; and the artificial sugars, such as lactulose (used as a laxative in chronic constipation).
SUH Sulphonylurea hypoglycemia (Chlorpropamide, Glibenclamide, Tolbutamide, etc).
SUI Secondary urinary incontinence; Secondary uterine inertia; Severe uncontrolled infection; Stress urinary incontinence; Suicide.
SUID Sudden unexplained infant death.
sui generis (L.). on its/ their own (kind/ momentum/ singularity/ way).
sulf sulfate (= sulph).
sulfa sulfonamide (= SU; Su; sulpha).
SULF-PRIM Sulfamethoxazole and trimethoprim.
sulph sulphate (see sulf).
sulpha sulphonamide (see sulfa).
sum let him take/ let it be taken/ take/ to be taken (L. sumantur; sumat; sume; sumendum; sumendus).
SUMA Sporadic ulcerating and mutilating acropathy.
SUMC Stanford University Medical College.
SUMEX Stanford University Medical Experiment(al Computer).
SUMEX-AIM Stanford University Medical Experimental Computer - Artificial Intelligence in Medicine (= "Dr. SUMEX").
SUMIT Streptokinase-urokinase myocardial infarct(ion) test/ trial (NHLI).
SUMMIT Stanford University Medical Media and Information Technologies.
sum tal take a similar one/ take one like this (L. sumat talem).
SUN Standard unit of nomenclature; Serum urea nitrogen.
S unit Sedimentation rate (Svedberg).
SUNY State University of New York.
SUO Single use only; Syncope of unknown origin.
SUP Schizo-unipolar; Start-up program; Supination (see supin); Symptomatic uterine prolapse.
Sup; sup Above (L. supra); Superficial; Superior; Superscript; Supination/tor (see supin); Supine (see supin); Supplement (see suppl); Suppository (see suppos); Suppressor bed (chromatography); Suppressor grid (electron tube).
sup- prefix meaning less or under (L.), e.g. suppurate = to fester or gather pus underneath.
sup cit cited above (L. supra citato) (see supra cit).
Super Superintendent (slang for) (see Supt).
super- prefix meaning above, beyond, or superior (L.).
Superl Superlative.
supin supination/ supinator/ supine (= SU; Sup; sup).
Supp Supplement(ary) (see suppl); Suppository (see suppos); Suppurative.
suppl supplement(ary) (= Sup; sup; Supp).
suppos suppository (= Sup; sup; Supp).
supra- prefix meaning above (L.).
supra cit cited above (L. supra citato) (= sup cit).
Supt Superintendent (= Super, slang for).
SUR Surgery/gical (see surg).
surf surface.
Surg Surgeon (journal).
surg surgeon/gery/gical.
Surgi Surgigator.
SURI Sonographic uterine receptivity index (e.g. preovulatory index) (Obs/Gyn).
SURS Solitary ulcer of rectum syndrome.
SUS Saybolt Universal Seconds; Silitek ureteral stent; Society of University Surgeons; Solitary ulcer syndrome; Stained urinary sediment; Suppressor sensitive (see SuS).
SuS Suppressor sensitive (= SS; SUS).

SuSBP Supine systolic blood pressure.
SUSM Stanford University School of Medicine.
susp suspend(ed)/pension.
SUTI Symptomatic urinary tract infection.
Sut Suture(s): I. A stitch or series of stitches made to secure tissue apposition; II. A type of fibrous joint in which the apposed surfaces are closely united:
Absorbable suture;
Albert's suture (deep intestinal suture - see Czerny's suture);
Appolito's suture (see Gely's suture);
Apposition suture (= Coaptation suture);
Approximation suture (a deep suture for securing apposition);
Atraloc suture;
Barrel knot suture (urethrotomy/ urethropexy);
Beclard's suture (a continuous through-and-through suture with two threads);
Bell's suture (made from within outward alternately - a form of glovers or lock-stitch suture);
Bolster suture (made over a roll of guaze or rubber tubing to lessen tension on skin);
Bozeman's suture (a form of button suture - see Button suture);
Bridle suture (ophthalmology);
Bunnell suture;
Buried suture (deep suture, concealed by the skin);
Button suture (passed through a button-like disk to prevent trauma of skin);
Catgut suture (CGS) (sheep catgut, for wound closure);
Chain suture (see Continuous suture);
Circular suture (applied all round the particular organ);
Clavate suture (see Quilled suture);
Coaptation suture (see Apposition suture);
Cobblers' suture (threaded through a needle at each end - see Taylor's suture);
Compound suture (see Quilled suture);
Connell suture (a U-shaped continuous suture used in intestinal anastomosis);
Continuous suture (= Chain suture; Uninterrupted suture);
Cushing suture (a continuous suture used in surgery of the gastrointestinal tract - see Inverting suture);
Czerny's suture (i. a deep intestinal suture {= Albert's s}, ii. suture uniting a ruptured tendon);
Czerny-Lembert suture (a combination of Czerny's and Lembert sutures - see Lembert suture);
Davis & Geck eye sutures (ophthalmology);
Deklene suture (cardiovascular);
Deknatel sutures;
Dermalon suture;
Double-armed suture;
Double # 2, 40-day chromic catgut suture;
Double-button suture (with two buttons, as in Button suture);
Dry suture (using adhesive plaster);
Dulox suture;
Dupuytren's suture (a continuous Lembert suture - see Lembert suture);
Duvergier's suture (stitching of intestine over a section of calf's trachea);
Emmet's suture (a series of double Lembert sutures);
Ethibond suture material;
Ethicon silk suture;
Ethiflex suture material;
Ethilon suture;
Everting suture (with eversion of the wound edges);
Figure-of-eight suture (follows the contours of the figure 8) (= Gussenbauer's, Hare-lip, India rubber, Pin, Rigal's, Rubber and Twisted sutures);
Frost suture;
Furnas suture (otoplasty) - also called Furniss suture;
Furrier's suture (for intestinal wounds);
Gaillard-Arlt suture (used in correction of entropion);
Gambee sutures;
Gely's suture (a continuous suture for repair of intestinal wounds) (= Appolito's suture);
GI pop-off silk suture;
Glovers's (see Bell's suture; Lock-stitch suture);
"Glue-in" sutures (used with suprapubic catheter placement);
Gould's suture (a reversed type of mattress

suture - see Mattress suture);
Gussenbauer's suture (a figure-of-eight suture used on the intestine - see Figure-of-eight suture);
Guy suture (ophthalmology);
Halstead suture (a modification of the Lembert suture);
Halstead type sutures;
Hare-lip suture (a figure-of-eight suture used in correction of hare-lip - see Figure-of-eight suture);
Harris's suture (used in intestinal anastomosis);
Heaney suture;
Hemostatic sutures control oozing of blood from raw areas;
Imbricating suture (general surgery);
India rubber suture (see Figure-of-eight suture; Rubber suture);
Interpalpebral suture;
Interrupted suture (with separate pieces of suture material, using different needles) (= Jobert's, Loop and Noose sutures);
Intradermic suture (below the skin surface);
Inverting suture (used in intestinal anastomosis, as in the Cushing and Lembert sutures);
Ivalon suture;
Jobert's suture (an interrupted suture used in a divided intestine - see Interrupted suture);
Kelly-Kennedy suture (obstetrics and gynecology);
Lace suture (a series of fine stitches);
Lead plate suture (see Plate suture);
Lead-shot tie suture;
Le Dentu's suture (an intestinal suture);
Le Fort's suture (for divided tendon);
Lembert suture (inverting suture used in gastrointestinal surgery - see Czerny-Lembert, Dupuytren's, Emmet's and Halsted sutures);
Lempert suture otolaryngology);
Littre's suture (used in operations for intestinal gangrene);
Living suture (prepared from the patient's freshly removed fascia);
Lock-stitch or Locking suture (a continuous hemostatics, used in intestinal surgery - see Bell's suture; Glovers' suture);
Loffler's suture (for intestinal wounds);
Loop suture (see Interrupted suture);
Lytle sutures (general surgery);
Marshall V suture (general surgery);
Mattress suture (continuous Quilt/ Quilted sutures; horizontal; reverse-Gould's suture; right-angle; vertical) (in which the sutures are made parallel with the edges of the wound);
Maunsell suture (of the mesenteric border of the divided intestine);
Maxon suture material (MSM - green monofilament polyglyconate);
McCannell suture (ophthalmology);
Mers suture;
Mersilene sutures;
Mild chromic suture;
Monofilament suture;
Moynihan suture (General Surgery);
Multifilament suture;
Nerve suture (material for uniting the ends of a divided nerve);
Nonabsorbable suture (material for closing wounds with nonabsorbable materials such as cotton, silk and stainless steel, or synthetic material such as nylon);
Noose suture (see Interrupted suture);
Novafil suture material (blue filament polybutester);
Over-and-over suture (in which equal tissue bites are taken on each side of the wound, and the edges approximated);
Palfyn's suture (for repairing intestinal wounds);
Pancoast's suture (a form of plastic suture - see Plastic suture);
Pare's suture (with cloth strips applied along the edges of the wound);
Parker-Kerr suture; PDS suture (polydioxanone);
Petit's suture (for intestinal wounds);
Pin suture (a figure-of-eight suture with the use of pins - see Figure-of-eight suture);
Plastic suture (in which a tongue is cut in the lip of the wound and a groove in the other, before apposition) (= Tongue-and-groove suture);
Plate suture (= Lead plate suture);
Polydek suture;
Polyglycolic suture;
Polypropylene sutures;
Pop-off sutures;

Preplaced suture (ophthalmology);
Pre-section suture (a stitch/ stitches made before the incision);
Primary suture (made immediately after a wound);
Prolene suture;
Purse-string suture (a type of inverting suture, as in appendectomy);
Quilled suture (a double-threaded suture made over quills or a soft catheter as in Clavate and Compound sutures);
Quilt suture,
Quilted suture (a continuous mattress suture);
Ramdohr's suture (a method of stitching the divided intestine);
Reinforcing suture (with use of exceptionally strong material, such as braided silk, stainless steel, etc. - see Retention suture);
Relaxation suture/ Relief suture(for temporary wound closure) (= Tension suture);
Reo Macrodex sutures;
Retention suture (a reinforcing suture for abdominal wounds);
Richardson angle suture;
Richter's suture (with the use of metallic loops - in closing intestinal wounds);
Rigal's suture (see Figure-of-eight & Rubber sutures);
Ritisch's suture (a method of enterorrhaphy, attaching the bowel wall to the exterior);
Rubber suture (a figure-of-eight suture using rubber bands instead of thread - see Figure-of-eight suture);
Saenger's suture (used in cesarean section with silver wire);
Secondary suture (suturing of a wound at least a week after the operation);
Seroserous suture (apposition of two serous surfaces);
Sewing ring suture (prosthetic device e.g. heart valve, lens implant, etc.;
Shirodkar sutures (in pregnant uterus to prevent abortion);
Shotted suture (with wire passed through a perforated shot);
Silkworm gut suture (from the entrails of the silkworm, for wound closure);
Silver wire suture (use of silver wire - see Saenger's suture);
Simon's suture (used in closing the lacerated perineum and ruptured sphincter ani) (= Triangular suture);
Sims' suture (= Shotted suture);
Staple suture (with use of U-shaped wires);
Sturmdorf suture;
Subcuticular suture (in skin closure);
Superficial suture (solely through the skin);
Surgaloy sutures;
Taylor's suture (in amputation of the cervix uteri with Cobblers' sutures);
Tension suture (see Relaxation, Relief sutures
Through-and-through suture (see Beclard's suture);
Tom Jones suture;
Tongue-and-groove suture (see Plastic suture);
Transfixion sutures (for tight closure of anatomic layers);
Transition sutures (from one anatomic area to another);
Triangular suture (see Simon's suture);
Twisted suture (see Figure-of-eight suture);
Tycron suture (urology);
U#256 suture material;
Uninterrupted suture (see Continuous suture);
Ureteroparietal suture (attaching the uterus to inner surface of the abdominal wall: performed in cesarean section);
V#226 suture;
VEST traction suture;
Vicryl suture;
VicrylSH suture material;
Viscero-parietal suture (stitching of a viscus to the abdominal wall);
Werner suture (obstetrics and gynecology);
Wolfler's suture (i. for a divided intestine; ii. for a divided tendon);
Worst medallion suture (ophthalmology);
Wysler suture (a seromuscular-seromuscular suture for approximating the peritoneal layers of the intestine).

SUUD Sudden unexpected and unexplained death.

SUV Single-use vial; Small unilamellar vesicle (see LSM).

SUX Succinylcholine (see SCh); Suction (see SZ).

SV Alcoholic spirit/ Spirits of wine (see sv);

Saphenous/ Scalp/ Splenic/ Subclavian vein; Saponification value; Sarcoma/ Satellite/ Simian (papova) virus; Selective vagotomy; Semilunar valve; Seminal vesicle; Severe (see sv); Sigmoid volvulus; Single vibration (see sv); Single ventricle; Sinus venosus; Slow virus (produces disease with a greatly delayed onset and protracted course); Snake venom; Southern Veterinarian (journal); Southwestern Veterinarian (AVMA journal); Spontaneous ventilation; Stroke volume (heart); Subjective vertigo; Subventricular; Supraventricular; Supravital (see sv); Ventriculus lateralis (thalamus).

Sv Sievert (= sv).

sv alcoholic spirit/ spirit(s) of wine (L. spiritus vini) (= SV); severe (= SV); sievert (see Sv); single vibration(s) (= SV); supravital (= SV).

S/V Surface/volume (ratio).

SV 40 Simian (vacuolating) virus 40 - a virus originally found in monkeys.

SVA Selective vagotomy and/ with antrectomy; Selective visceral angiography; Sequential ventriculoatrial (pacing); Snellen visual acuity; Social-vocational adjustment (in chronic depression); Subtotal villous atrophy; Supraventricular arrhythmia; Symptomatic ventricular arrhythmia.

SVAS Supravalvular/ Supraventricular aortic stenosis.

SVAT Supraventricular atrial tachycardia (= MAT; SAT).

SVB Saphenous vein bypass.

SVBG Saphenous vein bypass graft(ing) (= SVG).

SV/BSA Stroke volume/ Body surface area (ratio) (see SVI).

SVC Segmental venous capacitance; Selective venous catheterization; Slow vital capacity; Stovarsol Vaginal Compound - vaginal tablets containing acetarsol with carbohydrate, used in the local treatment of trichomonal vaginitis and idiopathic proctitis (a proprietary drug); Subclavian vein catheterization; Superior/ Suprahepatic vena cava.

SVCCS Superior vena cava compression syndrome (= SVCS).

SVCG Spatial vectorcardiogram (procedure/ cardiology).

SVCO Superior vena-caval obstruction.

SVCP Special Virus Cancer Program (= SCPV).

SVC-PA Superior vena cava to pulmonary artery (shunt).

SVCR Segmental venous capacitance ratio.

SVC-RPA Superior vena cava to right pulmonary artery (shunt).

SVCS Superior vena cava syndrome (see SVCCS).

SVD Serious/ Severe/ Significant valvular disease; Serious/ Severe vascular disease/ disorder; Single/ Small vessel disease; Singular value decomposition; Spontaneous vaginal/ vertex delivery; Stavudine (HIV reverse transcriptase inhibitor); Swine vesicular disease.

SVE Side-viewing endoscope; Slow volume encephalography; Soluble viral extract; Sterile vaginal examination; Streptococcus viridans endocarditis; Supraventricular ectopic (beat) (see SVPB).

SVEB Supraventricular ectopic beat (see SVPB).

S-ve SP Seronegative sex(ual) partner (see S-SP).

S+ve SP Seropositive sex(ual) partner (see S+SP).

SVET Survival and Ventricular Enlargement Trial.

SVF Simple virilizing form (of Congenital adrenal hyperplasia) (see CAH); Sudden vestibular failure.

SVG Saphenous vein graft (operation/ coronary bypass) (see SVBG).

SV GAL Brandy (L. spiritus vini gallici).

SVI Small volume infusion; Stroke volume index (ml/m^2) (= Stroke volume/ body surface area; SV/BSA); Superficial venous incompetence; Systemic viral infection.

SVIB Strong Vocational Interest Blank (psychology).

SVK Sunrise view of knee (seen on X-ray of bent knee, so the patella resembles the sun rising above the rest of the knee structures).

SVL Severe visual loss; Superficial vastus lateralis.

SVM Seminal vesicle microsome; Syncytiovascular membrane.

SVN Sinuvertebral nerve; Small volume nebulizer.

SvO$_2$ Venous oxygen saturation, i.e. O_2 sat. of the pulmonary artery.

SVOM Sequenced/ Sequential volitional oral movement.

SVP If you please/ please (Fr. s'il vous plaît); Selective vagotomy and/ with pyloroplasty; Senior vice president; Small volume parenteral (infusion); Spontaneous venous pulse; Spun vegetable protein; Standing venous pressure; Superior vascular plexus.

SVPB Supraventricular premature beat (= SVE; SVEB).

SVPC Supraventricular premature contraction.

SVR Rectified spirit of wine (see svr); Sequential vascular response; Supraventricular rhythm; Sustained virologic response (to medication); Systemic vascular resistance = (dyne/s/cm^{-5}) or 80 (MAP - RAP)/CO or 80 (Mean arterial pressure - right atrial pressure)/cardiac output.

svr alcohol/ rectified spirit of wine (L. spiritus vini rectificatus) (= 90% Alcohol; Rectified Spirit) (= SVR).

SVRI Systemic vascular resistance index.

SVS Slit ventricle syndrome; Society for Vascular Surgery; Systemic venous system.

SVT Sinoventricular tachycardia; Small vessel thrombosis; Snake-venom therapy; Subclavian vein thrombosis; Superficial venous thrombosis; Supraventricular tachyarrhythmia/ tachycardia; Sustained ventricular tachycardia.

svt concentrated alcohol/ proof spirit (L. spiritus vini tenuis).

SVV Systolic ventricular volume.

SW Sandwich; Seriously wounded; Short wave(s); Silent Worker (journal for the deaf); Sinewave; Slow/ Spike wave (see S-W); Soap and water (see S&W); Social/ Stroke work; Social Work (journal); Social worker; Southwest; Spiral/ Stab wound (see sw); Sterile water; Sturge-Weber (syndrome); Swiss Webster (mouse).

Sw Swine (veterinary medicine).

sw spiral/ stab wound (= SW).

S-W Slow-wave/ Spike-wave (= SW).

S/W Special warning(s).

S&W Soap and water (enema) (= SW).

SWA Seriously wounded in action; Silver-wire appearance (of retinal arteries); Social work aide/ assistant.

SWAC Salt-wasting adrenal crisis (as in Congenital adrenal hyperplasia) (see CAH).

SWC Submaximal working capacity.

SWCF Simeon Weight Clinics Foundation.

SWD Severe watery diarrhea; Short wave diathermy.

SWE Slow wave encephalography.

Swed Swedish.

Sweet Lucy Marijuana (see Cannabis).

SWFI Sterile water for injection (see SWI).

SWG Silkworm gut; Standard wire guage; Sudden weight gain.

SWHC Social Work in Health Care (journal).

SWI Sterile water for injection; Stroke work index (g.m/m^2) = Stroke volume index x (arterial pressure - pulmonary capillary wedge pressure) x 0.0136 = SVI x (AP - PCWP) x 0.0136; Surgical wound infection.

S&WI Skin and wound isolation.

SWIC Sidewall infusion cannula (Ophthalmology).

SWIFS Southwest Institute of Forensic Sciences.

SWIM Sperm-washing insemination method.

SWIORA Spinal cord injury without radiologic abnormality.

SWIR Selective wavelength infrared analyzer.

Swiss P Swiss Pharmacopeia (Pharmacopoea Helvetica).

SWIU Service Workers International Union.

SWL Significant/ Sudden weight loss (see USWL).

SWM Spatial working memory (remembering where things are/ rapidly lost in Alzheimer's disease).

SWMV Sine wave monophasic waveform (defibrillation) (see SMS).

SWN Salt-wasting nephropathy; Speech weighted noise.

SWOG Southwest Oncology Group.

SWP Small whirlpool.

SWR Serum Wassermann reaction (see STS-SWR); Severe water retention; Surface wrinkling retinopathy (Ophthalmology); Sustained weight reduction.

SWS Severe withdrawal syndrome; Sleep-

wake state (as in neonates, etc.); Slow-wave sleep; Spike-wave stupor; Steroid-wasting syndrome; Student ward secretary; Sturge-Weber syndrome.
SWT Sine-wave threshold; Social work technician; Stab wound of the throat; Standard walking time.
SWU Separative work unit (U-235 concentration plant); Septic work-up.
SWVP Saturated water-vapor pressure.
Sx; S_x Sign(s); Surgery; Symptom(s).
SXR Skull X-ray; A gene member of a family of proteins known as nuclear receptors.
Sxs Serological sex-specific (antigen).
SXT Sulfamethoxazole-trimethoprim (mixture).
SY Syphilis/litic.
sy- prefix meaning with (Gr.) (see syl-).
SYA Subacute yellow atrophy.
SYDS Stomach yin deficiency syndrome.
syl- prefix meaning with (Gr.) (= sy-; sym-).
Syl-ag-ol Pysillium, agar-agar, mineral oil (laxative) - proprietary drug.
Sym; sym Symmetrical/ry; Symptom(s) (= SM; Sympt; sympt).
sym- prefix meaning with (Gr.) (see syl-).
symb symbiosis; symbol(ic)/(s) (see Symbols).
SYMBIOSIS System for Medical and Biological Science Information Searching.
Symbols - used in or associated with: 1. Biology; 2. Calculation; 3. Chemistry; 4. Greek Alphabet; 5. Medicine and Pharmacy; 6. Numeration; 7. Signs of the Zodiac (see Table).

Symbols

1. Biology.

○, ⊙, ① Annual plant.
♂, ⊙⊙, ② Biennial plant.
♃ Perrenial herb.
Δ Evergreen plant.
⊙ Monocarpic plant, bearing fruit only once.
ℨ Shrub.
ʃ Tree-like shrub.
ℰ Tree.
⌒ Climbing plant.
♂, ♅, oo Male organism or cell; Staminate plant or flower.
♀ Female organism or cell; Pistillate plant or flower.
⚥ Hermaphrodite.
☿ Perfect, or hermaphroditic plant or flower.
❍ Individual, especially female, organism.
❑ Individual, especially male, organism.
♂♀ Unisexual; having male and female flowers on the same plant.
♂-♀ Monoecious; having male and female flowers on the same plant.
♂:♀ Dioecious; having male and female flowers on different plants.
♀ Polygamous; having hermaphroditic and unisexual flowers on the same and on different plants.
∞ Indefinite number, as of stamens, when there are more than twenty.
0 Locking, or absent, as a part.
) Turning or winding to the left.
(Turning or winding to the right.
× Crossed with; used as a hybrid.
P Parental (generation).
F Filial (generation); offspring.
F_1; F_2; F_3; etc. Offspring of the first, second, third, etc. filial generation.
+ Possessing a (specified) characteristic.
− Lacking a (specified) characteristic.
$\underline{*}$ Northern hemisphere.
$\overline{*}$ Southern hemisphere.
|* Old World.
*| New World.
°, ', " Feet, inches, lines.
', ", ''' Feet, inches, lines (in European usage).

2. Calculation.

+; ⊥; ⊕; P Plus, the sign of addition; Acid reaction; Excess; Positive; Present; Slight reaction/trace.
-; ⊖ ; N Minus, the sign of substraction; Absent; Alkaline reaction; Deficiency; Negative (= N; neg).
±; ∓ Plus or minus; Either positive or negative; Equivocal; Indefinite; Very slight trace.
× a) Multiplied by, as in 4 x 3 = 12; also indicated by a central dot, as in 4·3 = 12, or by placing the factors in immediate juxtaposition, as in: 6ab = 6 x a x b. b) Magnification.

c) By - used in dimensions, as in paper: 6 x 10 inches.
÷ Divided by, as in: x ÷ y. Other signs of division are: x : y = x/y.
= Equals; is equal to.
≠ Is not equal to.
+ reaction Acid reaction.
- reaction Alkaline reaction.
- Negative/ negative reaction.
± Very slight trace/ reaction.
+ Slight trace/reaction.
++ Trace/ noticable reaction.
+++ Moderate amount/ reaction.
++++ Large amount or pronounced reaction.
> Greater than.
< Less than.
≥ Is greater than or equal to.
⋝ Is equal to or greater than.
≮ Is not less than.
≤ Is less than or equal to.
⋜ Is equal to or less than.
≯ Is not greater than.
≎ Is equivalent to; applied to magnitude or quantities that are equal in area or volume, but are not of the same form.
≡ Is identical with.
≅ Approximately; congruent to.
∼ Approximate.
~ The difference between; used to designate the difference between two quantities, as in: x ~ y = the difference between x and y.
∝ Varies as; is directly proportional to, as in: x ∝ y; that is, x varies as y.
∺ Geometric proportions, as in: ∺ x:y::a:b; that is, the geometric proportion, x is to y, as a is to b.
: Is to; the ratio of; ratio.
:: As; equality/used between ratios; equals; proportionate to.
∞ Infinity; indefinitely great.
? Possible; questionable; question of.
l or L The factorial of, or the continued product of numbers from one upward, as in: 5l = 5L = 5 x 4 x 3 x 2 x 1.
∴ Therefore.
∵ Because; since.
... And so on; etcetera.
∠ Angle, as in ∠ PQR.
∟ Right angle.
⊥ Is perpendicular to, as in: AB ⊥ YZ = AB is perpendicular to YZ.
|| Parallel; is parallel to, as in: AB || YZ.
○ Circle; Circumference; 360°.
∩ Arc of a circle.
π pi - the 16th lower case (small) letter of the Greek alphabet; the ratio of circumference to diameter of a circle: 3.1415926536.
Δ Change, finite difference, or increment; Temperature (on anesthesia records); Triangle.
ΔS Entropic variation.
Δt Time interval.
24° Twenty-four hours.
□ Square.
▭ Rectangle.
▱ Parallelogram.
√ Square root.
$^3\surd$ Cube root, as in: $^3\surd 64 = 4$.
$^x\surd$ y is the index, expressing the degree of the required root of the number y, as in: $^6\surd 64$ = the 6th root of 64 = 2.
✓ c̄ Check with.
/ Per.
% Percent (= P).
1; 2; 3; etc. 1. Exponents, placed above and to the right of a quantity, indicate that it is raised to the first, second, third, etc. power, as in: 10^1, a^2, $(a + b)^3$; etc. 2. Exponents, placed above and to the right of a word, are used to refer the reader (of the book or article), to the equivalent number in the bibliography.
'; "; '": etc. Prime; double or second prime; triple or third prime; etc. are used to distinguish between different values of the same variable, as in: x'; x"; x'"; etc.
—— Vinculum, as in: a+b.
( ) Parentheses, as in: 2(a + b).
[ ] Brackets, as in: p[2(a = b)].
{ } Braces, as in: q + {12 + p[2(a + b)]}.
ƒ or F Function; function of, as in: ƒ(a) or F(a), a function of a.
d Differential of, as in: da.
δ Variation of, as in: δa.
Δ Finite difference, or increment.
D Differential coefficient, or derivative.
∫ Integral; integral of, indicating that the expression following it, is to be integrated, as

in: $\int p(x)qx$, indicating the indefinite integral of p(x) with respect to x.

$\int^a_b$ Definite integral, indicating the limits of integration, as in: $\int^a_b p(x)qx$, indicating the integral of p(x) with respect to x, between the limits of a and b.

Σ Sum; sum of; algebraic sum; when used to indicate the summation of finite differences, it has a sense similar to that of the symbol ∫.

@ At.

Π The continued product of all terms such as (those indicated).

π Pi = 3.14159265+; the ratio of the circumference of a circle to its diameter, of a semicircle to its radius, and of the area of a circle to the square of its radius.

e or ∈ The number 2.7182818+; the base of the Napierian system of logarithms, and the eccentricity of a conic section.

M The modules of a system of logarithms, especially of the common system of logarithms, where it is equal to 0.4342944819+.

g The acceleration of gravity.

1 or Ṫ One.

II ṪṪ Two.

1x Once.

2x; etc. Twice; etc.

° Degree(s), as in: 180°.

1° First degree; Primary.

* Asterisk.

2° Secondary; Second degree.

2^ndry Secondary.

' Foot, feet; Minute(s) of arc/time; Primary accent; Univalent.

x̄ Mean.

" Bivalent; Inch(es); Second(s) of arc/time; Secondary accent.

''' Line (1/12 inch); Trivalent.

Δt Time interval.

24° 24 hours.

h Hour(s).

m Minute(s) of time.

s second(s) of time.

Number; Pound.

£ Pound sterling.

$ Dollar.

₪ or nש New Shekel/ Shekel Hadash (Israeli currency).

σ 1/1000 of a second (millisecond); Standard deviation; Sigma.

3. Chemistry.

Elements. The symbol of each of the chemical elements (see under Elements), is formed of the initial or abbreviation of its English, Latin, Modern Latin, or Greek names, as in "Initials": C for Carbon (Eng., L. carbo), Au for Gold (L. aurum), K for Potassium (Modern L. kalium), and Ba for Barium (Gr. barys), or "Abbreviations": Mn for Manganese (Eng., L. manganum), Pb for Lead (L. plumbum), Pt for Platinum (Modern L. platina), and Tl for Thallium (Gr. thallos).

• Separate radicals, as in CH_3•CHO (= acetaldehyde; C_2H_4O), or the water of crystallization, as in: Na_2SO_3•$5H_2O$ (= sodium thiosulfate).

, Indicates elements which are interchangeable; for example: (Er,Y)PO_4 means ErPO_4 (Erbium phosphate) and YPO_4 (Yttrium phosphate) in proportions that vary.

( ) Parentheses - indicate a radical within a compound, as in $C_3H_5(NO_3)_3$, glyceryl trinitrate, or is used to set off elements that are interchangeable, as in the example for the preceding symbol.

[ ] Brackets - are used together with parentheses to indicate certain radicals as in: $Fe_3[Fe(CN)_6]_2$, ferrous ferricyanide, or in coordination formulas to indicate relationship to the central atom.

○ Benzene ring - is used in structural formulas, as in:

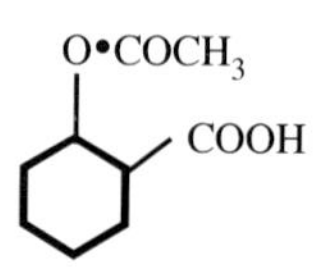

[= CH_3•CO_2•C_6H_4•COOH; $C_9H_8O_4$; Acetylsalicylic acid (Aspirin)].

$^+$; $^{++}$; $^{+++}$; etc. or $^{1+}$; $^{2+}$; $^{3+}$; etc. Indicate the unit charges of positive electricity, as in: Ca^{++}, a calcium ion with 2 positive charges.

$^-$; $^{--}$; $^{---}$; etc. or $^{1-}$; $^{2-}$; $^{3-}$; etc. Indicate the unit charges of negative electricity, as in: N^{---}, a nitrogen ion with 3 negative charges.

4. Greek Alphabet.

Letter	Name	Capital letter	Small letter	English transcription
1st	alpha	Α	α	a
2nd	beta	Β	β	b
3rd	gamma	Γ	γ	g
4th	delta	Δ	δ	d
5th	epsilon	Ε	ε	e
6th	zeta	Ζ	ζ	z
7th	eta	Η	η	ē
8th	theta	Θ	θ	th
9th	iota	Ι	ι	i
10th	kappa	Κ	κ	k
11th	lambda	Λ	λ	l
12th	mu	Μ	μ	m
13th	nu	Ν	ν; ν	n
14th	xi	Ξ	ξ	x
15th	omicron	Ο	ο	o
16th	pi	Π	π	p
17th	rho	Ρ	ρ	r
18th	sigma	Σ	σ, ς	s
19th	tau	Τ	τ	t
20th	upsilon	Υ	υ	y
21st	phi	Φ	φ; ϕ	ph
22nd	chi	Χ	χ	ch
23rd	psi	Ψ	ψ; ψ	ps
24th	omega	Ω	ω	ō

-; =; ≡; etc. Indicate 1) the same as the symbols immediately preceding, as in: N≡, and 2) a single, double, or triple band, as in: HC=CH, acetylene.

·; :; ⋮; etc. Indicate a single, double, triple, etc. bond as in: CH_2:CH·O·CH:CH_2 (= vinyl ether).

'; "; '"; etc. Indicate 1) a valence of one, two, three, etc., as in Fe''', trivalent iron, and 2) the unit charges of negative electricity, as in CO_3", a carbonate ion with 2 negative charges.

1-; 2-; 3-; etc., α-; β-; γ-; etc. Indicate one of the several possible positions of substituting groups in a parent compound, as in: 3-acetylpyridine or α-tocopherol.

\- Indicates levorotation, as in: -130°.

\+ 1) Means "with the addition of" or "together with", as in: $H_2SO_4 + Ca(OH)_2 = CaSO_4 + 2H_2O$. 2) Indicates dextrorotation, as in: +130°.

= Means "form" or "results in", as is used in chemical equations, as in: $HCl + NaHCO_3 = NaCl + CO_2 + H_2O$, i.e. one molecule each of hydrochloric acid and sodium bicarbonate, combine to form one molecule each of sodium chloride, carbon dioxide, and water.

→ To the right; results in (is due to); transfer to; yields/ causes.

← To the left.

→ or ← Indicates the direction of the reaction (in a chemical equation).

⇌ or ⇄ Indicates a reversible reaction, as in: $H_2O + CO_2 \rightleftarrows H_2CO_3$, i.e. one that can proceed in either direction, or in both direc-

6. Numeration.

Arabic	Greek symbol	Greek name	Roman numeral
0	...	...	...
1	α	alpha	I
2	β	beta	II
3	γ	gamma	III
4	δ	delta	IV or IIII
5	ε	epsilon	V
6	ς	sigma	VI
7	ζ	zeta	VII
8	η	eta	VIII or IIX
9	θ	theta	IX or VIIII
10	ι	iota	X
11	ια	iota alpha	XI
12	ιβ	iota beta	XII
13	ιγ	iota gamma	XIII or XIIV
14	ιδ	iota delta	XIV or XIIII
15	ιε	iota epsilon	XV
16	ις	iota sigma	XVI
17	ιζ	iota zeta	XVII
18	ιη	iota eta	XVIII or XIIX
19	ιθ	iota theta	XIX or XVIIII
20	κ	kappa	XX
30	λ	lambda	XXX
40	μ	mu	XL or XXXX
50	ν	nu	L
60	ξ	xi	LX
70	ο	omicron	LXX
80	π	pi	LXXX or XXC
90	♀	...	XC or LXXXX
100	ρ	rho	C
200	σ	sigma	CC
300	τ	tau	CCC
400	υ	upsilon	CD or CCCC
500	φ; Φ; ϕ	phi	D or IↃ
600	χ	chi	DC or IↃC
700	ψ	psi	DCC or IↃCC
800	ω	omega	DCCC or IↃCCC
900	...	...	CM or DCCCC or IↃCCCC
1,000	...	...	M or CIↃ
2,000	...	...	MM or CIↃCIↃ
5,000	...	...	IↃↃ
10,000	...	...	MↃ or CCIↃↃ
50,000	...	...	IↃↃↃ
100,000	...	...	MↃↃ or CCCIↃↃↃ or C̄
500,000	...	...	IↃↃↃↃ
1,000,000	...	...	M̄

After the sign IↃ for D or 500, when the character Ↄ is repeated, each repetition has the effect of multiplying IↃ (i.e. 500) by 10, as in:IↃ = 500; IↃↃ = 5,000; IↃↃↃ = 50,000; IↃↃↃↃ = 500,000. In writing numbers twice as great as these, C is placed as many times before the stroke I as the Ↄ is written after it, as in: CIↃ = 1,000; CCIↃↃ = 10,000; CCCIↃↃↃ = 100,000.
A line drawn over a numeral indicates thousands, as in: $\bar{C}$ = 100,000; $\bar{M}$ = 1,000,000.

tions at the same time, in a state of equilibrium.

↓ Indicates that the specified reaction product (after which it is written), appears as a precipitate.

↑ Indicates that the specified reaction product (after which it is written), appears as a gas.

≡ or ≎ Means "is equivalent to", and is used in quantitative equations to indicate the quantities of specified substances that will react with each other completely, so as to leave no excess matter.

↑ or ↗ Increase(s); Above; Elevated; Greater than; Rising.

↓ or ↘ Decrease(s); Below; Falling; Less than.

↑ Up.

4. Greek Alphabet. – see table on p. 749.

5. Medicine and Pharmacy.

↑↑ Extensor response - Babinski sign positive (dorsiflexion) (neurological examination); Testes undescended.

↓↓ Plantar response - Babinski sign negative (plantar flexion) (neurological examination);

Ⓜ Murmur.

℞ Take; of a prescription used at the beginning (L. recipe) (= Rp).

Rp Take (see ℞).

℥ Ounce(s).

℥ i One ounce.

℥ ij Two ounces.

℥ ss Half an ounce.

℥ iss. One ounce and a half.

f℥ A fluid ounce.

ʒ Drachm(s)/ Dram(s) - teaspoonful(s).

ʒi One drachm/ dram.

ʒii Two drachms/ drams.

ʒiss One drachm/ dram and a half.

ʒss Half a drachm/ dram.

fʒ A fluid drachm/ dram.

℈ Scruple; ℈ i = one scruple; ℈ii = two scruples; ℈ss = half a scruple; ℈iss = one scruple and a half.

♏ or ♍ Minim.

A; Å Angstrom unit.

$\bar{A}$; $\bar{A}\bar{A}$; $\bar{a}\bar{a}$ (Gr. ana).

C' Complement.

C A gallon (L. congius).

c; $\bar{c}$ With (L. cum).

© Copyright.

D; d A dose (L. dosis); Dextro (L.) - right.

do As before/ ditto/ the same (L. dictum).

E_0 Electroaffinity.

F1; F_1 First filial generation.

F2; F_2 Second filial generation.

L; l Laevo/ Levo (L.) - left.

lb Pound.

M Mix (L. misce).

O Female (also ♀); Pint (L. octarius); Respirations (on anesthesia records).

♂; OO Male.

⊙ Start of operation (on anesthesia records).

Q Energy unit or Quadrillion (= 10^{15} Btu or British thermal unit; 1.054 x 10^{18} joule).

® Registration/ Trade Mark; Right.

S Label/ Write (L. signa) - used in prescriptions to indicate the directions to be placed on the label of the medicine (see sig); Suction (on anesthesia records).

$\bar{s}$ Without (= s; Σ).

∨ Systolic blood pressure (on anesthesia records).

∧ Diastolic blood pressure (on anesthesia records).

° Pulse rate (on anesthesia records).

O Respirations (on anesthesia records).

Δ Average/ Average change; Temperature (on anesthesia records).

* Asterisk; Birth.

† Death; died; used in genealogies, reports, etc.
✡ Red Shield of David (Hebrew: Magen David Adom).
✚ Red Cross.
☾ Red Crescent.
Fracture (see Fract).
BB Fracture of both bones (see Fract BB).
Σ Sum/ Summation of series (L. sigma); Syphilis; Without (= s̄; s).
ΣST Sum of ST segment elevations (see SST; ΣST).
& And.
&c And others/ And so forth (L. et cetera).
© Copyrighted.
λ Lambda (= 0.001 ml; 10^{-6} liter); wave length.
μ Micro (prefix for 10^{-6}); micron (10^{-6} meter).
μc Microcurie (= μCi).
μch Microcurie-hour.
μCi Microcurie (see μc).
μEq Microequivalent.
μf Microfarad.
μg Microgram (= 1/1000 mgm).
μγ Microgamma (= 10^{-12} gram).
μIU Micro-international unit.
μj Microjoule (= 10^{-6} joule; mj).
μl Microliter (= 10^{-6} liter).
μμ Micromicron/ pico (= 10^{-12} meter; picometer; pm).
μM Micromolar (solution).
μmol Micromole.
μμg Micromicrogram; picogram (= γ,γ).
μR Microrad; microroentgen.
μs; μsec Microsecond.
μU Microunit.
μv Microvolt.
μw Microwatt.
μΩ Microhm.
mγ Milligamma.
mμ Millimicron.
mμc Millimicrocurie (= nanocurie).
mμg Millimicrogram (= nanogram).
mEq Milliequivalent.
mg; mgm Milligram.
mg% Milligrams per cent.
nM Nanomole (= 10^{-9} mole; nmol).
πif Interstitial fluid colloid osmotic pressure.
πp Plasma colloid osmotic pressure.
σ Millisecond (1/1000 of a second); sigma; standard deviation.
X^2 Chi square (statistical test).
Ω Ohm; omega.
QO_2 Oxygen consumption.
m- Meta-.
o- Ortho-.
p- Para-.
ss; s̄s̄ One-half (L. semis).
τ Life (time).
τ1/2 Half-life (time).
x/7 Days (Medical records and visit dates).
x/12 Months (Medical records and visit dates).
x/52 Weeks (Medical records and visit dates).
α, β, δ, θ Alpha, beta, delta, theta electroencephalograph waves.

6. Numeration – see table on p. 750.

7. Signs of the Zodiac.

Spring Signs:
1. ♈ Aries (the Ram).
2. ♉ Taurus (the Bull).
3. ♊ Gemini (the Twins).

Summer Signs:
4. ♋ Cancer (the Crab).
5. ♌ Leo (the Lion).
6. ♍ Virgo (the Virgin).

Autumn Signs:
7. ♎ Libra (the Balance).
8. ♏ Scorpio (the Scorpion).
9. ❆ Sagittarius (the Archer).

Winter Signs:
10. ✳ Capricorn (the Goat).
11. ♒ Aquarius (the Water Bearer).
12. ♓ Pisces (the Fish).

symp; sympat; sympath sympathetic.
symph symphysis.
Sympt; sympt Symptom (see Sym).
SYN Synovitis (see Syn; syn).
Syn; syn Syndrome (= Synd; synd); Synergistic; Synonym; Synovial (fluid); Synovitis (= SYN).
syn- prefix meaning union or with (Gr.).
Synd; synd Syndrome (see Syn; syn).
Syndrome X Angina pectoris associated with exercise, with a normal coronary arteriogram.
syndromy a combination of syndromes.

Syph; syph Syphilis (see Σ)/ Syphilitic/ Syphiloid/ Syphilology/ Syphilous.
SYR Syrian (hamster).
Syr; syr Syrup (L. syrupus); syringe.
SYS Stretching-yawning syndrome.
SyS Sign-your-site (procedure before surgery).
sys; syst system(ic); systole/lic.
SYS-BP Systolic blood pressure.
syst m systolic murmur.
SZ Streptozocin (see SZN); Suction (= SUX).
Sz Schizophrenia; Seizure.
SZMC Shaare Zedek Medical Center (Jerusalem, Israel).
SZN Streptozocin (= SZ).
SZT Streptozyme test/ titer (see ST).

T

T Absolute temperature; An electrocardiographic wave corresponding to the repolarization of the ventricles (wave); Life (time); Period (time); Period of Oscillation; Ribosylthymine; Tablespoon(ful); Taenia; Tamoxifen (see TAM); Tau - the 19th (Capital) letter of the Greek alphabet; T-bandage; T-bar (orthodontics); Telomere/ Terminal banding; Temperature; Temporal; Temporal electrode placement in electroencephalography; Temporary; Tender; Tension (intraocular) (see T+1; T-1; Tn; etc.); Tera- (prefix for 10^{12}), e.g. Tg = Teragram = 10^{12} gram (see tera-); Terminal; Tertiary; Tesla; Testicle(s); Testosterone; Tetra; Tetracycline; T-fiber (nerve cell); Theophylline; Therapy; Thoracic (in vertebral formulas); Thorax; Threatened (animal); Three (L. ter); Threonine; Thrombosis; Thrombus; Thymic-derived (lymphocyte); Thymidine; Thymine; Thymus (cell); Thymus-derived (lymphocyte) (= Thymic-d. l.); Thyroid; Tidal gas/ volume (respiration); Time; Tincture; T lymphocyte (= Thymic/ Thymus-derived l.); Tocopherol; Ton/ Tonne; Topical (drug administration); Torque; Total; Toxicity; Trace; Training (group); Transition (point); Transmittance (in spectrophotometry); Transverse; Treatment; Treponema (= Trep); Trichinella; Trichomonas (= Trich); Trichophyton; Tritium; Troy; Trypanosoma; Tryptamine; Tuberculin; Tuberculosis; Tumor; Turnkey system; T-wave (ventricular recharging/ recovery/ repolarization on the electrocardiogram (see above); Type.

t duration; Student t-test (of significance); teaspoon(ful); temperature; temporal; temporary; ter (L.) - three times; terminal; tertiary; test of significance; three/ three times (L. ter); time; tissue; ton/ tonne; topical; total; toxic; transfer; translocation; transverse.

τ Greek lower case letter tau; Symbol of life (time) of radioactive isotope; Relaxation time; Shear stress; Spectral transmittance; Transmission coefficient.

Θ Greek capital letter theta; Thermodynamic temperature.

θ Greek lower case letter theta; an angular coordinate variable; customary temperature; temperature interval.

T+ Increased tension.

T- Decreased tension.

T1/2; t1/2 Serum/ Terminal elimination half-life.

T1/2; $T_{1/2}$; τ1/2; $\tau_{1/2}$; t1/2; $t_{1/2}$ Symbol for half-life (time) of 50 radioactive isotope (see Symbols).

T1-T12 First to twelfth thoracic (dorsal) vertebrae.

T_1...T_{12} Thoracic nerve I through 12.

T_1 Spin-lattice or longitudinal relaxation time; Tricuspid first heart sound.

T+1; T+2; T+3 First, second, and third stages of increased intraocular tension.

T-1; T-2; T-3 First. second, and third stages of decreased intraocular tension.

$t^{-0.50}$; $t^{-1.7}$; etc. Rate of change of retention of injected radioactive material.

T 1 Time constant (in the order of seconds) - in MRI.

T 2 Time constant (in the order of milliseconds) - in MRI.

T-2 Dactinomycin, doxorubicin (Adriamycin), vincristine, and cyclophosphamide.

T_2 Diiodothyronine; Spin-spin or transverse relaxation time; Trichothecene toxin - a deadly poison prepared for use in chemical warfare, purported to have been used by the former Soviet regime in the form of "yellow rain" in their military operations in Afghanistan, Laos, and Cambodia; Tricuspid second heart sound.

T3 Tylenol with codeine 30 mg.

T_3 Resin uptake test; Triiodothyronine (free) (= TIT; TITh).

T_4 Cyclonite; Free thyroxine; Total thyroxine concentration (thyroxine, levothyroxine, tetraiodothyronine).

2,4,5-T 2,4,5-Trichlorophenoxyacetic acid - a herbicide.

T-7 Free thyroxine factor.

T-20 Enfuvirtide (a fusion inhibitor, anti-HIV drug, given by subcutaneous injections).

t_{50} half-life (see T1/2).

33-T-57 Methisazone (= Metisazone; N-Methylisatin β-Thiosemicarbazone) - a chemotherapeutic agent used in the prophylaxis of smallpox, and which appears to act by preventing the replication of the virus. Methisazone is suitable for mass (oral) administration in the event of an epidemic of smallpox and conveys immediate protection. Also used in the treatment of eczema vaccinatum and vaccinia gangrenosa.

T_{90} Time required for 90% mortality in a population of microorganisms, exposed to a toxic agent.

T-156 Hexazole.

T-1384 Netropsin.

T-1824 Azovan Blue (= Azovanum Caeruleum; Evans Blue; Evan's Blue) - a blue dye of low toxicity used intravenously for the determination of blood and plasma volumes.

T 1/2α Initial first half-life (of a drug in the plasma) (see T 1/2β).

TA Alkaline tuberculin; Arterial tension; Axillary temperature - see T(A); Tactile afferent; Takayasu/ Temporal arteritis; Teaching assistant; Technology assessment (see OTA); Teichoic/ Titrable/ Titratable acid; Terminal antrum; Test age; Therapeutic abortion; Thermal analysis; Thermochimica Acta (journal); Thermophilic Actinomyces; Thymic activity (see STA); Thymocytotoxic autoantibody; Thyroglobulin autoprecipitation; Thyroid antibody/ autoimmunity; Tibialis anterior; Tidal/ Trapped air (pulmonary); Total acidity/ alkaloids/ antibody; Toxic adenoma; Toxin-antitoxin (see T-A); Tracheal aspirate; Traction/ Traumatic alopecia (= PA - Pressure alopecia); Traffic accident; Trait anxiety; Transactional analysis; Transaldolase; Transantral; Transplantation/ Trophoblast antigen; Transpostion of the aorta; Transverse axis (approximately perpendicular to the mechanical axis but is sloped posteriorly in the sagittal plane (see MA - Mechanical axis); Triamcinolone acetonide; Tricuspid atresia; True anomaly; Truncus arteriosus; Tryptamine; Tryptophane acid (reaction); Tryptose agar; Tube agglutination; Tuberculin, alkaline; Tumor-associated (antigen) (see TAA).

Ta Tantalum (Z = 73) (see Elements - Tantalum); Tarsal; Temperature (dry bulb); Tonometry applanation.

T/A Time and amount.

T-A Thyroid antibodies (test for); Toxin-antitoxin (= TA).

T(A) Temperature, axillary (on temperature charts) (= TA).

T&A Tonsillectomy and adenoidectomy (= Adenotonsillectomy); Tonsillitis and adenitis (= Adenotonsillitis); Tonsils and adenoids.

ta- combining form meaning stretch or tension (Gr. ton-).

TAA Therapeutic alkylating agent; Thioacetamide; Thoracic aortic aneurysm; Tobacco-alcohol amblyopia (with progressive to permanent visual loss {PVL}, due to associated deficiency of vitamin B1); Topical anesthetic/ antibiotic/ antimicrobial agent; Total alcohol abstinence; Total ankle arthroplasty; Transverse aortic arch; Triamcinolone acetonide; Tumor-associated antibodies/(dy)/ antigen.

TAAF Thromboplastic activity of the amniotic fluid.

TA-AIDS Transfusion-associated acquired immunodeficiency syndrome.

TAAOO Transactions of the American Academy of Ophthalmology and Otolaryngology (journal).

TAAP Transactions of the Association of American Physicians (journal).

TAAT Transabdominal aspiration technique (Obs/Gyn).

TAB Technical Activities Board (IEEE); Technical Advisory Board (Dept. of Commerce); Technical Assistance Bureau (AID); Technology Assessment Board; Therapeutic abortion (see TAb); Total autonomic blockage; Trifluoroacetylbutyl (ester); Triple antibiotic (bacitracin, neomycin, and polymyxin); Typhoid-paratyphoid A and B (vaccine) (see TAB/Vac).

TAb Therapeutic abortion.

Tab; tab Capsule of LSD-25 (see LSD); Tablet (L. tabella) (= tbl).

TABC Total aerobic bacteria count; Typhoid-paratyphoid A, B, and C (vaccine) (see TABC/Vac).

TABCho Typhoid-paratyphoid A and B, and Cholera (vaccine) (see TABCho/Vac).

TABCho/Vac Typhoid-paratyphoid A and B, and Cholera Vaccine.

TABC/Vac Typhoid-paratyphoid A, B, and C Vaccine.

Tablesp Tablespoon(ful).

TABP Type A behavior pattern.

Tabs Tablets.

TABT Typhoid-paratyphoid A and B, and tetanus toxoid (combined vaccine) (see TABT/Vac).

TABTD Typhoid-paratyphoid A and B, tetanus toxoid, and diphtheria toxoid (combined vaccine) (see TABTD/Vac).

TABTD/Vac Typhoid-paratyphoid A and B, Tetanus (toxoid) and Diphtheria (toxoid) Vaccine.

TABT/Vac Typhoid-paratyphoid A and B, and Tetanus (toxoid) Vaccine.

TAB/Vac Typhoid-paratyphoid A and B Vaccine.

TAC Technical advisory committee; Terminal antrum contraction; Tetracaine, adrenaline, and codeine; Therapeutic abortion committee; Threaded acetabular component (Orthopedic implant); Time, amount and color; Time-activity curve; Topically applied corticosteroid; Total abdominal colectomy; Total aganglionosis coli; Total antioxidant control; Toxicology Advisory Committee (FDA); Triamcinolone cream; Tricarboxylic acid cycle (see KCAC).

tac- combining form meaning arrange (Gr. tak-).

TACE Chlorotrianisene [= Chlorotrian; Tri-p-anisylchloroethylene; l-Chloro-1,2,2-tri(para-methoxyphenyl)ethylene - a synthetic estrogen, which is not a steroid; it is slowly converted in the liver to an estrogenically active compound; Teichoic acid crude extract.

TACEI Triazole acetylcholinesterase inhibitor (an enzyme used in the treatment of Alzheimer's disease).

tachy tachycardia.

tachy- prefix meaning fast (Gr. tachys).

tact- combining form meaning touch (L. tactus).

TAD Test of auditory discrimination; Thoracic aortic disease; Thoracic asphyxiant dystrophy; Topically active/ administered/ applied drug; Total administered dose/ drug; Total area descriptor; Transient acantholytic dermatosis; Transverse abdominal diameter; Tricyclic antidepressant(s); Tricyclic antidepressant drug; Triple arthrodesis (surgical fusion of three joints).

TADA Time-amplitude domain analysis (heart sounds).

TADAC Therapeutic abortion, dilatation, aspiration, and curettage.

TADP Tumor Antigen Discovery Program.

TADPO 6-Thioguanine, Ara-C (Cytosine arabinoside), Daunorubicin, Prednisone and Oncovin (Chemotherapy).

TAE Transaminase elevation (in Liver disease); Transcatheter arterial embolization.

TAF Albumose-free tuberculin (Ger. Tuberculin Albumose Frei); Thymic activity factor; Tissue/ Tumor angiogenesic/sis factor; Toxin/ Toxoid-antitoxin floccules; Transient atrial fibrillation; Trypsin-aldehyde-fuchsin.

TAG Target-attaching globulin; Technical advisory group; Thymine, adenine, and guanine; Treatment Action Group (AIDS).

TAGH Triiodothyronine, aminoacids, glucagon, and heparin.

TAGVHD Transfusion-associated graft-versus-host disease (see AT).

TAH Topical antihistamine; Total abdominal/ Transabdominal hysterectomy; Total artificial heart; Transient angiolymphoid hyperplasia.

TAH BSO Total abdominal hysterectomy and bilateral salpingo-oophorectomy.

TAI International Atomic Time (see IAT); Test Anxiety Inventory; Transacromial incision (see inc).

TAICH Technical Assistance Informational Clearing House.

TAJ Treatment-associated jaundice.

TAL Tendon Achilles lengthening; Thymic alymphoplasia (see TAl); Total arm length.

TAl Thymic alymphoplasia (= TAL).

Tal Such a one (see tal).

tal a similar one or such a one (L. talis).

TALC Teaching aids of low cost.

talc talcum (powder).

tal dos such doses.

TALH Thick ascending limb of Henle's loop; Transient angiolymphoid hyperplasia.
TALL; T-ALL T-cell acute lymphoblastic leukemia.
TALLA T-cell acute lymphoblastic leukemia antigen.
TALROS Transactions of the American Laryngological, Rhinological, and Otological Society (journal).
TAM Tamoxifen (= T; TMX; TPF) (see PF; TPF); Technicon Autoanalyser Methodology; Teen-age mother; Terminologia Anatomica Nomenclature; Textbook of Alternative Medicine; Thermoacidurans agar, modified; Total active motion; Toxin-antitoxin/ Toxin-antitoxoid/ Toxoid-antitoxin/ Toxoid-antitoxoid mixture; Traditional Arab medicine; Transient abnormal myelopoiesis; Treatment-associated mortality.
TAMA Tumor-attacking monoclonal antibody.
TAME Toluenesulfonyl/ Toluenesulfotrypsin/ Tosyl arginine methyl ester.
TAMe Toxoid-antitoxin mixture esterase.
TAMG Thymoma-associated myasthenia gravis.
TAMIS Telemetric Automated Microbial Identification System.
TAML Therapy-related acute myelogenous leukemia.
TAN Terminologia Anatomica Nomenclature; Total adenine nucleotide; Total ammonia nitrogen.
tan tandem (translocation); tangent.
TANA Transactions of the American Neurological Association (journal).
TANI Total axial (lymph) node irradiation.
TANS Territorial Army Nursing Service.
TAO Thromboangiitis obliterans; Thyroid-associated ophthalmopathy; Triacetyloleandomycin; Troleandomycin (antibiotic).
Tao Taoist (religion).
TAOD Transantral orbital decompression (in Graves' ophthalmopathy, etc.
TAP Technology Assessment Panel (of Engineers Joint Council); Tension by applanation (Ophthalmology); Thermally activated polarization; Tonometry by applanation; Transesophageal atrial pacing.
TAP# Transacetabular pelvic fracture (see TAPF).
TAP 1, 2 Transporter-associated protein 1, 2 (gene) (with antigenic processing) (= TPA - Transport peptide antigen).
TAPF Transacetabular pelvic fracture (= TAP#).
TAPS Trial assessment procedure scale.
TAPVC Total anomalous pulmonary venous connection.
TAPVD Total anomalous pulmonary venous drainage.
TAPVR Total anomalous pulmonary venous return.
TAQW Transient abnormal Q wave (electrocardiography).
TAR Thoracic aortic rupture; Thrombocytopenia with absent radii (syndrome); Tissue-to-air ratio (radiation); Total abortion rate; Total ankle replacement; Transabdominal route; Transaxillary resection; Treatment authorization request; Trypsin-activated renin.
Tar Gum opium (see Papaver).
TARA Total articular replacement arthroplasty; Tumor-associated rejection antigen.
Ta reaction Tryptophane acid reaction.
TARS Threonyl-tRNA synthetase; Thrombocytopenia with absent radii syndrome.
tarso- combining form meaning edge of eyelid or instep (Gr. tarsos).
TAR syndrome Thrombocytopenia with absent radii syndrome (see TARS).
TART Thesaurus of Adverse Reaction Terms (see COSTART).
TAS Tetanus antitoxin serum; Therapeutic activities specialist; Thermal analysis system; Thoracoabdominal surgery/ syndrome; Total allergy syndrome (see MCS); Traumatic apallic syndrome; Typical absence seizures.
TASA Tumor-associated surface antigen.
TASAIO Transactions of the American Society for Artificial Internal Organs (journal).
TASC Treatment alternatives to street crime.
TASE; T'ASE; Tase Trytophan synthetase.
Taser A stun gun (Tom Swift and his Electric Rifle).

TASS Thyrotoxicosis - Addison disease - Sjögren syndrome - sarcoidosis (syndrome); Ticlopidine Aspirin Stroke Study.

TAT Tetanus antitoxin; Thematic Apperception/ Aptitude Test (psychology); Thrombin-antithrombin complex; Thromboplastin activation test; Till all taken; Total antitryptic activity; Toxin-antitoxin; Transacting transcriptional (regulation of virus replication); Transactivator; Transaxial tomography; Tray agglutination test; Tumor activity test; Turnaround time; Tyrosine aminotransferase.

TATA Pribnow (box); Tumor-associated transplantation antigen.

TATG Thioacetylthioglycolic acid.

TAT gene Transactivating gene - a regulatory gene of the AIDS virus (HIV-1) genome, that enhances viral protein synthesis through its action on a sequence in the LTR gene (see LTRs).

TAT mixture Toxin-antitoxin mixture.

TATR Tyrosine aminotransferase regulator.

TATST Tetanus antitoxin skin test.

Taur Taurine.

TAUS Transabdominal ultrasonogram/graph(y).

tauto- combining form meaning same (Gr. tautos).

TAV Trapped air volume.

TAX Transcriptional activator of expression (a gene) - an important factor in HTLV-1 leukemia.

Tax Taxonomy.

tax- combining form meaning arrange (Gr.).

TB Tailor's bunion (on the fifth digit of the foot); Taussig-Bind (syndrome); Term birth; Terminal bronchiole/ bronchus; Thromboxane B; Thymol/ Toluidine blue; Total base/ bilirubin/ body; Toxicity Bibliography (NLM journal); Tracheal bronchiolar (region); Tracheobronchitis; Trapezoid body; Travenol bag (used in abdominal surgery to pack the bowel out of operative field); Tub bath; Tubercle bacillus (see Tbc); Tuberculin (see Tuberculin); Tuberculosis (referred to as such in speaking) (see Tbc); Tumor-bearing.

Tb Tbilisi (phage); Terbium (Z = 65) (see Elements - Terbium); Tubercle bacillus; Tuberculosis (referred to as such in speaking) (see Tbc).

Tb Biological half-life; Body temperature.

tb tuberculosis (see Tbc).

T1/2β Terminal slow half-life (of a drug in the plasma) (see T1/2á).

TB 1-698 Thiacetazone (= TB 1/698; TBB 1-698; Amithiazone; Thioacetazone; Tibione) - a thiosemicarbazone compound used in the treatment of tuberculosis and leprosy.

TBA Team-based approach; Tertiary butylacetate; Testosterone-binding affinity; Thiobarbituric acid; Tick bite alopecia; To be absorbed/ added/ administered/ admitted/ announced; Total bile acids; Total body (surface) area; Trypsin-binding activity; Tubercle bacillus (see Tbc); Tuberculosis - probably active (see tba); Tumor-bearing animal.

tba Tuberculosis - probably active (radiography symbol) (= TBA).

TBAB Tryptose blood agar base.

TBAb Thyrotropin-blocking antibody.

TBAN Transbronchial aspiration needle.

TBARS Thiobarbituric acid-reactive substances; Thrombexane B acid reactive substance.

TBB Thymol-barbitural buffer; Transbronchial biopsy.

TBB 1-698 Tibione (see TB 1-698).

TBBM Total body bone minerals.

TBBP Type B behavior pattern.

TBC Tertiary butylcatechol; Thyroxine-binding coagulin; Total blood count; Total body calcium/ clearance; Tuberculosis (see Tbc).

Tbc Tubercle bacillus (= TB; Tb; TBA; tbc); Tuberculosis (= TB; Tb; tb; TBC; tbc).

tbc tubercle bacillus (see Tbc); tuberculosis (see Tbc).

TBCC Tom Baker Cancer Centre (Calgary, Canada).

TBD Thienobenzodiazepine; Tick-borne disease(s): Babesiosis; Erchlichiosis; Lyme disease; Rickettsial diseases such as Q fever, Tick typhus and Tsutsugamushi fever, etc.; Total body deficit/ density; Toxicology Data Base; Trophoblastic disease.

TBE Tick-borne encephalitis; Total breech extraction (see VAE); Transactions on Biomedical Engineering (IEEE); Tuberculin bacillin/llus emulsion (see Tuberculin - TBE; TBN).

TBF Total body fat.

TBFB Tracheobronchial foreign body.

TBFVL Tidal breathing flow-volume loops.

TBG Testosterone/ Thyronine/ Thyroxine-binding globulin; Thyroglobulin; Thyroid binding globulin; Total body gain; Tracheobronchography; Tris-buffered Gey's solution.

TBGA Thyroxine-binding prealbumin (see TBPA).

TBGE Thyroxine-binding globulin estimate.

TBGI Thyroid-/ Thyroxine-binding globulin index.

TBGP Total blood granulocyte pool.

TBH Total body hematocrit/ hemoglobin.

tBHP Terbutyl hydroperoxide.

TBHT Total-body hyperthemia.

TBI p-Aminobenzaldehyde thiosemicarbazone; Thyroid/ Thyroxine - binding index; Tick-borne illness/ infection (e.g. Lyme disease); Tooth-brushing instruction; Total body iron; Total-body irradiation (= TBX); Traumatic brain injury.

TBII Thyroid-stimulating hormone-binding inhibitory immunoglobulin.

TBIL Total body iron load/ loss.

T bili Total bilirubin.

TBK Total body potassium (kalium).

TBL Tetracycline bone labeling (Orthopedics); Total body load/ loss.

tbl tablespoon (15 ml) (see tbsp); tablet (see Tab; tab).

TBLB Transbronchial lung biopsy.

TBLC Term birth, living child.

TBLF Term birth, living female.

TBLI Term birth, living infant.

TBLM Term birth, living male.

TBM Tingible-body macrophage (tinged or stained macrophage containing nuclear debris - found in reactive atypia); Total body mass; Tracheobronchomalacia; Trachiobronchiomegaly; Trophoblastic/ Tubular basement membrane; Tuberculous meningitis.

TBN Travenol biopsy needle.

TBMN Thin basement membrane nephropathy.

TBN Tuberculin bacillin/ bacillus emulsion (see Tuberculin - TBN); Total body nitrogen.

TBNA Total body neutron activation; Transbronchial needle aspiration; Treated but not admitted.

TBNa Total body sodium.

TBNAA Total body neutron activation analysis.

TBP Bithionol (= Thiobisdichlorophenol); Terblanche procedure (decompression of the bile duct in treatment of adenocarcinoma); Testosterone/ Thyroid/ Thyroxine (= Tx) - binding protein; Therapeutic blood product(s); Time-bandwidth product; Total body photographs; Total bypass; Tributyl phosphate; Tuberculous peritonitis.

TBPA Thyroxine-binding prealbumin (= TBGA).

TBPC Transactions of British Pharmaceutical Conference (contained in YBP).

TBPT Total body protein turnover.

TBR Tight binding rate (of a drug); Total bed rest; Triple-bone resection (= Interscapulothoracic or Tikhoff-Linberg resection) (see TLP; TLR); Tumor-bearing rabbit.

TB-RD Tuberculosis - respiratory disease.

TB-RD Association Tuberculosis-Respiratory Diseases Association.

TBS Formylsuccinanilic acid thiosemicarbazone (tuberculostatic agent); Tachycardia-bradycardia syndrome; Target brain structure (for pacemakerlike implant); Tensile breaking strength (see MTS); Tertbutylphenyl salicylate; Tight building syndrome (= SBS); Total body scan/ solids/ solute/ surface; Total burn size; Trabecular bone surface; Tracheobronchial submucosa; Tracheobronchoscopy; Tribromosalicylamate/cylanilide; Tribromsalan; Triethanolamine-buffered saline (solution); Triple bypass surgery (see CABG); Truncated biphasic shock (used in cardiac arrest) (see SMS).

tbs tablespoon(ful) (see tbsp).

TBSA Total body/ burn surface area.

tbsp tablespoon(ful) (= tbs).

TBSV Tomato bushy stunt virus.

TBT Template bleeding time; Tolbutamide

test; Tracheobronchial toilet/ tract/ tree.
TBTT Tuberculin time test.
tbu tuberculosis, (activity) uncertain.
TBV Total blood volume; Transient blurred vision; Transluminal balloon valvuloplasty.
TB-VI Tuberculostat - 6 (solvoteben).
TB-Vis Isoniazid.
TBW Total body washout (used as a desperate "last-ditch" treatment in hepatic coma (= TW); Total body water/ weight (= TW).
TBX Thromboxane; Total body irradiation (X-rays) (see TBI).
TBX_2 Thromboxane B2.
TBZ Tetrabenazine (see Ro 1-9569); Thiabendazole.
TC Target/ Tumor cell; Tarlov cyst(s) (in the lumbosacral roots, found on the myelogram); Taurocholate; Technical committee; Temperature compensated/ compensation/ control; Teratocarcinoma; Tertiary cleavage; Tetracycline (see Tc; TCN); Thermal conductivity; Thermocouple; Thoracic cage; Throat/ Tissue culture; Thyrocalcitonin (see TCa); Till countermanded; To contain; Total calcium/ capacity (lung - PFT)/ cholesterol/ colonoscopy/ correction; Toxic concentration; Transcobalamin (see Tc); Transient channel (= T-type channel; almost absent in healthy ventricular tissue) (see LLC); Transplant(ing)/ Trauma center; Transverse colon; Treacher Collins (syndrome); True conjugate; Tuberculin contagiosum/ious (see Tuberculin); Tubo curarine (on anesthesia reports); Tumor of cerebrum; Type and crossmatch (see T&C); Tzanck cell(s) (found in pemphigus vulgaris and herpes virus infections).
Tc One trillion cycles; Technetium (Z = 43) (see Elements - Technetium); Tetracycline (= T; TC; TCN; TET); Transcobalamin (= TC).
tc transcutaneous; translational control.
T/C Telephone call; To consider.
t (°C) temperature on the Celsius scale.
T_c Cytotoxic T-cell (cell mediated) lymphocyte, a CD8 positive cell (which carries the CD8 protein within the surface membrane). It lyses virally infected cells at the sites of infection, and is activated by the Helper T-cell lymphocytes. It recognizes foreign material in association with HLA class I molecules (see Th); The generation time of a cell cycle.
T&C Turn and cough; Type and crossmatch (laboratory/ blood bank) (= TC; T&X).
TC I; TC II; etc Transcobalamin I, II, etc.
T&C #3 Tylenol with 30 mg codeine (= T3).
3TC Lamivudine (an antiviral drug - trade name "Epivir").
T_4(C) Serum thyroxine measured by column chromatography.
TC_{50} Medium toxic concentration.
^{99}Tc; ^{99m}Tc; Tc^{99m}; Tc 99m Radioactive technetium (99m).
TC 199 Mixture 199 - a complex synthetic nutrient medium, containing aminoacids, glucose, vitamins, accessory growth factors and salts, which has been used for the storage of bone marrow and other tissue cultures.
TCA Team conference assessment; T-cell activation; T-cell A (locus); Terminal cancer; Tetracyclic/ Tricyclic antidepressant (= TCAD); Texas Commission on Alcoholism; Thioguanine and cytarabine; Thyrocalcitonin (see TCa); Tissue Culture Association; Total cholic acid; Total circulating albumin; Total circulatory arrest; Transcervical administration (= TCI); Transcutaneous absorption; Tricalcium aluminate; Tricarboxylic/ Trichloracetic/ Trichloroacetic acid; Trichloroacetate; Tricuspid atresia; Tricyclic antidepressant.
TCa Terminal cancer; Thyrocalcitonin (= TC; TCA; TCT).
TCAB 3,3',4,4'-tetrachloroazobenzene.
TCABG Triple coronary artery bypass graft (= TCAG).
TCAC Tone count audiometric computer (audiometer).
TC/AC ratio Thoracic circumference/Abdominal circumference ratio (Obs).
TCAD Tetracyclic/ Tricyclic antidepressant (see TCA).
TCAE Transcatheter angiographic embolization (technique).
TCAG Triple coronary artery graft (see TCABG).
TCAOB 3,3',4,4'-tetrachloroazoxybenzene.
TCAP Trimethyl-cetyl-ammonium pen-

tachlorophenate (a fungicide).

TCAR T-cell antigen receptor.

TCAT Transcervical aspiration technique (Obs/Gyn).

TCB Technician Certification Board (AAIT); Tetrachlorobiphenyl; Tibial cast bracing (Orthopedics); Total cardiopulmonary bypass (transcatheter) biopsy; Tumor cell burden.

TCBF Total cerebral/ coronary blood flow.

TCBS Thiosulfate-citrate-bile salts (sucrose agar culture medium).

TCC Terminal complement complex; Thromboplastic cell component; Thymic carcinomatous component (of rhabdomyosarcoma) (see GCC; TMC); Transitional-cell carcinoma; Trichlorocarbanilide (= Triclocarban) - a nonirritant antibacterial agent particularly effective against gram-positive organisms. Used in soaps, solutions, powders, and ointments for the control of skin infections (= Tcc); Turkey-claw clamp (Orthopedics).

Tcc Triclocarban (see TCC).

TCCA Transitional cell cancer-associated (virus) (see TCCAV).

TCCAV Transitional cell cancer-associated virus (= TCCA virus).

TCCB Transitional cell carcinoma of the bladder.

TCCL T-cell chronic (lymphoblastic) leukemia (see TCCLL).

TCCLL T-cell chronic lymphoblastic leukemia (= TCCL).

TCD Thermal conductivity detector; Tissue culture dose; Transcarbamylase deficiency; Transverse cardiac diameter; Tumor cell death; Tumorocidal drug.

TCD; T-CD T (thymus) cell depletion (as in AIDS).

TCD_{50} Mean/ Median tissue culture dose (see $TCID_{50}$).

TCDB Turn, cough, and deep breathe (see TC&DB).

TC&DB Turn, cough, and deep breathe (= TCDB).

TCDC Taurochenodeoxycholate.

TCDD Tetrachlorodibenzodioxin (= 2,3,7,8-tetrachlorodibenzo-p-dioxin; Dioxin) - a poisonous industrial-chemical residue.

^{99m}Tc-DTPA Radioactive technetium - labeled diethylene thriamine penta acetic acid.

TCE T-cell enriched/ epitope; Tetrachlorodiphenyl ethane (a mosquito larvicide); Tissue culture experience (pregnancy - infant of diabetic mother) (Obstetrics); Trichloroethanol; Trichlorethylene.

T-cell Thymus-derived cell (lymphocyte).

TCES Transcutaneous cranial electrical stimulation.

TCESOM Trichloroethylene-extracted soybean oil meal.

TCET Transcerebral electrotherapy.

TCF Terminal cardiac failure; Tissue coding factor; Total coronary flow; Trapezoid compression frame (for # of the pelvis); Trillion cubic feet (= 10^{12} cu ft) (of gas).

T-CFC T-colony forming cell.

TCFDA Trade Correspondence of the Food and Drug Administration (journal).

TCF 2L Colonoscope (T = treatment; C = colon; F = flexible; 2 = double channel; L = long).

TCF 1S Sigmoidoscope (T = treatment; C = colon; F = flexible; 1 = single channel; S = short).

TCFU Tumor colony-forming unit.

TCG Trichorionic gestation (Obstetrics).

TCGF T-cell growth factor.

^{99m}TcGH Technetium - 99m - glucoheptonate.

TCH Thiopen-2-carboxylic acid hydrazide; Total circulating hemoglobin; Turn, cough, and hyperventilate.

TChE Total cholinesterase.

^{99m}Tc-HEDSPA Radioactive technetium - labeled 1-hydroxy-ethylidene-disodium phosphate (brain scanning agent).

tchg teaching.

T^cH_2O Tubular reabsorption of solute free water.

Tchr Teacher.

^{99m}Tc-HSA Serum albumin labeled with radioactive technetium.

TCI Thermodilution cardiac index; To come in (to hospital); Total cerebral ischemia; Transcervical injection (see TCA); Transient cerebral ischemia (see TCIE).

TCi Teracurie.

TCID Tissue culture infection/tious/tive or inoculated dose.

$TCID_{50}$ Median tissue culture infective dose (= 50% tissue culture infectious dose) - that quantity of a cytopathogenic agent (virus) that will produce a cytopathic effect in 50% of the cultures inoculated.
TCIE Transient cerebral ischemic episode.
TCIT T-cell immunotherapy.
TCK Thyroid cytokine (such as Interleukin-1, Tumor necrosis factor α, and Interferon-y).
TCKA Total condylar knee arthroplasty (see TCKP; TCKR).
TCKP Total condylar knee prosthesis (see TCKA; TCKR).
TCKR Total condylar knee replacement (Howmedica - see OI/OP).
TCL Terminal command language (computer); Thermochemiluminescence; Tibial collateral ligament; Total capacity of the lung; Transverse carpal ligament; Triglyceride-carrying lipoprotein; Tuberculoid leprosy (see LML; MBL; PBL).
TCL; T-CL T-cell leukemia (see TCCL; TCCLL; TCLL; T-CLL).
T-CLL T-cell chronic lymphatic leukemia.
TCLL; T-CLL T-cell lymphatic leukemia (see TCCL; TCCLL; TCL; T-CLL); T-cell lymphoblastic lymphoma.
TCLo; TC_{Lo} Lowest toxic concentration (published) (= Toxic c. low).
TCM T-cell-mediated (see OSTCMAD); Tissue culture medium; Traditional Chinese medicine; Transcutaneous monitor; Triazole carboxamide/ carboxyacid/ carboxylic acid metabolite (of Ribavirin).
TC 99m Technetium-99m (see 99 TC, etc.).
TCMA Transcortical motor aphasia.
TCMAD T-cell-mediated autoimmune disease (see OSTCMAD).
Tc-MAFH Technetium 99m-labeled macroaggregated ferrous hydroxide.
TCMH Tumor-direct cell-mediated hypersensitivity.
TCMP Thematic Content Modification Program.
TCMZ Trichloromethiazide.
TCN Terminal care need(s); Tetracycline (see TC).
TCNE Tetracyanoethylene.
TcNM Tumor with (lymph) node metastases (see TNM).
TCNQ Tetracyano-p-quinodimethane.
TCNS Transcutaneous nerve stimulation/ator.
TCNU Tauromustine.
TCNV Terminal contingent negative variation.
TCO Treatment crossover.
T_{CO} Transfer factor for carbon monoxide (see PFT).
T_{CO2} Total carbon dioxide.
$^{99m}Tc\ O4$ Technetium 99m (as the pertechnetate).
TCOM Texas College of Osteopathic Medicine; Transcutaneous oxygen monitor.
TCP Therapeutic class profile; Therapeutic continuous penicillin; Thrombocytopenia; Time-consuming procedure; Total circulating protein; Transcultural psychiatry; Tranylcypromine; Tricalcium phosphate; Trichlorophenol; Tricresyl phosphate (= Tri-o-cresyl phosphate) - an anti-esterase; Thrombocytopathy.
Tcp Teacup.
TCPA 2,4,5-Trichlorophenoxyacetic acid (see PAH).
TCPC Total contact plaster cast.
tcP_{CO2}; tcPCO2 Transcutaneous carbon dioxide pressure.
tcP_{O2}; tcPO2 Transcutaneous oxygen pressure.
TCPA Tetrachlorophthalic anhydride.
TCPP Thrombocytopenic purpura.
^{99}Tc-PP Polyphosphate labeled with radioactive (99m) technetium.
TCPPA Trichlorophenoxypropionic acid (see 2,4,5-TCPPA).
2,4,5-TCPPA 2-(2,4,5-trichlorophenoxy)propionic acid.
TCPS Total cavopulmonary shun; Twin-chorionic peak sign (or Lambda sign) - evidence of dichorionic twin pregnancies (= LS; TPS Obstetrics).
^{99m}Tc-PYP Stannous pyrophophate labeled with radioactive technetium.
TCR T-cell reactivity/ receptor/ rosette; Temperature coefficient of resistance; Thalamocortical relay; Total cytoplasmic ribosome; Translational clinical research.
tcRNA Translational control ribonucleic acid.
TCRP Total cellular receptor pool.

TCRV Total red cell volume.

TCS T-cell supernatant; Tethered cord syndrome; Tissue culture study; Tonic-clonic seizure; Total cellular/ coronary score; Treacher Collins syndrome.

TCSA Tetrachlorosalicylanilide.

TCSF T-colony stimulating factor.

TCSM T-cell surface molecule (= CD 154; CD 40 ligand).

TCT Therapeutic cloning technique (see CDT); Thrombin clotting time; Thyrocalcitonin (see TCa); Trachial cytotoxin; Traditional chemotherapy; Transitional cell tumor; Transmission computed tomography; Triple-combination therapy (see TDT).

Tct Tincture (see Tinct).

TCTS Tonic-clonic-type seizure (e.g. due to alcohol withdrawal).

TCu copper T (an IUD).

TCV Thoracic cage volume; Three concept view; Tissue culture vaccine (e.g. rabies v).

TCVA Thromboembolic cerebral vascular accident.

TD Takayasu's disease; Tangier disease (a peripheral neuropathy caused by α-lipoprotein deficiency, and resulting in dissociated sensory loss, with loss of pain and temperature sensation and preservation of tactile sensation); Tardive dyskinesia; T-cell dependent; Teacher of the deaf; Temporary/ Total disability; Temporary duty; Teratoma, differentiated; Terminal device; Tetanus-diphtheria (toxoid) (see Td); Tetrodotoxin; Therapeutic dietician; Therapy/ Treatment discontinued (see T/D); Thermal dilution; Thoracic duct; Three times/ Thrice daily (L. ter die) (see tid); Threshold of detectability/ discomfort; Threshold/ Titrated/ Total/ Toxic/ Tumor dose; Thymus-dependent (cells); Timed disintegration; To deliver; Tocopherol (Vitamin E) deficiency; Tone decay; Torsion dystonia (athetosis); Total discrimination; Totally disabled; Toxidrome (= Toxic syndrome); Tracheal/ Transverse (of heart) diameter; Tracking device/ dye; Transdermal; Traveler's diarrhea; Treating distance; Tropical Doctor (RSM journal); Twice-daily; Typhoid dysentery.

Td "Delayed" T-cell (cell mediated) lymphocyte, a CD4 subset positive cell, which produces lymphokines, leading to the activation of immune cells (see Th); Tetanus-diphtheria (toxoid) (= TD).

td three times/ thrice daily (L. ter die) (see tid).

T/D Therapy/ Treatment discontinued (= TD).

TD1 Thanatophoric dysplasia type I (characterized by short limbs, a narrow thoracic cage and curved femora, and with or without a cloverleaf skull) (see PLSDs - Obstetrics).

TD2 Thanatophoric dysplasia type II (characterized by short limbs, a narrow thoracic cage, straight femora, and a cloverleaf skull) (see PLSDs - Obstetrics).

T_D The time required to double the number of cells in a given population; Thermal death time.

T_4D; T4(D) Serum thyroxine (measured by displacement analysis).

TD_{50} Median toxic dose.

TDA Tax-deferred annuity; Tetradecenyl acetate; Thermodynamic analysis (laser irradiation); Thiazide-diuretic agent; Thyroid-stimulating hormone-displacing antibody; 2-Toluene diamine; Transfusion-dependent anemia; Two-dimentional analysis.

TDAO Thrombotic digital arterial occlusion.

TDB Third degree burn (see WSL); Toxicology Data Bank/ Base; Tropical Disease(s) Bulletin (journal).

T_{db} Temperature.

TDC Taurodeoxycholic acid; Thoracic disc collapse; Time-dependent change; Total dietary calories; Total drug concentration.

TDCH Three-dimensional color histogram (see VFI).

TDD Tegaderm dressing; Telecommunication device for the deaf; Tetradecadiene; Thoracic duct drainage; Thrice/ Total/ Twice daily dosage/ dose/ dosing; Total digitalizing dose; Toxic doses of drugs; Transdermal delivery; Tuberculous Diseases Diploma.

TDDD Total daily dose difference(s) (in drug medication).

TDDR Thrice/ Twice -daily dosing regimen.

TDE Tetrachlorodiphenylethane (= DDD; Dichlorodiphenyldichloro ethane) - an insecticide; Total daily energy (requirement).

TDENA Transdermal estradiol/ norethisterone

acetate.

TDF Testis determining factor - a sex gene found on the Y chromosome, that may trigger male sexual development in the embryo. Without the gene, the embryo becomes female; Thoracic duct fistula/ flow; Time/ Tumor dose fractionation; Tissue-damaging factor.

tdf tour de force (Fr.) - a feat of skill/ strength.

TDFC Total dietary fiber content.

TDH Threonine dehydrogenase; Traumatic dislocation of the hip (Orthopedics).

TDI Temperature difference integration/ator; Three-dimensional interlocking (hip); Toluene 2,4-diisocyanate; Total daily intake; Total dose infusion/ insulin.

TDK Tardive dyskinesia (see TD).

TDL Thoracic duct lymph; Thymus-dependent lymphocyte; Toxic dose level.

TDLo Lowest published toxic dose.

TDM Therapeutic drug monitoring; Therapeutic Drug Monitoring (journal, UK); Thrice/ Twice-daily medication (see TDDR; TDMR; TDR); Tocodynamometer (intrauterine catheter for measuring maternal contractions); Traditional diagnostic method(s).

TDMR Thrice/ Twice-daily medication regimen (= TDDR; TDM; TDR).

TDN Total digestible nutrients; Transdermal nitroglycerin (see TDNTG).

tDNA Transfer deoxyribonucleic acid.

TDNTG Transdermal nitroglycerin (= TDN).

TDO Tricho-dento-osseous (syndrome).

TDOL Tetradecanol.

TDOS Trichodento-osseous syndrome (frontal bossing, square jaw with small, pitted and widely spaced teeth - autosomal dominant, ectodermal dysplasia).

TDP Thermal death point; Thoracic duct pressure; Thymidine diphosphate; Les torsade des pointes or Torsades de pointes (Ventricular arrhythmia intermediary between ventricular tachycardia and fibrillation) (= TdP; TVF); Total degradation products; Transdermal patch (see TDS); Three/ Two-day period.

TdP Torsade de pointes.

TDR Teratogenic/ Therapeutic dose range; Thrice/ Twice-daily regimen (see TDDR; TDM; TDMR); Total daily/ dairy ration; Triple-drug regimen.

TdR Thymidine.

TDS Tardive Dyskinetic syndrome; Temperature, depth, salinity; Thiamine disulfide; Three-dimensional study; Total dissolved solids; Transcranial Doppler sonography; Transdermal Delivery System; Transdermal system; Transduodenal sphincteroplasty; Traumatic dislocation of the shoulder (joint); Two-dimensional study (Type of echocardiogram, done with M-mode echo).

tds take/ to be taken three times a day (L. ter die sumendum) (see tid).

TDSD Transient digestive system disorder.

TDT Tentative discharge tomorrow; Terminal deoxynucleotidyl transferase (an enzyme found in lymphoid precursors in lymphomas, etc.) (see TdT); Therapeutic drug trial; Thermal death time; Tone decay test; Triple-drug therapy (such as reverse transcriptase inhibitors, integrase inhibitors, and protease inhibitors, used in the treatment of AIDS); Tumor doubling time.

TdT Terminal deoxynucleotidyl transferase (= TDT).

TDTA Templin-Darley Test of Articulation.

TDTC Three-dimensional tissue culture.

TD toxoid Tetanus-diphtheria toxoid.

TDU Transcranial Doppler ultrasonogram/graph(y).

TDUS Three-dimensional ultra sonogram/aph(y)/ sound (Obstetrics).

TDV Tilting disc valve (Lillchei-Kaster aortic valve prosthesis).

TDWB Touch down weight bearing.

TDx Fluorescence polarization immunoassay.

TDy Temporary duty.

TDZ Thymus-dependent zone (of lymph node).

TE Echo-time; Expiratory time; Tennis elbow; Test ear; Tetanus (see Te); Tetracycline; Threshold energy; Thromboembolism; Thymus epithelium; Thyrotoxic exophthalmos; Tick-borne/ Toxoplasma encephalitis; Time estimation; Tissue engineering; Tissue-equivalent; Tonsillectomy; Tooth extracted; Total estrogen; Toxic epidermolysis; Trace element; Tracheoesophageal; Transepithelial;

Treadmill exercise; Trial (and) error (see T&E).
Te Effective half-life; Tellurium (Z = 52) (see Elements - Tellurium); Tetanic contraction; Tetanus (= TE).
T_E Expiratory phase time (see PFT - T_E).
T-e Erythrocyte triiodothyronine (see ET-3).
T&E Testing and evaluation; Training and experience; Trial and error (= TE).
TEA Temporal external artery; Tetraethylammonium; Thermal energy/ evolution analyzer; Thrombendarterectomy; Total elbow arthroplasty; Transdermal estradiol administration; Triethanolamine.
Tea Marijuana (see Cannabis).
TEAB Tetraethylammonium bicarbonate (buffer); Tetraethylammonium bromide (= Tetramone bromide; Tetrylammonium Br) - a ganglion-blocking agent, formerly used in the treatment of hypertension.
TEAC Tetraethylammonium chloride - a ganglion-blocking agent formerly used in the treatment of hypertension; Trolox equivalent antioxidant capacity.
TEACCH Treatment and Education of Autistic Children with Communication Handicap.
TEAE Treatment-emergent adverse event/ experience; Triethylaminoethyl (= Triethylammonioethyl).
TEAM Total Exposure Assessment Methology (of indoor air pollution; EPA study); Training in Expanded Auxillary Management.
teasp teaspoon(ful).
TEBG; TeBG Testosterone-estradiol binding globulin.
TEC Tamper-evident cap; Thromboembolic complication(s); Thyroid-eye clinic; Tissue-engineered cartilage; Total electron/ eosinophil count; Total exchange capacity; Transient erythroblastopenia of childhood; Transluminal extraction catheter.
T&EC Trauma and Emergency Center.
TECA Transluminal extraction catheter atherectomy.
Tecata Heroin (see Diamorph HCl).
tech technical/cian.
Technic (IOTT journal).
tect- combining form meaning cover (L. tectus).
TECV Traumatic epiphyseal coxa vara.
TED Tasks of Emotional Development; Threshold erythema dose; Thromboembolic disease/ disorder; Thyroid eye disease; Tissue equivalent dose; Transient endothelial dysfunction; Transmitted electron detector (SEM).
TEDK Treatment emergent dyskinesia.
TEDS Anti-embolism stockings.
TEE Thermic effect of exercise; Total estrogen excretion; Transesophageal echocardiography; Tri-exponential elimination (of a drug); Tyrosine ethyl ester.
TE excretion Total estrogen excretion (see TEE).
TEF Thermal effect of food; Tracheo-esophageal fistula; Trunk extension-flexion (unit).
T_{eff} Effective half-life (= Te).
T-E fistula Tracheo-esophageal fistula (see TEF).
TEFRA Tax Equity and Fiscal Responsibility Act.
TEFS Transmural electrical field stimulation.
TEG Thromboelastogram/graph; Triethyleneglycol.
teg- combining form meaning cover (L. tego).
TEH; TEHTN Treatment-emergent hypertension.
TEI Total energy intake; Transesophageal imaging.
TEIB Triethyleneiminobenzo quinone.
TEIR Transthoracic electric impedance respirogram (= TER).
TEL Telemetry (see tele); Tetraethyl lead.
tel- combining form meaning end (Gr. telos).
tele telemetry (= TEL).
tele- combining form meaning distant (Gr.).
Telex Automatic teletypewriter service by Western Union (= Tex).
TEM Roswell Park Memorial Institute (USA) code for experimental substances; Thermic effect of meal; Total energy measurement; Transmission electron micrograph(y)/ microscope/py; Treatment effect magnitude; Triethylenemelamine (= Tretamine; Triethanomelamine) - a cytotoxic drug used

in the palliative treatment of chronic leukemias and Hodgekin's disease.

TEMED Tetramethylethylenediamine.

temp temperature (= TPR); temple; temporary.

temp- combining form meaning time (L. tempus).

temp dex; temp dext (to the) right temple (L. tempori/ tempus dextro).

temp sinist (to the) left temple (L. tempori/ tempus sinistro).

TEMUR Tetramethylurea.

TEN Total enteral nutrition; Total excreted/tory nitrogen; Toxic epidermal necrolysis; Transepidermal neurostimulation.

Ten see Table.

ten tension (intraocular pressure).

ten- combining form meaning tight band (Gr. tenon).

Ten A 10-milligram amphetamine tablet (see Amphet).

Tenac Tenaculum.

TENS Telephone emergency-number service (911); Terminal electrode nerve stimulator; Transcutaneous electrical nerve/ electroneural stimulation (= Transneural stimulation) - a new widely used analgesic therapy.

tens- combining form meaning stretch (L. tensus).

TENTS Toxic epidermal necrolysis transition syndrome.

TEOAE Transiently evoked otoacoustic emission (see DPOAE).

TEP Terminal elimination phase (of a drug); Thromboembolic process; Thromboendophlebectomy; Tracheo-esophageal puncture; Traditional emergency personnel (in airports, casinos, etc.); Transesophageal pacing; Treatment-experienced patient; Tubal ectopic pregnancy.

TEPA Roswell Park Memorial Institute (USA) code for experimental substances; Triethylenephosphamide/phosphoramide (see TESPA).

TEPP Tetraethylpyrophosphate (= Ethyl pyrophosphate; Tetraethyl phosphoric anhydride) - an organophosphorus insecticide; Triethylene pyrophosphate.

TEPS Tardive extrapyramidal syndrome.

TER Teratogen; Thromboembolic risk; Total elbow replacement; Total endoplasmic reticulum; Transcapillary escape rate; Transthoracic electric (impedance) respirogram (see TEIR).

ter end; rub (L. tere); teratogenic; terminal; ternary; tertiary/ three times/ threefold (see tert).

TERA Transvascular escape rate of albumin.

tera- 10_{12} or one trillion times (symbol: T) (Gr. teras) (= T. Tera); prefix meaning large.

terato- prefix meaning monster (Gr. teras).

Teratol Teratology (TS journal).

TERB Terbutaline.

TERC Technical Education Research Center.

ter in die three times a day.

Ter leu Tertiary leucine.

term terminal/nate(d)/nation.

ter sim rub together (L. tere simul).

tert tertiary/ three/ three times/ threefold (L.) (= ter).

TES Tardive extrapyramidal syndrome; Testosterone-estradiol shunt; Thymic epithelial supernatant; Tissue Engineering Society (US); Total endoscopic score; Total enteral support (concentrated nutrition/ food supplement); Toxic epidemic syndrome; Trace elements supplement; Tracheo-esophageal shunt; Transcutaneous/ Transmural electrical stimulation; Treatment Emergent Symptoms; Trimethylaminoethane-sulfonic acid.

TEs Transposable elements (known today as transposons - anonymous, ex- cess, "junk", mobile, noncoding, nonfunctional elements of the DNA genetic code, also referred to as "jumping genes").

TE shunt Testosterone-estradiol shunt (see TES); Tracheo-esophageal shunt (see TES).

TESI Treatment-emergent symptom incidence.

TESPA Thiotepa (= Thiophosphamide; thio-TEPA; Triethylenethiophosphamide/phosphoramide; TSPA) - an alkylating agent used in the palliative treatment of neoplastic diseases.

test- combining form meaning testicle (L. testis).

TET Teacher of Electrotherapy; Tetracycline (see Tc); Thallium exercise test; Thermometric enthalpy titration; Thymic epithelial tumor; Topical estrogen therapy (= LET) for vaginal atrophy; Total ejection time;

Ten

Value	Latin	Symbol	American	British
10^{1}	deka-	da	ten	ten
10^{2}	hecto-	h	hundred	hundred
10^{3}	kilo-	k	thousand	thousand
10^{6}	mega-	M	million	million
10^{9}	giga-	G	billion	milliard
10^{12}	tero-	T	trillion	billion
10^{15}			quadrillion	
10^{18}	exa-		quintillion	trillion
10^{21}			sextillion	
10^{24}			septillion	quadrillion
10^{27}			octillion	
10^{30}			nonillion	quintillion
10^{33}			decillion	
10^{36}			undecillion	sextillion
10^{39}			duodecillion	
10^{42}			tredecillion	septillion
10^{45}			quattuordecillion	
10^{48}			quindecillion	octillion
10^{51}			sexdecillion	
10^{54}			septendecillion	nonillion
10^{57}			octodecillion	
10^{60}			novemdecillion	decillion
10^{63}			vigintillion	
10^{66}				undecillion
10^{72}				duodecillion
10^{78}				tredecillion
10^{84}				quattuordecillion
10^{90}				quindecillion
10^{96}				sexdecillion
10^{102}				septendecillion
10^{108}				octodecillion
10^{114}				novemdecillion
10^{120}				vigintillion
10^{303}			centillion	
10^{600}				centillion
10^{-1}	deci-	d		
10^{-2}	centi-	c		
10^{-3}	milli-	m		
10^{-6}	micro-	μ		
10^{-9}	nano-	n		
10^{-12}	pico-	p		
10^{-15}	femto-	f		
10^{-18}	atto-	a		
10^{-24}	avo-	A		

Total exchange(able) thyroxine; Transcranial electrostimulation therapy; Treadmill exercise test.

Tet Tetralogy (of Eisenmenger/ Fallot).

tet tetanus.

TETA Triethylenetetramine (polystyrene resin).

TETD Tetraethylthiuram disulfide.

Tet E Tetralogy of Eisenmenger.

Tet F Tetralogy of Fallot (= TF).

Tetra-D Tetracycline hydrochloride.

TETT Total extrathyreoidal thyreoidin (Tx).

Tet tox Tetanus toxoid.

TEV Tadpole edema virus; Talipes equinovarus.

TeV Trillion electron volt(s) (Te = [L.] teras; [Gr.] monster).

TEWL Transepidermal water loss.

Tex Automatic teletypewriter service by Western Union (see Telex).

Texas tea Marijuana (see Cannabis).

TF Free thyroxine; Tactile fremitus; Tail flick (reflex); Temperature/ Thymus/ Tissue-damaging/ Tolerance/ Transfer factor; Testicular feminization; Tetralogy of Fallot (see Tet F); T-fracture; Thymol flocculation; Till forbidden; To follow; Total flow; Transferrin (see Tf); Transformant of fibroblast (matrix); Transformation frequency; Transfrontal; Tube feeding; Tuberculin filtrate (see Tuberculin); Tubular fluid; Tuning fork.

Tf Transferrin (= TF; TFN).

T_f Free thyroxine (= TF); Freezing temperature.

t (°F) temperature on the Fahrenheit scale.

TFA Thyroid function abnormalities/ty; Total fatty acids; Trans-fatty acid(s) - found in partially hydrogenated oils; Transverse fascicular area; Trifluoroacetic acid (see TFAA); Trifluroacetamide.

TFAA Trifluoroacetic acid (= TFA).

T factor Tolerance factor (= TF).

TFAET Trifluoroacetyl ethanolamide.

TFAI Trifluoroacetyl-imidazole.

TFB Trifascicular block.

TFC Common form of transferrin.

TFCA Thyroid follicular cell adenoma.

TFCC Thyroid follicular cell carcinoma; Triangular fibrocartilage complex.

TFCN Thyroid follicular cell neoplasm.

TFD Target-film distance; Transcription factor decoy.

TFd Dialyzable transfer factor.

TFE Tetrafluor-ethylene (= Polytetrafluoroethylene; Teflon); Thyroid follicular epithelium.

T_{fem} Temperature of blood in femoral leg veins.

TFF Tube-fed food; Tube-feeding formula.

TFI Threefold increase; Total fat intake.

TFIS Tri-flow incentive spirometer (Respiratory therapy) (= TIS).

TFL Talo-fibular ligament (anterior/ inferior); Transferritin level; Trifluridine (= Trifluorothymidine).

TFM Testicular feminization male/ mutation; Total fluid movement; Truncal fat mass (= AFM).

TFMA 4-Trifluoromethylaniline (a metabolite of Leflunomide, a pyrimid- ine synthesis inhibitor [N-{4'-trifluoromethylphenyl}-5-methylisoxazole -4-carboxamide = $C_{12}H_9F_3N_2O_2$], used in the treatment of rheumatoid arthritis).

TFMC Trifluoro-methylhydroxymethylene camphorate.

TFMPP 1-(Trifluoromethylphenyl)-piperazine.

TFN Total fecal nitrogen; Transferrin (see Tf).

TFND Transient focal neurological defect/ disturbance.

TFNS Territorial Force Nursing Service.

TFP Tibial fixation plate (Orthopedic Implants); Treponemal false positive; Trigger finger phenomenon (STV or Stenosing tendovaginitis at the wrist and fingers) (Orthopedics); Tubular fluid plasma (= TF/P).

TF/P Tubular fluid plasma (see TFP).

TFPZ Trifluoroperazine.

TFR Total fertility rate; Total flow resistance; Trasferrin receptor.

TFS Testicular feminization syndrome; Thyroid function study; Transplantation-free survival; Tube-fed saline.

TFT Thrombus formation time; Thyroid flocculation test (see LFT iv); Tight filum terminale; Tissue-flap transplant(ation) (plastic surgery); Trifluorothymidine. Thyroid func-

tion test(s):
ATA: Anti-thyroglobulin antibodies;
FTI: Free thyroxine index;
NT4;
PBI: Protein-bound iodine;
T3: Triiodothyronine;
T4: Tetraiodothyroxine;
TA: Thyroid antibodies;
TBG: Thyroxine-binding globulin or Thyroglobulin;
TRH: Thyrotrophin-releasing hormone (test);
T3RU: T3 resin uptake (test) (= UTR);
TSH: Thyroid-stimulating hormone (level);
TSIg: Thyroid-stimulating immunoglobulin;
TS: Thyroid scanning;
TTS;
TT4;
URI: Uptake of radioactive iodine (^{132}I);
UTR: Uptake of triiodothyronine (T3) resin (see TFT - T3RU).

TFX Toxic effects.

TFZ Transformation zone (between the outer squamous cells and internal glandular cells, where the cervix merges into the uterus, or the anus into the anal canal).

TG Tendon graft; Testosterone glucuronide; Tetraglycine; Therapeutic Gazette (journal); Thermography; Thermogravimetry; Thioglucose; Thioglycolate; Thioguanine (see 6-TG); Thromboglobulin; Thyroglobulin (see Thg); Total gastrectomy; Toxic goiter; Transmissible gastroenteritis (see TGE); Treated group; Triacylglycerol; Trigeminal (neuralgia); Trigeminal ganglion; Triglyceride (see TGL); Tumor growth; Type genus (see Tg).

T/G Tubuloglomerular (balance).

T_G Tubular reabsorption of glucose.

Tg Generation time; Thyroglobulin (see Thg); Toxoplasma gondii; Type genus (= TG).

T_g Glass transition temperature.

tG_1 Time required to complete the G_1 phase of the cell cycle.

tG_2 Time required to complete the G_2 phase of the cell cycle.

6-TG Thioguanine (= TG; 6-Thioguanine; 2-Aminopurine-6-thiol hemihydrate) - a purine antagonist and cytotoxic drug, used in the management of leukemias. Also has been suggested for use as an immunosuppressive agent.

TG-9 Triethyleneglycol dipelargonate.

TGA Taurocholate gelatin agar; Teratogenic agent; Thermogravimetric analysis; Thyroglobin activity/ antibody (= see TgAb); Thyroid gland antibody; Total glycoalkaloids; Total gonadotropin activity; Transgenic animal; Transient global amnesia; Transposition of the great arteries; Tumor glycoprotein assay.

TgA Thyroglobin antibody (see TgAb).

TGAB Thyroglobin antibody (see TgAb).

TgAb Thyroglobin antibody (= TGA; TgA; TGAB).

TGAR Total graft area rejected.

TGB Thyroid-binding globulin (see TBG).

TGBG Dimethylglyoxal bis-guanylhydrazone.

TGC Time pain compensation; Topical glucocorticoid; Transgrow culture; Triglyceride chylomicron(s) (large lipid particles).

TGD Telfa guaze dressing; Thermal-green dye; Third-generation drug.

TGE Teratogenic effect; Theoretical growth evaluation; Transmissible gastroenteritis (virus) (= TG); Tryptone glucose extract (agar/broth culture medium).

TGF T-cell/ Transforming growth factor; Tubo/ Tubulo glomerular feedback; Tumor growth factor.

TGFA Triglyceride fatty acid(s).

TGF-β Transforming growth factor β - a member of the family of dimeric polypeptide growth factors that includes bone morphogenic proteins and activins, and one of the most potent regulators of the production and deposition of extracellular matrix. It decreases the production of enzymes that degrade the extracellular matrix, including collagenase, heparinase, and stromelysin, and increases the production of enzymes such as PAI-type I - Plasminogen-activator inhibitor type I, and tissue inhibitor of metalloprotease, thus upgrading the growth of extracellulr matrix. It has an important role in the spread of cancer. There are three isoforms, each encoded by a distinct, tissue-specific gene, TGF-β1, TGF-β2, and TGF-β3, and expressed through an mRNA (messenger RNA), which binds to three high-affinity cell-surface receptors, types I, II, and III respectively. TGF-β1 is expressed in endothelial, hematopoietic, and connective tissue cells; TGF-β is expressed in epithelial and neuronal cells, and TGF-β3 is expressed in mesenchymal cells (see CAP; ECMP).

TGF-β AS Transforming growth factor - beta anti-sense (a genetic deactivator of TGF-beta).

TGG Turkey gamma globulin.

TGH Toronto General Hospital.

TGID Transient gastrointestinal disorder/ disturbance.

TGL Triglyceride(s) (= TG; TGl); Triglyceride lipase.

TGl Triglyceride (see TGL); Tuberculin globin (in 10% salt solution) (see Tuberculin).

TGOC Third-generation oral contraceptive (containing a progestogen such as desogestrel, gestodene, etc.).

TGOM The Goals of Medicine: i. To Cure Sometimes; ii. TO Relieve Often; iii. To Comfort Always.

TGP Tobacco glycoprotein; Trigeminal pulse (or Trigeminy); Triglycidyl phophate.

TGR Teratogenic/ Thrombogenic risk.

6-TGR 6-Thioguanine riboside.

TGS Thermogravimetric system; Tincture of green soap; Transmission grid scan (converter).

TGSA Third-generation synthetic analogue.

TGT Thromboplastin generation test/ time; Tolbutamide-glucagon test.

TGTR Thromboplastin generation test reagent - used to detect stage I coagulation deficiencies.

TGV Thoracic gas volume (Plethysmograph); Transposition of the great vessels.

TGXT Thallium-graded exercise test.

TGY Tryptone (= Tryptophane peptone) glucose yeast (agar).

TGYA Tryptone glucose yeast agar.

TH Tension headache; Tetrahydrocortisol; T-helper (cell) (see Th); Theophylline; Thoracic/ax (see Th); Thrill (see Th); Thymic hormone (= Thymosin); Thyrohyoid (= Th); Thyroid hormone (thyroxine) (see Hormones - TH); Thyrotropic hormone (= THTH) (see Hormones - TTH); Topical hypothermia; Torcular Herophili; Total hysterectomy; Tyrosine hydroxylase.

T&H Type and hold.

TH# Transverse horizontal fracture (see THF).

T-H Take home (see THB).

Th T-helper (cell) (see above); Thenar (see th); Therapy; Thoracic/ax (= TH; Thor; thor); Thorium (Z = 90) (see Elements - Thorium); Thrill (= TH; Thr); Throat; Thursday; Thyrohyoid (see TH).

T_H; T_h; Th T-helper (cell/ cell-mediated lymphocyte) - a CD4 positive cell (which carries the CD4 protein within its surface membrane). It helps the B cell lymphocytes to make antibody, and activates the Tc, Td and Ts lymphocytes in controlling infection, by recognizing foreign antigen in association with HLA class II molecules (= TH) (see also Tc, Td, and Ts).

th thenar (= Th); thermie; thoracic; thyroid (see thr); transhepatic.

TH 1314 Ethionamide (= Ethioniamide) - a tuberculostatic agent used in conjunction with other drugs in the treatment of pulmonary and extrapulmonary tuberculosis.

TH 2132 Sulphasomizole (see M&B 4438).

TH 4114 Phenobutiodil - a contrast medium used in the X-ray examination of the biliary tract.

THA Tetrahydroaminoacridine (= Tacrine HCl) - a stimulant of the central nervous system, sometimes used in conjunction with narcotics such as morphine, to lessen respiratory depression without diminishing the analgesic effect. Has been tried in the treatment of Alzheimer's disease; Texas Hospital Association; Total hip arthroplasty; Total hydroxyapatite; Transient hemispheric attack; Treponema hemagglutination.

ThA Thoracic aorta.

THAL; Thal Thalassemia.

THAM Trometamol (= Tham-E; Trihydroxymethylaminometamine/aminomethane; TRIS; Trisaminomethane; Tris(hydroxymethyl)aminomethane; Tromethamine) - an organic amine base which has been used in the treatment of metabolic and respiratory acidosis.

Tham-E Tromethamine (see THAM).
TH&C Terpin hydrate and codeine (medication order) (= THC).
THB Take home bottle; Tetrahydro B (see THBP); Todd-Hewitt broth; Total heart beats.
THb Total hemoglobin.
THBI Thyroid hormone binding inhibitor.
THBP 7,8,9,10-Tetrahydrobenzo(a)-pyrene (= THB); Thyroid hormone-binding protein.
THC Terpin hydrate and codeine (see TH&C); Tetrahydrocannabinol (major active ingredient of marijuana) (see Cannabis); Tetrahydrocortisol; Tetrahydrocortisone (E) (see THE); Thiocarbanidin; Total hormone concentration; Total hydrocarbons; Toxin-hemaglutinin complex (Type A -*Clostridium* botulinum); Transhepatic cholangiogram; Transplantable hepatocellular carcinoma; Transtetrahydrocannabinol.
THCA α-Trihydroxy-5-β-cholestannic acid.
THC-CRC Tetrahydrocannabinol - cross-reacting cannabinoids.
THCF Topics in Health Care Financing.
ThCult Throat culture.
tHCY Total homocysteine (plasma).
THD Therapeutic/ Topical human dose (= HTD); Transverse heart diameter.
ThD Last element of the disintegration series derived from Thorium, a stable isotope of lead, with an atomic weight of 208 (see Elements - Thorium).
Thd Ribothymidine.
THDOC Tetrahydrodeoxycorticosterone.
THE Tetrahydrocortisone E; Tetrahydro-E; Thyroid hormone evaluation; Tonic hindlimb extension; Transhepatic embolization; Tropical hypereosinophilia.
the- combining form meaning put (Gr.).
thec- combining form meaning repository (Gr. theke).
thel- combining form meaning nipple (Gr. thele).
theor theoretical/ry.
ther therapeutic/py (see therap); thermometer (see therm).
therap therapeutic/py (= ther).
therap- combining form meaning treatment (Gr. therapeia).
ther ex therapeutic exercise.
therm thermal; thermometer (= ther).
therm- combining form meaning heat (Gr. therme).
THF Tetrahydrocortisone F; Tetrahydrofluorenone; Tetrahydrofolate; Tetrahydrofolic acid (see THFA); Tetrahydrofuran; Tetrahydro-F; Thymic humoral factor; Transverse horizontal fracture (= TH#).
THFA Tetrahydrofolic acid (= THF); Tetrahydrofurfuryl alcohol.
THFC Trishepatofluoro-propylhydroxymethylene camphorato.
Thg Thyroglobulin (= TG; Tg).
THH Telangiectasia hereditaria haemorrhagica.
THI Temperature-humidity index; Texas Heart Institute (Houston); Tinnitus Handicap Inventory; Transient hypogammaglobulinemia of infancy; Traumatic head injury; Trihydroxindole.
Thi Thiamine (see Vitamins - B_1).
thi- combining form meaning sulfur (see thio-).
T-1-HI Type 1 humoral immunity.
Thin Prep 2000 (system) A more efficient type of PAP smear, used in the diagnosis of early cancer of the cervix.
THIO Thioridazine (hydrochloride).
thio- combining form meaning sulfur (Gr. theion) (= thi-).
thio-TEPA Triethylene-thiophosphamide/phosphoramide (see TESPA).
THIP Tetrahydroisoxazolopyridinol.
THJ The Hearing Journal (US).
THJR Total hip joint replacement (see OI/OP).
THKAFO Trunk-hip-knee-ankle-foot orthosis.
THL Telogen hair loss (= Diffuse alopecia) (see ACT); Terminal half-life.
THM Total heme mass.
TH_2O Titrated water.
ThO_2 Thorium dioxide - used in radiography of the alimentary tract (see Elements - Thorium).
Thor Thorax (BMA journal).
Thor; thor Thoracic/ax (see Th).

thorac- prefix meaning chest (Gr. thorakos).
Thorotrast X-ray contrast media.
thou a thousandth; thousand.
THP Take home packs; Tamm-Horsfall protein (a mucoprotein found in urine, but not in plasma); Tau hyperphosphorylation (in Alzheimer's disease) (see Cdk 5); Tertiary hyperparathyroidism; Tetrahydropapaveroline; Tetrahydropyranyl; Tissue hydrostatic pressure; Total hip (replacement) (see THR); Total hip prosthesis (Muller-Charnley) (see OI/OP); Total hydroxyproline; Trihexphenidyl; Transformed hematopoietic progenitor.
THPA Tetrahydropteric acid.
THPP Thiamine pyrophophate (see ThPP); Trihydroxy propriophenone.
ThPP Thiamine pyrophophate (= THPP).
THPV Transhepatic portal vein.
THQ Tetrahydroxyquinone; Tetraquinone.
THR Target heart range (in bpm or beats per minute) - optimum heart rate range during exercise (= 220 - age, x 60% and 74%) e.g. For a person age 50 years: 220 - 50 = 170 x 60% and x 75% = range between 102 and 128 bpm; Threonine (= Thr); Total heart replacement; Total hip replacement (= THP) (see OI/OP); Training heart rate; Transhepatic resonance.
Thr Threonine (see THR); Thrill (see Th).
thr thyroid(ectomy) (= th).
Three D's of Pellagra Dementia, Dermatitis, and Diarrhea (see Vitamins - B Complex, PP).
Three-to-one I 3-1 Insulin (see Insulin - 3-1 I).
THRF Thyrotropic hormone - releasing factor (see Hormones - TRH).
-thrix suffix meaning hair (Gr.).
throm; thromb thrombosis/bus.
Thrombel Thrombelastograph.
thrombo- prefix meaning clot (Gr. thrombos).
Thruster Amphetamine pill (see Amphet).
THS Tetrahydro compound S (= Tetrahydro-11-deoxycortisol) (see Cpd S); Thrombohemorrhagic syndrome; Tolosa-Hunt syndrome (painful superior orbital fissure syndrome, caused by granulomatous tissue involving cranial nerves III, IV and VI); Total Hip System (see OI/OP).
THSC Totipotent hematopoietic stem cell.
THSR Tufts Health Science Review (journal).
THT Teacher of hydrotherapy; Time-honored tradition; Transient hypothyroidism.
THTH Thyrotropic hormone (see TH).
THTV Therapeutic home trial visit (Psychiatry).
THU Tetrahydrouridine.
THUG Thyroid uptake gradient.
Thumb Marijuana cigarette (see Cannabis).
TH urinary microprotein Tamm-Horstall urinary microprotein (see THP).
THVO Terminal hepatic vein obliteration.
Th X A radioactive element produced by disintegration of thorium, and an isotope of radium with a half-life of about 3 $^{2}/_{3}$ days; used in the treatment of superficial skin conditions.
Thx Thromboxane.
Thy Thymine.
thy thymectomy; thymus.
Thym; thym Thymol.
-thymia suffix meaning mind (Gr. thymos).
thymo- combining form meaning thymus gland (Gr. thymos).
thym turb thymol turbidity (laboratory/ chemistry).
thyr- combining form meaning shield (Gr. thyreos).
THz Terahertz.
TI Inversion time; Tannate insulin (see Insulin - TI); Temporal integration; Terminal ileum; Thalassemia intermedia; Therapeutic/ Thoracic/ Throbogenicity index; Threshold of intelligibility; Thymus-independent (cells); Thyroxine iodine (serum) (see T4 - I); Time interval; Tonic immobility; Total iron; Transient insomnia; Transischial; Translational inhibition; Transport index (shipper's assigned); Transverse diameter/ distance (between ischia); Tricuspid incompetence/ insufficiency; Tumor induction.
Ti Titanium (Z = 22) (see Elements - Titanium).
T_I Inspiration/tory (phase) time (see PFT - TI).
T_4-I Thyroxine iodine (serum) (= TI).
TIA Total inhibitory activity; Transient ischemic attack (= ICA; TICA); Tumor-

induced angiogenesis; Turbidimetric immunoassay.

TIAH Total implantation of artificial heart.

TIAS Transient ischemic attacks (cerebral) (see TIAs).

TIAs Transient ischemic attacks (cerebral) (= TIAS).

TIB Tibia (see Tib); Time in bed; Tumor immunology bank.

Tib Tibia (= TIB).

TIBC Total iron-binding capacity (blood) (= Fe/TIBC).

TIC Topical intranasal corticosteroid; Toxicology Information Center; Trypsin inhibitory capacity; Tubulo-interstitial cell; Tumor-inducing complex.

Tic (dental journal).

TICA Transient ischemic cerebral attack (see TIA).

TICAR Ticarcillin (disodium).

TICAS-RTCIP Taxonomic Intra-Cellular Analytic System - Real Time Cell Identification Processor.

Ticket LSD-25 (see LSD).

TID Time interval difference (imaging); Tissue-invasive disease; Titrated initial dose; Tobacco-inflicted disease (such as lung cancer).

tid three times a/ per day (L. ter in die) (= TD; td; tds).

TIDA Tuberoinfundibular dopaminergic system.

TIE Telomerase-inhibiting enzyme; Transient ischemic episode; Treatment initiation education; Tumor inhibitory effect(s) (of cytotoxic drugs).

TIF Tumor-inducing/ -inhibiting factor.

TIFA Todd insecticidal generator.

TIFF Tagged image file format.

TIG Tetanus immune globulin.

TIg Tetanus immunoglobulin.

Tiger Ayahuasca (a hallucinogenic beverage of Peruvian Indians).

TIG(H) Tetanus Immune Globulin (Human).

TIGR The Institute for Genomic Research (Rockville, Md, USA) (Craig Venter's private research facility).

TIH Time interval histogram; Tumor-induced hypercalcemia.

TII Topoisomerase (1) inhibitor (e.g. Irinotecan, used in metastatic colorectal cancer).

TIL Thyroid-infiltrating lymphocyte; Treatment-induced (= secondary) leukemia; Tumor-infiltrating leukocyte/ lymphocyte (anti-cancer T cells).

TIM Topoisomerase (an enzyme); Total-ion monitor(s); Transthoracic intracardiac monitor(ing); Triosephosphate isomerase.

TIMC Tumor-induced marrow cytotoxicity.

TIME Techniques to Improve Management Efficiency.

TIMI Thrombolysis in myocardial infarction.

TIMIS Thrombolysis in Myocardial Infarction Study (= TIMI).

TIMP Tissue inhibitor of metalloproteinases.

TIMP-2 Tissue inhibitor metalloproteinase, type 2 (a new anti-cancer drug).

TIMS The Institute of Management Science.

TIN Tubulointerstitial nephropathy.

tin three times a night/ nightly (L. ter in nocte).

Tinc; tinc tincture (see Tinct).

Tinct; tinct Tincture (= Tct; Tinc; tinc; Tr; tr).

$T_{3/4}$ ind Triiodothyronine to thyroxine index (laboratory/ endocrinology).

T_3 Index Triiodothyroxine index (laboratory/ endocrinology).

TINU Tubulointerstitial nephritis-uveitis (syndrome).

TIOH Thiazide-induced orthostatic hypotension.

TIP Terminal interphalangeal (joint); Terminally ill patient; Tetraiodophthalein (= Iodognost; Iodophthalein; Tetrothalein sodium) - a contrast medium which has been used (orally) in the X-ray examination of the biliary tract; Thermal inactivation point; Toxicology Information Program; Translation-inhibiting protein; Tumor-inhibiting principle.

TIPA Thrombin-induced platelet aggregation.

TIPI Time-insensitive predictive instrument.

TIPPS Tetraiodophenylphthalein sodium/ solution.

TIPS Tactical information (about) perilous situations.

TIQ Tetrahydroquinoline.

TIR Terminal innervation ratio; Total immunoreactive (insulin) (see Insulin - TIRI).
TIRF Toxin-induced renal failure.
TIRI Total immunoreactive insulin (see Insulin - TIRI).
TIR insulin See TIRI.
TIRR Texas Institute of Rehabilitation and Research.
TIS Tetracycline-induced steatosis; Transdermal infusion system; Tri-flow incentive spirometer (see TFIS); Trypsin-insoluble segment; Tumor in situ.
TISAB Total ionic strength adjustment buffer.
TISP Total immunoreactive serum pepsinogen.
TISS Therapeutic Intervention Scoring System.
TIT Therapy-induced tumor; Treponema immobilization test (see STS - TIT); Triiodothyronine (see T_3; TITh).
T_I/T_E Inspiratory - expiratory phase time ratio (PFT).
TITh Triiodothyronine (see T_3).
TITJLS Tower International TechnoMedical Institute Journal of Life Sciences.
Title XVIII Medicare (Social Security Act).
Title XIX Medicaid (Social Security Act).
titr titrate.
TIU Trypsin-inhibiting unit.
TIUV Total intra-uterine volume.
TIVC Thoracic inferior vena cava.
+tive positive.
TIW Three times a week.
TJ Marijuana (produced in Tijuana, Mexico) (see Cannabis); Tetrajoule; Thigh junction; Triceps jerk.
TJA Total joint arthroplasty.
TJN Twin jet nebulizer.
TJR Total joint replacement.
TJS Tom Jones suture (used in hysterectomy) (see Sut).
TK Thymidine kinase; Transketolase; Triose-kinase.
T(°K) Absolute temperature on the Kelvin scale.
TKA Total knee arthroplasty; Transketolase activity; Trochanter, knee, and ankle.
TKD Thymidine kinase deficiency; Tokodynamometer.
TKE Terminal knee extension.
TKF Terminal kidney failure (see ESRD; ESRF; TRF).
TKG Tokodynagraph.
TKI Tyrosine kinase inhibitor (used in cancer therapy).
TKLI Tachykinin-like immunoreactivity.
TKM Transgenic knockout mice/ mouse.
TKN Total Kjeldahl nitrogen.
TKNO To keep needle open.
TKO Technical knock-out; To keep open (intravenous therapy).
TKP Thermokeratoplasty; Total knee prosthesis (see OI/OP).
TKR Total knee replacement (see OI/OP).
TKRS Total knee replacement surgery (= TKR)/ System (see OI/OP).
TKS Total Knee System (Orthopedic Implants - see OI/OP).
TKVO To keep vein open.
tky turkey.
TL Team leader; Temporal lobe; Terminal limen; Tetrahedron Letters (journal); Thermolabile; Thermoluminescence; Threat to life; Threshold limit; Thymus-leukemia (antigen); Thymus lymphocyte/ lymphoma; Time lag/ lapse/ limit(ed); Tocolysis (abatement of contractions in premature labor - see TLA); Total lipids; Total lung (capacity); Trial leave; Tubal ligation.
Tl Thallium (Z = 81) (see Elements - Thallium).
T-L Thymus-dependent lymphocyte.
T/L Terminal latency.
^{201}Tl Radioactive thallium (= Thallium 201).
TLA Thrombolytic agent; Tissue lactase activity; T-lymphocyte antigen (e.g. CTLA-4 or the cytotoxic TLA gene); Tocolytic agent (for abatement of contractions in premature labor); Tongue-to-lip adhesion; Translaryngeal aspiration; Translumbar aortogram/ arteriogram; Transluminal angioplasty; Tube latex agglutination (test).
TLAA T-lymphocyte-associated antigen.
TLam Thoracic laminectomy.
TLC Teenage Living Center; Tender loving care; Tend with legal care; Thin-layer chromatography; Total L-chain concentration; Total lung capacity - the amount/ volume of

gas that is contained in the lung at the end of a maximal inspiration (see PFT); Total lung compliance (see PFT); Total lymphocyte count; Triple lumen catheter; Tumoral lipocalcinosis (Orthopedics).

TLD Thermoluminescence/ent detector/ dose/ dosimeter/ dosimetry; Third-line drug (see TLDT); Thoracic lymph(atic) duct; Tocolytic drug; Tumor lethal dose.

T/LD$_{100}$ Minimum dose causing 100% deaths or malformations.

TLDT Third-line drug therapy (in RA) - such as Immunosuppressant drugs (ISDs), Cytotoxic agents (CTAs) and Corticosteroids.

TLE Temporal lobe epilepsy; Thin-layer electrophoresis; Total lipid extract; Toxicologic effect.

TLEC Thin-layer electrochemistry.

TLF Total liver function.

TL frequency distributions Thorndike-Lorge frequency distributions.

TLG Thin-layer gel filtration.

TLGH Technetium labelled glucoheptonate (used in kidney scan).

TLHN Translocational hyponatremia (due to hyperglycemia, etc.).

TLI Thoracolumbar injury; Thymidine labeling index; Total lymphoid irradiation; Translaryngeal intubation; Trypsin-like immune (activity).

TLIA Trypsin-like immune activity.

TLIEF Thin-layer isoelectric focusing.

TLJ Thoracolumbar junction (see TLS).

TLL T-lymphoblastic lymphoma.

TLm Median tolerance limit.

TLN Telephone Lecture Network.

TLNB Term living newborn.

TLP Tikhoff-Linberg procedure (Classical interscapulothoracic resection) - see SCS; SGO; SGR); Time lapse photography (for digital microscopic imaging of cells); Transitional living programme; Translabyrinth procedure.

TLQ Total living quotient.

TLR Thoracolumbar region; Tikhoff-Linberg resection (of different amounts of clavicle, humerus, and scapular bones) (see TBR; TLP); Tonic labyrinthine reflex.

TLS Temporal lobe seizure (see CPE; TLE); Test(ing) for/ of/ the limit(s) for/ of sex (psychology); Thoracolumbosacral; Thoracolumbar spine; Tourette-like syndrome; Tumor/ Tumour lysis syndrome (featuring hyperuricemia, hyperkalemia, hypocalcemia, acute and respiratory failure).

TLSO Thoracolumbosacral orthosis.

TLSSO Thoracolumbosacral spinal orthosis.

TLT Third-line therapy/ treatment (e.g. for metastatic disease); Tryptophan load test.

TLV Threshold limit value (toxicology, formerly MAC); Total lung volume (see PFT - TLV).

TLW Total lung water.

TLX Trophoblast-lymphocyte cross-reactivity.

T-lymphocyte(s) Thymus-dependent/ derived lymphocyte(s) - responsible for specific cellular immunity.

TM Tantalum mesh (prosthetic eye); Technical manual; Tectorial/ Tympanic membrane; Temperature by mouth; Temporalis/ Trapezius muscle; Temporomandibular (joint); Tender midline; Tendomyopathy; Teres/ Thalassemia major; Tests and measurements; Thayer-Martin (medium); Time-motion; Tinnitus masker (hearing aid); Tobramycin (see TOB); Trabecular meshwork; Trademark; Traditional/ Traumatic/ Tropical medicine; Transatrial membranotomy; Transcendental meditation (see SCI); Transitional mucosa; Transmediastinal; Transmetatarsal; Transport mechanism (of the tubular cells of a nephron); Transport medium/ messenger (see tm); Transverse myelitis; True mean (see tm); Tuberculous meningitis; Tubular mass; Tumor (see Tu); Twitch movement.

Tm Thulium (Z = 69) (see Elements - Thulium); Transport maximum; Tubular maximum (excretory capacity of the kidneys) = Maximal tubular excretory capacity/ resorption = Maximum tubular clearance (= T_m); Tumor-bearing mice.

T$_m$ Melting/ Muscle temperature; Temperature midpoint; Tubular maximum excretory capacity/ resorption of the kidneys (see Tm).

tM Time required to complete the M phase of the cell cycle.

tm transport medium/ messenger (= TM); true

mean (= TM).

T-M Thayer-Martin (medium).

T&M Type and match (crossmatch).

TMA Tetramethylammonium; Texas Medical Association; Thermomechanical analyzer; Thrombotic microangiopathy; Thyroid microsomal antibody; Transcortical mixed aphasia; Transmetatarsal amputation; Trimellitic anhydride; Trimethoxyamphetamine; Trimethoxyphenyl aminopropane (a hallucinogen); Trimethylamine; Trimethylxanthine amphetamine.

TMAH Trimethylphenylammonium hydroxide (= Trimethylanilinium hydroxide).

TMAI Trimethylphenylammonium (anilinium) iodide.

TMAO Trimethylamine oxide.

TMAS Taylor Manifest Anxiety Scale.

T_{max}; tmax Maximum threshold/ time; Time of maximum concentration (e.g. plasma concentrations); Time to maximum/ peak plasma/ serum concentration/ level = Time of occurrence of - to Cmax.

TMB Transient monocular blindness; Transmural breathing; Trimethoxybenzoate.

TMBA Trimethoxybenzaldehyde.

TMC Teratomatous component (of rhabdomyosarcoma) (see GCC; TCC); Texas Medical Center (Houston); Thorough medical checkup; Transmural colitis; Triamcinolone; Triamcinolone and terramycin capsules; Tucson Medical Center (Arizona); Tulsa Medical College (Oklahoma).

TMCA Trifurcation of the middle cerebral artery; Trimethylcolchine acid.

TMCHD Transtetramethyl-cyclohexanediamine.

TMCS Trimethylchlorosilane.

TMCSL Transactions of the Medical-Chirurgical Society of London.

TM culture medium Thayer-Martin culture medium.

TMD Targeted maintenance dose; Total monthly dose; Traditional medical doctor; Transmissible mink disease; Trimethadione.

TMDI Theoretical maximum daily intake.

TMDS Tetramethyldisilazane.

t-MDS Therapy-related myelodysplasic syndrome.

TME Teacher of Medical Electricity; Thermolysin-like metalleondopeptidase; Total metabolizable energy; Transmissible mink encephalopathy (see Agent X); Transmural enteritis.

tme- combining form meaning cut (Gr.).

TMED Tetramethylethylenediamine.

TMET Treadmill exercise test.

TMF Transformed mink fibroblast; Transmitral flow.

TMG Thymomatous myasthenia gravis; Time mark generator; Torticollis muscularis congenita (Orthopedics); Tubular maximum (absorption rate for) glucose (see TM_g).

TM_g; Tm_G; T_{mg} Maximum tubular reabsorption rate for glucose = Maximum glucose reabsorption capacity (of kidney) = Tubular maximum absorption rate for glucose (Renal function test) = TMG.

TMH Taylor Manor Hospital (Maryland); Tetramethylammonium hydroxide; The Methodist Hospital (Texas Medical Center, Houston).

TMHN Tropical Medicine and Hygiene News (ASTMH journal).

TM-HSA Trimellityl-human serum albumin.

TMI Testing motor impairment; Threatened/ Transmural myocardial infarction/ ischemia; Transmural infarction; Tumor microsatellite instability (in colorectal cancer).

TMIC Toxic Materials Information Center.

TMIF Tumor-cell migratory inhibition factor.

TMIS Technicon Medical Information System.

TMJ Tarsal-metatarsal joint (= MTJ); Temporomandibular/ Trapeziometacarpal joint.

TMJD Temporomandibular joint disorder (see TMJS).

TMJ-PDS Temporomandibular joint - pain dysfunction syndrome (= TMJS).

TMJS Temporomandibular joint syndrome (see TMJ-PDS).

TML Terminal midline; Terminal motor latency; Tetramethyl lead.

TMLR Transmyocardial laser revascularization.

TMM Telemetric monitor(ing); Thayer-Martin medium (for culture of *Neisseria* gonorrheae

from the cervix); Torn medial meniscus.
Tmm McKay-Marg tension.
TMMG Teacher of Massage and Medical Gymnastics.
TMN Transient mild nausea.
TMNST Tethered median nerve stress test.
TMP Thallium myocardial perfusion; Thiamine/ Thymidine/ Thymolphthalein monophophate; Transmembrane potential(s)/ pressure/ protein (e.g. p185 - associated with cancer); Trimethoprim; Trimethylpsoralen.
TM_{PAH}; Tm_{pah} Maximum tubular excretory/ reabsorption capacity (of kidney), for para-aminohippuric acid (KFT).
TMPD Tetramethyl-p-phenylinediamine.
TMPDS Temporomandibular pain and dysfunction syndrome; Thiamine monophosphate disulfide.
TMP-SMX; TMP-SMZ Trimethoprim + sulfamethoxazole (= Cotrimoxazole; TRM-SMX; TRM-SMZ).
TMP/SMX Trimethoprim/Sulfamethaxazole.
TMR Tissue maximum ratio; Topical magnetic resonance; Trainable mentally retarded; Transmyocardial revascularization; Transverse metaphyseal radiolucency.
TMS Tandem mass spectometry; Tetramethylsilane; Thalium myocardial scintigraphy; 'Thousand-mile stare' (seen in coma and characteristic of PBD - Permanent brain damage); Thread mate system; Titanium modular spacer; Transcranial magnetic stimulation (a technique for temporarily inhibiting neural activity in the frontotemporal area of the brain); Trapezoidocephaly-multiple synostosis (syndrome); Trimethylsilane; Trimethylsilyl; Trimethysilane.
TMSDEA Trimethylsilyl-dimethylamine.
TMST Treadmill stem/ stress test.
TM studies Tympanometric studies.
TMT Tarsometatarsal; Telomerase test (blood test for cancer) (see CDM); Tetramethylthiuram (see TMTD); Trail-Making test; Treadmill test; Trimethyllin; Tympanic membrane temperature/ thermometer.
Tmt; tmt Treatment (see Trt).
TMTC Too many to count.
TMTD Tetramethylthiuram disulfide - an antibacterial and antifungal agent.
TMTX Trimethexate.
TMU Tetramethyl urea; Time and modifying unit(s); Tropical Medicine Unit (Department of State).
TMV Tobacco mosaic virus.
tMVIV Maximal venous incremental volume time (see MVIV).
tMVO Maximal venous outflow time (i.e. time of total emptying) (see MVO).
TMX Tamoxifen (see TAM).
TMZ Temazepam; Transformation zone.
TN Talonavicular; Tarsonavicular; Team nursing; Temperature normal; Toenail; Total negatives; Toxic neuropathy; Trigeminal/ Trochlear nucleus; Troponin; True negative.
Tn Normal (intraocular) tension; Thoron/ Thorium emanation (see Elements - Thorium); Transposition.
T/N Tar and nicotine.
T&N Tension and nervousness.
T_4N Normal(ized) serum thyroxine.
TNA Total nutrient admixture.
TNAS Tuberculosis Nursing Advisory Service.
TNB Term newborn; Tru-Cut needle biopsy.
TnBP Tri-(n-butyl)phosphate (an organic solvent).
TNBS Trinitrobenzene-sulfonic acid.
TNC The Nature Conservancy.
TN-C The calcium-binding subunit of troponin.
TND Term normal delivery.
TNE Tris sodium chloride EDTA buffer ("Tris Natrium EDTA").
t-NE Total norepinephrine.
TNEE Titrated norepinephrine excretion.
TNEMC Tufts, New England Medical Center.
TNF Trinitrofluorenone; True negative fraction; Tumor necrosing/is factor ("cachectin", a protein produced by macrophages in immune responce).
TNFRC Tumor necrosis factor-related cytokine (or TRANCE, responsible for osteoclast regeneration).
TNG Nitroglycerine (trinitrate).
tng tongue; training.
TNH Transient neonatal hyperammonemia.
TNI Total nodal irradiation.

TN-I The inhibitory subunit of troponin.

TNM Tumor (primary), nodes (regional), metastases - international cancer/ tumor grading or staging system, based on T (tumor), N (nodes), and M (metastasis) classification; Thyroid node metastases; Tumor node metastasis.

TNMR Tritium nuclear magnetic resonance.

TNN Tetanus neonatorum (= NNT).

T1No Tumor (earliest clinical phase), nodes (no positive disease).

TNP Total net positive (score); Treatment-naive patient.

TNP; TNP-470 A synthetic analogue of the fungal antibiotic fumagillin and an angiogenesis inhibitor, acting by blocking enzymes that instruct tumor blood-vessels to divide (see AAGT; AGI; AS).

TNR Tonic neck reflex; True negative rate.

TNS Total nasal symptoms; Total nuclear score; Transcutaneous nerve stimulation; Tumor necrosis serum.

TNSAP Topical nonsteroidal anti-pruritic.

TNT Tetranitroblue tetrazolium; Triamcinolone and nystatin; Trinitrotoluene (= 2,4,6-trinitrotoluene).

TN-T Tropomyosin-binding subunit of troponin.

TNTC Too numerous to count (laboratory report).

TNV The next virus; Tobacco necrosis virus.

TO Old/ Original tuberculin (see Tuberculin - TO); Oral temperature [see T(O)]; Table of organization; Target organ; Telephone order (see T/O); Theiler's Original (virus strain); Thoracic orthosis; Tincture of opium (L. tinctura opii) (see To); Total obstruction/ oestrogens; Tracheoesophageal; Transfer out; Tuberculin ober (Ger.) = Supernatant T (see Tuberculin - TO); Tubo-ovarian; Turned on; Turnover (number).

To Tincture of opium (L. tinctura opii) (= TO; to).

to tincture of opium (see To).

T_0 Total oestrogens (= TO).

T/O Telephone order (= TO).

T(O) Temperature, oral (= TO).

T&O Tubes and ovaries.

TO_2 Oxygen transport.

TOA Time of arrival; Tuberculin-original-alt (Ger) (see Tuberculin - TO); Tubo-ovarian abscess.

TOAP Thioguanine, oncovin, (cytosine) arabinoside, and prednisone.

TOB Tobramycin (= TM).

Tob Tobacco.

TOBEC Total body electrical conductivity.

TobRV Tobacco ringspot virus.

TOC Tag open cup (flash point test); Total organic carbon; Treatment of choice; Triphasic oral contraceptive.

TOCE Transcatheter oily chemoembolization.

TOCO Tocodynamometer.

TOCP Triorthocresylphosphate (= Tri-o-cresyl phosphate).

TOD Right eye tension (Tension - oculus dexter/ L.); Target organ damage; Therapeutic oral dose; Time-Oriented Data (Bank); Titanium optimized design (plate); Total oxygen demand.

Tod Heal Today's Health (journal).

TODS Toxic organic dust syndrome.

TOE Tracheoesophageal.

TOES Toxic oil epidemic syndrome (= TOS).

TOF Tetralogy of Fallot (see T of F); Time-of-flight (sequence); Total of four; Train of four (monitor); Tracheo-(o)esophageal fistula.

T of F Tetralogy of Fallot (= TOF).

TOFD Tardive orofacial dyskinesia (= OFD).

TOGV Transposition of the great vessels.

TOH Througout hospitalization; Transient osteoporosis of the hip; Tyrosine hydroxylase.

toko- prefix meaning childbirth (Gr. tokos).

TOL Trial of labor.

tol tolerance/ate(d).

TOLB; tolb Tolbutamide (= Tolglybutamide; D 860; U 2043; N- Butyl-N'-toluene-p-sulphonylurea) - a sulphonylurea compound, used orally in the treatment of adult (type B) diabetes mellitus.

TOM Threshold of octave masking; Tomorrow; Toxic oxygen metabolite; Transcutaneous oxygen monitor.

tom- combining form meaning a surgical cut (Gr.).

TOMHS Treatment of Mild Hypertension Study.

Tomog Tomogram/aphy.

TON Tonight.

Ton Aluminium silicate.

ton- combining form meaning stretch or tension (Gr.).

TONAR The oral/ nasal acoustic ratio.

Tongue-tie Ankyloglossia (a defect of the mouth in which the membrane under the tongue {frenulum linguae or lingual frenum} is too short, limiting tongue movement and impairing speech).

To Noc; tonoc Tonight (L. nocte).

TO number Turnover number.

Tooie Tuinal capsule.

TOP Temporal, occipital, and parietal (lobes of the brain); Termination of pregnancy; Toxic oxidation product.

top topical(ly).

Topi Peyote.

TOPO Trioctylphosphine oxide.

TOPO I Topoisomerase I (an enzyme found in rapidly growing tumors, which untwists supercoiled DNA, resulting in very malignant cancers).

TOPO II Topoisomerase II (an enzyme found in slow-growing cancers).

TOPS Take of pounds sensibly; Twin oligohydramnios/ polyhydramnios sequence (Obstetrics).

TOPT Thoraco-omphalopagus twins (see pagus).

TOPV Trivalent oral poliovaccine/ poliovirus vaccine.

TORCH (syndrome) microbial agents that cause clinically similar symptoms in the newborn: **T**. Toxoplasmosis, **O**. Others (congenital syphilis and viruses), **R**. Rubella, **C**. Cytomegalovirus, and **H**. Herpes simplex virus.

TORP Total ossicular reconstructive/ replacement prosthesis.

Torpedo Chloral hydrate drink (see Chloral hydrate).

torr mm Hg pressure.

tors- combining form meaning twist (L. torsus).

torsade de pointes French - "a pointed or twinging twisted cord" - used in reference to ECG findings in ventricular arrhythmia.

TOS Left eye tension (Tension - oculus sinister - L.); Target organ sensitivity; Thoracic outlet syndrome; Toxic oil syndrome (see TOES); Turnover study.

TOT Target organ toxicity; Total operating time.

ToT Tip-of-the-tongue (phenomenon) - not being able to remember an everyday word or phrase; especially common after the age of 60.

Tot; tot Total.

TotBili Total bilirubin.

Tot Prot Total protein.

TOUS Transmission oscillator ultrasonic spectrometer.

TOV Thrombosed oral varix; Trial of voiding.

TOWER Testing, orientation, and work evaluation in rehabilitation.

Tox; tox Toxic(ity); Toxin.

tox- combining form meaning poison (Gr. toxikon).

Toxicol Toxicology (journal).

TOXICON Toxicity/ Toxicology Information Contraversial/ Conversational On-Line Network.

Toxicon IST journal.

TOXLINE Toxicology Information On-Line (NLM) (data bank), i.e. On-Line References and Abstracts in the field of Toxicology and Pharmacology (NLM).

TOXLIT Toxicology Literature (data bank).

TOXNET Toxicology Network (NLM) (data bank).

TP A segment of the electrocardiogram; Telectronic pacemaker; Teleprocessing (of data); Temperature and pressure; Temperature probe; Temporal plane (= PT); Temporoparietal; Terminal phalanx; Testosterone propionate; Thal procedure (see HHR - Hiatal hernia repair); Therapeutic pass; Thick padding; Threshold potential; Thrombocytopenic purpura; Thrombophlebitis; Thymic/ Thymus polypeptide; Thymopentin; Thymus/ Total protein; Todd's paralysis; Toilet paper; Torsades de pointes; Total positives; Trainor procedure (for ptosis of the eyelids); Transforming principle (bacteriology); Transition/ Trigger point; Transmission pulse (ultrasound); Transpersonal psychology; Transplantation

Proceedings (TS journal); Transposon (see Tes); Transverse polarization/ process; Treating physician; Treatment period/ planning; Treponema pallidum (see Tp); Trigger point; Triphosphate; True positive; Tryptophan (see Tp); Tryptophan photo product; Tryptophan pyrrolase; Tube precipitin; Tuberculin precipitate/ation (= Calmette's tuberculin) (see Tuberculin - TP).

Tp Treponema pallidum (= TP); Tryptophan (a transmitter amine) (= TP).

T_p Physical half-life.

T + P Temperature and pulse (see T&P).

T&P Temperature and pulse (= T + P); Turn and position.

6-TP 6-Thiopurine.

TP 21 Thioridazine hydrochloride - a tranquillizing agent used mainly for the treatment of schizophrenia, and for the control of mania and agitation. Also used in the management of anxiety states, and in children with behavior problems (see TPS 23).

TPA Tachyphylaxis (diminished response in hemodynamic function); Tannic/ Tiaprofenic acid, polyphosphomolybdic acid, and aminoacid (staining technique); Terephthalic acid; 12-O-tetradecanoyl-phorbol-13-acetate; Third-party administrator; Thyroid peroxidase antibody (present in about 75% of patients with Graves' hyperthyroidism) (see GHT); Tissue plasminogen activator (see t-PA); Tissue/ Tumor(-derived) polypeptide antigen; Total parenteral alimentation; Transporter peptide antigen (see TAP 1, 2); Treponema pallidum agglutination.

tPA Tissue-type plasminogen activator antigen.

t-PA Tissue/ Tissue-type plasminogen activator (= TPA).

TPB Tetraphenyl borate; Tryptone phosphate broth.

TPBF Total pulmonary blood flow.

TPBS Three-phase (radionuclide) bone scanning.

TPC Technetium pertechnatate/ pyrophosphate scan; Telescoping plugged catheter; Telopeptide-poor collagen; Thromboplastic plasma component; Total patient care; Total plasma catecholamines/ cholesterol; Total/ Trough plasma concentration; Treponema pallidum complement (fixation test) (see STS - TPC).

TPCF Treponema pallidum complement fixation (test) (see STS - TPCF).

TPCK Tosylphenylethyl-chloromethyl-ketone (= N-Tosyl-L-phenylalanine chloromethyl ketone).

TPCV Total packed cell volume.

TPD Temporary partial disability; Thiamine propyl disulfide; Total progesterone deficiency; Transplant donor; Tripotassium phenolphthalein disulfate; Tropical pancreatic diabetes; Tumor-producing dose.

TPDS Tropical pancreatic diabetes syndrome.

TPE Therapeutic plasma exchange; Totally protected environment; Tropical pulmonary eosinophilia; Typhoid-paratyphoid enteritis.

T^{Pe} Expiratory pause time (see PFT).

TPEIA Time of postexpiratory inspiratory activity.

T Per/Vac Tetanus and Pertussis Vaccine (= Tetanus-Whooping-cough Prophylactic V).

TPEY Tellurite polymyxin egg yolk (agar).

TPF Tamoxifen - a cytotoxic drug added to PF (= L-phenyl-alanine mustard plus 5-fluoruracil), in order to enhance the effectiveness of the antimetabolite treatment of breast cancers after mastectomy (see PF; TAM); Terminal phalanx of a/ the finger (Orthopedics); Thymus permeability factor; Thymus to peak flow; Trained participating father; True positive fraction.

TPFA Treponema pallidum fluorescent antibody (test) (see FTA - ABS; STS - TPFA).

TPG Transmembrane potential gradient; Transplacental gradient; Tryptophan peptone glucose (broth); Tumor-promoting gene (= Oncogene).

TPGYT Trypticase-peptone-glucose-yeast extract-trypsin (medium).

TPH Thromboembolic pulmonary hypertension; Tibial peg hole(s) (Orthopedic Implants); Trained participating husband; Transplacental hemorrhage.

TPHA Treponema pallidum hemagglutination (test) (see STS - TPHA).

T PHOS Triple phosphate (crystals).

TPI Time period integrator; Transplacental

infection; Treponema pallida immobilization (test for syphilis) (see STS - TPI); Treponemal immobilization (test); Triosephosphate isomerase.

T^{Pi} Inspiratory pause time (see PFT).

TPIA Treponema pallidum immune adherence (test) (see STS - TPIA).

TPJ Tendoperiosteal junction.

TPK Tyrosyl protein kinase (see BCP; TPP).

TPL Threatening premature labour; Titanium proximal loading; Trough and peak levels (of antibiotics); Trough plasma level; Tyrosine phenol-lyase.

T plasty Tympanoplasty.

TPLV Transient pulmonary vascular lability (see TPVL).

TPM Temporary pacemaker; Thrombophlebitis migrans; Total particulate matter; Total passive motion; Triphenylmethane.

TPMT Thiopurine methyltransferase.

TPN Sandoz Pharmaceuticals (USA) code for experimental substances; Thalamic projection neuron; Total parenteral nutrition (intravenous therapy); Triphosphopyridine nucleotide (= NADP; Nicotinamide-adenine dinucleotide phosphate) (see Co-2).

TPNH Reduced triphosphopyridine nucleotide (= NADPH; Nicotinamide adenine dinucleotide phosphate - reduced form).

TPNX; TPnx Tension pneumothorax.

TPO Sandoz Pharmaceuticals (USA) code for experimental substances; Transplantable pig organ; Trial prescription order; Thrombopoietin; Thyroid/ Tryptophan peroxidase.

T point Transition point.

TPP Thiamine pyrophosphate (= Diphosphothiamine); Transplacental passage (see TPT); Transpulmonary pressure; Treadmill performance test; Triphenyl phosphite; Tyrosyl protein phosphorylation (in bone cells) (see BCP).

TP&P Time, place, and person.

TPPase Thiamine pyrophosphatase.

TPPD Thoracic-pelvic-phalangeal dystrophy.

TPPN Total peripheral parenteral nutrition.

TPPT ThinPrep Pap Test (a new, more accurate Papanicolaou test for de- tecting precancerous and cancerous lesions of the cervix (see APPSS).

TPPV Trans pars plana vitrectomy.

TPQ Threshold Planning Quantity.

TPR Temperature (see temp); Temperature, pulse, and respiration (vital signs); Testosterone production rate; Total peripheral/ pulmonary resistance; Total protein; Toxicological position report; Transplant recipient; True positive rate.

TPRF Totally preventable risk factor (such as alcohol intake, cigarette smoking, drugs and superfluous medication).

TPRI Total peripheral resistance index.

T PROT Total protein.

TPS Total protein synthesis; Traditional prostate surgery; Trypsin (= Tr); Tumor polysaccharide substance; Twin peak sign (see TCPS).

TPS 23 Mesoridazine (= Mesuridazine) - a metabolite of thioridazine used in the treatment of chronic schizophrenia and depression (see TP 21).

TPSE 2-(p-triphenyl)sulfonylethanol.

TPST True positive stress test.

TPT Tactual Performance Test (psychology); Tetraphenyl tetrazolium - a histological stain (see TPTZ); Thoracopagus twins (see pagus); Thyroid-parathyroid (vaccine) (see TPV); Time to peak tension; Total protein tuberculin (see Tuberculin - TPT); Toxoplasmosis test(s) = serological tests such as ELISA-IgG, IFA-IgM and RA latex slide test; Transplacental transfer (of drugs, medicines, etc.) (= TPP); Treadmill performance test; Typhoidparatyphoid (vaccine) (see TPV).

TPTE 2-(p-triphenyl)thioethanol.

TPTX Thyro-parathyroidectomized.

TPTZ Triphenyltetrazolium (chloride) (= Red Tetrazolium; TTC) - a color reagent used as a diagnostic test for bacteriuria. It is reduced by dividing bacteria to an insoluble red compound, triphenylformazon; Tripyridyltriazine.

TPV Tetanus-pertussis vaccine; Thyroid-parathyroid/ Typhoid-paratyphoid vaccine; Tipranavir (a PI anti-HIV drug - Boehringer-Ingelheim).

TP vaccine Thyroid-parathyroid/ Typhoid-paratyphoid vaccine (see TPV).

TPVL Total pulmonary vascular lability (= TPLV).

TPVR Total peripheral/ pulmonary vascular resistance.

TPZ Thioproperazine.

TQ Time questionnaire; Tocopherolquinone; Tourniquet.

TQM Total quality management.

TQR Total quadriceps resection (Orthopedics).

TR Reaction/ Recovery/ Reduction/ Repetition/ Response/ Retention time (see RT); Rectal temperature [see T(R)]; Residual tuberculin (see Tuberculin R/residue); Tabula rasa (cell); Teaching and research (see T&R); Terminal repeat; Tetrazolium reduction; Therapeutic radiology/ recreation/ regimen/ response; Theta rhythm (EEG); Thrombosis Research (UK journal); Time(d) release; To return; Total repair/ resistance/ response; Trachea(l)/eostmy/eotomy (see Trach); Transfusion reaction; Transmit-receive; Transplant recipient(s); Transplantation Reviews (journal); Tricuspid regurgitation; Tuberculin R (= New tuberculin) (see Tuberculin - TR); Tuberculin residue (see Tuberculin - TR); Tumor registry; Turbidity-reducing; Turnover ratio.

Tr Tincture (see Tinct); Trace (see tr); Traction (see Tract); Tragion; Transferrin; Treatment (see Trt); Tremor (see tr); Trypsin (see TPS).

tr tincture (see Tinct); trace (= Tr); traction (see Tract); transaldolase (see tra); trauma(tic) (see traum); treatment (see Trt); tremor (= Tr); triradial.

T(R) Temperature, rectal (on temperature records) (= TR).

T(°R) Absolute temperature on the Rankine scale.

T_r Radiologic half-life; Retention time (see RT; TR).

T&R Teaching and research (= TR); Tenderness and rebound.

TR 495 Methaqualone hydrochloride (see QZ 2).

TRA Therapeutic recreation associate; To run at; Total renin activity; Transaldolase (= see tra); Tumor-resistant antigen.

tra transaldolase (= tr; TRA); transfer.

TRAb Thyrotoxin receptor antibody; Thyrotropin-receptor antibody (see GHT; IgMI).

Trach; trach Trachea(l)/eostomy/eotomy (= TR).

Trach asp Tracheal aspiration.

trache- prefix meaning trachea (Gr. tracheia).

trachei- combining form meaning neck (Gr. trachelos).

Tract; tract Traction (= Tr; tr; Trx; trx).

tract- combining form meaning drag or pull (L. tractus).

TRAE Treatment-related adverse effect/ event.

Train; train Training (= Trg; trg).

TRAJ Time repetitive ankle jerk.

TRALI Transfusion-related acute lung injury (see TRALT).

TRALT Transfusion-related acute lung injury (= TRALI).

TRAM Treatment Rating Assessment Matrix; Treatment Received and Measured (basis); Treatment Response Assessment Method.

TRAMPCOL Thioguanine, Rubidomycin (daunorubicin), Ara-C (cytarabine), methotrexate, prednisolone, cyclophosphamide, Oncovin (vincristine), and L-asparaginase (combination drugs used in the treatment of the leukemias).

TRAMPE Tricho-rhino-auricular multiple phalangeal exostoses.

TRANCE Tumor and necrosis factor-related cytokine (see TNFRC).

Trans; trans Transact(ion); Transfer(ence); Transmission/mitted (see Transm); Transplant(ation)/(ed) (see Transpl); Transport(ation) (ed) (see Transpo); Transverse.

trans- prefix meaning through (L.).

trans D; trans d transverse diameter.

Transfus Transfusion (AABB journal).

Transm; transm Transmission/mitted (= Trans; trans).

Transpl Transplant(ation)/(ed) (= Trans; trans; transpl; TX); Transplantation (TS journal).

transpl transplant(ation)/(ed) (see Transpl).

Transpo Department of Transportation; Transport(ation)/(ed) (= Trans; trans; trans-

po).
transpo transport(ation)/(ed) (see Transpo).
trans sect transverse section.
TRAP Tartrate-resistant acid phosphatase; Thioguanine, Rubidomycin (daunorubicin), Ara-C (cytarabine), and prednisolone (anti-leukemia combination drugs); Transport and rapid accessioning for additional procedures; Twin reversed arterial perfusion (syndrome) (Obstetrics).
trap trapezius.
TRAS Transplanted renal artery stenosis.
trau; traum trauma(tic) (= tr).
trauma- prefix meaning wound (Gr.).
TRB Terbutalone.
TRBAb Thyrotropin-receptor-blocking antibody.
TRBF Total renal blood flow (kidney function test).
TRBM Texas Reports on Biology and Medicine.
TRC Anti-thyroglobulin antibody; Tanned red cell (tannic acid-treated red blood cell agglutination titers); Taste-receptor cell (taste bud in the tongue); Therapeutic residential center; Timed release capsule; Total renin concentration; Total respiratory conductance; Total ridge count; Transferrin receptor concentration; Transient reversible cardiomyopathy; Treatment-related change.
TRCA Tanned red cell agglutination.
TRCH Tanned red cell hemagglutination.
TRCHI Tanned red cell hemagglutination inhibition.
TRCHII Tanned red cell hemagglutination inhibition immuno-assay.
TRCV Total red cell volume.
TRD Therapy-related disease (see TRI); Thrombogenic rhythm disorder; Tongue-retaining device; Traction retinal detachment.
TRDN Transient respiratory distress of the newborn.
TRE Thymic reticuloendothelial (cell); Treatment-related effect (see TRUE); True radiation emission.
TREA Thoroughness, Reliability, Efficiency, and Analytic ability; Triethanolamine.
Tread Treadmill.
Treat; treat Treatment (see Trt).
Tren Trendelenburg (see Trend).
TREND Trial on Reversing Endothelial Dysfunction (study).
Trend Trendelenburg (position) (= Tren; TRND).
Trep Treponema (see T - Treponema).
TRF T-cell replacing factor; Terminal renal failure (see ESRD; ESRF; TKF); Thyrotropin-releasing factor (= Thyroid stimulating hormone releasing factor) (see Hormones - TRH); Transient risk factor; Tubular rejection fraction.
TRFC Total (sheep erythrocyte) rosette-forming cell(s).
TRG Tibial resection guide (Orthopedic Implants); Triglyceride(s) (= Trg; trg; TRIG; trig).
Trg; trg Training (see Train); Triglyceride(s) (see TRG).
TRH Tension-reducing hypothesis; Thyrotropin-releasing hormone (see Hormones - TRH).
TRH-ST Thyrotropin-releasing hormone stimulation test.
TRI Tetrazolium reduction inhibition; Therapy-related illness (= TRD); Thyroid Research Institute; Total response index (psychology); Touch Research Institute (anti-stress, massage program - Univ. of Miami, Florida); Toxic (Chemical) Release Inventory; Transplant-related illness/ infection; Tubuloreticular inclusion.
tri tricentric; trimester.
T_3RIA; T_3(RIA) Triiodothyronine radioimmunoassay.
T_4RIA; T_4(RIA) Thyroxine/ Tetraiodothyronine radioimmunoassay.
TRIAC Triiodothyroacetic acid.
Triazol 156 4-cyclohexyl 3-ethyl 1-2-4 triazol - a compound used as a convulsant in the treatment of schizophrenia.
TRIC; TrIC Trachoma-inclusion conjunctivitis (agent[s]) - a group of microorganisms, now classified under the genus Chlamydia.
TRICB Trichlorobiphenyl.
Trich Trichomonas (see T - Trichomonas).
trich- combining form meaning hair (Gr. trichos).
Trid; trid Three days (L. triduum).

TRIDEX 3-D time sequence radiography.
TRIG Triglyceride(s) (see TRG).
trig trigger; triglyceride(s) (see TRG); trigonum.
TRIM Thrombin Inhibition in Myocardial Ischmemia (substudy).
TRIMIS Tri-Service Medical Information System.
trip triplicate/ation.
trip- combining form meaning rub (Gr. tribo).
-tripsy suffix meaning crush (Gr. tripsis).
TRIS Trometamol (= Tris-hydroxymethyl-amino methane) (see THAM).
TRISS Trauma and Injury Severity Score.
TRIT; TrIT Triiodothyronine.
Trit Tritium.
trit triturate (grind) (L. tritura).
TRITC Tetrarhodamine isothiocyanate.
TRJ Therapeutic Recreation Journal.
TRK Roche Products Ltd (England) code for experimental substances; Transketolase.
Trk; trk Turkey.
TRL Triglyceride-rich lipoprotein (see CETRL).
TRLP Triglyceride-rich lipoprotein.
TRM Treatment-related moniliasis/ mortality.
TRMC Tetra/Tri methylrhodamino-isothiocyanate.
TRML; Trml Terminal.
TRM-SMX; TRM-SMZ Trimethoprim-sulfamethoxazole (see TMP-SMX; TMP-SMZ).
TRN Tegmental reticular nucleus.
tRNA Transfer ribonucleic acid.
TRND Trendelenburg (see Trend).
TRO Tissue reflectance oximetry; To return to office.
troc a lozenge (see troch).
TROCA Tangible reinforcement response orientation.
troch a lozenge, medicated tablet, or troche (Gr. trochos; L. trochiscus).
Trop; trop Tropical.
trop- combining form meaning react or turn (Gr.).
troph- combining form meaning nourish (Gr.).
tropi- combining form meaning change or turn (Gr. tropikos).
Trop Med Tropical Medicine.
TRP Test-result privacy; Tibial relocation plate (Orthopedic Implants); Total refractory period; Trichorhinophalangeal (syndrome); Tubular reabsorption of phosphate (see KFT).
Trp Tryptophan (see Tryp).
TRPA Tryptophan-rich prealbumin.
TRPD Toxicology Research Projects Directory (SSIE).
TrPl Treatment plan.
TRPS Trichorhinophalangeal syndrome.
TRPT Theoretical renal phosphate/ phosphorus threshold.
TRP Type I Tricho-rhino-phalangeal (syndrome) - type 1 (distinct facies with pear-shaped nose, fusinform proximal IP joints - an autosomal dominant, ectodermal dysplasia).
TRP Type II Tricho-rhino-phalangeal (syndrome) - type 2 (bulbous nose, thin upper lip, large protruding ears, exostoses, loose skin, etc. / sporadic inheritance of ectodermal dysplasia) (= LG - Langer-Giedion [syndrome]).
TRR Time-response relationship; Total respiratory resistance.
TRS Technamatic Radiology System; Therapeutic Recreation Specialist; Thyrotropin-receptor sequence(s); Total reduced sulfur; Total reducing sugars; Tubular renal secretion/ system (see RTS); Tubuloreticular structure; Tumor-related sign/ symptom.
TrS Trauma(tic) surgery.
TRSTMH Transactions of the Royal Society of Tropical Medicine and Hygiene (journal).
TRSV Tobacco ringspot virus.
TRT Testosterone/ Thyroid/ Thyroxine-replacement therapy; Thermoradiotherapy; Thoracic radiotherapy; Total reading time; Treatment (see Trt); Tumor radiation therapy (see RSP).
Trt; trt Treatment (= Tmt; tmt; Tr; tr; Treat; treat; TRT).
TRU Turbidity-reducing unit (= TR unit).
T_3RU Triiodothyronine resin uptake (laboratory/ endocrinology).
TRUE Treatment-related undesirable effect(s).
TR unit Turbidity-reducing unit (see TRU).
TRUS Transrectal ultrasonography.
TRUSP Transrectal ultrasound of the prostate.
Trustee (American Hospital Association jour-

nal).

TRV Tobacco rattle virus; Treatment-related vaginitis/(nosis)/ vulvovaginitis/(nosis) (see TRM).

Try; Tryp Tryptophan (= Trp).

Trx; trx Traction (see Tract).

TRZ Triazolam.

TS Tay-Sachs (disease/ syndrome); Technical Survey (journal); Temperature-sensitive; Temperature sensitivity; Temperature, skin (see Ts); Temporal stem; Tensile/ Triple strength; Teratology Society; Terminal sensation; Test solution; Thermal stability; Thoracic surgery; Thymidylate synthetase (enzyme, in DNA synthesis); Thyroid scanning; Time sharing (computer); Time-span; Tissue space; Today's Surgery (journal); Toe signs; Total solids (in urine); Tourette/ Toxic/ Turner syndrome; Toxic substance; Tracheal/ Tubular sound; Training school; Transferrin saturation (blood measurement; iron status) (= Serum iron/ IBC - Iron binding capacity) (see IS); Transitional sleep; Transplantation Society; Transsexual; Transverse section/ sinus; Traube's space (bounded by the left hepatic lobe, the left lung and the spleen); Trauma/ Treadmill score; Trendelenberg's sign; Trichostasis spinulosa; Tricuspid stenosis; Triple sugar (glucose, lactose, and sucrose); Tropical sprue; Trypticase soy (plate); T supressor (cell) (see Ts); Tuberous sclerosis; Tumor-/ Type-specific.

TS# Tibial shaft fracture (see TSF).

Ts Skin temperature (= TS); "Suppressor" T-cell (cell-mediated) lymphocyte, a CD 8 subset positive cell, taking part in the immunoregulation of autoimmune and other diseases. It carries the CD 8 protein within its surface membrane, and recognizes foreign antigen in association with HLA class I molecules (see Tc, Td and Th); Testosterone; Tosylate.

tS time required to complete the S phase of the cell cycle.

ts teaspoon(full) (see Tsp).

T_s Skin temperature (see Ts); T-cell suppressor (see Ts).

T-S Tay-Sachs (disease) (= TS; TSD).

T/S Thyroid/serum (ratio of radioiodine).

T + S Type and screen.

TSA Technical surgical assistance; Test of syntactic ability; Thyroid stimulating activity; Thyroxine-specific activity (see T4SA); Toluene sulfonic acid (test); Topical surface anesthetic; Total shoulder arthroplasty; Total systemic availability; Toxic shock antigen; Transcortical sensory aphasia; Trypticase-soy agar; Tumor-specific/ surface antigen; Type-specific antibody.

T_4SA Thyroxine-specific activity (= TSA).

TSAA Tissue-specific antioxidant action.

TSAb Thyroid-stimulating antibody.

TSAD Triscaphe arthrodesis (fusion of three bones at the wrist, including the scaphoid).

TSAG Trivalent sodium antimony gluconate.

TSAH Traumatic subarachnoid hemorrhage (= TSH).

Ts and Blues A mixture of Talwin (= pentozacine), a morphine-like pain-killing drug, and the blue antihistamine tablet Pyribenzamine, recently used as a cheap and artificial substitute to heroin. Quickly causes a heroin-like dependency. Used by addicts in the form of injections prepared from tablets. Frequently gives rise to seizures, strokes, and brain damage. This relatively new habit is especially prevalent in the big cities of the US such as New Orleans, Chicago and Detroit, etc.

TSAP Toxic-shock-associated protein.

Tsaph Temperature (of blood) in the saphenous vein.

TSAR Theophylline serum concentration.

TSAS Total severity assessment score.

TSAT Tube slide agglutination test.

TSB Total serum bilirubin; Transfer sliding board (for the immobilized patient); Trypticase/ Tryptone soy broth.

TSBA Total serum bile acids.

TSBB Transtracheal selective bronchial brushing.

TSC Technetium sulfur colloid; Thiosemicarbazide; Total static compliance; Transverse spinal sclerosis.

TSCA Toxic Substances Control Act.

TSCB Technetium sulfur colloid bleeding (study) - a radionuclide scan for gastrointestinal bleeding.

TSCS Tennessee Self-Concept Scale.
TSD Target-skin distance (X-rays); "Target stop date" (e.g. for total cessation of smoking); Tay-Sachs disease (see T-S); Tennessee School for the Deaf; Theory of signal detectability/ detection; Trans-synaptic degeneration.
TSE Tangent screen exam (for examining the central visual field); Testicular self-examination; Total skin examination; Total systemic exposure; Toxic side effect(s); Transmissible spongiform encephalopathy (a devastating prion-activated illness such as CJD or Creutzfeldt-Jakob disease); Transsphenoidal exploration; Trisodium edetate; Turbo spin echo (see MRT).
TSEB Total skin electron beam.
TSEC Taft Sanitary Engineering Center.
T sect Transverse (cross) section.
TSEM Transmission scanning electron microscope/py.
TSES Target Symptom Evaluation Scale.
T-set Tracheotomy set.
TSF Testicular feminization syndrome; Thrombopoiesis/etic/ stimulating factor; Thyroid-stimulating factor (an IgG antibody) (see TSAb); Tibial shaft fracture (= TS#); Total systemic flow; Triceps skinfold.
TSG Tumor-suppressing/ suppressor gene (a cancer-related, anti-oncogene e.g. pRB {retinoblastoma} and p53 proteins); Tumor-specific glycoprotein (see TSGP).
TSGP Tumor-specific glycoprotein (= TSG).
TSH Thyroid-stimulating hormone (thyrotropin) (see Hormones - TSH; TTH); Transient synovitis of the hip; Traumatic subarachnoid hemorrhage (see TSAH).
Ts-H43 Mutant strain of Mycoplasma pneumoniae.
TSHR Thyroid-stimulating hormone-receptor/ releasing (antibody, factor, hormone, mutant, etc.).
TSHRF; TSH-RF Thyroid-stimulating hormone-releasing factor (see Hormones - TSHRF).
TSH-RH Thyroid-stimulating hormone-releasing hormone (see Hs - TSH-RH).
TSI Telesensory Systems Inc. (devices for the blind); Thyroid stimulating immunoglobulin; Total serum iron; Transferrin saturation index (= Serum iron/ Iron binding capacity); Triple sugar iron (glucose, lactose and sucrose sugar iron agar) (= TSIA).
TSIA Total small intestine allotransplant(ation); Triple sugar iron agar (see TSI).
tSIDS Totally unexplained sudden infant death syndrome.
TSIg Thyroid-stimulating immunoglobulin.
TSIM Trimethylsilyl imidazole.
TSJ Trans-species jump (of viruses).
TSL Terminal sensory latency; Toxic Substances List (PHS).
TSM Type-specific M (protein).
TSN Tryptophan peptone sulfide neomycin (agar).
TSNS Ten State Nutrition Survey (HEW).
TSO Thoracic surgical oncology.
TSP Technical Support Package (NASA); Thrombin-sensitive protein; Tobacco-smoke pollution; Totally synthetic progestogen (e.g. levonorgestrel) - used as an emergency contraceptive in preventing fertilization or ovulation; also in inhibiting implantation by altering the endometrium); Total serum protein; Total suspended particulate; Transsulfuration pathway; Trisodium phosphate; Tropical spastic paraparesis (a neurological manifestation of adult T cell leukemia) (see HTLV1); Tumor suppressor protein.
Tsp Teaspoon(ful) (= ts; tsp).
tsp teaspoon(ful) (see Tsp).
TSPA Thiotepa (see TESPA).
TSPAP Total serum prostatic acid phosphatase.
TSPP Tetrasodium pyrophosphate.
TSR Temperature-sensitive resistor; Testosterone sterilized (female) rat; Theophylline sustained release; Thyroid/serum ratio (= T/S ratio); Total shoulder replacement; Total systemic resistance; Transsphenoidal resection (of a pituitary tumor).
T/S ratio Thyroid/serum ratio (see TSR).
TSRI The Scripps Research Institute (La Jolla, California).
TSS Tone-shock system (fear conditioning of the amygdala); Total severity score; Total

shoulder system (Neer II - Orthopedic Implants); Total suspended solids; Toxic shock syndrome (= Tampon shock syndrome) - a rare but sometimes fatal bacteria-related disorder affecting menstruating women (a staphylococcal toxemia), caused by introduction of the bacterium into the vagina by insertion of the absorbent pluglike hygienic device, the vaginal tampon, during the menstrual period; Transsphenoidal surgeon (see TSR); Tropical splenomegaly syndrome; Tuberculin skin sensitivity; Tubigrip support stocking (used in leg fractures, etc.) (Seton, Oldham, UK) (Orthopedics).

TSSA Tumor-specific cell surface antigen.

TSSE Toxic shock syndrome exotoxin.

TSSGA Transactions of the Southern Surgical and Gynecological Association (journal).

TSST Toxic shock syndrome toxin.

TSSU Theater sterile supply unit.

TST Thromboplastin screening test; Titmus stereocuity test; Titmus stereotest (= sTt - see DPT - Depth perception test); Topical skin therapeutic; Topical steroidal therapy/ treatment; Total sleep time; Transferrin saturation test (of blood - for hemochromatosis); Transient symptomatic therapy; Trans-scrotal testosterone; Treadmill stress test (= TT); Triple sugar (iron) test; Tuberculin/ Tumor skin test; Two-sided test.

TSTA Toxoplasmin skin test antigen; Tumor-specific tissue/ transplantation antigen.

TSU Tissue sugar urea (agar).

T_3SU Triiodothyronine serum uptake (laboratory/ endocrinology).

TSV 'Top-shelf' vertigo (with tilting of the head, and looking up and/ or down) (see BPPV; BPV); Total stomach volume.

TSY Trypticase soy yeast.

TT Tablet triturate; Tactile/ Twitch tension; Talking task; Tendon transfer; Terminal (deoxynucleotidyl) transferase; Testtube; Tetanus toxin/ toxoid; Tetrathionate (culture broth); Tetrazol; Thrombin/ Total/ Treadmill/ Turnover time; Thymol turbidity; Thyrotropin (see Hormones - TTH); Tibial tubercle; Tick typhus (= Fievre boutonneuse or Spotted fever - caused by *Rickettsia* conori and transmitted by ticks) (see SF - Spotted fever); Tilt table; Tine/ Token/ Tolerance/ Tuberculin test; Tonometry; Tooth treatment; Total thyroxine (see TT4); Toxomycosis titer; Tranquillity tank (a water tank, darkened and soundproof, for relaxing mental and physical tensions); Transient tachypnea; Transferred to; Transit time (of blood through the heart and lungs) (see MTT); Transthoracic; Transtracheal; Treadmill test (see TST); Tuberculin tested (milk); Tube thoracostomy; Tumor thrombus; Twenty Twenty (journal); Tzanck test (for diagnosis of herpes virus infections).

TT# Torsional tibial fracture (see TTF).

T/T Trace of ... /trace of ...

T&T Time and temperature; Tobramycin and ticarcillin; Touch and tone.

TT_2 Total diiodothyronine.

TT_3 Total triiodothyronine.

TT_4 Total thyroxine (= TT).

TTA Tetanus Toxoid Adsorbed (USP); Tetanus toxoid antibody; Timed therapeutic absence; Total toe arthroplasty; Transtrochanteric approach (hip surgery); Transtracheal aspirate/tion.

TTAP Threaded titanium acetabular prosthesis.

TTB Test-tube baby; Tetanus toxoid booster.

T_4TBP Thyroxine bound to protein.

TTC Thyrotoxic crisis; Toilet-trained child(ren); Trichloro-compound(s); Triphenyltetrazolium chloride (see TPTZ); T-tube cholangiogram.

TTCP Thrombotic thrombocytopenic purpura (see TTP).

TTC test See TPTZ.

TTD Tablet-treated diabetes/tic; Temporary total disability; Tetraethylthiuram disulfide (= Antabuse; Disulfiram; Ethyldithiourame) - a drug used in the treatment of chronic alcoholism; the ingestion of alcohol, even in small quantities, evokes an extremely unpleasant syndrome of systemic reactions in patients taking this drug, with flushing of the face, injection of the conjunctiva, sensation of heat, throbbing headache, accelerated pulse, and severe giddiness, which with larger doses of alcohol (in excess of 50 ml), may cause nausea, vomiting, sweating, accelerated and deepened respiration, a marked fall of blood-pressure, and collapse; Thiazide-type diuretic; Tissue tolerance dose; Transient tic disorder; Transverse thoracic diameter; Trichothiodystrophy; Trousseau tracheal dilator; Typical tennis elbow (see PINL).

TTE Time-to-event (see TTEA; TTED); Transient toxic effect; Typical tennis elbow (see PINL) (Orthopedics).

TTEA Time-to-event analysis.

TTED Time-to-event data.

TTF Tetrathiofulvalene; Time to treatment failure; Torsional tibial fracture (= TT#).

TTFD Thiamine tetrahydrofurfuryl disulfide.

TTG Tellurite, taurocholate, and gelatin; Third trimester of gestation.

TTGA Tellurite, taurocholate, and gelatin agar.

TTH Tension-type headache; Thyrotropic hormone (see Hormones - TTH); Tritiated thymidine (see TTh).

TTh Tritiated thymidine (= TTH).

TTI Tension-time/ Time-tension index; Transthoracic impedance; Transtracheal insufflation; Traumatic tension ischemia (of muscle and nerve) (Orthopedics).

TTJ Tibiotalar joint.

TTL Total thymus lymphocytes; Transistor-transistor logic; Troponin T level (see TTT).

TTLC True total lung capacity.

TTLD Terminal transverse limb defect.

TT leprosy Tuberculoid leprosy (caused by *Mycobacterium* leprae).

TTN Transient tachypnea of the newborn; Trichotillomania.

TTNA Transthoracic needle aspiration.

TTNB Transient tachypnea of the newborn (= TTN); Transthoracic needle biopsy.

TTO To take out; Transtracheal oxygen.

TTOD Tetanus toxoid outdated.

TTOT Transtracheal oxygen therapy.

T toxoid Tetanus toxoid.

TTP Third trimester of pregnancy (see LTP); Thrombotic thrombocytopenic purpura; Thymidine triphosphate; Time to peak.

TtP Trough-to-peak (ratio).

TTP; TtP Time to progression.

TTPA Tissue-type plasminogen activator; Triethylene thiophosphoramide.

TTR Therapeutic/Toxic ratio (= T/T ratio); Thyrotropin receptor; Transthoracic resistance; Transthyretin; Triceps tendon reflex; Triple therapy regimen (for *Helicobacter* pylori-associated PUD); Type/token ratio (= T/T ratio).

T/T ratio Therapeutic/Toxic ratio (see TTR); Type/token ratio (see TTR).

TTS Tarsal tunnel syndrome; Technetium tetracycline scan; Temporary threshold shift; Tetanus toxoid series (= FTS); Through the skin; Tilt table standing; Transdermal therapeutic system; Triple-therapy study (e.g. the use of azothioprine, corticosteroids, and cyclosporine in preventing acute organ transplant rejection); Twin transfusion syndrome.

TTT Taxoid/ Trastuzumab therapy (Cytotoxic, Herceptin therapy, used in the treatment ofmetastatic breast cancer); Thymol turbidity test (see LFT iv); Tilt table test (for cardiac function); Tolbutamide tolerance test; Total twitch time; Troponin T test (blood troponin T {more than 0.2 μg/l}, a marker of myocardial damage associated with MI); Tuberculin time test.

TTTS Twin-twin transfusion syndrome (Obstetrics).

TTTT Test tube turbidity test.

TTUTD Tetanus toxoid up-to-date.

TTV Tracheal transport velocity; Traditional tidal volume (ventilation in ALI & ARDS) (see LTV); Transfusion-transmitted virus; Tubovesicular typhoid vaccine (= TV).

TTVP Temporary transvenous pacemaker.

TTWB Touch toe weight bearing.

TTX Tetrodotoxin (highly lethal).

TU Thiouracil; Thyroid(al) uptake; Todd/ Toxic/ Toxin/ Transmission/ Tuberculin/ Turbidity unit; Transrectal ultrasound; Transurethral.

Tu Thulium (former chemical symbol, now abbreviated: Tm) (see Elements - Thulium); Tumor.

tu tuberculin unit (see TU).

T_3U Triiodothyronine uptake (resin sponge uptake).

Tu 1/2 Time required to excrete half of an injected substance in the urine.

TUA Transurethral absorption.

tuber- combining form meaning swelling (L.).

Tuberc Tubercle (BTA journal); Tuberculosis.

Tuberculin a sterile liquid containing the growth products of, or the specific substances from, the tubercle bacillus (= TB).
Tuberculins include:
AF: Albumose-free (tuberculin) (see Tuberculin - AFT).
AFT: Albumose-free tuberculin (= AF; TAF).
AT: Alkaline tuberculin (= TA).
BE: Bacillen emulsion (tuberculin) (see Tuberculin - BET).
BET: Bacillen emulsion tuberculin (= BE; TBE; TBN).
BF: Bouillon filtrate (tuberculin) (see Tuberculin - BFT).
BFT: Bouillon filtrate tuberculin (= BF; Denys' tuberculin).
HOT: Human old tuberculin (see Tuberculin - TO).
OT: Old tuberculin (= Tuberculinum pristinum) (see Tuberculin - TO).
PPD: Purified protein derivative (= Seibert's tuberculin).
PTO: Perisucht Tuberculin Original (Ger) (= Klemperer's tuberculin; Spengler's tuberculin).
TA: Alkaline tuberculin (see Tuberculin - AT).
TAF: Albumose-free tuberculin (see Tuberculin - AFT).
TB: Tuberculin.
TBE: Tuberculin bacillen emulsion (see Tuberculin - BET).
TBN: Tuberculin bacillen (emulsion) (see Tuberculin - BET).
TC: Tuberculin contagious (= Tuberculase; Tulase) (see Tuberculin - TX).
TF: Tuberculin filtrate.
TGl: Tuberculin globulin (in 10% salt solution).
TO: Tuberculin - original (Ger. alt) (= Koch's tuberculin; Human old tuberculin (HOT); Old tuberculin (OT); Original tuberculin; Supernatant tuberculin (Ger. Tuberculin Ober); Tuberculin-original-alt (TOA); Tuberculin ober (Ger.); Tuberculin oristinum.
TOA: Tuberculin-original-alt (Ger.) (see Tuberculin - TO).
TOT: A purified tuberculin used intradermally as a test for tuberculosis.
TP: Tuberculin precipitation (= Calmette's tuberculin; Purified tuberculin; Tuberculin precipitate).
TPT: Total protein tuberculin.
TR: Tuberculin residue (= Koch's tuberculin; New tuberculin; Rückstandtuberculin; Tuberculin residuum).
TV: Tuberculin volutin - a principle believed to exist in tubercle bacilli.
TX: von Behring's tuberculin (a derivative of Tuberculin contagious) (= TC).
TZ; Tz: Tubercle zymoplastische - the dried residue of the portions of the tubercle bacilli which are soluble in alcohol.

TUC Transitional urothelial cell (= "decoy cell") - found in urine of renal allograft patients with BK virus infection.

TUD Total urethral discharge.

TUDS Transurethral delivery system.

Tues Tuesday.

TUF Total ultrafiltration; Transurethral fulguration.

TUG Total urinary gonadotropin.

TUH Temple University Hospital (Philadelphia, Pennsylvania).

TUI Transurethral incision.

TUN Total urinary nitrogen.

TUNA Transurethral Needle Ablation (operation for BPH).

TUP Tranurethral prostactectomy (= TUPR; TUR; TURP).

TUPR Transurethral prostatic resection (see TURP).

T_3 uptake Triiodothyronine uptake.

T_4 uptake Thyroxine uptake.

TUR Transurethral resection (of prostate) (see TURP).

T_3 UR Triiodothyronine uptake ratio.

TURB Transurethral resection of bladder (tumor) (see TURBT).

turb turbid(ity).

TURBN Transurethral resection of the bladder neck.

TURBT Transurethral resection of bladder tumor (= TURB).

TURP Transurethral prostatectomy/ resection of the prostate (= TUR).

Turp Turpentine.

TURS Transurethral resection syndrome.
TURV Transurethral resection of valves.
TUS Therapeutic ultrasound; Transurethral suppository/ system.
tus; tuss cough (L. tussis).
TUSM Temple/ Tufts' University School of Medicine.
TUSRI Transperineal ultrasound-guided radioactive implant (= Brachytherapy see LRPB).
TUU Transurethroureterostomy.
TV Talipes varus; Television; Temporary visit; Terminal velocity; Tetrazolium violet (histological stain) (= VT); Thoracic/ True vertebra; Tickborne virus; Tidal/ Total volume (PFT); Toxic vertigo; Transvenous; Transverse; Transvestite; Trial visit; Trichomonas vaginalis (see Tv); Tricuspid valve; Trivalent; Truncal vagotomy; Tuberculin volutin (see Tuberculin - TV); Tubovesicular (typhoid) vaccine (see TTV).
Tv Trichomonas vaginalis (= TV).
T/V Touch - verbal.
TVA Tennessee Valley Authority; Thalidomide Victims Association (of Canada); Tricuspid valve anuloplasty (Cardiovascular surgery); Truncal vagotomy and/with antrectomy.
TVBD Trabecular vertebral bone density (see VBD).
TVC Timed vital capacity (PFT); Tinea versicolor (see PVC); Total viable cells; Total volume capacity (PFT); Transvaginal cone; Triple voiding cystogram (procedure/ urology); True vocal cords.
TVCD Triple vessel coronary disease (= TVD).
TVCT Timed vital capacity test (= VG) (see PFT).
TVD Transmissible virus dementia; Transthoracic ventricular defibrillation (see SMS; TBS); Transient visual disturbance(s); Triple vessel disease; Tropical venereal disease.
TVDALV Triple vessel disease with an abnormal left ventricle.
TVF Tactile vocal fremitus; Transient ventricular fibrillation (see TDP).
TVG Time-varied gain.
TVH Total vaginal hysterectomy; Turkey virus hepatitis.
TVI Transvaginal injection.
TVL Tenth-value layer (shielding from radiation); Transitory visual loss; Tunica vasculosa lentis.
TVM Tropical Veterinary Medicine.
TVN Tonic vibration response.
TVP Tensor veli palatini (muscle); Test of Visual Perception (assessing eye-motor coordination, figure ground perception, etc.); Textured vegetable protein; Transvenous pacemaker; Transvesicle prostatectomy; Tricuspid valve prolapse/ prothesis; Truncal vagotomy and/with pyloroplasty.
TVR Target-vessel revascularization (in acute myocardial infarction/ ischemia, coronary sclerosis, etc.); Tonic vibratory reflex; Total vascular resistance; Transvaginal route; Tricuspid valve replacement.
TV-R Television or radio.
TVRVV Tetravalent rotavirus vaccine (for prevention, control, and treatment of Traveler's diarrhea).
TVS Transvaginal scan(ning) (of the endometrium) (Obs/Gyn); Transvaginal sonogram/aph(y) (see TVUS).
TVSC Transvaginal sector scan.
TVSS Tactile Vision Substitution System; Transient voltage surge suppressor.
TVSI Transvaginal sonographic image.
TVT Transmissible venereal tumor; Transvaginal transducer (Gynecology/ Obstetrics); Tunica vaginalis testis.
TVU Total volume of urine (in 24 hours); Transvaginal ultrasonography (see TVUS).
TVUS Transvaginal ultrasonogram/graph(y)/ ultrasound.
TVV Total venous volume.
TW Tandem walking (in neurological examination); Tap water; Terminal web; Test weight; Total washout/ water/ weight (see TBW).
Tw Twist.
TWA Time-weighted average.
T_{WB} Wet bulb temperature.
TWBC Total white blood cells/ count.
TWD Thrice/ Twice-weekly dose; Total white and differential (cell count); Tracheal wall defect.

TWE Tap/ Tepid water enema.
Tween 80 Polysorbate 80.
Twenty-five LSD-25 (see LSD).
TWETC Tapwater enema till clear.
TWG Total weight gain.
TWHW ok Toe walking and heel walking all right.
Twist Marijuana (see Cannabis).
TWL Transepidermal water loss.
TWN Thin-walled needle (Cardiac catheterization).
TWR Total wrist replacement; Two-way radio.
TWS Tranquilizer withdrawal syndrome.
TWs Triphasic waves.
TWSb Antimony dimercaptosuccinate (= Friedheim's TWSb; Sulphantimon) - potassium salt, i.e. antimony potassium dimercaptosuccinate, a trivalent antimony compound used in the treatment of schistosomiasis.
TWSb/1 Antimony magnesium dimercaptosuccinate - used as in TWSb (see TWSb).
TWSb/6 Stibocaptate (= Antimony sodium dimercaptosuccinate) (see Ro4-1544/6).
TWT Travelling wave tube.
TWWD Tap water wet dressing.
TWX Teletype wire exchange (= Teletypewriter exchange service - AT&T).
TX Thromboxane; Thyroidectomized; Transplant(ation)/(ed) (see Transpl); Treatment (see Tx); von Behring's tuberculin (within cells of body - a derivative of contagious tuberculin) (see Tuberculin - TX).
Tx; T_x A derivative of contagious tuberculin (see Tuberculin - TX); Radioactive thyreoidin; Therapy; Traction (orthopedics) (= tx); Transfusion; Treatment (= TX); Tympanostomy.
tx traction (see Tx).
T&X Type and crossmatch (see T&C).
TXA; TxA Thromboxane A.
TXA2; TXA_2; TxA_2 Thromboxane A2 (A_2) - a powerful vasoconstrictor and prostaglandin, promoting platelet aggregation.
TXB2; TXB_2; TxB_2 Thromboxane B2 (B_2).
TXDS; TxDs Qualifying toxic dose (TSL - Toxic Substances List).
TXM Type and crossmatch (see T&C); T cell crossmatch.
Ty Type; Typhoid; Tyrosine (see Tyr).
TYCO #3 Tylenol with 30 mg codeine (see T&C #3).
Tyl Tylenol; Tyloma (callus).
Tymp Tympanic; Typanicity/any (with reference to auscultation of the abdomen/ chest); Tympanogram; Tympanum.
TympMemb Tympanic membrane.
TYMV Turnip yellow mosaic virus.
typ typical.
typ- combining form meaning type (Gr. typos).
Type 1 DM 'Juvenile' onset diabetes mellitus (see HDM; IDDM).
Type 2 DM 'Maturity' onset diabetes mellitus (see NIDDM).
Type IV HS Type IV hypersensitivity (see CHSR; CMIR).
typh- combining form meaning stupor (Gr. typhos).
typhl- combining form meaning cecum (Gr. typhlon), or blind (Gr. typhlos).
Tyr Tyrosine (= Ty).
TyRIA Thyroid radioisotope assay.
TYRs Traditional Yemenite remedies (used especially by elderly Jewish immigrants to Israel, such as: Amulets, Branding, Cupping, Foods rubbed into the skin, Henna applications, Herb ingestion, Herbal applications, Incantations, Massage, Scarification, etc.).
TZ; Tz Transition zone; Tuberculin zymoplastische (Ger.) - Zymoplastic tuberculin (the dried residue which is soluble in alcohol) (see Tuberculin - TZ).
TZn; Tzn Total estrogens after zinc treatment (i.e. Zn - HCl).
TZP Trizygotic pregnancy.

U

U Congenital limb absence; Eaton Laboratories (USA) and the Upjohn Co. (USA) code for experimental substances; Excretion; Hemolytic assay unit (whole complement); Internal energy; International Unit of enzyme activity; Mann-Whitney rank sum statistic; Part of ECG wave (an undulating deflection that follows the T wave); Potential difference (in volts); Ulcer; Ulna(r); Ultralente (insulin); Umbilicus; Uncertain; Uncle; Unerupted (tooth); Unit (= u) (in lab reports); Unitarian; Universalist; University; Unknown; Upper (= u); Uptake; Uracil; Uranium (Z = 92) (see Elements - Uranium); Urea; Ureter; Urethra; Uridine; Uridylic acid; Urinary concentration; Urine; Urologist/gy; Uterine/rus; U-virus (antigenetically related to the ECHO virus); Uvula; Vitamin U - antiulcer factor (see Vitamins - U); Volume velocity (= u).

u to be used (L. utendus); unified atomic mass unit; unit(s) (see U); upper (see U); velocity (see U).

υ Greek lower case letter "upsilon" - also "ypsilon" (see Symbols - 4).

Υ Greek capital letter "upsilon" - also "ypsilon".

U/ At umbilicus (level of).

1/U One finger breadth above the umbilicus.

U/1 One finger breadth below the umbilicus.

U/2 Upper half.

U/3 Upper third (with reference to long bones).

U_{24} 24-hour uptake.

U-235; U^{235}; ^{235}U Radioactive uranium (fissionable isotope) (see Elements - Uranium).

U 935 Amiquinsin hydrochloride (a hypotensive agent).

1592U89 Original preclinical name for Abacavir, an anti-HIV drug, first employed in therapy in 1997.

U 2,043 Tolbutamide (see D 860; TOLB).

U 6,987 Carbutamide (see BZ 55).

U 8,344 Uramustine (= Uracil mustard) - an alkylating agent chiefly used in the treatment of chronic lymphocytic leukemia and the malignant lymphomas.

U 12,504 Azepinamide - a sulfonylurea compound, a chlorinated analogue of tolozamide (U 17,835). Has been tried clinically as a hypoglycemic agent, but a relatively high incidence of jaundice has followed its use.

U 17,312 E Etryptamine acetate - a non-hydrazine monoamine oxidase inhibitor formerly used in the treatment of depression.

U 17,835 Tolozamide - a sulfonylurea used in the oral treatment of diabetes mellitus of the adult, maturity-onset, or stable (B) type.

U 18,396 Sulfamoxole (= Sulfadimethyloxazole) - a long-acting sulfonamide that has been used in the treatment of various infections.

U 19,920 A Cytarabine hydrochloride (= Cytosine arabinoside HCl) - an antiviral agent suggested for use in the topical treatment of herpes keratitis. It has also been reported to have antineoplastic properties.

UA Ultra-audible; Ultrasonic arteriography; Umbilical artery; Unaggregated; Unauthorized absence; Uncertain about; Unit of analysis; Unstable angina; Upper airways/ arm; Uric (see U/A; KFT)/ Uridylic/ Uronic acid; Urinalysis (see U/A; KFT); Urinary aldosterone; Urine aliquot; Uterine aspiration.

ua as far as/ up to (L. usque ad).

U/A Uric acid/ Urinalysis (= UA) (see KFT).

UAA Uniform Arbitration Act (malpractice legislation); Uridylyl-adenylyl-adenosine (A specific stop codon in the mRNA molecule, which determines the point of initiation of peptide chain synthesis) (see Codon; mRNA).

UAB University of Alabama - Birmingham (Medical Center).

UABF Umbilical artery blood flow (Obstetrics).

UABT Ultrasonic aspiration-biopsy transducer.

UAC Umbilical artery catheter; Under active; Upper airway congestion; Uterine aspiration curettage (Obstetrics and Gynecology).

UA/C Uric acid/ creatinine (ratio).

UACM University of Arizona College of Medicine.

UACR Urinary albumin/ candesartan ratio.

UAD Unipolar affective disorder (recurrent depressive disorder); Urinanalysis dip (test).
UADV Umbilical artery Doppler velocimetry (see DBFV).
UAE Unilateral absence of excretion; United Arab Emirates; Urinary/ne albumin excretion.
UAFV Umbilical artery flow velocity (see UAV).
UAG Universidad Autonomo de Guadalajara (University of Guadalajara, Mexico).
UAGA Uniform Anatomical Gift Act.
UAI Uncomplicated acute illness; Unprotected anal intercourse; Uterine activity interval.
U/Air Ultrasonic nebulization (air) therapy.
UAIT Uricosuric anti-inflammatory therapy/ treatment (for gout or hyperuricemia).
UAL Umbilical artery line; Up ad lib.
UAMC University of Alabama Medical Center.
U-AMY Urinary amylase.
UAN Uric acid nephropathy (see UANP)/ nitrogen (see KFT).
UANP Uric acid nephropathy.
UAO Upper airway obstruction; Uric acid output.
UAP Union of American Physicians; Unstable angina pectoris; Urinary acid/ alkaline phosphatase.
UAPF Upon arrival patient found.
UAR Upper abdominal region; Upper airway resistance; Uric acid riboside.
UAREP Universities Associated for Research and Education in Pathology (AFIP).
UARS Upper-airway resistance syndrome.
UAS Upper abdominal surgery; Upper airway symptoms; Upstream activation site; Uric acid synthesis.
UAT Up as tolerated; Upper alimentary tract (see UGIT).
UATLD Union Against Tuberculosis and Lung Disease (WHO).
UAU Uterine activity unit.
UAV Umbilical artery velocimetry (Obstetrics).
UAVC Univentricular atrioventricular connection.
UAW United Auto Workers.
UB Ultimobranchial (body)/ body; Unna boot; Upper back; Urinary bladder; Urine bilirubin (see LFT iv).
UB 82 Universal billing document (1982).
UBA Undenatured bacterial antigen.
UBB Upper body brace.
UBBC Unbound/ Unsaturated vitamin B_{12} binding capacity.
$UB_{12}BC$ Unbound/ Unsaturated B_{12} binding capacity (= UBBC).
UBBST Universal blood and body substance technique.
UBC University of British Columbia (brace); Unsaturated binding capacity; Urinary bladder carcinoma.
UBD Urinary bladder disorder.
UBF Umbilical blood flow (see UABF); Unknown black female; Uterine blood flow.
UBG; Ubg Urobilinogen.
UBH Unhurried bowel habits.
UBI Ultraviolet blood irradiation.
UBIP Ubiquitous immunopoietic polypeptide.
UBL Undifferentiated B-cell lymphoma.
UBM Unformed bowel movement(s); Unknown black male.
UBN Urobilin.
UBP Upright blood pressure; Ureteral back pressure; Urinary bladder papilloma.
UBR Undersea Biomedical Research (UMS journal).
UBS Ultra-broad spectrum (antibiotic); Urinary bladder stone.
13UBT (Carbon-13) Urea breath test for urease activity by Helicobacter pylori, in cases of duodenal ulcer) (see also HUT).
UC Ulcerative colitis; Ultracentrifugal/ge; Umbilical cholesterol/ cord (blood); Unchanged; Unclassifiable/fied; Unconscious; Undercover (narcotics agent); Undifferentiated/ Untreated cells; Unit clerk; Unsatisfactory condition; Urea clearance (test) (see KFT; UCl; UV/P); Urethral and cervical (see U&C); Urethral catheter(ization); Urinary catheter; Urine concentrate/ culture (see KFT); Usual and customary (see U&C); Uterine contraction(s).
U/C UICC/Cincinnati classification of radiographs of the pneumoconioses.
U&C Urethral and cervical (= UC); Usual and customary (= UC).
UCA Uniform compound amount (factor)

(medical accounting).

UCAD Uncontrolled/ Unstable coronary artery disease.

UCAIR University of California Association of Interns and Residents.

UCAR Union Carbide (Corporation).

UCB Ultimate clinical benefit; Umbilical cord blood; Unconjugated bilirubin; University of California at Berkeley.

UCB 3,412 Dixyrazine - a phenothiazine compound used in the management of various psychiatric disorders characterized by anxiety, agitation and aggression.

UCB 4,445 Buclizine hydrochloride - a piperazine compound with antihistaminic properties. Used mainly as an anti-emetic, but also in the symptomatic treatment of allergic conditions and vertigo.

UCBC Umbilical cord blood culture.

UCC Umbilical cord complication(s) (major cause of fetal death); United Cancer Council; United Church of Canada (member); Universal Copyright Convention.

UCCR Upstate Center Cancer Registry (New York Upstate Medical Center).

UCD Uncontrolled/ Unrecognized/ Unstable cardiac/ coronary (see UCAD) disease; Urea cycle disorder; Urine collection device; Usual childhood disease(s) (= UCHD).

UCDPN Uniform Code on Dental Practitioners and Nomenclature.

UCD-SMC University of California (Davis) - Sacramento Medical Center.

UCE Umbilical cord entanglement (see UCC); Uncontrolled epilepsy; Urea cycle enzymopathy; Urinary citrate excretion.

UCF Uncompensated cardiac failure (= UHF).

UCG Ultrasonic cardiography; Urinary chorionic gonadotropin (see Hormones - HCG).

UCH Ubiquitin carboxy-terminal hydrolase L1 (a gene implicated in the pathogenesis of Parkinson's disease).

UCHD Usual childhood disease(s) (see UCD).

UCHS Uncontrolled hemorrhagic shock.

UCI Uganda Cancer Institute; Umbilical coiling index (Obstetrics); Umbilical cord insertion; University of California at Irvine; Unusual/ Usual childhood illness(es); Urethral/ Urinary catheter in.

UCL Ulnar/ Upper collateral ligament; Umbilical cord ligation (Obstetrics); Uncomfortable loudness level; University College London (UK); Upper confidence limit(s); Urea clearance (see UCl).

UCl Urea clearance (test) (= UC; UCL) (see KFT; UV/P).

UCLA University of California at Los Angeles.

UCLH University College London Hospital (UK).

UCLP Unilateral cleft lip and palate.

UCMS University of Chicago Medical School.

UCNA Urologic Clinics of North America (journal).

UCO Unilateral cryptorchidism; Urethral/ Urinary catheter out(put).

UCOD Underlying cause of death.

UCP Uncoupling protein; United Cerebral Palsy; Urethral closure pressure; Urinary coproporphyrin/ C-peptide.

UCPA United Cerebral Palsy Association.

UCPRF United Cerebral Palsy Research Foundation.

UCPT Urinary coproporphyrin test.

UCR Unconditioned response; Uniform capital recovery (factor) - medical accounting; Urologic and Cutaneous Review (journal); Usual, customary, and reasonable (fees).

UCre Urinary creatinine.

UCS Ultimate compressive strength (of bone - orthopedics); Unconditioned stimulus; Unconscious (see ucs); Uncontrolled clinical study; Urinary collecting system; Uterine compression syndrome.

ucs unconscious (= UCS).

UCSD University of California at San Diego.

UCSF University of California at San Francisco.

UCST Urinary catecholamine secretion test (for pheochromocytoma).

UCT Umbilical cord twist (see UCI); Urea clearance test (see KFT).

UCTD; uCTD Unclassifiable/ Undifferentiated connective tissue disease.

UCU Urinary care unit.

UCV Uncontrolled variable.

UCVD Underlying/ Undetected cardiovascular

disease.

UCX Urine culture.

UD Ulcerative dermatosis; Ulnar deviation; Underdeveloped; Undesirable/ Urethral discharge; Undetermined; Unit dose; Uridine diphosphate (= UDP); Urology Digest (journal); Uroporphyrinogen decarboxylase; Uterine delivery/ distension; Uterus didelphys (two distinct uteri in same person).

ud as directed (L. ut dictum).

UDA Upward dose adjustment.

UDC Underdeveloped countries/ry; Uniform donor card (human organs for transplant); Universal decimal code (books); Ureteral/ Urethral dilatation catheter; Usual diseases of childhood.

UDCA Ursodeoxycholic acid.

UDD Upper digestive disorder(s) (such as GERD).

UDM Uncompensated diabetes mellitus.

UDMH Unsymmetric dimethylhydrazine.

UDN Ulcerative dermal necrosis; Updraft nebulizer.

UDO Undetermined origin.

UDP Unit dose pouch (for transdermal patches); Uridine diphosphate (see UD).

UDPG Uridine diphosphate glucose/ diphosphoglucose.

UDPGA Uridine diphosphate glucuronic/ diphosphoglucuronic acid.

UDPGal Uridine diphosphate galactose/ diphosphogalactose.

UDPGlc Uridine diphosphate glucose/ diphosphoglucose.

UDPGT Uridine diphosphate glucoronosyl/nyl transferase.

UDR-BMD Ultradistal radius bone mineral density.

UDRP Uridine diribose phosphate.

UDS Ultra-Doppler sonography; Unconditioned stimulus; unreduced dislocation of the shoulder; Unscheduled deoxynucleic acid synthesis; Urinary drop spectrometer; Urinary drug screen (= BDZS; BZE).

UDT Underwater demolition; Urine dipstick test(ing).

UDU Unconfirmed/ Uncomplicated/ Undetected/ Undiagnosed duodenal ulcer.

UE Uncertain/ Undetermined/ Unknown etiology; Under elbow; Uninvolved epidermis; Upper esophagus; Upper extremity (= U/ext; U ext; u/ext); Uterine evacuation.

UEA United Epilepsy Association, Inc; Upper extremity, arterial; Uranium Enrichment Association.

UEE Upper extremity edema.

UEG Ultrasonic encephalography; Unifocal eosinophilic granuloma.

UEI Universal Environmental Instruments Co.

UEL Upper explosive limit.

UEM Universal electron microscope.

UEMC Unidentified endosteal marrow cell.

UEMS Union of European Medical Specialists.

UEP Union of Pedo-psychiatrists; Unruptured ectopic pregnancy; Uterine endometrial peristalsis (Obs/Gyn).

UER Uneventful recovery.

UES Unstable endogenic secretion (of hormones e.g. progesterone, etc.); Upper esophageal segment/ sphincter/ stricture (= UOS)/ sphincter; Upper-extremity support.

uE_s; u^{Es} Unconjugated estriol.

UESP Upper esophageal sphincter pressure.

UET Upper extremity trauma.

U/ext; U ext; u/ext Upper extremity (see UE).

UF Ultrafiltrate/ filtration; Ultrafine; Ultrasonic frequency; United Fund; Universal feeder; Unknown factor; Until finished (prescription); Urinary formaldehyde.

UFA Unesterified (free) fatty acid.

UFB Unidentified foreign body; Urinary fat bodies.

UFC Urinary free cortisol.

UFCM University of Florida College of Medicine.

UFCT Ultrafast computed tomography; Urinary free cortisol test.

UFD Ultrasonic flow detector; Unilateral facet dislocation.

UFE Upper femoral epiphysis.

UFF Unusual facial features.

UFFI Urea formaldehyde foam insulation.

UFFVA United Fresh Fruit and Vegetable Association.

UFI Urea formic iodide - used externally as an antiseptic and fungistatic agent.

UFL Upper flammable limit.

UFN Until further notice.
UFO Unflagged order; Unidentified flying/ foreign object.
UFP Ultrafiltration pressure.
UFR Ultrafiltration rate; Urine filtration/ flow rate (see KFT - V).
uFSH Urinary follicle-stimulating hormone.
UFT Urine filtration/ flow time (see KFT - V).
UG Until gone; Urinary glucose; Urogastrone; Urogenital.
Ug; U_g Specific gravity of urine.
UGA Uridylyl guanylyl adenosine; Urogenital atrophy.
UGB Undiagnosed genital bleeding.
UGC Undergraduate clerk(ship); Urogenital cancer (see RCC; RPC).
UGD Urogenital diaphragm.
UGDH UDP-glucose dehydrogenase (an enzyme required for the production of hyaluronic acid and proteoglycans; UDP or Uridine diphosphate, a uracil riboside, is used in the treatment of muscular atrophy, degeneration or wasting) (see UDP).
UGDP University Group Diabetes Program/ Project.
UGF Unidentified growth factor.
UGH Uveitis-glaucoma-hyphema (syndrome).
UGH+ Uveitis-glaucoma-hyphema plus vitreous hemorrhage (syndrome).
UGI Upper gastrointestinal (tract); Upper gastrointestinal irritation.
UGIB Upper gastrointestinal bleeding.
UGIC Upper gastrointestinal complication(s).
UGIH Upper gastrointestinal hemorrhage.
UGIPUB Upper gastrointestinal perforation, ulcer, or bleed(ing).
UGIS Upper gastrointestinal series.
UGIT Upper gastrointestinal tract (= UAT).
UGITD Upper gastrointestinal tract disease/ disorder.
UGK Urine glucose ketones.
UGM Urine glucose monitoring.
UGP Urban general practitioner(s).
UGS Urogenital sinus/ system.
UGT Undifferentiated glial tumor; Upper genital tract; Uridine diphosphate (UDP)-glucuronosyl-transferase (gene promotor, associated with Gilbert's syndrome) (see FNS; GS); Urogenital tract.
UGT; UGTB Urogenital tuberculosis.
ugt urgent.
UGTI Upper genital tract infection.
UH Umbilical hernia; Unfavorable/ Unknown history; University Hospital; Upper half; Urban Health (journal).
UHA Ulnar-humeral articulation (see UHJ); Unipolar hemiarthroplasty (Orthopedics).
UHBI Upper hemibody irradiation.
UHCC Universal health care coverage (see NHCS); Unstable heart disease.
UHD Underlying hematologic disease (e.g. thalassemia, refractory anemia, or other myelodysplastic disorders); Unstable hemoglobin disease.
UHDDS Uniform Hospital Discharge Data Set.
UHE Upper humeral epiphysis (Orthopedics).
UHF Ultrahigh frequency; Uncompensated (see UCF)/ Unexplained/ Unspecified heart failure; United Hospital Fund.
UHG UnitedHealth Group (Insurance group - US).
UHI Universal health insurance.
UHJ Ulnar-humeral joint (= UHA).
UHL Universal hypertrichosis languinosa.
UHMW Ultrahigh molecular weight.
UHP University Health Plan.
UHR Underlying heart rhythm.
UHS Uncombable hair syndrome (Hair shaft irregularity - see HSA); Universal Head System (Hip prosthesis - see OI/OP).
UHSC University Health Sciences Center (Louisiana State, US); University health services clinic.
UHSM University of Hawaii School of Medicine.
UHT Ultrahigh temperature.
uHV Ultra high vacuum/ voltage (>765 kv).
UI Ultralente insulin (see Insulin - UI); Unemployment insurance; Urge/ Urinary incontinence; Uroporphyrin isomerase.
U/I Unidentified.
UIA Ultrasonic Industry Association; Unruptured intracranial aneurysm.
UIB Unemployment insurance benefit.
UIBC Unsaturated iron-binding capacity.
UIC University of Illinois, Chicago.

UICAO Unilateral internal carotid artery occlusion.
UICC Union Internationale Contre le Cancer (Fr.) - International Union Against Cancer.
UID Once daily (L. unus in die); Usual initial dose.
UIEP Urine immunoelectrophoresis.
UIF Undegraded insulin factor.
UI-LI Use it or lose it (male sex, especially in the elderly).
UIMC International Union of Railway Medical Services (Fr.).
U_{in} Inulin concentration (in urine).
UIP Usual interstitial pneumonia.
UIQ Upper inner quadrant.
UIS Unemployment Insurance Service (DOL); Urea infusion; Utilization Information Service.
U-i-S Uroporphyrinogen-i-synthetase.
uj microjoule (= 10^{-6} joule) (see μj).
UJA United Jewish Appeal.
UJC Universal joint cervix (laceration of the fascial layers in the broad and Mackenrodt ligaments, resulting in a "universal joint" type of total mobility of the cervix with minimal, if any, movement of the corpus uteri) (= AMS; MAS).
UJF United Jewish Fund.
UJI Uniform Jury Instructions.
UJT Unijunction transistor.
UK United Kingdom; Unknown (see unk); Urinary kallikrein (see UKa); Urine potassium (L. kalium); Urokinase (see UKase).
UK 738 Ethybenztropine hydrobromide (= Tropethydryline HBr; $C_{22}H_{27}NOHBr$) - a parasympatholytic drug much weaker than atropine. Used in the treatment of parkinsonism and other extrapyramidal disorders.
UK-92,480 Sildenafil ("Viagra" - Pfizer, US) (a new anti-impotency drug).
UKA Urokinase activity.
UKa Urinary kallikrein (= UK).
UKAEA United Kingdom Atomic Energy Authority.
UKAOC United Kingdom Air Operations Control.
UKase Urokinase (= UK).
UKCC United Kingdom Central Council (for Nursing, Midwifery and Health Visiting).
UKCCSG United Kingdom Children's Cancer Study Group.
UKD Underlying kidney damage/ disease (see URD).
UKM Urea kinetic modeling.
UKMC University of Kansas Medical Center.
UKPDS United Kingdom Prospective Diabetic Study.
UKWMO United Kingdom Warning and Monitoring Organization.
UL Ultrasonic (see US); Underwriters' Laboratories (Inc); Undifferentiated lymphoma; Upper limb/ limit (see U/L)/ lobe; Upper and lower (see U&L).
U/L Upper limit(s) (= UL); Upper and lower (see U&L).
U/l Units per liter.
U&L Upper and lower (= UL; U/L).
ULBW Ultralow birth weight.
ULD Upper limb defect.
ULDH Urinary lactate dehydrogenase.
ULF United Leukemia Fund.
ULG Upper limb girdle.
ULJ Unilocular joint (a synovial joint having only one cavity); Upper limb joint.
ULL Uncomfortable loudness level; Upper limb lesion.
ULLE Upper lid of left eye.
ULM Uteroleiomyoma.
ULN Upper limits of normal.
uln ulna(r).
ULNV Upper limit of normal value.
ULO Chlorphedianol hydrochloride (Ulone).
ulo- combining form meaning cicatrix/ scar (Gr. oule), or gingival/gum (Gr. oulon).
ULP Unilateral leg pain; Ultralow profile.
ULPB Ultra-low profile balloon (Coronary angiography).
ULPE Upper lobe pulmonary edema.
ULQ Upper left quadrant.
ULRE Upper lid of right eye.
ULS Underwriters' Laboratory Standard; Upper limb surgery.
ULSM University of Louisville School of Medicine (Kentucky).
ULT; UlT Ultrahigh temperature (pasteurization).
ult excessive/ last/ ultimate(ly) (L. ultimus).
ult praes last prescribed/ the last ordered (L.

ultimus praescriptus).
ultra- prefix meaning beyond or excess (L.).
ULV Ultralow volume.
ULytes Urine electrolytes.
UM Undulating membrane; Unmarried; Upper motor (neuron); Uracil mustard.
UMA Ulcerative mutilating acropathy; Unique mechanism of action; Urgent medical assessment; Urinary muramidase activity.
Umax; U_{max} Maximal/ Maximum urinary/ urine osmolality/ osmolarity.
UMB Ultra-micro bacterium; Ultrasound in Medicine and Biology (UK journal).
umb umbilical/cus.
umb ven umbilical vein.
UMC Unidimensional chromatography; Union Médicale du Canada (journal); University Medical Center.
UMCV-TO Ulnar motor conduction velocity across thoracic outlet.
UMD Unipolar major depression; Unipolar mood disorder.
UMDD Unipolar major depressive disorder.
UMDNS Universal Medical Device Nomenclature System.
UMF Upper mantle field (in radiation therapy).
UMI Uncomplicated myocardial infarction; Urinary meconium index.
UMK Unilateral multicystic kidney.
UMKC University of Missouri at Kansas City.
UML United Medical Laboratories.
U/ml Units per milliliter.
UML 491 Methysergide maleate (= Methysergid; Methylergonovine) - was once popular as a prophylactic agent in the management of severe recurrent migraine, but its use has now been greatly restricted due to increasing reports of retroperitoneal fibrosis, cardio-circulatory, skeleto-muscular, and other complications following its use for prolonged periods.
UMLS Unified Medical Language System.
UMMC University of Michigan Medical Center.
UMN Upper motor neuron.
UMND Upper motor neurone degeneration; Upper motor neuron dysfunction.
UMNFP Upper motor neurone facial palsy/ paralysis.
UMNI University of Miami neurospinal index.
UMNL Upper motor neuron lesion.
UMNP Upper motor neuron palsy/ paralysis/ paresis/ pathology (= UMNL; UMNW).
UMNW Upper motor neurone weakness (see UMNP).
UMP Unexplained muscle pain; Uridine-5-monophosphate; Uridylic acid.
UMPK Uridine monophosphate kinase.
UMS Undersea Medical Society; United Medical Service (Blue Shield); Urethral manipulation syndrome.
UMSM University of Maryland School of Medicine.
UMT Unexplained muscle tenderness; Units of medical time.
UMW Unexplained muscle weakness.
UN Ulnar nerve; Undernourished; Unilateral neglect; United Nations; United Nurses (Canada); Urea nitrogen (see KFT - BUN); Urinary nitrogen.
un- prefix meaning one (L. unus) (see uni-).
UNA Urinary nitrogen appearance.
UNa; U_{Na} Urinary sodium.
unacc unaccompanied.
UNAM National Union for the Future of Medicine (Fr.).
UNaV Urinary sodium volume (excretion).
UNB Ulnar nerve block; Unhibited neurogenic bladder.
UNC University of North Carolina; Ureteroneocystostomy.
UNCF United Nations Childrens Fund.
UnChChr United Church of Christ (member).
UNCND United Nations Commission on Narcotic Drugs.
uncomp uncompensated; uncomplicated.
uncon unconscious.
uncond unconditioned.
uncond ref unconditioned reflex.
uncor; uncorr uncorrected.
UnC S; Unc S Unconditioned stimulus (= UnS; US).
unct ointment (L. unctio) (see Ung); smeared (L. unctus).
UNCV Ulnar nerve conduction velocity.
UNDA Uniform Narcotic Drug Act (1932).

undet undetermined.
undet ori; undet orig undetermined origin.
UNDP United Nations Development Program.
UNDRO United Nations Disaster Relief Office.
UNE Urinary norepinephrine.
UNEA United Nations Environmental Agency.
UNEP United Nations Environmental Program.
UNESCO United Nations Educational, Scientific, and Cultural Organization.
UNFDAC United Nations Fund for Drug Abuse Control.
UNFPA United Nations Fund for Population Activities.
Ung; ung Ointment (L. unguentum) (= Oint; unct).
UNHCR United Nations High Commissioner for Refugees.
Uni Unitarian/ Universalist Church member.
uni- prefix meaning one (L. unus) (= un-).
UNICEF United Nations International Children's Emergency Fund.
UNIFIL United Nations Interim Forces In Lebanon.
unilat unilateral.
UNITAR United Nations Institute for Training and Research.
Univ University (= U).
univ universal(ist) (= U).
Univ Coll Hosp University College Hospital (London).
UNK; Unk; unk; unkn Not reported; Unknown (= UK).
UNL Ulnar nerve lesion; Upper normal limit.
UNMC University of Nebraska Medical Center.
unof; unoff unofficial.
UNOS United Network for/ of Organ Sharing.
UNP Ulnar nerve palsy/ paralysis/ paresis.
UNRRA United Nations Relief and Rehabilitation Administration.
UNRWA United Nations Relief and Works Agency.
UnS Unconditioned stimulus (see UnC S).
uns unsatisfactory/ unsaturated (see unsat); unsymmetrical (see unsym).
unsat unsatisfactory/ unsaturated (= uns).
UNSCEAR United Nations Scientific Committee on the Effects of Atomic Radiation.
unsym unsymmetrical (= uns).
UNT Untreated.
UNTS Unilateral nevoid telangiectasia syndrome.
UNUDHR United Nations Universal Declaration of Human Rights.
UNWFC United Nations World Food Conference (1974).
UNWM United Nations World Model (Wassily Leontief).
UNX Uninephrectomy.
UO Uncertain/ Undetermined/ Unexplained/ Unknown origin; Under observation (see u/o); Urethral orifice; Urinary output (= UOP).
u/o under observation (= UO).
UOA United Ostomy Association (Inc).
UOC University Obesity Center (UCLA).
UOH Uncontrolled/ Unwanted ovarian hyperstimulation (Gyn/Obs).
UOMS University of Oregon Medical School.
UOO Urinary outflow obstruction; Utricular otolith organ (in the vestibule of the inner/ internal ear).
UOP Universal Oil Products (Inc); Urinary output (see UO).
UOPOPCP Methylene-uridine triphosphate.
UOQ Upper outer quadrant (of the breast/ buttock).
UOR Univariate odds ratio.
UOS Upper oesophageal segment/ sphincter/ stricture (see UES).
UOsm Urinary osmolality.
$\mathbf{U_{osm}V}$ Osmol excretion.
UOT Uniovular twins (see MZT).
UOV Units of variance.
UP Ulcerative proctitis; Ultra(high) purity (helium); Under proof; Unexplained phenomenon; Unipolar; Universal precaution(s); Upright posture; Ureteropelvic; Uridine phosphorylase; Uroporphyrin (= URO).
U/P Urine/plasma (concentration ratio), e.g. of glucose.
√up check up.
UPA Urban planning aid; Uridylyl phosphate adenosine; Urokinase-type plasminogen activator (see scu-PA).

u-PA Urinary type plasminogen activator.
up ad lib ambulatory/ out of bed as desired/ patient may walk (L. ad libitum).
U_{pah} Para-aminohippurate concentration (in the urine).
UPBF Uteroplacental blood flow.
UPC Universal product code (retailing); Uteroplacental circulation.
UPD Urinary production.
Update (UK journal).
UPDRS Unified Parkinson's Disease Rating Scale.
UPE Urinary protein excretion.
UPEP Urinary protein electrophoresis.
UPET Urokinase - pulmonary embolism trial.
UPF Universal proximal femur (prosthesis).
UPG Uridylyl phosphate guanosine; Uroporphyrinogen (= URO).
UPGMA Unweighted pair group method with averages.
UPI Uteroplacental insufficiency/ ischemia.
UPJ Uteropelvic junction.
UPL Unusual position of limbs.
UPMC University of Pennsylvania Medical Center.
UPOR Usual place of residence.
UPP Urethral pressure profile.
Upper Amphetamine pill (see Amphet).
UPPP Uvulopalatopharyngoplasty.
UPPRA Upright peripheral plasma renin activity.
UPR Uncontrolled/ Unmanageable proliferative retinopathy.
UPRO Utah Professional Review Organization.
UPS Ultraviolet photoelectron spectroscopy; Uninterruptible power supply; United Parcel Service; Uroporphyrinogen synthetase (= URO-S); Uterine progesterone system.
UPs Ureidopenicillins (parenteral antibiotics including mezlocillin, azlocillin and piperacillin).
Ups Amphetamine pills (see Amphet).
UPSIT University of Pennsylvania Smell Identification Test.
UPSM University of Pennsylvania School of Medicine.
UPT Uniform Procedural Terminology; Uptake; Urine pregnancy test.
UPU Uridylyl phosphate uridine.
UPW Uniform present worth (factor) - in medical accounting.
UQ Ubiquinone; Upper quadrant/ quartile.
UQS Upper quadrant syndrome.
UR Unconditional/ Unconditioned reflex/ response; Unrelated; Upper respiratory (tract); Urea (see Ur); Ureter (see Uret); Urethra(l) (see Ureth); Uridine (see Urd); Urinal/nary/ne (see Ur); Urinary retention; Urologist/gy (see Urol); Utilization review.
Ur Urea (= UR); Ureter (see Uret); Urethral (see Ureth); Uridine (see Urd); Urinal/nary/ne (= UR); Urologist/gy (see Urol).
ur- prefix meaning urinary tract or urine (Gr. ouron) (= uro-).
URA; Ura Uracil.
URAI Unprotected receptive anal intercourse (in homosexuals).
Ur an; Ur anal Urine analysis.
urano- prefix meaning palate (Gr. ouranos).
URB Undiagnosed/ Unrecognized/ Unsuspected rectal bleeding.
URC Upper rib cage; Utilization review committee (hospital).
URD Underlying renal damage/ disease (= UKD); Undifferentiated/ Unspecified/ Upper respiratory disease.
Urd Uridine (= UR; Ur).
UREM Uncontrolled rapid eye movement (= Nystagmus - as demonstrated in Bard's sign).
Uret Ureter (= UR; Ur).
uretero- combining form meaning ureter (Gr. oureter).
Ureth; ureth Urethra(l) (= UR; Ur).
urethro- prefix meaning urethra (Gr. ourethra).
URF Unidentified reading frame; Uterine relaxing factor.
URI Upper respiratory illness/ infection.
-uria suffix meaning urine (Gr. ouron).
UR individuals Unrelated individuals.
UricA Uric acid.
urino- combining form meaning urine (L. urina).
url unrelated.
URMC University of Rochester Medical Center.
URN Upper range of normal.

U-RNA Uridylic acid ribonucleic acid.
URO Urologist/gy (see Urol); Uroporphyrin (see UP); Uroporphyrinogen (see UPG).
uro- prefix meaning urine (Gr. ouron) (see ur-).
UROB Urobilinogen.
UROGEN; URO-GEN; urogen Urogenital.
Urol Urologist/gy (= UR; Ur; URO); Urology (journal).
URO-S Uroporphyrinogen synthetase (see UPS).
URQ Upper right quadrant.
URS Ultrasonic renal scanning; Ureterorenoscope (Urology).
URT Upper respiratory tract.
URTI Upper respiratory tract infection.
URVD Unilateral renovascular disease.
US Ultrasonic (= UL); Ultrasound; Ultrasonogram/graphy; Unconditioned stimulus (see UnC S); Unique sequence; Unit secretary/ separator; United States; Upper segment/ strength; Ureteroscope/py; Urinary sugar; Urological Survey (journal); Usher syndrome.
us as mentioned above (L. ubi supra).
USA Unit services assistant; United States of America; United States Army; Unstable angina (see UA); Uricosuric agent (= USD).
USAAA United States Army Audit Agency.
USACE United States Army Corps of Engineers.
USACIP United States Advisory Committee on Immunization Practices (see ACIP).
USAEHA United States Army Environmental Health/ Hygiene Agency.
USAF United States Air Force.
USAFH United States Air Force Hospital.
USAFMJ United States Armed Forces Medical Journal.
USAFMSD United States Air Force Medical Service Digest (journal).
USAFRHL United States Air Force Radiological Health Laboratory.
USAFSAM United States Air Force School of Aerospace Medicine.
USAGH United States Army General Hospital.
USAH United States Army Hospital.
USAHC United States Army Health Clinic.
USAHSC United States Army Health Services Command.
USAID United States Agency for International Development.
USAIDR United States Army Institute of Dental Research.
USAMEDS; USAMedS United States Army Medical Service.
USAMRDC United States Army Medical Research and Development Command.
USAMRIID United States Army Medical Research Institute of Infectious Diseases.
USAN United States Adopted Names (Council) - drug nomenclature, a non-proprietary designation for any compound used as a drug.
USANC United States Adopted Names Council (see USAN).
USAP Unstable angina pectoris.
USARIEM United States Army Research Institute of Environmental Medicine.
USASI United States of America Standards Institute (see ANSI).
USAVB United States Army Veterinary Bulletin (journal).
USB Upper small bowel; Upper sternal border.
USBD Upper small bowel disease/ disorder (e.g. Coeliac/Crohn's disease).
USBLS United States Bureau of Labor Statistics (DOL).
USBS; USBuStand United States Bureau of Standards.
USC United States Code; University of South Carolina (Columbia); University of Southern California.
USCC United States Chamber of Commerce.
USCCTS United States - Canadian Communications Technology Satellite.
USCG United States Coast Guard.
USC:MHMR United States Congress: Mental Health, Mental Retardation (NASMHPD journal).
USCSM University of Southern California School of Medicine.
USCVD Unsterile controlled vaginal delivery.
USD Ultrasonographic diagnosis; United States Dispensary/ Dispensatory; University Science Development (program) (NSF);

Upper septal/tum defect; Uricosuric drug (see USA); Urinary system disorder.
USDA United States Department of Agriculture.
USDHEW United States Department of Health, Education, and Welfare.
USDHHS United States Department of Health and Human Services.
USDI United States Department of the Interior.
USDJ United States Department of Justice.
USDL United States Department of Labor.
USE Ultimate specific extension (Orthopedics); Ultrasonic/sound echography; Ultrasonography (see USG); Ultrasound examination; Undesirable/ Unwanted side-effect.
USES United States Employment Service (Manpower Administration - DOL).
USF Uniform sinking fund (factor, in medical accounting).
USFMG United States foreign medical graduate.
USFMS United States foreign medical student.
USFWS United States Fish and Wildlife Service (Dept. of the Interior).
USG Ultrasonography (= USE).
USGM United States Government Manual.
USGPO United States Government Printing Office.
USGS United States Geological Survey.
USH Usual state of health.
USHHSD United States Health and Human Services Department.
USHL United States Hygienic Laboratory.
USHMAC United States Health Manpower Advisory Council.
USHPR Act Uniformed Services Health Professions Revitalization Act.
USHR United States House of Representatives.
USI Unusual ski injuries/ry (Orthopedics); Urinary stress incontinence.
USIA United States Information Agency.
US-LS; US/LS Upper segment - lower segment (ratio, of body measurements); Upper strength - lower strength (ratio, of body muscles).
USLT Ultrasonic lithotriptor (Urology).
USM United States Medicine (journal); Useful surrogate marker; Uterine smooth muscle.
USMB United States Metric Board.
USMC United States Marine Corps.
USMG United States medical graduate.
USMH United States Marine Hospital.
USMLE United States Medical Licensing Examination.
USMS Utah State Medical Society.
USN Ultrasonic nebulizer; Unilateral spatial neglect; United States Navy.
USNCHS United States National Center for Health Statistics.
USNCMP United States National Committee for Medical Physics.
USNCUNESCO United States National Commission for the United Nations Educational, Scientific, and Cultural Organization (UNESCO).
USNF United States National Formulary (1965).
USNH United States Naval Hospital.
USNM United States Navy Medicine (journal).
USNMB United States Naval Medical Bulletin.
USO Ultimate survival outcome; Unilateral salpingo-oophorectomy.
USOC United States Olympic Committee.
USOE United States Office of Education (HEW).
USOS United States Occupational Standard (e.g. safe concentration of toxic substances).
USP United States Pharmacopeia (= USPhar); Unsafe sexual practice(s).
USPat United States patent.
USPC United States Pharmacopeial Convention Inc.
USPDI United States Pharmacopeia Drug Information.
USPhar United States Pharmacopeia (see USP).
USPhC United States Pharmacopeial Convention.
USPHS United States Public Health Service.
USPHSCS United States Public Health Service Clinical Society.
USPRS United States Pharmacopeia

Reference Standards/ Substances.

USPRSC United States Pharmacopeia Reference Standards Committee.

USPS United States Postal Service.

USPSRS United States Pharmacopeia Steroid Reference Substances.

USPSTF United States Preventive Services Task Force.

USPTA United States Physical Therapy Association.

USPU United States Pharmacopeia unit.

USR Ultrasonic renography; Unheated serum reagin (test for syphilis) (see STS-USR); United States Reserves.

USRC United States Reserve Corps.

USRDS United States Renal Data System.

USS Ultrasound scanning; United States Senate/ Service/ Ship/ Steamer/ Steamship; Unsafe sex (see SSP).

USSCt United States Supreme Court.

USSR Union of Soviet Socialist Republics (now defunct).

USSS United States Steamship (= USS).

UST Useful screening test.

ust burnt or calcined (L. ustus).

USTS United States Travel Service (DOC).

USUCVD Unsterile uncontrolled vaginal delivery.

USUHS Uniformed Services University of the Health Sciences (= FMC - FederaL Medical College).

USVB United States Veterans Bureau.

USVH United States Veterans Hospital.

USVMD Urine specimen volume measuring device.

USW Ultrashort waves.

USWL Unexplained significant weight loss (= SWL; UWL).

UT Ullrich-Turner (syndrome); Unna-Thost (syndrome); Untested; Untreated; Urinary tract; Urticaria.

uT Unbound testosterone.

UTA Uterine artery.

Utah Bio Utah Biomedical Laboratory.

UTB Urinary tract bleeding.

UTBG Unbound (unsaturated) thyroxine-binding globulin.

UTC Converted universal time; Unable to climax; Upper thoracic compression; Urinary tract cancer/ carcinoma.

UTCM University of Tennessee College of Medicine.

UTD Up to date; Urinary tract disease/ disorder.

ut dict as directed (L. ut dictum).

UTE Unexplained transaminase elevation; Urinary tract endoscopy; Uterotonic effect (of oxytocic drugs, etc.).

U teeth Unerupted teeth.

utend to be used (L. utendus).

utend mor sol to be used in the usual manner/ use as usual (L. utendus more solito) (= ut mor sol).

UTF Usual throat flora.

UTHSC University of Texas Health Science Center.

UTHSCD University of Texas Health Science Center at Dallas.

UTI Urinary tract infection; Urinary trypsin inhibitor; Utility type incision (see inc).

UTIc Catheter-associated urinary tract infection.

UTL Ultimate tensile load (Orthopedics); Unbalanced translocation (involving chromosomes).

UTLC Ultra-thin-layer chromatography.

UTLD Utah Test of Language Development.

UT level Upper tertile level.

UTMB University of Texas Medical Branch.

ut mor sol use as usual (see utend mor sol).

UTMU University of Tennessee Medical Units.

UTO Unable to obtain; Upper tibial osteotomy; Urinary tract obstruction.

UTP Unilateral tension pneumothorax; Uridine triphosphate (= Uridine-5-triphosphoric acid) - a derivative of uridine, uracil riboside, one of the four nucleosides present in ribonucleic acid. Used in the treatment of disorders such as muscular atrophy and muscular weakness.

UTR Untranslated region (of/ on the gene); Uptake of triiodothyronine resin.

UTS Ullrich-Turner syndrome; Ulnar tunnel syndrome; Ultimate tensile strength; Ultrasound; Unna-Thost syndrome; Uptake study.

UTSCC University of Texas System Cancer

Center.

UTSMS University of Texas Southwestern Medical School.

UTT Urinary tract tumor.

UTZ Ultrasound.

UU Unitarian - Universalist Church member; Urinary urea; Urine urobilinogen (see LFT iv).

UUA Uricosuric activity/ agent (e.g. Allopurinol).

UUB Undiagnosed uterine bleeding (see UUH); Unexplained uterine bleeding (see UUH).

UUH Unexplained uterine hemorrhage (= UUB).

UUI Urge urinary incontinence.

UUIE Urge urinary incontinence episode.

UUMC University of Utah Medicine Center.

UUN Urinary/ne urea nitrogen (see KFT).

UUO Unilateral urethral obstruction.

UUOM Ureaplasma urealyticum osteomyelitis.

UUP Urinary uroporphyrin.

UUT Unit under test.

UUU; uuu Uridylyl uridylyl uridine (= three consecutive nucleotides of uracil).

UV Ultraviolet (= uv); Umbilical vein; Uppsala virus (see Uv); Uretero-vesical; Urinary/ne volume.

Uv; U_v Uppsala virus (= UV).

uv ultraviolet (see UV).

UVA Ultraviolet application (therapy) (see UV-A); Undetermined/ Undiagnosed/ Unexplained ventricular arrhythmia(s); Univariate analysis; Ureterovesical angle.

UV-A Ultraviolet-A light/ pigmenting rays (in the 320-400 nm range) - they penetrate beyond the epidermis, and damage the dermal collagen (= UVA).

UVB Undiagnosed vaginal bleeding.

UVB; UV-B Ultraviolet-B light/ erythema-inducing rays (in the 290-320 nm range) - they do not penetrate the epidermis.

UVBF Umbilical vein blood flow.

UVC Ultraviolet-C (light) (see UV-C); Umbilical vascular cooling; Umbilical venous catheter.

UV-C Ultraviolet-C light/ partly pigmenting rays (= UVC).

UVCM University of Virginia College of Medicine.

UV_{cr} Creatinine clearance (urinary).

UVD Undiagnosed/ Unspecified visual disturbance.

UVER Ultraviolet-enhanced reactivation.

UVI Ultraviolet irradiation.

U-virus Virus antigenetically related to ECHO virus.

UVJ Ureterovesical junction.

UVL Ultraviolet light; Umbilical venous line.

UVM Universal vendor marking standard.

UVO Urinary volume output.

UVP Ultraviolet photometry.

UV/P Clearance ratio (mass of substance excreted in unit time/ concentration in plasma): U = concentration of solute in urine, V = volume of urine excreted in a unit of time, and P = concentration of substance in plasma (ratio = clearance of the substance in urine) (see U/P).

UVR Ultraviolet radiation; Ureterovesical reimplantation.

UV_{Ur} Uric acid excretion.

UW Unilateral weakness.

UWB; U/WB Unit of whole blood.

UWCM University of Wales College of Medicine (UK).

UWD Urbach-Wiethe disease.

UWF Unknown white female.

UWH University of Wisconsin Hospital.

UWL Unexplained/ Unintentional weight loss.

UWM Unknown white male; Unwed mother.

UWMS University of Wisconsin Medical School.

UWSC Unstimulated whole saliva collection.

UWSM University of Washington School of Medicine.

UX Uranium X, proactinium (see UX2).

ux wife.

UX_2 Proactinium; chemical element, better known by the symbol: Pa (Z = 91) (see Elements - Proactinium).

UYP Upper yield point.

V

V Antigen; Chest electrode (ECG) - unipolar; Coefficient of variation; ECG lead (Chest vs LL + LA + RA); Electrical potential (in volts); In electroencephalography - vertex sharp transient; Five (Roman numeral); Gas volume (see PFT - V); A logical binary relation that is true if any argument is true, and false otherwise; Luminous efficiency; Minute volume (see PFT - V); Potential energy (joules); Roman numeral five; Unipolar chest lead (ECG); Urinary/ne flow rate (UFR) (= Urine volume/ unit time) (see KFT - V_o); Vaccinate(d)/tion (see Vacc); Vaccine (see Vac); Vagina; Valine (see Val); Valve (see val); Vanadium (Z = 23) (see Elements - Vanadium); Variable; Variation; Varnish (dentistry); Vector; Vegetarian; Vein (L. vena) (= v); Velocity (= v); Vena (L.) - vein, e.g. V. lingualis/ the lingual vein; Venous (= v); Ventilation; Ventral (= v); Ventricle; Ventricular (fibrillation) (= v); Verb; Verbal (comprehension factor) (= v); Vertebra(l); Vertex/tical; Very (= v); Vestibular; Vibrio; Violet (an indicator color) (= v); Viral (antigen); Virgin; Virulence/nt (= v); Virus (= v); Virus (antigen); Vision (= v); Visual acuity; Voice; Volt (the unit of electromotive force in the MKS system of measurement, being the force necessary to cause one ampere of current to flow against one ohm of resistance) (= v); Voltage; Volume (= v); Volume of gas (see PFT - V); Vomiting.

v against (L. versus); of (Ger. von) (used in names); or (L. vel); rate of reaction catalyzed by an enzyme; see (L. vide); specific volume; valve (see V); vein (L. vena) (see V); velocity (see V); venous (see V); ventral/ricular (see V); verbal (see V); versus (L.) - against; very (see V); violet (see V); virulence/nt (see V); virus (see V); vision (see V); volt (see V); volume (see V).

$\dot{V}$ Volume of gas per unit of time (= Rate of gas flow) (= V) (see PFT - V).

$\bar{V}$; $\bar{v}$ Ventilation (L/min).

v- vicinal isomer.

V+ (substance) Kynurenine.

+V Positive vertical divergence.

V1 Chest lead with central electrode (= the central terminal) (ECG); The amount of blood leaving the leg in the first second (on the APG - Air plethysmography, recording) (see OF - Outflow fraction).

V1; V2; etc Precordial (Unipolar chest) leads (ECG).

V III Ventricular tertius (thalamus).

V_{60} 60% of control (of total lung capacity).

VA Alveolar aspiration (see PFT - VA); Alveolar ventilation (= V_A; $\dot{V}_A$; V_a; Volume of alveolar air); Nucleus latero-polaris of the thalamus; Vacuum aspiration; Vaginal atrophy; Valproic acid; Variant angina (see PVA; VSA); Vasodilator agent; Ventriclar aneurysm/ arrhythmia; Ventriculo-atrial; Ventroanterior; Vertebral artery; Veterans Administration (see VAd)/ Affairs; Vincent's angina (= NUG); Viral antigen (see Va); Visual activity/ acuity/ aid/ axis (= Va); Volt-ampere (see V/A); Volume-average; Volume of alveolar gas (see VA; PFT - VA).

Va Neon dilution volume; Viral antigen (= VA); Visual activity/ acuity/ aid/ axis (see VA).

va volt-ampere (see V/A).

V_A; $\dot{V}_A$; V_a Alveolar ventilation (= VA; Volume of alveolar gas) (see PFT - V_A).

V/A Volt/ampere (= VA; va).

VAA Vaccination Assistance Act; Veterans Affairs Administration.

VAB Van Allen (radiation) belt; Venoarterial bypass; Ventilator-associated barotrauma (see VALI); Vincristine, actinomycin D, and bleomycin; Violent antisocial behavior.

VAB III Vinblastine, Actinomycin D, Bleomycin, Cyclophosphamide and Cisplatin (Chemotherapy).

VAB IV Vinblastine, Actinomycin D, Bleomycin, Cyclophosphamide, Cisplatin, Chlorambucil and Doxorubicin (Chemotherapy).

VABP Venoarterial bypass pumping.

VAC Ventral anterior cingulate (brain); Ventriculo-atrial conduction; Vincristine, actinomycin D (doxorubicin), and cyclophosphamide; Virus capsid antigen; Volts (rms), alternating current.

Vac; vac Vaccinate(d)/tion (see Vacc); Vaccine (= V); Vacuum.

VAcc Visual acuity with correction.

Vacc; vacc Vaccinate(d)/tion (= V; Vac; vac).

vacc- combining form meaning cow (L. vacca).

VACO Veterans Administration Central Office.

VACS Veterans Administration Cooperative Study; Voice-activated camera system (= AESOP, used in robosurgery).

VACTEL Vertebral, Anal, Cardiac, Tracheo-Esophageal and Limb (defects) (see VACTERL).

VACTERL Acronym for a congenital syndrome, which has been associated with the administration of progestogens during pregnancy, consisting of: Vertebral abnormalities, Anal atresia, Cardiac abnormalities, Tracheo-esophageal fistula and/or Esophageal atresia, Renal agenesis and dysplasia, and Limb defects (= VACTEL).

VACV Valaciclovir (an anti-herpes drug).

VAD Vacuum-assisted delivery; Vascular/Venous access device; Venous admixture; Ventricular assist device; Vincristine, Adriamycin (doxorubicin), and dexamethasone; Vitamin A deficiency; Virus-adjusting diluent; Voluntary Aid Detachment (Britain).

VaD Vascular dementia (see HAAS).

VAd Veterans Administration (= VA).

VADRIAC Vincristine, Adriamycin (doxorubicin), and cyclophosphamide.

VAE Version and extraction (delivery of a baby in which a fetus being born head-first is turned and delivered foot-first) (= IDP or Internal podalic version; TBE or Total breech extraction).

VAERS Vaccine Adverse Event Reporting System (US).

$\dot{V}_A$/f Volume of gas entering the alveolar space (see PFT).

Vag; vag Vagina(l)/nitis.

VAG HYST; Vag Hyst Vaginal hysterectomy.

vagin- combining form meaning sheath (L. vagina).

Vag Pess Vaginal pessary.

Vag tab(s) Vaginal tablet(s).

VAH Vasoactive hormone; Vertebral ankylosing hyperostosis; Veterans Administration/Affairs Hospital; Virilizing adrenal hyperplasia; Vitreous asteroid hyalosis (multiple, small, yellow spheres consisting of calcium soaps seen in the vitreous, which usually do not affect visual acuity) (= AH).

VA-HIT Veterans Administration - HDL Intervention Trial.

VAHS Virus-associated hemophagocytic syndrome.

VAIN Vaginal intraepithelial neoplasm.

VAKT Visual association, kinesthetic, and tactile (reading ability).

Val Valine (= V).

val valve (= V).

VALE Visual acuity of left eye (see VAOS).

Valer Valerian.

VALG Veterans Administration Lung Cancer Group.

VALI Ventilator-associated lung injury (= VAB; VAP).

VAM Anesthetic (inhalation); Ventricular arrhythmia monitor.

VAMC Veterans Administration/ Affairs Medical Center.

VaMedMonth Virginia Medical Monthly (journal).

VAMIS Virginia Medical Information System (Service Center).

VAMP Vincristine, amethopterin, 6-mercaptopurine, and prednisone (cancer chemotherapy).

VAMS Visual Analogue Mood Scale.

VANCO/P Vancomycin - peak.

VANCO/T Vancomycin - trough.

VAOD Visual acuity of right eye (L. oculus dexter) (= VARE).

VA.OD.LP Visual acuity, right eye (L. oculus dexter) light perception (eye examination).

VAOS Visual acuity of left eye (L. oculus sinister) (= VALE).

VA.OS.LP with P Visual acuity, left eye (L. oculus sinister) light perception with projection (eye examination).

VAP Vaginal acid phosphatase; Vague abdominal pain; Variant angina pectoris; Venous access port; Ventilator-associated pneumonia (see VALI); Vincristine, asparaginase, and prednisone.

vap vapor.

$\dot{V}_A/\dot{Q}$; $\dot{V}a/\dot{Q}$; $\dot{V}_A/\dot{Q}_C$; Va/Qc; VAQT Ventilation/perfusion (ratio).

VAR Varicella (Chickenpox) (vaccine); Visual-auditory/ Visual-aural range.

Var; var Variable; Variance/nt; Variation; Variety; Various.

var varicose; volt-ampere reactive.

V-A/R Renal vein renin relative to arterial renin.

VARE Visual acuity of right eye (see VAOD).

varico- prefix meaning swollen or twisted (L. varix).

VARO Veterans Administration Regional Office.

VARTEC Virtual and Augmented Reality Technologies.

VAS Vascular (see vas); Ventriculoatrial shunt/ Ventriculoatriostomy (see AVS); Vertebral angiosarcoma (see MHE); Vertebral artery stenosis (with cerebral infarction); Vesicle attachment site; Viral arthritis syndrome; Visual acuity screening; Visual Analogue Scale.

vas vascular (= VAS; vasc).

vas- combining form meaning vessel (L.).

VASA Vascular successful aging.

VASAG Veterans Administration Surgical Adjuvant Group.

VASC Verbal/ Visual Auditory Screen (Test) for Children; Verbal/ Visual Auditory Screening of Children.

VAsc Visual acuity without correction.

vasc vascular (see vas).

VaSCAAP Virginia Sickle Cell Anemia Awareness Program.

vas dis vascular disease.

V-A shunt Ventricular-atrial shunt (for hydrocephalus).

vaso- prefix meaning blood vessel (L. vas).

VAS RAD Vascular radiology.

VAST Ventricular aneurysm septal tear.

vas vit glass vessel (L. vas vitreum).

VAT Value Added Tax; Variable antigen type; Vascular access thrombosis; Ventricular accommodation test; Ventricular activation time; Visual action time; Visual acuity test; Visual/ Vocational apperception test.

VAT:ADV Vocational Apperception Test: Advanced form.

VATER Vertebral defects, imperforate anus, tracheoesophageal fistula, and radial and renal dysplasia.

VATH Vinblastine, Adriamycin (doxorubicin), thiotepa, and Halotestin (fluoxymesterone).

VATS Veterans Administration (Medical Center) transference syndrome.

VATs Surface variable antigen.

VB Vaginal/ Viable birth; Vaginal bulb; Valence/ Venous blood; Van Buren (catheter); Ventrobasal; Veronal/ Virus buffer; Vertebral/ro basilar (artery); Veterinary Bulletin (UK); Vinblastine (see VBL); Voided bladder; Volta Bureau.

VB_1 First voided bladder (specimen).

VB_2 Second (midstream) voided bladder (specimen).

VBA Vertebrobasilar artery.

VBAC Vaginal birth after cesarean (section).

VBACS Vaginal birth after cesarean section (= VBAC).

VBAIN Vertebrobasilar artery insufficiency nystagmus.

VBAP Vincristine, carmustine, Adriamycin (doxorubicin) and prednisone.

VBC Vincristine, bleomycin, and cisplatin; Viral birth control (as in HAART).

VBD Vanishing bile duct; Veronal-buffered diluent; Vertebral body/ bone density (Orthopedics) (see TVBD); Vinblastine, bleomycin (= Blenoxane), and doxorubicin.

VBF Vertebral body fusion (Orthopedics).

VBG Vagotomy and Billroth gastroenterostomy; Venous blood gases; Vein/ Venous (aortocoronary artery) bypass graft; Vertical-banded gastroplasty.

VBI Vertebrobasilar insufficiency/ ischemia; Viral brain infection (e.g. dengue fever, Japanese encephalitis, yellow fever, etc.).

VBL Vinblastine (= VB; VLB) (cancer chemotherapy).

VBM Vertebrobasilar migraine.

VBMA Volwiler Body Movement Analysis.

VBOS Veronal-buffered oxalated saline (solution).

VBP Vagal body paraganglia; Vector-borne parasite/ pathogen/ protozoa(n) (e.g.

Leishmania, Trypanosoma); Venous blood pressure; Venous blood pooling (due to drug vasodilatation e.g. by glyceryl trinitrate, etc.); Ventricular premature beat (see PVB); Vinblastine, bleomycin, and platinum compd (cisplatin).

VBR Ventricular brain ratio; Vesiculobullous rash (skin).

VBS Veronal-buffered saline (medium/ solution); Vertebrobasilar system.

VB's disease Van Buren's disease.

VBS:FBS Veronal-buffered saline - fetal bovine serum.

VBT Vascular brachytherapy.

VC Color vision; Pulmonary capillary blood volume; Vacuum curettage; Vasoconstriction; Vena cava; Venereal case; Venous capacitance; Ventilatory capacity (see PFT); Ventral column; Ventricular contraction; Vertebral caval/ column; Veterinary Corps; Videocasette; Vincristine (cancer chemotherapy) (see VCr); Vinyl chloride (carcinogen); Visual acuity for color (= Color vision) - above; Visual capacity/ cortex; Vital capacity - the maximum amount of gas that can be expelled from the lungs by forceful effort after maximal inspiration (= Vit Cap; vit cap) (see PFT); Vocal cord; Voluntary closing (prosthesis)/ control; VP-etoposide and cisplatin.

V/C Ventilation/circulation (ratio); Voltage-to-current (conversion).

V_C Pulmonary capillary blood flow/ volume (see PFT).

V&C Vertical and centric (bite).

VCA Vaginal cesium/ cream applicator; Vancomycin, colistin, and anisomycin; Vasoconstrictive action/ activity; Viral capsid antigen (of Epstein-Burr virus).

VCA-EB Viral capsid antigen, Epstein-Barr.

VCAM Vascular-cell adhesion molecule (see CAM; ICAM).

VCAP Vincristine, cyclophosphamide, Adriamycin, and prednisone.

VCBF Vertebral compressive breaking force (and BMD - Bone mineral den- sity).

vCBF Venous cerebral blood flow.

VCC Vasoconstrictor center; Vena cava clamp (Satinsky); Venous cerebral circulation; Ventral cell column.

VCCA Velocity (of blood) in the common carotid artery.

VCD Vaginal contraceptive diaphragm; Vibrational circular dichroism; Virally-coded enzyme e.g. thymidine kinase (= VEE); Vocal cord dysfunction (psychoneurotic/ somatic dysfunction).

VCE Contractile-element velocity; Vagina, ectocervix, and endocervix; Ventrocaudalis externus (nucleus of thalamus).

VCEM Voluntary conjugate eye movement(s).

VCF Vena caval filter (Mobin-Udder); Vertebral compression/ crush fracture (physical signs - dorsal kyphosis, height loss, etc.).

VCFS Velo-cardio-facial syndrome; Vertebral crush fracture syndrome (Orthopedics) (see VCF).

VCG Vectorcardiogram/graphy; Voiding cystography/ cystourethrography.

VCI Velamentous cord insertion (Obstetrics); Ventrocaudalis internus (nucleus of thalamus); Volatile corrosion inhibitor.

V-cillin Penicillin V (proprietary name).

VC-K Eli Lilly & Co (Canada) code for experimental substances.

VC/kwt Vital capacity in milliliters per kilogram of body weight (see PFT).

VCl Vinyl chloride.

VCM Vinyl chloride monomer; Viral cardiomyopathy.

VCMP Vincristine, cyclophosphamide, melphalan, and prednisone.

VCN Vancomycin (hydrochloride), colistomethane (sodium), and nystatin (medium); Vibrio cholerae neuroaminidase (see VCNase).

VCNA Veterinary Clinics of North America (journal).

VCNase Vibrio cholerae neuroaminidase (= VCN).

VCO Voltage-controlled oscillator.

VCO; V_{CO} Endogenous production of carbon monoxide (see PFT - V_{CO}).

VCO_2; V_{CO2}; $\dot{V}_{CO2}$ Amount of carbon dioxide eliminated per minute (= Carbon dioxide output) (see PFT).

VCP Ventricor pacemaker; Veterinary Creolin-Pearson; VideoCassette Recorder; Vincristine, cyclophosphamide, and prednisone; Viral capsid protein; Virus cancer program (NIH); Visual comfort probability.

VCR Vasoconstriction rate; Video Cassette Recorder; Vincristine (see VCr); Volume clearance rate.

VCr Vincristine (= Oncovin) - used in cancer chemotherapy (= VC; VCR).

VCR-MTX-CF Vincristine, Methotrexate and Citrovorum factor (Chemotherapy).

VCS Vasoconstrictor substance; Vesicocervical space; Vision-correcting surgery.

VCSA Viral cell surface antigen.

VCSF Ventricular cerebrospinal fluid.

VCT Venous clotting time; Vital capacity test.

VCU Videocystourethrography; Voiding cystourethrogram/graphy (= VCUG) (see KFT - VCU).

VCUG Vesicoureterogram; Voiding cystourethrogram/graphy (see VCU; KFT - VCU).

VC utterance Vowel-consonant utterance.

VCV utterance Vowel-consonant-vowel utterance.

VD Vagotomy drainage; Valvular/ Vascular/ Venereal disease; Vanadium deuteride; Vapor density; Vasodilation/tor; Venous dilation/ distensibility; Ventricular dilator; Ventrodorsal; Vertical deviation/ divergence; Video-disk; Virus diarrhea; Voided/ Voiding (see Vd); Volume of dead space/ dialysate (total volume exchanged)/ distribution (see Vd).

Vd Apparent volume of distribution (= VD); Voided/ Voiding (= VD); Volume of dead space (see V_D).

vD van Deen (see vD's test).

vd double vibrations (cycles).

V_D; V_d Volume of dead space (physiologic dead air space) (= VD; Vd; VDA) (see PFT).

V&D Vomiting and diarrhea.

1-VD One vessel disease (coronary heart disease).

2-VD Two vessel disease (coronary heart disease).

3-VD Three vessel disease (coronary heart disease).

VDA Anatomic dead space (see V_D; PFT); Vasoconstrictive action/ activity; Venous digital angiogram; Videodimensional analyzer; Visual discriminatory acuity.

VDAC Voltage-dependent anion channel.

VDAG Vaginal delivery after cesarean.

VDAHD Vasodilator antihypertensive drug.

VDB van den Bergh (see VdB); Venereal Disease Branch (PHS); Ventilator-delivered breath.

VdB; vdB van den Bergh ('s test) (direct & indirect), for serum bilirubin (A.A. Himans van den Bergh, Dutch physician, 1869-1943) (= VDB) (see LFT iv).

VDBR Volume of distribution of bilirubin (see LFT iv).

VDC Vaccine Development Committee (NIH); Vasodilator center.

vdc volts - direct current (i.e. direct-current voltage).

VDCAC Venereal Disease Control Advisory Committee (HEW).

VDCC Venereal Disease Control Center (Center for Diseases Control, HEW).

VDD Atrial synchronous ventricular inhibited (pacemaker); Variable daily dose; Vasodilating/tory drug; Vitamin D-dependent.

VDDR Vitamin D-dependent rickets.

VDEL Venereal Diseases Experimental Laboratory (Britain).

VDEM Vasodepressor material (see VDM).

VDF Ventricular diastolic fragmentation.

VDFG Variable diode function generator.

VDG; VD-G Venereal disease - gonorrhea.

vdg voiding (see VD; Vd).

VDH Vascular disease of the heart.

VDI Vaginal dryness index (vaginal elasticity, moisture and epithelial integrity) (see VHI); Venereal disease information.

vdK's law van der Kolk's law.

VDL Vascular diagnostic laboratory; Vasodepressor lipid; Visual detection level.

VDM Vasodepressor material (a substance formed by the liver that stimulates secretion of antidiuretic hormone (= VDEM).

VD or M Venous distension or masses.

VDP Ventricular premature depolarization (see VPD); Vincristine, daunorubicin, and prednisone/ Vinblastine, decarbazine, and platinum compd (cisplatin) (both cancer chemotherapies); Volume-depleted patient.

VD_p; V_{Dp} Physiologic dead space volume (see PFT - VD_p).

VD_p/Vt ratio Physiologic dead space/tidal volume ratio (see VD/VT).

VDR Venereal disease reaction; Venous diameter ratio.

VDRL Venereal disease reaction level; Venereal Disease Research Laboratory (test for syphilis, originated by this laboratory) (see STS - VDRL).

VDRR Vitamin D-resistant rickets.

VDRS Verdun Depression Rating Scale.

VDRT Venereal disease reference test (Harris) (see STS - VDRT).

VDS Vasodilator substance; Venereal disease - syphilis (see VD-S); Vertebral disc space; Vindesine; Volume-deficiency shock.

VD-S Venereal disease - syphilis (= VDS).

Vdss; Vd_{ss} Volume of distribution (of a drug) (see Vss; V_{ss}).

Vdss/F Weight-adjusted apparent volume of distribution (of a drug).

vD's test van Deen's test - for blood in gastric juice (Izaak Abramson van Deen, Dutch physician, 1804-1869) (= vD).

VDT Vibration disappearance threshold; Vigorous diuretic therapy; Visual display terminal; Visual distortion test.

VDU Video display unit.

VDV Ventricular (end-)diastolic volume.

VDVD Veterinary Doctor and Veterinary Digest (UK journal).

vdV's test van der Velden's test (= Maly's test) - for free hydrochloric acid in gastric juice (van der Velden, German physician, 1851-1903).

VD/VT Ratio of dead space ventilation to total ventilation (= Dead space ventilation/total ventilation-ratio; Physiologic dead space/tidal volume-ratio) (= VD_p/Vt) (see PFT - VD/VT).

VE Vaginal examination; Velar elevation; Venezuelan/ Viral encephalitis; Venous emptying/ extension; Ventilation (see Ve); Ventilatory equivalent; Ventricular elasticity/ escape/ extrasystole; Verbal-emotional (stimulus); Vertex (= Vert); Vesicular exanthema; Veterinary Economics (journal); Visual efficiency; Vitamin E (see Vitamins - E); Vocational education/ evaluation; Volume ejection (see Ve period); Voluntary effort.

Ve Ventilation (= VE).

V_E Environmental variance; Volume of expired air (see $\dot{V}_E$).

$\dot{V}_E$ Respiratory minute volume (= V_E) (see PFT - $\dot{V}$E).

V&E Vinethene and ether (an anesthetic mixture of vinyl ether 25% w/w and anesthetic ether 75% w/w).

VEA Ventricular ectopic activity/ arrhythmia; Viral envelope antigen.

VEB Ventricular ectopic beat (see PVB).

VECG Vector electrocardiogram.

VECP Visually evoked cortical potential.

VED Vacuum erection device; Ventricular ectopic depolarization; Vital exhaustion and depression.

Ved Vedanta (religion).

VEDP Ventricular end-diastolic pressure.

VEE Vagina, ectocervix, and endocervix; Venezuelan equine encephalomyelitis; Virally encoded enzyme (see VCD).

VEEP Volunteer Enterprises Educational Program.

VEF Ventricular ejection fraction; Visually evoked field.

+veFH Positive family history (= PFH).

-veFH Negative family history (= NFH).

VEGAS Ventricular enlargement with gait apraxia syndrome.

VEGF Vascular endothelial growth factor.

vehic vehicle (L. vehiculum).

VEI Vaginal epithelial integrity (see VHI).

vel or (L.); velocity (see veloc).

veloc velocity (= vel).

Velsicol 1068 Chlordane (see CD 68).

VEM Vasoexcitor material.

Ven; ven Vein/ Venous (see V.).

veno- prefix meaning vein (L. vena).

vent ventilate/ation/ator; ventral; ventricle/cular (see ventric).

vent fib ventricular fibrillation.

Venti-mask Venturi mask - a displacable plastic mask which delivers measured oxygen concentrations by the Venturi mixing principle. Three separate masks (27%, 30%, and 35%) are available.

ventr ventral.
ventr- prefix meaning belly, or front of body (L. venter).
ventric ventricle/cular (= vent).
ventriculo- prefix meaning ventricle of brain/ heart (L. ventriculus).
V_{EO2}; Ve_{O2} Ventilatory equivalent for oxygen (see PFT - Ve_{O2}).
VEP Visco-elastic property (of mucus); Visually evoked potential.
Ve period Volume ejection period (= VE) (see PFT).
+vePT Positive pregnancy test (= PPT).
-vePT Negative pregnancy test (= NPT).
V_{equiv} Ventilatory equivalent for oxygen in liters (see PFT - V_{equiv}).
VER Ventricular escape rhythm; Visual evoked response.
Ver; ver Genuine (L. verus).
Verc Vervet (African green monkey kidney) cells.
Verda Verdamycin sulfate.
vers- combining form meaning turn (L. versus) (see vert-).
Vert; vert Vertebra(l)/(te); Vertex (see VE); Vertical.
vert- combining form meaning turn (L. verto) (see vers-).
Ves; ves Bladder (L. vesica); Vesicular (= Vesic); Vessel.
Vesic; vesic A blister (L. vesicula; vesicatorium); Vesicular (see Ves).
vesic- prefix meaning bladder (L. vesica).
vE's method van Ermengen's method.
vesp evening (L. vesper).
vest vestibular.
Ves ur; ves ur Urinary bladder (L. vesica urinaria).
VET; VeT Vestigial testis (rat).
Vet Veteran; Veterinarian/inary.
v et See also (L. vide etiam).
Vet Ad; Vet Admin Veterans Administration.
VetMB Bachelor of Veterinary Medicine.
VetMD Doctor of Veterinary Medicine.
Vet Med Veterinary medicine.
VETS Veterans Adjustment Scale.
Vet Sci Veterinary science.
Vetus (L.) Old.
Ve/V_{O2} 100 ml Ventilatory equivalent (see PFT - Ve/V_{O2} 100 ml).
VF Left leg electrode (ECG); Ventricular fibrillation/ fluid/ flutter; Verbal factor (comprehension factor, psychology) (see V factor); Variant/ Video/ Visual frequency (see Vf); Visual field (see Vf); Vitreous fluorophotometry; Vocal fremitus.
Vf Field of vision (= Visual field) (= VF; vf); Variant frequency (see V_f); Visual frequency (= VF).
vf visual field (see Vf).
V_f Variant frequency (= VF; Vf).
VFA Volatile fatty acid.
V factor Verbal comprehension factor (psychology) (= VF).
VFC Vaccines for Children (Program); Variable frequency clock; Ventricular function curve; Voltage-to-frequency converter.
VFD Visual feedback display; Visual field defect.
VFDF Very fast death factor.
VFF Voice fundamental frequency.
V-fFN Vaginal fetal fibronectin.
VFG Vascularized fibular graft (Orthopedics).
VFI Vascularization and flow indices (a combination-system of vascular indices called the TDCH or Three-dimensional color histogram, used in the assessment of circulatory changes in the umbilical vessels of the fetus, especially in multifetal pregnancies); Venous filling index; Visual field intact.
V fib Ventricular fibrillation.
VFL Visual field loss.
VFL; VFl Ventricular flutter.
VFM Vaginal fluid mucinase.
VFP Vascular/ Ventricular filling/ fluid pressure; Venous filling pressure (preload, to the ventricles); Vitreous fluorophotometry.
VFPN Volu-feed premie nipple.
VFR Vertebral fracture rate; Voiding flow rate.
VFRN Volu-feed regular nipple.
VFS Vaginal fluid sialidase; Vascular fibrous stroma (Orthopedics); Vascular fragility syndrome; Vertebral Fracture Study (see FIT).
VFT Venous filling time; Ventricular fibrillation threshold.
VFV Vaginal fluid volume (see VHI).
VG van Gieson (stain); Vein graft; Ventilated group; Ventricular gallop; Ventriculography;

Very good (see V/G); Vitalography (see PFT; TVCT); Volume of gas.

V_G Genetic variance.

V/G Very good (= VG).

VGCC Voltage-gated calcium channels.

VGH Very good health.

vGJ von Gies joint (a chronic syphilitic chondro-osteoarthritis).

VGK Von Graefe's knife (Ophthalmology).

VGM Venous graft myringoplasty; Ventriculogram.

VGP Viral glycoprotein.

VGS Ventricular gallop sound.

vG's method van Gehucten's method.

VH Vaginal hysterectomy; Velar height; Venous hematocrit; Ventricular hypertrophy; Vestibular hydrops (see RLV); Veterans Hospital; Viral hepatitis; Vitamins and Hormones (journal); Vitreous hemorrhage.

V_H Variable domain of heavy chain.

VHA Veterans Health Administration; Volatile halogenated anesthetic (e.g. Desflurane).

VHC Vertex hair count.

VHD Valvular heart disease; Viral hematodepressive disease.

VHDL Very high density lipoprotein.

VHEW Very heavily exuding wound.

VHF Very high frequency; Viral hemorrhagic fever; Visual half-field (eye examination).

VHI Vaginal health index (elasticity, fluid volume, pH, epithelial integrity and moisture of the vagina).

VHIB Voluntary Health Insurance Board.

VHL Vertex hair loss; von Hippel-Lindau (gene/ syndrome) - a tumor-suppressor gene that has been linked to kidney cancer.

VHLD Von Hippel-Lindau disease (see VHL).

VHN Vickers hardness number.

VHP Vasoactive hormone pathway.

VHR Ventricular heart rate.

VHS Value Health Services.

VI Roman numeral six (see Symbols - 6); Vaginal intercourse/ irrigation; Variable interval (reinforcement); Vascularization index (see VFI); Vastus intermedius; Vegetable insulin (see Insulin - VI; PI ii); Virgo intacta; Virulence/nt (see Vi); Viscosity/ Vitality/ Volume index; Visual impairment/ inspection; Volume indicator (sound).

Vi Virginium - a former name for the element now known as Francium (Fr) (Z = 87) (see Elements - Francium); Virulence/ Virulent (= VI).

vi See below (L. vide infra).

V_i Average urine output (see KFT - V_i).

VIA Vasoactive intestinal polypeptide; Virus inactivating agent - an agent present in the serous excretion of the nose which inactivates the influenza virus and certain other viruses; Virus infection-associated antgen.

VIB Flanders (Interuniversity) Institute for Biotechnology (Belgium); Venomous insect bite; Viral inclusion bodies/ body (or "decoy cells") - found in the urine and allograft tissue in patients suffering from nephropathy, and caused by reactivation of polyomavirus type BK (BK virus), due to severe renal-allograft dysfunction; Vitamin Information Bureau; Vocational interest blank.

Vib; vib Vibration.

VIBS Vocabulary, information, block design, similarities (psychology).

VIC Vasoinhibitory center; Voice intensity control(ler).

vic times (L. vices).

VICA Velocity (of blood) in the internal carotid artery.

VICC Vascular interstitial closed circuit.

VI-CTS Vibration-induced carpal tunnel syndrome.

VI-CVC Vagal-induced cardiovascular collapse.

VIC Virus-infected cardiocyte (see HMV)/ cell.

VID Videodensitometry; Visible iris diameter.

vid See (L. vide).

VIDA Ventricular impulse detector and alarm.

Vidarabine Adenine arabinoside (an anti-viral drug).

VIE Vascular ischemic event.

VIEN Vaginal intraepithelial neoplasia/sm (see VAIN; VIN).

VIF Virus-induced interferon.

VIG; VIg Vaccinia immunoglobulin (= Vaccinia-immune globulin).

VIGOR VIoxx Gastrointestinal Outcomes Research (US) (Vioxx [MSD] = Rofecoxib, a COX-2 inhibitor used in the treatment of osteoarthritis, rheumatoid arthritis, and other joint diseases).

VIIag Factor VII antigen (see Factor VII).

VIIIc Factor VIII clotting activity (see Factor VIII).

VIII_{vwf} von Willebrand factor (see vWF).

VILI Ventilator-induced lung injury (see EIS; HPAP; IPPH; SILI).

Villitis Bacterial infection within the placental villi (see Amnionitis; Chorioamnionitis; Funisitis).

VIM Video-intensification microscopy; Vimentin; Volunteers in Mission (United Presbyterian Church).

Vim Ventro-intermedius (= Intermediate ventral nucleus of thalamus).

VIN Vaginal/ Vulvar intra-epithelial neoplasm.

Vin; vin Vinyl; Wine (L. vinum).

VINITI All-Union Institute of Scientific and Technical Information (Moscow).

Vio-D Vitamin D_2 (see Vitamins - D_2).

VIP Variable incentive pay (Military Medical Services); Vasoactive intestinal peptide/ polypeptide (a neuropeptide); Vasoactive intracorpeal pharmacotherapy; Vasoinhibitory peptide; Venous independance plethysmography; Very important patient/ person; Vinblastine/ VP-etoposide, ifosfamide, and platinum compd (cisplatin); Viral-inactivation procedure; Volantary interruption of pregnancy.

VIPCON; ViPCon Visual perception confusion (diagnostic test).

VIPoma Vasoactive intestinal polypeptide-secreting tumor.

VIQ Verbal Intelligence Quotient.

VIR; Vir Viral/ Virology/ Virus.

vir green (L. viridis); virulent.

Virol Virology (journal).

VIS Vaginal irrigation smear; Venous insufficiency syndrome; Vertebral irritation syndrome; Virus inactivation study; Visible/ Vision/ Visual (see Vis); Visual information storage; Visual spectroscopy (see ViS).

ViS Visual spectroscopy (= VIS; Vis; vis).

Vis; vis Visible/ Vision/ Visual (= VIS); Visit(ed)/(ing)/(or); Visual spectroscopy (see ViS).

vis-à-vis French - compared with/ in relation to.

VISC Vitreous infusion suction cutter.

visc viscera(l); viscosity/ous.

viscero- combining form meaning viscera (L. viscus).

VISI Volar intercalated segment instability.

VISSR Visible infra-red spin-scan radiometer.

VISTA Volunteers in Service to America (see ACTION).

VIT Vaccine/ Venom immunotherapy; Vibration isolation table.

Vit Vitamin (see Vitamins).

vit vital; yolk of an egg (L. vitellus) (see Vitel).

vit- combining form meaning life (L. vita).

VITA Volunteers in Technical Assistance (to developing countries).

Vitamins (= Vit; Vits) A general term for a number of unrelated organic substances that occur in many foods in small amounts, and that are necessary for the normal metabolic functioning of the body. They may be fat-soluble or water-soluble.

Vitamin A: (= Anti-infective Vitamin; Antixerophthalmic Vitamin; Axerophthol; Axerophthylium; Retinol) Fat-soluble, unsaturated, aliphatic alcohol present in the liver oils of the cod, shark, and other fish, in butter, egg yolk, cheese and liver, as well as in many vegetable foods in most of which it exists as the plant pigment carotene, in three isomeric forms, alpha-, beta- and gamma-carotenes. It is also synthesized. Deficiency in the diet causes (i) inadequate production and regeneration of the visual purple with resulting night blindness, and (ii) disturbances in the epithelial tissue resulting in keratomalacia, xerophthalmia, and lessened resistance to infections through the epithelial surfaces.

Vitamin A_1: A form of vitamin A found in the eye tissues of marine fishes.

Vitamin A_2: Similar to vitamin A but with a different absorption spectrum in the ultraviolet. Found in the livers of freshwater fish.

Vitamin B complex: A group of water-soluble substances including thiamine, riboflavine, nicotinic acid (niacin), nicotinamide (niacin amide; nicotinic acid amide), the vitamin B_6

group (pyridoxine, pyridoxal, pyridoxamine, alpha and beta pyracin), biotin, pantothenic acid, folic acid, possibly para-aminobenzoic acid, inositol, vitamin B_{12}, and possibly choline. Nicotinic acid and nicotinamide are also known together, as the PP, P-P, pellagra-preventing, or antipellagra factor.

Vitamin B: A member of the vitamin B complex.

Vitamin B_1: (= Aneurine Hydrochloride; Aneur HCl; Aneurine Chloride Hydrochloride; Thiamine HCl; Thiamine Hydrochloridum; Thiaminium Chloride) Rich sources of this vitamin include peas, beans, oatmeal, whole wheat, enriched flour and bread, lean pork, etc., including the common foods such as milk, vegetables, and fruits. Deficiency of aneurine results in fatigue, anorexia, gastro-intestinal disturbances, tachycardia, and ultimately edema and cardiac failure of beri-beri.

Vitamin B_2: (= Riboflavine; Lactoflavin; Riboflav; Riboflavin; Riboflavinum; Vitamin G) The richest dietary sources of riboflavine are liver, kidneys, eggs, milk, yeast, and green vegetables. Deficiency in man is characterized by a well-defined syndrome, with angular stomatitis, glossitis, seborrhoeic follicular keratosis of the nasolabial skin, dermatitis of the ano-genital region, and "burning feet".

Vitamin B_3: (= i. Nicotinamide - see Vitamin PP. ii. Pantothenic Acid) Present in all living tissues; liver is one of the richest sources but meat, cereals and milk also contain this vitamin. It may be prepared synthetically. Deficiency symptoms in animals include dermatitis (anti-dermatitis factor of chicks), keratitis, adrenal hemorrhage and atrophy, depigmentation of hair and arrest of growth. Has been reported as an anti-grey hair factor in experimental animals. No accepted therapeutic use in human medicine.

Vitamin B_4: (= Biotin) A water-soluble factor from yeast, that prevents a specific paralysis in rats and chicks.

Vitamin B_5: A factor necessary to maintain growth in rats, and weight in pigeons.

Vitamin B_6: (= Pyridoxine Hydrochloride; Pyridox HCl; Pyridoxini Hydrochloricum; Pyridoxal HCl; Pyridoxamine HCl; Pyridoxium Chloride; Pyridoxol HCl; Adermine HCl; Alpha and Beta Pyracin) It occurs in yeast, liver, cereals, meat and other foods, and is also prepared synthetically. Pyridoxine, pyridoxal, and pyridoxamine which occcur in foodstuffs, are collectively known as vitamin B_6. In the body they are converted to pyridoxal phosphate which is the coenzyme for aminoacid decarboxylase and for transaminase. Has been used for convulsions in infants and in the treatment of anemia induced by pyridoxine deficiency; also as a prophylactic against peripheral neuritis, and in nausea and vomiting of pregnancy and irradiation sickness, but the evidence of its value in these conditions is not impressive. Has also been tried in the treatment of acute alcoholism for its excellent sobering-up effect when given intravenously.

Vitamin B_8: (= Adenylic acid; Adenosine Phosphate; AMP; Adenosine-5-phosphoric acid; 5'-Adenylic Acid; Phosphentaside) A nucleotide constituent of animal cells, concerned with the storage and release of energy. Has been used as a vasodilator in angina pectoris, and has been claimed to be of value in the treatment of disseminated sclerosis, porphyria, and in a variety of rheumatic and inflammatory conditions.

Vitamin B_{10}: A compound allied to Folic acid, which has an influence on feathering and on growth in chicks.

Vitamin B_{11}: Same as vitamin B_{10}.

Vitamin B_{12}: (= Cobalamine; Cobamin; Cyanocobal; Cyanocobalamine; Cyanocobalaminum; Cycobemin) A cobalt-containing substance, obtained from liver or separated from the products of metabolism of various microorganisms. A compound influencing erythropoiesis and representing the "anti-pernicious-anemia principle" of purified liver extracts. It is present in liver, kidney, milk, eggs, and muscle tissue, and is produced by bacterial synthesis in the colon. The intrinsic factor present in normal gastric secretion is essential for the absorption of cyanocobalamin from the alimentary tract.

This vitamin is effective in the treatment of pernicious anemia and its neurological complication, subacute combined degeneration of the spinal cord.

Vitamin B_{12a}: = Vitamin B_{12b}.

Vitamin B_{12b}: (= Hydroxycobalamine; Hydroxocobal; Hydroxocobalamin; Vitamin B_{12a}) In acid solutions hydroxocobalamin takes up a hydrogen ion which converts the hydroxyl to a coordinated water molecule, aquocobalamin. Hydroxocobalamin is more readily bound to serum protein than cyanocobalamin, and so has the advantage that a higher initial level and more prolonged serum levels of vitamin B_{12} may be obtained.

Vitamin B_{14}: A compound isolated from urine; said to check reproduction of cancer cells and to act as an anti-pernicious anemia factor.

Vitamin B_{15}: (= Pangamic acid) A water-soluble, amino derivative of glycuronic acid, originally discovered in the kernel of the apricot.

Vitamin B_{17}: Amygdalin, a cyanide-producing chemical found in bitter almonds and apricot pits, and thought by some to be a potential cure for cancer. Sold under the tradename, Laetrile

Vitamin B_c: (= Folic acid; Acid Folicum; Folacin; Folinsyre; Pteroylglutamic acid; Vitamin M) Identical with the Lactobacillus casei factor of the liver. It is present, free or combined (vitamin B_c conjugate) in liver, meat, yeast, cereals, spinach and other green leafy vegetables, and may be prepared synthetically. Folic acid is necessary for the normal production of red blood cells, including maturation of megaloblasts into normoblasts. A deficiency of free folic acid may result in: a) nutritional macrocytic anemia - from a diminished intake, b) sprue - from failure to absorb the conjugate, and c) pernicious anemia - from failure to break down or utilize the conjugate. Although it produces a hemopoietic response, folic acid fails to protect the onset of subacute combined degeneration of the spinal cord, and thus the use of cyanocobalamin (vitamin B_{12}) is essential in the treatment of pernicious anemia. Without folic acid the living cell cannot divide but is halted in the metaphase; this property underlies the use of folic acid antagonists in the treatment of neoplastic disease.

Vitamin B_c conjugate: = Combined Folic Acid (see Vitamin B_c).

Vitamin B_t: A vitamin necessary for the nutrition of the mealworm beetle, Tenebrio molitor.

Vitamin B_x: (= Para-aminobenzoic Acid; Aminobenzoic Acid; Amben; PAB; PABA; Pabacidum; p-Aminobenzoic acid; Vitamin H') Widely distributed in plant and animal tissue such as yeast, liver, and rice polishings. It was first recognized as an essential metabolite for certain microorganisms, and as such, a bacterial growth factor. Before the era of broad-spectrum antibiotics, para-aminobenzoic acid was used in the treatment of rickettsial infections and in particular, in typhus and Rocky Mountain spotted fever.

Vitamin C: (= Ascorbic Acid; Ascorb Acid; Acidum Ascorbicum; L-Ascorbic Acid; Cevitamic Acid) May be extracted from the juice of citrus fruits or vegetable sources such as rose hips and blackcurrents, and is prepared synthetically. Ascorbic acid is essential for the formation of collagen and intercellular material, and hence for the development of cartilage, bone, and teeth, and for the healing of wounds. Known also as the antiscorbutic vitamin, it is particularly useful nowadays in the prevention of infantile scurvy. It influences the formation of hemoglobin and erythrocyte maturation, and is used successfully in the treatment of familial idiopathic methemoglobinemia. Ascorbic acid is especially required in adolescence, pregnancy and lactation, infections, thyrotoxicosis, and postoperative states.

Vitamin D: Any one of the several related sterols possessing the property of preventing rickets. These substances are derivatives of sterols which acquire antirachitic properties when exposed to ultraviolet light. They may be prepared artificially by the irradiation of ergosterol and a few related sterols. Vitamin D is present naturally in the liver oils of various fish, in butter and egg yolk, and is produced in the body on exposure to sunlight. Its

deficiency causes rickets in children, and osteomalacia and osteoporosis in adults.
Vitamin D_1: A term formerly applied to an impure mixture of calciferol with another sterol.
Vitamin D_2: (= Calciferol; Calcif; Ergocalciferol; Ergocalciferolum; Irradiated Ergosterol; Vio-D; Viosterol) An antirachitic substance obtained from ergosterol, a sterol occurring in yeast, by ultraviolet irradiation. Another metabolite is Hydroxyergocalciferol (HEC).
Vitamin D_3: (= Cholecalciferol; Natural Vitamin D; Activated 7-dehydrocholesterol) The chief form of vitamin D present in fish-liver oils, or prepared by irradiation of 7-dehydrocholesterol, i.e. "activated" or rendered anti-rachitic. Used for the same purposes as calciferol. Patients who have become insensitive to calciferol may still respond to cholecalciferol. Metabolites of vitamin D_3 are Hydroxycholecalciferol (HCC), 25-Hydroxycholecalciferol (25-HCC) (peak IV metabolite of vitamin D_3), and 21, 25 HCC (peak V metabolite of vitamin D_3).
Vitamin E: (= Tocopherols) Alpha-tocopherol, one of the three tocopherols (alpha, beta, and gamma), occurring in the oil of soya bean, wheat germ, rice germ, cotton-seed, maize and other cereals, egg yolk and beef and in green leaves such as lettuce. Can be prepared synthetically. A vitamin necessary in the diet of rats to ensure reproduction. Has been used in the treatment of amyotrophic lateral sclerosis and other degenerative diseases. Also in the treatment of sterility; it was once called the "anti- sterility" vitamin, but clinical evidence has failed to substantiate this claim (IDO-E = d-alpha-tocopherol).
Vitamin F: A name given to a mixture of unsaturated fatty acids, including linoleic, linolenic, and arachidonic acids, which have been found essential for the growth of rats, and may be essential for man. They have been given to lower blood-cholesterol levels in patients with hypercholesterolemia, and have been used in atherosclerosis and coronary disease. These unsaturated fatty acids are also given by mouth or appleed externally in eczema and other skin diseases.
Vitamin G: Riboflavine (see Vitamin B_2).
Vitamin H: (= Biotin; Bios II; fH; Coenzyme R) A crystalline substance, widely distributed in plants and animals, the richest sources being liver, kidney, pancreas, yeast, milk and eggs. Widely distributed in living tissues; biotin was first recognized as a growth factor for yeast. Deficiency symptoms in humans resemble those of any type of B-group deficiency states - anorexia, lassitude, paraesthesia, and seborrhoeic dermatitis. Biotin is classified under the Vitamin B complex.
Vitamin H': = Para-aminobenzoic acid (see Vitamin B_x).
Vitamin J: A vitamin which is apparently necessary for development in guinea pigs.
Vitamin K: (= Anti-hemorrhagic factor; Coagulation vitamin). A group of naphthaquinone derivatives occurring in nature and fat-soluble, together with several synthetic preparations with vitamin K activity, some of these being water-soluble. These compounds promote clotting of the blood by increasing the synthesis of prothrombin by the liver. They occur naturally in alfalfa, spinach, cabbage, putrefied fish meal, hog-liver fat, egg yolk and hemp-seed. They have an antihemorrhagic activity with a specific effect on prothrombin deficiency. They are used in obstructive jaundice, in hemorrhagic states associated with intestinal diseases and with disease of the liver, and in hypoprothombinemia of the newborn, being given parenterally to the infant or to the mother during labor.
Vitamin K_1: (= Phytomenadione; Phytomenad; Phytonadione; Methylphytylnaphthochinonum) A naturally occurring naphthaquinone, vitamin K_1 is isolated from the chloroplasts of green plants (see Vitamin K). It is a fatsoluble vitamin, acting more rapidly than the synthetic vitamin-K analogues, such as Menaphthone (vitamin K_3) and Acetomenaphthone.
Vitamin K_2: A naturally occurring naphthaquinone of microbial origin, obtained from putrefying plant and animal material. Fat-soluble (see Vitamin K).

Vitamin K_3: (= Menadione; Menadionum; Menaph; Menaphthene; Menaphthone; Methylnaphthochinonum) A synthetic, fat-soluble, slower-acting, vitamin-K analogue, given by intramuscular injections in the treatment of multiple sclerosis and muscular dystrophy.
Vitamin L: A factor necessary for lactation in rats.
Vitamin L_1: Found in beef-liver extract.
Vitamin L_2: Found in yeast.
Vitamin M: = Folic acid (see Vitamin B_c).
Vitamin P: (= Trihydroxyethyl-rutocide; Vitamin X) The term "permeability-vitamin", together with its occurrence in paprika, gave rise to the name vitamin P. This is the flavone factor in lemon juice (citrin) and Hungarian red pepper, deficiency of which causes increased permeability of capillary walls. This factor is possibly a mixture of flavone, eriodictyol, hesperidin, and rutin; these are the water-soluble bioflavinoids obtained from citrus fruits and other vegetable sources. Vitamin P has been used in the treatment of apoplexy, thrombophlebitis, chronic venous insufficiency and Meniere's disease, and in conditions associated with increased capillary fragility, such as post- thrombotic syndromes.
Vitamin PP: (= Nicotinic acid; Acidum Nicotinicum; $C_6H_5NO_2$; $C_6H_6N_2O$; Niacin; Niacinamide; Nicotin Acid; Nicotinamide; Nicotinamidum; Nicotinic Acid Amide; Nicotylamide; Nikotinsaure; Pyridine-3-carboxyamide; Pyridine-3-carboxylic acid; Vitamin P-P). Also known as the pellagra-preventing factor, hence the name vitamin P-P. It belongs to the vitamin B complex and is prepared synthetically. It is found in rice-polishings, yeast, lean meats, and to a lesser extent in potatoes and vegetables. Deficiency produces pellagra, which is characterized by loss of appetite, lethargy, weakness, diarrhea, dermatitis, and mental changes. Used in the prevention and treatment of pellagra and for its vasodilator action, in the treatment of certain types of Meniere's disease and peripheral vascular disorders including chilblains, frostbite, and migraine. Also in arthritis, hypercholesterolemia, and ischemic heart disease.
Vitamin R: A vitamin necessary for proper development of chicks.
Vitamin S: A vitamin necessary for proper development of chicks.
Vitamin U: (= Anti-ulcer factor or vitamin; Cabagin) This substance is present in the juice of the white cabbage, and prevents the formation of experimental ulcers, and cures "histamine ulcers" in guinea-pigs. The dried juice, in doses of 2 g thrice daily, has been reported to have given good results in the treatment of peptic ulcer, chronic gastritis, and chronic cholangiohepatitis.
Vitamin V: A vitamin concerned in the development of chicks.
Vitamin X: A name formerly given to vitamin P (see Vitamin P).

Vit Cap; vit cap Vital capacity (see VC; PFT).

Vitel Yolk (L. vitellus) - of an egg (= vit).

vit ov sol dissolved in egg yolk (L. vitello ovi solutus).

vitr glass (L. vitreum).

Vits Vitamins (see Vitamins).

VIUP Viable intrauterine pregnancy.

vivi- combining form meaning alive (L. vivus).

viz namely (L. videlicet).

VJ Ventriculojugular (shunt); Veterinary Journal; Vogel-Johnson (agar).

VJC Ventriculojugular-cardiac.

VK Vervet (African green monkey) kidney cell(s).

VKC Vernal keratoconjunctivitis.

VKH Vogt-Koyanagi-Harada (syndrome) (see VKHS).

VKHS Vogt-Koyanagi-Harada syndrome.

VKP Vitallium knee prosthesis (Walldius).

VKT Vane Kindergarten Test.

VL Left arm electrode (ECG); Vascular laboratory; Ventralis lateralis (nucleus/ thalamus); Ventrolateral; Visceral leishmaniasis; Vision of the left eye (see VOS); Volunteer Leader (Amer Hosp Assoc journal).

V_L Variable domain of the light chain.

VLA Virus-like agent.

VBL Vincaleukoblastine (= Vinblastine; Velban; VB; VBL) (see VBL).

VLBR Very low birth rate.

VLBW Very low birth weight.

VLCD Very low caloric diet (less than 2,090 kJ/day).

VLCFA Very long chain (saturated) fatty acid - elevated in the fatal gastric disorder Adrenoleukodystrophy (ADL; ADLD; ALD); recently treated with the use of very-long-chain unsaturated fatty acids such as Oleic acid and Erucic acid.

VLD Very low density.

VLDL; VLDLP Very low density lipoprotein (a triglyceride) (see VLD-TG).

VLDL-C Very low density lipoprotein cholesterol.

VLD-TG Very low density triglyceride (see VLDL; VLDLP).

VLF Very low frequency.

VLG Ventral (nucleus) of the lateral geniculate (body).

VLH Ventrolateral nucleus of the hypothalamus.

VLI Very low incidence; Virus-like infection.

VLLB Viral Leukemia and Lymphoma Branch (NCI).

VLM Vastus lateralis muscle (see ALT); Visceral larva migrans.

VL nucleus Ventrolateral nucleus (of thalamus) (L. ventralis lateralis).

VLO Vastus lateralis obliquus (muscle).

VLP Vincristine, L-asparaginase, and prednisone; Virus-like particle.

VLPO Ventrolateral preoptic area (of the hypothalamus) - the "sleep" center on the ventral surface of the cerebrum, just behind the eyes.

VLR Vinleurosine.

VLS Vascular leak syndrome.

VLSI Very large scale integration.

VLU Venous leg ulcer.

VM Vasomotor; Valsalva's maneuver (see CRP); Ventralis medialus; Ventricular mass; Ventriculometry; Ventromedial; Vestibular membrane; Veterinary Medicine (journal); Viomycin; Viral myocarditis; Visual Medicine (journal); Voltmeter.

V/m Volts per meter.

VM 26 Teniposide.

VMA Vanillylmandelic acid (= Vanil/ Vanillin mandelic acid; VML; 3-Methoxy-4-hydroxymandelic acid) (laboratory/ endocrinology).

VMACHF Vasodilation in the Management of Acute Congestive Heart Failure (trial).

V_{MAX}; Vmax Maximal on-load/ Maximum velocity (of the contractile element); Maximal rate of depolarization.

$\dot{V}_{max}$ Maximal rate of airflow during forced expiration (see PFT).

$\dot{V}$max 75, $\dot{V}$max 50, $\dot{V}$max 25 Maximal expiratory flow at 75%, 50%, 25% of Vital capacity (VC).

VMB Vagally-mediated bradyarrhythmia.

VMBR Visuo-motor behavior rehearsal (see BI).

VMC Vasomotor center.

VMCF Vie Médicale au Canada Français (journal, formerly Laval Medical).

VMCP Vincristine, melphalan, cyclophosphamide, and prednisone.

VMCG Vector magnetocardiogram.

VMD Doctor of Veterinary Medicine.

vMDV Virulent Marek disease virus.

VMF Vasomotor flushing.

VMG Vaginal moisturizing gel (bioadhesive).

VMGT Visual Motor Gestalt Test.

VMH Ventromedial hypothalamic (neurons/ nuclei/ region/ syndrome).

VMI Vasomotor instability; Visual motor integration (= VSI).

VMIT Visual Motor Integration Test.

VML Vanillylmandelic acid (see VMA).

VMM Virginia Medical Monthly (journal); Voluntary muscle movement.

VMN Ventromedial nucleus.

VMO Vastus medialis obliquus (muscle).

VM&P Varnish makers' and painters' naphtha.

VMR Vasomotor rhinitis.

VMS Valid medical strategy; Video monitoring system; Visual memory span; Visual Motor Sequencing (test) (see VMST).

VM/SAC Veterinary Medicine/ Small Animal Clinician (journal).

VMST Visual Motor Sequencing Test.

VMT Vasomotor tonus; Ventilatory muscle training; Ventromedial tegmentum; Vitalometer testing (see PFT).

VMV Visna-maedi virus (gag p27).

VN Vesical neck; Vestibular neurectomy;

Vestibular/ Visceral nucleus; Virus neutralization/zing; Visiting Nurse; Vocational Nurse (also LPN; LVN); Vomeronasal.

VNA Virus neuraminidase (influenza A and B); Visiting Nurse Association.

VNAB Ventral noradrenergic bundle.

VNC Vesicle neck contracture.

VNDPT Visual Numerical Discrimination Pre-Test.

VNE Verbal-nonemotional (stimulus).

VNMP Vital Notes on Medical Periodicals (MLA journal).

VNO Vomeronasal organ.

VNS Varied/ Various neurological signs/ symptoms; Visiting nursing service.

VNTR Variable number of tandem repeats (regions or sequences in the human genome).

VO Verbal order (see V/O); Volume overload; Voluntary opening (prosthesis).

Vo Oral ventral (nucleus of thalamus) (ventro-oralis) (see Voi); Standard volume.

vo verbal order (see VO; V/O).

V_0 Urinary/ Urine output (in milliliters per hour) (see KFT - V_0).

V/O Verbal order (= VO).

VO2; VO_2; V_{O2} Oxygen uptake/ consumption (per minute) or Volume of oxygen utilization (at rest) (see PFT - VO2).

$\dot{V}_{O2\,max}$ Maximum oxygen consumption.

Voa Ventro-oralis anterior (thalamus).

VOC Volatile organic chemical.

Voc Vocational.

Vocab Vocabulary.

VOCC Voltage-operated calcium channel.

Voc Ed Vocational education.

VOCTOR Void on call to operating room.

VOD Veno-occlusive/ Venous occlusive disease; Viral ocular disease; Vision of right eye (L. viseo oculus dexter = VR).

Voi Oral ventral nucleus of the thalamus (L. ventro-oralis internus) (see Vo).

Vol; vol Volar; Volatile (L. volatilis); Volume(tric); Voluntary/teer.

vol% volume percent (= VPC).

VOM Veno-occlusive mechanism (of the corpora cavernosa); Vinyl chloride monomer; Volt-ohm-milliammeter (= Volt-ohmmeter).

VON Victorian Order of Nurses (Canada).

V-ONC Viral oncogene.

VOO Ventricular asynchronous (competitive, fixed-rate pacemaker).

VOP Venous occlusion plethysmograph(y).

VOP; Vop Ventro-oralis posterior (thalamus).

VOR Vestibulo-ocular reflex.

VOS Varicocele oligospermia; Villanueva osteochrome stain (Orthopedics); Vision of left eye (L. visio oculus sinister) (= VL).

vos dissolve(d) in egg yolk/ yolk of egg (L. vitello ovi solutus).

VOT Visual Organization Test; Voice-onset time.

VOU Vision of each eye (L. visio oculus uterque).

voxel volume element (in CT scanning).

VP Etoposide (see VP-16); Physiological/ Plasma volume (see Vp); Valvuloplasty; Vapor/ Venous pressure (see vp); Variable pitch; Variegata/te porphyria; Vascular permeability; Vasopressin; Velopharyngeal; Venipuncture; Ventral premammillary (nucleus); Ventricular pacing/ premature (beat) (see Vp); Ventriculo-peritoneal; Ventroposterior; Vertex potential; Veterinary Practice (UK journal); Vice president; Vincristine & prednisone (cancer chemotherapy); Viral/ Virus protein; Viviparous; Voges Proskauer (medium/ reaction/ test); Volume-pressure (see V/P); Vulnerable period.

Vp Peak voltage; Phenotype variance; Physiological/ Plasma volume (= VP); Ventricular pacing/ premature (beat) (= VP).

vp vapor/ venous pressure (= VP).

V/P Ventilation/perfusion (ratio) (= V&P); Volume-pressure (= VP).

V&P Vagotomy and pyrloroplasty; Ventilation and perfusion (see V/P).

VP-16 Etoposide (= VP).

VPA Valproic acid (an antiepileptic drug).

VPB Ventricular premature beat (see PVB); Veterinary Pharmaceuticals and Biologicals (publication).

VPC Vaginal fibronectin concentration (see CFC; PMF); Vapor-phase chromatography; Ventricular premature complex/ contraction (see PVB); Virus-producing cell; Volume of packed cells; Volume percent (see vol%).

VPCs Ventricular premature complexes/ contractions.

VPCT Ventricular premature contraction threshold.
VPD Vaccine-preventable disease; Vasoplastic disease; Ventricular premature depolarization (= VDP); Vincristine, Prednisolone and Daunorubicin (Chemotherapy).
VPDF Vegetable protein diet plus fiber.
VPE Vigorous physical exertion (see HPE).
VPF Vascular permeability factor.
VPG Velopharyngeal gap; Ventricular-pacing group (see PPG).
VPGSS Venous pressure gradient support stockings.
VPI Vapor phase inhibitor; Velopharyngeal insufficiency.
VPL Ventroposterolateral (nucleus of the thalamus) (= Ventral posterior lateralis - a caudal ventral nucleus of the thalamus).
VPLM Variable parameter lung model.
VPLS Ventilation-perfusion lung scan (using isotopes) (= IVPLS; VQ scan) (see PFT - V/Q).
VPM Ventilator pressure manometer; Ventroposteromedial (= Ventral posterior medialis - a caudal ventral nucleus of the thalamus).
vpm vibrations per minute.
V_{PM} Actual/ Physiologic maximal shortening velocity of the contractile element.
VPN Ventral pontine nucleus.
VPO Velopharyngeal opening; Veritical pendular oscillation.
VPP Viral porcine pneumonia.
VPPs Viral polyproteins.
VPR Voges-Proskauer reaction (see VP test); Volume/pressure ratio; Volume pressure response.
VPRBC Volume of packed red blood cells.
VPRC Volume of packed red cells.
VPRP Violence Prevention Research Program.
VPS Ventriculoperitoneal shunt (see V-P shunt); Visual pleural space.
vps vibrations per second.
V-P shunt Ventriculoperitoneal shunt (for hydrocephalus) (= VPS).
VPT Vibratory perception threshold.
VP test Voges-Proskauer test (bacteriology) (= VPR).
VPV; VPVN Volunteer Physicians for Vietnam (AMA).
VPW Ventral prostate weight.
V/Q Voice quality.
V/Q; $\dot{V}/\dot{Q}$; $\dot{V}$-$\dot{Q}$ Ventilation-perfusion (see PFT - $\dot{V}/\dot{Q}$).
VQ scan see VPLS; VQ.
VR Right arm electrode (ECG); Valve replacement; Variable ratio (of reinforcement); Vascular rejection/ resistance; Venous reflux/ return; Ventilation rate/ ratio; Ventral root; Ventricular rate/ rhythm; Verbal reprimand; Vesicular rosette; Veterinary Record (BVA journal); Veterinary Review (UK journal); Vision of right eye (see VOD); Vital records; Vocal resonance; Vocational rehabilitation; Volta Review (journal on deafness).
Vr Volume of relaxation.
vr venous rete (network of small veins); ventral root (of a spinal nerve).
V-R Vagotomy and antrectomy.
VR_1 First vocalized response.
VRA Visual reinforcement audiometry; Vocational Rehabilitation Administration (HEW).
VRBC Volume of red blood cell(s).
VRC Venous renin concentration; Vocational rehabilitation counselor.
VRCP Vitreoretinochoroidopathy.
VRD Ventricular radial dysplasia; Vitreoretinal degeneration (= GFD); von Recklinghausen's disease.
VRE Vancomycin-resistant Enterococcus; Virtual reality experience.
VRE; VR&E Vocational rehabilitation and education.
VRF Vascular risk factor (for heart disease, stroke, etc.); Violence Research Foundation.
VRI Viral replication inhibitor (e.g. Amantadine); Viral/ Virus respiratory infection.
VRII Variable rate insulin infusion.
VRL Ventral root, lumbar; Virus Reference Laboratory.
VRM Visual-recognition memory.
VR/min Ventricular rate per minute.
VRNA Viral ribonucleic acid.
VRNF Von Recklinghausen's neurofibromatosis (= RNF).

VROM Voluntary range of motion.
VRP Very reliable product.
VRPPC Vision Research Program Planning Committee.
VRR Vaccine-related risk; Ventral root reflex.
VRS Verbal rating scale.
VRT Variance of resident time; Vehicle rescue technician; Ventral root, thoracic; Virtual-reality technique/ therapy; Visual Retention Test.
VRU Viscosity reducing unit.
VRV Ventricular residual volume; Viper retro-virus.
VS Single vibration (see vs); Vaccination scar; Vaccine serotype; Vagal stimulation; Valvular stenosis; Vascustat (Vascular surgery); Vasospasm; Vectoroscope; Venesection/ Venisection (see Vs); Ventricular septum; Verbal scale (of IQ); Very sensitive (to antibiotic); Vesicular sound(s) (pulmonary); Vesicular stomatitis; Veterinary Surgeon; Vibration second (see vs)/ syndrome; Vicryl suture (see Sut); Visual storage; Vital sign(s) (see V/S); Vogt-Spielmeyer (syndrome); Volatile solid; Volumetric solution; Voluntary sterilization; Without glasses (L. vitreum sine).
Vs Venesection/ Venisection (L. venaesectio) (= VS).
vs against (L. versus); see above (L. vide supra); single vibration(s) (= VS); versus; vibration second(s) - the unit of measurement of sound waves (= VS; Vùs); vital signs (see V/S).
V/S Vital sign(s) (= VS; vs).
V·s Vibration second (see vs); Volt-second.
V ss Mean steady state volume of distribution (of a drug into the body (= Vd ss) tissues.
V x s Volts by seconds.
VSA Variant-specific surface antigen; Vasospastic angina (= VA - Variant angina); Volatile substance abuse (= 'solvent abuse'/ 'glue sniffing' etc.) such as Acetone (nail polish remover, polystyrene cements, etc.); Amyl, butyl and isobutyl nitrites; Butane; CHCs - Chlorinated hydrocarbons (found in cleaning fluids, paints, varnishes, lacquers and dyes); Petrol (gasoline); Propane; and Toluene-containing glues.
VsB Bleeding in the arm (L. venaesectio brachii).
VSBE Very short below-elbow (cast).
VSC Vital sign change(s); Voluntary surgical contraception.
VSD Ventricular septal defect; Virtually safe dose.
VSEPR Valence shell electron pair repulsion (theory of Gillespie and Nyholm).
VSFP Venous stop flow pressure.
VSG Variable/ Variant surface glycoprotein (genes on the coat or surface protein of the trypanosome parasite in blood).
VSHD Ventricular septal heart defect.
VSI Vagal/ Vagosplanchnic interaction (gastric, etc.); Visual (motor) integration (see VMI).
VSINC Virus Subcommittee of the International Nomenclature Committee.
VSM Vascular smooth muscle; Vital sign monitoring.
VSMF Visual search microfilm files (IHS).
VSMS Vineland Social Maturity Scale.
vsn vision.
VSO Vertical subcondylar oblique; Voluntary Service Overseas (British).
VSOK Vital signs all right/ normal/ OK.
VSP Variable spine plating; Ventricular synchronous pacing.
VSPC Virtual storage personal computing.
VSR Vasospastic reaction/ response; Venous stasis retinopathy; Visual-spatial response (e.g. driving reactions).
VSS Vital signs stable; Vital Statistics System (US).
VSs Vital signs (temperature, blood pressure, pulse and respiratory rate).
Vss; V_{ss} Mean steady volume of distribution (of a drug into the body tissue) (= Vdss; Vd_{ss}).
VST Ventral spinothalamic tract; Volume substitution therapy.
VSULA Vaccination scar on upper left arm.
VSURA Vaccination scar on upper right arm.
VSV Vesicular stomatitis virus; Virus-specific vaccine.
VSVE Volume substituted visco-elastic (eye surgery).
VSW Ventricular stroke work.

VSWR Voltage standing wave radio.

VT Tetrazolium violet (see TV); Tidal volume (see V\T); Total ventolation (see V/T); Vacuum tube/ tuberculin; Variable/ Venous time; Vasotonin; Venous thrombosis; Ventricular tachyarrhythmia/ tachycardia/ triggered (pacemaker); Verocytotoxin; Verotoxin; Vertical transmission (of disease, e.g. HIV, from mother to fetus) (see MFT); Veterinary Toxicology (ACVT journal); Vibration threshold; Videotape; Voice tube.

V_T; V_t; V\T Tidal volume (see PFT - V_T); Total ventilation (see PFT - V_T).

V&T Volume and tension (pulse pressure).

VTA Ventral tegmental area (of the brain); Ventricular tachyarrhythmia.

V tach Ventricular tachycardia.

VTD Ventricular tachydysrhythmia.

VTE Venous thromboembolism; Ventricular tachycardia event; Vicarious trial and error.

VTEA Venous thromboembolic accident (e.g. DVT, Pulmonary embolism, etc.) (see VTED).

VTEC Verotoxin-producing Escherichia coli.

VTED Venous thromboembolic disease.

VTEE Venous thromboembolic event (= VTE).

VTEP Venous thrombo-embolic process.

VTER Venous thromboembolic/ism risk (see VTEA; VTED).

V test Voluter test (radiology).

VTG; $\dot{V}_{TG}$; $\dot{V}_{tg}$ Volume thoracic gas/ Thoracic gas volume/ Total gas volume/ Respiratory trapped gas (see PFT - $\dot{V}_{TG}$).

VTI Vaginally transmitted infection (HIV - in AIDS, etc.); Volume-thickness index.

VTK Viral thymidine kinase (gene/ viral strain).

VTM Mechanical tidal volume; Virus transport medium.

VTOL Vertical take-off and landing.

VTP Versatrax pacemaker.

VTR Vagotomy retractor (Weinberg); Variable tandem repeats; Videotape recorder/ding or replay; Vesicular transport system.

VTS Vanishing twin syndrome (caused by total intrauterine reabsorption of the dead twin fetus) (Obstetrics); Vesicular transport system (see VTR).

VTSRS Verdun Target Symptom Rating Scale.

VTVM Vacuum tube voltmeter.

VTX; Vtx; vtx Vertex.

VU Varicose ulcer; Very urgent; Voltage unit (= vu); Voltmeter/ Volume unit (= vu).

vu voltage/ voltmeter/ volume unit (see VU).

VUC Vacuum-uterine-cannula.

vuls- combining form meaning pull or twitch (L. vulsus).

VUR Vesicoureteral reflex; Vesicoureteric reflux.

VUSM Vaginal ultrasound monitor(ing) (Obstetrics).

VUV Vacuum ultraviolet (spectroscopy).

VV Flow volume; Varicose veins (= vv); Venous volume (functional) (see FVV); Viper venom; Viral vector; Vulva and vagina (see V&V); Vulvovaginitis.

vv varicose veins (see VV); veins; vice versa (L.) - interchange sequence.

V-V Veno-venous (bypass).

V/V Ratio of volumes (see v/v).

v/v percent volume (of solute) in volume (of solvent) (= percent volume in volume; ratio of volumes; volume for volume; V/V).

V&V Vulva and vagina (= VV).

VVA Vulvovaginal atrophy.

VVAW Vietnam Veterans Against the War.

VVC Vulvovaginal candidosis/ complaint(s).

VVD Vaginal vertex delivery; Vulvovaginal disorder.

VVFR Vesicovaginal fistula repair.

VVI Ventricular inhibited (pacemaker); Vocal velocity index.

V/VI Grade 5 on a grade 6 basis.

vvMDV Very virulent Marek disease virus.

VVOR Visual vestibulo-ocular reflex.

VVP Viral vector protein.

VvP Virus-versus-protein (argument/ controversy/ debate) (see Prion; TSE).

VVR Vasovagal reaction.

VVS Vesicovaginal space; Vestibulo-vegetative syndrome.

VVT Varicose vein therapy (Cosm. surgery).

VVVA Vein-vein vascular anastomoses/mosis (between fetuses) (Obstetrics).

VW Vascular/ Vessel wall; von Willebrand's (disease) (see vWF).

vW von Willebrand (= VW).

v/w volume per weight.
vWA von Willebrand's assay (a clotting time test for the diagnosis of von Willebrand's disease) (see vWF).
VWD; vWD von Willebrand's disease (see vWF).
VWF Velocity waveform; Vibration-induced white finger; von Willebrand's factor (see vWF).
vWF; vWf von Willebrand's factor (= Ristocetin cofactor; VIII_{vwf}; VW; VWD; vWD; VWF; vWS; WF).
VWM Ventricular wall motion.
vWS von Willebrand syndrome (see vWF).
Vx Vertex.
V_x Vitrectomy.
VZ; V-Z Varicella-zoster (virus).
VZ/CF Varicella-zoster complement fixation.
VZIG; VZIg Varicella-zoster immune globulin/ immunoglobulin.
VZV Varicella-zoster virus (primary infection causes varicella or chickenpox; reactivation causes shingles or herpes zoster).

W

W Dominant spotting (mouse); Energy (electric - see w); Kendall coefficient of concordance; Section modulus; Series of small triangular incisions in plastic surgery; Tryptophan; Tungsten (Z = 74), also known as Wolfram (Ger.) or Wolframium (L.) (see Elements - Tungsten); Wallace Laboratories (USA); Ward; Warner-Lambert Pharmaceutical Co (USA) code for experimental substances; Water (see w); Watt (see w); Weber (test); Week (see w); Wehnelt (a unit of hardness of roentgen rays); Weight (see w); West; White (see Wh); Whole response (Rorschach); Wide (see w); Widow (ed)/(er); Width; Wife (= w); Wilcoxson (rank sum statistic); Wistar (rat); With (see w); Wolfram/ Wolframium (see W - Tungsten); Word fluency (psychology); Work; Wound.

w velocity (m/s); (= W); water; watt (a unit of electric power, being the work done at the rate of 1 joule per second. It is equivalent to a current of 1 ampere under a pressure of 1 volt); week; weight; while; white (see Wh); wide; wife (see W); with.

W+ Weakly positive.

W 5 A leukocyte antigen.

W 27 An antigen associated with rheumatoid variants.

W 37 Buformin (see DBV).

^{185}W Radioactive tungsten.

W 583 Mebutamate - a depressant of the central nervous system; a methylpentane derivative, chemically and pharmacologically related to meprobamate. Has been suggested for use as an adjunct in the treatment of hypertension.

W 713 Tybamate - a methylpentane derivative chemically related to meprobamate. A minor tranquillizer, reported to be more effective than meprobamate in the treatment of anxiety and tension, with less pronounced sedative effects than the latter drug.

W 1206 Fencamfamin hydrochloride - a stimulant of the central nervous system, of value in the treatment of fatigue and depression following debilitating illness. It has no anorectic action.

W 1760A Namoxyrate (= Namol Xenyrate) - an analgesic compound, reported to be similar to codeine in clinical effectiveness.

W 3395 Alphasone acetonide - a topical anti-inflammatory agent.

WA When/ While/ Wide awake; White adult; Wiskott-Aldrich (syndrome); Woman's auxiliary.

W/A Watt/ampere.

W&A Weakness and atrophy.

wa when/ while/ wide awake (see WA).

WAA Well-adjusted adult.

WAACP World Association of Anatomic and Clinical Pathology.

WAADA Women's Auxiliary to the American Dental Association.

WAADS Women's Auxiliary of the Alaska Dental Society.

WAAMA Women's Auxiliary to the American Medical Association (= WAB).

WAB Western Aphasia Battery; Women's Auxiliary Branch (AMA) (see WAAMA).

WAC Women's Army Corps; World Alzheimer Congress (2000).

WaC Wait-and-see (approach/ policy).

WADT Wepman Auditory Discrimination Test.

WAF Weakness, atrophy, and fasciculation; White adult female.

WAGR Wilms' (tumor), aniridia, genitourinary (abnormalities) and (mental) retardation.

WAIS Wechsler/ Wexler Adult Intelligence Scale.

WAIS-R Revised Wechsler Adult Intelligence Scale.

WAK Wearable artificial kidney.

WAM White adult male.

WAMD Wet age-related macular degeneration (very severe, exudative type) (see DAMD).

WAME World Association of Medical Editors.

WAP Wandering atrial pacemaker.

WAR Wassermann antigen reaction; Without additional reagents; Without any regret(s); Women Against Rape.

WARDA West African Rice Development Association (Liberia).

WARDS Welfare of Animals used for Research in Drugs and Therapy.

WARF Warfarin (= Antiresistant/ DDT; Butyl-p-chlorobenzenesulfonamide) - an insecticide and rodenticide. Mixed with dicophane (equal parts), it has a synergistic insecticidal effect on dicophane-resistant strains of mosquitoes; Wisconsin Alumni Research Foundation.

WAS Weekend athlete syndrome; Weekly activities/vity summary; Wiskott-Aldrich syndrome; Withdrawal (Abstinence) Syndrome.

WaS Wait-and-see.

Was Wassermann test (see Wass; STS - WR).

WASACP World Association of Societies of Anatomic and Clinical Pathology (CIOMS) (see WAACP).

WASAMA Women's Auxiliary to the Student American Medical Association.

WASC Western Association of Schools and Colleges (California, USA).

WASP Weber Advanced Spatial Perception (test); White, Anglosaxon, and Protestant; Wiskott-Aldrich syndrome protein (causing immunodeficiency with thrombocytopenia and eczema) (see WA; WAS); World Association of Societies of Pathology.

Wass Wassermann (reaction/ test) (= Was) (see STS - WR).

WAT Word association test.

WaT Wear-and-tear.

Water Methamphetamine (see Amphet).

WATFOR A computer programming language (Waterloo College Fortran).

WATS Wide Area Telecommunications System; Wide area telephone service.

WAVMISID World Association of Veterinary Microbiologists, Immunologists, and Specialists in Infectious Diseases.

WAWPF William Alanson White Psychiatric Foundation.

Wax E Montanglycol wax (see MGW).

WB Methaqualone (= Wall-banger) (see QZ 2); Waist belt; Washable base; Washed bladder; Water-based; Water bottle; Wechsler-Bellevue (Scale) (psychological test); Weight-bearing; Well baby; Western blot (assay); Wet bulb (temperature); Whole blood; Whole body (count); Willowbrook (virus); Wilson-Blair (agar); World Bank.

Wb Weber (= We); Well-being.

WBA Wax bean agglutinin; Whole body activity.

Wb/A Webers/ampere.

WBAA Whole-blood antibody assay (= WBT).

WBAPTT Whole blood activated partial thromboplastin time.

WBAT Weight bearing as tolerated.

WBB Weight-bearing bone.

WBC Well baby care/ clinic; White blood cell; White/ Whole blood cell count.

WBC/hdf White blood cells per high dry field (see KFT).

WBC/hpf White blood cells per high power field (see KFT).

WBCNI White blood cell nuclear imaging (labelled imaging) - for use in detecting abscesses in IBD - Inflammatory bowel disease, PGI - Prosthetic graft infection and OM - Osteomyelitis.

WBCT Whole-blood clotting time.

WBD Whole-body dosage (of radiation) (see CNSS).

WBDS Whole-body digital scanner.

WBE Weight-bearing exercise; Whole-body extract (insect).

WBF Whole-blood folate.

WBG Wide based gait.

WBGT Wet bulb global/be temperature.

WBH Whole-blood hematocrit; Whole-body hyperthermia.

WBI Whole-body imaging/ irradiation; Whole-bowel irrigation (= GL - Gut lavage; WGL).

WBJ Weight-bearing joint (such as hip, knee, etc.).

WBL Water-based lubricant.

WBld Whole blood.

Wb/m^2 Weber per square meter.

WBN Wellborn nursery; Whirlybird needle (Otolaryngology); Whole-blood nitrogen.

WBP Weight-bearing phase (Orthopedics).

WBPTT Whole-blood partial thromboplastin time.

WBQC Wide base quad cane.

WBR Whole-body radiation.

WBRS Ward Behavior Rating Scale.

WBRT Whole-blood recalcification time.

WBS Web-based service (e-mail) (see NCD); Wechsler-Bellevue Scale; Weight-bearing surface; Whole-blood serum; Whole-body scan; Wiedemann-Beckwith syndrome; Withdrawal body shakes.

WB scale Wechsler-Bellevue scale (see WBS).

WBT Western blot test (antibody serum test for HIV infection, Lyme disease, etc.); Wet bulb temperature; Whole-blood test (see WBAA).

WBTF Waring Blender tube feeding.

WBTT Weight bearing to tolerance.

WBUS Weeks by ultrasound.

WbW Woman-by-woman (basis of medication or treatment).

WC Ward clerk/ confinement; Water closet (toilet); Weber-Christian (disease/ syndrome); Wernicke's encephalopathy; Wet compress(es); Wheel chair (see W/C); White cell casts/ count (see WCC); White child/ count; Whooping cough; Wild caught (animal); Will call; Work capacity; Workmen's compensation (see W-C); Writer's cramp (seen in ataxic or spastic hand, benign essential tremor, carpal tunnel syndrome, joint disease, Parkinson's disease, torsion dystonia or athetosis, etc.).

W/C Wheel chair (= WC; wc).

WC' Whole complement.

W-C Workmen's compensation (= WC).

wc wheel chair (see W/C).

WCA Worst-case/ course analysis.

WCB Workmen's compensation board.

WCBA Woman/ Women of childbearing age.

WCC Walker's carcinosarcoma cells; Well child care; White cell casts/ count (= WC); Wound Care Center.

WCCN World Congress on Clinical Nutrition.

WCD Wales Council for the Disabled; Weber-Christian disease (see RFNNSP); Well-controlled disease; White cell differential; Wound cavity dressing.

WCDS; WCDs White cell differentials.

WCE Work capacity evaluation.

WCF Wind-chill factor.

WCI Worse-case incidence.

WCL Wenckebach cycle length; Whole cell lysate.

w/cm² watts per square centimeter.

WCMC Westchester County Medical Center (New York Medical College).

WCMG West Coast Medical Group.

WCN Walthard cell nest(s).

WCNS World Congress of Neurological Sciences.

WCP Watering-can perineum (caused by urethral stricture and fistulae, as in schistosomiasis of the urinary tract) (see SHI); Woman/ Women of Childbearing Potential.

WCPTB World Confederation for Physical Therapy Bulletin (journal).

WCRF World Cancer Research Fund.

WCRP Women's Cancer Research Program (UCLA).

WCS Weber-Christian syndrome; Weck-cel sponge (eye surgery); Well-conducted/ controlled study; White clot syndrome; Wisconsin Card Sort (test); Worst-case scenario.

WCSG Western Cancer Study Group.

WCSH World Conference on Smoking and Health.

WCST Wisconsin Card Sorting Test.

WCTU Women's Christian Temperance Union.

WCVR World Commission on Vocational Rehabilitation.

WD Wallerian degeneration; Washington Developments (Am Hosp Assn journal); Water deficit (= Total body water [TBW] x [1 - {140 ÷ serum sodium concentration}]); Weil's disease (a severe form of leptospirosis caused by the spirochaete, *Leptospira* icterohemorrhagica and characterized by jaundice, renal failure and hemorrhages); Well defined/ developed/ differentiated (see w/d); Wet dressing; Whipple's disease (see ILD); Whitney Damon (dextrose); Wilson's disease (Progressive lenticular degeneration; Dermatitis exfoliativa); With disease; Without dyskinesia; Wolman's disease; Wrist disarticulation/ drop.

W/D Warm and dry; Withdrawal.

Wd Ward; Word; Wound(ed) (= wd).

wd well defined/ developed/ differentiated (see w/d); wound(ed) (see Wd).

w/d well defined/ developed/ differentiated (=

WD; wd).

W → D Wet to dry.

W4D Worth four-dot (test).

WDA Wildlife Disease Association.

WDCC Well-developed collateral circulation.

WDF White divorced female.

WDHA Watery diarrhea, with hypokalemia and achlorhydria (syndrome).

WDHH Watery diarrhea-hypokalemia-hypochlorhydria.

WDI Warfarin Dose Index.

WDL Well-differentiated lymphocyte.

WDLL Well-differentiated lymphatic lymphoma.

WDM White divorced male.

WDMF Wall-defective microbial forms.

WDMS World Directory of Medical Schools (WHO).

WDR Weekly dosing regimen.

WDRC Wide dynamic range compression (hearing aid circuit/ sound amplification).

WDS Watery diarrhea syndrome (see WDHA); Wet dog shakes (syndrome).

Wds Wounds.

WDT Water deprivation test (Dashe) (see DWD).

WDWN; WD/WN Well developed and well nourished.

WDWN-BF Well-developed, well-nourished black female.

WDWN-BM Well-developed, well-nourished black male.

WDWN-WF Well-developed, well-nourished white female.

WDWN-WM Well-developed, well-nourished white male.

WDXS Wavelength dispersive X-ray spectrometer (SEM).

WE Wage earner; Wax ester; Weekend (see W/E); Wernicke encephalopathy; Western encephalitis/ encephalomyelitis (see WEE); Wound of entry.

We Weber (see Wb).

W/E Weekend (= WE).

WEA Well-established association.

WECP Wernicke's encephalopathy (ataxia, confusion, ophthalmoplegia, peripheral neuropathy) caused by thiamine (vitamin B1 deficiency, as in alcoholism.

WED Water and electrolyte depletion; Water-excretion defect (see RWE).

Wed Wednesday.

Wedge A flat LSD-25 tablet (see LSD).

WEE Wakefulness-enhancing effect; Western equine encephalitis/ encephalomyelitis (= WE).

Weed Marijuana (see Cannabis).

WEF War emergency formula (Britain).

WEFT Witkin Embedded Figures Test.

WEP Water-extended polyester (collimator); Weekend pass.

WER Wheal erythema reaction.

Wes Wesleyan (Church member).

WESDR Wisconsin Epidemiologic Study of Diabetic Retinopathy (US).

WEUP Willful exposure to unwanted pregnancy.

WEX Well-established xenograft (e.g. of breast carcinoma).

WF von Willebrand factor (see vWF); Walsh function; Weil-Felix (reaction) (see WFR); White female (see W/F); Wistar-Furth (rat).

W/F; wf White female (= WF).

WFA World Federation of Anesthesiologists (see WFSA).

WFC Wet field cautery (eye surgery); World Food Conference.

WFCC World Federation of Culture Collections.

WFE Williams flexion exercise.

WFEB Worchester Foundation for Experimental Biology (Massachusetts).

WFI Water for injection.

WFL Within function limits.

WFMH World Federation for Mental Health.

WFMHB World Federation for Mental Health Bulletin (journal).

WFN World Federation of Neurology (CIOMS).

WFNS World Federation of Neurological Surgeons/ Neurosurgical Societies.

WF-O Will follow in office.

WFOT World Federation of Occupational Therapists.

WFP World Food Program (FAO).

WFPMM World Federation of Proprietary Medicine Manufacturers.

WFR Weil-Felix reaction (= WF); Wheal-and-

flare reaction.
WFS World Future Society; Waterhouse-Friderichsen syndrome (the malignant or fulminating form of meningococcal meningitis).
WFSA World Federation of Societies of Anesthesiologists (CIOMS) (see WFA).
WFT Weil-Felix test (*Bacillus* proteus OXK agglutinins in scrub typhus and *Bacillus* proteus OX2 and OX19 agglutinins for other rickettsial diseases) (= WFR).
WfW Weight-for-weight (basis/ ratio).
WG Water/ Wire guage; Wegener's granulomatosis; Wild Geronimo (barbiturate dissolved in an alcoholic drink) (see Barb); Wright-Giemsa (stain).
WGA Weekly Government Abstracts (NTIS); Wheat germ agglutinin.
WGH Western General Hospital (Edinburgh).
WGL Whole-gut lavage (see WBI).
WGS Whole-genome scan(ning).
WGTA Wisconsin General Test Apparatus (for monkeys).
WH Walking heel (cast); War on Hunger (AID journal); Well healed/ hydrated; Werdnig-Hoffmann (syndrome); Whole homogenate; World Hospitals (IHF journal); Wound healing.
Wh White (= W; w; wh).
wh watt-hour (see w-hr); whisper(ed); white (see Wh).
w-h watt-hour (see w-hr).
WHA Warm and humid air; World Health Assembly/ Association.
WHAP Woman's Health and Abortion Project.
WHC Women's Health Center (UCLA).
wh ch wheel chair; white child.
WHCOA White House Conference On Aging.
WHD Werdnig-Hoffman disease (acute progressive infantile spinal muscular atrophy).
WHE Whole human embryo (cell).
Wheat Marijuana (see Cannabis).
WHF World Heart Federation/ Forum; Wurzburg Hearing Field.
WHHL Watanabe hereditary hyperlipidemic (rabbit).
WHHMC West Hills Hospital & Medical Center (California).
WHI Women's Health Initiative.
WHIMS Women's Health Initiative Memory Study (NIH).
White Amphetamine (benzedrine pill) (see Amphet).
White lady Cocaine (see Erythroxylum); Heroin (see Diamorph HCl).
WHML Wellcome Historical Medical Library.
WHO World Health Organization (UN); Wrist-hand orthosis.
WHOI Woods Hole Oceanographic Institution.
WHOIRP World Health Organization International Reference Preparation.
WHP Water-hammer pulse; Wheeler halving procedure (Ophthalmology).
Whp; whp; Whpl; whpl Whirlpool (procedure/ physical therapy).
WHPB Whirlpool bath.
WHR Waist/Hips (girth) ratio.
w-hr; whr watt-hour - a unit of electrical energy or work, equal to the wattage multiplied by the time in hours (= wh; w-h).
WHRC World Health Research Center.
WHS Werdnig-Hoffmann syndrome; Women's Health Study.
WHSP White House Science Presence.
WH syndrome Werdnig-Hoffmann syndrome (see WHS).
WHT Walsh-Hadamard transform.
WHV Woodchuck hepatic virus.
WHVP Wedged hepatic vein/ venous pressure.
WI Human embryonic lung cell line; Ventricular demand pacing; Walk-in (patient); Water ingestion; Wistar Institute (rat).
W/I Within.
W&I; W + I Work and interest.
WI-38 Human diploid cells.
WIA Wounded in action.
WIAB Wistar Institute of Anatomy and Biology.
WIC Women, infants, and children - special supplemental food program for pregnant women, infants, and children (USDA).
WICHE Western Interstate Commission for Higher Education.
Wid Widow(ed)/(er) (= W).
WIG Welfare Inspector General (New York State Department of Social Services).

WIH Whitely Index of Hypochondriasis.
WIHM Wellcome Institute for the History of Medicine.
WIMJ West Indian Medical Journal.
WIN See Win; World of Irish Nursing (INO journal).
WIn Work Incentive (Program) (DOL).
Win Winthrop Laboratories (USA) code for experimental substances (= WIN).
Win 1258-2 Hydroxychloroquine sulfate (see SN 16,168).
Win 5047 Chlorbetamide - an acetamide derivative used as an amebicide and also in the treatment of hookworm infestation. Much more effective in intestinal amebiasis than in the hepatic form of the disease.
Win 5063-2 Thiamphenicol (see CB 8053).
Win 5494 Amotriphene hydrochloride - a dimethylamino-propene derivative, with similar effects on the heart as quinidine sulfate, but also causes coronary vaso-dilatation. Has been used in the treatment of cardiac arrhythmias.
Win 8077 Ambenonium chloride (= Ambestigmine chloride) - an anti-cholinesterase with actions similar to those of physostigmine (eserine), but like neostigmine its nicotinic actions are more pronounced, and its muscarinic actions less pronounced than those of physostigmine. Used in the treatment of myasthenia gravis. It has a longer duration of action than neostigmine.
Win 8851-2 Sodium tyropanoate - an iodine-containing contrast medium used in the radiographic examination of the biliary tract. Its actions and uses are similar to those of iopanoic acid (Iopan).
Win 9154 Inositol Nicotinate (= Inositol Niacinate; Mesoinositol; Hexanicotinate) - a peripheral vasodilator used in the treatment of Raynaud's disease, acrocyanosis and chilblains, and has been also given in the treatment of conditions accompanied by intermittent claudication. Inositol is also included in the vitamin B complex (see Vitamins - B complex).
Win 9317 Propatylnitrate (see ETTN).
Win 10,448 Quinocide hydrochloride (see CN 1115).
Win 14,833 Stanozolol (= Androstanazole; Methylstanazole) - a sex hormone with anabolic and androgenic actions similar to those of methandienone. Used in conditions characterized by protein and bone wasting, in the treatment of osteoporosis, crush fractures due to corticosteroid treatment, to alleviate the low backache of the menopause, and in chronic debilitating diseases (see Hormones - AH ii).
Win 18,320 Nalidixic acid - a synthetic antibacterial agent used in the treatment of infections of the genitourinary tract.
Win 18,501 Oxypertine hydrochloride - a tranquillizing drug used in the treatment of schizophrenia.
Win 20,228 Pentazocine (see NIH 7958).
Win 20,740 Cyclazocine - a cyclopropylbenzazocine narcotic analgesic, reported to be 40 times as potent as morphine.
WIO Wright Institute of Otology.
WIPI Word Intelligibility Picture Identification.
WIS Weakened immune system; Wechsler Intelligence Scale; Weizman Institute of Science (Rehovot, Israel).
WISC Wechsler Intelligence Scale for Children.
WISC-R Wechsler Intelligence Scale for Children - Revised.
WIST Whitaker Index of Schizophrenic Thinking.
WITT Wittenborn (Psychiatric Rating Scale).
W-J Woodcock-Johnson (Psychoeducational Battery).
WJC World Jewish Congress.
WJM Western Journal of Medicine (Calif Med Assoc journal).
WJP Watson-Jones procedure (in ligament reconstruction); Wrist joint prosthesis (see OI/OP).
WJSOG Western Journal of Surgery, Obstetrics and Gynecology.
WK Week (see wk); Wernicke-Korsakoff (disease/ syndrome); Wilson-Kimmelstiel (disease).
wk weak; week (= WK); work.
WKD Wilson-Kimmelstiel disease.
WKE Well-known exception.

W/kg Watts per kilogram.
WKS Wernicke-Korsakoff syndrome.
WKT Work Knowledge Test (psychology).
WKY Wistar-Kyoto (rat).
WL Waistline; Waiting list; Wallenstein Laboratory (culture medium); Warner-Lambert Pharmaceutical Co. (USA) and White Laboratories, Inc. (USA) code for experimental substances; Waterload (see WL test); Wavelength (= wl; Weight loss; White lady (= Heroin) (see Diamorph HCl); Withdrawal; Working level; Workload.
wl wavelength (see WL).
WLE Wide local excision.
WLF Whole lymphocytic fraction; Wild Life Fund.
WL/F/L Wood's lamp/filter/light (an ultraviolet light used to detect fluorescein in blood vessels, bacterial and other infections, etc.
WLI Weight-length index; Whiplash injury.
WLM White light microscopy; Working level month (radon).
WL medium Wallenstein Laboratory medium (= WL).
WLN Wiswesser Line Notation.
WLR Wrist laceration repair.
WLS Wet lung syndrome; Whip-lash syndrome (cervical).
WLT Waterload test (= WL test); White line of Toldt (fascial line in pelvis); Whole lung tomography.
WL test Waterload test (procedure/ endocrinology) (= WL).
WM Waldenström's macroglobulinemia; War Medicine; Ward manager; Warm and moist; Wernicke-Mann (hemiplegia); Wet mount; White male (see W/M); Whole milk (see wm); Wilson-Mikity (syndrome); World Medicine (journal).
wm white male (see W/M); whole milk (= WM); whole mount (in microtechnic).
W/M; w/m White male (= WM; wm).
w/m² watts per square meter.
WMA Wall motion abnormality; Wholesome Meat Act (1967); World Medical Association (CIOMS).
WMC Weight-matched control.
WMD Weekly maintenance dose.
WME Williams' medium E; World Medical Electronics (journal).
WMF White married/ middle-aged female.
WMG Welsh Medical Gazette (journal).
WMI Wildlife Management Institute; Willie-Meyer incision (Breast surgery) (see inc); Wintrobe method of indices hematocrit).
WMJ World Medical Journal (WMA).
WMM White married/ middle-aged male.
Wmn Woman/ Women.
WMO Ward Medical Officer; World Metereological Organization.
WMP Weight management program; World Medical Periodicals.
WMR Work metabolic rate; World Medical Relief.
WMS Wechsler Memory Scale.
WMSC Women's Medical Specialists Corps.
WMT Weekly maintenance therapy.
WMX Whirlpool, massage, and exercise.
WN Well-nourished (see w/n).
Wn Work weight where "n" equals "number of pounds".
w/n; wn well-nourished (= WN).
WNC Waist and neck circumference; Wasting of the nerve contour (in carpal tunnel syndrome).
wnd wound.
WNE West Nile encephalitis.
WNF; wnf Well-nourished female.
WNL Within normal limits.
WNLS Weighted non-linear least squares.
WNM; wnm Well-nourished male.
WNPW Wide, notched P wave.
WNV West Nile virus.
WO Wash out; Water-in-oil (see W/O); Written order (see W/O).
wo weeks old; without (see w/o).
W/O Water-in-oil (emulsion) (= WO); Written order (= WO).
w/o without (= wo).
WOB Work of breathing.
WOE Wound of entry.
WOG World Organization of Gastroenterology (CIOMS).
WOMAC Western Ontario and MacMaster/ McMaster (Universities).
WOP Wash-out period (see WOW); Without pain.
WOPT Whole organ pancreas

transplant(ation).

W or A Weakness or atrophy.

WOS West of Scotland (Study, of the effect of Pravastatin on CHD).

WOSCOPS West of Scotland Coronary Prevention Study.

WOT Wash-out technique (gastric lavage); Whole-organ transplant.

WOU Women's outpatient unit.

WOW Wash-out week (see WOP)

WOWS Weak opiate withdrawal scale.

WOX Wound of exit (= WX).

WP Weakly positive; Weather permitting; Wedge pressure; Wet pack (= WPk); Wettable powder (= wp); Whirlpool; White phosphorus/ pulp; Wies procedure (surgery for entropion); Word processor; Working point.

wp wettable powder (see WP).

W/P Water/powder (ratio).

WPA World Psychiatric Association (CIOMS).

WPB Whirlpool bath.

WPC World Population Conference.

wpc watts per candle.

WPCA Water Pollution Control Act.

WPCF Water Pollution Control Federation.

WPCU Weighted patient care unit.

WPFM Wright peak flow meter.

WPIC Western Psychiatric Institute and Clinic.

WPk Ward's pack (mechanical tissue pack - dentistry); Wet pack (see WP).

WPM Words per minute.

WPP Word-processing program.

WPPA World Population Plan of Action (UN).

WPPSI Wechsler Preschool and Primary Scale of Intelligence.

WPRS Wittenborn Psychiatric Rating Scale.

WPS Wasting pig syndrome; Withdrawal precipitated seizure; Workplace stress; World Population Society.

WPW Wolff-Parkinson-White (syndrome).

WQA Water Quality Association.

WR Warner-Lambert Pharmaceutical Co (USA) code for experimental substances; Wassermann reaction (see STS - WR); Water retention; Weak/ Whole response; Weakly reactive; Whispered rehearsal; Widal/ Wiping reaction; Work rate.

Wr Wrist; Writhe.

WRA Wellness-related activity.

Wr a A very rare blood group antigen.

WRAIR Walter Reed Army Institute of Research (US Army).

WRAMC Walter Reed Army Medical Center (US Army).

WRAML Wide Range Assessment of Memory and Learning.

WRAT Wide Range Achievement Test.

WRC Washed red cells; Water-retention coefficient.

WRD Work-related disability.

WRE Whole ragweed extract.

W-response Whole response.

WRF Walsh-Rademacher function.

WRGH Walter Reed General Hospital (US Army hospital).

WRH Weight-regulating hormone (leptin).

WRHL Washington Report on Health Legislation (journal).

WRK Woodward's reagent K.

WRLTC Washington Report on Long Term Care (journal).

WRMH Washington Report on Medicine and Health (journal).

WRMT Woodcock Reading Mastery Test.

WRP Weight-reducing pill; Weight reduction program (= WRR).

WRR Weight reduction regime(n) (see WRP).

WRRI Walter Reed Research Institute.

WRS Weight reduction strategy; Wiedemann-Rautenstrauch syndrome.

WRS; WRSs Word recognition score(s).

WRST Wilcoxon's rank-sum test (statistical analysis).

WRVP Wedged renal vein pressure.

WS A Rorschach response; Waardenburg/ Waldenström's/ Warkany/ West/ Williams syndrome; Waddell's sign (a complex of abnormal neurological findings); Walsh spectroscopy; Ward secretary; Warthin-Starry (stain); Washine Chemical Corp (USA) code for experimental substances; Water soluble/ swallow; Werner's syndrome (growth ceases by age 12, with greying of hair at temples and progressive alopecia and sclerosis of skin, ulcers on legs and generalized arteriosclerosis - an autosomal recessive, congenital hypotrichosis) (= Pangeria; PAS); Wilderness/ Wildlife Society (The); Wilder's silver (stain); Withdrawal syndrome (see AS); Wolfram syndrome (a rare neurodegenerative disorder, associated with two copies of a mutant gene on chromosome 4 and characterized by diabetes, optic nerve atrophy, hallucinations and progressive dementia); Work simplification.

ws; w/s; W·s watt-second (joule) (= w-sec).

W&S Wound and skin.

WSA Water-soluble agent (see WSD)/ antibiotic.

WSAT Willner-Scheerer Analogy Test.

WSB Wheat-soy blend.

WSC Weeping/ Wet skin condition.

WSCPS West of Scotland Coronary Prevention Study.

WSCS Wisconsin Sleep Cohort Study (US).

WSD Water soluble drug (= WSA; WSP); Water Supply Division (EPA); Widespread serious disease; Wool sorters' disease (= Pulmonary anthrax).

WSDM Whey soy drink mix.

w-sec watt-second (see ws).

WSepF White separated female.

WSepM White separated male.

WSF White single female.

W shunt Waterston shunt.

WSI Waardenburg syndrome type I; Water safety instructor (Red Cross).

WSL Wesselsbron (virus); Whole skin loss (3rd degree burn).

WSM White single male.

WSMA Washington State Medical Association.

WSMS Wyoming State Medical Society.

WSMSA Washington Standard Metropolitan Statistical Area.

WSND Wide spectrum neoplastic disease.

WSP Water soluble product (see WSD); Wearable speech processor; Withdrawal seizure prone.

WSPID World Society for Paediatric Infectious Diseases (Congress of the)

WSR Westergren sedimentation rate; Withdrawal seizure resistant.

W/sr Watts per steradian.

WSRT Wilcoxson Sign Rank Test (a statistical evaluation test for non-parametric ordinal data).

WST Wirt stereo test (Ophthalmology).

WSV Water-soluble vitamin (Bx, C, etc.).

WT Walking tank; Wall thickness; Water temperature; Welch's test (a parametric t. in statistical analysis) (see PMT); Whitaker test (see PVP); Wild type (strain); Wilms' tumor; Wisdom teeth/ tooth; Work therapy.

wt weight; white.

WTA Well-tolerated antibiotic.

WTB Whistling-type breathing.

WTC World Trade Center, New York City. The twin towers were levelled to ground zero by international terrorists on the morning of September 11, 2001.

WTE Water-tight equipment (MET - 501); Whole time equivalent.

WTF Weight transferral frequency.

WtH Waist-to-hip (ratio).

wt. per mil weight per milliliter.

WTS Whole tomography slice; Wild-type sequence (as opposed to mutant sequence, in genes).

WtW White-to-white (measurement) - of the conjunctiva, giving the transverse diameter of the anterior chamber, which determines the size of the lens implant to be used.

WU Wood unit (of resistance to blood flow in the pulmonary circulation; elevated in patients with mitral valve disease, chronic lung disease, etc.).

W/U; w/u Workup.

WUC Wake-up call.

WUMS Washington University Medical School/ Service.

W unit Wohlgemuth/ Wroblewski unit.

WV Walking ventilation; Whispered/ring voice.

Wv Variable dominant spotting (mouse).

W/V; w/v Weight/volume/ Percent weight in volume/ Weight by volume (solution)/ Weight per volume/ Weight of solute in volume of solution.

WVA World Veterinary Association.

WVMJ West Virginia Medical Journal.

WVSMA West Virginia State Medical Association.

WW Weight Watchers; Wet weight; Window

width; Word from Washington (UCPA journal).

W/W; w/w Weight of solute in weight of solvent (= percent weight/solution concentration by weight/weight-to-weight ratio).

WWAC Walk with aid of cane.

WWE Wasp waist effect (hourglass appearance); World-wide epidemic.

W & We Water and Wastes Engineering (journal).

WWF World Welfare Fund.

WWHPC Worldwide health and personal care.

WWI World War 1 (or First World War); Worldwatch Institute.

WWidF White widowed female.

WWidM White widowed male.

WWII World War 2 (or Second World War).

W/wo With or without.

WWU Weighted work units (of DRGs - Division of Research Grants, NIH).

WWW World Weather Watch; World Wide Web (Internet).

WX Wound of exit (see WOX).

WxB Wax bite.

WxP Wax pattern.

WY Women years.

Wy Wyeth Laboratories (USA) code for experimental substances.

Wy 401 Ethoheptazine citrate (= Heptacyclazine citrate) - an analgesic, chemically allied to pethidine, employed in the treatment of moderately severe pain, particularly that associated with musculo-skeletal disorders.

Wy 806 Oxethazaine (= Oxetacaine) - a surface anesthetic, poorly absorbed from mucous membranes. Has been given by mouth in conjunction with antacids for the symptomatic relief of heartburn and indigestion.

Wy 1359 Propiomazine hydrochloride - a phenothiazine derivative and a depressant of the central nervous system. A rapidly-acting tranquillizer, it is usually given by intramuscular injection to produce sedation before and during surgical and obstetric procedures.

Wy 1485 Chlormethiazole edisylate (see SCTZ).

Wy 2445 Carfenazine maleate (= Carphenazine m) - a phenothiazine tranquillizing drug, also exhibiting anti-emetic, hypotensive, and anticholinergic properties. Has been used in the long-term management of chronic schizophrenia.

Wy 3277 Nafcillin sodium (= Nafcillinium natricum; Sodium nafcillin) - a penicillin-derived antibiotic, given chiefly by intramuscular injection in infections caused by benzylpenicillin-resistant staphylococci.

Wy 3467 Diazepam (see LA 111).

Wy 3498 Oxazepam - a benzodiazepine derivative, a tranquillizer related chemically to chlordiazepoxide. It has been used in the treatment of anxiety states, and behavior disorders associated with cerebral arteriosclerosis and senile brain diseases.

WZa Wide zone alpha (hemolysis).

X

X Across; Androgenic (zone); Break; Chromosome (the female X chromosome in humans); Cross or transverse (with reference to selections); Crossbite; Cross out/ Delete; Cross section; Except (see X); Exophoria distance; Experiment; Extra; Factor (unidentified); Female sex chromosome; Fever (X Fever of Montana USA, a tick-borne disease, described as being due to a rickettsia group of microorganisms); Homeopathic symbol for the decimal scale of potencies; Ionization exposure (rate); Kienbock's unit (of X-ray dosage/ exposure); Magnification; Match (cross-match - laboratory/ blood bank); Multiplication times; Multiply; Reactance; Removal of; Respirations (anesthesia chart); Roman numeral ten; Start of anesthesia; Ten (10) - Roman numeral; "Times" (multiplication sign); Translocation between two X chromosomes; Transverse; Unknown quantity; X ray/ unit (roentgen) (= x); Xylene; Xylocaine (see XYLO); Zone (X zone - inner zone of the adrenal cortex in young mammals).

x except; extremity; horizontal axis of a rectangular coordinate system or a cylindrical lens; mole fraction; multiplication times; roentgen (rays) (see X); sample mean (see $\bar{X}$); unknown factor; xanthene (see Xan).

$\bar{\mathbf{X}}$ Except (= X); Sample mean (mathematics) (see Symbols - 2).

Χ Chi. the 22nd letter of the Greek alphabet.

Ξ Greek (14th) capital letter "xi" (see Symbols - 4).

ξ Greek (14th) lower case letter "xi" (see Symbols - 4).

X + # Xiphoid plus number of fingerbreadths.

X^2 Chi-square(d) (statistic; test or measure goodness of fit).

X3 Orientation as to time, place, and person.

x3; x4; etc. 3 times, 4 times; etc.

x2d; x3d; x4d; etc. for 2/ 3/ 4 days, etc. (medication order).

X 1497 Methicillin sodium (see BRL 1241).

X 5079 C An antimicrobial polypeptide produced by the growth of a species of Streptomyces, with antifungal properties, and active against Blastomyces and Histoplasma, but ineffective against Candida and Coccidioides. Used by parenteral injection in the treatment of aspergillosis, blastomycosis, histoplasmosis, mycetoma, and sporotrichosis.

XA Xanthurenic acid; Xylene-alcohol (mixture) (see X-A).

Xa Chiasma (= xma); Thrombotic activity.

X-A Xylene-alcohol (mixture) - a larvacide, for killing insect larvae (= XA).

Xaa Unknown amino acid.

Xam Examination.

Xan Xanthine (= x).

Xanth Xanthomatosis.

xanth- combining form meaning blond or yellow (Gr. xanthos).

xantho- prefix meaning yellow (Gr. xanthos).

Xao Xanthosine.

Xb Bacillus X.

XBD Xanthine bronchodilator (e.g. Aminophylline, Theophylline, etc.).

XBI Xenogeneic bone implant (Orthopedics).

XBT Xylose breath test.

XC; Xc Excretory cystogram (see KFT - XC); X-/ Sex chromosome.

X-CGD X-linked chronic granulomatous disease.

X-chromosome Sex chromosome (see XC; Xc).

XCT X-ray (transmission) computed tomography.

XD Times daily; X-linked dominant (chromosome); Xenodiagnosis (Gr. xenos = stranger/ foreigner) - diagnosis of a disease, made by finding in the feces, the infective forms of the organism involved (such as *Trypanosoma* cruzi), by feeding the patient clean laboratory-fed ('stranger') bugs, such as the triatomid bugs of the *Reduiviidae* family in the early stages of Chagas' disease.

X2d Times two days.

XDH Xanthine dehydrogenase.

XDP Xanthine diphosphate; Xeroderma pigmentosum (an autosomal recessive, hereditary hypotrichosis, with absence of hair, defect of DNA excision repair, extreme photosensitivity, pigmentation, atrophy, keratoses

and malignancies (= XP).
XDR Transducer.
Xe Electric susceptibility; Xenon (Z = 54) (see Elements - Xenon).
Xe^{133} Radioactive xenon (chemical symbol).
XECT Xenon-enhanced computed tomography.
X-ed Crossed.
XEF Excess ejection fraction.
XEM Xonics electron mammography.
xeno- prefix meaning strange (Gr. xenos).
XERG Xonics electron radiography.
xero- prefix meaning dry (Gr. xeros).
XES X-ray energy spectrometer/metry/ spectroscope/py (dispersive).
XF X-factor or heme - the non-protein, insoluble, iron protoporphyrin constituent of hemoglobin, and various other respiratory (animal and vegetable) pigments.
X factor An unidentified factor; heme (see XF).
Xfb Cross-linked fibrin.
XG Xenograft (animal-organ transplant).
Xg Blood group.
XGP Xanthogranulomatous pyelonephritis.
X-l HIMS X-linked hyper-IgM syndrome (see HIM; HIgMS).
x-iog radiography.
XIP X-ray-induced polypeptide.
xiph- prefix meaning sword (Gr. xiphos) (see xipho-).
xiphi- see xipho-.
xipho- combining form denoting relationship to the xiphoid process (Gr xiphos = sword) (= xiph-; xiphi-).
XIT X-irradiation therapy/ treatment.
XKO Not knocked out.
XL Excess lactate; Extended-Release (tablet); Extra large; X-linked (inheritance); Xylose-lysine (agar base).
XL; X-L Cross/ X-linked.
X-LA X-linked agammaglobulinemia.
XLAS X-linked aqueductal stenosis.
XLD Xylose, lysine, deoxycholate/ desoxycholate (agar).
X-leg Cross leg/ Cross-legged.
X-LG X-linked gene.
XLH X-linked hypophosphatemia.
XLI X-linked icthyosis.
X-LID X-linked immunodeficiency.
XLJR X-linked juvenile retinoschisis.
XLMR X-linked mental retardation (= XMR).
XLP X-linked lymphoproliferative (syndrome).
XLR X-linked recessive (gene).
XLRD X-linked recessive disease.
XLS X-linked (recessive) lymphoproliferative syndrome.
XM Crossmatch (blood) (= X-mat; X-match; X-matching).
xm Magnetic susceptibility.
Xm Maternal chromosome X.
xma chiasma (see Xa).
X-mas Christmas (factor).
X-mat; X-match Crossmatch (see XM).
X-matching Cross matching (see XM).
XMM Xeromammography.
XMP Xanthine monophosphate.
XMR X-linked mental retardation (see XLMR).
xMS Excessive mucus secretion.
XN Night blindness.
Xn Christian.
XO Presence of only one sex chromosome (symbol meaning only one chromosome is present); Turner's syndrome (sex-chromosome abnormality); Xanthine oxidase.
XOI Xanthine oxidase inhibitor (e.g. allopurinol).
XOM Extraocular movements.
XOR Exclusive operating room.
X-organ Neurocirculatory organ in crustaceans.
XP Xanthogranulomatous pyelonephritis; Xeroderma pigmentosum (see XDP)
Xp Paternal/Short arm of chromosome X.
Xp- Deletion of short arm of chromosome X.
X5P Xylulose 5-phosphate.
XPA Xeroderma pigmentosum group A.
XPC Xeroderma pigmentosum group C.
XPD Xeroderma pigmentosum group D (a body protein critical in the repairing of damaged DNA).
XPS X-ray photoelectron/ photoemission spectroscopy.
Xq Long arm of chromosome X.
Xq- Deletion of long arm of chromosome X.
XR Extended-release (capsule/ tablet) (= XL);

Xeroradiography; X-linked recessive (chromosome/ inheritance); X-ray.
X-ray(s) Roentgen ray(s) (see XR).
XRC X-ray cardiogram/graph(y).
XRD X-ray diffraction.
XRF X-ray fluorescence (spectroscopy).
XRFS X-ray fluorescence spectroscopy.
XRG Xero-/ Xonics radiography.
XRMP Xeroradiography mammographic positioner.
XRMR X-linked recessive mental retardation.
XRS X-ray sensitivity.
XRT X-ray technician/ therapy.
XS Cross-section (= Transverse s.; X-sect); Excess(ive); Xiphisternum.
×s Electric susceptibility.
XSA Cross-section area.
XSCID X-linked severe combined immunodeficiency.
X-sect; X section Cross/ Transverse section (see XS).
XS-LIM Exceeds limits (of procedure).
XSP Xanthoma striatum palmare.
XSS Xomed Silastic splint(s) (Otolaryngology).
XT Exotropia (eye examination).
X(T) Intermittent exotropia.
Xta Chiasmata.
Xtab Cross-tabulating/ion.
Xtal Crystal.
XTE Xeroderma, talipes, and enamel defect (syndrome).
X-TEP Crossed immunoelectrophoresis.
XTM Xanthoma tuberosum multiplex.
XTP Xanthosine triphosphate.
XU Excretory urogram (see KFT - XU); X-ray unit (= Siegbahn - 1.002063 x 10^{-13} meter).
XULN Times upper limit of normal.
XuMP Xylulose monophophate.
XV Fifteen.
XVS Xenon ventilation scan (see PLS).
XX Double strength; Sex-linked chromosome present in females (Normal female chromosome type); Twenty.
46, XX 46 chromosomes, 2 X chromosomes (normal female).
XXL Xylocaine.
XXX Thirty.
XX/XY Sex karyotypes.
49, XXXXY 49 chromosomes, 4 X and 1 Y chromosomes (XXXXY syndrome).
XXY A 49th chromosome present in some individuals; Klinefelter's syndrome (see 47, XXY).
47, XXY 47 chromosomes, 2 X and 1 Y chromosomes (Klinefelter's syndrome) (= XXY).
XXYY A 49th chromosome present in some individuals.
XY Sex-linked chromosome present in males (Normal male chromosome type).
46, XY 46 chromosomes, 1 X and 1 Y chromosome (normal male).
47 XY, + 21 47 chromosomes, male, additional No: 21 chromosome (Down syndrome).
XYL Xylocaine (see XYLO).
Xyl Xylose.
XYLO Xylocaine (= X; XYL).
xylo- prefix meaning wood (Gr. xylon).
XYY A 49th chromosome present in some individuals.
47, XYY 47 chromosomes, 1 X and 2 Y chromosomes (XYY syndrome).

Y

Y A coordinate axis in a plane; Cartilage; Male sex chromosome; Dysentery bacillus; Ligament; Tyrosine; Y-angle; Yard; Year; Yellow (= Yel); Yield; Young; Yttrium (Z = 39) (see Elements - Yttrium); Yersinia.

y The vertical axis of a rectangular coordinate system; year (see Y).

Υ; υ Upsilon (Greek 20th upper & lower case letters - also "ypsilon").

^{90}Y Radioactive yttrium.

YA Yersinia arthritis.

Y/A Years of age.

YACP Young adult chronic patient.

YAD Young-adult death.

YAD; YADH Yeast alcohol dehydrogenase.

YAG Yttrium, aluminium, garnet (laser medium) (see LASER).

Yage Ayahuasca - a narcotic drink, known as Ayahuasca in Bolivia, Ecuador and Peru, containing the principles harmine and harmaline (which include the alkaloids, banisterine, telepathine and yageine).

YAP Young adult patient.

YARU Yale Arbovirus Research Unit.

YAVIS Youthful, attractive, verbal, intelligent and successful (psychological rating scale).

Ya Yan Tzu The Chinese species of the plant Brucea; its seeds are used in treating amebic dysentery.

YB Yoon Band (fallope ring).

Yb Ytterbium (Z = 70) (see Elements - Ytterbium).

YBP Year-book of Pharmacy and Transactions of British Pharmaceutical Conference.

YC Y-chromosome.

YCB Yeast carbon base.

YCC Youth Conservation Corps (USDA, USDI).

yd yard.

yd^2 square yard (see sq yd).

yd^3 cubic yard (see cu yd).

YDV Yeast-derived (hepatitis B) vaccine.

YDYES Yin deficiency yang excess syndrome.

YE Yeast extract; Yellow enzyme.

YEC *Yersinia* enterocolitica (a gram negative coccobacillus causing among other ailments, AIE **-** Acute infective enterocolitis and ERA **-** Enteropathic reactive arthritis); *Yersinia* enterocolitis (gram negative coccobacilli infection).

YEH; YEH$_2$ Reduced yellow enzyme.

YEI Yersinia enterocolitica infection.

Yel Yellow (see Y).

Yellow Yellow jacket (nembutal capsule) (see Barb).

Yel/Vac Yellow Fever Vaccine.

Yen Somnolence during withdrawal of morphine or heroin.

Yerba 1) Marijuana (see Cannabis), or 2) Herb, e.g. Yerba santa (Sp.) = "Sacred herb" or Eriodictyon.

Yerbine An alkaloid prepared from Ilex paraguayensis, resembling caffeine.

Yerli A fine quality of Turkish opium (see Papaver).

YF Yellow fever (caused by a mosquito-borne flavivirus).

YFC Young febrile child(ren).

YFI Yellow fever immunization.

YFMD Yellow fever membrane disease.

YFV Yellow-fever vaccination/ vaccine/ virus.

Yh 1 Phenylimino-oxo-oxazolidine (see PIO).

YJV Yellow jacket venom.

YKHC Yukon-Kuskokwin Health Corporation.

-yl a chemical suffix signifying a radical, particularly a univalent hydrocarbon radical (Gr. yle = a substance).

YLC Youngest living child.

-ylene a chemical suffix denoting a bivalent hydrocarbon radical.

YM Yeast and mannitol.

Y_{max} Maximum yield.

Y/N Yes/no.

YNB Yeast nitrogen base.

Y-NHH Yale - New Haven Hospital (Connecticut).

YNS Yellow nail syndrome.

YO; Y/O; y/o Years old.

YOB Year of birth.

Yopo Hallucinogenic snuff prepared from the plant, Piptadenia.

YORA Younger-onset rheumatoid arthritis.

Y-organ Moulting gland in crustaceans.
YP Yeast phase; Yield pressure.
YPA Yeast, peptone, and adenine sulfate.
YPLL Years of potential life lost.
YRD Yangtze River disease.
yr(s) year(s).
YS; ys Yellow spot (on retina); Yolk sac.
YSC Yolk sac carcinoma.
YSI Yellow Springs Instrument Co (Ohio).
YSKV Yale SK virus (poliovirus strain).
YST Yolk sac tumor; Yukon standard time.
YT; Yt; yt Former symbol for the chemical element, Yttrium, now Y (Z = 39) (see Elements - Yttrium).
YTD Year to date.
YUSM Yale University School of Medicine
Y-V Y-V (anoplasty).

Z

Z Acoustic independence; Atomic number (of the 106 known chemical elements) - the number of protons in the atomic nucleus (= z) (see Table; see also Elements); Complex impedance; Contraction (Ger. Zuckung); Glutamic acid; Glutamine; Impedance; Intermediate disk (Ger. Zwischenscheibe) - the disk that separates sarcomeres (= Z-disk); Ionic charge number; No effect; Point formed by a line perpendicular to the nasion-menton line through the anterior nasal spine; Proton number; Section modulus; Standard score (statistic); Standardized (normal) deviate (= z); Zeitschrift (German journal/ periodical); Zero (= z); Zone; Z-shaped incision in plastic surgery.

z algebraic unknown or space coordinate; atomic number (see Z - Atomic number; Elements); axis of a three-dimensional rectangular coordinate system; catalytic amount; standard normal deviate (see Z); zero (see Z).

Z Greek capital letter "zeta".

ζ Greek lower case letter "zeta".

Z'; Z" Increasing degrees of contraction.

ZA Zinc arginate.

ZAF Atomic number, absorption, and fluorescence correction factors in quantitative X-ray spectroscopy.

ZAM Zeiss Axiophot Microscope (Zeiss New York, New York).

ZAP Zymosan-activated plasma (rabbit).

ZAP-70 Zeta-associated protein 70 (gene).

ZAPF Zinc adequate pair-fed.

ZAS Zymosan-activated autologous serum.

Zazen Zen meditation.

ZB Zebra body.

ZCD Zinc chloride poisoning.

ZD Zero defects/ discharge; Zinc deficiency.

ZDC Zinc dibenzyl-dithiocarbamate.

ZDDP Zinc dialkyldithiophosphate.

Z-disk Intermediate disk (Ger. Zwischenscheibe) (see Z).

Z-DNA Ziz-zag (left-handed helical) deoxyribonucleic acid.

ZDO Zero differential overlap.

ZDS Zinc depletion syndrome; Zung Depression Scale (psychological test).

ZDV Zero dead volume (tubing connector); Zidovudine (= AZT) (HIV reverse transcriptase inhibitor) (see RTI).

ZE Zollinger-Ellison (syndrome) (see ZES); Zone electrophoresis.

ZEC Zinsser-Engman-Cole (syndrome).

ZEEP Zero end-expiratory pressure.

ZEG Zero economic growth.

Zen Bud Zen Buddhism (religion).

zero-mid Xomed (see XSS).

ZES Zollinger-Ellison syndrome (a triad comprising i. atypical, fulminating, or intractable peptic ulcers; ii. extreme gastric hyperacidity, and iii. non-beta cell, non-insulin-secreting islet cell tumors, which might be single or multiple, small or large, benign or malignant).

Z-ESR Zeta erythrocyte sedimentation rate.

ZES Zollinger-Ellison syndrome.

ZETT Zollinger-Ellison type tumor (of pancreas).

ZF Zero frequency; Zona fasciculata.

ZFF Zinc Fume Fever.

ZG Zero gas; Zona glomerulosa; Zymogen granule(s).

ZGM Zinc glycinate marker.

ZHG Zoster hyperimmune globulin (see ZIG).

ZI Zyplast implant (see SDCI).

Zidovudine Azidothymidine (see AZT).

ZIFT Zygote intrafallopian tube transfer.

ZIG; ZIg Zoster immmune/immuno globulin - a specific globulin (= ZHG).

ZIP Zoster immune plasma.

ZIPP Zinc Oxide and Iodoform Paste (= Past Zinc Oxid et Iodof), namely Zinc Oxide 4, Iodoform 4, and Liquid Paraffin 5 (parts by weight) Paste - used as a mild antiseptic and application to wounds and abscesses.

ZK Zuelzer-Kaplan (syndrome).

zla; zl^a Symbol for isotope with atomic number Z and atomic weight a.

ZLS Zimmerman-Laband syndrome.

ZM Cell membrane (see ZW).

Zm Zygomaxillare.

ZMA Zinc meta-arsenite.

ZMC Zygomatic.

ZN Zeitschrift für Naturforschung (Ger.) -

Z - atomic number

Atomic No.	Name	Symbol	Atomic weight
1	Hydrogen	H	1.00797
2	Helium	He	4.0026
3	Lithium	Li	6.939
4	Beryllium	Be	9.0122
5	Boron	B	10.811
6	Carbon	C	12.01115
7	Nitrogen	N	14.0069
8	Oxygen	O	15.994
9	Fluorine	F	18.9984
10	Neon	Ne	20.183
11	Sodium	Na	22.9898
12	Magnesium	Mg	24.312
13	Aluminium	Al	26.9815
14	Silicon	Si	28.086
15	Phosphorus	P	30.9738
16	Sulfur	S	32.064
17	Chlorine	Cl	35.453
18	Argon	Ar	39.944
19	Potassium	K	39.102
20	Calcium	Ca	40.08
21	Scandium	Sc	44.956
22	Titanium	Ti	47.90
23	Vanadium	V	50.942
24	Chromium	Cr	51.996
25	Manganese	Mn	54.9380
26	Iron	Fe	55.847
27	Cobalt	Co	58.9332
28	Nickel	Ni	58.71
29	Copper	Cu	63.54
30	Zinc	Zn	65.37
31	Gallium	Ga	69.72
32	Germanium	Ge	72.59
33	Arsenic	As	74.9216
34	Selenium	Se	78.96
35	Bromine	Br	79.909
36	Krypton	Kr	83.80
37	Rubidium	Rb	85.47
38	Strontium	Sr	87.62
39	Yttrium	Y	88.905
40	Zirconium	Zr	91.22
41	Niobium	Nb	92.906
42	Molybdenum	Mo	95.94
43	Technetium	Tc	99
44	Ruthenium	Ru	101.07
45	Rhodium	Rh	102.905
46	Palladium	Pd	106.4
47	Silver	Ag	107.870
48	Cadmium	Cd	112.40
49	Indium	In	114.82
50	Tin	Sn	118.69

Atomic No.	Name	Symbol	Atomic weight
51	Antimony	Sb	121.75
52	Tellurium	Te	127.60
53	Iodine	I	126.9044
54	Xenon	Xe	131.30
55	Caesium	Cs	132.905
56	Barium	Ba	137.34
57	Lanthanum	La	138.91
58	Cerium	Ce	140.12
59	Praseodymium	Pr	140.907
60	Neodymium	Nd	144.24
61	Promethium	Pm	147
62	Samarium	Sm	150.35
63	Europium	Eu	151.96
64	Gadolinium	Gd	157.25
65	Terbium	Tb	158.924
66	Dysprosium	Dy	162.50
67	Holmium	Ho	164.930
68	Erbium	Er	167.26
69	Thulium	Tm	168.934
70	Ytterbium	Yb	173.04
71	Lutetium	Lu	174.97
72	Hafnium	Hf	178.49
73	Tantalum	Ta	180.948
74	Tungsten	W	183.85
75	Rhenium	Re	186.2
76	Osmium	Os	190.2
77	Iridium	Ir	192.2
78	Platinum	Pt	195.09
79	Gold	Au	196.967
80	Mercury	Hg	200.59
81	Thallium	Tl	204.37
82	Lead	Pb	207.19
83	Bismuth	Bi	208.980
84	Polonium	Po	210
85	Astatine	At	211
86	Radon	Rn	222
87	Francium	Fr	223
88	Radium	Ra	226
89	Actinium	Ac	227
90	Thorium	Th	232.038
91	Protactinium	Pa	231
92	Uranium	U	238.03
93	Neptunium	Np	237
94	Plutonium	Pu	242
95	Americium	Am	243
96	Curium	Cm	247
97	Berkelium	Bk	247
98	Californium	Cf	249
99	Einsteinium	Es	254
100	Fermium	Fm	253

Atomic No.	Name	Symbol	Atomic weight
101	Mendelevium	Md	256
102	Nobelium	No	254
103	Lawrencium	Lw	257
104	Kurchatovium	Ku	?
105	Hahnium	Ha	?
106	Seaborgium	?	?
88/89	Mesotherium 1	Ms-Th or MSTh	226/227
89/90	Mesothorium 2	Ms-Th or MSTh	226/227

Journal of Nature Research.

Zn Zinc (Z = 30) (see Elements - Zinc).

ZNA Mixture of dill wood and monosodium glutamate.

$ZnBr_2$ Zinc bromide.

$ZnCl_2$ Zinc chloride.

$ZnCO_3$ Zinc carbonate.

^{65}ZnDTPA Radioactive zinc diethylenetriamine pentacetate.

^{65}ZnEDTA Radioactive zinc edathauril (see EDTA).

ZnG Zinc gluconate.

ZN6-Na Sodium Fusidate (= Sod Fusid) - the hemihydrate of the sodium salt of Fusidic acid, an antimicrobial substance produced by the growth of Fusidium coccineum. Highly active against gram-positive bacteria and gram-negative cocci.

ZnO Zinc oxide.

ZnO_2 Zinc peroxide (= ZPO).

ZnOE Zinc oxide and eugenol (= ZOE).

ZnPP Zinc protoporphyria.

ZnPT Zinc Pyridinethione (= Pyrithione Zinc) - a bactericide and fungicide, claimed to be of value in the treatment of dandruff.

ZNS Ziehl-Neelsen stain.

$ZnSO_4$ Zinc sulfate.

ZO Zichen-Oppenheim (syndrome); Zuelzer-Ogden (syndrome).

zo- prefix meaning animal (Gr. zoon) (see zoo-), or life (Gr. zoe), e.g. zoetic - pertaining to life.

ZOA Zionist Organization of America.

ZOE Zinc oxide and eugenol (see ZnOE).

ZOK Zero-order kinetics.

zoo- prefix meaning animal (Gr. zoon), e.g. zoology - the biology of animals (= zo-).

Zoochem Zoochemistry.

Zool Zoological/gy.

ZP Revlon Inc (USA) code for experimental substances; Zirconium phosphate (see ZrP).

Z-P Z-plasty (plastic surgery) (see Z-plasty).

ZPA Zone of polarizing activity.

ZPC Zero point of change; Zopiclone.

ZPG Zero population growth.

ZPI Zinc-protamine insulin (see Insulin - PZI).

Z-plasty A plastic operation for the relaxation of contractures, in which a Z-shaped incision is made, the middle bar of the Z being over the contracted scar (= Z-P).

ZPM Zitron pacemaker.

ZPO Zinc peroxide (see ZnO_2).

ZPP Zinc protoporphyrin.

ZPT Zinc pyrithione.

Z purple Marijuana grown in Zacatecas, Mexico (see Cannabis).

ZR Zona reticularis.

Zr Zirconium (Z = 40) (see Elements - Zirconium).

^{95}Zr Radioactive zirconium.

ZrO_2 Zirconium dioxide (= Zirconium Oxide; Zirconia; Zirconic Anhydride) - used as a radiopaque medium in roentgenography of the digestive tract, and in an ointment for treating poison ivy dermatitis.

ZrP Zirconium phosphate (= ZP).

ZS Zellweger syndrome.

ZSB Zero stools since birth.

ZSFT Zinc sulfate flocculation test (see LFT iv).

ZSR Zeta sedimentation rate/ ratio.

ZS-RDS Zung Self-Rating Depression Scale.

ZRSS Zeus Robotic Surgical System.

ZS Zieve's syndrome (acute gross fatty changes in the liver, hemolysis and pancreatitis).

Z-technique Inserting trocar beneath the fascia in laparascopy.

Z-test Zulliger test.

Z-track Method of administering intramuscular medication.

ZTS Zymosan-treated serum.

Z-TSP Zephiran-trisodium phosphate.

ZTT Zinc turbidity test (see LFT iv).

ZUDC Zurich University Dermatology Clinic.

ZVT Zehlenverbindungstest.

ZW Cell wall (see ZM).

Zy Zygion.

ZyC Zymosan complement.

zyg zygotene.

zyg- prefix meaning joined (Gr. zygon).

zym- prefix meaning ferment (Gr. zyme) (see zymo-).

zymo- combining form denoting relationship to an enzyme or to fermentation (Gr. zyme) (= zym-).

Zz Ginger (L. zingibar).

ISBN 0-444-51265-9

9 780444 512659